Basic & Clinical Pharmacology

Basic & Clinical Pharmacology

Edited by

BERTRAM G. KATZUNG, MD, PhD

Professor of Pharmacology
Department of Pharmacology
University of California, San Francisco

LANGE Medical Publications

LMP

Los Altos, California 94022

Lange Medical Publications

Drawer L, Los Altos, California 94022

International Standard Book Number: *0-87041-260-4*
Library of Congress Catalogue Card Number: *82-83463*

Basic & Clinical Pharmacology **$23.50**

A Concise Medical Library for Practitioner and Student

Current Medical Diagnosis & Treatment 1982 (annual revision). Edited by M.A. Krupp and M.J. Chatton. 1113 pp.	1982
Current Pediatric Diagnosis & Treatment, 7th ed. Edited by C.H. Kempe, H.K. Silver, and D. O'Brien. 1106 pp, *illus.*	1982
Current Surgical Diagnosis & Treatment, 5th ed. Edited by J.E. Dunphy and L.W. Way. 1138 pp, *illus.*	1981
Current Obstetric & Gynecologic Diagnosis & Treatment, 4th ed. Edited by R.C. Benson. 1038 pp, *illus.*	1982
Harper's Review of Biochemistry (formerly **Review of Physiological Chemistry**), 18th ed. D.W. Martin, Jr., P.A. Mayes, and V.W. Rodwell. 614 pp, *illus.*	1981
Review of Medical Physiology, 10th ed. W.F. Ganong. 628 pp, *illus.*	1981
Review of Medical Microbiology, 15th ed. E. Jawetz, J.L. Melnick, and E.A. Adelberg. 553 pp, *illus.*	1982
Basic & Clinical Immunology, 4th ed. Edited by D.P. Stites, J.D. Stobo, H.H. Fudenberg, and J.V. Wells. 775 pp, *illus.*	1982
Basic Histology, 3rd ed. L.C. Junqueira and J. Carneiro. 504 pp, *illus.*	1980
Clinical Cardiology, 3rd ed. M. Sokolow and M.B. McIlroy. 763 pp, *illus.*	1981
General Urology, 10th ed. D.R. Smith. 598 pp, *illus.*	1981
General Ophthalmology, 9th ed. D. Vaughan and T. Asbury. 410 pp, *illus.*	1980
Correlative Neuroanatomy & Functional Neurology, 18th ed. J.G. Chusid. 476 pp, *illus.*	1982
Principles of Clinical Electrocardiography, 11th ed. M.J. Goldman. 438 pp, *illus.*	1982
Handbook of Obstetrics & Gynecology, 7th ed. R.C. Benson. 808 pp, *illus.*	1980
Physician's Handbook, 20th ed. M.A. Krupp, L.M. Tierney, Jr., E. Jawetz, R.L. Roe, and C.A. Camargo. 774 pp, *illus.*	1982
Handbook of Pediatrics, 13th ed. H.K. Silver, C.H. Kempe, and H.B. Bruyn. 735 pp, *illus.*	1980
Handbook of Poisoning: Prevention, Diagnosis, & Treatment, 11th ed. R.H. Dreisbach. About 640 pp.	1982

Lithographed in USA

Table of Contents

Preface

This book succeeds *Review of Medical Pharmacology,* by Frederick H. Meyers, Ernest Jawetz, and Alan Goldfien. The seven editions of "Meyers' Pharmacology" were widely admired and accepted, and it is my hope that *Basic & Clinical Pharmacology* will achieve the same degree of utility for students in the health professions.

Although no single book can satisfy every reader's needs, *Basic & Clinical Pharmacology* has been designed to provide information needed by students in the health sciences and a variety of health professionals. Each chapter offers a concise and current presentation of both basic pharmacology and relevant information regarding the clinical use of drugs. This has required some flexibility in the organization of individual chapters but permits the inclusion of far more useful material than would otherwise be possible.

The sections on clinical pharmacology provide an introduction to the practical use of the drugs covered and, more importantly, provide the reader with some concepts regarding therapeutic strategies, choice of drug, monitoring of therapeutic responses, and other principles that are missing from the sources of information traditionally used by students and house officers on clinical services.

While no attempt has been made to discuss every drug or even every useful drug, the authors have, I believe, covered examples of all the *important and useful* drugs, plus those newer agents whose importance is not yet known but whose promise is sufficient to command current attention.

I invite the reader to write to me regarding their experiences in using this book and to send notes on any factual errors uncovered. Please address letters to me at the Department of Pharmacology, University of California, San Francisco, CA 94143, USA.

I wish to express my thanks to all who helped prepare *Basic & Clinical Pharmacology* and to the authors of *Review of Medical Pharmacology* for providing both example and inspiration.

Bertram G. Katzung, MD, PhD

San Francisco
November, 1982

The Authors

David F. Altman, MD
Assistant Clinical Professor of Medicine, Department of Medicine, University of California, San Francisco.

Michael J. Aminoff, MD
Associate Professor of Neurology, Department of Neurology, University of California, San Francisco.

Charles E. Becker, MD
Associate Professor of Medicine, Department of Medicine, University of California, San Francisco.

Leslie Z. Benet, PhD
Professor and Chairman, Department of Pharmacy, School of Pharmacy, University of California, San Francisco.

Neal L. Benowitz, MD
Associate Professor of Medicine and Clinical Pharmacology, Department of Medicine, University of California, San Francisco.

Barry A. Berkowitz, PhD
Director of Biological Research, Biological Research Laboratories, Smith Kline & French Laboratories, Philadelphia.

Daniel D. Bikle, MD, PhD
Assistant Professor of Medicine, Department of Medicine, and Co-Director, Special Diagnostic and Treatment Unit, University of California, San Francisco.

Henry R. Bourne, MD
Professor of Medicine and Pharmacology, Departments of Medicine and Pharmacology, and Chief, Division of Clinical Pharmacology, University of California, San Francisco.

Homer A. Boushey, MD
Associate Professor of Medicine, Department of Medicine, University of California, San Francisco.

Alan Burkhalter, PhD
Professor of Pharmacology, Department of Pharmacology, University of California, San Francisco.

Neal Castagnoli, Jr., PhD
Professor of Chemistry and Pharmaceutical Chemistry, Department of Pharmaceutical Chemistry, University of California, San Francisco.

John F. Catchpool, MB, BS (Lond), LRCP, MRCS, MD
Research Associate in International Health, Department of International Health, University of California, San Francisco.

Kanu Chatterjee, MB, FRCP
Lucie Stern Professor of Cardiology, Professor of Medicine, Cardiology Division, Department of Medicine, University of California, San Francisco.

Martin S. Cohen, MD
Assistant Professor of Pediatrics in Residence, Department of Pediatrics, and Chief, Pediatric Clinical Pharmacology Unit, University of California, San Francisco.

Maria Almira Correia, PhD
Associate Professor of Pharmacology in Residence, Department of Pharmacology, University of California, San Francisco.

Betty J. Dong, PharmD
Associate Clinical Professor of Pharmacy, Division of Clinical Pharmacy, University of California, San Francisco.

Oscar L. Frick, MD, PhD
Professor of Pediatrics, Department of Pediatrics, University of California, San Francisco.

Alan Goldfien, MD
Professor of Obstetrics and Gynecology and Medicine, Departments of Obstetrics and Gynecology and Medicine, University of California, San Francisco.

Robert S. Goldsmith, MD, DTM&H
Professor of Tropical Medicine and Epidemiology, Department of Epidemiology and International Health, University of California, San Francisco.

Marc E. Goldyne, MD, PhD
Assistant Professor in Residence, Dermatology and Medicine, Departments of Dermatology and Medicine, University of California, San Francisco.

Francis S. Greenspan, MD
Clinical Professor of Medicine and Radiology, Department of Medicine, and Chief, Thyroid Clinic, University of California, San Francisco.

Philip D. Hansten, PharmD
Associate Professor of Clinical Pharmacy, Department of Pharmacy, Washington State University College of Pharmacy, Pullman, Washington.

Brian B. Hoffman, MD
Assistant Professor of Medicine and Pharmacology, Department of Medicine, Division of Clinical Pharmacology, Stanford University School of Medicine, Stanford, California.

Nicholas H.G. Holford, MSc, MRCP (UK)
Assistant Professor of Medicine and Pharmacy, Departments of Medicine and Pharmacy, University of California, San Francisco.

Leo E. Hollister, MD
Professor of Medicine and Psychiatry, Stanford University School of Medicine, Palo Alto Veterans Administration Hospital, Palo Alto, California.

Michael J. Holtzman, MD
Cardiovascular Research Institute and Department of Medicine, University of California, San Francisco.

Luc M. Hondeghem, MD, PhD
Associate Professor of Pharmacology, Department of Pharmacology, University of California, San Francisco.

Ernest Jawetz, MD, PhD
Professor of Microbiology and Medicine, Department of Microbiology, University of California, San Francisco.

John P. Kane, MD, PhD
Professor of Medicine, Department of Medicine, University of California, San Francisco.

John H. Karam, MD
Associate Professor of Medicine in Residence, Metabolic Research Unit, University of California, San Francisco.

Bertram G. Katzung, MD, PhD
Professor of Pharmacology, Department of Pharmacology, University of California, San Francisco.

Mary Anne Koda-Kimble, PharmD
Associate Clinical Professor of Pharmacy, Division of Clinical Pharmacy, School of Pharmacy, University of California, San Francisco.

David C. Klonoff, MD
Clinical Instructor in Medicine, Department of Medicine, University of California, San Francisco.

Nancy M. Lee, PhD
Associate Research Pharmacologist, Department of Pharmacology, University of California, San Francisco.

Paul W. Lofholm, PharmD
Associate Clinical Professor of Pharmacy, School of Pharmacy, University of California, San Francisco.

Lisa A. Lybecker, RPh
College of Pharmacy, University of Cincinnati, Cincinnati.

Howard I. Maibach, MD
Professor of Dermatology, Department of Dermatology, University of California, San Francisco.

Mary J. Malloy, MD
Associate Clinical Professor of Pediatrics, Department of Pediatrics, University of California, San Francisco.

Jay W. Mason, MD
Assistant Professor of Medicine, Department of Medicine, Cardiology Division, and Director, Cardiac Arrhythmia Study Unit, Stanford University School of Medicine, Stanford, California.

Ronald D. Miller, MD
Professor and Vice Chairman of Anesthesia, Professor of Pharmacology, Department of Anesthesia, University of California, San Francisco.

John Mills, MD
Associate Professor of Medicine, Microbiology, and Clinical Pharmacy, University of California, San Francisco, and Chief, Infectious Disease Section, San Francisco General Hospital, San Francisco.

Roger A. Nicoll, MD
Professor of Pharmacology and Physiology, Department of Pharmacology, University of California, San Francisco.

Kent R. Olson, MD
Clinical Toxicology Fellow, San Francisco General Hospital, San Francisco, and Emergency Physician, Garden of Eden Hospital, Castro Valley, California.

William W. Parmley, MD
Professor of Medicine, Department of Medicine, Cardiology Division, University of California, San Francisco, and Chief of Cardiology, H.C. Moffitt Hospital, San Francisco.

William H. Pitlick, PhD
Research Scientist and Health Scientist Administrator, Epilepsy Branch, National Institutes of Health, Bethesda, Maryland.

Roger J. Porter, MD
Chief, Epilepsy Branch, National Institutes of Health, Bethesda, Maryland.

Ian A. Reid, PhD
Professor of Physiology, Department of Physiology, University of California, San Francisco.

Curt A. Ries, MD
Associate Clinical Professor of Medicine, Hematology-Oncology, Department of Medicine, University of California, San Francisco.

James M. Roberts, MD
Associate Professor of Obstetrics and Gynecology and Reproductive Sciences, Department of Obstetrics and Gynecology, and Associate Staff, Cardiovascular Research Institute, University of California, San Francisco.

Dirk B. Robertson, MD
Clinical Instructor in Dermatology, Department of Dermatology, University of California, San Francisco.

Sydney E. Salmon, MD
Professor of Hematology-Oncology, Department of Hematology-Oncology, and Professor of Medicine, Department of Internal Medicine, and Director, University of Arizona Cancer Center, University of Arizona School of Medicine, Tucson.

Daniel V. Santi, MD, PhD
Professor of Biochemistry and Pharmaceutical Chemistry, Departments of Biochemistry and Biophysics and Pharmaceutical Chemistry, University of California, San Francisco.

Alan C. Sartorelli, PhD
Professor and Chairman, Department of Pharmacology, Yale University School of Medicine, New Haven, Connecticut.

Martin A. Shearn, MD
Chief, Department of Medicine, Kaiser-Permanente Medical Center, Oakland, California, and Clinical Professor of Medicine, University of California, San Francisco.

Anthony Trevor, PhD
Professor of Pharmacology and Toxicology, Department of Pharmacology, University of California, San Francisco.

Robert T. Wall, MD
Internist, Hematologist, Charleston Hematology-Oncology University Center, Charleston, South Carolina, and Assistant Professor, Department of Medicine, Stanford University School of Medicine, Stanford, California.

David G. Warnock, MD
Associate Professor of Medicine in Residence, Division of Nephrology, Department of Medicine, University of California, San Francisco.

August M. Watanabe, MD
Professor of Medicine and Pharmacology, Departments of Medicine and Pharmacology, Indiana University School of Medicine, Indianapolis.

E. Leong Way, PhD
Professor of Pharmacology and Toxicology, Department of Pharmacology, University of California, San Francisco.

Walter L. Way, MD
Professor of Anesthesia and Pharmacology, Department of Anesthesia, University of California, San Francisco.

Introduction | 1

Bertram G. Katzung, MD, PhD

Pharmacology can be broadly defined as the science dealing with interactions between living systems and molecules, especially chemicals introduced from outside the system. This definition thus includes **medical pharmacology**—the science of materials used to prevent, diagnose, and treat disease—as well as the important role played by chemicals in the environment that *cause* disease and the use of certain chemicals as molecular probes for the study of normal biochemistry and physiology. **Toxicology** is that branch of pharmacology that deals with the undesirable effects of chemicals in biologic systems.

What is or is not a **drug** can be broadly or narrowly defined. For our purposes, a drug will be any small molecule that, when introduced into the body, alters the body's function by interactions at the molecular level. There is clearly some overlap with endocrinology in this definition. This is as it should be, since hormones are properly considered drugs whether introduced from outside the body ("exogenous") in any amount or released internally in increased amounts by administration of a stimulant agent. Poisons are drugs whether administered with criminal or suicidal intent or encountered inadvertently in the environment.

Drugs vary in molecular size. Molecules as small as carbon monoxide and methanol and as large as thrombolytic enzymes fall within the above functional definition. However, the great majority of drugs fall into the molecular weight range of 100–1000. There is a practical reason for this: As noted below, a drug is often introduced for reasons of convenience into a part of the body remote from the target tissue. To be absorbed and distributed to the target organ, the drug molecule must be capable of diffusion (or transport by carrier mechanisms). With some exceptions, molecules within the narrow range of MW 100–1000 are capable of convenient administration and efficient absorption and distribution.

Drugs also vary in their chemical nature. On the one hand, there are highly reactive alkylating agents such as mechlorethamine; on the other, "inert" anesthetic gases such as xenon. The various classes of organic compounds—carbohydrates, proteins, and lipids—are all represented. Many drugs are weak acids or weak bases. This fact has important implications for the way they are handled by the body, since the pH differences between different compartments of the body may alter the degree of ionization of such compounds (see below).

Drug-Body Interactions

The interactions between a drug and the biologic system are conveniently divided into 2 classes: **pharmacodynamic** interactions, the effects of the drug on the body; and **pharmacokinetic** interactions, the way in which the body handles the drug. The quantitative aspects of pharmacodynamics—the drug receptor concept and dose-response relationships—are discussed in Chapter 2. The principles of pharmacokinetics—absorption, distribution, metabolism, and excretion—are presented in Chapter 3. Some of the introductory concepts used in discussing these interactions are presented in this chapter.

Drug Permeation

As noted above, movement of drug molecules—into the body from the site of administration (absorption), between different parts of the body (distribution), and out of the body (excretion)—are important characteristics of any useful therapeutic agent. Because the body is protected from the outside world and is itself internally compartmentalized by membrane barriers to the free movement of water and solute, permeation of drug molecules across membranes plays a role in all 3 of these processes.

There are 4 major mechanisms by which drugs move across barriers.

A. Aqueous Diffusion: This is a pathway of limited capacity across most barriers, eg, the epithelial lining of the surfaces of the body, such as the cornea, gut, and bladder. Because these cells are connected by tight junctions, only molecules small enough (less than MW 100–150, eg, Li^+, methanol) to pass through very small aqueous pores permeate these barriers by the aqueous route. In contrast, most capillaries have very large pores between cells that allow molecules as large as MW 20,000–30,000 to pass. The capillaries of most of the brain lack these pores, but they are found in a few areas of the central nervous system: the pituitary gland, the pineal gland, the median eminence, the area postrema, and the choroid plexus.

B. Lipid Diffusion: Movement across cell membranes by solution in the lipids of the membrane, with passive transfer across the lipid driven by a concentration gradient, is one of the most important mechanisms of drug permeation. Obviously, a high degree of lipid solubility relative to aqueous solubility (often quantitated as the octanol/water or olive oil/water partition coefficient) will favor this mode of permeation. However, since drugs must first be in aqueous solution to gain access to the lipid membrane, too low a level of water solubility is undesirable.

A great many drugs are weak acids or weak bases. Such molecules are relatively *more water-soluble when ionized (polar) and more lipid-soluble when un-ionized*. Because the pH of the environment will determine the degree of ionization according to the Henderson-Hasselbalch equation, the ability of such molecules to permeate lipid barriers is a function of the local pH.

For weak acids, eg, phenobarbital,

$$HA \rightleftharpoons H^+ + A^- \quad \ldots(1)$$

and

$$\log\left(\frac{\text{Protonated form}}{\text{Unprotonated form}}\right) = pK_a - pH \quad \ldots(2)$$

The pKa of phenobarbital is 7.4 (Table 1–1). Therefore, if phenobarbital is being excreted in an acid urine, more of the drug will be protonated (un-ionized) and readily reabsorbable by permeation across the lipid membranes of renal tubular cells. In an alkaline urine, more of the drug will be dissociated (ionized), poorly soluble in lipid, and more rapidly excreted. The magnitude of this effect can be estimated by applying the Henderson-Hasselbalch equation:

For pH 6.4:

$$\log\left(\frac{HA}{A^-}\right) = 7.4 - 6.4 = 1$$

$$\text{antilog } (1) = 10 \quad \ldots(3)$$

Therefore, the ratio of readily reabsorbed (protonated) to poorly reabsorbed (dissociated) phenobarbital is 10 when the urine pH is 6.4.

For pH 8.0:

$$\log\left(\frac{HA}{A^-}\right) = 7.4 - 8.0 = -0.6$$

$$\text{antilog } (-0.6) = 0.25 \quad \ldots(4)$$

Therefore, in alkaline urine, most of the phenobarbital is dissociated (charged) and therefore readily excreted. In treating a patient who has taken an

Table 1–1. Ionization constants of some common drugs.

Drug	pKa*	Drug	pKa*	Drug	pKa*
Weak acids		**Weak bases (cont'd)**		**Weak bases (cont'd)**	
Acetazolamide	7.2	Amphetamine	9.8	Methadone	8.4
Ampicillin	2.5	Atropine	9.7	Methamphetamine	10.0
Aspirin	3.5	Bupivacaine	8.1	Methyldopa	10.6
Chlorothiazide	6.8, 9.4†	Caffeine	0.8	Methysergide	6.6
Chlorpropamide	5.0	Chlordiazepoxide	4.6	Metoprolol	9.8
Cromolyn	2.0	Chloroquine	10.8, 8.4†	Morphine	7.9
Ethacrynic acid	3.5	Chlorpheniramine	9.2	Nicotine	7.9, 3.1†
Furosemide	3.9	Chlorpromazine	9.3	Norepinephrine	8.6
Ibuprofen	4.4	Cocaine	8.5	Pentazocine	9.7
Levodopa	2.3	Codeine	8.2	Phenylephrine	9.8
Methotrexate	4.8	Cyclizine	8.2	Physostigmine	7.9, 1.8†
Methyldopa	2.2, 9.2†	Desipramine	10.2	Pilocarpine	6.9, 1.4†
Penicillamine	1.8	Diazepam	3.3	Pindolol	8.8
Pentobarbital	8.1	Dihydrocodeine	8.8	Procainamide	9.2
Phenobarbital	7.4	Diphenhydramine	9.0	Procaine	9.0
Phenytoin	8.3	Diphenoxylate	7.1	Promazine	9.4
Propylthiouracil	8.3	Ephedrine	9.6	Promethazine	9.1
Salicylic acid	3.0	Epinephrine	8.7	Propranolol	9.4
Sulfadiazine	6.5	Ergotamine	6.3	Pseudoephedrine	9.8
Sulfapyridine	8.4	Fluphenazine	8.0, 3.9†	Pyrimethamine	7.0
Tolbutamide	5.3	Guanethidine	11.4, 8.3†	Quinidine	8.5, 4.4†
Warfarin	5.0	Hydralazine	7.1	Scopolamine	8.1
Weak bases		Imipramine	9.5	Strychnine	8.0, 2.3†
Albuterol (salbutamol)	9.3	Isoproterenol	8.6	Terbutaline	10.1
Allopurinol	9.4, 12.3†	Kanamycin	7.2	Theophylline	0.7
Alprenolol	9.6	Lidocaine	7.9	Thioridazine	9.5
Amiloride	8.7	Metaraminol	8.6	Tolazoline	10.6

*The pK_a is that pH at which the concentrations of the ionized and un-ionized forms are equal.
†More than one ionizable group.

overdose of phenobarbital, alkalinizing the urine is one method of hastening elimination of the drug.

For weak bases, eg, pyrimethamine, an antimalaria drug:

$$H^+ + RNH_2 \rightleftharpoons RN^+H_3 \quad \ldots(5)$$

and, as before,

$$\log\left(\frac{\text{Protonated form}}{\text{Unprotonated form}}\right) = pK_a - pH \quad \ldots(6)$$

The pKa of pyrimethamine is 7.0 (Table 1–1). Therefore, at pH 8.0, the ratio of the protonated to the unprotonated form is 0.1; at pH 7.0, the ratio is 1; and at pH 6 it is 10. However, the protonated form of a base is the ionized, poorly lipid-soluble form. Thus, in contrast to phenobarbital, more of the pyrimethamine is in the more lipid-soluble form in alkaline environments than in acid ones.

Most weak bases used in pharmacology are substituted amines. Because the nitrogen atom can form bonds with one, 2, 3, or 4 carbon atoms, we can speak of primary, secondary, tertiary, and quaternary amines. Pyrimethamine is a primary amine, since only one of the nitrogen bonds is to a carbon atom. Secondary and tertiary amines can also acquire a proton and become charged, as in the example given above. Quaternary amines, on the other hand, are permanently charged, since the carbon-nitrogen bond is not subject to change by physiologic pH alterations.

The degree of ionization of weak electrolytes is not the only factor that influences lipid solubility, but it is especially important in those body compartments in which the pH may change. For instance, the gastric pH may vary between 1.5 and 7 and the pH of the urine between 5.5 and 8. For drugs that have moderately high lipid solubility in the un-ionized form (and which therefore permeate very readily), changes of pH of this magnitude can have considerable clinical significance. For example, phenobarbital is cleared 7 times more rapidly into alkaline urine than into acid urine. Mecamylamine, an antihypertension drug and a weak base, is cleared almost 80 times more rapidly into acidic than into alkaline urine.

C. Via Special Carriers (Facilitated Diffusion): A few classes of drugs are transported by special carriers in the membranes of cells. Such carriers include those for amino acids in the "blood-brain barrier" and those for weak acids in the proximal convoluted tubule of the kidney.

D. Pinocytosis: Drugs of exceptionally large size (over MW 1000) can enter cells only by pinocytosis—the process of engulfing extracellular material within membrane vesicles. This is of importance for only a few drugs, most of them proteins. Botulinus toxin is an example.

E. Factors Influencing Permeation: For most mechanisms of permeation, the rate of drug transfer is a function of the surface area available for transfer and, in the case of a passive process, of the concentration gradient driving it. Thus, transfer across the lipid barrier of organs with very large surface areas (lung, small intestine) is usually much faster than across small areas (stomach). The concentration gradient depends upon processes on both sides of the membrane. In a typical example of drug absorption from a site of subcutaneous administration, the amount of drug administered will determine the concentration on one side. The rate of removal of drug will determine the concentration on the other side. Thus, a high blood flow will rapidly replace blood in which drug has dissolved with blood containing no drug, thereby maintaining a high concentration gradient. Vasodilator substances are typically absorbed very rapidly, whereas vasoconstrictor drugs are absorbed more slowly because they modify blood flow in opposite directions.

Absorption of Drug Into the Body

Use of a drug almost always involves transfer of the agent into the bloodstream. Exceptions include topical application for local effect on the skin or mucous membranes and oral administration of drugs that act from within the intestinal lumen such as antacids and laxatives. However, even when the site of therapeutic action is in one of these locations, absorption into the bloodstream may occur and may have undesirable (nontherapeutic) effects.

In addition to the factors described above that affect drug permeation, absorption into the blood is significantly influenced by the **route of administration.** In addition to the intravenous route, which bypasses the absorption process, the important routes of administration are oral, inhalational, topical, transdermal, subcutaneous, intramuscular, and buccal (sublingual). Less commonly, the intra-arterial, intrathecal, and rectal routes may be used.

The **oral route** is most commonly used because of its convenience and, for most drugs, efficiency of absorption. The large surface area of the gastrointestinal tract, the mixing of its contents, and the differences in pH at different levels favor effective absorption of drugs given in this way. However, the acids and enzymes secreted by the patient and the biochemical activity of the resident microbiologic flora also have the capacity to destroy a drug before it is absorbed. Some penicillins are inactive when given orally because they are rapidly inactivated by gastric acid. Polypeptide hormones such as insulin are hydrolyzed in the intestine and therefore must be given **parenterally** (by a nongastrointestinal route).

Because the gut is lined by epithelium with tight junctions, absorption of most drugs is by lipid diffusion. Thus, the basic rules of lipid permeation described above apply.

The **inhalational route** of administration, in addition to its obvious role in the use of gaseous anesthetics and other therapeutic gases, can be used for pharmacologic agents that vaporize readily, eg, amyl nitrite, and for drugs that can be deposited in solution in fine aqueous droplets, eg, certain ergot derivatives. Because of the very large surface area of the alveolar membrane and the high blood flow through the lungs, therapeutic gases of suitable solubility characteristics are rapidly absorbed from the lungs.

The airway itself is an important target of drugs used in asthma; the use of aerosols for delivery to the bronchi constitutes a type of topical administration.

The **topical route** includes application, for local effect, to the skin, the eye, the nose and throat, and the vaginal surface. (Drugs are occasionally used topically in the rectum for their anti-inflammatory effect. More often, the rectal route is used as an alternative to oral administration, for systemic effects.) The **transdermal route** utilizes application of drugs to the skin for systemic effects. Prolonged blood levels of some drugs can be achieved by this method because they are slowly absorbed. The skin constitutes a multilayered lipid barrier with special pharmacokinetic features as discussed in Chapter 61. The basic principles of lipid permeation apply to the skin and to the other body surfaces mentioned above.

The **buccal route** is an important one for drugs that must be self-administered but are too rapidly inactivated by the liver to be useful after ingestion. Some drugs are so rapidly metabolized by the liver that when absorbed from the stomach and small intestine into the portal circulation they are more than 90% inactivated before reaching the systemic circulation. Blood flow through the buccal mucosa is high, and venous drainage is into systemic veins, not the portal circulation. Therefore, drugs such as nitroglycerin are effective in much lower dosage when placed under the tongue than when swallowed.

When drugs must be given by **injection,** several options are available. The **intravenous route** is the most direct and bypasses the absorption barriers. It is also the most hazardous, because a very high concentration of drug is delivered to the target organs very rapidly. Drugs in aqueous solution injected **intramuscularly** are often absorbed fairly rapidly. "Depot" injections of drug dissolved in oil can be used to provide a slowly absorbed reservoir of drug. Some formulations provide significant levels of drug for weeks after a single injection. Some drugs cannot be given by this route because they cause pain and tissue damage at the site of injection. **Subcutaneously** injected drugs are usually more slowly absorbed. Irritating substances are particularly painful when given by this route, and large volumes are not feasible unless they contain hyaluronidase, an enzyme that facilitates the spread of the injected solution through the tissue. The **intra-arterial** and **intrathecal routes** are special ones used to achieve high drug concentrations in specific target organs.

Distribution of Drug Within the Body

Once a drug has been absorbed into the blood, it may be distributed to different physical compartments of the body (Table 1–2). If avidly bound to plasma proteins, it may remain in the vascular compartment until eliminated. Small water-soluble molecules may be freely distributed in the total body water. Drugs that are highly lipid-soluble (eg, DDT) are ultimately distributed to fat. Drugs that are not tightly bound to cells or proteins within the blood leave the vascular compartment, at a rate and to an extent governed by the permeability principles outlined above. Certain ions, especially the heavy metals and fluoride, are sequestered in bone (Table 1–2).

Table 1–2. Physical volumes (in L/kg) of examples of body compartments into which drugs may be distributed.

Compartment and Volume		Examples
Total body water	0.6*	Small water-soluble drugs; ethanol.
Extracellular water 0.2		Larger water-soluble drugs; mannitol.
Blood 0.08 Plasma 0.04		Strongly plasma protein-bound drugs and very large drugs; heparin.
Fat	0.2–0.35	Highly lipid-soluble drugs; DDT.
Bone	0.07	Certain ions; lead, fluoride.

*An average figure. Total body water in a young lean male might be 0.7 L/kg; in an obese woman, 0.5 L/kg.

Such compartments of the body, since they constitute actual physical entities, may be considered *real* volumes of potential distribution. However, many drugs are not simply dissolved in these volumes but bind to cell surfaces and intercellular macromolecules. If the volume in which a drug is dissolved is computed by dividing the total amount of drug present by the measured concentration, the *apparent* volume of distribution is obtained. Because some drugs are almost 100% bound by tissue structures, leaving only a small amount in solution, the apparent volume of distribution may be extremely large—much larger than the total volume of the body (Chapter 3, Part 1). Although the apparent volume of distribution is obviously an abstract rather than a real entity, it is nevertheless more useful than the real volume of distribution for purposes of pharmacokinetic calculation.

The most important of the principles that determine drug distribution are protein binding, blood flow, membrane permeation, and tissue solubility.

In the blood, drugs may bind to albumin and several other serum proteins. The degree to which this occurs is usually measured as the percentage of total drug in the blood that is not dialyzable, ie, is bound to large molecules (Table 3–1). Binding sites on these molecules are sometimes referred to as **inert binding sites** to differentiate them from **receptor binding sites,** since binding to albumin brings about no specific pharmacologic response, whereas (by definition) binding to the drug receptor alters the function of the cell that contains the receptor site. Binding to nonreceptor proteins also takes place outside the vascular compartment and may account for a significant fraction of the total drug in the body.

Drug molecules bound to inert binding sites are not available for diffusion or interaction with recep-

Table 1–3. Blood flow to some important tissues of the body (based on a 70-kg human).

Tissue	Mass (kg)	Blood Flow (mL/min)	Flow (Percent of Cardiac Output)
Brain	1.4	750	13.9
Heart	0.3	250	4.7
Liver	2.9	1500	27.8
Kidneys	0.3	1260	23.3
Skeletal muscle	34.4	840	15.6
Skin	4.0	462	8.6
Placenta and fetus (term)	3.8	500	9
Whole body	70	5400	100

tors. They are, however, in equilibrium with free drug, so that alterations in the concentration of free drug will result in changes in the amount (but not the percentage) bound.

Nonreceptor protein binding sites are not very specific—eg, many weak acids with different pharmacologic effects bind to the same or closely related plasma protein sites. Therefore, different drugs may compete for the same binding sites. This can have important consequences if a high percentage of a potent drug ("A") is bound, since the binding sites must be loaded to achieve a therapeutic concentration of free drug in the plasma. Addition of a second drug ("B") that competes for the same inert binding site (but not the receptor site) may cause a marked increase in the concentration of free "A" and thus precipitate toxicity (Appendix I).

Blood flow determines how rapidly drug molecules are delivered to a given tissue and how effectively the concentration gradient between blood and tissue is maintained. Therefore, drugs equilibrate rapidly between the blood and organs with a high blood flow (Table 1–3). If the drug is very soluble or bound in the cells of these organs—eg, lipid-soluble drugs in the brain—then a very high concentration may be achieved at the steady state. Conversely, if an organ is sufficiently massive, eg, skeletal muscle, large amounts of drug may be distributed to it without ever reaching a very high concentration.

Elimination of Drugs From the Body & Termination of Drug Effect

Termination of drug effect is sometimes dependent upon excretion from the body. More commonly, termination of effect is the result of **biotransformation** to inactive products that are then excreted. A few drugs are given in a pharmacologically inactive ("prodrug") form and metabolized into another form that is pharmacologically active. Therefore, drug excretion and drug metabolism must be considered separately, as in Chapter 3.

The major organs for drug excretion are the kidneys, the liver, the gastrointestinal tract, and the lungs. Other minor routes of drug excretion are sweat and milk.

A. Kidneys: Drugs are excreted by the kidneys by 2 processes, glomerular filtration and tubular secretion, and reabsorbed usually by passive diffusion. Glomerular filtration is a passive, nonsaturable process that removes molecules up to the size of small proteins. Therefore, drugs that are effectively bound to plasma protein are poorly filtered; and conversely, drugs that are not bound are cleared from the blood at a rate approximately equal to creatinine clearance (Chapter 3, Part I). Some drugs are actively secreted by special mechanisms located in the mid segment of the proximal convoluted tubule. Drugs that are weak acids, including many diuretic drugs, are secreted in this manner and may compete with endogenous acids such as uric acid for the carrier. Active secretion is a saturable process.

Once in the tubular urine, the drug is exposed to the lipid membrane of the nephron; highly lipid-soluble molecules will be rapidly reabsorbed; more water-soluble ones are likely to be excreted. Metabolism of many drugs results in a less lipid-soluble product (Chapter 3, Part II); such metabolites are less likely than the parent drug to be reabsorbed from the tubular lumen.

B. Liver: The liver is the most important organ for drug metabolism. Bile may contain higher concentrations of metabolites than of the parent molecule, especially if the metabolite is sufficiently polar to be reabsorbed poorly from bile. A few drugs appear to be actively secreted into the bile, eg, certain cardiac glycosides, antibiotics, and quaternary ammonium cholinergic blocking agents.

Drugs and their metabolites that are secreted into bile are carried by the biliary ducts and the common duct to the duodenum. Some may then be absorbed from the lumen of the intestine and, via the enterohepatic circulation, appear again unchanged in the blood.

C. Gastrointestinal Tract: The walls of the stomach and intestines constitute large lipid membranes across which drugs can be transferred from blood to lumen. This passive diffusion is occasionally of importance when a weakly basic drug is present in very high concentration in the blood, eg, after self-administration of a large dose of morphine. Any morphine that diffuses into the acidic environment of the stomach would be almost 100% ionized (pK_a 7.9, pH 1.5–2.5) and poorly reabsorbed. Such trapped drug could then be removed by lavage. (If the morphine were not removed from the stomach, it would pass into the more alkaline environment of the intestine and be promptly reabsorbed.)

D. Lungs: The lungs are the most important route of excretion of gaseous anesthetics but a relatively unimportant route for most other drugs.

E. Minor Routes: Inconsequential amounts of drugs are excreted by the sweat and salivary glands. Similarly, the amount of drug excreted in milk is usually a small fraction of the total excreted. However, for the nursing infant, the drug in the milk may constitute a significant dose (Chapter 60).

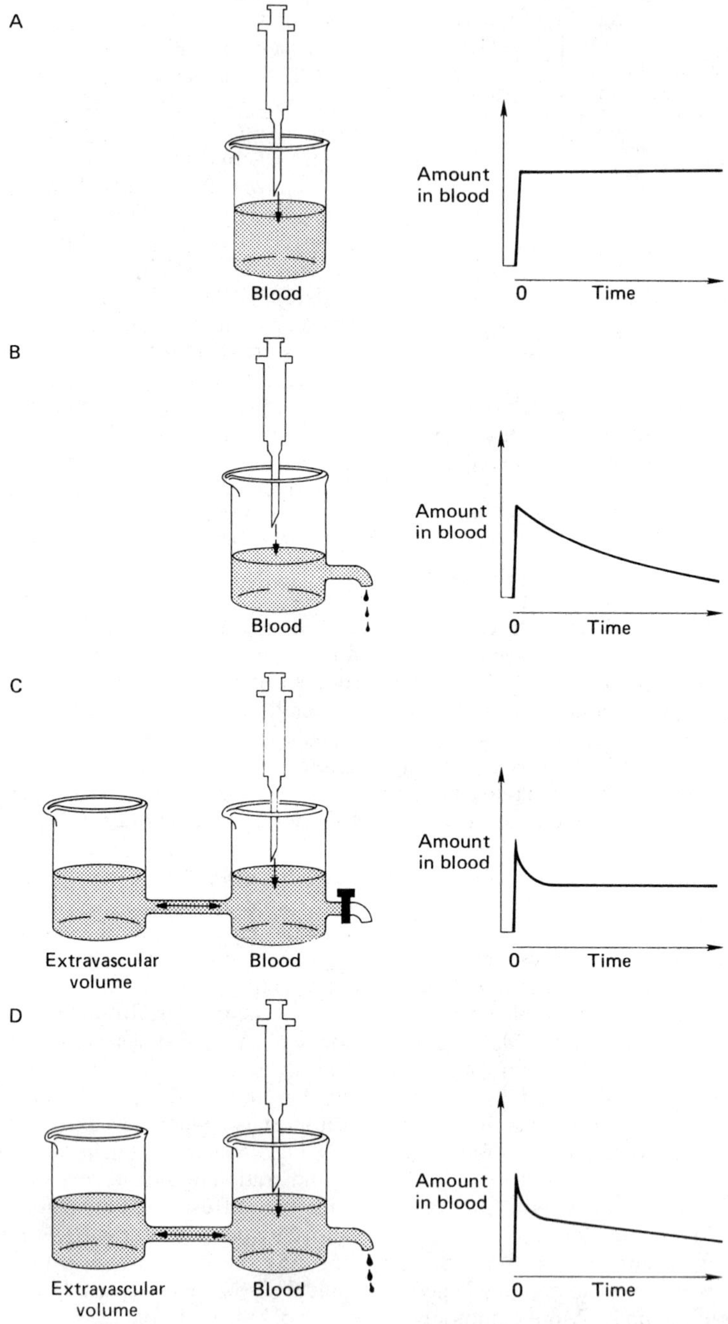

Figure 1–1. Models of drug distribution and elimination. The effect of adding drug to the blood by rapid intravenous injection is represented by expelling a known amount of the agent into a beaker. The time course of the amount of drug in the beaker is shown in the graphs at the right. In the first example *(A)*, there is no movement of drug out of the beaker, so the graph shows only a steep rise to maximum followed by a plateau. In the second example *(B)*, a route of elimination is present, and the graph shows a slow decay after a sharp rise to a maximum. Because the level of material in the beaker falls, the "pressure" driving the elimination process also falls, and the slope of the curve decreases, approaching the steady state asymptotically. This is an exponential decay curve. In the third model *(C)*, drug placed in the first compartment (blood) equilibrates rapidly with the second compartment (extravascular volume) and the amount of drug in "blood" declines logarithmically to a new steady state. The fourth model *(D)* illustrates a more realistic combination of elimination mechanism and extravascular equilibration. The resulting graph shows an early distribution phase followed by the slower elimination phase. These curves can be linearized by plotting the logarithm of the amount of drug against time.

History of a Single Drug Administration

As will be emphasized in Chapters 2 and 3, the most important factor determining the intensity of pharmacologic response is the concentration of drug at the receptor sites in the target tissue. It would be desirable to monitor this concentration to guide the adjustment of dosage, interpretation of treatment failure, etc, but direct tissue measurements are not often feasible in clinical practice. Therefore, blood (or plasma) concentrations are usually measured when pharmacokinetic studies are done.

The pharmacokinetic history of a drug dose, determined by repeatedly measuring its blood concentration after a single administration, provides useful information for developing a concept or "model" about how the body handles the drug. In their simplest form, such models can be thought of as systems of compartments into which the drug is placed at the time of administration or into which it diffuses. Fig 1–1 illustrates these concepts. For many drugs, the history of concentration in the blood is fairly well predicted by a 2-compartment model like that shown in Fig 1–1D. Many other drugs exhibit more complex curves when analyzed in this way. A few drugs display simpler kinetic behavior. For example, a drug that is retained within the vascular compartment does not manifest a distribution phase. If such a drug were to enter the body and be neither metabolized nor excreted, it might produce the graph shown in Fig 1–1A.

Drug Groups

The proper use of a drug requires an understanding of its pharmacokinetic properties and its pharmacodynamic interactions. To learn each pertinent fact about each of the many hundreds of drugs mentioned in this book is impractical, and, fortunately, unnecessary. Therapeutic agents fall naturally into about 50 or 60 groupings on the basis of similarities in therapeutic effects or mechanisms of action. Thus, if the major pharmacodynamic and pharmacokinetic features of a prototype drug are learned, the characteristics of many of the other agents in the same drug group can often be inferred.

Information Sources

The references at the end of each chapter in this book were selected to provide information specific to those chapters. Three textbooks (listed alphabetically below) provide more general discussions and references:

Bowman WC, Rand MJ: *Textbook of Pharmacology,* 2nd ed. Blackwell Scientific, 1980. [A large textbook with a chemical and comparative pharmacology orientation.]

Gilman AG, Goodman LS, Gilman A: *Goodman and Gilman's The Pharmacological Basis of Therapeutics,* 6th ed. Macmillan, 1980. [A large textbook with a medical orientation.]

Goldstein A, Aronow L, Kalman SM: *Principles of Drug Action,* 2nd ed. Wiley, 1974. [A specialized text emphasizing general principles: receptor concepts, dose-response principles, pharmacokinetics, biochemical toxicology.]

Specific questions relating to basic or clinical research are best answered by searching the general pharmacology journals and the clinical specialty serials. Two periodicals can be recommended as useful sources of current information about drugs: *The New England Journal of Medicine,* which publishes much original drug-related research as well as frequent reviews of topics in pharmacology; and *The Medical Letter on Drugs and Therapeutics,* which publishes critical reviews of new and old therapies, mostly pharmacologic.

Other sources of information pertinent to the USA should be mentioned: the "package insert," a summary of information the manufacturer is required to place in the prescription sales package; *Physicians' Desk Reference* (PDR), which is basically a compendium of package inserts published annually with supplements; and *Facts and Comparisons,* a more complete loose-leaf drug information service with monthly updates. The package insert consists of a brief description of the chemical and physical characteristics of the drug product, a description of its pharmacology, and lists of approved indications, contraindications, warnings, precautions, and adverse reactions. Information on the recommended dosage and the effects of overdosage are also provided. While this brochure contains much practical information, it is also used as a device to shift liability for untoward drug reactions from the manufacturer onto the practitioner. Therefore, the manufacturer typically lists every toxic effect ever reported, no matter how rare. A disadvantage of PDR is that it is industry-oriented rather than professionally oriented. Since only those drugs are described that their manufacturers want to pay to have included, it is inevitable that some drugs the physician or pharmacist may want information about will not be found.

• • •

References

Bowman WC, Rand MJ: Pages 40.1–40.28 in: *Textbook of Pharmacology,* 2nd ed. Blackwell Scientific, 1980.

Seeman P, Sellars EM, Roschlau WHE: Pages 1–89 in: *Principles of Medical Pharmacology,* 3rd ed. Univ of Toronto Press, 1980.

2 | Drug Receptors & Pharmacodynamics

James M. Roberts, MD, & Henry R. Bourne, MD

The therapeutic and toxic effects of drugs result from their interactions with molecules in the patient. In most instances, drugs act by associating with specific macromolecules in ways that alter their biochemical or biophysical activity. This idea, now almost a century old, is embodied in the terms **receptive substances** and **receptor:** the component of a cell or organism that interacts with a drug and initiates the chain of biochemical events leading to the drug's observed effects.

Initially, the existence of receptors was inferred from observations of the chemical and physiologic specificity of drug effects. Thus, Ehrlich noted that certain synthetic organic agents had characteristic antiparasitic effects while other agents did not, although their chemical structures differed only slightly. Langley noted that curare did not prevent electrical stimulation of muscle contraction but did block contraction triggered by nicotine. From these simple beginnings, receptors have now become the central focus of investigation of drug effects and their mechanisms of action (pharmacodynamics). The receptor concept, extended to endocrinology, immunology, and molecular biology, has proved essential for explaining many complexities of biologic regulation. Drug receptors are now being isolated and characterized as macromolecules, thus opening the way to precise understanding of the molecular basis of drug action.

In addition to its usefulness for explaining biology, the receptor concept has immensely important practical consequences for the development of drugs and for making therapeutic decisions in clinical practice. These consequences—explained more fully in later sections of this chapter—form the basis for understanding the actions and clinical uses of drugs described in every chapter of this book. They may be briefly summarized as follows:

(1) Receptors largely determine the quantitative relations between dose or concentration of drug and pharmacologic effects. The receptor's affinity for binding a drug determines the concentration of drug required to form a significant number of drug-receptor complexes, and the total number of receptors often limits the maximal effect a drug may produce.

(2) Receptors are responsible for selectivity of drug action. The molecular size, shape, and electrical charge of a drug determine whether—and with what avidity—it will bind to a particular receptor among the vast array of chemically different binding sites available in a cell, animal, or patient. Accordingly, changes in the chemical structure of a drug can dramatically increase or decrease the new drug's affinities for different classes of receptors, with resulting alterations in therapeutic and toxic effects.

(3) Receptors mediate the actions of pharmacologic antagonists. Many drugs and endogenous chemical signals, such as hormones, regulate the function of receptor macromolecules as **agonists;** ie, they change the function of a macromolecule as a more or less direct result of binding to it. Pure pharmacologic **antagonists,** however, bind to receptors without directly altering the receptors' function. Thus, the effect of a pure antagonist on a cell or in a patient depends entirely upon its preventing the binding and blocking the biologic actions of agonist molecules. Some of the most useful drugs in clinical medicine are pharmacologic antagonists.

MACROMOLECULAR NATURE OF DRUG RECEPTORS

It is still true that the chemical structures and even the existence of receptors for most clinically useful drugs can only be inferred from the chemical structures of the drugs themselves. By noting which chemical groups are required for specific pharmacologic effects of chemical congeners of a drug, pharmacologists imagine the complementary shape and distribution of electrical charge of the receptor site. In recent years, however, investigators have begun to characterize drug receptors in biochemical terms. Most of these receptors turn out to be proteins, presumably because the polypeptide structure provides the necessary diversity and specificity of shape and charge.

The best-characterized drug receptors are **regulatory proteins,** which mediate the actions of endogenous chemical signals such as neurotransmitters, autacoids, and hormones. This class of receptors mediates effects of many of the most useful therapeutic agents, which either mimic actions of endogenous agonists or, acting as antagonists, prevent responses to endogenous chemical signals. Although the physiologist or endocrinologist may think of these regulatory proteins as the only class of receptors, virtually any kind of protein molecule may serve as a receptor for a drug. Other classes of proteins that have been clearly identified as drug receptors include **enzymes,** which may be inhibited (or, less commonly, activated) by binding a drug (eg, tetrahydrofolate reductase, the receptor for the antineoplastic drug methotrexate); **transport proteins** (eg, Na^+,K^+-ATPase, the membrane receptor for cardioactive digitalis glycosides); and **structural proteins** (eg, tubulin, the receptor for colchicine, an anti-inflammatory agent).

Of the membrane-bound proteins that serve as receptors for neurohormones and drugs, the nicotinic cholinergic receptor is the best-characterized (see Chapter 5). This receptor is an oligomer composed of 4 peptide subunits with molecular weights ranging from 40,000 to 65,000. All 4 peptides span the membrane's lipid bilayer, but only one peptide binds acetylcholine, the neurotransmitter. The binding of acetylcholine triggers opening of a transmembrane channel or pore through which sodium ions penetrate from the extracellular fluid into the cell, an event that initiates an action potential in the nerve or muscle cells that are targets for nicotinic stimulation. The function of the 3 remaining subunits of the nicotinic receptor is the subject of intensive investigation. These subunits somehow transduce the binding of a cholinergic ligand into opening the ion channel and probably constitute the channel itself. Thus, the nicotinic receptor, a single oligomeric protein molecule, performs 2 distinct functions as a receptor: (1) specific recognition of a drug or regulatory ligand (binding of acetylcholine), and (2) initiation of a biochemical event (opening of the sodium channel) that leads to the characteristic response of the cell (a propagated action potential).

RELATION BETWEEN DRUG CONCENTRATION & RESPONSE

The relation between dose of a drug and the clinically observed response may be quite complex. In carefully controlled in vitro systems, however, the relation between concentration of a drug and its effect is often simple and can be described with mathematical precision. We will analyze this simple, idealized relation first because it underlies virtually all of the more complex relations between dose and effect that occur when drugs are given to patients.

Concentration-Effect Curves & Receptor Binding of Agonists

Even in intact animals or patients, responses to low doses of a drug usually increase in direct proportion to dose. As doses increase, however, the incremental response diminishes; finally, doses may be reached at which no further increase in response can be achieved. In idealized or in vitro systems, the relation between drug concentration and effect is described by a hyperbolic curve (Fig 2–1A), according to the following equation:

$$E = \frac{E_{max}[C]}{[C] + K_{act}}$$

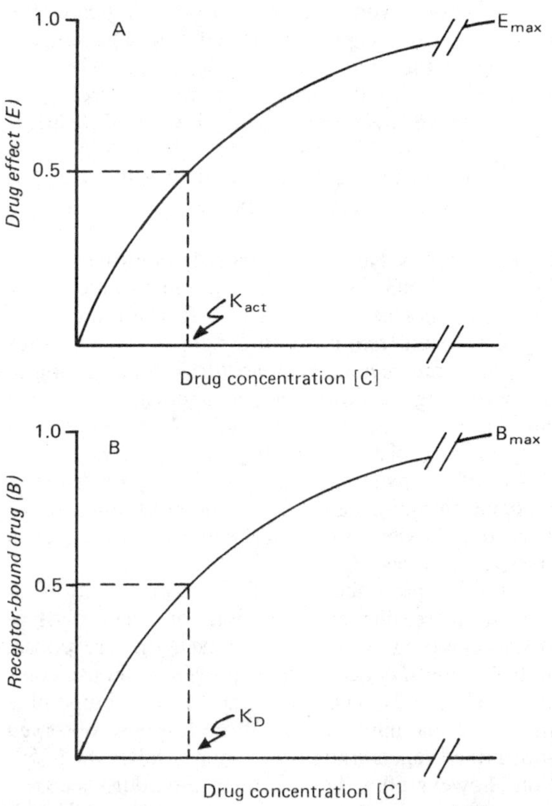

Figure 2–1. Relations between drug concentration and drug effect *(A)* or receptor-bound drug *(B)*. The drug concentrations at which effect or receptor occupancy are half-maximal are denoted K_{act} and K_D, respectively.

where E is the effect observed at concentration C, E_{max} is the maximal response that can be produced by the drug, and K_{act} is the concentration of drug that produces half-maximal effect. This K_{act} concentration is often called the EC50 (concentration for 50% of maximal effect).

The resemblance of this hyperbolic relation to the mass action law that predicts association between 2 molecules of a given affinity suggested that drug agonists act by binding to ("occupying") a distinct class of biologic molecules with a characteristic affinity for the drug—the receptor. With the advent of radioactive receptor ligands, including both agonists and antagonists, this occupancy assumption has been amply confirmed for a number of drug-receptor systems. In these systems, the relation between drug bound to receptors (B) and the concentration of free (unbound) drug (C) depicted in Fig 2–1B is described by an analogous equation:

$$B = \frac{B_{max}[C]}{[C] + K_D}$$

in which B_{max} indicates the concentration of bound drug at infinitely high concentrations of free drug, and K_D (the equilibrium dissociation constant) indicates the concentration of free drug at which half-maximal binding is observed. The value of B_{max} indicates the total number of receptors in the cell or tissue available for binding the drug, while the K_D characterizes the receptor's affinity for binding the drug in a reciprocal fashion: If the K_D concentration is low, binding affinity is high, and vice versa.

Note also that the K_{act} and K_D may be identical but need not be so, as discussed below.

Competitive & Noncompetitive Antagonists

Receptor antagonists act by binding to the receptor but do not activate it. The effects of these antagonists result from preventing agonists (other drugs or endogenous regulatory molecules) from binding to and activating receptors. Such antagonists are divided into 2 classes depending on whether or not they compete with agonists for binding to receptors. The 2 classes of receptor antagonism produce quite different concentration-effect and concentration-binding curves in vitro and exhibit important practical differences in therapy of disease.

In the presence of a fixed concentration of agonist, increasing concentrations of a **competitive antagonist** progressively inhibit the agonist response; high antagonist concentrations prevent response completely (Fig 2–2). The concentration of a competitive antagonist that inhibits 50% of the response observed with a fixed concentration of agonist is called the IC50. Note, however, that the IC50 of an antagonist is different for every concentration of agonist used. This is because the inhibition is competitive, so that high enough concentrations of agonist can overcome the effect of any fixed concentration of antagonist. (The converse is also true.) As a result, in the presence of a fixed concentration of competitive antagonist, an agonist concentration-effect curve (Fig 2–3A) has the same E_{max} as does the curve seen in the absence of antagonist; however, concentrations of agonist required for producing any given level of effect are increased, and the curve is shifted to the right.

In an idealized system, the response elicited by mixtures of various concentrations of agonist (C) and competitive antagonist (I) can be predicted on the basis of the K_{act} for the agonist and the antagonist's dissociation constant (K_I), according to the following equation:

$$E = \frac{E_{max}[C]}{[C] + K_{act}(1 + \frac{[I]}{K_I})}$$

Conversely, in a carefully controlled in vitro system, this mathematical relationship allows experimental determination of the K_I of a competitive antagonist.*

*K_I can be determined by measuring responses to mixtures of known concentrations of agonist and antagonist. For example, an experiment can be designed to determine the IC50 of a competitive antagonist at a fixed concentration (C) of agonist. If the K_{act} of the agonist is known from other experiments,

$$K_I = \frac{IC50}{1 + [C]/K_{act}}$$

K_I values derived from such experiments agree with those determined by direct measurements of binding of radiolabeled competitive antagonists to receptors.

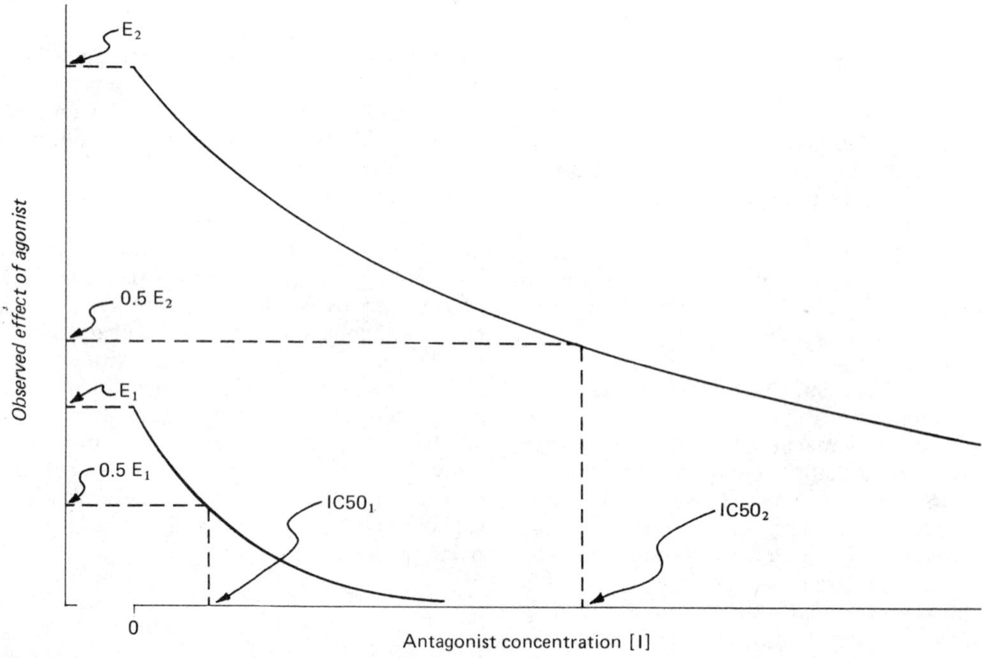

Figure 2–2. Increasing concentrations of a competitive antagonist progressively diminish the response to a fixed concentration of agonist. The IC50 concentration of antagonist is greater if the concentration of agonist is greater (upper versus lower curve).

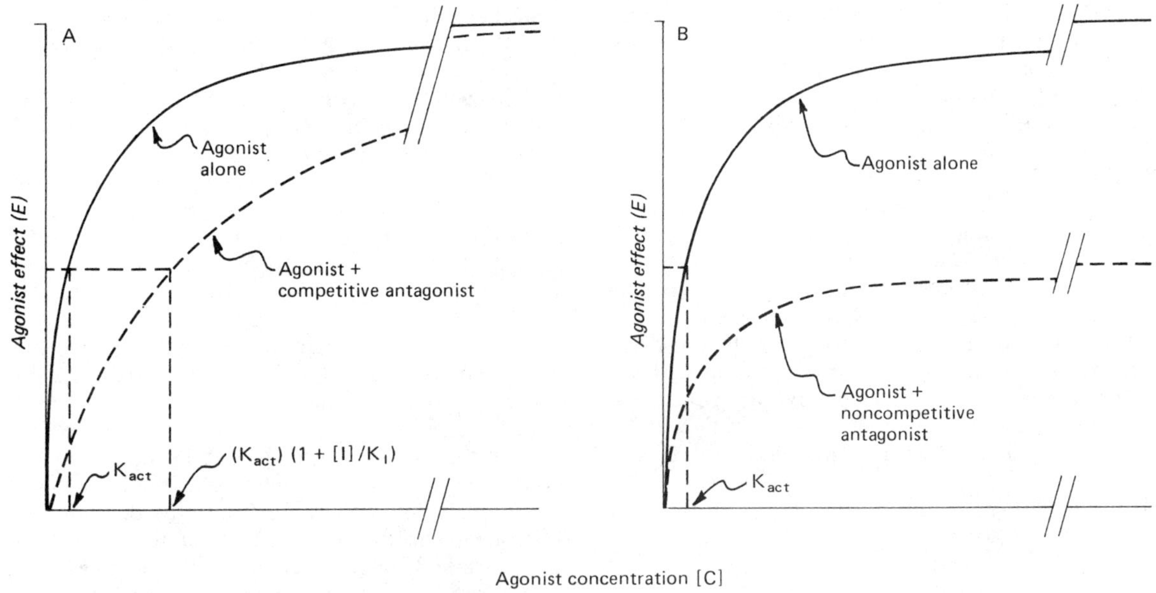

Figure 2–3. Changes in agonist dose-effect curves produced by a competitive antagonist *(A)* or by a noncompetitive antagonist *(B)*. In the presence of a competitive antagonist, higher concentrations of agonist are required to produce a given effect; thus, the agonist concentration required for half-maximal effect in the presence of [I] concentration of an antagonist is the product of the K_{act} times (1 + $[I]/K_I$). High agonist concentrations can overcome inhibition by a competitive antagonist. This is not the case with a noncompetitive antagonist, which reduces the maximal effect the agonist can achieve, although it may not change the K_{act}.

For the clinician, this mathematical relationship has 2 important therapeutic implications:

(1) The degree of inhibition produced by a competitive antagonist depends upon the concentration of unbound antagonist. Thus, the extent and duration of action of such a drug will depend upon its concentration in plasma and will be critically influenced by the rate of its metabolic clearance or excretion. Different patients receiving a fixed dose of propranolol, for example, exhibit a wide range of plasma concentrations, owing to differences in clearance of the drug. As a result, the effects of a fixed dose of this competitive antagonist of norepinephrine may vary widely in patients, and the dose must be varied accordingly.

(2) The equation defines another important source of variability in clinical response to a competitive antagonist, ie, the concentration of agonist that is competing for binding to receptors. Here also propranolol provides a useful example: When this competitive β-adrenergic antagonist is administered in doses sufficient to block the effect of basal levels of the neurotransmitter norepinephrine, resting heart rate is decreased. However, the increase in release of norepinephrine and epinephrine that occurs with exercise, postural changes, or emotional stress may suffice to overcome competitive antagonism by propranolol and increase heart rate. Consequently, the physician who devises a dosage regimen for a competitive antagonist must always consider possible changes in endogenous agonist that could influence therapeutic response.

The second class of receptor antagonists acts in a noncompetitive fashion; ie, after administration of a **noncompetitive antagonist,** high concentrations of agonist cannot completely overcome the antagonism, and maximal agonist response cannot be obtained (Fig 2–3B). In general, noncompetitive antagonists act in an irreversible or nearly irreversible fashion. Affinity of such an antagonist for a receptor may be so high that, for practical purposes, the receptor is unavailable for binding of agonist. Other antagonists in this class produce irreversible effects because after binding to the receptor they form covalent bonds to the receptor.

Therapeutically, noncompetitive antagonists present distinctive advantages and disadvantages. Once the noncompetitive antagonist has occupied the receptor, it need not be present in unbound form to inhibit agonist responses. Consequently, the duration of action of such an irreversible antagonist is relatively independent of its own rate of clearance and more dependent upon the rate of turnover of receptor molecules.

Phenoxybenzamine, an irreversible α-adrenergic antagonist, is used to reduce the increased blood pressure caused by catecholamines released from pheochromocytoma, a tumor of the adrenal medulla. If administration of phenoxybenzamine lowers blood pressure, blockade will be maintained even when the tumor episodically releases very large amounts of catecholamine. In this case, the ability to prevent responses to varying and high concentrations of agonist is a therapeutic advantage. If overdose occurs, however, a real problem may arise. If the α-adrenergic blockade cannot be overcome, excess effects of the drug must be antagonized "physiologically," eg, by using a pressor agent that does not act via α-adrenergic receptors.

Partial Agonists

Based on the maximal pharmacologic response that occurs when all receptors are occupied, agonists can be divided into 2 classes: **Partial agonists** produce a lower maximal response, at full receptor occupancy, than do **full agonists** (Fig 2–4A). As compared to full agonists, partial agonists produce concentration-effect curves that resemble curves observed with full agonists in the presence of a noncompetitive antagonist that irreversibly blocks receptor sites (compare Figs 2–4A and 2–3B). Nonetheless, radioligand-binding experiments have demonstrated that partial agonists may occupy all receptor sites (Fig 2–4B) at concentrations that will fail to produce a maximal response comparable to that seen with full agonists (Fig 2–4A). In addition, the failure of partial agonists to produce a "full" maximal response is not due to decreased affinity for binding to receptors. Such drugs compete, frequently with high affinity, for the full complement of receptors. Indeed, the partial agonists' ability to occupy the total receptor population is indicated by the fact that partial agonists competitively inhibit the responses produced by full agonists.

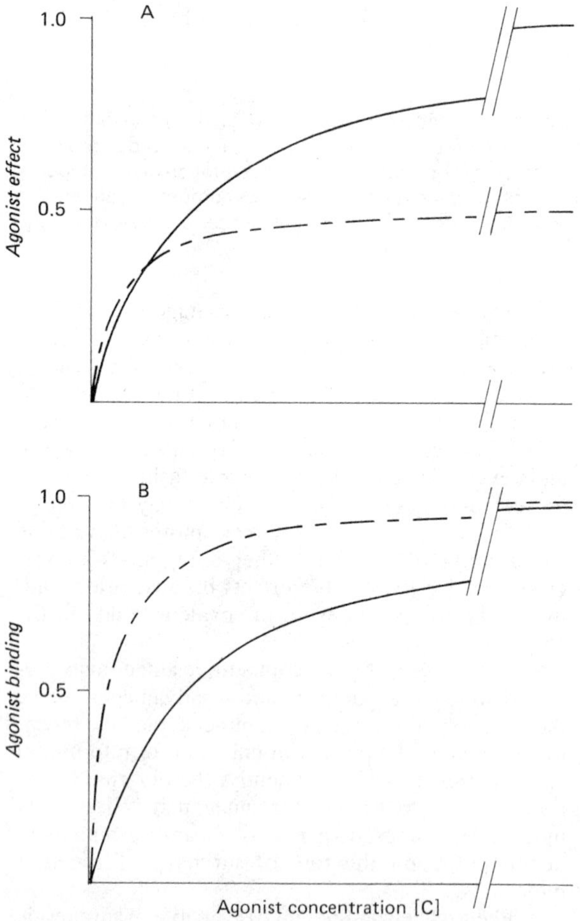

Figure 2–4. Comparison of a full agonist (solid lines) and a partial agonist (broken lines) with respect to effect *(A)* or receptor binding *(B)* at different agonist concentrations. In this example, the receptor has a higher affinity for the partial agonist than for the full agonist, so that a higher concentration of the latter is required for half-maximal binding. At high concentrations, however, the partial agonist produces a smaller maximal response than does the full agonist.

The precise molecular mechanism that accounts for blunted maximal responses to partial agonists is not known. It is simplest to imagine that the partial agonist produces an effect on receptors that is intermediate between the effect produced by a full agonist and that produced by a competitive antagonist. The full agonist changes receptor conformation in a way that initiates subsequent pharmacologic effects of receptor occupancy, while the "pure" competitive antagonist produces no such change in receptor conformation; in this view, the partial agonist changes receptor conformation, but not to the extent necessary to result in full efficacy of the occupied receptor.

To express this idea, pharmacologists refer to the **efficacy** (or "maximal efficacy") of a drug as a way of indicating the relation between pharmacologic response and occupancy of receptor sites. Efficacy for a full agonist is considered to be 1.0, while the efficacy of a pure antagonist is zero. Partial agonists have efficacies between zero and 1.0. The reader will see that many drugs used as competitive antagonists are in fact weak partial agonists.

Receptor-Effector "Coupling" & Spare Receptors

Whatever its actual nature, the conformational change that occurs when a receptor is occupied by an agonist is only one of several steps necessary for expression of a full pharmacologic response. The transduction process between occupancy of receptors and drug response is often termed "coupling." The efficiency of receptor-effector coupling is determined by the ionic environment and by specific cellular components ("coupling factors," some of which have been biochemically identified for the actions of certain drugs), in addition to the receptor itself. Thus, agonist-receptor interactions presumably result in full or "tight" coupling of full agonists to response, in less tight coupling of partial agonists, and in "uncoupling" of pure antagonists. However, it is possible for even full agonists to become "uncoupled" from responses as the result of changes in coupling processes that take place distal to the receptor.

High efficiency of receptor-effector coupling may also be interpreted as the result of **spare receptors.** Receptors are said to be "spare" for a given pharmacologic response when the full maximal response can be elicited by an agonist at a concentration that does not result in occupancy of the full complement of available receptors. Experimentally, spare re-

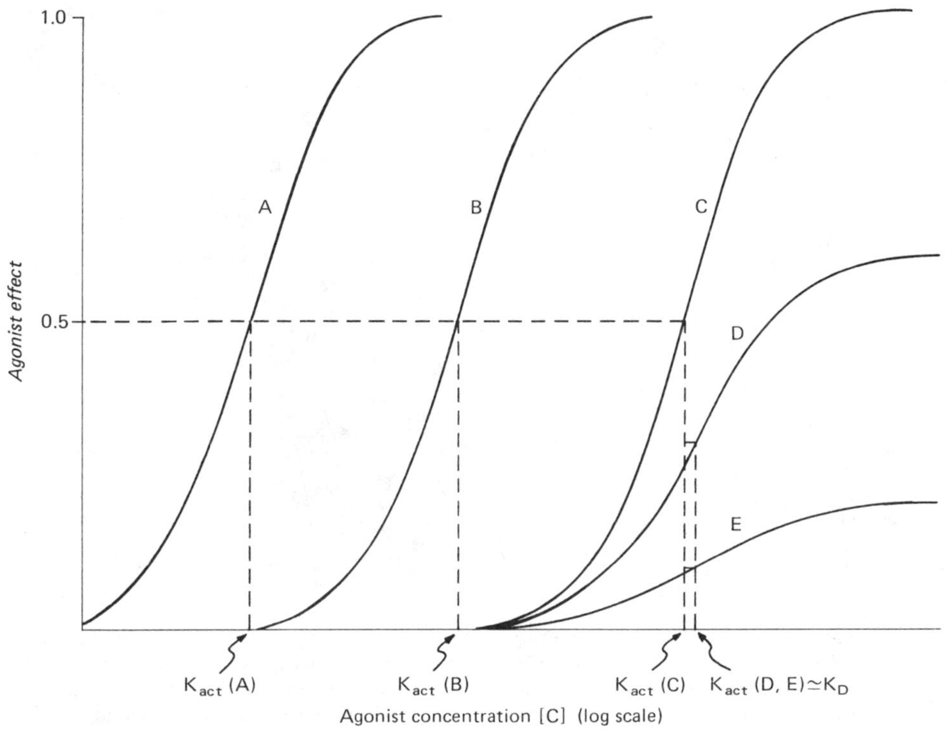

Figure 2–5. Experimental demonstration of spare receptors, using different concentrations of a noncompetitive (irreversible) antagonist. Curve A shows agonist response in the absence of antagonist. After treatment with a low concentration of antagonist (curve B), the curve is shifted to the right; maximal responsiveness is preserved, however, because the remaining available receptors are still in excess of the number required. In curve C, produced after treatment with a larger concentration of antagonist, the available receptors are no longer "spare"; instead, they are just sufficient to mediate an undiminished maximal response. Still higher concentrations of antagonist (curves D and E) reduce the number of available receptors to the point that maximal response is diminished. The apparent K_{act} of the agonist in curves D and E may approximate the K_D that characterizes the binding affinity of the agonist for the receptor.

ceptors may be demonstrated by using noncompetitive (irreversible) antagonists to prevent binding of agonist to a proportion of available receptors and showing that high concentrations of agonist can still produce an undiminished maximal response (Fig 2–5). Thus, a maximal inotropic response of heart muscle to β-adrenergic amines can be elicited even under conditions where up to 90% of the β-adrenergic receptors are occupied by a quasi-irreversible antagonist. Accordingly, myocardium is said to contain a large proportion of spare receptors.

Note, however, that spare receptors are not qualitatively different from nonspare ones. They are not "hidden" or unavailable, and they can be coupled to response. Fig 2–6 depicts one way of explaining how maximal response can occur without full occupancy of receptors. This will happen if the concentration or amount of a cellular component other than the receptor limits the coupling of receptor occupancy to response.

The spare receptor concept should help explain how the sensitivity of a cell or tissue to a particular concentration of agonist may depend not only on the affinity of the receptor for binding an agonist (characterized by the K_D) but also on the total concentration of receptors. Sensitivity may be expressed in terms of K_{act} or EC50, the concentration of agonist that results in half-maximal response. The K_D of the agonist-receptor interaction determines what fraction (B/B_{max}) of total receptors will be occupied at a given free concentration (C) of agonist, regardless of the receptor concentration:

$$\frac{B}{B_{max}} = \frac{[C]}{[C] + K_D}$$

In a tissue with 90% spare receptors, however, half-maximal response will occur at an agonist concentration (the K_{act}) that results in occupancy of only 5% of the receptors. Thus, K_{act} is considerably lower than K_D. If the receptor concentration in this tissue is then doubled, the concentration of free agonist that results in 5% occupancy of total receptors will be the same, because receptor affinity has not changed. Now, however, 5% occupancy (equivalent in number of receptors to 10% occupancy before receptors were doubled) will result in a maximal response; correspondingly, the K_{act} will be reduced. Thus, it is possible to change the sensitivity of tissues with spare receptors by changing

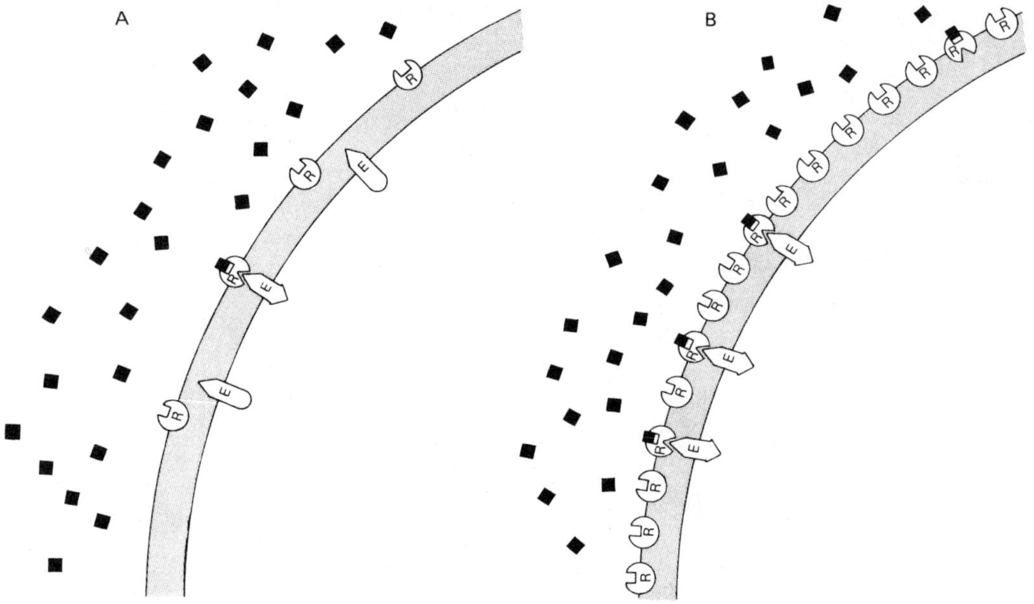

Figure 2–6. Spare receptors increase sensitivity to drug. In membrane A *(left),* the free concentration of agonist (■) is one-third the K_D concentration; this is sufficient to bind 25% of the 4 receptors (R) present, resulting in the formation of one agonist-receptor complex. (*Note:* Before going on, verify for yourself that free agonist at a concentration (C) one-third the K_D will occupy one-fourth of the total receptors. Remember that $B/B_{max} = [C]/[C] + K_D$.) Agonist occupancy of this one receptor changes its conformation so that it binds to and activates an effector molecule (E), resulting in a response. Because one of 3 effectors is stimulated by agonist-receptor complex, the response is 33% of maximum. In membrane B *(right),* the receptor concentration has been increased to 16, but the K_D for binding of agonist to receptors remains unchanged. As a result, the same free concentration of drug (one-third K_D) occupies 25% of the receptors. Now, however, this is *four* activated receptors, which results in activation of all 3 effectors and produces 100% response. Note that membrane B has one receptor that is occupied by drug but has no available effector molecule. This receptor is "spare," as are all the unoccupied receptors that could bind agonist at higher free agonist concentrations.

the receptor concentration. (Note, in passing, that changing the number of receptors does not usually change the free concentration of drug achieved by administering a given dose. This is because the concentration of receptors in a tissue is usually very small relative to effective concentrations of drugs.)

An important biologic consequence of spare receptors is that they allow agonists with low affinity for receptors to produce full responses at low concentrations, to the extent that K_{act} is lower than K_D. This is important because ligands with low affinity (high K_D) dissociate rapidly from receptors, allowing rapid termination of biologic responses. High binding affinity (low K_D), on the other hand, would result in slow dissociation of agonist from receptor and correspondingly slower reversal of a biologic response.

Other Mechanisms of Pharmacologic Antagonism

Not all of the mechanisms of pharmacologic antagonism involve interactions of drugs or endogenous ligands at a single type of receptor. Indeed, **chemical antagonists** need not involve a receptor at all. Thus, one drug may antagonize the actions of a second drug by binding to and inactivating the second drug. For example, protamine, a protein that is positively charged at physiologic pH, is used clinically to counteract the effects of heparin, an anticoagulant that is negatively charged; in this case, one drug antagonizes the other simply by binding it and making it unavailable for interactions with proteins involved in formation of a blood clot.

The clinician often uses drugs that take advantage of **physiologic antagonism** between endogenous regulatory pathways. Many physiologic functions are controlled by opposing regulatory pathways. For example, several catabolic actions of the glucocorticoid hormones lead to increased blood sugar, an effect that is physiologically opposed by insulin. Although glucocorticoids and insulin act on quite distinct receptor-effector systems, the clinician must sometimes administer insulin to oppose the hyperglycemic effects of glucocorticoid hormones, whether the latter are elevated by endogenous synthesis (eg, an inoperable tumor of the adrenal cortex) or as a result of glucocorticoid therapy.

In general, use of a drug as a physiologic antagonist produces effects that are less specific and less easy to control than are the effects of a receptor-specific antagonist. Thus, for example, to treat bradycardia caused by increased vagal tone associated with the acute pain of a myocardial infarction, the physician could use isoproterenol, a β-adrenergic agonist that increases heart rate by mimicking sympathetic stimulation of the heart. However, use of this physiologic antagonist would be less rational—and potentially more dangerous—than would use of a receptor-specific antagonist such as atropine (a competitive antagonist at the muscarinic receptors through which vagal stimuli slow heart rate).

CLASSIFICATION OF RECEPTORS

As we have seen, the existence of a specific drug receptor is usually inferred from studying the **structure-activity relationship** of a group of structurally similar congeners of the drug that mimic or antagonize its effects. Thus, if a series of related agonists exhibits identical relative potencies in producing 2 distinct effects, it is likely that the 2 effects are mediated by similar or identical receptor molecules. In addition, if the same molecular species of receptor mediates both effects, a competitive antagonist will inhibit both responses with the same K_I; a second competitive antagonist will inhibit both responses with its own characteristic K_I. Thus, studies of the relation between structure and activity of a series of agonists and antagonists can identify a species of receptor that mediates a set of pharmacologic responses.

Exactly the same experimental procedure can show that observed effects of a drug are mediated by different species of receptors. In this case, effects mediated by different receptors may exhibit different orders of potency among agonists, and different K_I values for each competitive antagonist.

Evidence that a particular drug acts via 2 or more distinct receptors usually presents an important therapeutic opportunity, because it suggests the possibility of developing new drugs that will exhibit enhanced selectivity for one receptor over the other. Such opportunities have been extensively exploited with the receptors for histamine, acetylcholine, and norepinephrine. Thus, for example, β-adrenergic antagonists can block cardioacceleration produced by norepinephrine without preventing catecholamine regulation of arteriolar constriction, which is mediated by α-adrenergic receptors. Similarly, α-adrenergic agonists can induce vasoconstriction without stimulating β receptors in the heart (see Chapter 7). Clinical uses of receptor-selective drugs are described in many chapters of this book (see Chapter 5 for cholinergic receptors; Chapter 14 for histamine receptors). In each case, the endogenous autacoid or neurotransmitter produces multiple effects in the intact patient, and it is therapeutically advantageous to stimulate or block one set of effects without substantially affecting others. This principle is illustrated in Fig 2–7.

RELATION BETWEEN DRUG DOSE & CLINICAL RESPONSE

We have dealt with receptors as molecules and shown how receptors can quantitatively account for the relation between dose or concentration of a drug and pharmacologic responses, at least in an idealized system. When faced with a patient who needs treatment, the physician must make a choice among a variety of possible drugs and devise a dosage regimen that is likely to produce maximal benefit and minimal toxicity. Because the patient is never an idealized system, the physician will not have precise information about

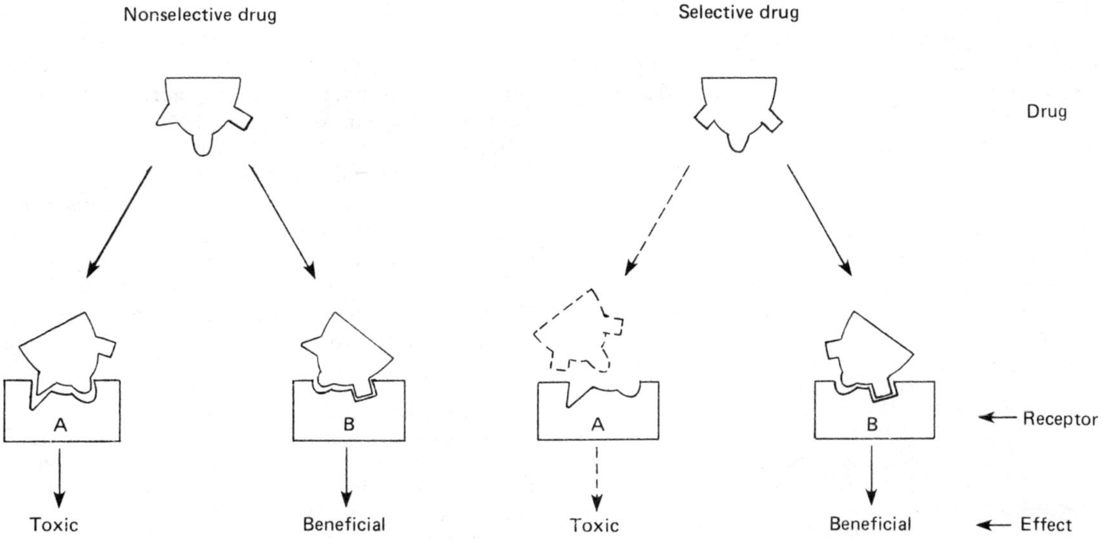

Figure 2–7. Receptor selectivity. Receptors A and B mediate toxic (unwanted) or beneficial (therapeutic) effects, respectively. A nonselective drug binds equally well to both types of receptor, while a selective drug binds with higher affinity to receptor B than to receptor A.

the physicochemical nature of the receptors involved, the number of receptors, or their affinity for drugs. Nonetheless, in order to make rational therapeutic decisions, the physician must understand how drug-receptor interactions underlie the relations between dose and response in nonideal patients, the nature and causes of variation in pharmacologic responsiveness, and the clinical implications of selectivity of drug action.

Dose & Response in Patients

A. Graded Dose-Response Relations: To choose among drugs and to determine appropriate doses of a drug, the physician must know the relative **pharmacologic potency** and **maximal efficacy** of the drugs in relation to the desired therapeutic effect. These 2 important terms, often confusing to students and clinicians, can be explained by reference to Fig 2–8, which depicts graded dose-response curves that relate log dose of 4 different drugs to the magnitude of a particular therapeutic effect, eg, lowering of blood pressure in a hypertensive patient or increasing urinary excretion of sodium in a patient with congestive heart failure.

1. Potency–Drugs A and B are said to be more potent than drug C because of their relative positions along the **dose axis** of Fig 2–8. Potency thus refers to the range of doses over which a drug produces increasing responses. Accordingly, drug B is actually more potent than drug A, because the increasing effects of B occur over a lower range of doses even though some doses of A can produce a larger quantitative effect. Potency of a drug depends in part on the affinity (K_D) of receptors for binding the drug and in part on the efficiency with which drug-receptor interaction is coupled to response. Both affinity and coupling efficiency contribute to the K_{act} or EC50 of a particular drug-response relation in vitro, as described above. When a drug is administered to a patient, its potency also depends upon its ability to reach the relevant receptors. Thus, a drug's potency may depend upon its route of administration, absorption, distribution through the body, and clearance from the blood or from its site of action.

While the potency of a drug clearly is important for determining the dose to be used, there is no reason to consider the relative potencies of 2 drugs in deciding which one to administer to a patient. (Low potency would only be important if the drug had to be administered in inconveniently large amounts.)

For therapeutic purposes, the potency of a drug should be stated in dosage units, usually in terms of a particular therapeutic end point (eg, 50 mg for mild sedation, 1 μg/kg/min for an increase in heart rate of 25 beats/min). Relative potency, the ratio of equieffective doses (0.2, 10, etc), may be used in comparing one drug with another.

2. Maximal efficacy–This parameter reflects the limit of the dose-response relation on the **response axis.** Drugs A and C in Fig 2–8 have equal maximal efficacy, while both have greater maximal efficacy than does drug B. The maximal efficacy (sometimes referred to simply as **efficacy**) of a drug is obviously crucial for making clinical decisions. It may be determined by the drug's mode of interactions with receptors (as with partial agonists, described above)* or by characteristics of the receptor-effector system involved. Thus, diuretics that act on one portion of the nephron may produce much greater excretion of fluid and electrolytes than diuretics that act elsewhere. In addition, the efficacy of a drug for achieving a therapeutic end point (eg, increased cardiac contractility) may be limited by the drug's propensity to cause a toxic effect (eg, fatal cardiac arrhythmia) even if the drug could otherwise produce a greater therapeutic effect.

B. Shape of Dose-Response Curves: While the responses depicted in curves A, B, and C of Fig 2–8 approximate the shape of a simple Michaelis-Menten relation (transformed to a logarithmic plot), some clinical responses do not. Extremely steep dose-response curves (eg, curve D) may have important clinical consequences if the upper portion of the curve represents an undesirable extent of response (eg, coma caused by a sedative-hypnotic). Steep dose-response curves in patients could result from cooperative interactions of several different actions of a drug (eg, effects on brain, heart, and peripheral vessels, all contributing to lowering of blood pressure). Such steep dose-response curves could also be produced by a receptor-effector system in which most receptors must be occupied

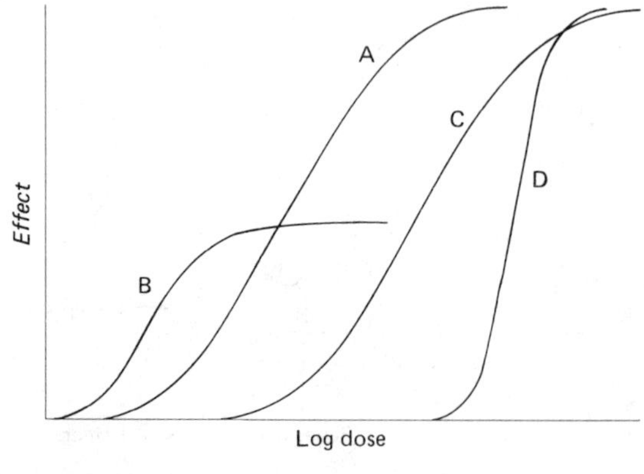

Figure 2–8. Graded dose-response curves for 4 drugs, illustrating different pharmacologic potencies and different maximal efficacies.

*Note that "maximal efficacy," used in a therapeutic context, does not have exactly the meaning the term implies in the more specialized context of drug-receptor interactions, described earlier in this chapter. In an idealized in vitro system, efficacy refers to the relative maximal efficacy of agonists and partial agonists that act via the same receptor. In therapeutics, efficacy refers to the extent or degree of an effect that can be achieved in the intact patient. Thus, therapeutic efficacy may be affected by the characteristics of a particular drug-receptor interaction, but it also depends upon a host of other factors, noted in the text.

before any effect is seen or by unusual pharmacokinetic properties of a drug that create a threshold dose below which little or no drug can reach the receptors responsible for its action (see Chapter 3).

C. Quantal Dose-Effect Curves: Despite their usefulness for characterizing the actions of drugs, graded dose-response curves of the sort described above have certain limitations in their application to clinical decision-making. For example, such curves may be impossible to construct if the pharmacologic response is an either/or event, such as prevention of convulsions, arrhythmia, or death. Furthermore, the clinical relevance of a quantitative dose-response relationship in a single patient, no matter how precisely defined, may be limited in application to other patients, owing to the great potential variability among patients in severity of disease and responsiveness to drugs.

Some of these difficulties may be avoided by determining the dose of drug required to produce a specified magnitude of effect in a large number of individual patients or experimental animals and plotting the cumulative frequency distribution of responders versus the log dose (Fig 2–9). The specified quantal effect may be chosen on the basis of clinical relevance (eg, relief of headache) or for preservation of safety of experimental subjects (eg, using low doses of a cardiac stimulant and specifying an increase in heart rate of 20 beats/min as the quantal effect), or it may be an inherently quantal event (eg, death of an experimental animal). For most drugs, the doses required to produce a specified quantal effect in individuals are lognormally distributed; ie, a frequency distribution of such responses plotted against the log of the dose produces a gaussian normal curve of variation (Fig 2–9). When these responses are summated, the resulting cumulative frequency distribution constitutes a quantal dose-effect curve (or dose-percent curve) of the proportion or percentage of individuals who exhibit the effect plotted as a function of log dose (Fig 2–9).

The quantal dose-effect curve is often characterized by stating the **median effective dose** (ED50), the dose at which 50% of individuals exhibit the specified quantal effect. Similarly, the dose required to produce a particular toxic effect in 50% of animals is called the **median toxic dose** (TD50). If the toxic effect is death of the animal, a **median lethal dose** (LD50) may be experimentally defined. Such values provide a convenient way of comparing the potencies of drugs in experimental and clinical settings: Thus, if the ED50s of 2 drugs for producing a specified quantal effect are 5 and 500 mg, respectively, then the first drug can be said to be 100 times more potent than the second for that particular effect. Similarly, one can obtain a valuable index of the selectivity of a drug's action by comparing its ED50s for 2 different quantal effects in a population (eg, cough suppression versus sedation for opiate drugs; increase in heart rate versus increased vasoconstriction for adrenergic amines; anti-inflammatory effects versus sodium retention for corticosteroids; etc).

Quantal dose-effect curves may also be used to generate information regarding the margin of safety to

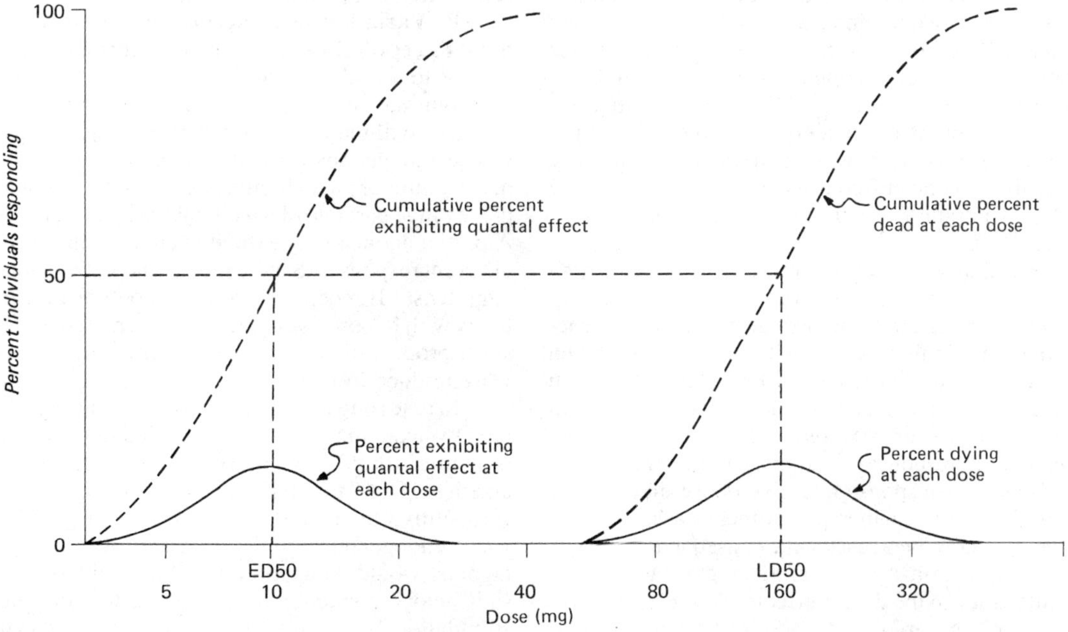

Figure 2–9. Quantal dose-effect curves. Solid curves indicate the frequency distribution of doses of drug required to produce a specified effect; ie, the curves show the percentage of animals that required a particular dose to exhibit the effect. Dashed lines indicate the cumulative frequency distribution of responses, which are lognormally distributed.

be expected from a particular drug used to produce a specified effect. One measure, which relates the dose of a drug required to produce a desired effect to that which produces an undesired effect, is the **therapeutic index.** In animal studies, the therapeutic index is usually defined as the ratio of the TD50 to the ED50 for some therapeutically relevant effect. The clinical usefulness of a drug usually relates to a much more conservative definition of therapeutic index and critically depends upon the severity of the disease under treatment. Thus, for the treatment of headache the physician might require a very large therapeutic index, defined as the ratio of the dose required to cause serious toxicity in a very small percentage of subjects (TD0.001) to the dose required to ameliorate headache in a very large proportion of subjects (ED99). For treatment of a lethal disease, such as Hodgkin's lymphoma, an acceptable therapeutic index might be defined less stringently.

Finally, note that the quantal dose-effect curve and the classic graded dose-response curve summarize somewhat different sets of information, although both appear sigmoid in shape on a semilogarithmic plot (compare Figs 2–8 and 2–9). Critical information required for making rational therapeutic decisions can be obtained from each type of curve: Both curves provide information regarding the **potency** and **selectivity** of drugs; the graded dose-response curve indicates the **maximal efficacy** of a drug; and the dose-effect curve indicates the potential **variability** of responsiveness among individuals.

Variation in Drug Responsiveness

Individuals may vary considerably in their responsiveness to a drug; indeed, a single individual may respond differently to the same drug at different times during the course of treatment. Occasionally, individuals exhibit an unusual or **idiosyncratic** drug response, one that is infrequently observed in most patients. These idiosyncratic responses are usually caused by genetic differences in metabolism of the drug or by immunologic mechanisms, including allergic reactions.

Quantitative variations in drug response are in general more common and more clinically important: An individual patient is **hyporeactive** or **hyperreactive** to a drug in that the intensity of effect of a given dose of drug is diminished or increased in comparison to the effect seen in most individuals. (***Note:*** The term **hypersensitivity** usually refers to allergic or other immunologic responses to drugs.) With some drugs, the intensity of response to a given dose may change during the course of therapy; in these cases, responsiveness usually decreases as a consequence of continued drug administration, producing a state of relative **tolerance** to the drug's effects. When responsiveness diminishes rapidly after administration of a drug, the response is said to be subject to **tachyphylaxis.**

The general clinical implications of individual variability in drug responsiveness are clear: The physician must be prepared to change either the dose of drug or the choice of drug, depending upon the response observed in the patient. Even before administering the first dose of a drug, the physician should consider factors that may help in predicting the direction and extent of possible variation in responsiveness. These include the propensity of a particular drug to produce tolerance or tachyphylaxis as well as the effects of age, sex, body size, disease state, and simultaneous administration of other drugs.

Four general mechanisms may contribute to variation in drug responsiveness among patients or within an individual patient at different times. The classification described below is necessarily artificial in that most variation in clinical responsiveness is caused by more than one mechanism. Nonetheless, the classification may be useful because certain mechanisms of variation are best dealt with according to different therapeutic strategies:

A. Alteration in Concentration of Drug That Reaches the Receptor: Patients may differ in the rate of absorption of a drug, in distributing it through body compartments, or in clearing the drug from the blood (see Chapter 3). Any of these pharmacokinetic differences may alter the concentration of drug that reaches relevant receptors and thus alter clinical response. These pharmacokinetic differences can often be predicted on the basis of age, weight, sex, disease state, or liver and kidney function of the patient, and such predictions may be used to guide quantitative decisions regarding an initial dosing regimen. Repeated measurements of drug concentrations in blood during the course of treatment are often helpful in dealing with the variability of clinical response caused by pharmacokinetic differences among individuals.

B. Variation in Concentration of an Endogenous Receptor Ligand: This mechanism contributes greatly to variability in responses to pharmacologic antagonists. Thus, propranolol, a β-adrenergic antagonist, will markedly slow the heart rate of a patient whose endogenous catecholamines are elevated (as in heart failure or pheochromocytoma) but will not affect the resting heart rate of a well trained marathon runner. A partial agonist may exhibit even more dramatically different responses: Saralasin, a weak partial agonist at angiotensin II receptors, lowers blood pressure in patients with hypertension caused by increased angiotensin II production and raises blood pressure in patients who produce low amounts of angiotensin.

In assessing clinical response to antagonist drugs, the physician must always make a judgment about the probable stimulation of receptors by endogenous agonists. Thus, unsatisfactory response to a dose of a competitive antagonist might be due to greatly elevated endogenous agonist, and a larger dose of antagonist would be appropriate. Alternatively, the unsatisfactory response might be due to low rates of stimulation by agonist; this would suggest that the diagnosis is wrong and that a different mode of therapy, rather than more drug, is indicated.

C. Alterations in Number or Function of Receptors: Experimental studies have documented changes in drug responsiveness caused by increases or decreases in the number of receptor sites or by alterations in the efficiency of coupling of receptors to distal effector mechanisms. Although such changes have not been rigorously documented in human beings, it is likely that they account for much of the individual variability in response to some drugs, particularly those that act at receptors for hormones, biogenic amines, and neurotransmitters. In some cases, the change in receptor number is caused by other hormones; for example, thyroid hormones increase both the number of β-adrenergic receptors in rat heart muscle and the cardiac sensitivity to catecholamines. Similar changes probably contribute to the tachycardia of thyrotoxicosis in patients and may account for the usefulness of propranolol, a β-adrenergic antagonist, in ameliorating symptoms of this disease.

In other cases, the agonist ligand itself induces a decrease in the number ("down regulation") or coupling efficiency of its receptors. Receptor-specific desensitization mechanisms presumably act physiologically to allow cells to adapt to changes in rates of stimulation by hormones and neurotransmitters in their environment. These mechanisms may contribute to tachyphylaxis or tolerance to the effects of some drugs, particularly the biogenic amines and their congeners. Recent investigations suggest, in addition, that similar adaptive mechanisms may be responsible for so-called "overshoot" phenomena that follow withdrawal of certain drugs (propranolol, opiates, some antihypertensive agents, etc). Thus, for example, an antagonist may actually raise the number of receptors in a cell by preventing down regulation caused by endogenous agonist; when the antagonist is withdrawn, the elevated receptor number allows an exaggerated response to physiologic concentrations of agonist.

Therapeutic strategies required to deal with receptor-specific changes in drug responsiveness vary according to the clinical situation. In some cases, the dose of an agonist must be increased to achieve a continuing satisfactory response, while in other cases different or additional drugs should be administered. Cessation of treatment with certain drugs should be gradual and carefully monitored.

D. Changes in Components of Response Distal to Receptor: Although a drug initiates its actions by binding to receptors, the response observed in a patient depends on the functional integrity of biochemical processes in the responding cell and physiologic regulation by interacting organ systems. Clinically, changes in these postreceptor processes represent the largest and most important class of mechanisms that cause variation in responsiveness to drug therapy.

Before initiating therapy with a drug, the physician should be aware of patient characteristics that may limit the clinical response. These characteristics include the age, sex, and general health of the patient and—most importantly—the severity and pathophysiologic mechanism of the disease. Once treatment is begun, the most important potential cause of failure to achieve a satisfactory response is that the diagnosis is wrong or physiologically incomplete. Thus, congestive heart failure will not respond satisfactorily to agents that increase myocardial contractility if the underlying pathologic mechanism is unrecognized stenosis of the mitral valve rather than myocardial insufficiency. Conversely, drug therapy will always be most successful when it is accurately directed at the pathophysiologic mechanism responsible for the disease.

When the diagnosis is correct and the drug is appropriate, treatment may still not produce an optimal result. An unsatisfactory therapeutic response can often be traced to compensatory mechanisms in the patient that respond to and oppose the beneficial effects of the drug. Compensatory increases in sympathetic nervous tone and fluid retention by the kidney, for example, can contribute to tolerance to antihypertensive effects of a vasodilator drug. In such cases, additional drugs may be required to achieve a useful therapeutic response.

Clinical Selectivity: Beneficial Versus Toxic Effects of Drugs

Although we classify drugs according to their principal actions, it is clear that *no drug causes only a single, specific effect.* Why is this so? It is exceedingly unlikely that any kind of drug molecule will bind to only a single molecular species of receptor, if only because the number of potential receptors in a patient is astronomically large. (Consider that the human genome codes for approximately 10^4 different peptide gene products and that the chemical complexity of each of these peptides is sufficient to provide many different potential binding sites.) Even if the chemical structure of a drug allowed it to bind to only one kind of receptor, the biochemical processes controlled by such receptors would take place in multiple cell types and would be coupled to many other biochemical functions; as a result, the patient and the physician would probably perceive more than one drug effect.

Accordingly, drugs are only *selective*—rather than specific—in their actions, because they bind to one or a few types of receptor more tightly than to others, and because these receptors control discrete processes that result in distinct effects. As we have seen, selectivity can be measured by comparing binding affinities of a drug to different receptors or by comparing ED50s for different effects of a drug in vivo. In drug development and in clinical medicine, selectivity is usually considered by separating effects into 2 categories: **beneficial or therapeutic effects** versus **toxic effects.** Pharmaceutical advertisements and physicians occasionally use the term **side-effect,** implying that the effect in question is insignificant or occurs via a pathway that is to one side of the principal action of the drug; such implications are frequently erroneous.

It is important to recognize that the designation of a particular drug effect as either therapeutic or toxic is a value judgment and not a statement about the phar-

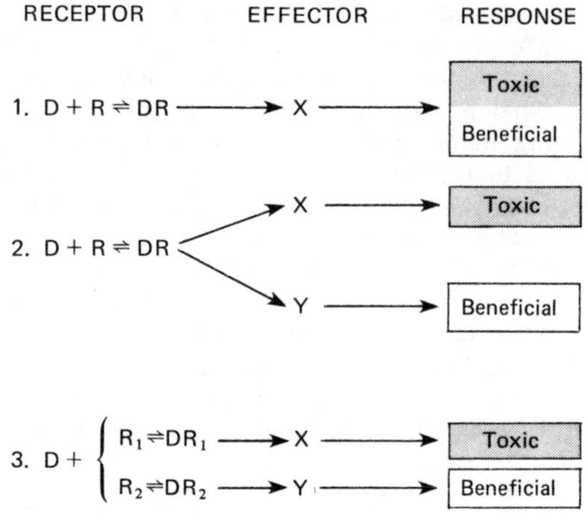

Figure 2–10. Possible relations between the therapeutic and toxic effects of a drug, based on different receptor-effector mechanisms. Therapeutic implications of these different relations are discussed in the text.

macologic mechanism underlying the effect. As a value judgment, such a designation depends on the clinical context in which the drug is used.

It is only because of their selectivity that drugs are useful in clinical medicine. Thus, it is important, both in the management of patients and in the development and evaluation of new drugs, to analyze ways in which beneficial and toxic effects of drugs may be related, in order to increase selectivity and usefulness of drug therapy. Fig 2–10 depicts 3 possible relations between the therapeutic and toxic effects of a drug based on analysis of the receptor-effector mechanisms involved.

A. Beneficial and Toxic Effects Mediated by the Same Receptor-Effector Mechanism: Much of the serious drug toxicity in clinical practice represents a **direct pharmacologic extension** of the therapeutic actions of the drug. In some of these cases (bleeding caused by anticoagulant therapy; hypoglycemic coma due to insulin), toxicity may be avoided by judicious management of the dose of drug administered, guided by careful monitoring of effect (measurements of blood coagulation or serum glucose) and aided by ancillary measures (avoiding tissue trauma that may lead to hemorrhage; regulation of carbohydrate intake). In still other cases, the toxicity may be avoided by not administering the drug at all, if the therapeutic indication is weak or if other therapy is available (eg, sedative-hypnotics ordinarily should not be used to treat patients whose complaints of insomnia are due to underlying mental depression).

In certain situations, a drug is clearly necessary and beneficial but produces unacceptable toxicity when given in doses that produce optimal benefit. In such situations, it may be necessary to add another drug to the treatment regimen. For example, guanethidine (Chapter 9) lowers blood pressure in essential hypertension by inhibiting cardiovascular stimulation by sympathetic nerves; as an inevitable consequence, patients will suffer from symptoms of postural hypotension if the dose of drug is large enough. (Note that postural hypotension has been called a "side-effect" of guanethidine, although in fact it is a direct effect, closely related to the drug's principal therapeutic action.) Appropriate management of such a problem takes advantage of the fact that blood pressure is regulated by changes in blood volume and tone of arterial smooth muscle in addition to the sympathetic nerves. Thus, concomitant administration of diuretics and vasodilators may allow the dose of guanethidine to be lowered, with relief of postural hypotension and continued control of blood pressure.

B. Beneficial and Toxic Effects Mediated by Identical Receptors But in Different Tissues or by Different Effector Pathways: Examples of drugs in this category include digitalis glycosides, which may be used to augment cardiac contractility but also produce cardiac arrhythmias, gastrointestinal effects, and changes in vision (all probably mediated by inhibition of Na^+,K^+-ATPase in cell membranes); methotrexate, used to treat leukemia and other neoplastic diseases, which also kills normal cells in bone marrow and gastrointestinal mucosa (all mediated by inhibition of the enzyme tetrahydrofolate reductase); and congeners of glucocorticoid hormones, used to treat asthma or inflammatory disorders, which also can produce protein catabolism, psychosis, and other toxicities (all thought to be mediated by similar or identical glucocorticoid receptors). In addition to these and other well-documented examples, it is likely that "side-effects" of many drugs are mediated by receptors identical to those that produce the recognized beneficial effect.

Three therapeutic strategies are used to avoid or mitigate this sort of toxicity. *First,* the drug should always be administered at the lowest dose that produces acceptable benefit, recognizing that complete abolition of signs or symptoms of the disease may not be achieved. *Second* (as described above for guanethidine), adjunctive drugs that act through different receptor mechanisms and produce different toxicities may allow lowering the dose of the first drug, thus limiting its toxicity (eg, use of other immunosuppressive agents added to glucocorticoids in treating inflammatory disorders). *Third,* selectivity of the drug's actions may be increased by manipulating the concentrations of drug available to receptors in different parts of the body. Such "anatomic" selectivity may be achieved, for example, by aerosol administration of a glucocorticoid to bronchi or by selective arterial infusion of an antimetabolite into an organ containing tumor cells.

C. Beneficial and Toxic Effects Mediated by Different Types of Receptors: Therapeutic advantages resulting from new chemical entities with improved receptor selectivity were mentioned earlier in this chapter and are described in detail in later chapters. Such drugs include the α- and β-adrenergic agonists and antagonists, the H_1 and H_2 antihistamines, nicotinic and muscarinic blocking agents, and receptor-selective steroid hormones. All of these receptors are grouped in functional families, each responsive to a small class of endogenous agonists. The receptors—and their associated therapeutic uses—were discovered by analyzing effects of the physiologic chemical signals—catecholamines, histamine, acetylcholine, and corticosteroids.

A number of other drugs were discovered in a similar way, although they may not act at receptors for known hormones or neurotransmitters. These drugs were discovered by exploiting toxic or side-effects of other agents, observed in a different clinical context. Examples include quinidine, the sulfonylureas, thiazide diuretics, tricyclic antidepressants, monoamine oxidase inhibitors, and phenothiazine antipsychotics among many others.

It is likely that some of these drugs will eventually be shown to act via receptors for endogenous agonists, as was recently established for morphine, a potent analgesic agent. Morphine has been shown to act on receptors physiologically stimulated by the opioid peptides. Pharmacologists are now beginning to subclassify the opioid receptors, in a fashion reminiscent of earlier studies of adrenergic and cholinergic reactions.

Thus, the propensity of drugs to bind to different classes of receptor sites is not only a potentially vexing problem in treating patients—it also presents a continuing challenge to pharmacology and an opportunity for developing new and more useful drugs.

• • •

References

Baxter JD, Funder JW: Hormone receptors. *N Engl J Med* 1979;**301**:1149.

Goldstein A, Aranow L, Kalman SM: *Principles of Drug Action: The Basis of Pharmacology,* 2nd ed. Wiley, 1974.

Heidman T, Changeux J-P: Structural and functional properties of acetylcholine receptor in its purified and membrane-bound states. *Annu Rev Biochem* 1978;**47**:317.

Iversen LL, Iversen SD, Snyder SH (editors): *Handbook of Psychopharmacology*. Vol 2: *Principles of Receptor Research*. Plenum Press, 1975.

Lefkowitz RJ: Direct binding studies of adrenergic receptors: Biochemical, physiologic, and clinical implications. *Ann Intern Med* 1979;**91**:450.

Roberts JM: Receptors and transfer of information into cells. *Semin Perinatol* 1981;**5**:203.

Snyder SH: Receptors, neurotransmitters and drug responses. *N Engl J Med* 1979;**300**:465.

Williams LT, Lefkowitz RJ: *Receptor Binding Studies in Adrenergic Pharmacology*. Raven Press, 1978.

3 | Pharmacokinetics: I. Absorption, Distribution, & Excretion

Leslie Z. Benet, PhD

When a clinician prescribes a drug and the patient takes it, their main concern is with the effect on the patient's disease. However, as illustrated in Fig 3–1, several processes are going forward from the time a dose is administered until the appearance of any therapeutic effect. These pharmacokinetic processes, defined in Chapter 1, determine how rapidly and in what concentration and for how long the drug will appear at the target organ. The 3 steps shown at the top of Fig 3–1—**input, distribution,** and **loss**—are the major pharmacokinetic variables. In most cases, input will consist of absorption from the most convenient site that meets the requirements for speed and completeness of absorption. For most drugs, oral administration is appropriate, and measurable concentrations of the drug in the blood result. The pattern of the concentration-time curve in the blood is a function of the input, distribution, and loss factors. In this chapter, we will examine the quantitative aspects of these relationships.

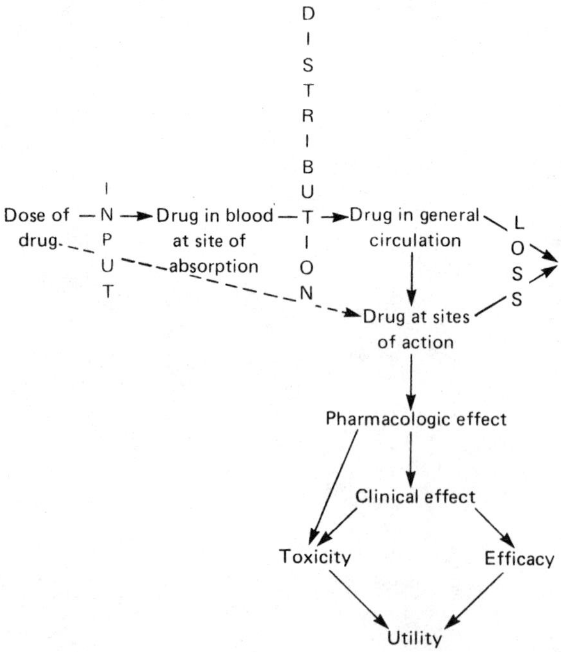

Figure 3–1. A schematic representation of the dose-effect relationships of a drug. (Modified and reproduced, with permission, from Benet LZ: Effect of route of administration and distribution on drug action. *J Pharmacokinet Biopharm* 1978;**6**:559.)

A fundamental hypothesis of pharmacokinetics is that a relationship exists between a pharmacologic or toxic effect of a drug and the concentration of the drug in a readily accessible site of the body (eg, blood). This hypothesis has been documented for many drugs (Table 3–1), although for some drugs no clear relationship has been found between pharmacologic effect and plasma or blood concentrations. In most cases, the concentration of drug in the general circulation will be related to its concentration at the site of action. The drug will then elicit a number of pharmacologic effects at the site of action. These pharmacologic effects may include toxic effects in addition to the desired clinical effect. The clinician then must balance the toxic potential of a particular dose of a drug with its efficacy to determine the utility of that agent in that clinical situation. Pharmacokinetics plays its role in the dose-efficacy scheme by providing the quantitative relationship between drug efficacy and drug dose, with the aid of measurements of drug concentrations in various biologic fluids. The importance of pharmacokinetics in patient care rests upon the improvement in drug efficacy that can be attained when the measurement of drug levels in the general circulation is added to traditional methods of predicting the dose of the drug. Knowledge of the relationship between efficacy and drug concentration measurements allows the clinician to take into account the various pathologic and physiologic features of a particular patient that make him or her different from the normal individual in responding to a dose of the drug.

PHARMACOKINETIC VARIABLES

Several pathologic and physiologic processes dictate dosage adjustment in individual patients (eg, heart failure, renal failure). They do so by modifying specific pharmacokinetic parameters. The 2 basic variables are **clearance,** the measure of the ability of the body to eliminate the drug, and **volume of distribution,** the measure of the apparent space in the body available to contain the drug.

Volume of Distribution

As briefly introduced in Chapter 1, volume of distribution (V_d) relates the amount of drug in the body to the concentration of drug (C) in blood or plasma:

$$V_d = \text{Amount of drug in body} \div C \qquad \ldots(1)$$

Volume of distribution is defined in terms of blood or plasma concentrations, depending upon the fluid measured. The plasma volume of a normal 70-kg man is 3 L, blood volume about 5.5 L, extracellular fluid outside plasma 12 L, and total body water about 42 L. However, many drugs exhibit volumes of distribution, according to equation (1), far in excess of these known body fluid volumes. For example, when 500 μg of digoxin is in the body of a healthy young 70-kg male, a plasma concentration of 0.78 ng/mL would be expected. Dividing the amount of drug in the body by the plasma concentration yields a volume of distribution for digoxin of 645 L—about 9 times the total body volume of a 70-kg man. This serves to emphasize that volume of distribution does not represent a real volume but must be considered as the size of the pool of body fluids that would be required if the drug were distributed equally throughout all portions of the body. In fact, digoxin, which is relatively hydrophobic, is distributed into muscle and adipose tissue, leaving a very small amount of drug in the plasma. Volume of distribution can change as a function of several variables, including the patient's age, sex, and disease. For example, the same 500 μg of digoxin in a middle-aged patient with congestive heart failure might yield a concentration of 1 ng/mL, corresponding to a 500-L volume of distribution.

Depending on the pK_a of the drug, the degree of plasma protein binding, the partition coefficient of the drug in the fatty tissues, and the degree of binding to other tissues within the body, volume of distribution may vary widely. For example, plasma volumes of distribution ranging from 8 to 1300 L/70 kg are represented in Table 3–1. The antimalarial quinacrine has been reported to exhibit an apparent volume of distribution approaching 50,000 L. For a drug extensively bound to plasma proteins but not to tissue proteins, most of the amount in the body will be retained in the blood, and the volume of distribution will have a lower limit of approximately 7 L, as exemplified by furosemide and warfarin in Table 3–1. In contrast, drugs such as imipramine, nortriptyline, and propranolol have high volumes of distribution even though over 90% of the drug in the blood is bound to plasma proteins. These drugs are even more extensively bound to tissue protein than to plasma protein. If plasma protein binding is more sensitive to pathologic changes than tissue binding, we might expect to see a linear relation between V_d and the unbound fraction in plasma, as has been shown for propranolol in patients with liver disease (Fig 3–2).

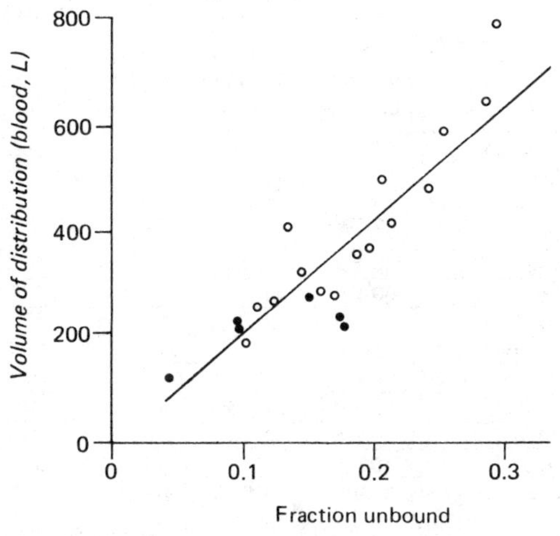

Figure 3–2. The volume of distribution (blood) of (+)–propranolol varies with the unbound fraction. The observations were made in 6 control subjects (●) and 15 patients (o) with chronic liver disease after an intravenous bolus (40 mg) of (+)–propranolol. (Modified and reproduced, with permission, from Branch RA, Jones J, Read AE: A study of factors influencing drug disposition in chronic liver disease, using the model drug (+)–propranolol. *Br J Clin Pharmacol* 1976;**3**:243.)

Clearance

Drug clearance principles are similar to the clearance concepts of renal physiology, in which creatinine or urea clearance is defined as the rate of elimination of the compound in the urine relative to the plasma drug concentration (UV ÷ P). At the simplest level, clearance of a drug is the rate of elimination by all routes relative to the concentration of drug in any biologic fluid:

$$CL = \text{Rate of elimination} \div C \qquad \ldots(2)$$

Clearance (CL) is usually defined as blood clearance (CL_b), plasma clearance (CL_p), or clearance based on unbound or free drug concentration (CL_u), depending on the concentration measured for the right side of equation (2) (C_b, C_p, or C_u).

In Table 3–1, the plasma clearance of amikacin is reported as 77 mL/min, with 98% of the drug excreted in the urine unchanged. In other words, the kidney is able to remove this drug from approximately 77 mL of plasma per minute. Since clearance is usually constant in a stable patient, the rate of elimination of amikacin will depend on the concentration of drug in the plasma as required by equation (2). Propranolol is cleared at a rate of 270 mL/min, almost exclusively by nonrenal routes, especially the liver. In this case, the liver is able to remove this drug from 270 mL of plasma per minute. For the drugs listed in Table 3–1, the highest plasma clearance is that for imipramine: 1400 mL/min, a value almost twice as high as the plasma flow to the liver, the dominant organ of elimination for this drug. However, since this drug distributes readily into red blood cells ($C_{rbc} \div C_p \simeq 2.7$), the amount of drug

Table 3–1. Pharmacokinetic and pharmacodynamic parameters for selected drugs.*

Drug	Oral Availability (percent)	Urinary Excretion (percent)	Bound in Plasma (percent)	Clearance (mL/min/70 kg)	Volume of Distribution (L/70 kg)	Half-Life (hours)	Effective† Concentrations	Toxic† Concentrations
Acetaminophen	63 ± 5	3 ± 1	0–15	350 ± 100	67 ± 8	2.0 ± 0.4	10–20 µg/mL	> 300 µg/mL
Amikacin		98	4	77 ± 14	15 ± 6	2.3 ± 0.4		
Amoxicillin	93 ± 10	52 ± 15	18	370 ± 90	29 ± 13	1.0 ± 0.1		
Ampicillin	25–70	90 ± 8	18	270 ± 50	20 ± 5	1.3 ± 0.2		
Aspirin	68 ± 3	1.4 ± 1.2	49	650 ± 80	11 ± 2	0.25 ± 0.3	See Salicylic Acid.	
Cephalexin	90 ± 9	96	14 ± 3	300 ± 80	18 ± 2	0.90 ± 0.18		
Cephalothin		52	71 ± 3	470 ± 120	18 ± 8	0.57 ± 0.32		
Chloramphenicol	75–90	5 ± 1	53 ± 5	250 ± 120	64	2.7 ± 0.8		
Chlordiazepoxide	100	< 1	96.5 ± 1.8	26 ± 4	21 ± 2	9.9 ± 2.5	> 0.7 µg/mL	
Cimetidine	62 ± 6	77 ± 6	19	840 ± 210	150 ± 70	2.1 ± 1.1	1.0 µg/mL	
Clonidine	75 ± 4	62 ± 11		210 ± 84	150 ± 30	8.5 ± 2.0	1 ng/mL	
Diazepam	100	< 1	98.7 ± 0.2	27 ± 4	77 ± 20	20–90	> 600 ng/mL	
Digitoxin	> 90	33 ± 15	90 ± 2	3.2 ± 1.6	36 ± 13	6.9 ± 2.7 days	> 10 ng/mL	> 35 ng/mL
Digoxin	60–75	72 ± 9	25 ± 5	130 ± 67	640 ± 200	42 ± 19	> 0.8 ng/mL	> 2 ng/mL
Disopyramide	83 ± 11	55 ± 6	30–70	90 ± 50	55 ± 18	7.8 ± 1.6	3 ± 1 µg/mL	
Erythromycin	18–45	10–15	72 ± 3	420 ± 170	50 ± 14	1.1–3.5		
Ethambutol	77 ± 8	79 ± 3	20–30	600 ± 60	110 ± 14	3.1 ± 0.4		> 10 µg/mL
Furosemide	40–60	66 ± 7	98.8 ± 0.2	140 ± 30	7.7 ± 1.4	1.5 ± 0.1		
Gentamicin		> 90	< 10	90	18	2–3		
Hydralazine	20–60	11–14	87	420–1100	110 ± 21	1.8–3.0	1 µg/mL	
Imipramine	47 ± 21	0–2	89–94	1400 ± 700	1050 ± 420	13 ± 3	> 225 ng/mL	> 1 µg/mL
Indomethacin	98	15 ± 8	90	110 ± 14	65 ± 37	2.6 ± 11.2	0.5–3 µg/mL	> 6 µg/mL
Lidocaine	35 ± 11	2 ± 1	51 ± 8	640 ± 170	77 ± 28	1.8 ± 0.4	1.2–6 µg/mL	> 6 µg/mL
Lithium	100	95 ± 15	0	25 ± 8	55 ± 24	22 ± 8	> 0.7 mEq/L	> 2 mEq/L
Meperidine	52 ± 3	4–22	58 ± 9	1200 ± 350	290 ± 90	3.2 ± 0.8		
Methotrexate	65	94	45 ± 14	105	28	8.4		0.9 µg/mL
Morphine	20–33	6–10	35 ± 2	1100 ± 140	220 ± 50	3.0 ± 1.2	65 ng/mL	
Nortriptyline	51 ± 5	2 ± 1	94.5 ± 0.6	500 ± 130	1300 ± 300	31 ± 13	50–139 ng/mL	
Phenobarbital	> 80	24 ± 5	51	6.5 ± 3	62 ± 23	4.4 ± 1.0 days	10–25 µg/mL	> 30 µg/mL
Phenytoin	98 ± 7	2	89 ± 23	Dose-dependent	45 ± 3	Dose-dependent	> 10 µg/mL	> 20 µg/mL
Prazosin	57 ± 10	< 1	93 ± 2	210 ± 20	42 ± 9	2.9 ± 0.8		
Procainamide	83 ± 16	67 ± 8	16 ± 5	350–840	130 ± 20	3.0 ± 0.6	3–5 µg/mL	> 9 µg/mL
Propranolol	36 ± 10	< 1	93 ± 1	840 ± 210	270 ± 40	3.9 ± 0.4	20 ng/mL	
Quinidine	70 ± 17	18 ± 5	89 ± 1	330 ± 130	190 ± 80	6.2 ± 1.8	2–5 µg/mL	> 8 µg/mL
Salicylic acid	100		Dose-dependent	Dose-dependent	12 ± 2	Dose-dependent	150–300 µg/mL	
Sulfamethoxazole	100	30 ± 1	62 ± 5	22 ± 3	15 ± 1.4	8.6 ± 0.3		
Sulfisoxazole	100	53 ± 9	88–92	23 ± 3.5	10.5 ± 1.4	5.9 ± 0.9		
Tetracycline	77	48	65 ± 3	130	91	9.9 ± 1.5		
Theophylline	96 ± 8	8	56 ± 4	48 ± 21	35 ± 11	8.1 ± 2.4	> 5 µg/mL	> 20 µg/mL
Tobramycin		90	< 10	77	18 ± 6	2.2 ± 0.1		
Tolbutamide	93 ± 10	0	93 ± 1	21 ± 3	11 ± 2	5.9 ± 1.4	80–240 µg/mL	
Trimethoprim	100	53 ± 2	70 ± 5	150 ± 40	130 ± 15	11 ± 1.4		
Valproic acid	100	< 5	93 ± 4	8.4 ± 2.8	9.1 ± 2.8	16 ± 3	55–100 µg/mL	
Warfarin	100	0	99	3.2 ± 1.7	7.7 ± 0.7	37 ± 15	2.2 ± 0.4 µg/mL	

*The values in this table represent the parameters determined when the drug is administered to healthy normal volunteers or to patients who are generally free from disease except for the condition for which the drug is being prescribed. The values presented here are adapted and updated from Benet LZ, Sheiner LB: Design and optimization of dosage regimens: Pharmacokinetic data. Pages 1675–1737 in: *Goodman and Gilman's The Pharmacological Basis of Therapeutics,* 6th ed. Gilman AG, Goodman LS, Gilman A (editors). Macmillan, 1980. This source may be consulted for the effects of disease states on the pertinent pharmacokinetic parameters.
†No pharmacodynamic values are given for antibiotics since these vary depending upon the infecting organism.

delivered to the excretory organ is considerably higher than plasma flow indicates. The clearance measured in terms of blood concentration is in the physiologic range of blood flow measurements. Thus, like volume of distribution, *plasma* clearance may assume proportions that are not "physiologic." A drug that is concentrated in the red blood cells (eg, mecamylamine) can manifest a plasma clearance of tens of liters per minute. However, if blood concentration is used to define clearance, the maximum clearance possible is equal to the sum of blood flows to the various organs of elimination. For a drug eliminated solely by the liver, blood clearance is therefore limited by the flow of blood to that organ, approximately 1500 mL/min (Table 1–3). It is important to note the additive character of clearance. Elimination of drug from the body may involve processes occurring in the kidney, the lung, the liver, and other organs. Dividing the rate of elimination at each organ by a concentration of drug (eg, plasma concentration) yields the respective clearance at that organ. Added together, these separate clearances equal total systemic clearance:

$$\frac{\text{Rate of elimination}_{\text{kidney}}}{C_p} = CL_{\text{renal}} \qquad \ldots(3a)$$

$$\frac{\text{Rate of elimination}_{\text{liver}}}{C_p} = CL_{\text{liver}} \qquad \ldots(3b)$$

$$\frac{\text{Rate of elimination}_{\text{other}}}{C_p} = CL_{\text{other}} \qquad \ldots(3c)$$

$$CL_{\text{renal}} + CL_{\text{liver}} + CL_{\text{other}} = CL_{\text{systemic}} \qquad \ldots(3d)$$

The example provided in equations (3a–d) indicates that the drug is eliminated by liver, kidney, and other tissues and that these routes of elimination account for all of the pathways by which the drug leaves the body. "Other" tissues of elimination could include the lungs, salivary glands, sweat glands, partition into the gut, and additional sites of metabolism, eg, hydrolysis in blood or muscle.

The 2 major sites of drug elimination are the kidneys and the liver. Clearance of unchanged drug in the urine represents renal clearance. Within the liver, drug elimination occurs via biotransformation of parent drug to one or more metabolites, or excretion of unchanged drug into the bile or both. The pathways of biotransformation are discussed later in this chapter. For most drugs, clearance is constant over the plasma or blood concentration range encountered in clinical settings, ie, elimination is not saturable, and the rate of drug elimination is directly proportionate to concentration (equation [2]). For drugs that exhibit saturable or dose-dependent elimination (eg, phenytoin, salicylic acid), clearance will vary depending on the concentration of drug that is achieved (Table 3–1). Dosage adjustments with such drugs are more complex than those for drugs with nonsaturable elimination and are discussed in Chapter 63.

A further definition of clearance is useful in understanding the effects of physiologic and pathologic variables on drug elimination, particularly with respect to a specific organ. The rate of elimination of a drug by a single organ can be defined in terms of the blood flow entering and exiting from the organ and the concentration of drug in the blood. The rate of presentation of drug to the organ is the product of blood flow and entering drug concentration ($Q \times C_i$), while the rate of exit of drug from the organ is the product of blood flow and exiting drug concentration ($Q \times C_o$). The difference between these rates at steady state is the rate of drug elimination:

$$\text{Rate of elimination} = Q \times C_i - Q \times C_o \qquad \ldots(4)$$

Dividing equation (4) by concentration of drug entering the organ of elimination (C_i), an expression for organ clearance of drug is obtained:

$$CL_{\text{organ}} = \frac{Q \times C_i - Q \times C_o}{C_i} \qquad \ldots(5a)$$

$$= Q \times \frac{C_i - C_o}{C_i} = Q \times ER \qquad \ldots(5b)$$

As shown in equation (5b), the expression $(C_i - C_o) \div C_i$ can be referred to as the extraction ratio (ER) of the drug.

The concepts developed in equations (5a) and (5b) have important implications for drugs that are eliminated by the liver. Consider a drug that is efficiently removed from the blood by hepatic processes. The concentration of drug in the blood leaving the liver will be small; the extraction ratio will approach unity; and clearance of the blood will be limited by hepatic blood flow. Drugs highly extracted by the liver (eg, hydralazine, imipramine, lidocaine, meperidine, morphine, nortriptyline, propranolol; Table 3–1) are restricted in their rate of elimination not by intrahepatic processes but by the rate at which they can be transported in the blood to hepatic sites of elimination. The availability of drugs that are highly extracted by the liver is sensitive to small changes in the hepatic extraction ratio. For a drug that is completely absorbed from the gastrointestinal tract and enters the liver without biotransformation, the systemic availability of the drug (F) is diminished by the extent of hepatic extraction:

$$F = 1 - ER \qquad \ldots(6)$$

Small changes in ER for a highly extracted drug can result in dramatic changes in availability, as will be discussed in the following section.

Clearance is probably the most important pharmacokinetic term to be considered in defining a rational drug dosage regimen. In most cases, the clinician would like to maintain steady-state drug concentrations within a known therapeutic range (Table 3–1). Steady state will be achieved when the dosing rate (rate of active drug entering the systemic circulation) equals the rate of drug elimination. Therefore,

$$\text{Dosing rate} = CL \times C_{ss} \qquad \ldots(7)$$

Thus, if the desired steady-state concentration (plasma or blood) is known, the clearance value in that patient will dictate the dosing rate.

Two additional pharmacokinetic variables, half-life and bioavailability, must be considered when designing appropriate drug dosage regimens.

Half-Life

Half-life ($t_{1/2}$) is an expression of the relationship between volume and clearance. For the simplest case (and the most useful in designing drug dosage regimens), the body may be considered as a single compartment (as illustrated in Fig 1–1B) of a size equal to the volume of distribution (V_d). However, the organs of elimination can only clear drug from the blood or plasma in direct contact with the organ. Thus, the time course of drug in the body will depend on both the volume of distribution and the clearance:

$$t_{1/2} = 0.693\ V_d \div CL \qquad \ldots(8)$$

Half-life is a useful kinetic parameter in that it indicates the time required to attain steady state or to decay from steady-state conditions after a change (ie, starting or stopping) a particular rate of drug administration (the dosing regimen). However, as an indicator of either drug elimination or distribution, it has little value. Early studies of drug pharmacokinetics in diseased subjects were compromised by reliance on drug half-life as the sole measure of alterations in drug disposition. Disease states can affect both of the physiologically related parameters, volume of distribution and clearance; thus, the derived parameter, $t_{1/2}$, will not necessarily reflect the expected change in drug elimination.

Bioavailability

Bioavailability is defined as the fraction of unchanged drug reaching the systemic circulation following administration by any route. For an intravenous dose of the drug, bioavailability is equal to unity. For a drug administered orally, bioavailability may be less than unity for several reasons. The drug may be incompletely absorbed. It may be metabolized in the gut, the gut wall, the portal blood, or the liver prior to entry into the systemic circulation. It may undergo enterohepatic cycling with incomplete reabsorption following elimination into the bile. Biotransformation of some drugs in the liver following oral administration is an important factor in the pharmacokinetic profile, as discussed below. Data on bioavailability following oral drug administration are set forth in Table 3–1 as percentages of dose available to the systemic circulation.

Absorption, Bioavailability, & Routes of Administration

In addition to the definition given above, bioavailability is often used to indicate the *rate* at which an administered dose reaches the general circulation. The difference between the 2 definitions of bioavailability—ie, the extent and the rate of availability—is illustrated in Fig 3–3. This figure depicts the concentration-time curve for a hypothetical drug prepared in 3 different dosage formulations. Dosage forms A and B are designed so that the drug is absorbed into the blood at the same rate but twice as fast as in dosage form C. The times at which drug concentrations reach a peak are identical for dosage forms A and B and occur earlier than the peak time for dosage form C. In general, the relative order of peak times following the administration of different dosage forms of the drug thus corresponds to the rates of availability of the drug from the various dosage forms. The extent of availability may be measured by using either drug concentration in the blood or drug amounts in the urine. The area under the blood concentration-time curve (area under the curve, AUC) for a drug is a common measure of the extent of availability. In Fig 3–3, the areas under curves A and C are identical and twice as great as the area under curve B. For most drugs, drug clearance is linear (a constant function of concentration), and the relative areas under the curve or the total amounts of unchanged drug excreted in the urine quantitatively describe the relative availability of the drug from the different dosage forms. However, even in nonlinear cases, where clearance is dose-dependent, the relative areas under the curve will yield a measurement of the rank order of availability from different dosage forms or from different sites of administration.

Since there is usually a minimum effective concentration (mec) of drug in the blood (Fig 3–3) that is necessary to elicit a clinical effect (note Effective Concentrations in Table 3–1), both the rate and the extent of input or availability can affect the clinical efficacy of a drug. In many cases, the duration of pharmacologic effect is a function of the length of time the blood concentration curve is above the minimum effective concentration, and the intensity of the effect is usually a function of the height of the blood level curve above the minimum effective concentration.

Thus, for the 3 different dosage forms depicted in Fig 3–3, there would be significant differences in the levels of clinical effectiveness. Dosage form B would require twice the dose to attain blood levels equivalent to those of dosage form A. Table 3–1 contains only measures of the extent of availability following oral dosing. No measures of the rate of availability are provided, since the fractional *extent* (F) is more useful than the *rate* of availability to estimate the amount of drug in the body. Differences in rate of availability may become important for drugs given as a single dose, such as a hypnotic used to induce sleep. In this case, drug from dosage form A would reach its minimum effective concentration earlier than from

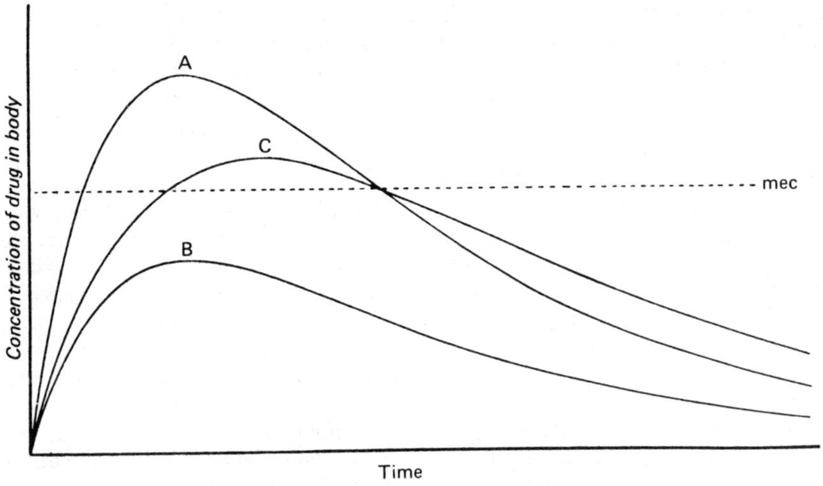

Figure 3–3. Blood concentration-time curves illustrating how changes in the rate and extent of drug availability can influence both the duration of action and the efficacy of a dose of a drug. The dotted line indicates the minimum effective concentration (mec) of the drug in the body. ***Case A:*** Drug is absorbed and is available rapidly and completely. This product will produce a prompt and prolonged response. ***Case B:*** Drug is absorbed at the same rate as in case A but is only half as available. There will be no clinical response, since the mec is not reached. ***Case C:*** Drug is absorbed at half the rate shown in cases A and B but is 100% available. The formulation produces a delayed and less prolonged response when compared to case A. (Modified and reproduced, with permission, from Benet LZ: Input factors as determinants of drug activity: Route, dose, dosage regimen, and the drug delivery system. Chap 2, pp 9–23, in: *Principles and Techniques of Human Research and Therapeutics.* McMahon FG Jr [editor]. Futura, 1974.)

dosage form C; concentrations from A would also reach a higher level and remain above the minimum effective concentration for a longer period. In a multiple dosing regimen, dosage forms A and C would yield the same average blood level concentrations, although dosage form A would show somewhat greater maximum and lower minimum concentrations.

Extraction Ratio & the First-Pass Effect

For most drugs, disposition or loss from the biologic system is independent of input, where disposition is defined as what happens to the active drug after it reaches a site in the circulation where drug concentration measurements can be made. Although disposition processes may be independent of input, the inverse is not necessarily true, since disposition can markedly affect the extent of availability. Drug absorbed from the stomach and the intestine must pass through the liver before reaching a site in the circulation that can be sampled for measurement. Thus, if a drug is metabolized in the liver or excreted in bile, some of the active drug absorbed from the gastrointestinal tract will be inactivated by hepatic processes before the drug can reach the general circulation and be distributed to its sites of action. If the metabolizing or biliary excreting capacity of the liver is great, the effect on the extent of availability will be substantial (first-pass effect). As stated in equation (6), the systemic availability of a drug metabolized in the liver will be decreased by the hepatic extraction ratio when the drug is given orally (ie, $F = 1 - ER$ for a drug completely absorbed and eliminated only by hepatic processes). Thus, if the hepatic clearance for a drug is large ($ER = CL_{liver} \div Q_{liver}$), the extent of availability for this drug will be low when it is given by a route that yields first-pass metabolic effects. This decrease in availability is a function of the physiologic site from which absorption takes place, and no amount of dosage form modification can improve the fractional availability. Of course, therapeutic blood levels may still be reached by this route of administration if larger doses are given. However, in this case, the levels of the drug metabolites will be increased significantly over those that would occur following intravenous administration, especially if the drug has a large volume of distribution. Therefore, the toxicity potential and elimination kinetics of the metabolites must be thoroughly understood before a decision to administer a large oral dose is made.

Drugs with high extraction ratios will show marked intersubject variability in bioavailability because of variations in hepatic function or blood flow or both. Consider a drug with an extraction ratio of 0.95 that falls to 0.90 as a result of hepatic impairment. In this instance, the bioavailability of the drug will double, from 0.05 to 0.10. These relationships can explain the marked variability in plasma or blood drug concentrations that occurs among individuals given similar doses of a highly extracted drug. Small variations in hepatic extraction between individuals will result in large differences in availability and plasma drug concentrations. These considerations are also pertinent for hepatic disease states accompanied by significant intrahepatic or extrahepatic circulatory shunting and in the presence of surgically created anastomoses between the portal system and the systemic venous circulation. For drugs that are highly extracted by the liver, shunting of blood past hepatic sites of elimination will result in substantial increases in drug availability, whereas for drugs that are poorly extracted by the liver (for which the difference in equations [4] and [5] between entering and exiting drug concentration is small), shunting of blood past the liver will cause little change in drug availability. Drugs in Table 3–1 that are poorly extracted by the liver are chlordiazepoxide, diazepam, digitoxin, phenytoin, theophylline, tolbutamide, and warfarin.

The first-pass effect can be avoided to a great extent by use of sublingual tablets and to some extent by use of rectal suppositories. The capillaries in the lower and mid sections of the rectum drain into the inferior and middle hemorrhoidal veins, which in turn drain into the inferior vena cava, thus bypassing the liver. However, suppositories tend to move upward in the rectum into a region where veins that lead to the liver, such as the superior hemorrhoidal, predominate. In addition, there are extensive anastomoses between the superior and middle hemorrhoidal veins; thus, only about 50% of a rectal dose can be assumed to bypass the liver. The lungs represent a good temporary clearing site for a number of drugs, especially basic compounds, as a result of partition into lipid tissues. The lungs also provide a filtering function for particulate matter that may be given by intravenous injection. The lung may serve as a site of first-pass loss by excretion and possible metabolism for drugs administered by nongastrointestinal ("parenteral") routes.

THE USE OF PHARMACOKINETICS IN DESIGNING A DOSAGE REGIMEN

The "dosage" of a drug represents a decision about 4 variables: (1) the amount of drug to be administered at one time; (2) the route of administration; (3) the interval between doses; and (4) the period of time over which drug administration is to be continued. The choice of the route of administration and the implications of this choice upon the extent and rate of drug availability were discussed in the previous section. Most patterns of administration fall into 2 classes, both of which may be described using pharmacokinetic principles: (1) continuous input by intravenous infusion (or any route that delivers drug at a constant rate), and (2) a series of intermittent drug doses, usually of equal size and given at approximately equally spaced intervals.

Maintenance Dose

In most clinical situations, drugs are administered in such a way as to maintain a steady state of drug in the body. Thus, calculation of the appropriate maintenance dose is a primary goal. To maintain the chosen steady state, all that is needed is to adjust dosage so that the rate of drug input (dosing rate) equals the rate of drug loss, ie, rate in = rate out. This relation was previously defined at steady state in equation 7:

$$\text{Dosing rate} = CL \times C_{ss} \qquad \ldots(7)$$

Dosing rate is also defined as the product of the extent of availability (F) and the dose divided by the dosing interval. Thus, if the clinician can specify the desired plasma drug concentration and knows the clearance and availability for that drug in a particular patient, the appropriate dosing rate can be calculated.

Example: A steady-state plasma theophylline concentration of 15 μg/mL is desired to relieve acute bronchial asthma in a patient. If the patient is a nonsmoker and otherwise normal except for the asthmatic condition, we may use the mean clearance given in Table 3–1, ie, 48 mL/min/70 kg. Since the drug will be given as an intravenous infusion, F = 1.

$$\text{Dosing rate} = CL_p \times C_{p,ss}$$

$$= \frac{48\ \text{mL}}{\text{min}/70\ \text{kg}} \times 15\ \mu\text{g/mL}$$

$$= 720\ \mu\text{g/min}/70\ \text{kg}$$

Therefore, in this patient, the proper infusion rate would be 0.72 mg/min, or 43.2 mg/h/70 kg. The drug might also be given as a series of bolus intravenous doses every 2 or 4 hours, for example. If the acute bronchial attack is relieved, the clinician might then want to maintain this plasma level using oral theophylline at intervals of 8, 12, or even 24 hours. When a series of multiple doses is given, the concentration term in equation (7) becomes the average of plasma concentrations over the dosing interval, $C_{p,avg}$ (Fig 3–4).

$$\frac{F \times \text{Dose}}{\text{Dosing interval}} = CL_p \times C_{p,avg}$$

$$\text{Dose} = (43.2\ \text{mg/h}/70\ \text{kg}) \times (\text{Dosing interval})$$

$$\simeq 85\ \text{mg every 2 hours, or 340 mg every 8 hours, or 1020 mg every 24 hours}$$

Note that the steady-state plasma level upon continuous infusion or the average plasma level following multiple dosing depends only on the primary disposition parameter, clearance. The values for volume of distribution and half-life are not needed to determine the average plasma concentration for a given dosing rate or for the reverse, determining the dosing rate for a desired plasma steady-state concentration.

Although the above equations are most useful in estimating the average drug concentrations, Fig 3–4 shows that at different dosing intervals the plasma level time curves will have different maximum and minimum values even though the average level will always be 15 μg/mL. If the clinician chose to infuse theophylline at a continuous rate of 720 μg/min, the

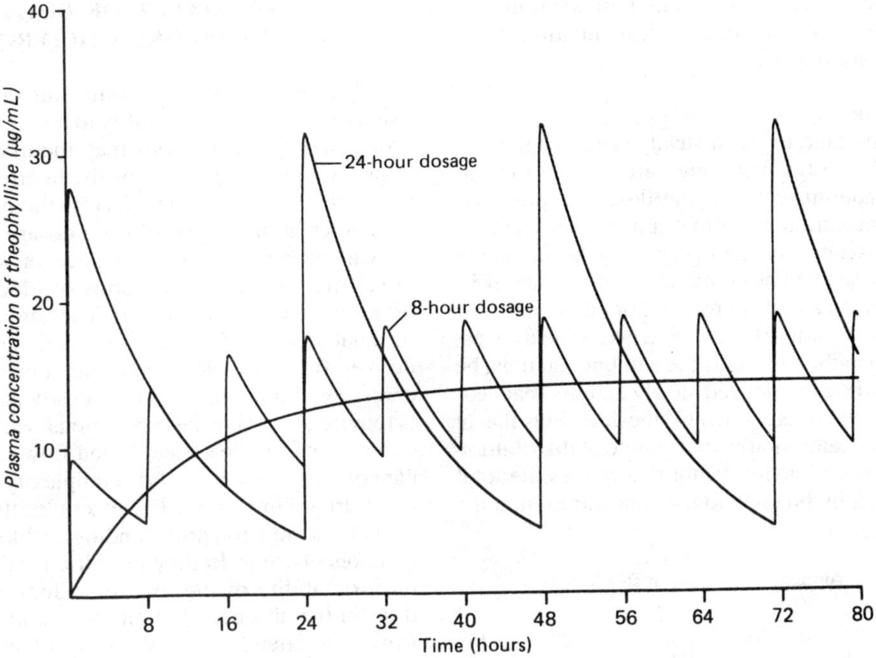

Figure 3–4. Relationship between frequency of dosing and maximum and minimum plasma concentrations, when a steady-state theophylline plasma level of 15 μg/mL is desired. The smoothly rising line shows the plasma concentration achieved with an intravenous infusion of 43.2 mg/hour. The doses for 8-hourly administration are 340 mg; for 24-hourly administration, 1020 mg. In each of the 3 cases, the mean steady-state plasma concentration is 15 μg/mL.

level of 15 μg/mL would be maintained continuously. However, with intermittent dosing, eg, at intervals of 2, 8, or 24 hours, the maximum and minimum levels would differ. A simplified way of calculating these maximum (Cp,ss_{max}) and minimum (Cp,ss_{min}) values is given in equations (9) and (10):

$$Cp,ss_{max} = \frac{F \times \text{Dose} \div V_d}{\text{Fraction lost in a dosing interval}}$$

$$= \frac{1020 \text{ mg}/35 \text{ L}}{0.88} = 33.1\ \mu\text{g/mL} \quad \ldots(9)$$

$$Cp,ss_{min} = Cp,ss_{max} \times \text{Fraction remaining after dosing interval}$$

$$= (33.1\ \mu\text{g/mL})\ (0.12) = 4\ \mu\text{g/mL} \quad \ldots(10)$$

The calculations in equations (9) and (10) were made assuming oral doses of 1020 mg per 24 hours of a drug with a half-life of 8 hours and an oral availability of about 1 (Table 3–1) and a patient with a V_d of 35 L. The denominator of equation (9), the fraction lost in a dosing interval, may be easily calculated when one knows the half-life. For example, a 24-hour dosing interval was chosen for theophylline; assuming a half-life of 8 hours, 50% of the dose would be lost in the first 8 hours, 75% in 16 hours, and 88% in 24 hours. Therefore, only 12% would remain at the end of the 24-hour dosing interval. Thus, with this dosing regimen, a maximum level of 33.1 and a minimum level of 4 μg/mL would be achieved. This would not be a good dosing scheme, since potentially toxic levels (> 20 μg/mL) would be maintained for over 5 hours, and levels below the minimum effective concentration (5 μg/mL) would be expected over 3 hours during each 24-hour dosing interval. A better choice would be 340 mg every 8 hours, where the fraction lost in a dosing interval would be 0.5, and maximum and minimum levels at steady state would be 19.4 and 9.7 μg/mL, respectively. However, in both cases, the average drug concentration would still be 15 μg/mL. In the above example, the fraction of drug eliminated from the body was derived from the simple relationship that states that 50% of the amount *remaining* to be eliminated is eliminated in each successive half-life. Thus, it takes 5 half-lives after cessation of therapy for a drug to be almost entirely (97%) eliminated from the body. It is interesting to note that this same relationship also applies to drug accumulation within the body toward a plateau that occurs with multiple dosing and constant rates of intravenous infusion (Fig 3–4).

In contrast to estimates of dosage rates and average steady-state levels, which may be determined independently of any pharmacokinetic model, using only clearance (equation [7]), the determination of maximum and minimum steady-state levels requires pharmacokinetic model assumptions. Equations (9) and (10) assume that the drug follows a one-compartment body model (Fig 1–1B) and that the absorption rate is much faster than the elimination rate.

For the calculation of estimated maximum and minimum concentrations in a clinical situation, these assumptions are reasonable.

Loading Dose

When the time to reach steady state is appreciable, as it is for drugs with long half-lives, it may be desirable to administer a loading dose that promptly raises the concentration of drug in plasma to the projected steady-state value. In theory, only the amount of the loading dose need be computed, not the rate of its administration; to a first approximation, this is so. The amount of drug required to achieve a given steady-state concentration in the *plasma* is the amount that must be in the *body* when the desired steady state is reached. (For intermittent dosage schemes, the amount is that at the average concentration). The volume of distribution (V_d) is the proportionality factor that relates the total amount of drug in the body to the concentration in the plasma ($C_{p,ss}$):

$$\text{Loading dose} = \text{Amount in the body at steady state}$$

$$= C_{p,ss} \times V_d \qquad \text{...(11)}$$

For the theophylline example above, the loading dose would be 525 mg (15 μg/mL × 35 L). For most drugs, the loading dose can be given as a single dose by the chosen route of administration. Up to this point, we have ignored the fact that some drugs follow complicated multicompartment pharmacokinetics, eg, the distribution process of Fig 3–1, illustrated by the 2-compartment model in Fig 1–1D. This is justified in the great majority of cases where pharmacokinetics is used as a tool in developing drug dosage regimens and in elucidating or predicting the effects of physiologic or pathologic changes in the patient. However, in some cases the distribution phase may not be ignored, particularly in connection with the calculation of loading doses. If the rate of absorption is rapid relative to distribution (this is always true for intravenous bolus administration), the concentration of drug in plasma that results from an appropriate loading dose can initially be considerably higher than desired. Severe toxicity may occur, albeit transiently. This may be particularly important, for example, in the administration of antiarrhythmia drugs, where an almost immediate toxic response is obtained when plasma concentrations exceed a particular level. Thus, while the estimation of the amount of a loading dose may be quite correct, the rate of administration can sometimes be crucial in preventing excessive drug concentrations, and slow administration of an intravenous drug (over minutes rather than seconds) is almost always wise. For intravenous doses of theophylline, initial injections should be given over a 20-minute period to avoid the possibility of high plasma levels during the distribution phase.

THE EFFECT OF DISEASE ON PHARMACOKINETIC PROCESSES

Disease states may modify all of the variables listed in Table 3–1. The ability to predict or understand how pathologic conditions may modify drug kinetics requires an understanding of the interrelationship between the variables. Clearance is the most important parameter in the design of drug dosage regimens. As shown in equation (5), clearance of an eliminating organ may be defined in terms of blood flow to the organ and the extraction ratio. The concepts embodied in equations (2), (5), and (7) are statements that can be derived from consideration of mass balance of a drug across an eliminating organ at steady state. No model is required to derive these equations. However, simple expressions for clearance, blood flow, and extraction cannot account for the full complexity of hepatic or renal drug elimination. For example, these equations do not account for drug binding to blood and tissue components, nor do they permit an estimation of the intrinsic ability of the liver or kidney to eliminate a drug in the absence of limitations imposed by blood flow. To extend the relationship of equation (5) to include expressions for protein binding and intrinsic clearance, it is necessary to formulate a model to describe organ elimination of drugs. The simplest model relating the extraction ratio to physiologic parameters is the so-called venous equilibration or well-stirred model. This approach assumes that the unbound drug concentration leaving the organ is equal to the unbound concentration inside the organ and that the intrinsic ability to metabolize or clear drug (CL_{int}) is equal to the rate of elimination divided by the unbound concentration in the organ. The clearance (with respect to blood concentration) for the eliminating organ then becomes

$$CL = Q \times \frac{fu \times CL_{int}}{Q + fu \times CL_{int}} \qquad \text{...(12)}$$

where fu is the unbound fraction of drug in blood and Q is the blood flow.

Equation (12) demonstrates that when the capability of the eliminating organ to metabolize the drug is large in comparison to the rate of drug presentation to the organ ($fu \times CL_{int} >> Q$), the clearance will approximate the organ blood flow:

$$CL \simeq Q \qquad \text{...(13)}$$

ie, drug elimination is limited by blood flow rate, and the compound is called a high-extraction-ratio drug. On the other hand, when the metabolic capability is small in comparison to the rate of drug presentation ($Q >> fu \times CL_{int}$), the clearance will be proportionate to the unbound fraction of drug in blood and the intrinsic clearance, ie,

$$CL \simeq fu \times CL_{int} \qquad \text{...(14)}$$

The drug is then called a low-extraction-ratio drug. When the capability for elimination is of the same order of magnitude as the blood flow, clearance is dependent upon the blood flow as well as on the intrinsic clearance and plasma protein binding (equation [12]). Equation (12) clarifies a number of important experimental results. For example, enzyme induction or hepatic disease may change the rate of imipramine metabolism in an isolated hepatic microsomal enzyme system, but no change in clearance is found in the whole animal with similar hepatic changes. This is explained by the fact that imipramine is a high-extraction-ratio drug and clearance is limited by blood flow rate (equation [13]), so that changes in CL_{int} due to enzyme induction or liver disease have no effect on clearance. Also, although imipramine is highly protein-bound (Table 3–1), changes in protein binding due to disease or competitive binding should have no effect on clearance even though volume of distribution is changed. In the latter case, a change in volume of distribution with no change in clearance will result in a change in half-life (equation [8]), although the elimination mechanisms have not been altered.

The differences between clearance and half-life are important in defining the underlying mechanisms for the effect of a disease state on drug disposition. For example, the half-life of diazepam increases with age (Fig 3–5). One explanation for this change is that the ability of the liver to metabolize this drug decreases as a function of age. However, when clearance is plotted against age for 20 normal individuals (Fig 3–6), it is apparent that there is no correlation with age.

The increasing half-lives illustrated in Fig 3–5 actually result from changes in the volume of distribution with age; the metabolic processes responsible for eliminating the drug are fairly constant. Although many reports indicate that hepatic impairment can reduce clearance and prolong half-life, there is some evidence that hepatic disease can also increase clearance and shorten half-life. For example, the clearance

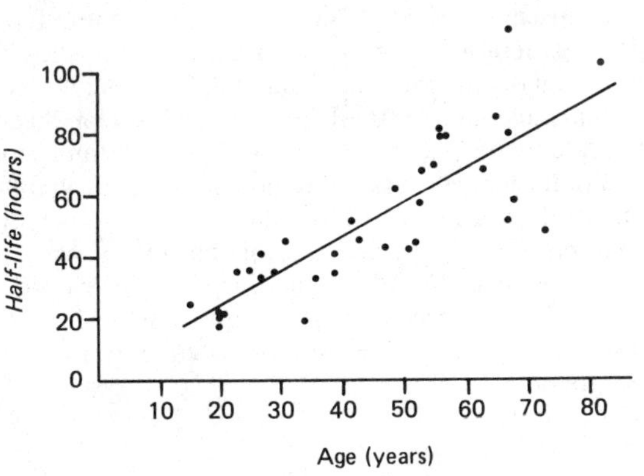

Figure 3–5. Correlation of diazepam half-life and age. (Modified and reproduced, with permission, from Klotz U et al: The effects of age and liver disease on the disposition and elimination of diazepam in adult man. *J Clin Invest* 1975;**55**:347.)

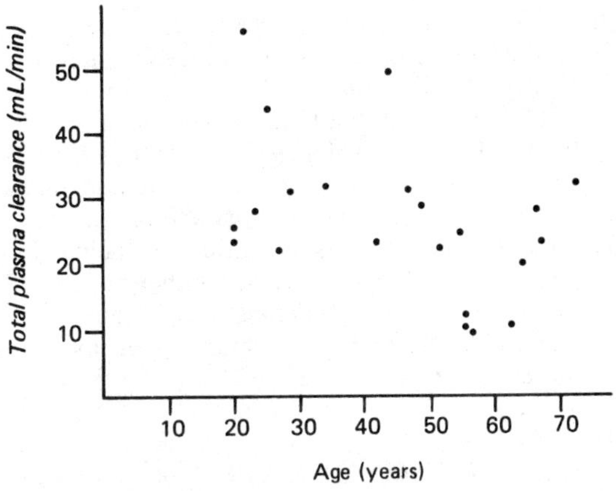

Figure 3–6. Relationship of plasma clearance of diazepam with age. (Modified and reproduced, with permission, from Klotz U et al: The effects of age and liver disease on the disposition and elimination of diazepam in adult man. *J Clin Invest* 1975;**55**:347.)

of tolbutamide may increase and its half-life decrease with no change in volume of distribution in individuals with acute viral hepatitis during the acute phase of illness in comparison to the recovery period. Tolbutamide is a low-extraction-ratio drug, and its hepatic clearance may be described by equation (14). The explanation for the observations appears to be a decrease in the unbound fraction of drug in plasma (fu) in the absence of a change in CL_{int}. The half-life is changed, since total clearance is changed without a change in volume of distribution. For many drugs, volume of distribution would be expected to increase as the free fraction of drug in plasma increases (Fig 3–2). However, the volume of distribution for tolbutamide is quite small (11 L/70 kg from Table 3–1), and the majority of the distribution space is related to blood volume, which is independent of fu.

Pharmacokinetic changes in renal disease may also be explained in terms of clearance concepts. However, since the net renal excretion of a drug is determined by filtration, active secretion, and reabsorption, the treatment of renal clearance is more complicated than that described above. Renal clearance can be described by the following equation:

$$CL_{renal} = (CL_{RF} + CL_{RS}) \times (1 - FR) \quad \ldots(15)$$

where CL_{RF} is renal filtration clearance, CL_{RS} is real secretion clearance, and FR is the fraction of drug filtered and secreted that is reabsorbed. The rate of filtration depends upon the volume of fluid that is filtered in the glomerulus and the unbound concentration of drug in plasma, because proteins and drugs bound to proteins are not filtered. The volume filtered is usually estimated from inulin or creatinine clearance. The renal filtration can usually be expressed as

$$CL_{RF} = fu \times CL_{cr} \quad \ldots(16)$$

where CL_{cr} is the creatinine clearance.

The secretion of drug in the kidney will depend on the relative binding of drug to the active transport carriers in relation to the binding to plasma proteins, the degree of saturation of these carriers, transfer of the drug across the tubular membrane, and the rate of delivery of the drug to the secretory site. With a model that combines these factors, the influence of changes in protein binding, blood flow, and number of functioning nephrons may be predicted and explained in a manner analogous to the examples given above for hepatic elimination.

ADJUSTMENT OF THE DOSAGE REGIMEN FOR THE INDIVIDUAL PATIENT

Attainment of an appropriate maintenance dosage regimen often requires adjustment for that patient. It is reasonable to assume that the usual recommended dose of a drug has been determined from appropriate experience with many "typical" cases. If a particular patient being treated is not expected to differ from the "typical" one with respect to *sensitivity* to the drug, one may adjust the usual maintenance dosage regimen on the basis of the patient's clearance of the drug. This requires computation or measurement of clearance for the patient (and bioavailability, if it will differ from usual) by the methods described below, and use of the following equation:

$$\text{Dosing rate}_{patient} = \text{Dosing rate}_{typical} \times \frac{CL_{patient}}{CL_{normal}} \quad \ldots(17)$$

At the corrected dosing rate, the patient's mean steady-state concentration of drug will be identical to that achieved in the presumably successful treatment of a "typical" patient.

When an intermittent regimen is adjusted for an individual patient, one may choose to alter the dose given per dosing interval, the dosing interval, or both. As a rule, adjustment of the amount of each dose, not the interval, is preferred. Adjustments of dosage are usually made to compensate for smaller-than-usual clearances. If the amount of each dose is reduced to compensate for reduced clearance, then fluctuations about the mean steady-state concentration will be smaller. For most drugs, a more constant concentration-time profile is not only acceptable but desirable.

Estimates of clearance must often be adjusted when patients have alterations in renal function. The quantities required for this adjustment are the fraction of normal renal function remaining and the fraction of drug usually excreted unchanged in the urine. The latter parameter appears in Table 3–1; the former can be estimated as the ratio of the patient's creatinine clearance to a normal creatinine clearance (100–120 mL/min/70 kg). If creatinine clearance has not been measured, it may be estimated from measurements of the concentration of creatinine in serum, using one of several different equations and nomograms (see Chapter 63).

Example: Renal clearance of digoxin in a patient with depressed renal function (CL_{cr} = 30 mL/min/70 kg) may be estimated as follows (see values in Table 3–1):

$$\begin{aligned} CL_{renal,\,normal} &= CL \times \text{Fraction excreted unchanged} \\ &= (130\ \text{mL/min/70 kg}) \times (0.72) \\ &= 94\ \text{mL/min/70 kg} \end{aligned} \quad \ldots(18)$$

$$\begin{aligned} CL_{renal,patient} &= \frac{CL_{cr,patient}}{CL_{cr,normal}} \times CL_{renal,\,normal} \\ &= \frac{30}{120} \times 94\ \text{mL/min/70 kg} \\ &= 24\ \text{mL/min/70 kg} \end{aligned} \quad \ldots(19)$$

$$\begin{aligned} CL_{patient} &= CL_{renal} + CL_{nonrenal} \\ &= 24 + 36 = 60\ \text{mL/min/70 kg} \end{aligned} \quad \ldots(3d)$$

Nonrenal clearance in equation (3d) was estimated as the difference between total and renal clearance in the normal person, which is assumed not to change in the patient with renal impairment. The oral dosing rate in a normal patient could be calculated using equation (7), assuming that an average plasma level of 1.2 ng/mL was desired and F = 0.65 (see Table 3–1). This would result in a dosing rate of 240 ng/min, or 0.35 mg/d for a 70-kg patient with normal renal function. Substituting this usual dosing rate into equation (17) along with the normal clearance (130 mL/min/70 kg; Table 3–1) and the calculated patient clearance of 60 mL/min from equation (3d), and assuming no change in F, yields a patient dosing rate of 0.16 mg/d. The above calculations provide a first estimate of the dosing rate. As described in greater detail in Chapter 63, drug level monitoring for drugs such as digoxin will allow the clinician to adjust the dose more accurately in a case like this one.

References

Benet LZ: Effect of route of administration and distribution on drug action. *J Pharmacokinet Biopharm* 1978;**6:**559.

Benet LZ (editor): *The Effect of Disease States on Drug Pharmacokinetics.* American Pharmaceutical Association, 1976.

Benet LZ, Sheiner LB: Design and optimization of dosage regimens: Pharmacokinetic data. Pages 1675–1737 in: *Goodman and Gilman's The Pharmacological Basis of Therapeutics,* 6th ed. Gilman AG, Goodman LS, Gilman A (editors). Macmillan, 1980.

Bennett WM et al: Drug therapy in renal failure: Dosing guidelines for adults. (2 parts.) *Ann Intern Med* 1980;**93:**62, 286.

Evans WE, Schentag JJ, Jusko WJ (editors): *Applied Pharmacokinetics: Principles of Therapeutic Drug Monitoring.* Applied Therapeutics, 1980.

Klotz U et al: The effects of age and liver disease on the disposition and elimination of diazepam in adult man. *J Clin Invest* 1975;**55:**347.

Oie S, Benet LZ: Altered drug disposition in disease states. Chap 29, pp 277–287, in: *Annual Reports in Medicinal Chemistry.* Vol 15. Hess HJ (editor). Academic Press, 1980.

Rowland M, Benet LZ, Graham GG: Clearance concepts in pharmacokinetics. *J Pharmacokinet Biopharm* 1973;**1:**123.

Sheiner LB, Rosenberg BG, Marathe VV: Estimation of population characteristics of pharmacokinetic parameters from routine clinical data. *J Pharmacokinet Biopharm* 1977;**5:**445.

Wagner JG: *Fundamentals of Clinical Pharmacokinetics.* Drug Intelligence, 1975.

Wilkinson GR, Shand DG: A physiologic approach to hepatic drug clearance. *Clin Pharmacol Ther* 1975;**18:**377.

Williams RL, Benet LZ: Drug pharmacokinetics in cardiac and hepatic disease. *Annu Rev Pharmacol Toxicol* 1980;**20:**389.

Williams RL et al: Influence of acute viral hepatitis on disposition and plasma binding of tolbutamide. *Clin Pharmacol Ther* 1977;**21:**301.

3 | Pharmacokinetics: II. Drug Biotransformation

Maria Almira Correia, PhD, & Neal Castagnoli, Jr., PhD

Humans are daily exposed to a wide variety of foreign compounds called **xenobiotics**—substances absorbed across the lungs or skin or, more commonly, ingested either unintentionally as compounds present in food and drink or deliberately as drugs for therapeutic or "recreational" purposes. Exposure to environmental xenobiotics may be inadvertent and accidental and may even be inescapable. Some xenobiotics are innocuous, but many can provoke biologic responses both pharmacologic and toxic in nature. Biologic responses often depend on conversion of the absorbed or ingested substance into an active metabolite. The discussion that follows is applicable to xenobiotics in general as well as to drugs and to some extent to endogenous compounds.

WHY IS DRUG BIOTRANSFORMATION NECESSARY?

Renal excretion plays a pivotal role in terminating the biologic activity of a few drugs, particularly those that have small molecular volumes or possess polar characteristics such as functional groups fully ionized at physiologic pH. Most drugs do not possess such physicochemical properties. Pharmacologically active organic molecules tend to be highly lipophilic and remain un-ionized or only partially ionized at physiologic pH. They are often strongly bound to plasma proteins. Such substances are not readily filtered at the glomerulus. The lipophilic nature of renal tubular membranes also facilitates the reabsorption of hydrophobic compounds following their glomerular filtration. Consequently, most drugs would have a prolonged duration of action if termination of their action depended solely on renal excretion. An alternative process that may lead to the termination or alteration of biologic activity is metabolism. In general, lipophilic xenobiotics are transformed to more polar and hence more readily excretable products. The role metabolism may play in the inactivation of lipid-soluble drugs can be quite dramatic. For example, lipophilic barbiturates such as thiopental and phenobarbital would have half-lives greater than 100 years if it were not for their metabolic conversion to more water-soluble compounds.

Metabolic products are often less active than the parent drug and may even be inactive. However, some biotransformation products have enhanced activity or toxic properties, including mutagenicity, teratogenicity, and carcinogenicity. This observation undermines the once popular theory that drug-biotransforming enzymes evolved as a biochemical defense mechanism for the detoxification of environmental xenobiotics. It is noteworthy that the synthesis of endogenous substrates such as steroid hormones, cholesterol, and bile acids involves many enzyme-catalyzed pathways associated with the metabolism of xenobiotics. The same is true of the formation and excretion of endogenous metabolic products such as bilirubin, the end catabolite of heme. Finally, drug-metabolizing enzymes have been exploited through the design of pharmacologically inactive prodrugs that are converted in vivo to the pharmacologically active species.

THE ROLE OF BIOTRANSFORMATION IN DRUG DISPOSITION

Most metabolic biotransformations occur at some point between absorption of the drug into the general circulation and its renal elimination. A few transformations occur in the intestinal lumen or intestinal wall. In general, all of these reactions can be assigned to one of 2 major categories, called phase I and phase II reactions (Fig 3–7).

Phase I reactions usually convert the parent drug to a more polar metabolite by introducing or unmasking a functional group (–OH, $-NH_2$, –SH). Often these metabolites are inactive, although in some instances activity is only modified.

If phase I metabolites are sufficiently polar, they may be readily excreted. However, many phase I products are not eliminated rapidly and undergo a subsequent reaction in which an endogenous substrate such as glucuronic acid, sulfuric acid, acetic acid, or an amino acid combines with the newly established functional group to form a highly polar conjugate. Such conjugation or synthetic reactions are the hallmarks of phase II metabolism. A great variety of drugs undergo these sequential biotransformation reactions, although in some instances the parent drug may already possess a functional group that may form a conjugate directly. For example, the hydrazide moiety

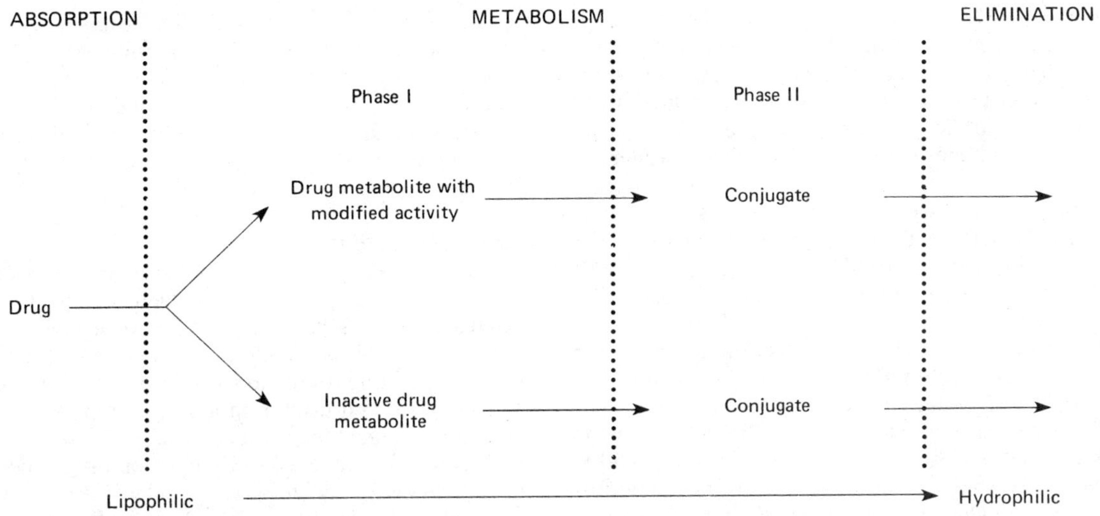

Figure 3–7. Phase I and phase II reactions in drug biodisposition.

of isoniazid is known to form an N-acetyl conjugate—in a phase II reaction—that is a substrate for a phase I type reaction, namely, hydrolysis to isonicotinic acid (Fig 3–8). Thus, phase II reactions may actually precede phase I reactions.

WHERE DO DRUG BIOTRANSFORMATIONS OCCUR?

Although every tissue has some ability to metabolize drugs, the liver is the principal organ of drug metabolism. Other tissues that display considerable activity include the gastrointestinal tract, the lungs, the skin, and the kidneys. Following oral administration, many drugs (eg, isoproterenol, meperidine, pentazocine, morphine) are absorbed intact from the small intestine and transported first via the portal system to the liver, where they undergo extensive metabolism. This process has been called a **first-pass effect.** Some orally administered drugs (eg, clonazepam, chlorpromazine) are more extensively metabolized in the intestine than in the liver. Thus, intestinal metabolism may contribute to the overall first-pass effect. First-pass effects may so greatly limit the bioavailability of orally administered drugs that alternative routes of administration must be employed to achieve therapeutically effective blood levels. The lower gut harbors intestinal microorganisms that are capable of many biotransformation reactions.

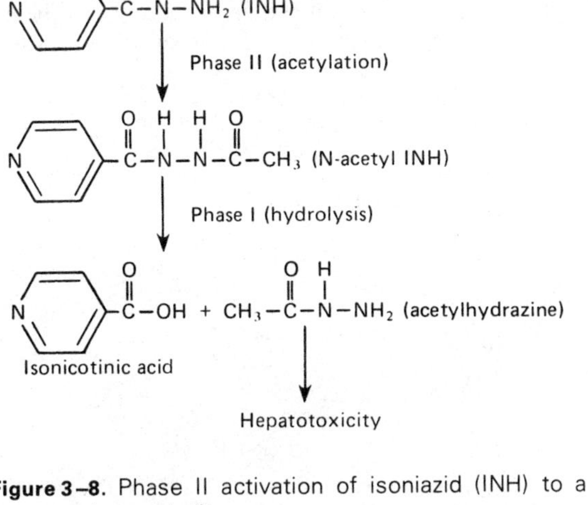

Figure 3–8. Phase II activation of isoniazid (INH) to a hepatotoxic metabolite.

Although drug biotransformation in vivo can occur by spontaneous, noncatalyzed chemical reactions, the vast majority are catalyzed by specific cellular enzymes. At the subcellular level, these enzymes may be located in the endoplasmic reticulum, mitochondria, cytosol, lysosomes, or even the nuclear envelope or plasma membrane.

MICROSOMAL MIXED FUNCTION OXIDASE SYSTEM

Many drug-metabolizing enzymes are located in the lipophilic membranes of the endoplasmic reticulum of the liver and other tissues. When these lamellar membranes are isolated by homogenization and fractionation of the cell, they are re-formed into vesicles called **microsomes.** Microsomes retain most of the morphologic and functional characteristics of the intact membranes, including the rough and smooth surface features of the rough (ribosome-studded) and smooth (no ribosomes) endoplasmic reticulum. Whereas the rough microsomes tend to be dedicated to protein synthesis, the smooth microsomes are relatively rich in enzymes responsible for oxidative drug metabolism. In particular, they contain the important class of enzymes known as the mixed function oxidases (MFO), or monooxygenases. The activity of this enzyme system requires both a reducing agent (NADPH) and molecular oxygen; in a typical reaction, one molecule of oxygen is consumed (reduced) per substrate molecule, with one oxygen atom appearing in the product and the other in the form of water.

In this oxidation-reduction process, 2 microsomal enzymes play a key role. The first of these is a flavoprotein, NADPH-cytochrome P-450 reductase. One mole of this enzyme (molecular weight ~ 80,000) contains 1 mol each of flavin mononucleotide (FMN) and flavin adenine dinucleotide (FAD). Because cytochrome c can serve as an electron acceptor, the enzyme is often referred to as NADPH-cytochrome c reductase. The second microsomal enzyme is a hemoprotein called cytochrome P-450 and serves as the terminal oxidase. The name cytochrome P-450 is derived from the spectral properties of this hemoprotein. In its reduced (ferrous) form, it binds carbon monoxide to give a ferrocarbonyl adduct that absorbs maximally in the visible region of the electromagnetic spectrum at 450 nm. As with other naturally occurring heme-containing proteins, the iron present in this molecule is complexed with protoporphyrin IX. Over half of the heme synthesized in the liver is committed to hepatic cytochrome P-450 formation. The relative abundance of cytochrome P-450, as compared to that of the reductase in the liver, contributes to making cytochrome P-450 heme reduction the rate-limiting step in hepatic drug oxidations.

Microsomal drug oxidations require cytochrome P-450, cytochrome P-450 reductase, NADPH, and molecular oxygen. A simplified scheme of the oxidative cycle is presented in Fig 3–9. Briefly, oxidized (Fe^{3+}) cytochrome P-450 combines with a drug substrate to form a binary complex (step ①). NADPH donates an electron to the flavoprotein reductase, which in turn reduces the oxidized cytochrome P-450-drug complex (step ②). A second electron is introduced from NADPH via the same flavoprotein reductase, which serves to reduce molecular oxygen and to form an "activated oxygen"-cytochrome P-450-substrate complex (step ③). This complex in turn transfers "activated" oxygen to the drug substrate to form the oxidized product (step ④).

The potent oxidizing properties of this activated oxygen permit oxidation of a large number of substrates. Substrate specificity is very low for this enzyme complex. High solubility in lipids is the only common structural feature of the wide variety of structurally unrelated drugs and chemicals that serve as substrates in this system (Table 3–2).

Enzyme Induction

An interesting feature of some of these chemically dissimilar drug substrates is their ability, on repeated administration, to "induce" cytochrome P-450 by enhancing the rate of its synthesis or reducing its rate of degradation. Induction results in an acceleration of metabolism and usually in a decrease in the pharmacologic action of the inducer and also of coadministered drugs. However, in the case of drugs metabolically transformed to reactive intermediates, enzyme induction may exacerbate drug-mediated tissue toxicity.

Various substrates appear to induce forms of cytochrome P-450 having different molecular weights and exhibiting different substrate specificities and immunochemical and spectral characteristics. The 2 isozymes that have been most extensively studied are (1) cytochrome P-450b, or LM_2 (for liver microsomal form 2), which is induced by treatment with phenobarbital; and (2) cytochrome P-448 (cytochrome P_1-450, or P-450c, or LM_4), which is induced by polycyclic aromatic hydrocarbons, of which 3-methylcholanthrene is a prototype. Environmental pollutants are capable of inducing cytochrome P-450. For example, exposure to benzo(a)pyrene, present in tobacco smoke, charcoal-broiled meat, and other organic pyrolysis products is known to induce cytochrome P-448 and to alter the rates of drug metabolism in both experimental animals and in humans.

Enzyme Inhibition

Other drug substrates may inhibit cytochrome P-450 enzyme activity. A well-known inhibitor is proadifen (SK&F 525-A; 2-[diethylamino]ethyl-2,2-diphenylvalerate). This compound binds avidly to the cytochrome molecule and thereby competitively inhibits the metabolism of potential substrates. Some

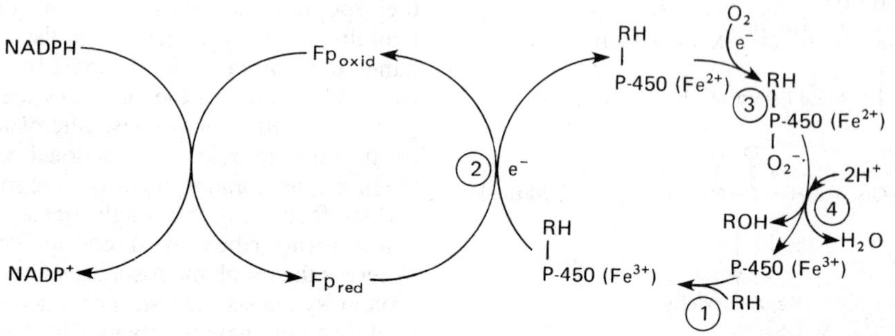

Figure 3–9. Cytochrome P-450 cycle in drug oxidations. (RH = parent drug; ROH = oxidized metabolite; Fp = flavoprotein; e⁻ = electron.)

Table 3–2. Phase I reactions.

Reaction Class	Structural Change	Drug Substrates
Oxidations		
Cytochrome P-450 – dependent oxidations:		
Aromatic hydroxylations	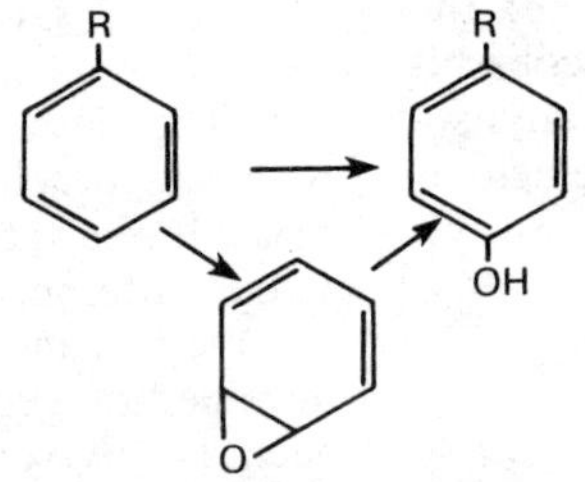	Acetanilid, propranolol, phenobarbital, phenytoin, phenylbutazone, amphetamine, warfarin, 17α-ethinylestradiol, naphthalene, benzpyrene.
Aliphatic hydroxylations	$RCH_2CH_3 \rightarrow RCH_2CH_2OH \rightarrow RCH(OH)CH_3$	Amobarbital, pentobarbital, secobarbital, chlorpropamide, ibuprofen, meprobamate, glutethimide, phenylbutazone.
Epoxidation	$RCH{=}CHR \rightarrow R{-}CH{-}CH{-}R$ (H O H; O bridging the two C)	Aldrin.
Oxidative dealkylation		
N-Dealkylation	$RNHCH_3 \rightarrow RNH_2 + CH_2O$	Morphine, ethylmorphine, benzphetamine, aminopyrine.
O-Dealkylation	$ROCH_3 \rightarrow ROH + CH_2O$	Codeine, *p*-nitroanisole.
S-Dealkylation	$RSCH_3 \rightarrow RSH + CH_2O$	6-Methylthiopurine, methitural.
N-Oxidation		
Primary amines	$RNH_2 \rightarrow RNHOH$	Aniline, chlorphentermine.
Secondary amines	$(R_1)(R_2)NH \rightarrow (R_1)(R_2)N{-}OH$	2-Acetylaminofluorene, acetaminophen.
Tertiary amines	$(R_1)(R_2)(R_3)N \rightarrow (R_1)(R_2)(R_3)N \rightarrow O$	Nicotine, methaqualone.
S-Oxidation	$(R_1)(R_2)S \rightarrow (R_1)(R_2)S{=}O$	Thioridazine, cimetidine, chlorpromazine.
Deamination	$RCH(NH_2)CH_3 \rightarrow R{-}C(OH)(NH_2){-}CH_3 \rightarrow R{-}C(=O)CH_3 + NH_3$	Amphetamine, diazepam.
Desulfuration	$(R_1)(R_2)C{=}S \rightarrow (R_1)(R_2)C{=}O$	Thiopental.
	$(R_1)(R_2)P{=}S \rightarrow (R_1)(R_2)P{=}O$	Parathion.
Dechlorination	$CCl_4 \rightarrow [CCl_3^{\bullet}] \rightarrow CHCl_3$	Carbon tetrachloride.
Cytochrome P-450 – independent oxidations:		
Amine oxidases	$RCH_2NH_2 \rightarrow RCHO + N_2$	Phenylethylamine, epinephrine.
Dehydrogenations	$RCH_2OH \rightarrow RCHO$	Ethanol, chloral hydrate.
Reductions		
Azo reductions	$RN{=}NR_1 \rightarrow RNH{-}NHR_1 \rightarrow RNH_2 + R_1NH_2$	Prontosil, tartrazine.
Nitro reductions	$RNO_2 \rightarrow RNO \rightarrow RNHOH \rightarrow RNH_2$	Nitrobenzene, chloramphenicol, clorazepam, dantrolene.
Carbonyl reductions	$RC(=O)R' \rightarrow RCH(OH)R'$	Metyrapone, methadone, naloxone.
Hydrolyses		
Esters	$R_1COOR_2 \rightarrow R_1COOH + R_2OH$	Procaine, succinylcholine, aspirin, clofibrate, methylphenidate.
Amides	$RCONHR_1 \rightarrow RCOOH + R_1NH_2$	Procainamide, lidocaine, indomethacin.

substrates irreversibly inhibit cytochrome P-450 via covalent interaction of a metabolically generated reactive intermediate that may react with either the apoprotein or the heme moiety of the cytochrome. A growing list of such inhibitors includes the steroids ethinylestradiol, norethindrone, and spironolactone; the anesthetic agent fluroxene; the barbiturates secobarbital and allobarbital; the analgesic sedatives allylisopropylacetylurea, diethylpentenamide, and ethchlorvynol; the solvent carbon disulfide; and propylthiouracil.

PHASE II REACTIONS

Parent drugs or their phase I metabolites that contain suitable chemical groups often undergo coupling or conjugation reactions with an endogenous substance to yield drug conjugates (Table 3–3). In general, conjugates are polar molecules that are readily excreted and often inactive. Conjugate formation involves high-energy intermediates and specific transfer enzymes. Such enzymes (transferases) may be located in microsomes or in the cytosol. They catalyze the coupling of an activated endogenous substance (such as the uridine 5′-diphosphate [UDP] derivative of glucuronic acid) with a drug (or endogenous compound), or of an activated drug (such as the S-CoA derivative of benzoic acid) with an endogenous substrate. Because the endogenous substrates originate in the diet, nutrition plays a critical role in the regulation of drug conjugations.

Drug conjugations were once believed to represent terminal inactivation events and as such have been viewed as "true detoxification" reactions. However, this concept must be modified, since it is now known that certain conjugation reactions (O-sulfation of N-hydroxyacetylaminofluorene and N-acetylation of isoniazid) may lead to the formation of reactive species responsible for the hepatotoxicity of the drug.

CLINICAL RELEVANCE OF DRUG METABOLISM

The dose and the frequency of administration required to achieve effective therapeutic blood and tissue levels vary in different patients because of individual differences in drug distribution and rates of drug metabolism and elimination. These differences are determined by genetic factors and nongenetic variables such as age, sex, liver size, liver function, circadian rhythm, body temperature, and nutritional and environmental factors such as concomitant exposure to inducers or inhibitors of drug metabolism. The discussion that follows will summarize the most important variables relating to drug metabolism that are of clinical relevance.

Individual Differences

Individual differences in metabolic rate depend on the nature of the drug itself. Thus, within the same population, steady-state plasma levels may reflect a 30-fold variation in the metabolism of one drug and only a 2-fold variation in the metabolism of another. Genetic factors that influence enzyme levels account for some of these differences. Succinylcholine, for example, is metabolized only half as rapidly in persons with genetically determined defects in pseudocholinesterase as in normals. Analogous pharmacogenetic differences are seen in the acetylation of isoniazid and the hydroxylation of warfarin. Environmental factors also contribute to individual variations in drug metabolism. Cigarette smokers metabolize some drugs more rapidly than nonsmokers. Industrial workers exposed to some pesticides metabolize certain drugs more rapidly than nonexposed individuals. Such

Table 3–3. Phase II reactions.

Type of Conjugation	Endogenous Reactant	Transferase (Location)	Types of Substrates	Examples
Glucuronidation	UDP glucuronic acid.	UDP-glucuronyl transferase (microsomes).	Phenols, alcohols, carboxylic acids, hydroxylamines, sulfonamides.	Nitrophenol, morphine, acetaminophen, diazepam, N-hydroxydapsone, sulfathiazole, meprobamate.
Acetylation	Acetyl-CoA.	N-Acetyl transferase (cytosol).	Amines.	Sulfonamides, isoniazid, clonazepam, dapsone, mescaline.
Glutathione conjugation	Glutathione.	GSH-S-transferase (cytosol, microsomes).	Epoxides, arene oxides, nitro groups, hydroxylamines.	Ethacrynic acid, bromobenzene.
Glycine conjugation	Glycine.	Acyl-CoA glycine transferase (mitochondria).	Acyl-CoA derivatives of carboxylic acids.	Salicylic acid, benzoic acid, nicotinic acid, cinnamic acid, cholic acid, deoxycholic acid.
Sulfate conjugation	Phosphoadenosyl phosphosulfate.	Sulfotransferase (cytosol).	Phenols, alcohols, aromatic amines.	Estrone, aniline, phenol, 3-hydroxycoumarin, acetaminophen, methyldopa.
Methylation	S-Adenosylmethionine.	Transmethylases (cytosol).	Catecholamines, phenols, amines, histamine.	Dopamine, epinephrine, pyridine, histamine, thiouracil.

differences make it difficult to determine effective and safe doses of drugs that have narrow therapeutic indices.

Drug-Drug Interactions During Metabolism

Many substrates, by virtue of their relatively high lipophilicity, are retained not only at the active site of the enzyme but remain nonspecifically bound to the lipid membrane of the endoplasmic reticulum. In this state, they may induce microsomal enzymes; depending on the residual drug levels at the active site, they also may competitively inhibit metabolism of a simultaneously administered drug. Such drugs include various sedative-hypnotics, tranquilizers, anticonvulsants, and insecticides (see Table 3–4 and Appendix I). Patients who routinely ingest barbiturates, other sedative-hypnotics, or tranquilizers may require considerably higher doses of warfarin or dicumarol, when being treated with these oral anticoagulants, to maintain a prolonged prothrombin time. On the other hand, discontinuation of the sedative may result in reduced metabolism of the anticoagulant and bleeding—a toxic effect of the enhanced plasma levels of the anticoagulant. Similar interactions have been observed in individuals receiving various combination drug regimens such as tranquilizers or sedatives with contraceptive agents, sedatives with anticonvulsant drugs, and even alcohol with hypoglycemic drugs (tolbutamide).

It must also be noted that an inducer may enhance not only the metabolism of other drugs but also its own metabolism. Thus, continued use of a drug may result in one form of tolerance—progressively reduced effectiveness due to enhancement of its own metabolism.

Table 3–4. Partial list of drugs that enhance drug metabolism in humans.

Inducer	Drug Whose Metabolism is Enhanced
Phenobarbital and other barbiturates*	Coumarin anticoagulants Barbiturates Phenytoin Digitoxin Quinine Desmethylimipramine Chlorpromazine Phenylbutazone Cortisol Testosterone Estradiol Doxorubicin Chloramphenicol
Glutethimide	Glutethimide Warfarin Antipyrine
Phenylbutazone	Aminopyrine Digitoxin Cortisol
Phenytoin	Digitoxin Dexamethasone Cortisol
Griseofulvin	Warfarin
Ethchlorvynol	Warfarin
Chlorcyclizine	Steroid hormones

*Secobarbital is an exception. See Table 3–5 and text.

Table 3–5. Drugs that inhibit drug metabolism in humans.

Inhibitor	Drugs Whose Metabolism is Inhibited
Allopurinol, chloramphenicol, isoniazid	Tolbutamide Dicumarol Probenecid Antipyrine
Dicumarol	Phenytoin
Cimetidine	Warfarin Chlordiazepoxide Diazepam
Diethylpentenamide	Diethylpentenamide
Disulfiram	Phenytoin Warfarin Antipyrine Ethanol
Ethanol	Methanol Chlordiazepoxide? Diazepam?
Nortriptyline	Antipyrine
Oral contraceptives	Antipyrine
Phenylbutazone	Tolbutamide Phenytoin
Secobarbital	Secobarbital

Conversely, simultaneous administration of 2 or more drugs may result in impaired elimination of the more slowly metabolized drug and prolongation or potentiation of its pharmacologic effects (Table 3–5). Both competitive substrate inhibition and irreversible substrate-mediated enzyme inactivation may augment plasma drug levels and lead to toxic effects from drugs with narrow therapeutic indices. For example, it has been shown that dicumarol inhibits the metabolism of the anticonvulsant phenytoin and leads to the expression of side-effects such as ataxia and drowsiness. Similarly, allopurinol both prolongs the duration and enhances the chemotherapeutic action of mercaptopurine by competitive inhibition of xanthine oxidase. Consequently, to avoid bone marrow toxicity, the dose of mercaptopurine is usually reduced in patients receiving allopurinol. Cimetidine, a drug used in the treatment of peptic ulcer, has been shown to potentiate the pharmacologic actions of anticoagulants and sedatives. The metabolism of chlordiazepoxide has been shown to be inhibited by 63% after a single dose of cimetidine; such effects are reversed within 48 hours after withdrawal of cimetidine. For such interactions to occur, drug metabolism must be rate-limiting, ie, must follow zero-order kinetics (see Chapter 3, Part I). Elimination of most drugs proceeds, however, by exponential (first-order) kinetics, thus greatly reducing the probability of such metabolically dependent interactions.

Impairment of metabolism may also result if a simultaneously administered drug irreversibly inactivates a common metabolizing enzyme, as is the case with secobarbital or novonal (diethylpentenamide) overdoses. These compounds, in the course of their metabolism by cytochrome P-450, inactivate the enzyme and result in impairment of their own metabolism and that of other cosubstrates.

Interactions Between Drugs & Endogenous Compounds

Various drugs require conjugation with endogenous substrates such as glutathione, glucuronic acid, and sulfuric acid for their inactivation. Consequently, different drugs may compete for the same endogenous substrates, and the faster-reacting drug may effectively deplete endogenous substrate levels and impair the metabolism of the slower-reacting drug. If the latter has a steep dose-response curve or a narrow margin of safety, potentiation of its pharmacologic and toxic effects may result.

Diseases Affecting Drug Metabolism

Acute or chronic diseases that affect liver architecture or function markedly affect hepatic metabolism of some drugs. Such conditions include fat accumulation, alcoholic hepatitis, active or inactive alcoholic cirrhosis, hemochromatosis, chronic active hepatitis, biliary cirrhosis, and acute viral or drug hepatitis. Depending on their severity, these conditions impair hepatic drug-metabolizing enzymes, particularly microsomal oxidases, and thereby markedly affect drug elimination. For example, the half-lives of chlordiazepoxide and diazepam in patients with liver cirrhosis or acute viral hepatitis are greatly increased, with a corresponding prolongation of their effects. Consequently, these drugs may cause coma in patients with liver disease when given in ordinary doses.

Liver cancer has been reported to impair hepatic drug metabolism in humans. For example, aminopyrine metabolism is slower in patients with malignant hepatic tumors than in normal controls. These patients also exhibit markedly diminished aminopyrine clearance rates. Studies with biopsy specimens of livers from patients with hepatocellular carcinoma also indicate impaired ability to oxidatively metabolize drugs in vitro. This is associated with a correspondingly reduced cytochrome P-450 content.

Cardiac disease, by limiting blood flow to the liver, may impair disposition of those drugs whose metabolism is flow-limited (Table 3–6). These drugs are so readily metabolized by the liver that hepatic clearance is essentially equal to liver blood flow. Pulmonary disease may affect drug metabolism as indicated by the impaired hydrolysis of procainamide and procaine in patients with chronic respiratory insufficiency and the increased half-life of antipyrine in patients with lung cancer. Impairment of enzyme activity or defective formation of enzymes associated with heavy metal poisoning or porphyria also results in reduction of hepatic drug metabolism. For example, lead poisoning has been shown to increase the half-life of antipyrine in humans.

Table 3–6. Rapidly metabolized drugs whose hepatic clearance is blood flow-limited.

Alprenolol	Lidocaine
Amitriptyline	Meperidine
Chlormethiazole	Morphine
Desipramine	Pentazocine
Imipramine	Propoxyphene
Isoniazid	Propranolol
Labetalol	Verapamil

Although the effects of endocrine dysfunction on drug metabolism have been well explored in experimental animal models, corresponding data for humans with endocrine disorders are scanty. Thyroid dysfunction has been associated with altered metabolism of some drugs and of some endogenous compounds as well. Hypothyroidism increases the half-life of antipyrine, digoxin, methimazole, and practolol, whereas hyperthyroidism has the opposite effect. A few clinical studies in diabetic patients indicate no apparent impairment of drug metabolism, as reflected by the half-lives of antipyrine, tolbutamide, and phenylbutazone. In contrast, the metabolism of several drugs is impaired in male rats treated with diabetogenic agents such as alloxan or streptozocin. These alterations are abolished by administration of insulin, which has no direct influence on hepatic drug-metabolizing enzymes. Malfunctions of the pituitary, adrenal cortex, and gonads markedly impair hepatic drug metabolism in rats. On the basis of these findings, it may be supposed that such disorders could significantly affect drug metabolism in humans. However, until sufficient evidence is obtained from clinical studies in patients, such extrapolations must be considered tentative.

Age & Sex

Increased susceptibility to the pharmacologic or toxic activity of drugs has been reported in very young and old patients as compared to young adults. Although this may reflect differences in absorption, distribution, and elimination, differences in drug metabolism cannot be ruled out—a possibility supported by studies in other mammalian species indicating that drugs are metabolized at reduced rates during the prepubertal period and senescence. Slower metabolism could be due to reduced activity of metabolic enzymes or reduced availability of essential endogenous cofactors. Similar trends have been observed in humans, but incontrovertible evidence is yet to be obtained.

Sex-dependent variations in drug metabolism have been well documented in rats but not in other rodents. Young adult male rats metabolize drugs much faster than mature female rats or prepubertal male rats. These differences in drug metabolism have been clearly associated with androgenic hormones. A few clinical reports suggest that similar sex-dependent differences in drug metabolism also exist in humans.

METABOLISM OF DRUGS TO TOXIC PRODUCTS

It is becoming increasingly evident that metabolism of drugs and other foreign chemicals may not always be an innocuous biochemical event leading to detoxification and elimination of the compound. Indeed, several compounds have been shown to be metabolically transformed to reactive intermediates that are toxic to various organs. Such toxic reactions may not be apparent at low levels of exposure to parent compounds when alternative detoxification mechanisms are not yet overwhelmed or compromised and the availability of endogenous detoxifying cosubstrates (glutathione, glucuronic acid, sulfate) is not limited. However, when these possibilities are exhausted, the toxic pathway may prevail, resulting in overt organ toxicity or carcinogenesis. The number of specific examples of such drug-induced toxicity is expanding rapidly. An example is acetaminophen (paracetamol)-induced hepatotoxicity (Fig 3–10). This analgesic antipyretic drug is quite safe in therapeutic doses (1.2 g/d). It normally undergoes glucuronidation and sulfation to the corresponding conjugates, which together comprise 95% of the total excreted metabolites. The alternative cytochrome P-450-dependent glutathione (GSH) conjugation pathway accounts for the remaining 5%. When acetaminophen intake far exceeds therapeutic doses, the glucuronidation and sulfation pathways are saturated, and the cytochrome P-450-dependent pathway becomes increasingly important. Little or no hepatotoxicity results as long as glutathione is available for conjugation. However, with time, hepatic glutathione is depleted faster than it can be regenerated, and accumulation of a reactive and toxic metabolite occurs. In the absence of intracellular nucleophiles such as glutathione, this reactive metabolite (thought to be an N-hydroxylated product or an N-acetylbenzoiminoquinone) reacts with nucleophilic groups present on cellular macromolecules such as protein, resulting in hepatotoxicity (Fig 3–10).

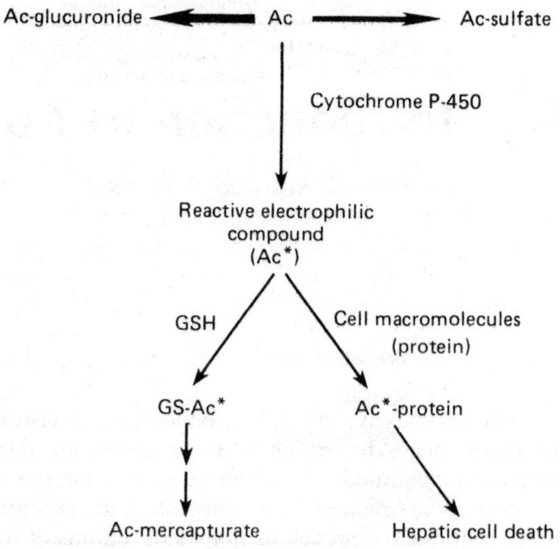

Figure 3–10. Metabolism of acetaminophen (Ac) to hepatotoxic metabolites. (GSH = glutathione; GS = glutathione moiety; Ac* = reactive intermediate.)

The chemical and toxicologic characterization of the electrophilic nature of the reactive acetaminophen metabolite has led to the development of effective antidotes—cysteamine and acetylcysteine (Mucomyst). Administration of acetylcysteine (the safer of the two) within 24 hours following acetaminophen overdosage has been shown to protect victims from fulminant hepatotoxicity and death.

Similar mechanistic interpretations can be invoked to explain the nephrotoxicity of phenacetin and the hepatotoxicity of aflatoxin and of benzo(a)pyrene, a pyrolytic product of organic matter present in cigarette tar and smoke and in smoked foods.

• • •

References

Hodgson E, Guthrie FE (editors): *Introduction to Biochemical Toxicology*. Elsevier/North Holland, 1980.

Jenner P, Testa B (editors): *Concepts in Drug Metabolism*. Part B of: *Drugs and the Pharmaceutical Science Series*. Vol 10. Marcel Dekker, 1981.

La Du BN, Mandel G, Way EL (editors): *Fundamentals of Drug Metabolism and Drug Disposition*. Williams & Wilkins, 1971.

Testa B, Jenner P (editors): *Drug Metabolism: Chemical and Biological Aspects*. Marcel Dekker, 1976.

4 | Introduction to Autonomic Pharmacology

Bertram G. Katzung, MD, PhD

The nervous system and the endocrine system are the major means by which body functions are controlled and integrated. They have several properties in common, including high-level integration in the brain, ability to influence processes in distant regions of the body, and extensive use of negative feedback. The major difference between the nervous and endocrine systems is in the mode of transmission of information. In the case of the endocrine system, transmission is largely chemical, via blood-borne hormones (see Chapter 34). The nervous system, on the other hand, relies primarily on rapid electrical transmission of information over nerve fibers. However, between nerve cells—and between nerve cells and their effector cells—signals are usually carried by chemical rather than electrical impulses. This chemical transmission takes place through the release of small amounts of transmitter or "neuromediator" substances from the nerve terminals into the region of the synapse. The chemical transmitter crosses the synaptic cleft by diffusion and activates (or inhibits) the postsynaptic cell by binding to a specialized receptor molecule.

Within the nervous system, one can discern 2 major functional subdivisions. The **autonomic division,** as the term implies, is largely independent in that its activities are not under direct conscious control. It is concerned primarily with visceral functions—cardiac output, blood flow to various organs, digestion, elimination, etc—necessary for life. The other major division of the nervous system, the **somatic division,** is largely nonautomatic and is concerned with consciously controlled functions such as locomotion as well as respiration and posture. Autonomic pharmacology is the study of those drugs that affect the autonomic nervous system itself or autonomic receptors on the effector cells controlled by the autonomic nervous system (cardiac muscle, smooth muscle, and glands). To understand the selectivity and actions of these drugs, it is necessary to understand the autonomic nervous system at the anatomic, biochemical, and functional levels.

ANATOMY OF THE AUTONOMIC NERVOUS SYSTEM
(See Figure 4–1.)

The autonomic nervous system lends itself to division on anatomic grounds into 2 major portions: the **sympathetic (thoracolumbar)** division and the **parasympathetic (craniosacral)** division. Both divisions originate in nuclei within the central nervous system and give off preganglionic fibers that exit from the brain stem or spinal cord. The sympathetic division contains discrete motor ganglia lying principally in 2 chains on either side of the spinal column; the parasympathetic division consists largely of groups of motor ganglia distributed diffusely in the walls of the organs innervated. The 2 divisions are further differentiated by the fact that their preganglionic efferent fibers originate in different portions of the central nervous system. The parasympathetic preganglionic fibers leave the central nervous system via cranial nerves (especially the third, seventh, ninth, and tenth) and the third and fourth sacral spinal roots. The sympathetic preganglionic axons leave the central nervous system via the thoracic and lumbar roots. In addition to these clearly defined peripheral motor portions of the autonomic nervous system, there are large numbers of afferent—sensory—fibers that impinge on important integrating centers in the hypothalamus and medulla to evoke the motor activity carried to the effector cells by the efferent fibers described above.

It is important to remember that the terms sympathetic and parasympathetic are anatomic ones and do not depend on the type of transmitter chemical released from the nerve endings nor on the kind of effect—excitatory or inhibitory—evoked by nerve activity.

NEUROTRANSMITTER CHEMISTRY OF THE AUTONOMIC NERVOUS SYSTEM

A different classification of autonomic nerve cells can be based on the transmitter molecules released from their terminal boutons and varicosities. A large number of peripheral autonomic nervous system fibers synthesize and release acetylcholine; they are **cholinergic** fibers. These include all preganglionic efferent autonomic fibers and the somatic (nonautonomic)

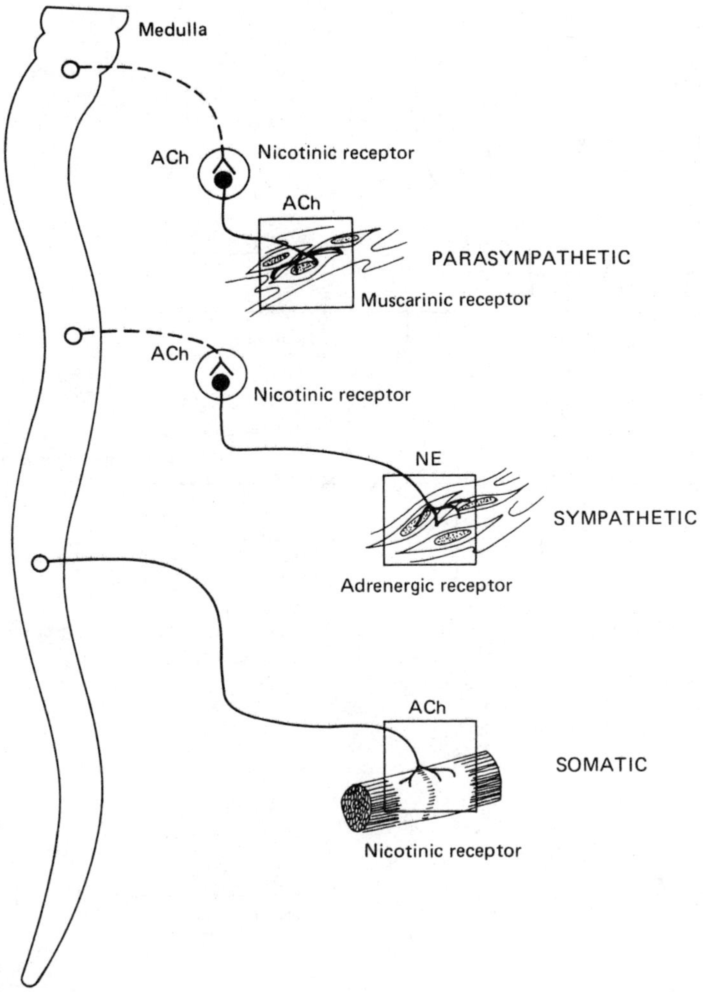

Figure 4–1. Schematic diagram comparing some anatomic and pharmacologic features of autonomic and somatic motor nerves. Because most parasympathetic ganglia are in or near the wall of the innervated organ, parasympathetic preganglionic nerves are long and postganglionic ones are short. Conversely, sympathetic ganglia are near the spinal cord; therefore, preganglionic fibers are short and postganglionic fibers long. Only the primary transmitter substances are shown: ACh = acetylcholine; NE = norepinephrine.

motor fibers to skeletal muscle as well. Thus, almost all efferent fibers leaving the central nervous system are cholinergic. In addition, all parasympathetic postganglionic and a few sympathetic postganglionic fibers are cholinergic. In contrast, most postganglionic sympathetic fibers release norepinephrine (noradrenaline); they are **noradrenergic** (often called simply "adrenergic") fibers. These chemical characteristics are presented schematically in Fig 4–1.

The terminals of cholinergic neurons contain large numbers of small membrane-bound vesicles concentrated near the synaptic portion of the cell membrane. These clear vesicles contain acetylcholine in high concentration and vasoactive intestinal polypeptide (Chapter 15), which is apparently a cotransmitter. Most of the acetylcholine is synthesized in the cytoplasm from choline and acetyl-CoA through the catalytic action of the enzyme choline acetyltransferase (Fig 4–2). Acetyl-CoA is synthesized in mitochondria, which are present in large numbers in the nerve ending. Choline is transported by a membrane carrier mechanism from the extracellular fluid into the neuron terminal. Synthesis is thus a rather simple process and is capable of supporting a very high rate of synaptic release. Vesicular storage of acetylcholine is accomplished by the packaging of "quanta" of acetylcholine molecules (usually 1000–50,000 molecules per quantum) in membranes cycled in from the neuronal surface. Release of transmitter occurs when an action potential reaches the terminal and triggers sufficient influx of calcium ions to "destabilize" the storage vesicles. Fusion of the vesicular membranes with the terminal membrane occurs, with exocytotic expulsion of several hundred quanta of acetylcholine

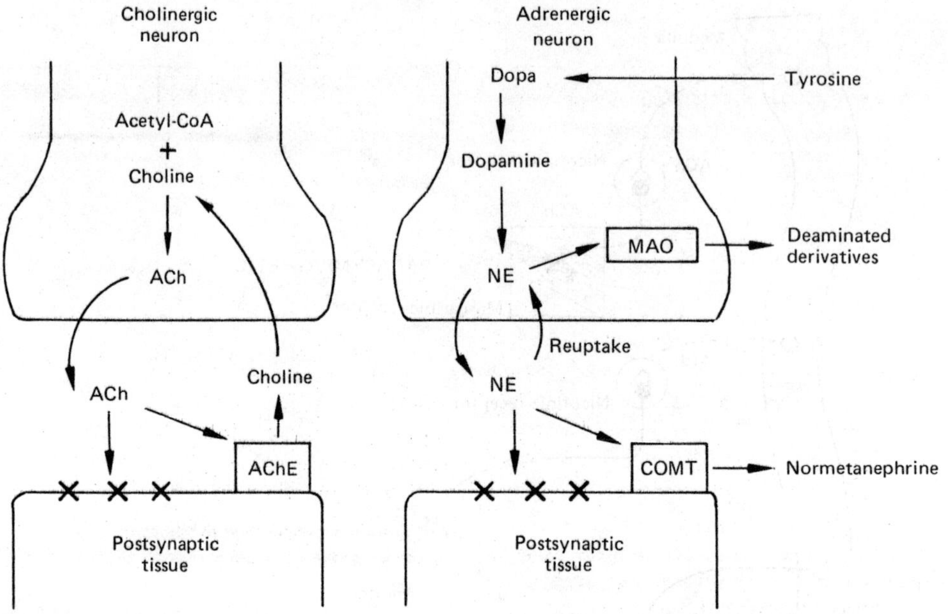

Figure 4–2. Comparison of the biochemical events at cholinergic endings with those at adrenergic endings. ACh = acetylcholine; AChE = acetylcholinesterase; NE = norepinephrine; X = receptor. Note that monoamine oxidase (MAO) is intracellular, so that some norepinephrine is being constantly deaminated in adrenergic endings. Catechol-O-methyltransferase (COMT) acts on norepinephrine after it is secreted. (Reproduced, with permission, from Ganong WF: *Review of Medical Physiology,* 10th ed. Lange, 1981.)

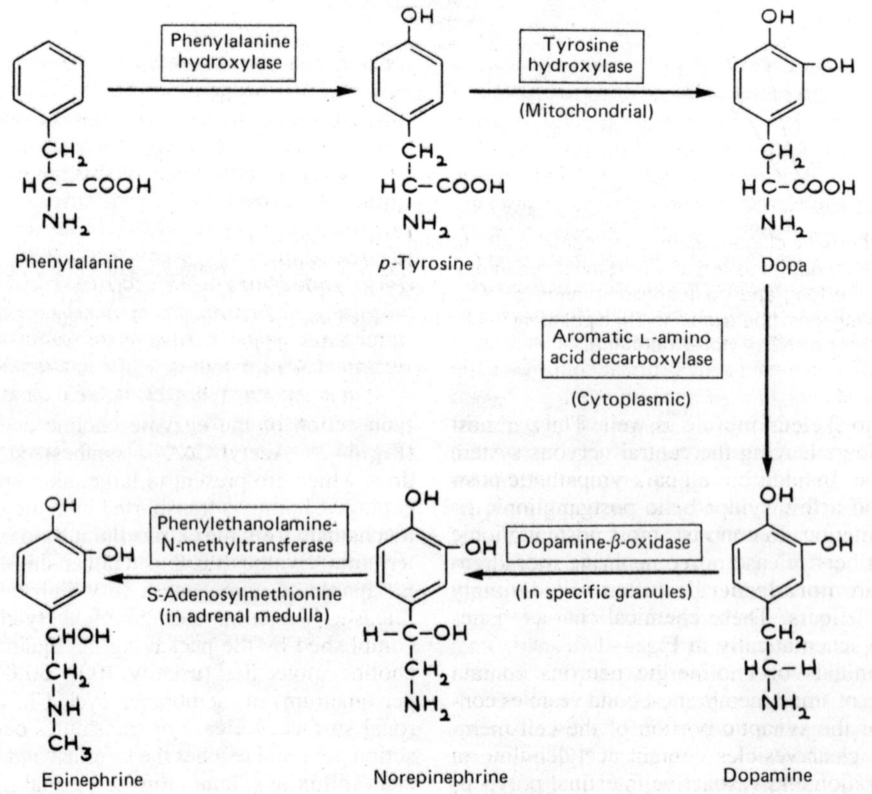

Figure 4–3. Biosynthesis of catecholamines. Dopa, dihydroxyphenylalanine; dopamine, dihydroxyphenylethylamine. (Modified and reproduced, with permission, from Meyers FH, Jawetz E, Goldfien A: *Review of Medical Pharmacology,* 7th ed. Lange, 1980.)

molecules and cotransmitter into the synaptic cleft. The physiologic role of the polypeptide cotransmitter is not known.

After release from the presynaptic terminal, acetylcholine molecules may bind to and activate a cholinergic receptor. Eventually (and usually very rapidly), all of the acetylcholine released will diffuse within range of an **acetylcholinesterase** molecule. Acetylcholinesterase (AChE) very efficiently splits acetylcholine into choline and acetate, neither of which has significant potency, and thereby terminates the action of the transmitter (Fig 4–2). Most cholinergic synapses are richly supplied with acetylcholinesterase; the half-life of acetylcholine in the synapse is therefore very short. In addition, acetylcholinesterase is found in other tissues, eg, red blood cells. (Another cholinesterase with a lower specificity for acetylcholine, butyrocholinesterase [pseudocholinesterase], is found in blood plasma, liver, glia, and many other tissues.)

Adrenergic neurons also store their transmitter substances in membrane-bound vesicles (Fig 4–2), but the synthesis of the adrenergic transmitters is more complex than that of acetylcholine, as indicated in Fig 4–3. In the adrenal medulla and certain areas of the brain, norepinephrine is further converted to epinephrine. In noradrenergic neurons, a portion of the norepinephrine is apparently not stored in vesicles but exists in a protected form in the neuronal cytoplasm; this secondary pool is not released by nerve action potentials but may be expelled by the action of certain indirect-acting sympathomimetic drugs such as tyramine. Several important transport mechanisms in the noradrenergic nerve terminal are potential sites of drug action. The first, located in the terminal cell membrane, actively transports norepinephrine and similar molecules into the cell cytoplasm. It can be inhibited by such agents as cocaine and the tricyclic antidepressants. The second high-affinity carrier for catecholamines is located in the wall of the storage vesicle itself and can be inhibited by a different class of drugs, the reserpine alkaloids.

Release of the vesicular content from noradrenergic nerve endings is believed to be similar to the calcium-dependent process described above for cholinergic terminals. In addition to the primary transmitter (norepinephrine), ATP, dopamine-β-hydroxylase, and certain polypeptides are also released into the synaptic cleft. It is not known whether any of these cotransmitters play a significant role in adrenergic transmission.

Norepinephrine and epinephrine can be metabolized by several enzymes, as shown in Figs 4–4 and 4–5. Because of the high activity of monoamine oxidase in the mitochondria of the nerve terminal, there is a significant turnover of norepinephrine even in the resting terminal. Since the metabolic products are excreted in the urine, an estimate of catecholamine turnover can be obtained from laboratory analysis of total metabolites (sometimes referred to as "total VMA and metanephrines") in a 24-hour urine sample.

Table 4–1. Autonomic receptor types.

Name	Typical Locations
Cholinergic	
Muscarinic	Parasympathetic effector cells: smooth muscle, cardiac muscle, exocrine glands; brain.
Nicotinic	Autonomic ganglia, skeletal muscle neuromuscular end-plate, spinal cord.
Adrenergic	
$Alpha_1$	Postsynaptic effector cells, especially smooth muscle.
$Alpha_2$	Presynaptic adrenergic nerve terminals, platelets, lipocytes.
$Beta_1$	Postsynaptic effector cells, especially heart; lipocytes, brain, presynaptic noradrenergic nerve terminals.
$Beta_2$	Postsynaptic effector cells, especially smooth muscle.
Dopaminergic	Brain and postsynaptic effectors, especially vascular smooth muscle of the splanchnic and renal vascular beds.

However, metabolism is not the primary mechanism for termination of action of norepinephrine physiologically released from noradrenergic nerves. Termination of noradrenergic transmission results from several processes including simple diffusion away from the receptor site (with ultimate metabolism in the plasma or liver) and reuptake into the nerve terminal **(uptake I)** or into perisynaptic glia or smooth muscle cells **(uptake II).**

Less is known about the biochemical nature of autonomic receptors than of transmitters, but this field is one of the most active research areas in pharmacology. Historically, indirect structure-activity analyses, with careful comparisons of the potency of series of autonomic analogs, led to the definition of different autonomic receptor subtypes (Table 4–1). Development of selective blocking drugs has led to the naming of subclasses within these major types, eg, within the adrenergic class, α_1 and α_2 receptors differ in both agonist and antagonist selectivity. Specific examples of such selective drugs are given in the chapters that follow. More recently, much progress has been made in isolating and purifying receptor proteins. Detailed characterization of the peptide sequences of these proteins and their 3-dimensional conformations should lead to the development of even more specific agonists and antagonists.

FUNCTIONAL ORGANIZATION OF AUTONOMIC ACTIVITY

A basic understanding of the interactions of autonomic components with each other and with their effector organs is essential for an appreciation of the actions of autonomic drugs, especially because of their significant "reflex" effects.

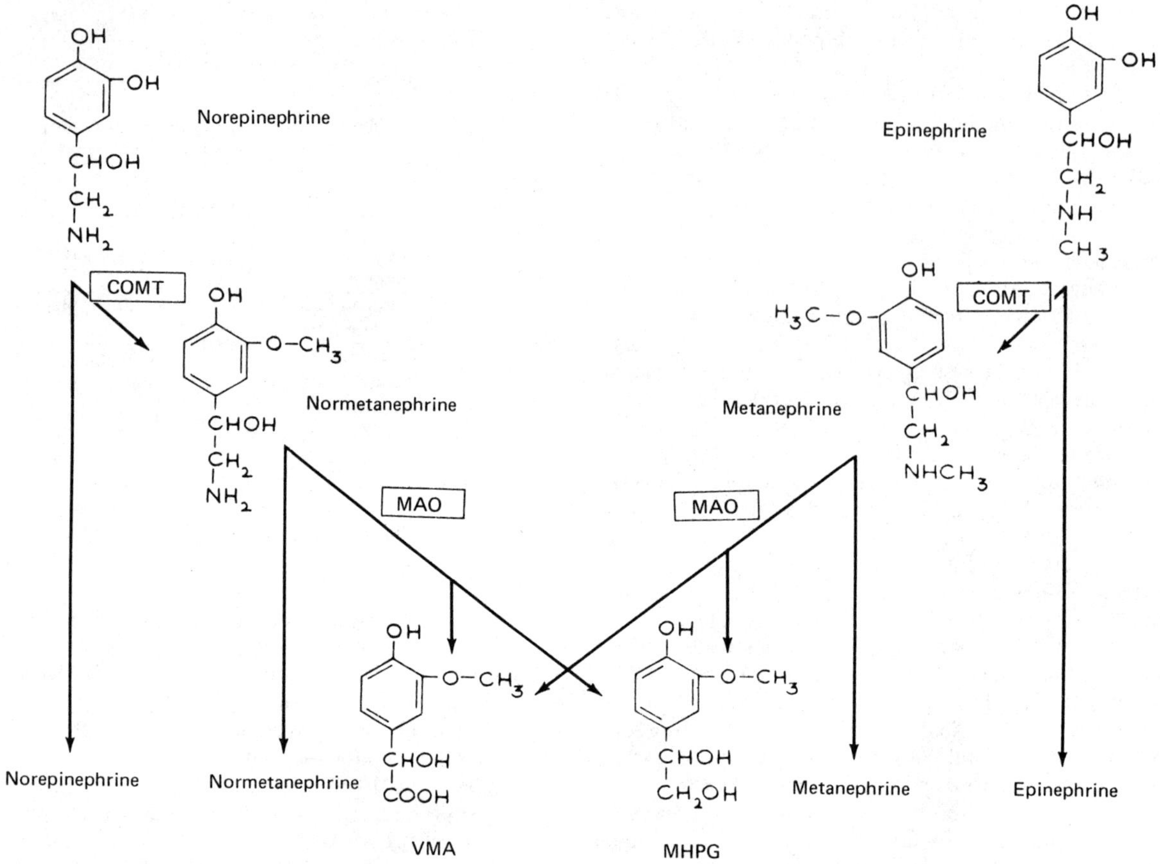

Figure 4–4. Metabolism of free catecholamines. Urinary excretion products appear on the lowest line. Excretion products may be conjugated with glucuronide or sulfate. COMT = catechol-O-methyltransferase; VMA = 3-methoxy-4-hydroxymandelic acid; MHPG = methoxyhydroxyphenylglycol; MAO = monoamine oxidase. (Modified and reproduced, with permission, from Meyers FH, Jawetz E, Goldfien A: *Review of Medical Pharmacology,* 7th ed. Lange, 1980.)

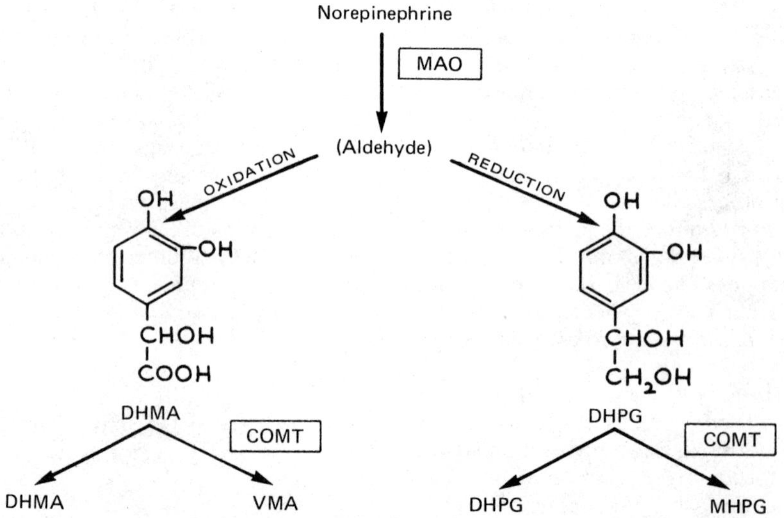

Figure 4–5. Metabolism of norepinephrine of storage pool and central nervous system. Urinary excretion products are shown in lowest line. Excretion products may be conjugated with glucuronide or sulfate. MAO = monoamine oxidase; DHMA = dihydroxymandelic acid; DHPG = dihydroxyphenylglycol; COMT = catechol-O-methyltransferase; VMA = 3-methoxy-4-hydroxymandelic acid; MHPG = methoxyhydroxyphenylglycol. (Modified and reproduced, with permission, from Meyers FH, Jawetz E, Goldfien A: *Review of Medical Pharmacology,* 7th ed. Lange, 1980.)

Central Integration

At the highest level—midbrain and medulla—the 2 divisions of the autonomic nervous system and the endocrine system are integrated with each other and with information from higher central nervous system centers. These interactions are such that early investigators called the parasympathetic system a **trophotropic** one (ie, leading to growth) and the sympathetic system an **ergotropic** one (ie, leading to energy expenditure) that was activated for "fight or flight." While such terms offer little insight into the mechanisms involved, they do provide simple descriptions applicable to many of the actions of the systems (Table 4–2). For example, slowing of the heart and stimulation of digestive activity are typical energy-conserving trophotropic actions of the parasympathetic system. In contrast, cardiac stimulation, increased blood sugar, and cutaneous vasoconstriction are responses produced by sympathetic discharge that are suited to fighting or surviving attack.

At a more subtle level of interactions in the brain stem, medulla, and spinal cord, there are important cooperative interactions between the parasympathetic and sympathetic systems. For some organs, sensory fibers in the parasympathetic system exert reflex control over motor outflow in the sympathetic system. Thus, the sensory baroreceptor fibers in the glossopharyngeal nerve have a major influence on sympathetic outflow from the vasomotor center. This example is developed in greater detail below. Similarly,

Table 4–2. Direct effects of autonomic nerve activity on some organ systems.

Organ	Effect of: Sympathetic Action*	Sympathetic Receptor†	Parasympathetic Action	Parasympathetic Receptor†
Eye				
Iris				
Radial muscle	Contracts	α	...	...
Circular muscle	...	...	Contracts	M
Ciliary muscle	[Relaxes]	β	Contracts	M
Heart				
Sinoatrial node	Accelerates	β	Decelerates	M
Ectopic pacemakers	Accelerates	β	...	...
Contractility	Increases	β	Decreases (atria)	M
Vascular smooth muscle				
Skin splanchnic vessels	Contracts	α_1	...	M‡
Skeletal muscle vessels	Relaxes	β_2	...	...
	[Contracts]	α_1	...	...
	Relaxes	M§	...	...
Bronchiolar smooth muscle	Relaxes	β_2	Contracts	M
Gastrointestinal tract				
Smooth muscle				
Walls	Relaxes	β_2	Contracts	M
Sphincters	Contracts	α	Relaxes	M
Secretion	...	...	Increases	M
Myenteric plexus	Inhibits	α	...	...
Genitourinary smooth muscle				
Bladder wall	Relaxes	β_2	Contracts	M
Sphincter	Contracts	α	Relaxes	M
Uterus, pregnant	Relaxes	β_2	...	...
	Contracts	α	...	...
Penis, seminal vesicles	Ejaculation	α	Erection	M
Skin				
Pilomotor smooth muscle	Contracts	α	...	...
Sweat glands				
Thermoregulatory	Increases	M	...	...
Apocrine (stress)	Increases	α	...	...
Metabolic functions				
Liver	Gluconeogenesis	α/β_2**	...	...
Liver	Glycogenolysis	α/β_2	...	...
Fat cells	Lipolysis	α_2, β_1††	...	...

*Less important actions are in brackets.
†Specific receptor type: α = alpha, β = beta, M = muscarinic.
‡Most vascular smooth muscle has uninnervated muscarinic receptors.
§Vascular smooth muscle in skeletal muscle has sympathetic cholinergic dilator fibers.
**Depends on species.
††Alpha$_2$ inhibits; β_1 stimulates.

parasympathetic sensory fibers in the wall of the urinary bladder significantly influence sympathetic inhibitory outflow to that organ.

Cardiovascular Reflexes

The reflexes that control or are controlled by autonomic nerve activity are particularly important in understanding cardiovascular responses to autonomic drugs. As indicated in Fig 4–6, the primary controlled variable in cardiovascular function is **mean arterial pressure.** Changes in any variable contributing to mean arterial pressure (eg, peripheral vascular resistance) will evoke homeostatic secondary responses that tend to compensate for the directly evoked change. The homeostatic response may sometimes be sufficient to prevent any change in mean arterial pressure. A slow infusion of norepinephrine provides a useful example. This agent produces direct effects on both vascular and cardiac muscle. It is a powerful vasoconstrictor and, by increasing peripheral vascular resistance, tends to increase mean arterial pressure. In the absence of reflexes, its effect on the heart is also stimulatory—ie, it increases heart rate and contractile force. However, in a subject with intact reflexes, the negative feedback baroreceptor response to increased mean arterial pressure causes decreased sympathetic outflow to the heart and a powerful increase in parasympathetic (vagus nerve) discharge at the cardiac pacemaker. As a result, the *net* effect of ordinary pressor doses of norepinephrine is to produce a marked increase in peripheral vascular resistance, a moderate increase in mean arterial pressure, and a consistent *slowing* of heart rate. Bradycardia is thus a reflex or compensatory response elicited by an autonomic drug and is *the exact opposite of the drug's direct action;* yet it is completely predictable if the integration of cardiovascular function by the autonomic nervous system is understood.

Presynaptic Regulation

The principle of negative feedback control is also found at the presynaptic level of autonomic function. While not yet as completely understood as the baroreceptor reflex, an important presynaptic feedback inhibitory control mechanism has been shown to exist in noradrenergic fibers. A special receptor, located on the presynaptic nerve terminals and designated α_2, is activated by norepinephrine and similar molecules; activation diminishes further release of norepinephrine from the nerve ending. Conversely, a presynaptic beta receptor may facilitate the release of norepinephrine. Selective activation of α_2 receptors by a drug might be expected to reduce sympathetic effects by attenuating endogenous norepinephrine release.

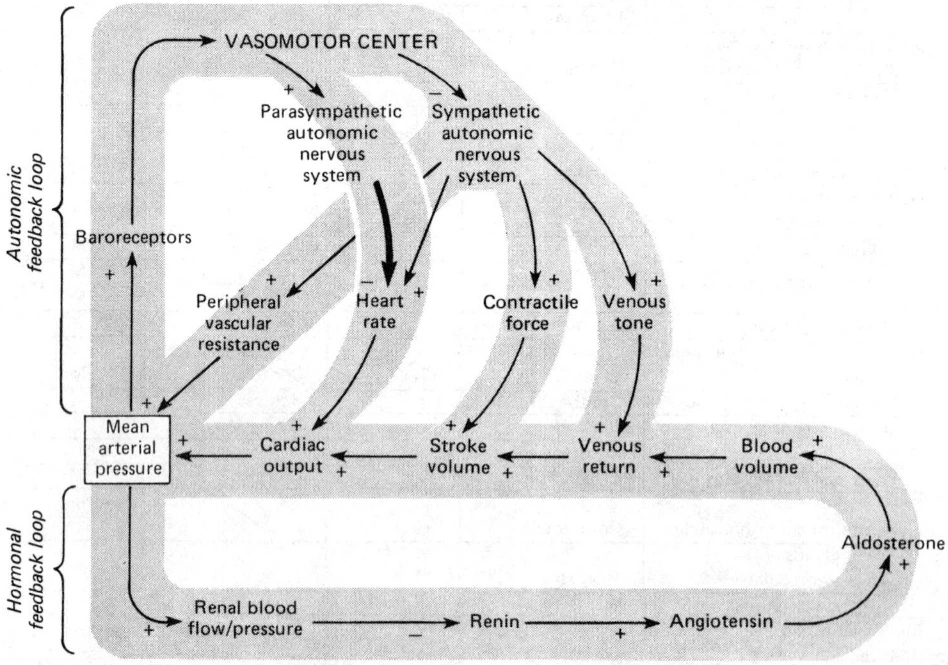

Figure 4–6. Autonomic and hormonal control of cardiovascular function. Note that at least 2 feedback loops are present, the autonomic nervous system loop and the hormonal loop. In addition, each major loop has several components. Thus, the sympathetic autonomic nervous system directly influences the 4 major variables peripheral vascular resistance, heart rate, force, and venous tone. The vagus directly influences heart rate. Angiotensin II directly increases peripheral vascular resistance (not shown), and the sympathetic autonomic nervous system probably directly increases renin secretion (not shown). The plus and minus signs on the arrows indicate the direction of change in the variables pointed to when activity along the arrow is increased.

Certain antihypertension drugs may act in this way (clonidine, α-methylnorepinephrine, the active metabolite of methyldopa; see Chapter 9). Inhibitory control of transmitter release is not limited to inhibition by the transmitter itself. Evidence also strongly implicates prostaglandins and polypeptides in the regulation of norepinephrine release. Presynaptic regulation by a variety of chemicals probably occurs in all nerve fibers.

Postsynaptic Regulation

Postsynaptic regulation can be considered from 2 perspectives: modulation by the prior history of activity (which may up- or down-regulate receptor number; see Chapter 2) and modulation of any given postsynaptic event by other temporally associated events. The first mechanism has been well documented in several autonomic receptor-effector systems. The second mechanism usually involves modulation of each primary transmitter-receptor event by secondary events, which are evoked by the same or other transmitters acting on different receptors.

Ganglionic transmission is a good example of this hierarchy. The postganglionic cells are activated (depolarized) as a result of binding of an appropriate ligand (acetylcholine or nicotine) to a nicotinic cholinergic receptor. The primary spike response (fast excitatory postsynaptic potential; EPSP) evoked by this event is often followed by a small and slowly developing but relatively long-lasting hyperpolarizing afterpotential—an inhibitory postsynaptic potential (IPSP). This in turn is followed by a small, slow excitatory postsynaptic potential. These slow potentials serve to modulate the responsiveness of the postsynaptic cell to subsequent primary excitatory presynaptic nerve activity. (See Chapter 18 for further examples.)

Table 4–3. Steps in autonomic transmission: Effects of drugs.

Process	Drug Example	Site	Action
Action potential propagation	Local anesthetics, tetrodotoxin[1], saxitoxin.[2]	Pre- and postganglionic nerve axons.	Block sodium channels; block conduction.
Transmitter synthesis	Hemicholinium.	Cholinergic nerve terminals: membrane.	Blocks uptake of choline and slows synthesis.
	α-Methyltyrosine.	Adrenergic nerve terminals and adrenal medulla: cytoplasm.	Blocks synthesis.
Transmitter storage	Carbachol.	Cholinergic terminals: vesicles.	Promotes release.
	Reserpine.	Adrenergic terminals: vesicles.	Promotes depletion.
Transmitter release	Many.[3]	Nerve terminal membrane receptors.	Modulate release.
	Mg^{2+}, Ca^{2+} influx inhibitors.	Nerve terminal membrane Ca^{2+} channels.	Reduce transmitter release.
	Botulinus toxin.	Cholinergic vesicles.	Prevents release.
	Latrotoxin.[4]	Cholinergic vesicles.	Causes explosive release.
	Tyramine, amphetamine.	Adrenergic nerve terminals.	Promote release.
Transmitter uptake after release	Cocaine, tricyclic antidepressants.	Adrenergic nerve terminals.	Inhibit uptake; increase transmitter effect on postsynaptic receptors.
	6-Hydroxydopamine.	Adrenergic nerve terminals.	Destroys the terminals.
Receptor activation/blockade	Norepinephrine.	Receptors at adrenergic junctions.	Binds α receptors; causes contraction.
	Phentolamine.	Receptors at adrenergic junctions.	Binds α receptors; prevents activation.
	Isoproterenol.	Receptors at adrenergic junctions.	Binds β receptors; activates adenylate cyclase.
	Propranolol.	Receptors at adrenergic junctions.	Binds β receptors; prevents activation.
	Nicotine.	Receptors, cholinergic junctions (autonomic ganglia, neuromuscular end-plates).	Binds nicotinic receptors; opens ion channel in postsynaptic membrane.
	Tubocurarine.	Neuromuscular end-plates.	Prevents activation.
	Bethanechol.	Receptors, parasympathetic effector cells (smooth muscle, cardiac muscle, glands).	Binds muscarinic receptors; activates guanylate cyclase.
	Atropine.	Receptors, parasympathetic effector cells.	Binds muscarinic receptors; prevents activation.
Enzymatic inactivation of transmitter	Neostigmine.	Cholinergic synapses (acetylcholinesterase).	Inhibits enzyme; prolongs and intensifies transmitter action.
	Tranylcypromine.	Adrenergic nerve terminals (monoamine oxidase).	Inhibits enzyme; increases stored transmitter pool.

[1] Toxin of puffer fish, California newt.
[2] Toxin of Gonyaulax (red tide organism).
[3] Norepinephrine, dopamine, acetylcholine, angiotensin II, various prostaglandins, etc.
[4] Black widow spider venom.

PHARMACOLOGIC MODIFICATION OF AUTONOMIC FUNCTION

Because the transmission of information involves different mechanisms in different segments of the autonomic nervous system, some drugs produce highly specific effects while others are nonselective in their actions. A summary of the steps in transmission of impulses, from the central nervous system to the autonomic effector cells, is presented in Table 4–3. Drugs such as local anesthetics are very nonselective in their action, since they act on a process that is common to all neurons. On the other hand, drugs that act on the biochemical processes involved in transmitter synthesis and storage are more selective, since the biochemistry of adrenergic transmission is very different from that of cholinergic transmission. Activation or blockade of effector cell receptors offers the maximum flexibility and selectivity of effect: adrenergic receptors are easily distinguished from cholinergic ones. Furthermore, several subgroups can be selectively activated or blocked within each major type.

The next 4 chapters provide the information needed to take advantage of this useful diversity of autonomic processes.

• • •

References

Burnstock G: Neurotransmitters and trophic factors in the autonomic nervous system. *J Physiol (London)* 1981;**313:**1.

Central integration of cardiovascular control. Central cardiovascular control: A distributed neural network. (Symposium.) Manning JW (chairman). *Fed Proc* 1980;**39:**2485.

Complexities of transmission in autonomic ganglia. (Symposium.) Volle RL (chairman). *Fed Proc* 1980;**39:**2980.

Glick G, Braunwald E: Relative roles of the sympathetic and parasympathetic nervous systems in the reflex control of heart rate. *Circ Res* 1965;**16:**363.

Guyton AC et al: Relative importance of venous and arterial resistances in controlling venous return and cardiac output. *Am J Physiol* 1959;**196:**1008.

Higgins CB, Vatner SF, Braunwald E: Parasympathetic control of the heart. *Pharmacol Rev* 1973;**25:**119.

Hokfelt T et al: Peptidergic neurones. *Nature* 1980;**284:**515.

Langer SZ: Presynaptic receptors and modulation of neurotransmission: Pharmacological implications and therapeutic relevance. *Trends Neurosci* 1980;**3:**110.

Langer SZ: Presynaptic regulation of the release of catecholamine. *Pharmacol Rev* 1980;**32:**337.

Miyamoto MD: The actions of cholinergic drugs on motor nerve terminals. *Pharmacol Rev* 1977;**29:**221.

Pumplin DW, Reese TS: Action of brown widow spider venom and botulinum toxin on the frog neuromuscular junction examined with the freeze-fracture technique. *J Physiol (London)* 1977;**273:**443.

Simpson LL: The origin, structure, and pharmacological activity of botulinum toxin. *Pharmacol Rev* 1981;**33:**155.

Starke K: Presynaptic receptors: A numerous family. Pages 9–17 in: *Progress in Pharmacology*. Vol 3, No. 4. von Zwieten PA, Schoenbaum E (editors). Gustav Fischer Verlag, 1980.

Watanabe AM et al: Cardiac autonomic receptors: Recent concepts from radiolabeled ligand-binding studies. *Circ Res* 1982;**50:**161.

Cholinergic Receptor Stimulants | 5

August M. Watanabe, MD

The cholinergic receptor stimulants comprise a large group of drugs that mimic acetylcholine. The effects of acetylcholine cover a broad spectrum, depending upon the receptor type—muscarinic or nicotinic—that is activated. There is a correspondingly wide spectrum of potential actions for other molecules (''cholinomimetics'') that activate cholinergic receptors. Thus, one important basis for classification of these agents is their *spectrum* of action and another is their *mechanism* of action, since some cholinergic drugs directly bind to (and activate) cholinergic receptors while a second important group acts indirectly by inhibiting the hydrolysis of endogenous acetylcholine (Fig 5–1).

SPECTRUM OF ACTION OF CHOLINERGIC DRUGS

In some of the first studies of the parasympathetic nervous system, Sir Henry Dale found that the alkaloid **muscarine** mimicked the effects of parasympathetic nerve discharge, ie, the effects were **parasympathomimetic.** Direct application of muscarine to ganglia and to autonomic effector tissues (smooth muscle, heart, exocrine glands) showed that the parasympathomimetic action of the alkaloid was mediated only by receptors at the effector cells, not those in the ganglia. Therefore, by convention, the effects of acetylcholine itself and of other cholinergic drugs at autonomic neuroeffector junctions are referred to as parasympathomimetic effects, mediated by muscarinic receptors.

In contrast, the alkaloid **nicotine** was found to stimulate autonomic ganglia and skeletal muscle neuromuscular junctions but to have little effect on autonomic effector cells when applied in low concentrations. The receptors involved were therefore labeled nicotinic. When it was later demonstrated that acetylcholine is the physiologic transmitter substance at both muscarinic and nicotinic receptors, it was recognized that both receptors are subtypes of cholinergic receptors.

Muscarinic receptors are located on plasma membranes of cells of organs innervated by parasympathetic nerves as well as on some tissues that are not innervated by parasympathetic nerves (Table 4–1). Nicotinic receptors are located on plasma membranes of parasympathetic and sympathetic postganglionic cells in autonomic ganglia and also on membranes of muscles innervated by somatic motor fibers (Fig 4–1). Because of the multiple sites of action of acetylcholine and the fact that it has both excitatory and inhibitory effects, unselective cholinergic stimulants can produce very diffuse and marked alterations in organ system function. Fortunately, drugs are available that have a degree of selectivity, so desired effects can be achieved while avoiding or minimizing unde-

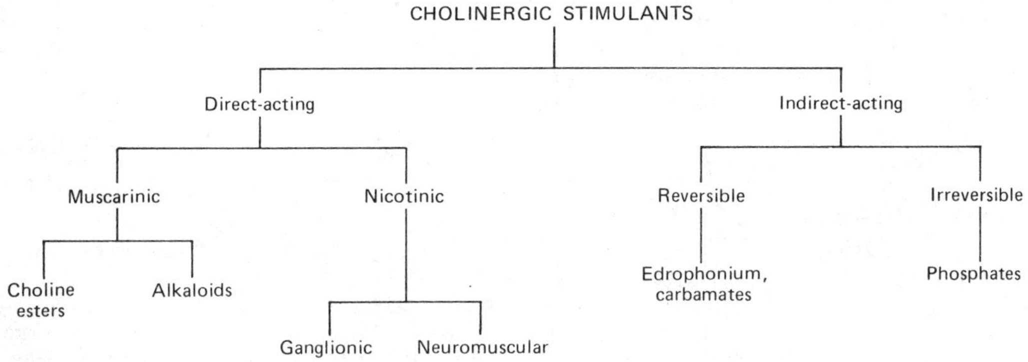

Figure 5–1. The major classes of cholinergic receptor stimulants.

sired side-effects. This selectivity of action is based on several factors. Thus, some drugs stimulate muscarinic receptors selectively, whereas others selectively activate nicotinic receptors. Some agents stimulate nicotinic receptors in ganglia preferentially, whereas others act preferentially on nicotinic receptors at neuromuscular junctions. Organ selectivity can also be achieved by utilizing appropriate routes of administration ("pharmacokinetic selectivity"). For example, muscarinic stimulants can be administered topically to the external surface of the eye to modify ocular function while minimizing systemic effects.

MODE OF ACTION OF CHOLINERGIC DRUGS

The cholinergic stimulant drugs can also be divided into 2 major categories on the basis of their mode of action: direct and indirect (Fig 5–1). The direct-acting agents directly bind to and activate the muscarinic or nicotinic cholinergic receptors. The indirect-acting agents produce their primary effects by inhibiting the action of acetylcholinesterase, which hydrolyses acetylcholine to choline and acetic acid (Fig 4–2). By inhibiting acetylcholinesterase, the indirect-acting drugs increase the concentration of endogenous acetylcholine in the synaptic clefts and neuroeffector junctions, and the excess acetylcholine in turn stimulates cholinergic receptors to evoke increased responses.

Some cholinesterase inhibitors, even in low concentration, also inhibit butyrocholinesterase (pseudocholinesterase), and most inhibit this enzyme when they are present in high concentrations. However, since this enzyme is not important in the physiologic termination of action of synaptic acetylcholine, inhibition of its action plays little role in the action of indirect-acting cholinergic stimulants. Some cholinesterase inhibitors also have a modest direct action as well; this is especially true of some quaternary carbamates, eg, neostigmine, that activate neuromuscular nicotinic cholinergic receptors.

Metoclopramide, a new drug with cholinergic effects, appears to act by increasing tissue responsiveness to background cholinergic activity, yet it is not a cholinesterase inhibitor. Because its mechanism of action is not yet defined and because its use is largely restricted to gastrointestinal indications, it is discussed in Chapter 62.

BASIC PHARMACOLOGY OF THE DIRECT-ACTING CHOLINERGIC STIMULANTS

The direct-acting cholinomimetic drugs can be divided on the basis of chemical structure into esters of choline (including acetylcholine) and alkaloids (such as muscarine and nicotine). A few of these drugs have a high degree of specificity for the muscarinic or for the nicotinic receptor. Many have effects on both receptors; acetylcholine is typical.

Chemistry & Pharmacokinetics

A. Structure: Four important esters of choline that have been studied extensively are shown in Fig 5–2. Because they contain the quaternary ammonium group, they are permanently charged and relatively insoluble in lipids. Many naturally occurring and synthetic cholinergic drugs that are not choline esters have been identified; a few of these are shown in Fig 5–3.

B. Absorption, Distribution, and Metabolism: The choline esters all have similar absorption and distribution characteristics, dominated by their low lipid solubility; they are poorly absorbed and poorly distributed into the central nervous system. Although they are all hydrolyzed in the gastrointestinal tract (and inactive by the oral route), they differ markedly in their susceptibility to hydrolysis by cholinesterase in the

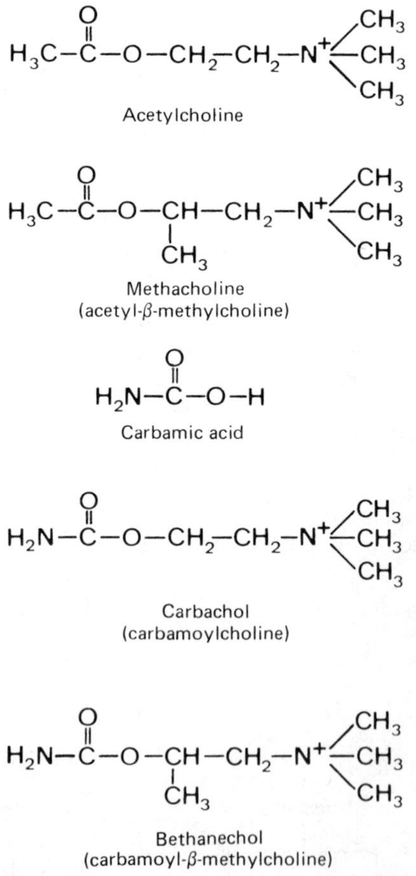

Figure 5–2. Molecular structures of 4 choline esters and carbamic acid. Acetylcholine and methacholine are acetic acid esters of choline and β-methylcholine, respectively. Carbachol and bethanechol are carbamic acid esters of the same alcohols.

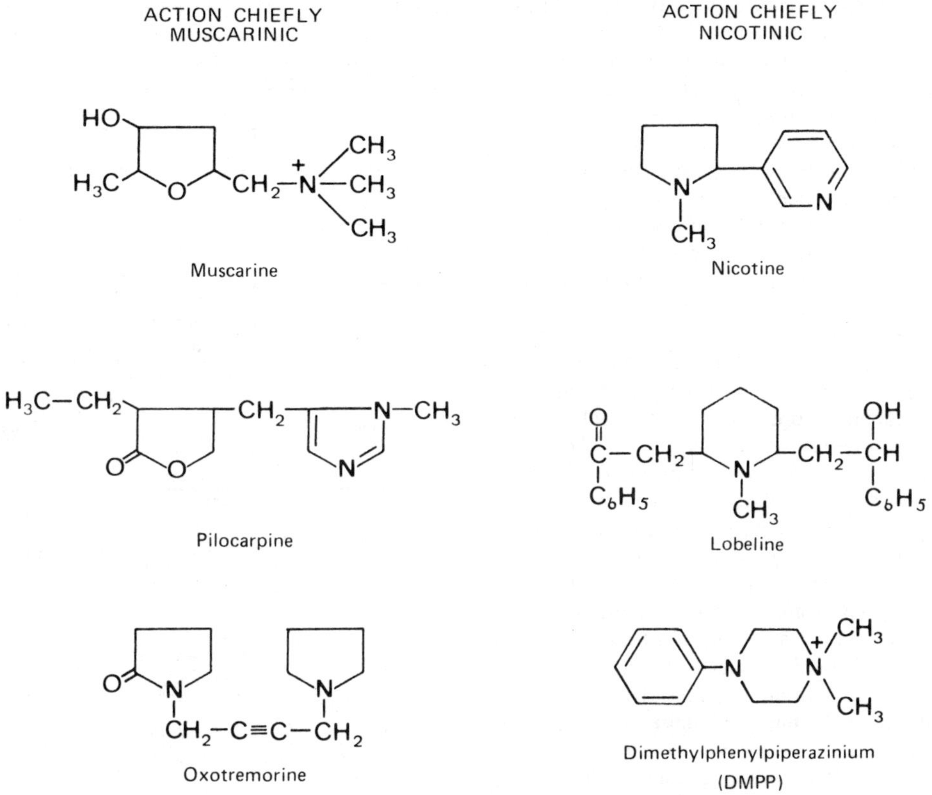

Figure 5–3. Structures of some cholinergic alkaloids and synthetic analogs.

body. Acetylcholine is very rapidly hydrolyzed, as described in Chapter 4; large amounts must be infused intravenously to achieve levels high enough to produce detectable effects. A large intravenous bolus injection has a brief effect, typically 5–20 seconds, whereas intramuscular and subcutaneous injection produce only local effects. Methacholine is at least 3 times more resistant to hydrolysis and produces systemic effects even when given subcutaneously. The carbamic acid esters, carbachol and bethanechol, are completely resistant to hydrolysis by cholinesterase and have correspondingly longer durations of action. Presence of the β-methyl group (methacholine, bethanechol) reduces the potency of these drugs at the nicotinic receptor (Table 5–1).

The tertiary cholinergic alkaloids (pilocarpine, nicotine, lobeline; Fig 5–3) are well absorbed from most sites of administration. Nicotine is sufficiently lipid-soluble to be absorbed across the skin. Muscarine, a quaternary amine, is less completely absorbed from the gastrointestinal tract than the tertiary amines but is nevertheless toxic when ingested, eg, in mushrooms. Excretion of these amines is chiefly by the kidneys. Clearance of tertiary amines can be accelerated by acidification of the urine. Oxotremorine is an extremely potent synthetic muscarinic agonist that has been used as a research tool. It is well distributed into the central nervous system. Lobeline is a plant derivative with lower potency than nicotine but a similar spectrum of action. Dimethylphenylpiperazinium (DMPP) is a potent synthetic nicotinic stimulant with little access to the central nervous system.

Table 5–1. Properties of choline esters.

Choline Ester	Susceptibility to Cholinesterase	Muscarinic Action	Nicotinic Action
Acetylcholine chloride	++++	+++	+++
Methacholine chloride	+	++++	+
Carbachol chloride	None	++	+++
Bethanecol chloride	None	++	None

Pharmacodynamics

A. Mechanism of Action: The subcellular or biochemical mechanism by which muscarinic stimulants alter cellular function is not well established. Several cellular events occur when muscarinic receptors are activated, one or more of which might serve as "second messengers" for muscarinic activation. Muscarinic agonists can increase cellular concentrations of cGMP, presumably by activating guanylate cyclase, which catalyses the conversion of GTP to cGMP. The role of cGMP in cellular regulation has not, however, been established. The activation of muscarinic receptors also increases potassium flux across cell membranes. However, it is not yet known whether alterations in potassium channels are directly coupled to muscarinic receptors or if one or more intervening "messengers" are involved in mediating the change in ion flux. Muscarinic agonists also accelerate the turnover of inositol phospholipids in membranes of cells that possess muscarinic receptors. However, what role this effect has in mediating muscarinic actions remains to be established. Finally, it has been shown in certain organs such as heart that muscarinic receptors are coupled to adenylate cyclase in an inhibitory manner; muscarinic agonists reduce cardiac cAMP levels.

The mechanism of nicotinic receptor activation has been studied in great detail, taking advantage of 3 factors: The receptor is present in extremely high concentration in the membranes of the electric organs of electric fish; α-bungarotoxin, a component of certain snake venoms, is tightly bound to the receptors and readily labeled as a marker for isolation procedures; and activation of the receptor results in easily measured electrical and ionic changes in the cells involved. The nicotinic receptor appears to be a pentamer of 4 types of glycoprotein subunits with a total molecular weight of about 250,000. It has one or 2 cholinergic receptor sites that, when activated by a nicotinic agonist, cause a conformational change in the protein that allows sodium and potassium ions to diffuse rapidly down their concentration gradients. Thus, the primary effect of nicotinic receptor activation is depolarization of the nerve cell or neuromuscular end-plate bearing the receptor.

If activation of the nicotinic receptor is prolonged, effector response is abolished; ie, the postganglionic neuron stops firing and the skeletal muscle cell relaxes. Furthermore, the continued presence of the nicotinic agonist prevents recovery of the postjunctional membrane. In this way, a state of "depolarizing blockade" is induced that is refractory to reversal by other agonists.

B. Organ System Effects: Most of the direct organ system effects of muscarinic cholinergic stimulants are readily predicted from a knowledge of the effects of parasympathetic nerve stimulation (Table 4–2) and the distribution of muscarinic receptors. Effects of a typical agent such as acetylcholine are listed in Table 5–2. The effects of nicotinic agonists are similarly predictable from a knowledge of the physiology of the autonomic ganglia and skeletal muscle motor end-plate.

1. Eye–Muscarinic agonists instilled into the conjunctival sac cause contraction of the smooth muscle of the iris sphincter (miosis) and of the ciliary muscle (accommodation). As a result, the iris is pulled away from the angle of the anterior chamber, and the trabecular meshwork at the base of the ciliary muscle is opened up. Both effects facilitate the outflow of aqueous humor into the canal of Schlemm, which drains the anterior chamber.

2. Cardiovascular system–The primary cardiovascular effects of muscarinic agonists are reduction in peripheral vascular resistance and changes in heart rate. The direct effects shown in Table 5–1 are modified by important homeostatic reflexes, as described in Chapter 4 and depicted in Fig 4–6. Intravenous infusions of minimal effective doses of acetylcholine in humans (eg, 20–50 μg/min) cause vasodilatation, resulting in a reduction in blood pressure, often accompanied by a reflex increase in heart rate. Larger doses of acetylcholine produce bradycardia and decreased conduction velocity through the atrioventricular node in addition to the hypotensive effect.

The direct cardiac actions of muscarinic stimulants include an important increase in membrane potassium permeability in atrial muscle cells and probably in the cells of the sinoatrial and atrioventricular nodes as well. In addition, cholinergic stimulants decrease the slow inward calcium current in atrial and nodal cells of at least some species. Both of these actions could contribute to the observed slowing of pacemaker rate and the hyperpolarization and decreased contractility of atrial cells. As noted above, the direct slowing of sinoatrial rate and atrioventricular conduction that is produced by muscarinic agonists is often opposed by reflex sympathetic discharge, elicited by the decrease in blood pressure. Therefore, the

Table 5–2. Effects of direct-acting cholinergic receptor stimulants. Only the direct effects are indicated; homeostatic responses to these direct actions may be important (see text).

Organ	Response
Eye	
Sphincter muscle of iris	Contraction (miosis).
Ciliary muscle	Contraction for near vision.
Heart	
Sinoatrial node	Decrease in rate (negative chronotropy).
Atria	Decrease in contractile strength (negative inotropy). Decrease in refractory period.
Atrioventricular node	Decrease in conduction velocity (negative dromotropy).
Ventricles	Small decrease in contractile strength.
Vessels	
Arteries	Dilatation.
Veins	Dilatation.
Lung	
Bronchial muscle	Contraction (bronchoconstriction).
Bronchial glands	Stimulation.
Gastrointestinal tract	
Motility	Increase.
Sphincters	Relaxation.
Secretion	Stimulation.
Urinary bladder	
Detrusor	Contraction.
Trigone and sphincter	Relaxation.
Glands	
Sweat, salivary, lacrimal, nasopharyngeal	Secretion.

net effect on heart rate depends on local concentrations of the agonist in the heart and in the vessels and on the level of reflex responsiveness. Effects on the ventricle are largely indirect and result from changes in vascular pressures and muscarinic modulation of adrenergic transmission in the ventricles.

The precise mechanism by which muscarinic stimulants bring about vascular smooth muscle relaxation is poorly understood. Preparations of isolated strips of vascular smooth muscle prepared in the traditional way are usually *contracted* by acetylcholine and its congeners even though the same vessels can be shown to dilate in intact animals. A possible explanation for this paradox has recently become available through the observation that isolated vascular strips relax like their counterparts in the intact animal if care is taken to avoid damaging or removing the intima of the vessel. This and other evidence suggest that the effect of muscarinic vasodilators may be to facilitate production of an endogenous vasodilator substance or to inhibit the production of a vasoconstrictor by the intima of the vessels.

The cardiovascular effects of all of the choline esters are similar to those of acetylcholine, the main difference being in their potency and duration of action. Because of the resistance of methacholine, carbachol, and bethanechol to acetylcholinesterase, substantially lower doses given intravenously are sufficient to produce effects similar to those of acetylcholine, and the duration of action of these synthetic choline esters is longer. The cardiovascular effects of most of the cholinomimetic natural alkaloids and synthetic analogs are also generally similar to those of acetylcholine. Pilocarpine is an exception. When given intravenously, it often produces hypertension after a brief initial hypotensive response. The longer-lasting hypertensive effect can be traced to ganglionic discharge caused by activation of slow excitatory postsynaptic potentials (Chapter 4). This effect, like the hypotensive effect, can be blocked by atropine, an antimuscarinic drug.

3. Respiratory system–The smooth muscle of the bronchial tree is contracted by muscarinic stimulants. In addition, the glands of the tracheobronchial mucosa are stimulated to secrete. This combination of effects can occasionally cause symptoms, especially in individuals with respiratory impairment.

4. Gastrointestinal tract–Administration of muscarinic agonists, like stimulation of the parasympathetic nervous system, causes an increase in secretory and motor activity of the gut. The salivary and gastric glands are strongly stimulated; the pancreas and small intestinal glands less so. Peristaltic activity is increased throughout the gut, and most sphincters are relaxed. Stimulation of contraction in this organ system has been shown to involve depolarization of the smooth muscle cell membrane and increased calcium influx.

5. Genitourinary tract–Muscarinic agonists stimulate the detrusor muscle and relax the trigone and sphincter muscles of the bladder, thus promoting voiding. The human uterus is not notably sensitive to muscarinic agonists.

6. Miscellaneous secretory glands–Muscarinic agonists stimulate the secretory activity of sweat, lacrimal, and nasopharyngeal glands.

7. Central nervous system–The central nervous system contains both muscarinic and nicotinic receptors, the brain being relatively richer in muscarinic sites and the spinal cord containing a preponderance of nicotinic sites. The physiologic role of these receptors is discussed in Chapter 18. In spite of the smaller ratio of nicotinic:muscarinic receptors in the brain, nicotine and lobeline (Fig 5–3) have important effects on the brain stem and cortex. The mild alerting action of nicotine absorbed from inhaled tobacco smoke is the best-known of these effects. In larger concentrations, nicotine induces tremor, emesis, and stimulation of the respiratory center. At still higher levels, nicotine causes convulsions, which may terminate in fatal coma. The lethal effects on the central nervous system and the fact that nicotine is readily absorbed form the basis for the use of nicotine as an insecticide. Dimethylphenylpiperazinium (DMPP), a synthetic nicotinic stimulant (Fig 5–3), is relatively free of these central effects because it does not cross the blood-brain barrier.

8. Peripheral nervous system–The autonomic ganglia are important sites of nicotinic synaptic action. All of the nicotinic agents shown in Fig 5–3 are capable of causing marked activation of the nicotinic receptors, resulting in firing of action potentials in the postganglionic neurons. The action is the same on both parasympathetic and sympathetic ganglia. The initial response therefore often resembles simultaneous discharge of both parasympathetic and sympathetic nervous systems. In the case of the cardiovascular system, the effects of nicotine are chiefly sympathomimetic. Dramatic hypertension is produced by parenteral injection of nicotine; sympathetic tachycardia may alternate with a vagally mediated bradycardia. In the gastrointestinal and urinary tracts, the effects are largely parasympathomimetic: nausea, vomiting, diarrhea, and voiding of urine are commonly observed.

A second class of nicotinic sites consists of receptors on sensory nerve endings—especially certain chemosensitive nerve endings in the coronary arteries and the carotid and aortic bodies. Activation of these nerve endings elicits complex medullary responses, including respiratory stimulation and vagal discharge.

9. Neuromuscular junction–The nicotinic receptors on the neuromuscular end-plate apparatus are similar but not identical to the receptors in the autonomic ganglia. Therefore, both types respond to acetylcholine and nicotine. (However, as discussed in Chapter 6, they differ in their structural requirements for nicotinic blocking drugs.) When applied directly (by iontophoresis or by intra-arterial injection), an immediate depolarization of the end-plate results, caused by an increase in permeability to sodium ions. Depending on the synchronization of depolarization of end-plates throughout the muscle, the contractile response will vary from disorganized fasciculations of independent motor units to a strong contraction of the entire muscle. Depolarizing nicotinic agents that are not rapidly hydrolyzed (like nicotine itself) cause rapid development of depolarization blockade, discussed further in Chapter 6. In the case of skeletal muscle, this block is manifested as flaccid paralysis.

BASIC PHARMACOLOGY OF THE INDIRECT-ACTING CHOLINERGIC STIMULANTS

The actions of acetylcholine released from autonomic and somatic motor nerves are terminated by enzymatic destruction of the molecule. Hydrolysis is accomplished by the action of acetylcholinesterase, a protein with a molecular weight of about 320,000, which is present in high concentrations in cholinergic synapses. The indirect-acting cholinergic agonists have their primary effect at the active site of this enzyme, although some also have direct actions at nicotinic cholinergic receptors. By far the most important use of these chemicals is as insecticides; a few have therapeutic applications. The chief differences between members of the group are chemical and pharmacokinetic—their pharmacodynamic properties are almost identical.

Chemistry & Pharmacokinetics

A. Structure: The commonly used cholinesterase inhibitors fall into 3 chemical groups: (1) simple alcohols bearing a quaternary ammonium group, eg, edrophonium; (2) carbamic acid esters of alcohols bearing quaternary or tertiary ammonium groups (carbamates, eg, neostigmine); and (3) organic derivatives of phosphoric acid (organophosphates, eg, isoflurophate). Examples of the first 2 groups are shown in Fig 5–4. Edrophonium, neostigmine, and ambenonium are synthetic quaternary ammonium agents used in medicine. Physostigmine is a naturally occur-

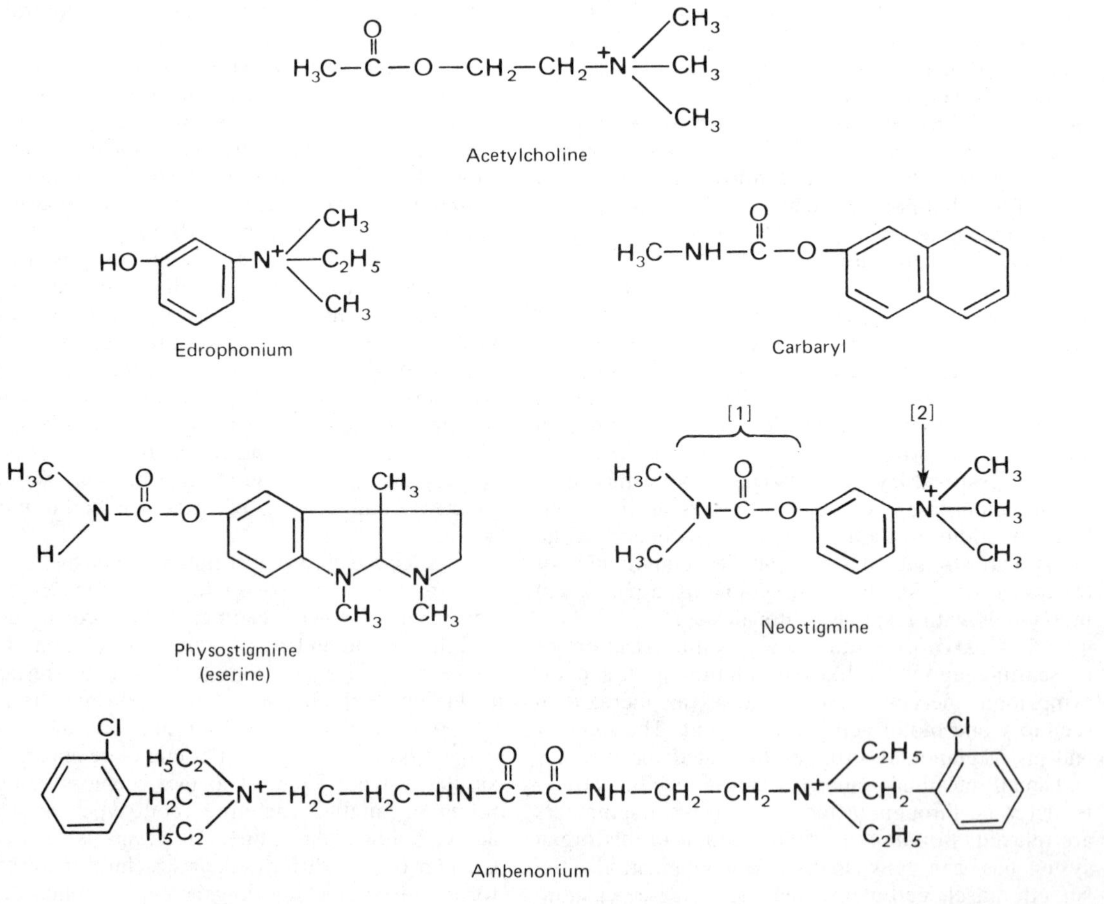

Figure 5–4. Cholinesterase inhibitors. Neostigmine exemplifies the typical compound that is an ester of carbamic acid ([1]) and a phenol bearing a quaternary ammonium group ([2]). Physostigmine, a naturally occurring carbamate, is a tertiary amine. Acetylcholine is shown in the same orientation (acid left, alcohol right) for reference. Edrophonium and ambenonium are not esters but bind to the active site of the enzyme.

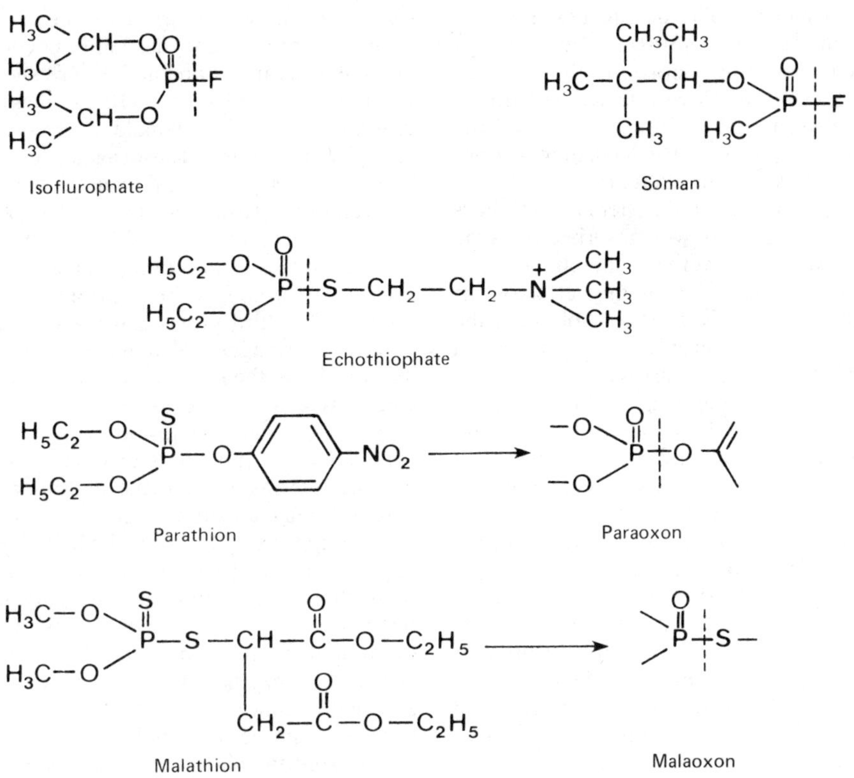

Figure 5–5. Structures of some organophosphate cholinesterase inhibitors. The dashed lines indicate the bond that is hydrolyzed in binding to the enzyme.

ring tertiary amine of greater lipid solubility that is also used in therapeutics. Carbaryl (carbaril) is typical of a large group of carbamate insecticides designed for very high lipid solubility, so that absorption into the insect and distribution to the central nervous system is very rapid.

A few of the estimated 50,000 organophosphates are shown in Fig 5–5. Many of the organophosphates (echothiophate is an exception) are highly lipid-soluble liquids. Isoflurophate (diisopropylfluorophosphate, DFP) was one of the first organophosphates synthesized and is one of the best-studied. It is still available for clinical use but has been superseded by better agents. Soman is an extremely potent "nerve gas." Echothiophate, a thiocholine derivative, is of clinical interest because it retains the very long duration of action of other organophosphates but is more stable in aqueous solution. Parathion and malathion are thiophosphate insecticides that are inactive as such; they are converted to the phosphate derivatives in animals and plants. They are somewhat more stable than compounds like isoflurophate and soman, making them more suitable for use as insecticides.

B. Absorption, Metabolism, and Distribution: Absorption of the quaternary carbamates from the conjunctiva, skin, and lungs is predictably poor, since their permanent charge renders them relatively insoluble in lipids. Similarly, much larger doses are required for oral administration than for parenteral injection. Distribution into the central nervous system is negligible. Physostigmine, in contrast, is well absorbed from all sites and can be used topically in the eye (Table 5–3). It is distributed into the central nervous system and is more toxic. However, even nonpolar carbamates used as insecticides are poorly absorbed across the skin—the ratio of dermal:oral lethal doses for this group is much higher than the ratios for the or-

Table 5–3. Uses and duration of action of cholinesterase inhibitors used in therapeutics.

	Uses	Approximate Duration of Action
Alcohols		
Edrophonium	Myasthenia gravis, ileus, arrhythmias	5–15 minutes
Carbamates and related agents		
Neostigmine	Myasthenia gravis, ileus	½–2 hours
Pyridostigmine	Myasthenia gravis	3–6 hours
Physostigmine	Glaucoma	½–2 hours
Ambenonium	Myasthenia gravis	4–8 hours
Demecarium	Glaucoma	4–6 hours
Organophosphates		
Isoflurophate	Glaucoma	100 hours
Echothiophate	Glaucoma	100 hours

ganophosphate pesticides. The carbamates are relatively stable in aqueous solution but can be metabolized by nonspecific esterases in the body, as well as by cholinesterase. However, the half-life of their effect is determined by the stability of the inhibitor-enzyme complex (see Mechanism of Action, below), not by metabolism or excretion.

The organophosphate cholinesterase inhibitors (except for echothiophate) are well absorbed from the skin, lung, gut, and conjunctiva—thereby making them dangerous to humans and highly effective as insecticides. They are relatively less stable than the carbamates when dissolved in water and thus have a limited half-life in the environment (as compared to the other major class of insecticides, the halogenated hydrocarbons, eg, DDT). Echothiophate is highly polar and more stable than most other organophosphates. It can be made up in aqueous solution for ophthalmic use and retains its activity for weeks.

The thiophosphate insecticides (parathion, malathion, and related compounds) are very lipid-soluble and are rapidly absorbed by all routes. They must be activated in the body by conversion to the oxygen analogs (Fig 5–5), a process that occurs rapidly in both insects and vertebrates. Malathion and certain other organophosphate insecticides are also rapidly metabolized by other pathways to inactive products in birds and mammals, but not in insects; these agents are therefore considered safe enough for sale to the general public. Unfortunately, fish are not able to detoxify malathion, and significant die-offs have occurred from the heavy use of this agent on and near waterways. Parathion is not detoxified effectively in vertebrates; therefore, it is considerably more dangerous to humans and livestock and is not available for general public use.

All of the organophosphates except echothiophate are fully distributed to all parts of the body, including the central nervous system. Poisoning with these agents therefore includes an important component of central nervous system toxicity.

Pharmacodynamics

A. Mechanism of Action: Acetylcholinesterase is an extremely active enzyme. In the initial step, acetylcholine binds to the enzyme active site and is hydrolyzed, yielding free choline and the acetylated enzyme. In the second step, the covalent acetyl-enzyme bond is split, with the addition of water. The entire process takes place in approximately 150 microseconds.

All of the cholinesterase inhibitors exert their pharmacologic effects by inhibiting acetylcholinesterase and thereby increasing the concentration of endogenous acetylcholine in the vicinity of cholinergic receptors. However, the molecular details of their interaction with the enzyme vary, resulting in 3 distinct groups.

The first group, of which edrophonium is the major example, consists of quaternary alcohols. These agents bind reversibly (by means of electrostatic forces) to the active site, thus preventing access by acetylcholine. The enzyme-inhibitor complex does not involve a covalent bond and is correspondingly short-lived (on the order of 2–10 minutes). The second group consists of carbamate esters, eg, neostigmine and physostigmine. These agents undergo a 2-step hydrolysis sequence analogous to that described for acetylcholine. However, the covalent bond of the carbamylated enzyme is considerably more resistant to the second (hydration) process, and this step is correspondingly prolonged (on the order of 30 minutes to 6 hours). The third group consists of the organophosphates. These agents also undergo initial binding and hydrolysis by the enzyme, resulting in a phosphorylated active site. The covalent phosphorus-enzyme bond is extremely stable and hydrolyzes in water at a very slow rate (hundreds of hours). After the initial binding-hydrolysis step, the phosphorylated enzyme complex may undergo a process called **aging.** This process apparently involves the breaking of one of the oxygen-phosphorus bonds of the inhibitor and results in further strengthening of the phosphorus-enzyme bond. The rate of aging varies with the particular organophosphate compound. Once aging has occurred, the enzyme-inhibitor complex cannot be split, even with oxime compounds. If given before aging has occurred, strong nucleophiles like pralidoxime are able to split the phosphorus-enzyme bond and can be used as "cholinesterase regenerator" drugs for organophosphate insecticide poisoning (Chapter 6).

Because of the marked differences in duration of action, the organophosphate inhibitors are sometimes referred to as "irreversible" cholinesterase inhibitors, relegating edrophonium and the carbamates to the category of "reversible" inhibitors. In fact, the molecular mechanisms of action of the 3 groups do not support this simplistic description, but the terms are frequently used.

B. Organ System Effects: The most prominent pharmacologic effects of cholinesterase inhibitors are on the cardiovascular and gastrointestinal systems, the eye, and the skeletal muscle neuromuscular junction. Because the primary action is to potentiate the action of endogenous acetylcholine, the effects are similar (but not always identical) to the effects of the direct-acting cholinergic agonists.

1. Central nervous system–In low concentrations, the lipid-soluble cholinesterase inhibitors cause diffuse activation of the EEG and a subjective alerting response. In higher concentrations, they cause generalized convulsions, which may be followed by coma and respiratory arrest.

2. Eye, respiratory tract, gastrointestinal tract, urinary tract–The effects of the cholinesterase inhibitors on these organ systems, all of which are well innervated by the parasympathetic nervous system, are qualitatively quite similar to the effects of the direct-acting cholinergic agonists.

3. Cardiovascular system–The cholinesterase inhibitors can increase activation in both sympathetic and parasympathetic ganglia supplying the heart and at the cholinergic receptors on those presynaptic nerve endings and neuroeffector cells (cardiac and vascular smooth muscles) that receive cholinergic innervation.

In the heart, the effects on the parasympathetic limb predominate. Thus, administration of cholinesterase inhibitors such as edrophonium, physostigmine, or neostigmine leads to effects on the heart that mimic the effects of vagal nerve activation. Heart rate decreases, conduction velocity through the atrioventricular junction diminishes, atrial contractility decreases, and cardiac output falls. The fall in cardiac output is contributed to by the bradycardia, decreased atrial contractility, and some reduction in ventricular contractility. The latter effect probably occurs as a result of presynaptic muscarinic modulation of sympathetic activity. When administered to patients who have undergone cardiac transplantation (which causes degeneration of the nerve endings in the transplanted heart), the same drugs have no effect. These results indicate that the effects of these drugs are dependent on endogenous acetylcholine released from vagal nerve endings.

The effects of cholinesterase inhibitors on vascular smooth muscle and on blood pressure are less marked than the effects of direct-acting muscarinic agonists. This is because indirect-acting drugs can modify the tone of only those vessels that are innervated by cholinergic nerves and because the net effects on vascular tone may represent activation of both the parasympathetic and sympathetic nervous systems. Since few vascular beds receive cholinergic innervation (Chapter 4), the cholinergic effect is minimal. Furthermore, although activation of cholinergic nerves (at ganglia and neuroeffector junctions) would tend to lower vascular resistance and blood pressure, activation of sympathetic ganglia would tend to oppose these hypotensive effects.

The *net* cardiovascular effects of moderate doses of cholinesterase inhibitors therefore consist of modest bradycardia, a fall in cardiac output, and no change or a modest fall in blood pressure. Large (toxic) doses of these drugs cause more marked bradycardia and hypotension.

4. Neuromuscular junction–The cholinesterase inhibitors have important therapeutic and toxic effects at the skeletal muscle neuromuscular junction. Low (therapeutic) concentrations moderately prolong and intensify the actions of physiologically released acetylcholine. This results in increased strength of contraction, especially in muscles weakened by curarelike neuromuscular blocking agents or by myasthenia gravis. At higher concentrations, the accumulation of acetylcholine may result in fibrillation of muscle fibers. Antidromic firing of the motor neuron may also occur, resulting in fasciculations that involve an entire motor unit. With marked inhibition of acetylcholinesterase, membrane depolarization becomes sustained and neuromuscular blockade may ensue.

Some quaternary carbamate cholinesterase inhibitors, eg, neostigmine, have an additional *direct* nicotinic agonist effect at the neuromuscular junction. This may contribute to the effectiveness of these agents in the therapy of myasthenia.

CLINICAL PHARMACOLOGY OF THE CHOLINERGIC STIMULANTS

The major therapeutic uses of the cholinergic stimulants are for diseases of the eye (glaucoma, accommodative esotropia), the gastrointestinal and urinary tracts (postoperative atony, neurogenic bladder), the neuromuscular junction (myasthenia gravis, curare-induced neuromuscular paralysis), and the heart (certain atrial arrhythmias). Cholinesterase inhibitors are also used in the treatment of atropine overdosage.

Clinical Uses

A. The Eye: Glaucoma is a disease characterized by increased intraocular pressure. There are 2 types of acquired glaucoma: primary, which can be subdivided into narrow-angle and open-angle types; and secondary, eg, caused by surgical procedures. Muscarinic stimulants and cholinesterase inhibitors can reduce intraocular pressure by facilitating outflow of aqueous humor and possibly also by diminishing the rate of its secretion. Of the direct agonists, methacholine (20%), carbachol (up to 3%), and pilocarpine (up to 4%) have been used for treatment of glaucoma. Among the cholinesterase inhibitors, physostigmine, demecarium, echothiophate, and isoflurophate have been extensively studied (Table 5–3).

Acute narrow-angle glaucoma is a medical emergency that is usually treated initially with drugs but frequently requires surgery for permanent correction. Initial therapy often consists of a combination of a direct muscarinic agonist and a cholinesterase inhibitor (eg, pilocarpine plus physostigmine). Once the intraocular pressure is controlled and the danger of loss of vision is diminished, the patient can be prepared for corrective surgery (iridectomy). Open-angle glaucoma and some cases of secondary glaucoma are chronic diseases that are not amenable to surgical correction. Consequently, therapy is based on long-term pharmacologic management that relies heavily on the use of cholinergic stimulating drugs as well as epinephrine, the beta-adrenergic blocking drugs, and acetazolamide. Of the cholinergic stimulants, the ones in current favor include pilocarpine (as drops, or a long-acting plastic film reservoir of drug [Ocusert] placed in the conjunctival sac) and physostigmine (drops). Longer-acting agents (demecarium, echothiophate) are reserved for cases in which control of the intraocular pressure cannot be achieved with other cholinergic or noncholinergic agents.

Accommodative esotropia (strabismus caused by hypermetropic accommodative error) in young children is sometimes diagnosed and treated with cholinergic agonists. Dosage is similar to or higher than that used for glaucoma.

B. Gastrointestinal and Urinary Tracts: In clinical disorders that involve depression of smooth muscle activity *without obstruction,* cholinergic agonists with direct or indirect muscarinic effects may be helpful. These disorders include postoperative ileus (atony or paralysis of the stomach or bowel following surgical manipulation) and congenital megacolon. Urinary retention may occur postoperatively or postpartum or may be secondary to spinal cord injury or disease (neurogenic bladder). Cholinergic agonists are also sometimes used to increase the tone of the lower esophageal sphincter in patients with reflux esophagitis. Of the choline esters, bethanechol is the most widely used for treatment of these disorders. For gastrointestinal problems, it is usually administered orally in a dose of 10–25 mg 3–4 times daily. In patients with urinary retention, bethanechol can be given subcutaneously in a dose of 5 mg and repeated in 30 minutes if necessary. Of the cholinesterase inhibitors, neostigmine is the most widely used for these applications. For paralytic ileus or atony of the urinary bladder, neostigmine can be given subcutaneously in a dose of 0.5–1 mg. If patients are able to take the drug by mouth, neostigmine can be given orally in a dose of 15 mg. In all of these clinical situations, the clinician must be absolutely certain that there is no mechanical obstruction to outflow prior to using the cholinergic agonist. Otherwise, the drug may exacerbate the problem and may even cause perforation as a result of increased pressure.

C. Neuromuscular Junction: Myasthenia gravis is a disease of the skeletal muscle neuromuscular junctions. An autoimmune process causes production of antibodies that decrease the number of functional nicotinic cholinergic receptors on the postjunctional end-plate. The characteristic symptoms of weakness and fatigability that remit with rest and worsen with exercise may affect any skeletal muscle but most often involve the small muscles of the hand, neck, and extremities. Frequent findings are ptosis, diplopia, difficulty in speaking and swallowing, and extremity weakness. Severe disease may affect all the muscles, including those necessary for respiration. The disease resembles the neuromuscular paralysis produced by d-tubocurarine and similar nondepolarizing neuromuscular blocking drugs (Chapter 24). Patients with myasthenia are exquisitely sensitive to the action of curariform drugs and other drugs that interfere with neuromuscular transmission, eg, aminoglycoside antibiotics.

Cholinesterase inhibitors—but not direct-acting cholinergic agonists—are extremely valuable in the therapy of myasthenia. (Some patients also respond to immunosuppressant therapy such as adrenocorticosteroids and cyclophosphamide).

Edrophonium is frequently used as a diagnostic test for myasthenia. Two milligrams are injected intravenously after obtaining baseline measurements of muscle strength. If no reaction occurs after 45 seconds, an additional 8 mg may be injected. Some clinicians divide the 8-mg dose into 2 doses of 3 and 5 mg given at 45-second intervals. If the patient has myasthenia gravis, an improvement in muscle strength that lasts about 5 minutes will usually be observed.

Edrophonium is also used to assess the adequacy of treatment with the longer-acting cholinesterase inhibitors in patients with documented myasthenia gravis. If excessive amounts of drug have been used, patients may become paradoxically weak because of nicotinic depolarizing blockade of the motor end-plate. These patients may also exhibit symptoms of excessive stimulation of muscarinic receptors (abdominal cramps, diarrhea, increased salivation, excessive bronchial secretions, miosis, bradycardia). Small doses of edrophonium (1–2 mg intravenously) will produce no relief or even worsen weakness if the patient is receiving excessive cholinesterase inhibitor therapy. On the other hand, if the patient improves with edrophonium, an increase in cholinesterase inhibitor dosage may be indicated. Clinical situations in which severe myasthenia (myasthenic crisis) must be distinguished from excessive drug therapy (cholinergic crisis) usually occur in very ill myasthenic patients and must be managed in hospital with adequate emergency and support systems (eg, mechanical ventilators) available.

Chronic long-term therapy of myasthenia gravis is usually accomplished with neostigmine, pyridostigmine, or ambenonium. The doses are titrated to optimum levels based on changes in muscle strength. These agents are relatively short-acting and therefore require frequent dosing (every 2–4 hours for neostigmine and every 3–6 hours for pyridostigmine and ambenonium; Table 5–3). Sustained-release preparations are available but should be used only at night and if needed. Longer-acting cholinesterase inhibitors such as the organophosphate agents are not used, because the dose requirement in this disease changes too rapidly to permit smooth control with long-acting drugs.

If muscarinic side-effects are prominent, they can be controlled by the administration of antimuscarinic drugs such as atropine. Frequently, tolerance to the muscarinic effects of the cholinesterase inhibitors develops, so atropine treatment is not required.

Neuromuscular blockade is frequently produced as an adjunct to surgical anesthesia, using nondepolarizing neuromuscular relaxants such as curare, pancuronium, and newer agents (Chapter 24). Following the surgical procedure, it is usually desirable to reverse this pharmacologic paralysis promptly. This can be easily accomplished with cholinesterase inhibitors; neostigmine and edrophonium are the drugs of choice. They are given intravenously or intramuscularly for prompt effect.

D. Heart: The short-acting cholinesterase inhibitor edrophonium has been used for treatment of supraventricular tachyarrhythmias, particularly paroxysmal supraventricular tachycardia. By potentiating the effects of endogenous acetylcholine released at the atrioventricular junction, atrioventricular conduction velocity is diminished, the number of supraventricular impulses conducted into the ventricles may be reduced, and an excessive ventricular rate may be slowed. Edrophonium may also convert the abnormal supraventricular tachyarrhythmia into normal sinus rhythm. Edrophonium usually is given intravenously in a dose of 5–10 mg (0.15 mg/kg) administered over 30 seconds. Carotid sinus massage should be performed after giving the drug if the ventricular rate has not slowed.

E. Antimuscarinic Drug Intoxication: Atropine intoxication is potentially lethal in children (Chapter 6) and may cause prolonged severe behavioral disturbances in adults. The tricyclic depressants, when taken in overdosage (often with suicidal intent), also cause severe muscarinic blockade (Chapter 27). Because the muscarinic receptor blockade produced by all of these agents is competitive in nature, it can be overcome by increasing the amount of endogenous acetylcholine present at the cholinergic neuroeffector junctions. Physostigmine is frequently the most appropriate drug for this application, because it enters the central nervous system and reverses the central as well as the peripheral signs of muscarinic blockade. Physostigmine salicylate is given in intravenous boluses of 0.5–2 mg repeated at 5- to 10-minute intervals until an effect is noted.

Toxicity

The toxic potential of the cholinergic stimulants varies markedly depending on the absorption of the drug, its access to the central nervous system, and its metabolism.

A. Direct-Acting Muscarinic Stimulants: Drugs such as pilocarpine and the choline esters cause predictable signs of muscarinic excess when given in overdosage. These effects include nausea, vomiting, diarrhea, salivation, sweating, cutaneous vasodilatation, and bronchial constriction. The effects are all blocked competitively by atropine and its congeners.

Certain mushrooms, especially those of the genus *Inocybe,* contain muscarinic alkaloids. Ingestion of these mushrooms causes typical signs of muscarinic excess within 15–30 minutes. Treatment is with atropine, 1–2 mg parenterally. (*Amanita muscaria,* the first source of muscarine, contains very low concentrations of the alkaloid.)

B. Direct-Acting Nicotinic Stimulants: Nicotine itself is the only common cause of this type of poisoning. The acute toxicity of the alkaloid is well defined but much less important than the chronic effects associated with smoking. In addition to its occurrence in tobacco, nicotine is also used in a number of insecticides.

1. Acute toxicity–The fatal dose of nicotine is approximately 40 mg, or 1 drop of the pure liquid. This is the amount of nicotine in 2 regular cigarettes. Fortunately, most of the nicotine in cigarettes is destroyed by burning or escapes via the "side-stream" smoke. Ingestion of nicotine insecticides and of tobacco by infants and children is usually followed promptly by vomiting, limiting the amount of the alkaloid absorbed.

The toxic effects of a large dose of nicotine are simple extensions of the effects described previously. The most dangerous are (1) central stimulant actions, which cause convulsions and may progress to coma and respiratory arrest; (2) skeletal muscle end-plate depolarization, which may lead to depolarization-blockade and respiratory paralysis; and (3) hypertension and cardiac arrhythmias.

Treatment of nicotine poisoning is largely symptom-directed. Muscarinic excess resulting from parasympathetic ganglion stimulation can be controlled with atropine. Central stimulation is usually treated with parenteral anticonvulsants such as diazepam. Neuromuscular blockade is not responsive to pharmacologic treatment and may require mechanical respiration.

Fortunately, nicotine is metabolized and excreted relatively rapidly. Patients who survive the first 4 hours usually recover completely if hypoxia and brain damage have not occurred.

2. Chronic nicotine toxicity–The health costs of tobacco smoking to the smoker and its socioeconomic costs to the general public are still incompletely understood. It is clear that among the preventable diseases, the financial costs of tobacco-associated diseases are exceeded only by those associated with alcohol abuse. Unfortunately, the fact that the most important of these diseases are delayed in onset reduces the health incentive to stop smoking. Furthermore, the fact that society—through private or national health insurance programs—subsidizes the extraordinary cost of tobacco-associated diseases reduces the personal financial incentive to control smoking in addicted users.

It is not known to what extent nicotine contributes to the well-documented adverse effects of chronic tobacco use. It appears highly probable that nicotine contributes to the elevated risk of vascular disease and sudden coronary death associated with smoking. It is also probable that nicotine contributes to the high incidence of ulcer recurrences in smokers with peptic disease.

C. Cholinesterase Inhibitors: The acute toxic effects of the cholinesterase inhibitors, like those of the direct-acting agents, are direct extensions of their pharmacologic actions. The major source of such intoxications is pesticide use in agriculture and in the home. Approximately 100 organophosphate and 20 carbamate cholinesterase inhibitors are available in pesticides and veterinary vermifuges used in the USA.

Acute intoxication must be recognized and treated promptly in patients with heavy exposure. The dominant initial signs are those of muscarinic excess: miosis, salivation, sweating, bronchial constriction, vomiting, and diarrhea. Central nervous system involvement usually follows rapidly, accompanied by peripheral nicotinic effects, especially depolarizing nicotinic blockade. Therapy always includes (1) maintenance of vital signs—respiration in particular may be impaired; (2) decontamination to prevent further absorption—this may require removal of all clothing and washing of the skin in cases of exposure to dusts and sprays; and (3) atropine parenterally in large doses, given as often as required to control signs of muscarinic excess (Chapter 6). Therapy often also includes treatment with pralidoxime as described in Chapter 6.

Chronic exposure to certain organophosphate compounds, including some organophosphate cholinesterase inhibitors, causes neuropathy associated with demyelination of axons. Triorthocresylphosphate, an additive in lubricating oils, is the prototype agent of this class. The effects are not caused by cholinesterase inhibition.

• • •

References

Burnstock G: Neurotransmitters and trophic factors in the autonomic nervous system. *J Physiol (London)* 1981;**313:**1.

Drachman DH: Myasthenia gravis. (2 parts.) *N Engl J Med* 1978;**298:**136, 186.

DuBois KP: Toxicological evaluation of the anticholinesterase agents. Pages 833–859 in: *Cholinesterase and Anticholinesterase Agents*. Koelle GB (editor). *Handbuch der Experimentellen Pharmakologie*. Vol 15. Springer-Verlag, 1963.

Finkbeiner AE, Bissada NK, Welch LT: Uropharmacology: Choline esters and other parasympathomimetic drugs. *Urology* 1977;**10:**83.

Furchgott RF: The requirement for endothelial cells in the relaxation of arteries by acetylcholine and some other vasodilators. *Trends Pharmacol Sci* 1981;**2:**173.

Granacher RP, Baldessarini RJ: Physostigmine: Its use in acute anticholinergic syndrome with antidepressant and antiparkinson drugs. *Arch Gen Psychiatr* 1975;**32:**375.

Havener WH: Pages 318–335 in: *Ocular Pharmacology*, 4th ed. Mosby, 1978.

Hobbiger F: Pharmacology of anticholinesterase drugs. Pages 487–581 in: *Neuromuscular Junction*. Vol 42. Zaimis E (editor). *Handbuch der Experimentellen Pharmakologie*. Springer-Verlag, 1976.

Karczmer AG: Pharmacology, toxicology, and therapeutic properties of anticholinesterase agents. Pages 163–322 in: *Physiological Pharmacology*. Vol 3. Root WS, Hoffman FG (editors). Academic Press, 1967.

Kosterlitz HW: Effects of choline esters on smooth muscle and secretions. Pages 97–161 in: *Physiological Pharmacology*. Vol 3. Root WS, Hoffman FG (editors). Academic Press, 1967.

Levy MN, Martin PJ: Neural control of the heart. Pages 581–620 in: *Handbook of Physiology: The Cardiovascular System I*. American Physiological Society, 1979.

Molitor H: A comparative study of the effects of five choline compounds used in therapeutics: Acetylcholine chloride, acetyl-beta-methylcholine chloride, carbaminoyl choline, ethyl ether beta-methylcholine chloride, carbaminoyl beta-methylcholine chloride. *J Pharmacol Exper Ther* 1936;**58:**337.

Raftery MA et al: Acetylcholine receptor: Complex of homologous subunits. *Science* 1980;**208:**1454.

Richelson E, El-Fakahamy E: The molecular basis of neurotransmission at the muscarinic receptor. *Biochem Pharmacol* 1981;**30:**2887.

Wieland T: Poisonous principles of mushrooms of the genus *Amanita*. *Science* 1968;**159:**946.

Cholinergic Receptor Antagonists | 6

Bertram G. Katzung, MD, PhD

Just as cholinergic agonists are divided into muscarinic and nicotinic subgroups on the basis of their specific receptor affinities, so the antagonists acting on these receptors fall into 2 major families: the **antimuscarinic** and **antinicotinic** agents. Muscarinic receptors are apparently very similar throughout the body; only limited selectivity for different muscarinic receptors has been achieved through modification of chemical structure. Nicotinic receptors, on the other hand, are readily divided on the basis of differential blockade into 2 subgroups: ganglion-blocking and neuromuscular blocking agents.

This chapter presents the general pharmacology of the muscarinic receptor-blocking drugs and some aspects of the ganglion-blocking nicotinic antagonists. The neuromuscular nicotinic antagonists are discussed in Chapter 24.

I. BASIC PHARMACOLOGY OF THE MUSCARINIC RECEPTOR–BLOCKING DRUGS

Because the effects of parasympathetic autonomic discharge can be blocked by muscarinic antagonists, they are often called parasympatholytic drugs. However, they do not "lyse" parasympathetic nerves, and they have some effects that are not predictable from block of the parasympathetic nervous system. For these reasons, the term "antimuscarinic" is preferable.

Naturally occurring compounds with antimuscarinic effects have been known and used for millenia as medicines, poisons, and cosmetics. The prototype of these drugs is **atropine.** Many similar plant alkaloids are known, and hundreds of synthetic antimuscarinic compounds have been prepared.

Chemistry & Pharmacokinetics

A. Source and Chemistry: Atropine and its naturally occurring congeners are tertiary ammonium alkaloid esters of tropic acid (Fig 6–1).

Atropine (hyoscyamine) is found in the plant *Atropa belladonna,* or deadly nightshade, and in *Datura stramonium,* also known as Jimson (Jamestown) weed or thorn apple. **Scopolamine** (hyoscine) occurs in *Hyoscyamus niger,* or henbane. Scopolamine is the *l*(–) stereoisomer and is obtained as such from the plant. Naturally occurring atropine is *l*(–)-hyoscyamine, but the compound readily racemizes, so the commercial material is racemic *d,l*-hyoscyamine. The *l*(–) isomers of both alkaloids are at least 100 times more potent than the *d*(+) isomers.

Semisynthetic tertiary ammonium analogs are produced by esterifying a natural base, eg, tropine, the base in atropine, with different acids. Thus, homatropine is the mandelic acid ester of tropine. A variety of fully synthetic molecules have antimuscarinic effects; the tertiary members of these classes (Fig 6–2) are often used for their effects in the eye or the central nervous system. Many antihistaminic (Chapter 14), antipsychotic (Chapter 26), and antidepressant (Chapter 27) drugs have similar structures and, predictably, significant antimuscarinic effects.

Quaternary ammonium antimuscarinic agents have been developed to reduce central nervous system effects. These drugs include both semisynthetic and synthetic molecules (Fig 6–2).

B. Absorption: The natural alkaloids and most tertiary antimuscarinic drugs are well absorbed from the gut and across the conjunctival membrane. When applied in a suitable vehicle, some, eg, scopolamine, are even absorbed across the skin (transdermal route). In contrast, only 10–30% of a dose of a quaternary antimuscarinic drug is absorbed after oral administra-

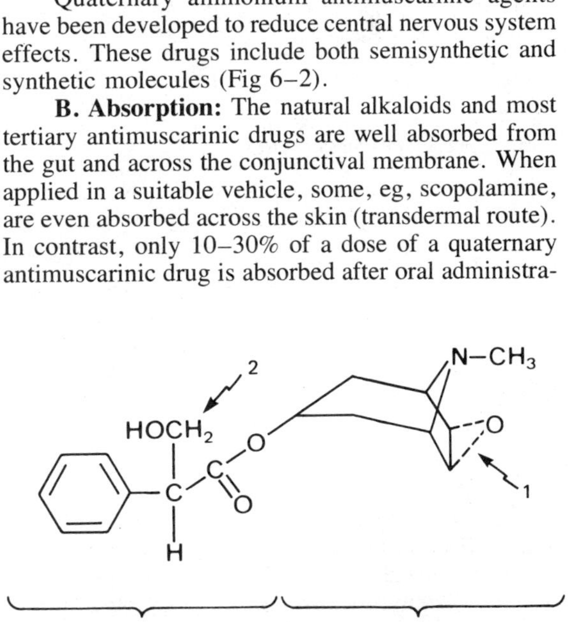

Figure 6–1. The structure of atropine (oxygen at 1 is missing) or scopolamine (oxygen present). In homatropine, the hydroxymethyl at 2 is replaced by a hydroxyl group.

Quaternary amines for gastrointestinal applications (peptic disease, hypermotility):

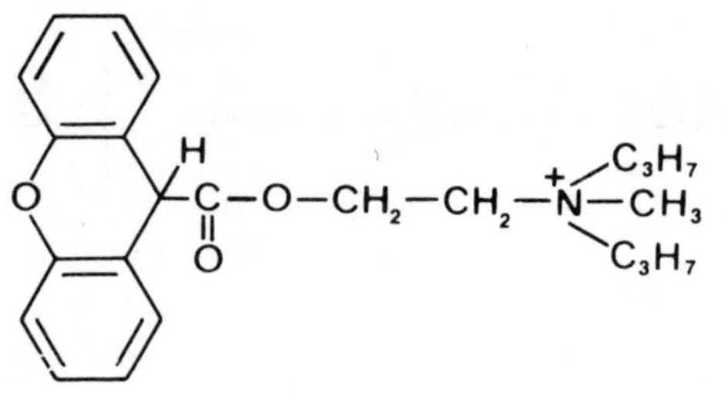

Propantheline

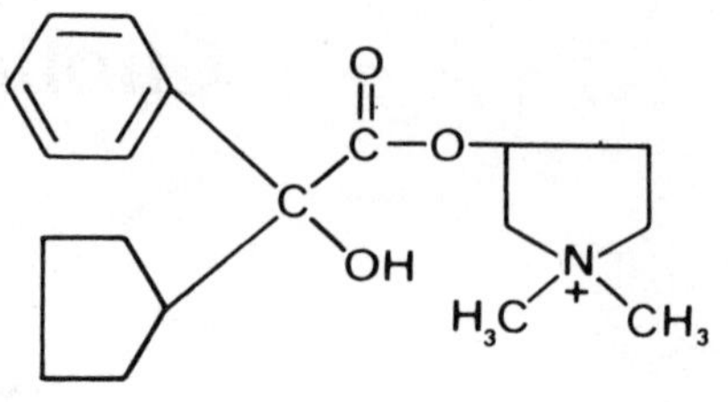

Glycopyrrolate

Quaternary amine for use in asthma:

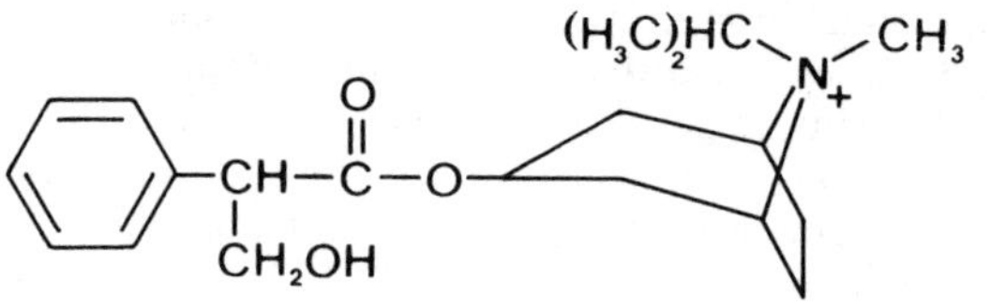

Ipratropium

Tertiary amines for peripheral applications:

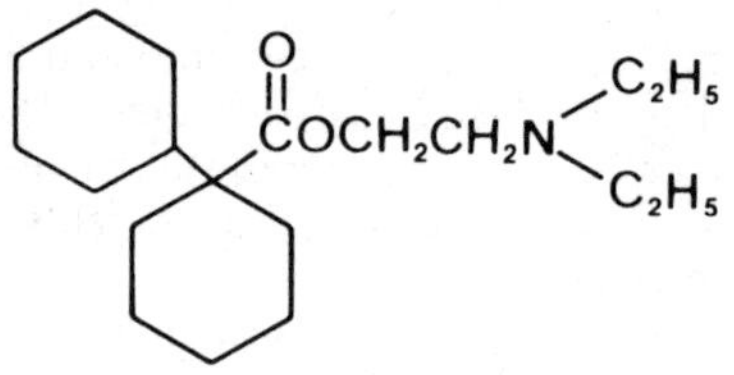

Dicyclomine
(peptic disease, hypermotility)

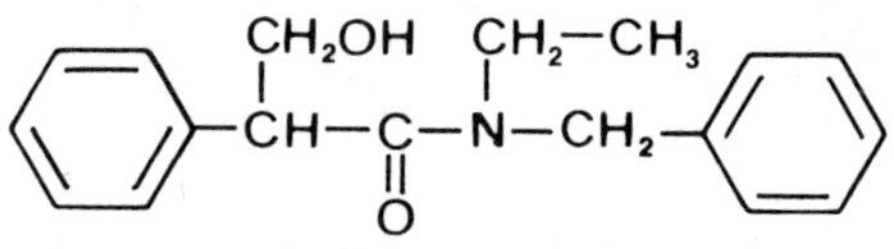

Tropicamide
(mydriatric, cycloplegic)

Tertiary amine for Parkinson's disease:

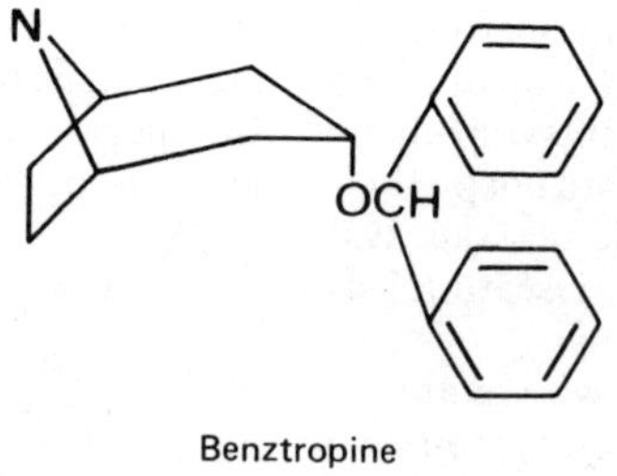

Benztropine

Figure 6–2. Structures of some semisynthetic and synthetic antimuscarinic drugs.

tion, reflecting the decreased lipid solubility of the charged molecule.

C. Distribution: Atropine and the other tertiary agents are widely distributed after absorption. Significant levels are achieved in the central nervous system within 30 minutes to 1 hour and may limit the dose tolerated when the drug is taken for its peripheral effects. The quaternary derivatives are very poorly taken up by the brain and therefore are relatively free of these central nervous system side-effects.

D. Metabolism and Excretion: Atropine disappears rapidly from the blood after administration. About 80% of the dose is excreted in the urine, with a half-life of 2 hours. Most of the rest appears in the urine with a half-life of 13–38 hours. About a third of the dose is excreted unchanged, with some free tropine base and some glucuronide metabolites accounting for a portion of the remainder. The effect of the drug on parasympathetic function declines rapidly in all organs except the eye. Effects on the iris and ciliary muscle persist for 48–72 hours.

Certain species, notably rabbits, have a specific enzyme—atropine esterase—that confers almost complete protection against the toxic effects of atropine.

Pharmacodynamics

A. Mechanism of Action: Atropine causes reversible blockade of the actions of acetylcholine at muscarinic receptors—ie, blockade by a small dose of atropine can be overcome by a larger concentration of acetylcholine or equivalent muscarinic agonist. This suggests competition for a common binding site. The interaction may not be so simple, however, since in vitro studies suggest that in some tissues there may be 3 separate sites (or 3 different states) for agonist binding but only one for antagonists. Furthermore, antagonist binding appears to involve a 2-step process from the initial rapidly reversible antagonist-receptor complex to a more slowly reversible complex. In any case, the result of binding to the muscarinic receptor is to reverse or prevent the actions described in Chapter 5 such as the synthesis of cGMP that are evoked by acetylcholine and other muscarinic agonists.

The effectiveness of antimuscarinic drugs varies with the tissue under study and with the source of agonist. The tissues most sensitive to atropine are the salivary, bronchial, and sweat glands. Secretion of acid by the gastric parietal cells is the least sensitive. Smooth muscle autonomic effectors and the heart are intermediate in responsiveness. In many tissues, antimuscarinic agents are much more effective in blocking exogenously administered cholinergic agonists than endogenously released acetylcholine.

Atropine is highly selective in its action. Its potency at nicotinic receptors is much lower than at muscarinic receptors; in clinical use, actions at nonmuscarinic receptors are generally undetectable. Most synthetic antimuscarinic drugs are considerably less specific. The overlap of side-effects of the antihistamine and antidepressant drugs has been mentioned. Furthermore, quaternary antimuscarinic drugs have more antinicotinic effects than atropine and can produce some of the symptoms of ganglionic blockade.

B. Organ System Effects:

1. Central nervous system–In the doses usually used clinically, atropine has mild stimulant effects on medullary centers, especially the vagal nucleus, and a slower, longer-lasting sedative effect. The central vagal stimulant effect is frequently sufficient to cause bradycardia, which is later supplanted by tachycardia as the drug's antimuscarinic effects at the sinoatrial node become manifest. Scopolamine has more marked sedative effects, producing drowsiness when given in recommended dosages and amnesia in sensitive individuals. In toxic doses, atropine and scopolamine cause excitement, agitation, hallucinations, and coma.

The tremor of Parkinson's disease is reduced by centrally acting antimuscarinic drugs, and atropine—in the form of belladonna extract—was one of the first drugs used in the therapy of this disease. As discussed in Chapter 25, parkinsonian tremor and rigidity seem to result from an excess of cholinergic activity and a deficiency of dopaminergic activity in the basal ganglia-striatal system. Thus, the combination of an antimuscarinic agent with a dopaminergic drug (levodopa) may provide a more effective therapeutic approach than either drug alone.

Vestibular disturbances, especially motion sickness, appear to involve muscarinic cholinergic transmission. Scopolamine is often effective in preventing or reversing these disturbances.

2. Eye–The pupillary constrictor muscle is dependent on muscarinic cholinergic activation. This activation is effectively blocked by topical atropine and other tertiary antimuscarinic drugs and results in unopposed sympathetic dilator activity and **mydriasis.** Dilated pupils were apparently considered cosmetically desirable during the Renaissance and account for the name belladonna (Italian, "beautiful lady") applied to the plant and its active extract.

The second important ocular effect of atropine is paralysis of the ciliary muscle, or **cycloplegia.** The result of cycloplegia is loss of the ability to accommodate; the fully atropinized eye cannot focus for near vision.

Both mydriasis and cycloplegia are therapeutically useful in ophthalmology. They are also potentially hazardous, since acute glaucoma may be precipitated in patients with a narrow anterior chamber (Chapter 5).

A third (less important) ocular effect of antimuscarinic drugs is reduction of lacrimal secretion. Patients occasionally complain of dry or "sandy" eyes when receiving large doses of antimuscarinic drugs.

3. Cardiovascular system–The atria of the heart are heavily innervated by parasympathetic (vagal) nerve fibers, and the sinoatrial node is therefore sensitive to muscarinic receptor blockade. The effect in the isolated, innervated, and spontaneously beating heart is a clear blockade of vagal slowing and a relative tachycardia. In patients, tachycardia is seen consistently when moderate to high therapeutic doses are given. However, as noted above, lower doses cause central vagal *stimulation* and may result in initial bradycardia before the effects of peripheral vagal block become manifest. The same mechanisms operate in the control of atrioventricular node function; in the presence of high vagal tone, administration of atropine can significantly reduce the P–R interval of the ECG. Muscarinic effects on atrial muscle are similarly blocked, but except in atrial flutter and fibrillation these effects are of no clinical significance. The ventricles, because of a much lower degree of control by muscarinic mechanisms, are relatively unaffected by antimuscarinic drugs at therapeutic levels. In toxic concentrations, the drugs can cause intraventricular conduction block by an unknown mechanism.

The blood vessels receive little or no direct innervation from the parasympathetic nervous system. However, as noted in Chapter 4, sympathetic cholinergic nerves cause vasodilatation in the skeletal muscle vascular bed. This vasodilatation can be blocked by atropine. Furthermore, almost all vessels contain muscarinic receptors that mediate vasodilatation (Chapter 5). These receptors respond to circulating direct-acting muscarinic agonists, and they are readily blocked by antimuscarinic drugs. At toxic doses, and in a few patients at normal doses, antimuscarinic agents cause cutaneous vasodilatation, especially in the blush area. The mechanism is unknown.

The net cardiovascular effects of atropine in patients with normal hemodynamics are not dramatic: tachycardia may occur, but there is little effect on blood pressure. However, the effects of administered direct-acting muscarinic stimulants (Chapter 5) are easily prevented.

4. Respiratory system–Both smooth muscle and secretory glands of the airway receive vagal innervation and contain muscarinic receptors. Even in normal individuals, some bronchodilatation and reduction of secretion can be measured after administration of atropine. The effect is much more dramatic in patients with airway disease, although the antimuscarinic drugs are not as useful as the beta-adrenergic stimulants in the treatment of asthma (Chapter 17). Nevertheless, the antimuscarinic agents are valuable in some patients with asthma. In addition, they are frequently used prior to administration of inhalant anesthetics to reduce the accumulation of secretions in the trachea and the possibility of laryngospasm.

5. Gastrointestinal tract–Blockade of muscarinic receptors has dramatic effects on motility and some of the secretory functions of the gut. However, since local hormones and noncholinergic neurons also modulate gastrointestinal function, even complete muscarinic block cannot totally abolish activity in this organ system. As in other tissues, exogenously administered muscarinic stimulants are more effectively blocked than the effects of parasympathetic (vagal) nerve activity.

The effects of antimuscarinic blockade on salivary secretion are marked; dry mouth is a frequent symptom in patients taking antimuscarinic drugs for Parkinson's disease or peptic ulcer. Gastric secretion is blocked less effectively: the volume and amount of acid and mucin are all reduced, but large doses of atropine may be required. Basal secretion is blocked more effectively than that stimulated by food, nicotine, or alcohol (Chapter 62). Pancreatic and intestinal secretion is little affected by atropine; these processes are primarily under hormonal rather than vagal control.

Motility of gastrointestinal smooth muscle is more broadly affected than is secretory activity in the gut. In general, the walls of the viscera are relaxed, and both tone and propulsive movements are diminished. Therefore, gastric emptying time is prolonged, and intestinal transit time is lengthened. Diarrhea due to overdose with parasympathomimetic agents is readily eliminated, and even that caused by noncholinergic agents can usually be temporarily controlled. However, intestinal "paralysis" induced by antimuscarinic drugs is temporary; local mechanisms will usually reestablish at least some peristalsis after 1–3 days of antimuscarinic drug therapy.

Several of the synthetic antimuscarinic agents are said to have "spasmolytic" activity in excess of their antimuscarinic effects. This is the result of selection of agents, through screening tests in isolated tissue, that relax the gut in the absence as well as the presence of cholinergic stimulants.

6. Genitourinary tract–Smooth muscle of the ureters and bladder wall is relaxed by the antimuscarinic action of atropine and its analogs. This action is useful in the treatment of spasm induced by mild inflammatory conditions, but it also poses a hazard of precipitating urinary retention in elderly men, who may have prostatic hypertrophy (see Clinical Pharmacology). The antimuscarinic drugs have no significant effect on the uterus.

7. Sweat glands–Thermoregulatory sweating is suppressed by atropine. The muscarinic receptors on eccrine sweat glands are innervated by sympathetic cholinergic fibers and are readily accessible to antimuscarinic drugs. In adults, body temperature is elevated by this effect only if large doses are administered, but in infants and children even ordinary doses may cause "atropine fever."

II. CLINICAL PHARMACOLOGY OF THE ANTIMUSCARINIC DRUGS

Therapeutic Applications

A. Central Nervous System Disorders:

1. Parkinson's disease–As described in Chapter 25, the treatment of Parkinson's disease is often an exercise in polypharmacy, since no single agent is fully effective over the (usually prolonged) course of the disease. Most of the large number of antimuscarinic drugs promoted for this application (Table 25–1) were developed before levodopa became available. Their use is accompanied by all of the adverse effects described below, but the drugs remain useful in the attempt to control the disease in many patients.

2. Motion sickness–Certain vestibular disorders respond to antimuscarinic drugs (and to antihistaminic agents with antimuscarinic effects). Scopolamine is one of the oldest remedies for seasickness and is still as effective as any more recently introduced agent. It can be given by injection as well as by mouth. A new dosage form, the transdermal patch, has recently been approved for use and results in significant blood levels over 24–48 hours. Unfortunately, useful doses usually cause significant sedation and dry mouth.

B. Ophthalmologic Disorders: Accurate measurement of refractive error in uncooperative patients,

Table 6–1. Antimuscarinic drugs used in ophthalmology.

Drug	Preparation	Duration of Mydriasis (days)	Duration of Cycloplegia (days)
Atropine	Drops, ointment, 0.5%, 1%, 2%, and 3%	7–10	7–12
Scopolamine	Drops, ointment, 0.2%, 0.25%, and 0.3%	3–7	5–7
Homatropine	Drops, 1%, 2%, and 5%	1–3	1–3
Cyclopentolate (Cyclogyl)	Drops, 0.5%, 1%, and 2%	1	1
Tropicamide (Mydriacyl)	Drops, 0.5% and and 1%	¼	¼

eg, young children, requires ciliary paralysis. In addition, ophthalmoscopic examination of the retina is greatly facilitated by mydriasis. Therefore, antimuscarinic agents, administered topically as eye drops or in ointment form, are extremely helpful in doing a complete examination. For adults and older children, the shorter-acting drugs are preferred (Table 6–1). For younger children, the greater efficacy of atropine is sometimes necessary, but the possibility of antimuscarinic poisoning is correspondingly increased. Loss of drug from the conjunctival sac via the nasolacrimal duct into the nasopharynx is diminished by the use of atropine ointment.

Antimuscarinic drugs should never be used for mydriasis unless cycloplegia or prolonged action is required. The alpha-adrenergic stimulant drugs, eg, phenylephrine, produce a short-lasting mydriasis that is usually sufficient for funduscopic examination (Chapter 6).

A second ophthalmologic use is to prevent synechia formation in uveitis and iritis. The longer-acting preparations, especially homatropine, are valuable for these indications.

C. Gastrointestinal Disorders: A major application of the antimuscarinic drugs is in the treatment of peptic ulcer and hypermotility of the gut. This subject is discussed in some detail in Chapter 62. The quaternary semisynthetic and synthetic agents (Table 6–2) are favored for this purpose, since central nervous system side-effects are diminished. Unfortunately, large doses are required to effectively reduce gastric acid secretion, which means that patients with peptic ulcer will have dry mouth, blurred vision, and urinary hesitancy when these drugs are used as the principal treatment. Fortunately, when combined with cimetidine, much lower doses can be useful and side-effects correspondingly diminished.

In the treatment of common traveler's diarrhea and other mild or self-limited conditions of hypermotility, the antimuscarinic agents, especially in combination with an opioid antidiarrheal drug, are extremely useful. The classic combination of atropine with diphenoxylate, a nonanalgesic congener of meperidine, is available under many names in both tablet and liquid form.

D. Cardiovascular Disorders: Marked vagal discharge sometimes accompanies the pain of myocardial infarction and may result in sufficient depression of sinoatrial or atrioventricular node function to impair cardiac output. Rare individuals without other detectable cardiac disease have hyperactive carotid sinus reflexes and may experience faintness or even syncope as a result of vagal discharge in response to pressure on the neck, eg, from a tight collar. Such individuals may benefit from the judicious use of atropine or a related antimuscarinic agent.

E. Respiratory Disorders: The use of atropine became part of routine preoperative medication when anesthetics such as ether were used, because these irritant anesthetics caused a marked increase in bronchial secretion and were associated with frequent episodes of laryngospasm. These hazardous effects were prevented by preanesthetic injection of atropine or scopolamine. The latter drug also produced significant amnesia for the events associated with surgery and obstetric delivery, a side-effect that was considered desirable. On the other hand, urinary retention and intestinal hypomotility following surgery could be significantly exacerbated by the use of the antimuscarinic drug.

With the advent of effective and nonirritant inhalational anesthetics such as halothane and enflurane, it would seem that the major reason for the routine use of antimuscarinic drugs as preanesthetic medication has been eliminated.

Inhalation of smoke from burning leaves of *Datura stramonium* has been used for centuries as a remedy for bronchial asthma. "Asthmador" cigarettes

Table 6–2. Antimuscarinic drugs used in gastrointestinal and genitourinary conditions.

Drug	Usual Dose (mg)
Quaternary amines	
Anisotropine (Valpin)	50
Clidinium (Quarzan)	2.5
Diphemanil (Prantal)	100
Glycopyrrolate (Glycobarb, Robinul)	1
Hexocyclium (Tral)	25
Isopropamide (Darbid)	5
Mepenzolate (Cantil)	25
Methantheline (Banthine)	50
Methscopolamine (Pamine)	2.5
Oxyphenonium (Antrenyl)	5
Propantheline (Pro-Banthine)	15
Tridihexethyl (Pathilon)	25
Tertiary amines	
Atropine	0.4
Dicyclomine (Bentyl, etc)	20
Methixene (Trest)	1
Oxyphencyclimine (Daricon)	10
Scopolamine	0.4
Thiphenamil (Trocinate)	400

containing *D stramonium* were available without prescription for this application until recently. As described in Chapter 16, the hyperactive neural bronchoconstrictor reflex present in most individuals with asthma is mediated by the vagus, acting on muscarinic receptors on bronchial smooth muscle cells. **Ipratropium** (Fig 6–2), a synthetic analog of atropine, is being studied as an inhalational drug for use in asthma. The aerosol route of administration provides the obvious advantages of maximal concentration at the bronchial target tissue with minimal systemic effects. This application is discussed in greater detail in Chapter 17.

F. Cholinergic Poisoning: Severe cholinergic excess is an important medical emergency, especially in rural communities where the use of cholinesterase inhibitor insecticides is common, and in cultures where wild mushrooms are eaten.

As noted in Chapter 5, both the nicotinic and the muscarinic effects of the cholinesterase inhibitor insecticides can be life-threatening. To reverse the muscarinic effects, a tertiary (not quaternary) amine drug must be used (preferably atropine), since the central nervous system effects as well as the peripheral effects of the organophosphate insecticides must be treated. Huge doses of atropine may be needed to combat the muscarinic effects of agents like parathion: 1–2 mg of atropine sulfate may be given intravenously every 5–15 minutes until signs of effect (dry mouth, reversal of miosis) appear. The drug may have to be repeated many times, since the acute effects of the anticholinesterase agent may last for 24–48 hours.

A second class of compounds, capable of regenerating active enzyme from the organophosphorus-cholinesterase complex, is also available for the treatment of organophosphorus insecticide poisoning. These **oxime** agents include pralidoxime (PAM), diacetylmonoxime (DAM), and obidoxime.

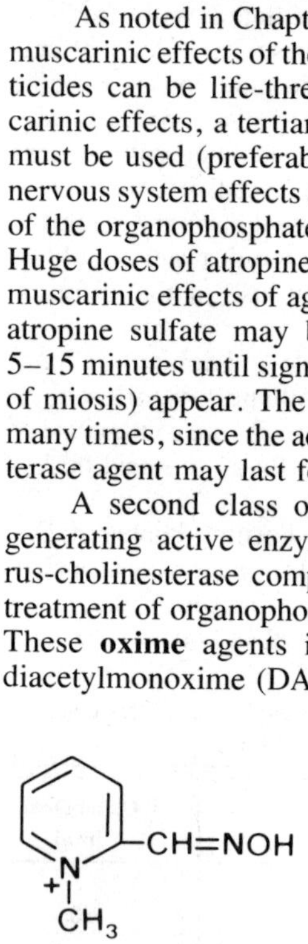

Pralidoxime

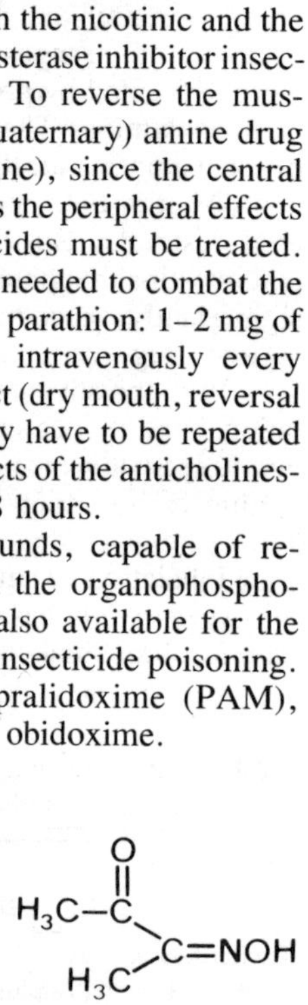

Diacetylmonoxime

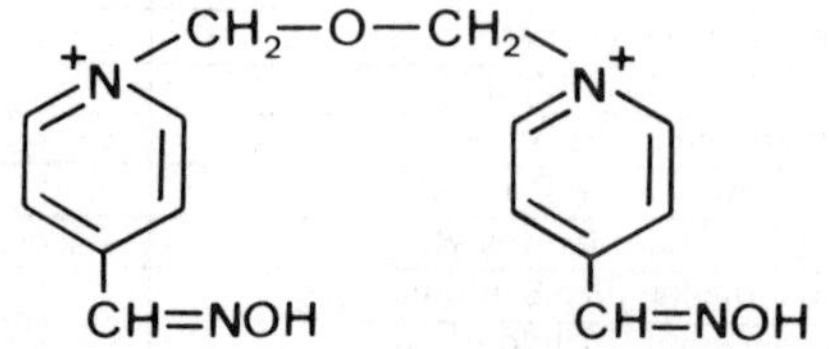

Obidoxime

The oxime group (=NOH) has a very high affinity for the phosphorus atom, and these drugs are able to hydrolyze the phosphorylated enzyme if the complex has not "aged" (Chapter 5). Obidoxime is the most potent of these oximes. Pralidoxime is the most extensively studied of the 3 agents shown above and the only one available for clinical use in the USA. It is most effective in regenerating the cholinesterase associated with skeletal muscle neuromuscular junctions. Because of its positive charge, it does not enter the central nervous system and is ineffective in reversing the central effects of organophosphate poisoning. Diacetylmonoxime, on the other hand, does cross the blood-brain barrier and, in experimental animals, can regenerate some of the central nervous system cholinesterase. The effect of the oximes on cholinesterase carbamylated by the reversible cholinesterase inhibitors is controversial.

Pralidoxime is administered by intravenous infusion, 1–2 g given over 15–30 minutes. In high doses, pralidoxime can induce neuromuscular weakness and a variety of other side-effects. Further details of the treatment of anticholinesterase toxicity are given in Chapter 58.

Mushroom poisoning has traditionally been divided into rapid-onset and delayed-onset types. The rapid-onset type is usually apparent within 15–30 minutes following ingestion of the mushrooms. It is often characterized entirely by signs of muscarinic excess: nausea, vomiting, diarrhea, vasodilatation, reflex tachycardia (occasionally bradycardia), sweating, salivation, and sometimes bronchoconstriction. Although *Amanita muscaria* contains muscarine (the alkaloid was named after the mushroom), numerous other alkaloids, including *antimuscarinic* agents, are found in this fungus. In fact, ingestion of *A muscaria* may produce signs of atropine poisoning, not muscarine excess. Other mushrooms cause rapid-onset poisoning of the muscarinic excess type. Parenteral atropine, 1–2 mg, is effective treatment in such intoxications.

Delayed-onset mushroom poisoning, usually caused by *Amanita phalloides,* manifests its first symptoms 6–12 hours after ingestion. Although the initial symptoms usually include nausea and vomiting, the mechanism involves hepatic and renal cellular injury. Atropine is of no value in this form of mushroom poisoning (see Chapter 58).

G. Other Applications: Atropine and quaternary antimuscarinic drugs have been used in the treatment of urinary urgency caused by minor inflammatory bladder disorders. This approach does provide some symptomatic relief, although it is no substitute for specific antimicrobial therapy if cystitis is caused by infection. The antimuscarinic agents have also been used in urolithiasis to relieve the ureteral smooth muscle spasm caused by passage of the stone. However, their usefulness in this condition is debatable.

Hyperhidrosis is sometimes reduced by the antimuscarinic agents. However, relief is incomplete at best.

Adverse Effects

Because of the broad range of antimuscarinic effects, treatment with atropine or its congeners directed at one organ system almost always induces undesirable effects in other organ systems. Thus, mydriasis and cycloplegia are "adverse" effects when an antimuscarinic agent is being used to reduce gastrointestinal secretion or motility, even though they are "therapeutic" effects when the drug is used in ophthalmology.

At higher concentrations, atropine causes block of all parasympathetic functions; these are predictable from the organ system effects described above. However, even in gram quantities, atropine is a remarkably safe drug *in adults*. Atropine poisoning has occurred as a result of attempted suicide, but recent cases are more apt to be due to attempts to induce hallucinations. Poisoned individuals manifest dry mouth, mydriasis, tachycardia, hot and flushed skin, agitation, and delirium. Body temperature is frequently elevated.

Unfortunately, children are much more sensitive to the hyperthermic effects of atropine. Although accidental administration of over 400 mg has been followed by recovery, deaths have followed doses as small as 2 mg. Therefore, atropine should be considered a highly dangerous drug when overdose occurs in infants or children.

The pharmacologic treatment of overdose with atropine and its tertiary congeners in both children and adults consists of giving **physostigmine** (Chapter 5). This tertiary cholinesterase inhibitor reverses muscarinic blockade in the central nervous system as well as the periphery. Given slowly intravenously (1–4 mg in adults; 0.5–1 mg in children), physostigmine is relatively safe and effective. Severe hyperthermia in children should also be treated with cooling blankets (but not aspirin).

Poisoning caused by high doses of the quaternary antimuscarinic drugs is associated with all of the peripheral signs of parasympathetic blockade but few or none of the central nervous system effects of atropine. These more polar drugs may cause significant ganglionic blockade, however, with marked orthostatic hypotension (see below). Treatment of the antimuscarinic effects can be carried out with a quaternary cholinesterase inhibitor such as neostigmine. Reversal of hypotension may require the administration of a sympathomimetic drug such as phenylephrine or methoxamine.

Contraindications

Contraindications to the use of antimuscarinic drugs are relative, not absolute. Obvious muscarinic excess, especially that caused by cholinesterase inhibitors, can always be treated with atropine.

Antimuscarinic drugs are contraindicated in patients with glaucoma, especially narrow-angle glaucoma. Even systemic use of moderate doses may precipitate angle closure (and acute glaucoma) in patients with shallow anterior chambers.

In elderly men, atropine should always be used with caution, and probably never in those with a history of prostatic hypertrophy.

Because the antimuscarinic drugs slow gastric emptying, they may increase symptoms in patients with *gastric* ulcer. If a stomach ulcer is to be treated pharmacologically, antacids and cimetidine are preferred (see Chapter 62).

III. BASIC & CLINICAL PHARMACOLOGY OF THE GANGLION-BLOCKING DRUGS

These agents block the action of acetylcholine and similar agonists at the nicotinic receptors of both parasympathetic and sympathetic autonomic ganglia. Because of their ability to block all autonomic outflow, the ganglion-blocking drugs are still important and useful in pharmacologic and physiologic research.

However, their lack of selectivity confers such a broad range of undesirable side-effects that they have been almost abandoned for clinical use. Their major remaining therapeutic application is for blood pressure control.

Chemistry & Pharmacokinetics

All of the ganglion-blocking drugs of interest are synthetic amines. The first to be recognized as having this action was **tetraethylammonium (TEA).** Because of its very short duration of action, **hexamethonium ("C6")** was developed and was soon introduced into clinical medicine as the first effective drug for management of hypertension. As shown in Fig 6–3, there is an obvious relationship between the structures of the normal agonist acetylcholine and the nicotinic antagonists tetraethylammonium and hexamethonium. It is interesting that decamethonium, the "C10" analog of hexamethonium, is an effective neuromuscular depolarizing blocking agent.

Because the quaternary ammonium compounds are poorly and erratically absorbed after oral administration, **mecamylamine,** a secondary ammonium compound, was developed to improve the degree and extent of absorption from the gastrointestinal tract. **Trimethaphan,** a short-acting ganglion blocker, is inactive by the oral route and is given by intravenous infusion (Chapter 9).

Pharmacodynamics

A. Mechanism of Action: As noted above, the nicotinic receptors of the ganglia, like those of the skeletal muscle neuromuscular junction, are subject to both depolarizing and nondepolarizing blockade. Nicotine itself, carbamylcholine, and even acetylcholine (if given with a cholinesterase inhibitor) can produce depolarizing ganglion block.

Blockade by agonists such as nicotine is associated with depolarization like that produced by an ordinary synaptic volley of impulses, except that the duration of depolarization is greatly prolonged. Initially, the postsynaptic cell is prevented from re-

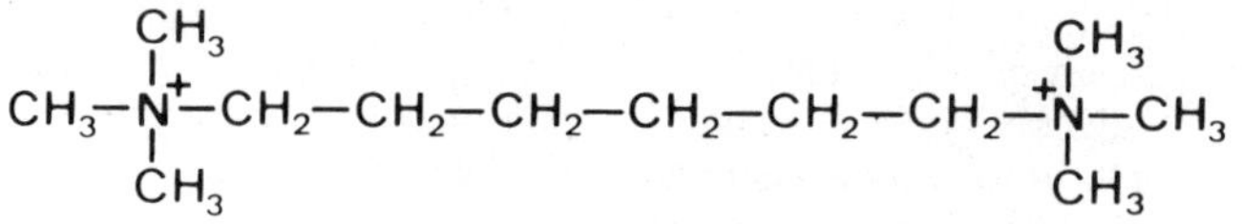

Hexamethonium

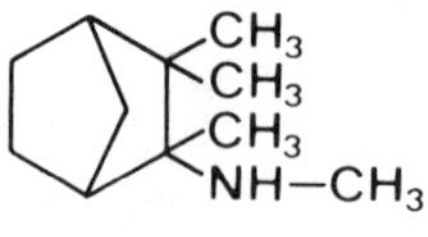

Mecamylamine

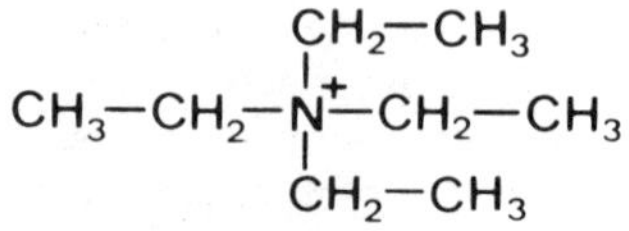

Tetraethylammonium

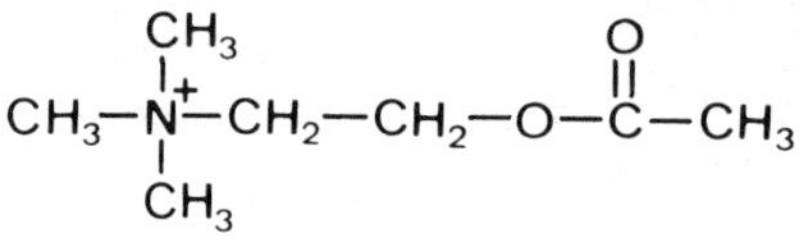

Acetylcholine

Figure 6–3. Some ganglion-blocking drugs. Acetylcholine is shown for reference. The structure of trimethaphan is shown in Fig 9–4.

polarizing and firing again by the sustained receptor activation. Subsequently, the cell becomes desensitized—by an unknown mechanism—and may repolarize, but it remains unable to respond to normal synaptic signals until the nicotinic agonist is removed.

All of the drugs presently used as ganglion blockers are nondepolarizing agents that bind to the nicotinic receptor without activating it. Because the many other receptors on the postganglionic neuron body (see Chapter 4) merely modulate the response to nicotinic receptor activation, block of the nicotinic receptor alone is usually sufficient to completely block ganglionic transmission.

B. Organ System Effects:

1. Central nervous system–The quaternary ammonium agents and trimethaphan are devoid of central effects because they do not cross the blood-brain barrier. Mecamylamine readily enters the central nervous system. Sedation, tremor, choreiform movements, and mental aberrations have all been reported as effects of the latter drug.

2. Eye–Because the ciliary muscle receives significant innervation only from the parasympathetic nervous system, the ganglion-blocking drugs cause a predictable cycloplegia with loss of accommodation. The effect on the pupil is not so easily predicted, since the iris receives both sympathetic innervation (mediating pupillary dilation) and parasympathetic innervation (mediating pupillary constriction). Because parasympathetic tone is usually dominant, ganglionic blockade usually causes moderate dilatation of the pupil.

3. Cardiovascular system–The blood vessels receive chiefly vasoconstrictor fibers from the sympathetic nervous system; therefore, ganglion blockade causes a very important decrease in arteriolar and venomotor tone. The blood pressure may drop precipitously, because both peripheral vascular resistance and venous return are decreased (see Fig 4–6). Hypotension is especially marked in the upright position (orthostatic hypotension), because postural reflexes that normally prevent venous pooling are blocked.

Cardiac effects include diminished contractility and, because the sinoatrial node is usually dominated by the parasympathetic nervous system, a moderate tachycardia.

4. Gastrointestinal tract–Secretion is reduced, although not enough to effectively treat peptic disease. Motility is profoundly inhibited, and constipation may be marked.

5. Other systems–Genitourinary smooth muscle is partially dependent on autonomic innervation for normal function. Ganglion blockade therefore causes hesitancy in urination and may precipitate urinary retention in men with prostatic hypertrophy. Sexual function is impaired in that both erection and ejaculation may be prevented by moderate doses.

Thermoregulatory sweating is blocked by the ganglion-blocking drugs. However, hyperthermia is not a problem except in very warm environments, because cutaneous vasodilatation is usually sufficient to maintain a normal body temperature.

6. Response to autonomic drugs–Because the effector cell receptors (muscarinic cholinergic, alpha-adrenergic, and beta-adrenergic) are not blocked, patients receiving ganglion-blocking drugs are fully responsive to autonomic drugs acting on the effector cell receptors. In fact, responses may be exaggerated, because homeostatic reflexes, which normally moderate autonomic responses, are absent.

Clinical Applications & Toxicity

Because of the availability of more selective autonomic blocking agents, the applications of the ganglion blockers are limited to the lowering of blood pressure. The great efficacy of trimethaphan, when aided by the orthostatic hypotensive effect of venous pooling, is valuable in the treatment of hypertensive emergencies. Controlled hypotension can be of value in neurosurgery to reduce bleeding in the operative field. The short, controllable effect of trimethaphan lends itself to this application as well. Trimethaphan has also been used in acute pulmonary edema to reduce pulmonary vascular pressure.

The toxicity of the ganglion-blocking drugs is limited to the autonomic effects already described. For most patients, these effects are intolerable except for acute use.

• • •

References

Antimuscarinic Drugs

Becker CE et al: Diagnosis and treatment of *Amanita phalloides-type mushroom poisoning. West J Med* 1976;**125:**100.

Birdsall NJM, Burgen SAV, Hulme EC: The binding of agonists to brain muscarinic receptors. *Mol Pharmacol* 1978;**14:**723.

Bowers J, Forbes J, Freston J: Effect of nighttime anisatropine methylbromide (AMB) on duodenal ulcer healing: A controlled trial. *Gastroenterology* 1977;**72:**1032.

Crowell EB, Ketchum JS: The treatment of scopolamine-induced delirium with physostigmine. *Clin Pharmacol Ther* 1967;**8:**409.

Duvoisin RC: Cholinergic-anticholinergic antagonism in parkinsonism. *Arch Neurol* 1967;**17:**124.

Epstein SE, Redwood DR, Smith ER: Atropine and acute myocardial infarction. *Circulation* 1972;**45:**1273.

Feldman M et al: Effect of low-dose propantheline on food-stimulated gastric acid secretion. *N Engl J Med* 1977;**297:**1427.

Fordtran JS: Placebos, antacids and cimetidine for duodenal ulcer. *N Engl J Med* 1978;**298:**1081.

Glick G, Braunwald E: Relative roles of the sympathetic and parasympathetic nervous systems in the reflex control of heart rate. *Circ Res* 1965;**16:**363.

Gowdy JM: Stramonium intoxication: Review of symptomatology in 212 cases. *JAMA* 1972;**221:**585.

Greenblatt DJ, Shader RI: Anticholinergics. *N Engl J Med* 1973;**288:**1215.

Kalser SC, McLain PL: Atropine metabolism in man. *Clin Pharmacol Ther* 1970;**11:**214.

Petrie GR, Palmer KNV: Comparison of aerosol ipratropium bromide and salbutamol in chronic bronchitis and asthma. *Br Med J* 1975;**1:**430.

Richelson E, El-Fakahany E: The molecular basis of neurotransmission at the muscarinic receptor. *Biochem Pharmacol* 1981;**30:**2887.

Rumack BH: Anticholinergic poisoning: Treatment with physostigmine. *Pediatrics* 1973;**52:**449.

Shader RI, Greenblatt DJ: Belladonna alkaloids and synthetic anticholinergics: Uses and toxicity. Pages 103–147 in: *Psychiatric Complications of Medical Drugs.* Shader RI (editor). Raven Press, 1972.

Yamamura HI, Snyder SH: Muscarinic cholinergic receptor binding in the longitudinal muscle of the guinea pig ileum with (^{3}H) quinuclidinyl benzilate. *Mol Pharmacol* 1974;**10:**861.

Ganglion-Blocking Drugs

Mason DFJ: Ganglion-blocking drugs. Pages 363–387 in: *Physiological Pharmacology: A Comprehensive Treatise.* Vol 3. Root WS, Hoffman FG (editors). Academic Press, 1967.

Salem MR: Therapeutic uses of ganglionic blocking drugs. *Int Anesthesiol Clin* 1978;**16:**171.

Stone CA et al: Ganglionic blocking properties of 3-methylaminoisocamphane hydrochloride (mecamylamine): A secondary amine. *J Pharmacol Exp Ther* 1956;**117:**169.

Volle RL: Ganglionic transmission. *Am Rev Pharmacol* 1969;**9:**135.

Wang HH, Tim LMP, Katz RL: A comparison of the cardiovascular effects of sodium nitroprusside and trimethaphan. *Anesthesiology* 1977;**46:**40.

7 | Adrenergic Receptor–Activating Drugs

Brian B. Hoffman, MD

The sympathetic nervous system is an important regulator of the activities of organs such as the heart and peripheral vasculature (see Chapter 4), especially in responses to stress. The ultimate effects of sympathetic stimulation are mediated by release of norepinephrine from nerve terminals that serve to activate the adrenergic receptors on postsynaptic sites. Also, in response to stress, the adrenal medulla releases norepinephrine, which is transported in the blood to target tissues. Drugs that partially or completely mimic the actions of epinephrine or norepinephrine—**sympathomimetics**—would be expected to have a wide range of effects. An understanding of the pharmacology of these agents is thus a logical extension of what we know about the physiologic role of the catecholamines. Some of these drugs act directly on adrenergic receptors; others act indirectly, their actions dependent on the release of endogenous catecholamines. Both types of sympathomimetics ultimately cause activation of adrenergic receptors, leading to some of the characteristic effects of catecholamines.

I. BASIC PHARMACOLOGY OF ADRENERGIC RECEPTOR–ACTIVATING DRUGS

Identification of Adrenergic Receptors

The effort to understand the molecular mechanisms by which catecholamines act has a long and rich history. A great conceptual debt is owed to the work of Langley and Ehrlich 75–100 years ago putting forth the hypothesis that drugs have their effects by interacting with specific "receptive" substances. Ahlquist, in 1948, rationalized a large body of observations by his conjecture that catecholamines acted via 2 principal receptors. He termed these receptors alpha and beta. Alpha receptors are those that exhibit the potency series epinephrine ≥ norepinephrine >> isoproterenol. Beta receptors have the potency series isoproterenol > epinephrine ≥ norepinephrine. Ahlquist's hypothesis was dramatically confirmed by the development of drugs that specifically antagonize alpha or beta receptors (see Chapter 8). Subsequently, it was found that there are at least 2 subtypes of beta receptors, designated β_1 and β_2. Beta$_1$ and β_2 receptors are operationally defined by their affinities for epinephrine and norepinephrine: β_1 receptors have approximately equal affinity for epinephrine and norepinephrine, whereas β_2 receptors have a higher affinity for epinephrine than for norepinephrine.

Table 7–1. Relative selectivity of agonists for adrenergic receptors.*

	Receptor
Alpha-agonists	
Phenylephrine, methoxamine	α_1-selective
Epinephrine, norepinephrine	$\alpha_1 \sim \alpha_2$
Clonidine, α-methylnorepinephrine	α_2-selective
Beta-agonists	
Norepinephrine, dobutamine, prenalterol	β_1-selective
Isoproterenol, epinephrine	$\beta_1 \sim \beta_2$
Fenoterol, albuterol (salbutamol), terbutaline	β_2-selective

More recently, it has been recognized that there are also at least 2 subgroups of alpha receptors (α_1 and α_2). The subtypes of alpha receptors are defined by their affinities for alpha receptor-blocking drugs such as prazosin (see Chapters 8 and 9).

Examples of adrenergic agonists that are relatively selective for these receptor subgroups are listed in Table 7–1 along with some nonselective agents. **Selectivity** means that a drug may preferentially activate one subgroup of receptors at concentrations too low to activate another subgroup. For example, norepinephrine preferentially activates β_1 receptors as compared to β_2 receptors. However, selectivity is not usually absolute, and at higher concentrations related classes of receptor may also be occupied by the drug. As a result, the subclassification of adrenergic receptors is clinically important only for drugs that have relatively marked selectivity.

Molecular Mechanisms of Adrenergic Action

The mechanisms by which alpha receptors affect cell function are not well understood. Certain α_2 receptors—such as those in fat cells—probably inhibit the activity of adenylate cyclase: activation leads to a fall in cAMP concentration. Other alpha receptors, such as those in vascular smooth muscle, do not regu-

Catecholamine + Beta receptor —Activates→ Adenylate cyclase ——→ cAMP —Activates→

Protein kinase —Activates→ Phosphorylase kinase —Activates→ Glycogen phosphorylase

Figure 7–1. Activation of liver glycogen phosphorylase by cAMP. Interaction of a catecholamine or related sympathomimetic drug with beta receptors in liver leads to enhanced cAMP synthesis. The cAMP binds to a subunit of protein kinase. Consequently, protein kinase activates phosphorylase kinase, which in turn activates glycogen phosphorylase.

late adenylate cyclase activity. These receptors seem to utilize calcium ion as an essential mediator of their effects.

Beta receptors activate adenylate cyclase, causing increased conversion of ATP to cAMP. cAMP is the major "second messenger" of beta-receptor activation. For example, in the liver of many species, beta-receptor activation increases cAMP synthesis, which leads to a cascade of events culminating in the activation of glycogen phosphorylase (Fig 7–1). Additional details are given in Chapter 34. In the heart, beta-receptor activation increases the influx of calcium across the cell membrane and its sequestration inside the cell.

Chemistry & Pharmacokinetics

Beta-phenylethylamine may be considered the parent compound from which sympathomimetic drugs are derived (Fig 7–2). This compound consists of a benzene ring with an ethylamine side chain. Substitutions may be made (1) on the terminal amino group, (2) on the benzene ring, and (3) on the α or β carbons. Substitution by –OH groups at the 3 and 4 positions yields sympathomimetic drugs collectively known as **catecholamines.** The effects of modification of β-phenylethylamine are to modify the affinity of the drugs for alpha and beta receptors as well as to influence the intrinsic ability to activate the receptors. Sympathomimetic drugs may activate both alpha- and beta-adrenergic receptors; however, the relative alpha-receptor versus beta-receptor activity spans the range from almost pure alpha activity (methoxamine) to almost pure beta activity (isoproterenol).

A. Substitution on the Amino Group: Increasing the size of alkyl substituents tends to increase beta-receptor activity. For example, methyl substitution on norepinephrine, yielding epinephrine, enhances activity at β_2 receptors. Beta activity is further enhanced with isopropyl substitution (isoproterenol). Beta$_2$-selective agonists generally require a large amino substituent group. The larger the substituent on the amino group, the lower the activity at alpha receptors; eg, isoproterenol is very weak at alpha receptors.

B. Substitution on the Benzene Ring: Maximal alpha and beta activity is found with catecholamines (drugs having –OH groups at the 3 and 4 positions). The absence of one or the other of these groups, particularly the hydroxyl at C3, without other substitutions on the ring may dramatically reduce the potency of the drugs. For example, phenylephrine (Fig 7–3) is

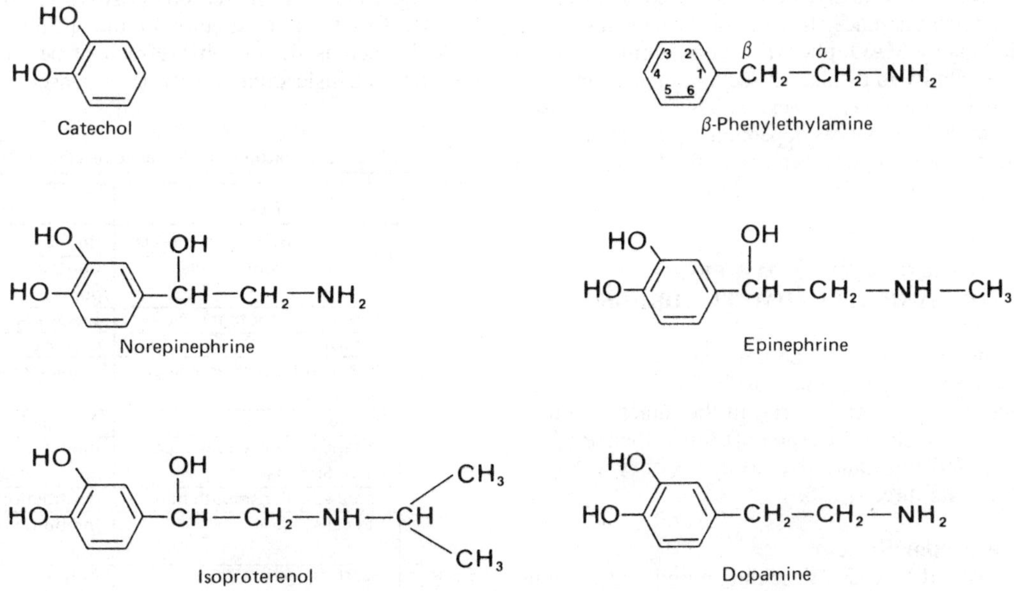

Figure 7–2. Phenylethylamine and some important catecholamines. These compounds are derivatives of β-phenylethylamine. Catechol is shown for reference.

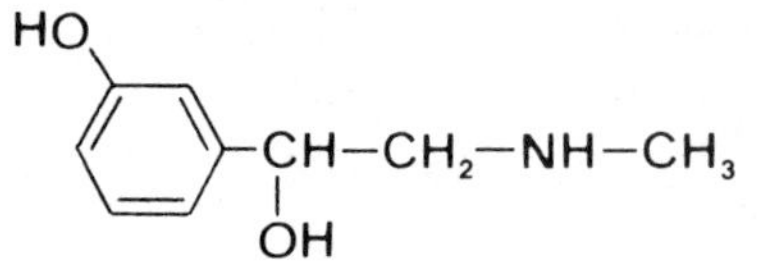

Phenylephrine

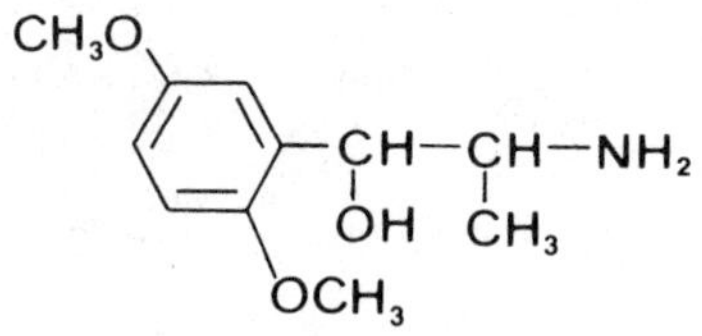

Methoxamine

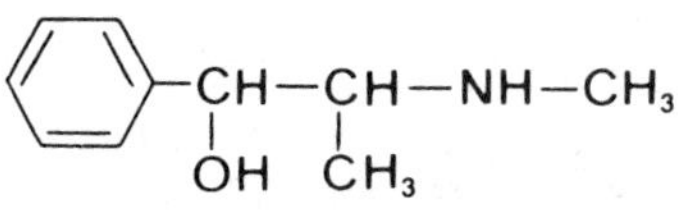

Ephedrine

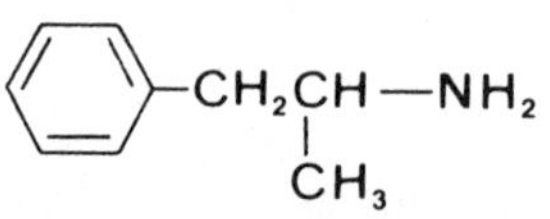

Amphetamine

Figure 7–3. Some examples of noncatecholamine sympathomimetic drugs.

much less potent than epinephrine; indeed, beta activity is almost negligible except at high concentrations. However, catecholamines are subject to inactivation by catechol-O-methyltransferase (COMT), an enzyme found in gut and liver (Chapter 4). Therefore, absence of one or both –OH groups on the phenyl ring increases the bioavailability after oral administration and prolongs the duration of action. Furthermore, absence of ring –OH groups increases the distribution of the molecule into the central nervous system. For example, ephedrine (Fig 7–3) is orally active, has a prolonged duration of action, and produces central nervous system effects not observed with the catecholamines.

C. Substitution on the Alpha Carbon: Substitutions at this site block oxidation by monoamine oxidase (MAO) and prolong the action of such drugs, particularly for noncatecholamines. Ephedrine and amphetamine are examples of α-substituted compounds (Fig 7–3). Alpha-methyl compounds are also called phenylisopropylamines. In addition to their resistance to oxidation by MAO, phenylisopropylamines have an enhanced ability to displace catecholamines from storage sites in noradrenergic nerves. Therefore, at least a portion of their activity is dependent upon the presence of normal norepinephrine stores in the body; they are *indirectly* acting sympathomimetics.

ORGAN SYSTEM EFFECTS OF SYMPATHOMIMETIC DRUGS

General outlines of the cellular actions of sympathomimetics are presented in Tables 4–2 and 7–2. The net effect of a given drug in the intact organism depends on its relative receptor affinity (alpha or beta), intrinsic activity, and the compensatory reflexes evoked by its direct actions.

Cardiovascular System

A. Blood Vessels: Vascular smooth muscle tone is regulated by adrenergic receptors; consequently, catecholamines are important in controlling peripheral vascular resistance and venous capacitance. Alpha receptors increase arterial resistance, whereas β_2 receptors promote smooth muscle relaxation. There are major differences in responsiveness of anatomically distinct vessels to catecholamines. The skin vessels predominantly constrict in the presence of catecholamines, as do the splanchnic vessels. Vessels in skeletal muscle may constrict or relax, depending on whether alpha or beta receptors are activated. Thus, the overall effects of a sympathomimetic drug on blood vessels depend on the relative activities at alpha and beta receptors and the anatomic sites of the vessels affected (Table 7–3).

B. Heart: Direct effects on the heart are determined largely by β_1 receptors, although β_2 and to a lesser extent α receptors have also been implicated. Beta-receptor activation results in increased calcium influx in cardiac cells. This has both electrical and mechanical consequences (Fig 7–4). Pacemaker activity, both normal (sinoatrial node) and abnormal (eg, Purkinje fibers), is increased (positive chronotropic effect). Conduction velocity in the atrioventricular node is increased, and the refractory period is decreased. Intrinsic contractility is increased (positive

Table 7–2. Distribution of adrenergic receptor subtypes.

Type	Tissue	Actions
$Alpha_1$	Most vascular smooth muscle.	Contraction.
	Pupillary dilator muscle.	Contraction (dilates pupil).
	Pilomotor smooth muscle.	Erects hair.
	Rat liver.	Glycogenolysis.
$Alpha_2$	Postsynaptic CNS adrenergic receptors.	Probably multiple.
	Platelets.	Aggregation.
	Adrenergic and cholinergic nerve terminals.	Inhibition of transmitter release.
	Some vascular smooth muscle.	Contraction.
	Fat cells.	Inhibition of lipolysis.
$Beta_1$	Heart, fat cells, CNS.	Activates adenylate cyclase.
$Beta_2$	Respiratory, uterine, and vascular smooth muscle.	Activates adenylate cyclase.

Table 7–3. Cardiovascular response to sympathomimetic amines.
(↑ = increase; ↓ = decrease; 0 = no change.)

	Phenyl-ephrine	Epi-nephrine	Isopro-terenol
Vascular resistance (tone)			
Cutaneous, mucous membranes (α)	↑↑	↑↑	0
Skeletal muscle (β_2, α)	↑	↓	↓↓
Renal (α)	↑	↑	↓
Splanchnic (α)	↑↑	↓ or ↑[1]	↓
Total peripheral resistance	↑↑↑	↓ or ↑[1]	↓↓
Venous tone	↑	↑	↓
Cardiac			
Contractility (β_1)	0 or ↑	↑↑↑	↑↑↑
Heart rate (predominantly β_1)	↓↓ (vagal reflex)	↑ or ↓	↑↑↑
Stroke volume	0 or ↓	↑	↑
Cardiac output	↓	↑	↑↑
Blood pressure			
Mean	↑↑	↑	↓
Diastolic	↑↑	↓ or ↑[1]	↓↓
Systolic	↑↑	↑↑	↑
Pulse pressure	0	↑↑	↑↑

[1] Small doses decrease, large doses increase.

inotropic effect), and relaxation is accelerated. As a result, the twitch response of isolated cardiac muscle is increased in tension but abbreviated in duration. In the intact heart, intraventricular pressure rises and falls more rapidly, and ejection time is decreased. These direct effects are easily demonstrated in the absence of reflexes evoked by changes in blood pressure, eg, in isolated myocardial preparations and in patients with ganglionic blockade. In the presence of normal reflex activity, the direct effects may be dominated by a reflex response to blood pressure changes.

C. Blood Pressure: The effects of sympathomimetic drugs on blood pressure can be explained on the basis of their effects on the heart, the peripheral vascular resistance, and the venous return (Fig 4–6). Stimulation of beta receptors in the heart tends to increase cardiac output. A relatively pure beta-agonist such as isoproterenol also decreases peripheral resistance. The net effect is to maintain systolic blood pressure while permitting a fall in diastolic pressure owing to enhanced diastolic runoff (Fig 7–5). A relatively pure alpha-agonist such as phenylephrine increases peripheral resistance and venous tone. The first effect directly increases blood pressure. A marked slowing of heart rate may result from the baroreceptor reflex thus evoked. However, cardiac output may not diminish in proportion to this slowing, because increased venous return will tend to increase stroke volume. The effects of drugs with both alpha and beta effects (eg, epinephrine and norepinephrine) are discussed below).

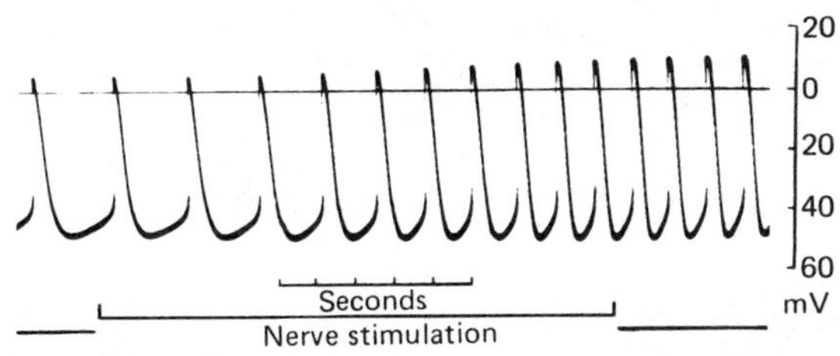

Figure 7–4. Effect on the cardiac pacemaker of sympathetic stimulation releasing catecholamines. Note the increased slope of diastolic depolarization. These effects are typical of β_1-stimulant drugs. (Reproduced, with permission, from Hutter O, Trautwein W: Vagal and sympathetic effects on the pacemaker fibers in the sinus venosus of the heart. *J Gen Physiol* 1956;**39**:715.)

Eye

The radial pupillary dilator muscle of the iris contains alpha receptors; activation by drugs such as phenylephrine causes mydriasis. Alpha and beta stimulants also have important effects on intraocular pressure via poorly understood mechanisms. Beta stimulants relax the ciliary muscle to an insignificant degree, causing a minor decrease in accommodation.

Respiratory Tract

Bronchial smooth muscle contains β_2 receptors that cause relaxation. Activation of these receptors thus results in bronchodilation (Table 7–2 and Chapter 17). The blood vessels of the upper respiratory mucosa contain α receptors; the decongestant action of alpha stimulants is clinically useful (see part II of this chapter).

Gastrointestinal Tract

Relaxation of gastrointestinal smooth muscle can be brought about by both α- and β-stimulant agents. Beta receptors appear to be located directly on the smooth muscle cells and mediate relaxation via hyperpolarization and decreased spike activity in these cells. Alpha stimulants are thought to decrease muscle activity *indirectly* by acting presynaptically to reduce the release of acetylcholine and possibly other stimulants.

Genitourinary Tract

The human uterus contains α and β_2 receptors. The fact that the beta receptors mediate relaxation can be clinically useful in pregnancy (see part II). The bladder base and urethral sphincter contain α receptors that mediate contraction and therefore promote continence. The β_2 receptors of the bladder wall mediate relaxation. Ejaculation is dependent upon normal α-adrenergic activity.

Exocrine Glands

The salivary glands contain adrenergic receptors that regulate the secretion of amylase and water. How-

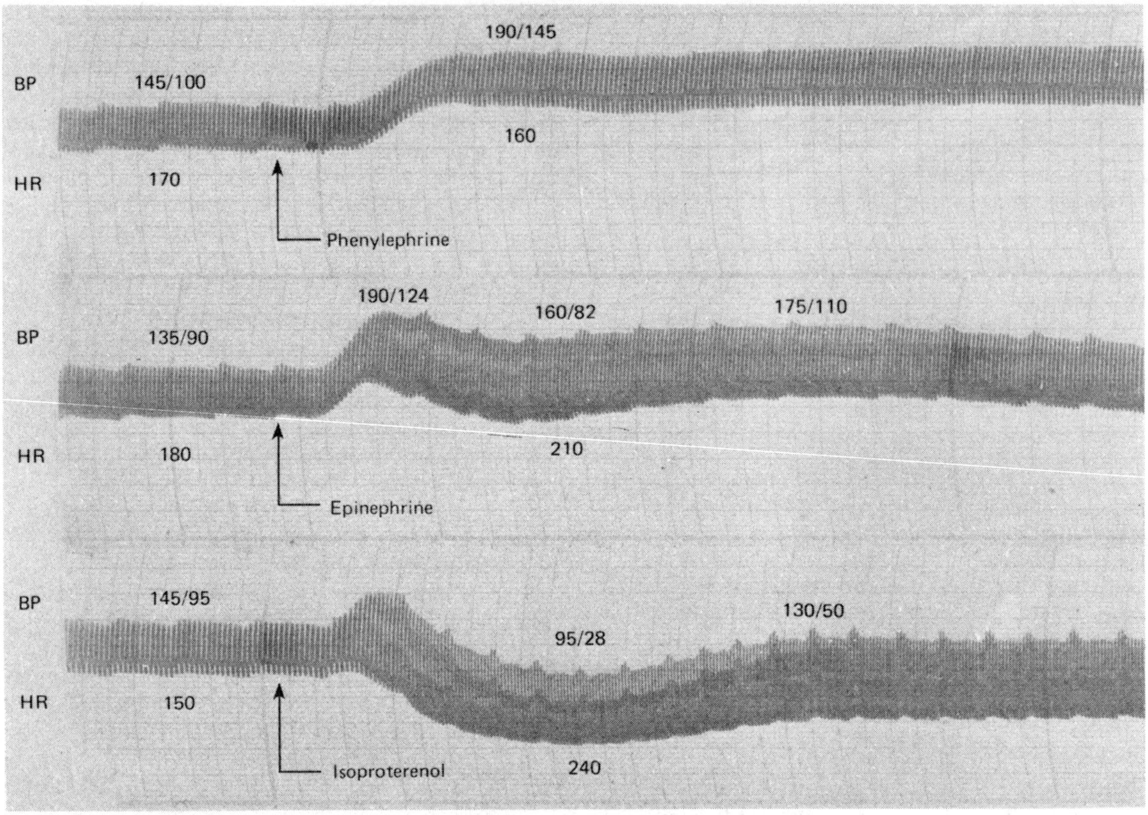

Figure 7–5. Effects of an alpha-selective (phenylephrine), beta-selective (isoproterenol), and nonselective (epinephrine) sympathomimetic, given as an intravenous bolus injection to a dog. (BP = blood pressure; HR = heart rate.) Reflexes are blunted but not eliminated in this anesthetized animal.

ever, certain sympathomimetic drugs—eg, clonidine, an α_2-selective agonist used in the treatment of hypertension—produce symptoms of dry mouth. The mechanism of this effect is uncertain; it is likely that central nervous system effects are responsible, although other (peripheral) effects may contribute.

The apocrine sweat glands, located on the palms of the hands and a few other areas, respond to alpha stimulants with increased sweat production. These are the nonthermoregulatory glands usually associated with psychologic stress. (The diffusely distributed, thermoregulatory eccrine sweat glands are regulated by cholinergic receptors.)

Metabolic Effects

Sympathomimetic drugs have important effects on intermediary metabolism. Activation of β_1-adrenergic receptors in fat cells leads to increased lipolysis. Human lipocytes also contain α_2 receptors that inhibit lipolysis by decreasing intracellular cAMP. Sympathomimetic drugs enhance glycogenolysis in the liver, which leads to increased glucose release into the circulation. In the human liver, the effects of catecholamines are probably mediated by beta receptors, although alpha receptors may also play a role.

Effects on Endocrine Function

Catecholamines are important endogenous regulators of hormone secretion from a number of glands. Insulin secretion is stimulated by beta receptors and inhibited by α_2 receptors. Similarly, renin secretion is stimulated by β and inhibited by α_2 receptors; indeed, beta-receptor antagonist drugs may lower plasma renin at least in part by this mechanism. Adrenergic receptors also regulate the secretion of parathormone, calcitonin, thyroxine, and gastrin; however, the physiologic significance of these control mechanisms is unclear.

SPECIFIC SYMPATHOMIMETIC DRUGS

Catecholamines

Epinephrine is a very potent vasopressor; the mechanism responsible for the rise in systolic blood pressure that occurs after epinephrine release or administration relates to its positive inotropic and chronotropic actions on the heart (predominantly β_1 receptors) and the vasoconstriction induced in many vascular beds (α receptors). Epinephrine also activates β_2 receptors in certain vessels, leading to their dilatation. Consequently, total peripheral resistance may actually fall, explaining the fall in diastolic pressure that is sometimes seen with epinephrine injection (Fig 7–5).

Norepinephrine and epinephrine have similar effects on β_1 receptors in the heart; however, norepinephrine is comparatively less potent at α receptors. More importantly, norepinephrine has relatively little effect on β_2 receptors. Consequently, norepinephrine increases peripheral resistance and both diastolic and systolic blood pressure. Compensatory vagal reflexes tend to overcome the direct positive chronotropic effects of norepinephrine; however, the positive inotropic effects are maintained.

Isoproterenol is an extremely potent beta-receptor agonist, having little effect on alpha receptors. The drug has positive chronotropic and inotropic actions; because isoproterenol activates beta receptors almost exclusively, it is a potent vasodilator. These actions lead to a marked increase in cardiac output associated with a fall in diastolic and mean arterial pressure and a lesser decrease or a slight increase in systolic pressure (Table 7–3; Fig 7–5).

Dopamine, the immediate metabolic precursor of norepinephrine, activates β_1 receptors in the heart. At low doses it has relatively little effect on peripheral resistance. However, at higher rates of infusion, it activates vascular alpha receptors, leading to vasoconstriction. Thus, high concentrations may mimic the actions of epinephrine. More importantly, it dilates renal and splanchnic resistance vessels by activating **dopamine receptors** that are not blocked by α- or β-blocking drugs. Similar dopamine receptors are found in the central nervous system and autonomic ganglia. The effect on renal blood flow is clinically useful. (See Shock in part II.)

Dobutamine is a relatively β_1-selective synthetic catecholamine; it is discussed below.

Other Sympathomimetics

These agents are of interest because of pharmacokinetic features (oral activity, distribution to the central nervous system) or because of relative selectivity for specific receptor subclasses.

Phenylephrine has been described above as an example of a relatively pure α-agonist (Table 7–3; Fig 7–5). It acts directly on the adrenergic receptors. Because it is not a catechol derivative (Fig 7–3), it is not inactivated by COMT and has a much longer duration of action than the catecholamines. It is an effective mydriatic and decongestant and can be used to raise the blood pressure (see part II).

Methoxamine. The pharmacologic actions of methoxamine are similar to those of phenylephrine, since it is predominantly a direct-acting alpha-receptor agonist. It may cause prolonged increase in blood pressure due to vasoconstriction; it also causes a vagally mediated bradycardia. Methoxamine is available for parenteral use; clinical applications are discussed below.

Ephedrine occurs in various plants and has been used in China for over 2000 years; it was introduced into western medicine approximately 60 years ago as the first orally active sympathomimetic drug. Because it is a noncatechol phenylisopropylamine (Fig 7–3), it has high bioavailability and a long duration of action. As is the case with many other phenylisopropylamines, a significant fraction of the drug is excreted unchanged in the urine. Since its pK_a is greater than 9, its excretion can be accelerated by acidification of the urine.

Ephedrine acts primarily through the release of stored catecholamines; in addition, it has some direct actions on adrenergic receptors. It is nonselective and mimics epinephrine in its spectrum of effects. Because it gains access to the central nervous system, it causes a mild amphetaminelike stimulation that is not seen with the catecholamines.

Clinically, ephedrine is utilized when a prolonged duration of effect is desired, particularly after oral administration. The main applications are in asthma, as a nasal decongestant, and as a pressor agent. These uses are discussed in more detail in part II.

Amphetamines. Amphetamine is a phenylisopropylamine (Fig 7–3) that is important because of its use and misuse as a central nervous system stimulant (see Chapter 29). Its pharmacokinetics are similar to those of ephedrine, but amphetamine enters the central nervous system even more readily and has a much more marked stimulant effect on mood and alertness and a depressant effect on appetite. Its peripheral actions are mediated primarily through the release of catecholamines. **Methamphetamine** (N-methylamphetamine) is very similar to amphetamine with an even higher ratio of central to peripheral actions. **Phenmetrazine** (see Fig 29–1) is a variant phenylisopropylamine with amphetaminelike effects. It has been promoted as an anorexiant (see part II) and is also a popular drug of abuse. **Methylphenidate** is an amphetamine variant with major pharmacologic effects and abuse potential similar to those of amphetamine.

Hydroxyamphetamine (4-hydroxyamphetamine) enters the central nervous system very poorly but has peripheral effects by virtue of its ability to release stored catecholamines. Its highly specialized application illustrates how knowledge of a drug's basic mechanism of action can be applied to clinical problems. Horner's syndrome is a condition resulting from interruption of the sympathetic nerves to the face, including the eye, in which it causes miosis. The syndrome can be caused by either preganglionic or postganglionic lesions. Because a postganglionic lesion leads to degeneration of the adrenergic nerve endings and loss of stored catecholamines in the iris, the abnormally constricted pupil in such a case will not dilate in response to an indirect-acting sympathomimetic (hydroxyamphetamine), but it does respond to phenylephrine, which acts directly on the alpha receptors. In contrast, a patient with a preganglionic lesion will show a normal response to both drugs, since the postganglionic fibers remain intact.

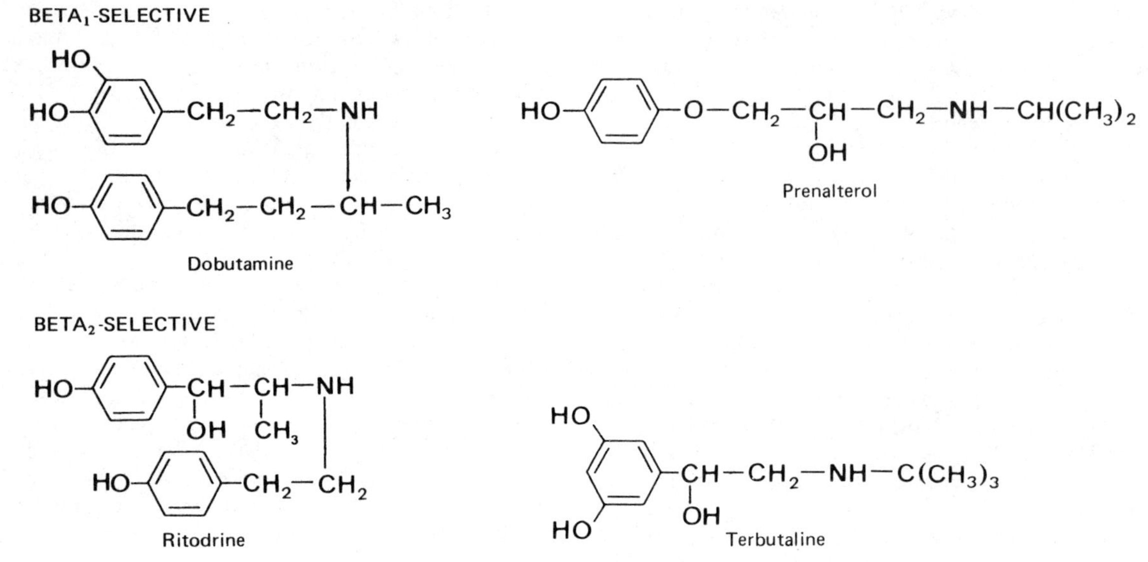

Figure 7–6. Examples of β_1- and β_2-selective agonists.

Receptor-Selective Adrenergic Agonists

Alpha$_2$-selective agonists are used in the treatment of hypertension. Clonidine and methyldopa are discussed in Chapter 9.

Beta-selective agonists have become important because of the separation of β_1 and β_2 effects that has been achieved. Although this separation is incomplete, it is sufficient to reduce side-effects in several clinical applications.

Beta$_1$-selective agents include dobutamine and prenalterol (Fig 7–6). Because they are less effective in activating vasodilator β_2 receptors, they may increase cardiac output with less reflex tachycardia than occurs with nonselective β-agonists such as isoproterenol. These agents are currently under study for the treatment of congestive heart failure and cardiogenic shock (see part II).

Beta$_2$-selective agents have achieved an important place in the treatment of asthma and are discussed in Chapter 17. An additional application is as uterine relaxants in premature labor (ritodrine; see part II). Some examples of drugs currently in use are shown in Figs 7–6 and 17–3; many more are available or under investigation.

Special Sympathomimetics

Cocaine is a local anesthetic with a sympathomimetic action that results from inhibition of transmitter reuptake at noradrenergic synapses (Chapter 4). It readily enters the central nervous system and produces an intense response that has made it a very heavily abused drug (Chapter 29).

Tyramine is a normal byproduct of tyrosine metabolism in the body and is also found in high concentrations in fermented foods such as cheese, beer, and wine. It is readily metabolized by MAO and is normally inactive if ingested. If administered parenterally, it has an indirect sympathomimetic action caused by the release of stored catecholamines. Thus, its spectrum of action is similar to that of norepinephrine. In patients treated with MAO inhibitors—used as antidepressants (see Chapter 27), tyramine may reach the systemic circulation and can be converted to octopamine, a false transmitter, and stored in sympathetic nerve endings (Chapters 5, 9, and 27).

II. CLINICAL PHARMACOLOGY OF ADRENERGIC RECEPTOR-ACTIVATING DRUGS

The rationale for the use of sympathomimetic drugs in therapy rests on a knowledge of the physiologic effects of catecholamines on tissues. Selection of a particular sympathomimetic drug from the host of compounds available depends upon such

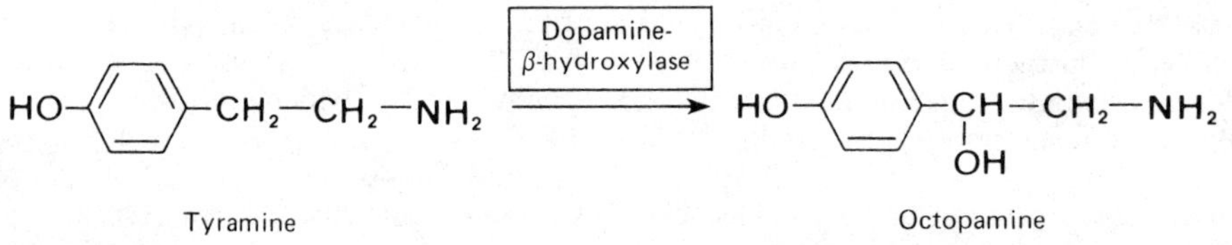

factors as whether activation of α, β_1, or β_2 receptors is desired; the duration of action desired; and the preferred route of administration. The adverse effects of these drugs are generally understandable in terms of their known physiologic effects.

Cardiovascular Applications

A. Conditions in Which Blood Flow or Pressure Is to Be Enhanced: Hypotension may occur in a variety of settings such as volume contraction, cardiac arrhythmias, adverse reactions to medications such as antihypertensive drugs, and infection. If cerebral and cardiac perfusion is maintained, hypotension itself does not usually require vigorous direct treatment. Rather, placing the patient in the recumbent position and ensuring adequate fluids—while the primary problem is determined and treated—is usually the correct course of action. The use of sympathomimetic drugs merely to elevate a blood pressure that is not an immediate threat to the patient may increase morbidity (see p 80). Sympathomimetic drugs may be utilized in a hypotensive emergency to preserve cerebral and coronary blood flow. Such situations might arise in severe hemorrhage, spinal cord injury, or overdose of antihypertensive or central nervous system depressant medications. The treatment is usually of short duration while indicated fluids or blood are being administered. Direct-acting alpha-agonists such as norepinephrine, phenylephrine, or methoxamine can be utilized in this setting if vasoconstriction is desired.

Shock is a complex acute cardiovascular syndrome that results in a critical reduction in perfusion of vital tissues and a wide range of systemic effects. Shock is usually associated with hypotension, an altered mental state, oliguria, and metabolic acidosis. If untreated, shock usually progresses to a refractory deteriorating state and death. The 3 major mechanisms responsible for shock are hypovolemia, cardiac insufficiency, and altered vascular resistance. Volume replacement and treatment of the underlying disease are the mainstays of the treatment of shock. While sympathomimetic drugs have been utilized in virtually all forms of shock, their efficacy is unclear. In most forms of shock, vasoconstriction mediated by the sympathetic nervous system is already intense. Indeed, efforts aimed at reducing rather than increasing peripheral resistance may be more fruitful.

Cardiogenic shock, usually due to massive myocardial infarction, has a poor prognosis. Mechanical perfusion and emergency cardiac surgery have been utilized in some settings. Optimal fluid replacement requires monitoring of pulmonary capillary wedge pressures. Positive inotropic agents such as dopamine or dobutamine may have a role in this situation. In low to moderate doses, these drugs may increase cardiac output and, compared with norepinephrine, cause relatively little peripheral vasoconstriction. Isoproterenol increases heart rate and work more than either dopamine or dobutamine.

Unfortunately, the patient with shock may not respond to general therapeutic maneuvers; the temptation is then great to use vasoconstrictors to maintain adequate blood pressure. While coronary perfusion may be improved, this gain may be offset by increased myocardial oxygen demands as well as more severe vasoconstriction in blood vessels to the abdominal viscera. Therefore, the goal of therapy in shock should be to optimize tissue perfusion, not blood pressure.

B. Conditions in Which Blood Flow Is to Be Reduced: Reduction of regional blood flow is desirable for achieving hemostasis in surgery, for reducing diffusion of local anesthetics away from the site of administration, and for reducing mucous membrane congestion. In each instance, alpha-receptor activation is desired, and the choice of agent depends upon the maximal efficacy required, the desired duration of action, and the route of administration.

Effective pharmacologic hemostasis, often required in facial, oropharyngeal, and nasopharyngeal surgery, requires drugs of high efficacy that can be administered by local application in high concentrations. Epinephrine is usually applied topically in nasal packs (epistaxis) or in a gingival string (gingivectomy). **Cocaine** is still sometimes used for nasopharyngeal surgery, because it combines a hemostatic effect with local anesthesia.

Combining alpha-agonists with local anesthetics greatly prolongs the duration of infiltration nerve block; the total dose (and the probability of toxicity) can therefore be reduced. **Epinephrine,** 1:200,000, is the favored agent for this application. It should *not* be combined with local anesthetics used for *spinal* anesthesia.

Mucous membrane decongestants reduce the discomfort of hay fever and, to a lesser extent, the common cold. Unfortunately, rebound hyperemia may follow the use of these agents, and repeated topical use of high concentrations may result in ischemic changes in the mucous membrane. Favored topical agents include phenylephrine and phenylpropanolamine in nasal sprays and ophthalmic drops. A longer duration of action, at the cost of much lower local concentrations and greater cardiac and central nervous system effects, can be achieved by the oral administration of agents such as ephedrine or one of its isomers, pseudoephedrine.

C. Cardiac Applications: Episodes of **paroxysmal atrial tachycardia** may be treated with alpha receptor-activating drugs such as phenylephrine or methoxamine. These drugs cause marked vasoconstriction, leading to a rise in blood pressure; the rise in blood pressure promotes a reflex vagal discharge that may convert the arrhythmia to sinus rhythm. The drugs should be given by slow intravenous infusion; caution must be utilized to prevent a dangerous rise in systolic blood pressure to greater than about 160 mm Hg. While these drugs are often effective in terminating this rhythm disturbance in patients who are hypotensive, generally safer alternatives may exist, such as the use of verapamil or edrophonium.

Catecholamines such as isoproterenol and epinephrine have also been utilized in the temporary emergency management of **complete heart block** and **cardiac arrest.** However, electronic pacemakers are both safer and more effective in heart block and should be inserted as soon as possible if there is any indication of continued high-degree block.

Congestive heart failure may respond to the positive inotropic effects of drugs such as dobutamine and prenalterol. Good results have also been reported following the use of β_2-selective agents used to reduce afterload by decreasing vascular resistance. These applications are discussed in Chapter 11.

Respiratory Applications

One of the most important uses of sympathomimetic drugs is in the therapy of bronchial asthma. This use is discussed in Chapter 17.

Anaphylaxis

Anaphylactic shock and related acute hypersensitivity reactions affect both the respiratory and the cardiovascular systems. The syndrome of bronchospasm, mucous membrane congestion, angioedema, and cardiovascular collapse usually responds rapidly to subcutaneous administration of **epinephrine,** 0.3–0.5 mg (0.3–0.5 mL of 1:1000 epinephrine solution). This drug is the agent of choice because of its great efficacy at α, β_1, and β_2 receptors; stimulation of all of these is helpful in reversing the pathophysiologic process. Glucocorticoids and antihistamines may occasionally be useful as secondary therapy in anaphylaxis; however, epinephrine is the initial treatment.

Ophthalmic Applications

Phenylephrine is an effective mydriatic agent frequently used to facilitate examination of the retina. It is also a useful decongestant for minor allergic hyperemia of the conjunctival membranes. The diagnostic use of hydroxyamphetamine has been described above.

Glaucoma responds to a variety of sympathomimetic and sympathoplegic drugs. **Epinephrine** and beta-blocking agents are among the most important therapies. Topical epinephrine (1–2% solution) lowers intraocular pressure apparently both by decreasing aqueous humor formation and by increasing aqueous outflow.

Genitourinary Applications

As noted above, β_2-selective agents relax the pregnant uterus. **Ritodrine, terbutaline,** and similar drugs have been used to suppress premature labor. In spite of some β_1 effects (tachycardia, arrhythmias), they seem to be superior to ethanol and can be used chronically if the initial response is favorable.

Central Nervous System Applications

The amphetaminelike sympathomimetics have a mood-elevating (euphoriant) effect; this effect is also the basis for the widespread abuse of this subgroup. The amphetamines also have an alerting, sleep-deferring action that is manifested by improved attention to repetitive tasks and by acceleration and desynchronization of the EEG. A therapeutic application of this effect is in the treatment of narcolepsy. The anorexiant effect of these agents is easily demonstrated in experimental animals. In obese humans, although an encouraging initial response may be observed, it is generally agreed that no long-term improvement in weight control can be achieved with amphetamines alone. A final application of the CNS-active sympathomimetics is in the **hyperkinetic syndrome** of children, a poorly defined and overdiagnosed behavioral syndrome consisting of short attention span, hyperkinetic physical behavior, and learning problems. Some patients with this syndrome respond well to low doses of the amphetaminelike drugs.

TOXICITY OF SYMPATHOMIMETIC DRUGS

The adverse effects of adrenergic agonists are primarily extensions of their receptor effects in the cardiovascular and central nervous systems.

Adverse cardiovascular effects seen with pressor agents include marked elevations in blood pressure, which may cause cerebral hemorrhage. Increased cardiac work may precipitate severe angina or myocardial infarction. Beta-stimulant drugs frequently cause tachycardia and, more significantly, may provoke serious ventricular arrhythmias. Sympathomimetic drugs may lead to myocardial damage, particularly after prolonged infusion. Special caution is indicated in elderly patients or those with hypertension or coronary artery disease. If an adverse effect requires urgent reversal, then a specific adrenergic antagonist should be used (see Chapter 8). For example, extravasation into subcutaneous tissues of norepinephrine being given by the intravenous route may lead to marked ischemia that can be reversed by alpha-adrenergic antagonists.

Central nervous system toxicity is rarely observed with catecholamines or drugs such as phenylephrine. Phenylisopropylamines commonly cause restlessness, tremor, insomnia, and anxiety. In very high doses, a paranoid state may be induced. Therapy is discussed in Chapter 29.

• • •

References

Day MD: *Autonomic Pharmacology*. Churchill Livingstone, 1979.

Goldberg LI: Dopamine: Clinical uses of an endogenous catecholamine. *N Engl J Med* 1974;**291:**707.

Himms-Hagen J: Sympathetic regulation of metabolism. *Pharmacol Rev* 1967;**19:**367.

Hoffman BB, Lefkowitz RJ: Alpha-adrenergic receptor subtypes. *N Engl J Med* 1980;**302:**1390.

Langer SZ: Presynaptic receptors and modulation of neurotransmission: Pharmacologic implications and therapeutic relevance. *Trends Neurosci* 1980;**3:**110.

Langer SZ: Presynaptic regulation of the release of catecholamines. *Pharmacol Rev* 1980;**32:**337.

Melmon KL: The endocrinologic function of selected autacoids: Catecholamines, acetylcholine, serotonin and histamine. Pages 515–588 in: *Textbook of Endocrinology*. Williams RH (editor). Saunders, 1981.

Minneman KP, Pittman RN, Molinoff PB: β-Adrenergic receptor subtypes: Properties, distribution, and regulation. *Annu Rev Neurosci* 1981;**4:**419.

Tarazi RC: Sympathomimetic agents in the treatment of shock. *Ann Intern Med* 1974;**81:**364.

Wurtman RJ: Catecholamines. (3 parts.) *N Engl J Med* 1965;**273:**637, 693, 746.

8 | Adrenergic Receptor–Blocking Drugs

Brian B. Hoffman, MD

Since catecholamines play a role in a variety of important physiologic responses, drugs that antagonize adrenergic receptors have obvious pharmacologic applications. The classification of adrenergic receptors into alpha and beta types has been discussed in Chapter 7. The present chapter deals with drugs whose major effect is to antagonize the action of catecholamines by occupying either alpha or beta receptors, thus preventing their activation by the catecholamines.

In general, alpha-adrenergic blocking drugs have been very useful in the experimental exploration of autonomic nervous system function; surprisingly, they have thus far had only limited clinical application. Even though these drugs effectively block the vasoconstricting effect of catecholamines, their use in hypertension—with the exception of prazosin—has been of little consequence. The place of alpha-adrenergic antagonists in the treatment of peripheral vascular disease is uncertain. In contrast, the beta receptor-blocking drugs have been found useful in a wide variety of clinical conditions.

I. BASIC PHARMACOLOGY OF ADRENERGIC RECEPTOR–BLOCKING DRUGS

ALPHA RECEPTOR–BLOCKING AGENTS

Alpha-receptor antagonists may be classified into 2 general categories: reversible and irreversible. Reversible antagonists may dissociate from the alpha receptor; irreversible drugs do not. Phentolamine and tolazoline are examples of reversible antagonists (Fig 8–1). Prazosin and labetalol, drugs used primarily for their antihypertensive effects, as well as several ergot derivatives (Chapter 14), are also reversible alpha-adrenergic blockers. Phenoxybenzamine, an agent related to the nitrogen mustards, forms a reactive ethyleneimonium intermediate (Fig 8–1) that covalently binds to the alpha-receptor site, resulting in irreversible blockade. Fig 8–2 illustrates the effects of a reversible drug in comparison with those of an irreversible agent.

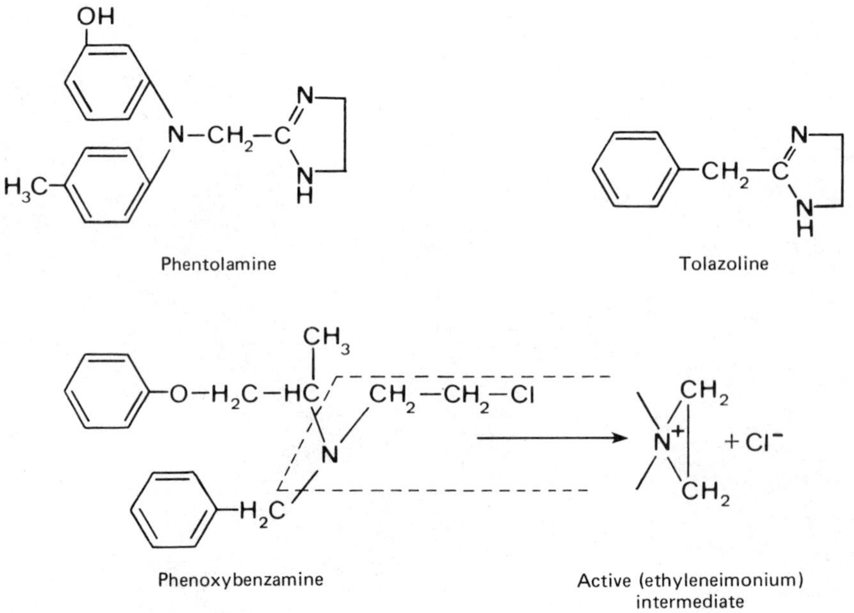

Figure 8–1. Structure of several alpha-adrenergic blocking drugs.

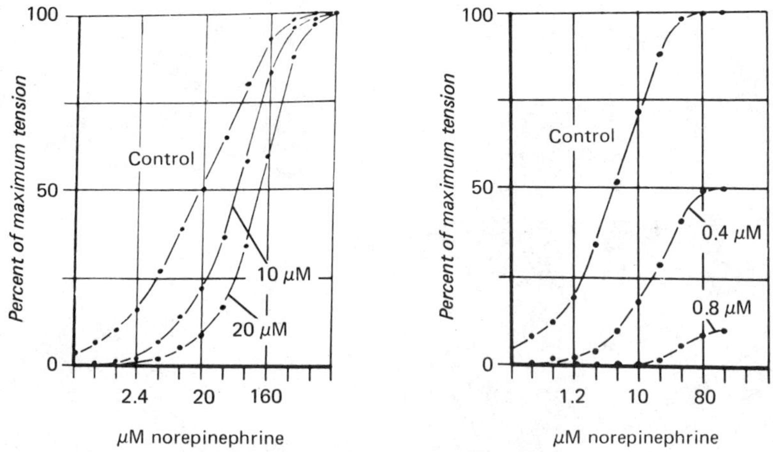

Figure 8–2. Dose-response curves to norepinephrine in the presence of 2 different α-adrenergic receptor-blocking drugs. The tension produced in isolated strips of cat spleen, a tissue rich in alpha receptors, was measured in response to graded doses of norepinephrine. ***Left:*** Tolazoline, a reversible blocker, shifted the curve to the right without decreasing the maximum response when present at concentrations of 10 and 20 μM. ***Right:*** Dibenamine, an analog of phenoxybenzamine and irreversible in its action, reduced the maximum response attainable at both concentrations tested. (Modified and reproduced, with permission, from Bickerton RK: The response of isolated strips of cat spleen to sympathomimetic drugs and their antagonists. *J Pharmacol Exp Ther* 1963; **142**:99.)

Pharmacologic Effects

A. Cardiovascular Effects: Because arteriolar and venous tone are determined to a large extent by alpha-adrenergic receptors on vascular smooth muscle, alpha-adrenergic blocking drugs cause a lowering of peripheral vascular resistance and blood pressure (Fig 8–3). They can prevent the pressor effects of usual doses of alpha-agonists; indeed, in the case of agonists with both α and β_2 effects (eg, epinephrine), they convert a pressor to a depressor response (Fig 8–3). This change in response is called **epinephrine reversal.** By inhibiting adrenergic-mediated venoconstriction, alpha-blockers may cause postural hypotension and reflex tachycardia. Tachycardia may be more marked with agents that block α_2 presynaptic receptors in the heart (Table 8–1), since the augmented release of norepinephrine will further stimulate beta receptors in the heart. Chronic use of alpha-antagonists may result in a compensatory increase in blood volume.

B. Other Effects: Minor effects that signal the blockade of alpha receptors in other tissues include reduced pupillary dilator tone, decreased adrenergic sweating, and nasal stuffiness. However, individual agents may have additional non-alpha-blocking effects that are far more important (see below).

Table 8–1. Relative selectivity of antagonists for adrenergic receptors.

	Receptor
Alpha-antagonists	
Prazosin, phenoxybenzamine	α_1-selective*
Phentolamine	$\alpha_1 = \alpha_2$
Yohimbine, tolazoline	α_2-selective*
Beta-antagonists	
Metoprolol, acebutalol, alprenolol, atenolol	β_1-selective*
Propranolol, timolol, nadolol, pindolol	$\beta_1 = \beta_2$
Butoxamine	β_2-selective*

*Selective means a *relatively higher* affinity for this receptor.

SPECIFIC AGENTS

Phentolamine, an imidazoline derivative, is a potent competitive antagonist of alpha receptors. Phentolamine causes a reduction in peripheral resistance, through both alpha-receptor blockade and an additional nonadrenergic action on vascular smooth muscle. The cardiac stimulation induced by phentolamine may be in part reflex; however, a component of this stimulation is not dependent on baroreceptor activity. Alpha$_2$-receptor blockade may be involved. Phentolamine is about equally potent at α_1 and α_2 receptors. Phentolamine also inhibits responses to serotonin. Phentolamine is an agonist at muscarinic and H_1 and H_2 histamine receptors.

Phentolamine is poorly absorbed after oral administration. The principal adverse effects are related to cardiac stimulation, which may cause severe tachycardia, arrhythmias, and angina. Gastrointestinal stimulation may cause diarrhea and increased gastric acid production.

Tolazoline is similar to phentolamine. It is somewhat less potent, but better absorbed from the gastrointestinal tract. It is rapidly excreted in the urine.

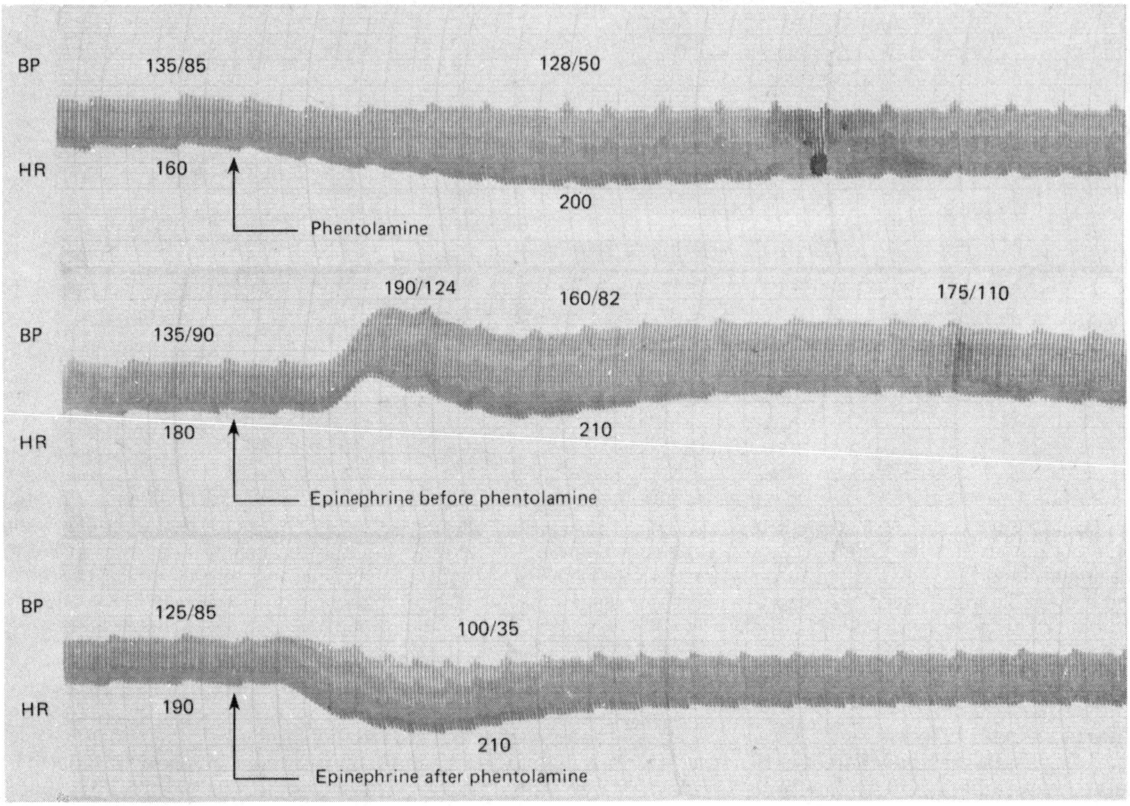

Figure 8–3. *Top:* Effects of phentolamine, an α-adrenergic blocking drug, on blood pressure in an anesthetized dog. Epinephrine "reversal" is demonstrated by tracings showing the response to epinephrine before *(middle)* and after *(bottom)* phentolamine. All drugs given intravenously. (BP = blood pressure; HR = heart rate.)

Tolazoline has limited clinical applications in peripheral vasospastic disease and in the treatment of pulmonary hypertension in newborn infants with respiratory distress syndrome.

Ergot derivatives—eg, ergotamine, dihydroergotamine—cause reversible alpha-receptor blockade. However, most of the clinically significant effects of these drugs are the result of other actions (Chapter 14).

Phenoxybenzamine, because it binds covalently to alpha receptors, causes irreversible blockade of long duration (14–48 hours). It is somewhat selective for α_1 receptors, but less so than prazosin. The drug inhibits reuptake of released norepinephrine by presynaptic adrenergic nerve terminals. Phenoxybenzamine blocks histamine (H_1), acetylcholine, and serotonin receptors as well as alpha receptors. Its clinical application is mainly in the treatment of pheochromocytoma.

The pharmacologic actions of phenoxybenzamine are primarily related to antagonism of alpha receptor-mediated events. Most importantly, phenoxybenzamine blocks adrenergic vasoconstriction. While phenoxybenzamine causes relatively little fall in blood pressure in supine individuals, it will reduce blood pressurr when sympathetic tone is high, eg, as a result of upright posture or because of reduced blood volume. Cardiac output may be increased because of reflex effects and because of presynaptic effects on cardiac sympathetic nerves.

Phenoxybenzamine is absorbed after oral administration, though bioavailability is low. It may be used intravenously but not by other parenteral routes, because it is too irritating. The drug is usually given orally, starting with low doses of 10–20 mg/d and progressively increasing the dose until the desired effect is achieved. Less than 100 mg/d is usually sufficient to achieve adequate alpha-receptor blockade.

The adverse effects of phenoxybenzamine derive from its alpha receptor-blocking action; the most important are postural hypotension and tachycardia. Nasal stuffiness and inhibition of ejaculation also occur. Since phenoxybenzamine enters the central nervous system, it may cause less specific effects, including fatigue, sedation, and nausea.

Prazosin is a relatively new drug effective in the management of hypertension (Chapter 9). It was originally thought to be a direct-acting vasodilator, but it is now clear that the major pharmacologic action of prazosin is that of an extremely potent alpha-receptor antagonist. It is highly selective for α_1 receptors, having relatively low affinity for α_2 receptors. This may partially explain the relative absence of tachycardia seen with prazosin compared to phentolamine and phenoxybenzamine. Prazosin leads to relaxation of both arterial and venous smooth muscle.

Prazosin is extensively metabolized in humans; because of metabolic degradation by the liver, only about 50% of the drug is available after oral administration. The half-life is normally about 3 hours.

OTHER ALPHA-ADRENERGIC RECEPTOR ANTAGONISTS

Other alpha-blockers include **yohimbine** (α_2-selective) and **trimazosin** (similar to prazosin but less potent). While yohimbine does not have an established clinical role, theoretically it could be useful in autonomic insufficiency by promoting neurotransmitter release by presynaptic blockade of α_2 receptors. Neuroleptic drugs such as chlorpromazine and haloperidol are potent alpha-receptor antagonists. While not used clinically to block alpha receptors, this action may contribute to the adverse effects of these drugs (eg, hypotension).

BETA RECEPTOR–BLOCKING DRUGS

Drugs in this category share the common feature of antagonizing the effects of catecholamines at beta-adrenergic receptors. Beta-blocking drugs occupy

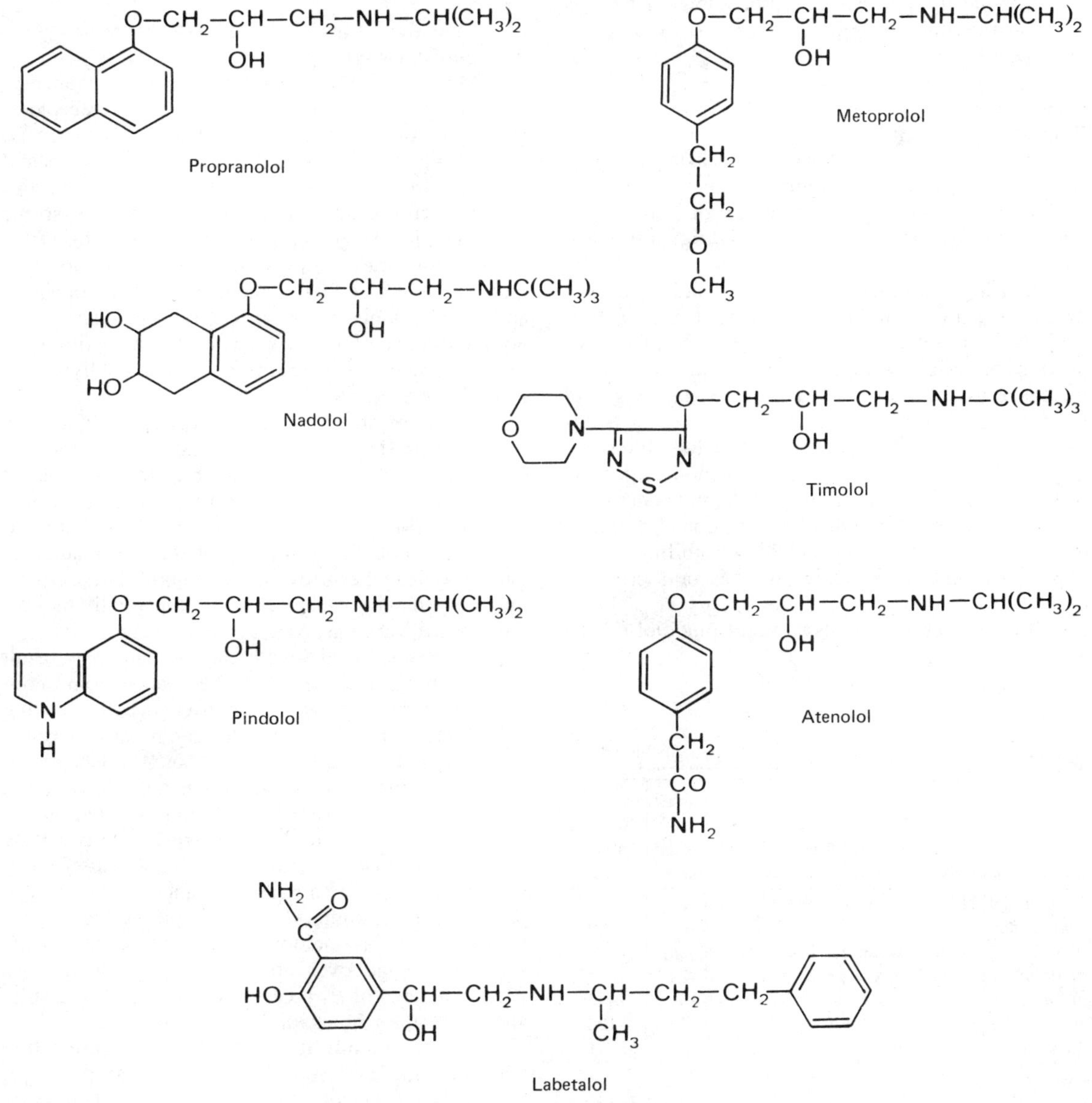

Figure 8–4. Structures of some beta-receptor antagonists.

beta-adrenergic receptors and competitively reduce receptor occupancy by catecholamines and other beta-agonists. Most beta-adrenergic blocking drugs in clinical use are pure antagonists; ie, the occupancy of a beta receptor by such a drug causes no activation of the receptor. However, certain beta receptor-blocking drugs cause partial activation of the receptor, albeit less than the full agonists epinephrine and norepinephrine. Another major difference among the many beta receptor-blocking drugs relates to their relative affinities at β_1 and β_2 receptors. Some of these antagonists have a higher affinity for β_1 than for β_2 receptors, and this selectivity for β_1 receptors may have important clinical implications. Other major differences among beta-antagonists relate to their pharmacokinetic characteristics and nonspecific membrane-stabilizing effects.

Chemically, the beta-receptor antagonist drugs (Fig 8–4) resemble isoproterenol (Fig 7–2), a potent beta-receptor agonist.

Pharmacokinetic Properties of the Beta-Receptor Antagonists

A. Absorption: Most of the drugs in this class are well absorbed after oral administration; peak concentrations occur 1–3 hours after ingestion. Sustained-release preparations of some of the drugs are available.

B. Bioavailability: Propranolol undergoes extensive hepatic (''first-pass'') metabolism; its bioavailability is relatively low (Table 8–2). The proportion of drug reaching the systemic circulation increases as the dose is increased, suggesting that hepatic extraction mechanisms may become saturated. A major consequence of the low bioavailability of propranolol is that intravenous injection of the drug leads to much higher drug concentrations than are achieved after oral administration of the same dose. There is great individual variability in the plasma concentrations achieved after oral propranolol. Bioavailability is limited to varying degrees for all of the beta-antagonists except pindolol (Table 8–2).

Table 8–2. Properties of several beta-adrenergic blocking drugs.

	Selectivity	Partial Agonist Activity	Local Anesthetic Activity	Elimination Half-Life (hours)	Bioavailability (percent)
Propranolol	None	None	+++	3.5–6	~30*
Metoprolol	β_1	None	+	3–4	50
Timolol	None	None	None	4–5	50
Nadolol	None	None	None	14–24	33
Atenolol	β_1	None	None	6–9	40
Pindolol	None	++	+	3–4	100
Labetalol	None	None	+	5	†

*Bioavailability is dose-dependent.

†Few data available, but bioavailability is low and dose-dependent.

C. Distribution and Clearance: The beta-antagonists are rapidly distributed and have large volumes of distribution. Propranolol crosses the blood-brain barrier. Most beta-antagonists are rapidly eliminated, with half-lives in the range of 2–5 hours. Propranolol and metoprolol are extensively metabolized in the liver, with little unchanged drug appearing in the urine. Pindolol and atenolol are less completely metabolized. Nadolol is excreted unchanged in the urine and has the longest half-life of any available beta-blocker (up to 24 hours). Nadolol's half-life is prolonged in renal failure. The elimination of drugs such as propranolol may be prolonged in the presence of liver disease, diminished hepatic blood flow, or hepatic enzyme inhibition. It is notable that the clinical effects of these drugs are often prolonged well beyond the time predicted from half-life data.

Pharmacodynamics of the Beta-Adrenergic Antagonist Drugs

Most of the effects of these drugs are related to occupancy and blockade of beta-adrenergic receptors. However, some actions may be related to other effects, including partial agonist activity at beta receptors and local anesthetic action.

A. Effects on the Cardiovascular System: Beta-blocking drugs *lower* blood pressure. This effect is the result of several factors, some of them not fully understood. These factors include effects on the heart and blood vessels, the renin-angiotensin system, and possibly the central nervous system. The action is of major clinical importance in the treatment of hypertension (Chapter 9).

Beta-receptor antagonists have prominent effects on the heart (Fig 8–5). The negative inotropic and chronotropic effects are predictable from the role of adrenergic receptors in regulating these functions. Slowed atrioventricular conduction with increased P–R interval on the ECG is a related result of adrenergic blockade in the atrioventricular node. These effects may be clinically valuable but are potentially hazardous. In the vascular system, beta-receptor blockade opposes β_2-mediated vasodilatation. This may result initially in a rise in peripheral resistance from unopposed alpha receptor-mediated effects. Beta-blocking drugs antagonize the release of renin caused by the sympathetic nervous system. As noted in Chapter 9, the relation between the effects on renin release and those on blood pressure is still being debated.

B. Effects on the Respiratory Tract: Blockade of the β_2 receptors in bronchial smooth muscle may lead to an increase in airway resistance, particularly in patients with asthma. $Beta_1$ receptor-selective antagonists such as metoprolol or atenolol may have some advantage over nonselective beta-antagonists when blockade of β_1 receptors in the heart is desired and β_2-receptor blockade is undesirable.

C. Effects on the Eye: Several nonselective beta-blocking agents reduce intraocular pressure, especially in glaucomatous eyes. The mechanism of this action is poorly understood. Because of in-

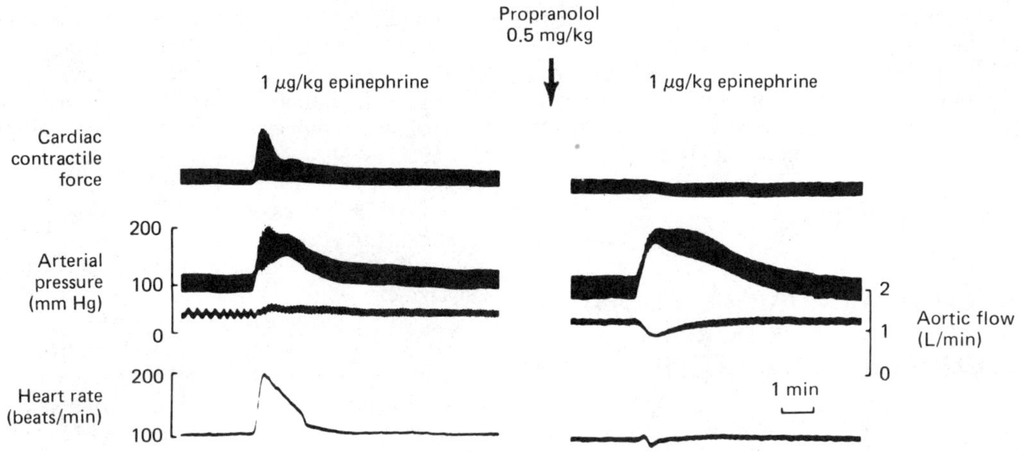

Figure 8–5. The effect in an anesthetized dog of the injection of epinephrine before and after propranolol. In the presence of a beta receptor-blocking agent, epinephrine no longer augments the force of contraction (measured by a strain gauge attached to the ventricular wall) nor increases cardiac rate. Blood pressure is still elevated by epinephrine because vasoconstriction is not blocked. (Reproduced, with permission, from Shanks RG: The pharmacology of beta sympathetic blockade. *Am J Cardiol* 1966;**18**:312.)

terspecies differences and differences in technique, many of the experimental data cannot be explained on the basis of a single mechanism of action. The mechanism usually reported is decreased aqueous humor production, but increased outflow has also been described. The site of action is also controversial, since unilateral topical application of a beta-antagonist may result in significant lowering of pressure in both eyes.

D. Metabolic and Endocrine Effects: Beta-antagonists such as propranolol inhibit sympathetic nervous system stimulation of lipolysis. The effects on carbohydrate metabolism are less clear, although glycogenolysis in the liver is at least partially inhibited after beta blockade. However, glucagon is the primary counterregulatory hormone employed to combat hypoglycemia. It is unclear to what extent beta-antagonists impair recovery from hypoglycemia, although caution is advised about their use in insulin-dependent diabetics. This may be particularly important in diabetics with inadequate glucagon reserve.

E. Effects Not Related to Beta Blockade: Partial beta-agonist activity was significant in the first beta-blocking drug synthesized, dichloroisoproterenol. It has been suggested that retention of some intrinsic sympathomimetic activity is desirable to prevent untoward effects such as precipitation of asthma. One of the currently available drugs, pindolol, is a partial beta-agonist. It is not yet clear whether partial agonism is clinically valuable.

Local anesthetic action, also known as "membrane-stabilizing" action, is a prominent effect of several beta-blockers. This action is the result of typical local anesthetic blockade of sodium channels and can be demonstrated in neurons, heart muscle, and skeletal muscle membrane. However, it is unlikely that these effects are important after systemic administration, since the concentration usually achieved by that route is too low for the anesthetic effects to be very evident.

SPECIFIC AGENTS
(See Table 8–2.)

Propranolol is the prototype beta-blocking drug. The spectrum of its actions shown in Table 8–2 is most remarkable for the degree of local anesthetic effect. In fact, propranolol is as potent as procaine in blocking nerve action potentials. It is also remarkable for its low and dose-dependent bioavailability, the result of extensive first-pass metabolism in the liver.

Metoprolol and atenolol are representatives of the β_1-selective group of drugs. As noted in part II of this chapter, these agents may be safer in patients who experience severe bronchoconstrictive responses to propranolol.

Nadolol is unusual because of its very long duration of action; its spectrum of action is similar to that of timolol.

Timolol is a nonselective agent with no local anesthetic activity. It has excellent ocular hypotensive effects.

Pindolol is of interest because it has considerable beta-agonist activity. Nevertheless, it is effective in the major cardiovascular applications of the beta-blocking group (hypertension and angina).

Selective β_2-blocking drugs have not been actively sought because there is no obvious clinical application for them. An agent reported to possess some selectivity for the β_2 receptors is butoxamine.

Labetalol is a reversible adrenoreceptor antagonist with affinity for both alpha and beta receptors.

Its affinity for alpha receptors is less than that of phentolamine, but labetalol is α_1-selective. Its nonselective beta-blocking potency is somewhat less than that of propranolol. Hypotension induced by this agent is accompanied by less tachycardia than occurs with phentolamine and similar alpha-blockers.

II. CLINICAL PHARMACOLOGY OF THE ADRENERGIC RECEPTOR–BLOCKING DRUGS

As noted above, the alpha-receptor antagonists have limited clinical applications. The best-defined of these uses are described below. The toxic effects of the alpha-receptor blockers were descrbed in part I of this chapter. In contrast, the applications of beta-receptor-blocking agents are many; a more detailed discussion of these uses and the toxicity associated with clinical use follows here.

APPLICATIONS OF THE ALPHA RECEPTOR–BLOCKING DRUGS

Pheochromocytoma

The major clinical use of both phenoxybenzamine and phentolamine is in the management of pheochromocytoma. Pheochromocytoma is a tumor usually found in the adrenal medulla that releases a mixture of epinephrine and norepinephrine. Patients have many signs of catecholamine excess, including hypertension, tachycardia, and arrhythmias.

The diagnosis of pheochromocytoma is usually made on the basis of chemical assay of circulating catecholamines and urinary excretion of catecholamine metabolites, especially 3-hydroxy-4-methoxymandelic acid, metanephrine, and normetanephrine. Infusion of phentolamine has been advocated as a diagnostic test in patients suspected of harboring a pheochromocytoma, since patients with this tumor often manifest a greater-than-average drop in blood pressure in response to alpha-blocking drugs. However, measurement of circulating catecholamines and of urinary catecholamines and their metabolites is a more reliable and safer diagnostic approach. Provocative testing for pheochromocytoma by infusion of drugs such as histamine may cause dangerous blood pressure elevation if performed improperly. Unavoidable release of stored catecholamines sometimes occurs during operative manipulation of pheochromocytoma; the resulting hypertension may be controlled with phentolamine or nitroprusside.

Alpha-receptor antagonists are also useful in the preoperative management of patients with pheochromocytoma. Administration of phenoxybenzamine in the preoperative period will prevent precipitation of acute hypertensive episodes during studies undertaken to localize the tumor and will tend to reverse chronic changes resulting from excessive catecholamine secretion such as plasma volume contraction, if present. Furthermore, the patient's operative course may be simplified. Oral doses of 10–20 mg/d may be increased at intervals of several days until hypertension is controlled. Some physicians prefer to treat pheochromocytoma patients with phenoxybenzamine for many weeks before surgery, whereas others operate sooner. Beta-blocking drugs may be required after alpha-receptor blockade has been instituted to reverse the cardiac effects of excessive catecholamines. Beta-antagonists should not be employed prior to establishing effective alpha-receptor blockade, since unopposed beta-receptor blockade can cause blood pressure elevation from increased vasoconstriction. Phenoxybenzamine may be very useful in the chronic treatment of patients with inoperable or metastatic pheochromocytoma.

Hypertensive Emergencies

The alpha-adrenergic blocking drugs have limited application in the management of hypertensive emergencies. They are most useful when increased blood pressure reflects excess circulating levels of alpha-agonist agents. Phentolamine can be used to control blood pressure in this circumstance, which may result from pheochromocytoma, overdosage of sympathomimetic drugs, or clonidine withdrawal. However, other drugs are generally preferable (Chapter 9).

Peripheral Vascular Disease

Although many alpha receptor-blocking drugs have been tried for treatment of peripheral vascular occlusive disease, there is no evidence that the effects are significant when morphologic changes limit flow in the vessels. Occasionally, individuals with Raynaud's syndrome and other conditions involving excessive reversible vasospasm in the peripheral circulation do receive significant benefit from phentolamine, tolazoline, or phenoxybenzamine.

Local Vasoconstrictor Excess

Phentolamine is also useful to reverse the intense local vasoconstriction caused by inadvertent infiltration of alpha-agonists into subcutaneous tissue during intravenous administration. The alpha-antagonist is administered by local infiltration into the ischemic tissue.

APPLICATIONS OF THE BETA RECEPTOR–BLOCKING DRUGS

Hypertension

Many of the beta-adrenergic drugs have proved to be effective and well tolerated in hypertension. While many hypertensive patients will respond to a beta-blocker used alone, the drug is most often used with either a diuretic or vasodilator (Chapter 9). In spite of the short half-life of many beta-antagonists, these drugs may be administered once or twice daily and still have an adequate therapeutic effect. Labetalol, a competitive alpha- and beta-antagonist, is effective in hypertension, although its ultimate role is yet to be determined.

Ischemic Heart Disease

Beta-adrenergic blockers reduce the frequency of anginal episodes and improve exercise tolerance in many patients with angina (Chapter 10). These actions relate to the blockade of cardiac beta receptors, resulting in decreased cardiac work and reduction in oxygen demand. Recent large-scale prospective studies indicate that the long-term use of timolol, propranolol, or metoprolol in patients who have had acute myocardial infarction may prolong survival. Studies in experimental animals suggest that use of beta-receptor antagonists during the acute phase of a myocardial infarction may limit infarct size. Preservation of ischemic myocardium in humans has not been convincingly demonstrated.

Cardiac Arrhythmias

Beta-antagonists are effective in the treatment of both supraventricular and ventricular arrhythmias (Chapter 12). In cases of sinus tachycardia and supraventricular ectopic beats, the underlying disease should be treated rather than merely using a beta-antagonist. By increasing the atrioventricular nodal refractory period, beta-antagonists will slow ventricular response rates in atrial flutter and fibrillation. These drugs can also reduce ventricular ectopic beats, particularly if the ectopic activity has been precipitated by catecholamines.

Other Cardiovascular Disorders

Beta-receptor antagonists have been found to increase stroke volume in some patients with obstruction cardiomyopathy. This beneficial effect is thought to result from the slowing of ventricular ejection and decreased outflow resistance.

Glaucoma

Systemic administration of beta-blocking drugs was found serendipitously to reduce intraocular pressure in patients with glaucoma. Subsequently, it was found that topical administration also reduces intraocular pressure. Timolol has been favored for local use in the eye, because it lacks local anesthetic properties and is a pure antagonist. The mechanism by which timolol suppresses intraocular pressure is unclear, but it may relate to decreased production of aqueous humor. Timolol appears to have an efficacy comparable to that of epinephrine or pilocarpine in open-angle glaucoma. While the maximal daily dose applied locally (1 mg) is small compared with the systemic doses commonly used in the treatment of hypertension or angina (10–60 mg), sufficient timolol may be absorbed from the eye to cause serious adverse effects on the heart and airways in susceptible individuals.

Hyperthyroidism

Adrenergic excess is an important aspect of the pathophysiology of hyperthyroidism (Chapter 36), especially in relation to the heart. The beta-antagonists have salutary effects in this condition. The beneficial effects presumably relate to adrenergic blockade and inhibition of peripheral conversion of thyroxine to triiodothyronine. The latter action may vary from one beta-antagonist to another. Propranolol is particularly efficacious in thyroid storm; it has been used cautiously in patients with this condition to control supraventricular tachycardias that often precipitate congestive heart failure.

Neurologic Diseases

Several studies suggest a beneficial effect of propranolol in reducing the frequency and intensity of migraine headache. The mechanism is not known. Since adrenergic stimulation may enhance certain tremors, it is not surprising that beta-antagonists have been found to reduce a variety of tremors. The somatic manifestations of anxiety may dramatically respond to low doses of propranolol, particularly when taken prophylactically. Propranolol is also of benefit in treating alcohol withdrawal.

Schizophrenia and the central nervous system manifestations of acute porphyria have also been reported to be alleviated by propranolol. However, most of the evidence for these effects is anecdotal.

CHOICE OF A BETA-BLOCKING DRUG

Propranolol is the standard against which all newer beta-antagonists promoted for systemic use should be measured. In many years of very wide use, it has proved to be a safe and effective drug for many indications. It is not clear that any of the newer beta-receptor blockers are superior to propranolol except in patients with significant asthma, who may be better managed with the β_1-selective agents metoprolol and atenolol. However, since the selectivity demonstrated by these drugs is far from complete, the risk of worsening airway obstruction is still significant. Since it is possible that some actions of a "beta-receptor antagonist" may relate to some other effect of the drug, these drugs should not be considered interchangeable for all applications. For example, only beta-antagonists known to be effective in hyperthyroidism or in prophylactic therapy after myocardial infarction should be used for those indications. It is possible that the beneficial effects of one drug in these settings might not be shared by another drug in the same class. The possible advantages and disadvantages of beta-blockers that are partial agonists have not been clearly defined in clinical settings.

CLINICAL TOXICITY OF THE BETA-RECEPTOR ANTAGONIST DRUGS

A variety of minor toxic effects have been reported for propranolol. Central nervous system effects include sedation, sleep disturbances, and depression. Rash, fever, and other manifestations of drug allergy are rare. Experience with the newer members of this group is too limited to permit comparison of the incidence of toxic effects.

The major adverse effects of beta-receptor antagonist drugs relate to the predictable pharmacologic consequences of beta blockade. $Beta_2$-receptor blockade associated with the use of nonselective agents commonly causes worsening of preexisting asthma and other forms of airway obstruction without having these consequences in normal individuals. Indeed, relatively trivial asthma may become severe after beta blockade. While β_1-selective drugs may have less effect on airways than nonselective beta-antagonists, they must be used very cautiously, if at all, in patients with reactive airways.

Beta-receptor blockade depresses myocardial contractility and excitability. In patients with abnormal myocardial function, cardiac output may be dependent on sympathetic drive. If this stimulus is removed by beta blockade, cardiac decompensation may ensue. Great caution must be exercised in using beta-receptor antagonists in patients with myocardial infarction or compensated congestive heart failure. While an adverse cardiac effect of a beta-antagonist may be overcome directly with isoproterenol or with glucagon (glucagon stimulates the heart via glucagon receptors that are not blocked by beta-antagonists), neither of these methods is without hazard. A very small dose of a beta-antagonist (eg, 10 mg of propranolol) may provoke severe cardiac failure in a susceptible individual.

A much-studied but still unanswered question relates to possible hazards of abruptly discontinuing beta-antagonist therapy after chronic use. Evidence suggests that patients with ischemic heart disease may be at increased risk if beta blockade is suddenly interrupted. The mechanism of this effect is uncertain but might involve "up regulation" of the number of beta receptors. Until better evidence is available regarding the magnitude of the risk, prudence dictates the gradual tapering rather than abrupt cessation of dosage when these drugs are discontinued.

Similarly, the true incidence of hypoglycemic episodes provoked or exacerbated by beta-blocking agents is unknown. Nevertheless, it would be inadvisable to use beta-antagonists in diabetics, particularly those with inadequate glucagon reserve, if reasonable alternatives are available.

Beta blockade may mask clinical signs of developing hyperthyroidism. With the increasing number of patients taking these medications for prolonged periods, this issue may become of more concern.

• • •

References

Berthelsen S, Pettinger WA: A functional basis for classification of alpha adrenergic receptors. *Life Sci* 1977;**21:**595.

Cambridge D, Davey MJ, Massingham R: The pharmacology of antihypertensive drugs with special reference to vasodilators, alpha-adrenergic blocking agents and prazosin. *Med J Aust* 1977;**2(Suppl 1):**2.

Conolly ME, Kersting F, Dollery CT: The clinical pharmacology of beta-adrenoceptor-blocking drugs. *Prog Cardiovasc Dis* 1976;**19:**203.

Frishman WH: β-Adrenoceptor antagonists: New drugs and new indications. *N Engl J Med* 1981;**305:**500.

Frishman WH: *Clinical Pharmacology of the Beta-Adrenoceptor Blocking Drugs*. Appleton-Century-Crofts, 1980.

Frishman WH: Nadolol: A new β-adrenoceptor antagonist. *N Engl J Med* 1981;**305:**678.

Hoffman BB, Lefkowitz RJ: Alpha-adrenergic receptor subtypes. *N Engl J Med* 1980;**302:**1390.

Langer SZ: Presynaptic receptors and modulation of neurotransmission: Pharmacological implications and therapeutic relevance. *Trends Neurosci* 1980;**3:**110.

Minneman KP, Pittman RN, Molinoff PB: β-Adrenergic receptor subtypes: Properties, distribution, and regulation. *Annu Rev Neurosci* 1981;**4:**419.

Nickerson M: The pharmacology of adrenergic blockade. *Pharmacol Rev* 1949;**1:**27.

Norwegian Multicenter Study Group: Timolol-induced reduction in mortality and reinfarction in patients surviving acute myocardial infarction. *N Engl J Med* 1981;**304:**801.

Potter DE, Rowland JM: Adrenergic drugs and intraocular pressure. *Gen Pharmacol* 1981;**12:**1.

Antihypertensive Agents | 9

Neal L. Benowitz, MD, & Henry R. Bourne, MD

By some estimates, the arterial blood pressure of 15% of American adults is elevated to a degree that requires medical treatment. Sustained arterial hypertension damages blood vessels in kidney, heart, and brain and leads to an increased incidence of renal failure, coronary disease, and stroke. Effective pharmacologic lowering of blood pressure has been shown to prevent damage to blood vessels and to substantially reduce morbidity and mortality rates. Many effective drugs are available. Knowledge of their antihypertensive mechanisms and sites of action allows accurate prediction of efficacy and toxicity. As a result, rational use of these agents, alone or in combination, can lower blood pressure with minimal risk of toxicity in most patients.

HYPERTENSION & REGULATION OF BLOOD PRESSURE

Diagnosis

The diagnosis of hypertension is based on repeated, reproducible measurements of elevated blood pressure. The diagnosis serves primarily as a prediction of consequences for the patient; it seldom includes a statement about the cause of hypertension.

Epidemiologic studies indicate that the risks of damage to kidney, heart, and brain are directly related to the extent of blood pressure elevation. Even mild hypertension (diastolic blood pressure ≥ 90 mm Hg) in young or middle-aged adults increases the risk of eventual end organ damage. The risks—and therefore the urgency of instituting therapy—increase in proportion to the magnitude of blood pressure elevation. The risk of end organ damage at any level of blood pressure or age is greater in black people and relatively less in premenopausal women than in men. Other positive risk factors include a family history of hypertension, smoking, hyperlipidemia, diabetes, and manifestations of end organ damage at the time of diagnosis.

It should be noted that the diagnosis of hypertension depends on measurement of blood pressure and not upon symptoms reported by the patient. In fact, hypertension is usually asymptomatic until overt end organ damage is imminent or has already occurred.

Etiology of Hypertension

A specific cause of hypertension can be established in perhaps no more than 10% of patients. It is important to consider specific causes in each case, however, because some of them are amenable to definitive surgical treatment: renal artery constriction, coarctation of the aorta, pheochromocytoma, Cushing's disease, and primary hyperaldosteronism.

Patients in whom no specific cause of hypertension can be found are said to have **essential hypertension.*** In most cases, elevated blood pressure is associated with an overall increase in resistance to flow of blood through arterioles, while cardiac output is usually normal. Meticulous investigation of autonomic nervous system function, baroreceptor reflexes, the renin-angiotensin-aldosterone system, and the kidney have failed to identify a primary abnormality as the cause of increased peripheral vascular resistance in essential hypertension.

Elevated blood pressure is usually caused by a combination of several abnormalities (multifactorial). Epidemiologic evidence points to genetic inheritance, psychologic stress, and environmental and dietary factors (increased salt intake) as perhaps contributing to the development of hypertension. Increase in blood pressure with aging does not occur in populations with low daily sodium intake. Patients with labile hypertension appear more likely than normal controls to have blood pressure elevations after salt loading.

Normal Regulation of Blood Pressure

According to the hydraulic equation, arterial blood pressure (BP) is directly proportionate to the product of the rate of blood flow (cardiac output, CO) and the resistance to passage of blood through precapillary arterioles (peripheral vascular resistance, PVR):

$$BP = CO \times PVR$$

Physiologically, in both normal and hypertensive individuals, blood pressure is maintained by moment-

*The adjective originally was intended to convey the now abandoned idea that blood pressure elevation was *essential* for adequate perfusion of diseased tissues. The term now serves as a reminder that we know "essentially" very little about the cause of this kind of hypertension.

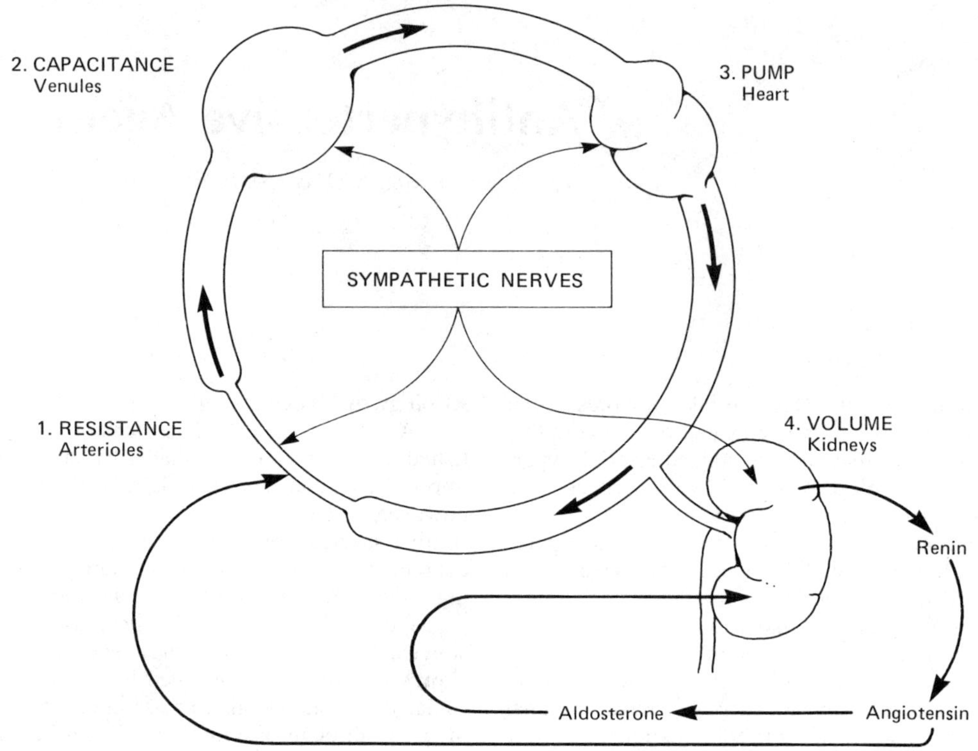

Figure 9–1. Anatomic sites of blood pressure control.

to-moment regulation of cardiac output and peripheral vascular resistance, exerted at 3 anatomic sites (Fig 9–1): arterioles, postcapillary venules (capacitance vessels), and heart. A fourth anatomic control site, the kidney, contributes to maintenance of blood pressure by regulating the volume of intravascular fluid. Baroreflexes, mediated by sympathetic nerves, act in combination with humoral mechanisms, including the renin-angiotensin-aldosterone system, to coordinate function at these 4 control sites and to maintain normal blood pressure.

Blood pressure in an untreated hypertensive patient is controlled by the same mechanisms that are operative in normotensive subjects. Regulation of blood pressure in hypertensives differs from normal in that the baroreceptors and the renal blood volume-pressure control systems appear to be "set" at a higher level of blood pressure. All antihypertensive drugs act by interfering with these normal mechanisms, which are reviewed below.

A. Postural Baroreflex: (Fig 9–2.) Baroreflexes are responsible for rapid, moment-to-moment adjustments in blood pressure, such as in transition from a reclining to an upright posture. Carotid baroreceptors sense the reduction in arterial pressure caused by pooling of blood below the heart; via vasomotor centers in the brain stem, the reflex acts through sympathetic nerve endings to increase peripheral vascular resistance (constriction of arterioles) and cardiac output (direct stimulation of the heart and constriction of capacitance vessels, which increases venous return to the heart), thereby restoring normal blood pressure. The same baroreflex acts in response to any event that lowers arterial pressure, including a primary reduction in peripheral vascular resistance (eg, caused by a vasodilating agent) or a reduction in intravascular volume (eg, due to hemorrhage or to loss of salt and water via the kidney).

B. Renal Response to Decreased Blood Pressure: Via control of blood volume, the kidney is primarily responsible for long-term blood pressure control. A reduction in renal perfusion pressure causes intrarenal redistribution of blood flow and increased reabsorption of salt and water. In addition, decreased pressure in renal arterioles as well as sympathetic neural activity (via β-adrenergic receptors) stimulates production of renin, which increases production of angiotensin II (see Fig 9–1 and Chapter 15). Angiotensin II causes (1) direct constriction of resistance vessels and (2) stimulation of aldosterone synthesis in the adrenal cortex, which increases renal sodium absorption and intravascular blood volume.

Therapeutic Implications

Because antihypertensive therapy is not usually directed at a specific cause, it necessarily depends upon interfering with normal physiologic mechanisms that regulate blood pressure. The risk of toxicity from treatment is high, because hypertension is treated, in effect, by creating another disease.

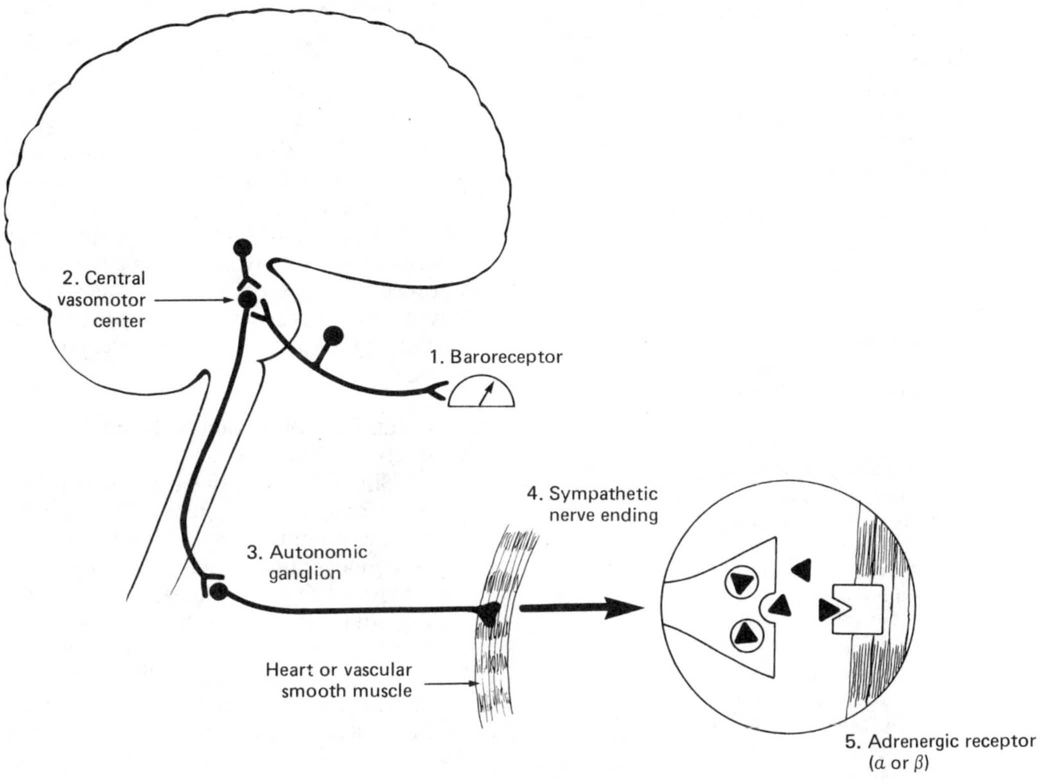

Figure 9–2. Baroreceptor reflex arc.

Antihypertensive therapy is administered to an asymptomatic patient, for whom it provides no direct relief from discomfort; instead, the benefit of lowering blood pressure lies in preventing disease and death at some future time. The natural human tendency to weigh present inconvenience and discomfort more heavily than future benefit means that a major problem—perhaps *the* major problem—in antihypertensive therapy is that of providing consistent, effective drug therapy over many years ("patient compliance").

It is essential to balance the risks of toxicity from drug treatment against the risks of not treating, which are proportionate to the extent of blood pressure elevation before treatment and vary according to the characteristics of individual patients. Accordingly, no single mode of treatment will be suitable for more than a small proportion of hypertensive patients.

I. BASIC PHARMACOLOGY OF ANTIHYPERTENSIVE AGENTS

All antihypertensive agents act at one or more of the 4 anatomic control sites depicted in Fig 9–1 and produce their effects by interfering with normal mechanisms of blood pressure regulation. A useful classification of these agents categorizes them according to the principal regulatory site or mechanism on which they act (Table 9–1). Because of their common mechanisms of action, drugs within each category tend to produce a similar spectrum of toxicities. The categories include the following:

(1) Diuretics, which lower blood pressure by depleting the body of sodium and reducing blood volume.

(2) Sympatholytic agents, which lower blood pressure by reducing peripheral vascular resistance, inhibiting cardiac function, and increasing venous pooling in capacitance vessels. (The latter 2 effects reduce cardiac output.) These agents are further subdivided according to their putative sites of action in the sympathetic reflex arc (see below).

(3) Direct vasodilators, which reduce pressure by relaxing vascular smooth muscle, thus dilating resistance vessels and—to varying degrees—increasing capacitance as well.

(4) Agents that block production or action of angiotensin and thereby reduce peripheral vascular resistance and (potentially) blood volume.

In contrast to many diseases, hypertension is often most effectively treated by a combination of 2 or more drugs, each acting by a different mechanism. The rationale for polypharmacy is that each of the drugs

Table 9–1. Classification of antihypertensive agents.

Diuretics
Low maximal efficacy
Thiazides
Phthalimidines
High maximal efficacy
Furosemide (Lasix)
Ethacrynic acid (Edecrin)
Potassium-sparing
Spironolactone (Aldactone)
Amiloride (Midamor)
Triamterene (Dyrenium)
Sympatholytic agents
Act on central nervous system
Methyldopa (Aldomet)
Clonidine (Catapres)
Act on autonomic ganglia
Trimethaphan (Arfonad)
Act on postganglionic sympathetic neuron
Guanethidine (Ismelin)
Reserpine
Monoamine oxidase inhibitors
Receptor blockers
β-Adrenergic receptors
Propranolol (Inderal)
Nadolol (Corgard)
Metoprolol (Lopressor)
Labetolol (Trandate)
α-Adrenergic receptors
Prazosin (Minipress)
Phentolamine (Regitine)
Phenoxybenzamine (Dibenzyline)
Vasodilators
Hydralazine (Apresoline)
Minoxidil (Loniten)
Diazoxide (Hyperstat)
Nitroprusside (Nipride)
Nifedipine (Adalat, Procardia)
Verapamil (Calan, Isoptin)
Inhibitors of renin-angiotensin system
Saralasin (Sarenin)
Captopril (Capoten)

acts on one of a set of interacting, mutually compensatory regulatory mechanisms for maintaining blood pressure. Thus, partial impairment of one regulatory mechanism increases the antihypertensive effect of impairing regulation by another mechanism. This is particularly important when the toxicity of one agent is a direct extension of its beneficial pharmacologic effect. Similarly, a drug that interferes with one regulatory mechanism may be limited in its effectiveness by the normal compensatory response of a second mechanism. Finally, in some circumstances, a normal compensatory response accounts for the toxicity of an antihypertensive agent, and the toxic effect can be prevented by administering a second type of drug.

Thus, when hypertension does not respond adequately to a regimen of one or 2 drugs, a second or third drug from a different class is usually added. The order of addition is generally similar to the order of classes listed above.

DRUGS THAT ALTER SODIUM & WATER BALANCE

Dietary sodium restriction has been known for many years to decrease blood pressure in hypertensive patients. With the advent of diuretics, sodium restriction was thought to be less important. Recently, there has been renewed interest in dietary control of blood pressure as a relatively nontoxic therapeutic and even preventive measure. Several studies have shown that even modest dietary sodium restriction lowers blood pressure (although to varying extents) in most individuals.

Mechanisms of Action & Hemodynamic Effects of Diuretics

Diuretics lower blood pressure primarily by depleting body sodium stores. The vasodilatation observed when intravenous diuretics are administered in the treatment of acute pulmonary edema is of doubtful antihypertensive usefulness over the long term. Initially, diuretics reduce blood pressure by reducing blood volume and cardiac output; peripheral vascular resistance may increase. After 6–8 weeks, cardiac output returns to normal while peripheral vascular resistance declines. Sodium is believed to contribute to vascular resistance by increasing vessel stiffness and neural reactivity. These effects are reversed by diuretics or sodium restriction.

Diuretics are effective in lowering blood pressure by 10–15 mm Hg in most patients, and diuretics alone often provide adequate treatment for mild or moderate essential hypertension. In more severe hypertension, diuretics are used in combination with sympatholytic and vasodilator drugs to control the tendency towards sodium retention caused by these agents. Vascular responsiveness—ie, the ability to either constrict or dilate—is diminished by sympatholytic and vasodilator drugs, so that the vasculature behaves like a pipe with a constant diameter. As a consequence, blood pressure becomes exquisitely sensitive to blood volume. Thus, in severe hypertension, when multiple drugs are used, blood pressure may be well controlled when blood volume is 95% of normal but much too high when blood volume is 105% of normal.

Selection of Diuretics

The sites of action within the kidney and the pharmacokinetics of various diuretic drugs are discussed in Chapter 13. Thiazide diuretics are appropriate for most patients with mild or moderate hypertension and normal renal and cardiac function. More powerful diuretics (eg, those acting on the loop of Henle) are necessary in severe hypertension, when multiple drugs with sodium-retaining properties are used; in renal insufficiency, when glomerular filtration rate is less than 30 or 40 mL/min; and in cardiac failure or cirrhosis, where sodium retention is marked.

Potassium-sparing diuretics are useful both to avoid excessive potassium depletion, particularly in patients taking digitalis, and to enhance the natriuretic effects of other diuretics.

Dosing Considerations

Although the pharmacokinetics and pharmacodynamics of the various diuretics differ, their common therapeutic end point in treating hypertension is daily natriuresis. However, it must be recognized that in steady-state conditions (as in long-term management of hypertension), daily sodium excretion is equal to dietary sodium intake. Diuretics are necessary to oppose the tendency toward sodium retention in a relatively sodium-depleted patient. Although thiazide diuretics are more natriuretic at higher doses (up to 100–200 mg of hydrochlorothiazide), when used as a single agent, lower doses (25–50 mg) exert as much antihypertensive effect as do higher doses. Thus, a threshold amount of body sodium depletion may be necessary for antihypertensive efficacy. In contrast to thiazides, the dose-response range for loop diuretics is many times greater than the usual therapeutic dose.

Toxicity of Diuretics

In the treatment of hypertension, the most important adverse effect of diuretics (except for potassium-sparing diuretics) is potassium depletion. Although mild degrees of hypokalemia are tolerated well by many patients, hypokalemia may be hazardous in persons taking digitalis or those who have chronic arrhythmias. Potassium loss is coupled to reabsorption of sodium, and restriction of dietary sodium intake will therefore minimize potassium loss.

DRUGS THAT ALTER SYMPATHETIC NERVOUS SYSTEM FUNCTION

In patients with moderate to severe hypertension, every effective drug regimen includes an agent that inhibits function of the sympathetic nervous system. Drugs in this group are classified according to the site at which they impair the sympathetic reflex arc (Fig 9–2). This neuroanatomic classification explains prominent differences in cardiovascular effects of drugs and allows the clinician to predict interactions of these drugs with one another and with other drugs.

Most importantly, the subclasses of drugs exhibit different patterns of potential toxicity. Thus, drugs that lower blood pressure by actions on the central nervous system tend to cause sedation and mental depression and may produce disturbances of sleep, including nightmares. Drugs that act by inhibiting transmission through autonomic ganglia produce toxicity from inhibition of parasympathetic regulation, in addition to profound sympathetic blockade. Drugs that act chiefly by reducing release of norepinephrine from sympathetic nerve endings cause effects that are similar to those of surgical sympathectomy, including inhibition of ejaculation, and hypotension that is increased by exercise and upright posture. Drugs that block postsynaptic adrenergic receptors produce a more selective spectrum of effects depending on the class of receptor to which they bind.

A few of the drugs to be discussed appear to act at more than one anatomic site, although each (probably) works by a single biochemical mechanism. No clinically useful drug acts primarily on baroreceptors. The **veratrum alkaloids** lower blood pressure by increasing sensitivity of baroreceptors, but they are of only academic interest because they produce erratic therapeutic effects and cause unacceptable toxicity in patients.

Finally, we should note that *all* of the agents that lower blood pressure by altering sympathetic function can elicit compensatory effects through mechanisms that are not dependent on adrenergic nerves. Thus, the antihypertensive effect of any of these agents used alone may be limited by retention of sodium and expansion of blood volume. For these reasons, sympatholytic antihypertensive drugs are most effective when used concomitantly with a diuretic.

Centrally Acting Sympatholytic Drugs

Mechanism & Sites of Action

Methyldopa and clonidine reduce sympathetic outflow from vasopressor centers in the brain stem but allow these centers to retain their sensitivity to baroreceptor control. Accordingly, the antihypertensive and toxic actions of these drugs are generally less dependent on posture than are the effects of drugs such as guanethidine that act directly on peripheral sympathetic neurons.

Methyldopa (L-α-methyl-3,4-dihydroxyphenylalanine) is an analog of L-dopa and is converted to α-methylnorepinephrine; this pathway, illustrated in Fig 9–3, directly parallels the synthesis of norepinephrine from dopa (see Chapter 4). Alpha-methylnorepinephrine is stored in adrenergic nerve granules, where it stoichiometrically replaces norepinephrine, and is released by nerve stimulation to interact with postsynaptic adrenergic receptors. However, this replacement of norepinephrine by a false transmitter in peripheral neurons is *not* responsible for methyldopa's antihypertensive effect, because the α-methylnorepinephrine released is an effective agonist at the α-adrenergic receptors that mediate peripheral sympathetic constriction of arterioles and venules. Direct electrical stimulation of sympathetic nerves in methyldopa-treated animals produces sympathetic responses similar to those observed in untreated animals.

Indeed, methyldopa's antihypertensive action appears to be due to stimulation of central α-adrenergic receptors by α-methylnorepinephrine, based on the following evidence: (1) Much lower doses of methyldopa are required to lower blood pressure in animals when the drug is administered centrally by cerebral intraventricular injection rather than intravenously.

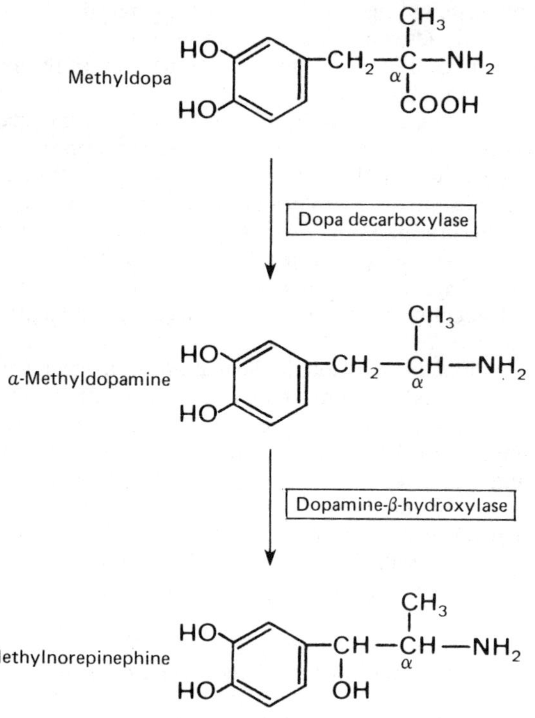

Figure 9–3. Metabolic activation of methyldopa.

(2) Alpha-adrenergic antagonists, administered centrally, block the antihypertensive effect of methyldopa, whether the latter is given centrally or intravenously. (3) Potent inhibitors of dopa decarboxylase, administered centrally, block methyldopa's antihypertensive effect, thus showing that metabolism of the parent drug is necessary for its action.

The antihypertensive action of **clonidine,** a 2-imidazoline derivative (Fig 9–4), was discovered in the course of testing the drug for use as a topically applied nasal decongestant. After intravenous injection, clonidine produces a brief rise in blood pressure followed by more prolonged hypotension. The pressor response is due to direct stimulation of α-adrenergic receptors in arterioles. The drug is classified as a partial agonist at α receptors because it also inhibits pressor effects of other α-agonists.

Considerable evidence indicates that the hypotensive effect of clonidine is exerted at α-adrenergic receptors in the medulla of the brain. In animals, the hypotensive effect of clonidine is prevented by central administration of α-adrenergic antagonists. Clonidine reduces sympathetic and increases parasympathetic tone, resulting in blood pressure lowering and bradycardia. These observations suggest that clonidine sensitizes brain stem pressor centers to inhibition by baroreflexes.

Thus, studies of clonidine and methyldopa suggest that normal regulation of blood pressure involves central adrenergic neurons that modulate baroreceptor reflexes. Both drugs bind more tightly to α_2- than to α_1-adrenergic receptors. Alpha$_2$-adrenergic receptors are located presynaptically on membranes of peripheral vascular sympathetic neurons, where they inhibit norepinephrine release (see Chapter 7). It is possible that clonidine and α-methylnorepinephrine act in the brain to reduce norepinephrine release onto relevant receptor sites.

METHYLDOPA

Methyldopa is useful in the treatment of mild to moderately severe hypertension. It lowers blood pressure chiefly by reducing peripheral vascular resistance; there is little change in heart rate or cardiac output in most patients.

Most cardiovascular reflexes remain intact after administration of methyldopa, and blood pressure reduction is not markedly dependent upon maintenance of upright posture. Postural (orthostatic) hypotension sometimes occurs, particularly in volume-depleted patients. One potential advantage of methyldopa is that it causes reduction in renal vascular resistance, perhaps owing to reduced efficacy of α-methylnorepinephrine as a vasoconstrictor in renal arterioles.

Pharmacokinetics & Dosage

Owing to extensive first-pass metabolism (primarily O-sulfate conjugation by the gastrointestinal mucosa), the bioavailability of methyldopa is low, averaging 25%, and varies among individuals. About two-thirds of the drug that reaches plasma is cleared by renal excretion, with a terminal elimination half-time of 2 hours. Impaired renal function results in reduced drug clearance. Although there are no studies in this regard, some clinicians report greater efficacy and toxicity and recommend using lower doses in patients with renal failure.

An oral dose of methyldopa produces its maximal antihypertensive effect in 4–6 hours, and the effect can persist for up to 24 hours. Because the effect depends upon accumulation of a metabolite, α-methylnorepinephrine, the action persists long after the parent drug has disappeared from the circulation.

The maximal efficacy of methyldopa in lowering blood pressure is limited. In most patients, a dose of 2 g or less will produce maximal reduction in hypertension; if this result is not satisfactory, higher doses will usually not result in greater effects. The usual therapeutic dose is about 1–2 g/d orally in divided doses. In many patients, once-daily therapy is effective.

Toxicity

Most of the undesirable effects of methyldopa are referable to the central nervous system. Of these, the most frequent is overt sedation, particularly at the onset of treatment. With long-term therapy, patients may complain of persistent mental lassitude and impaired mental concentration. Nightmares, mental depression, vertigo, and extrapyramidal signs may occur

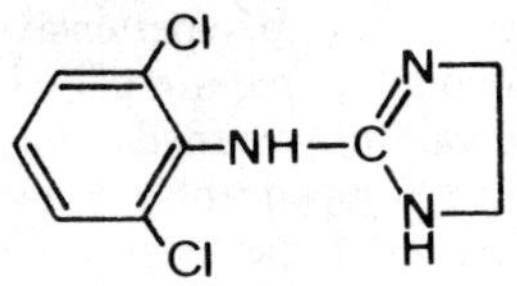

Clonidine

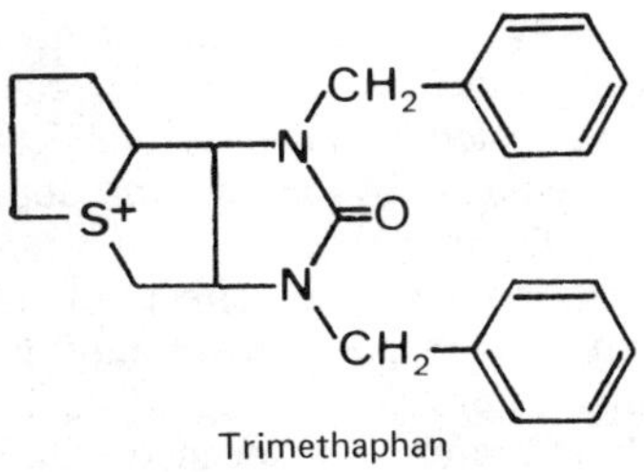

Trimethaphan

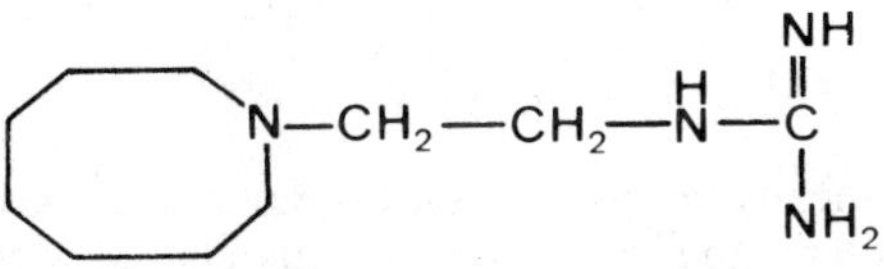

Guanethidine

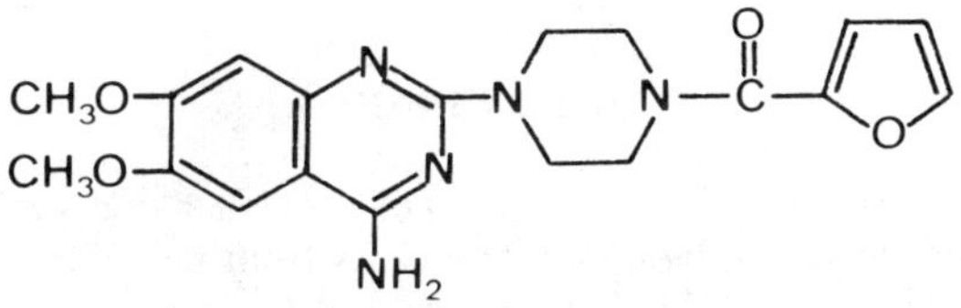

Prazosin

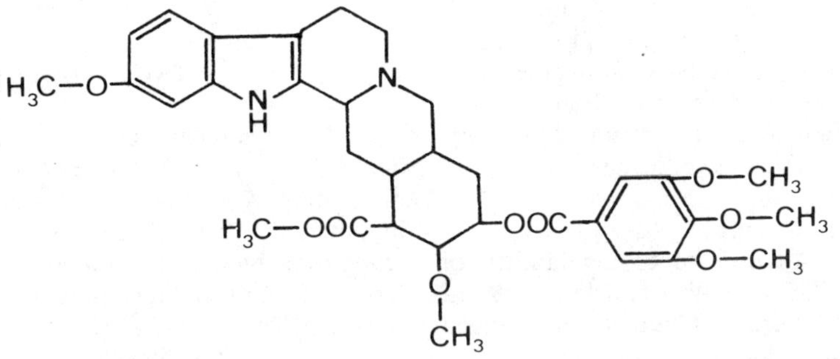

Reserpine

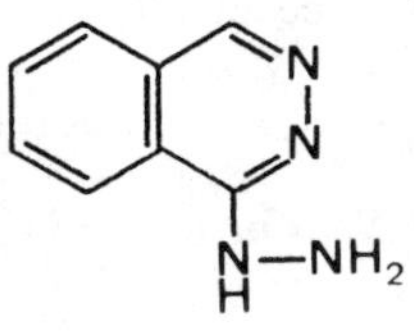

Hydralazine

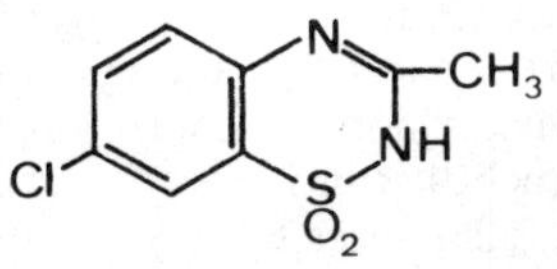

Diazoxide

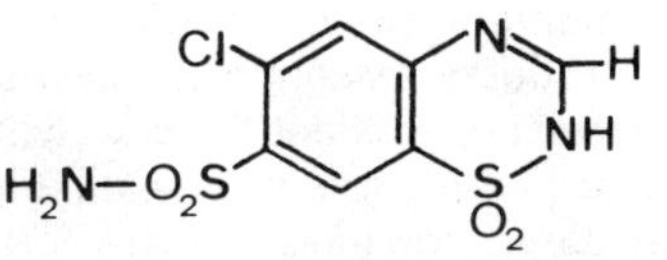

Chlorothiazide

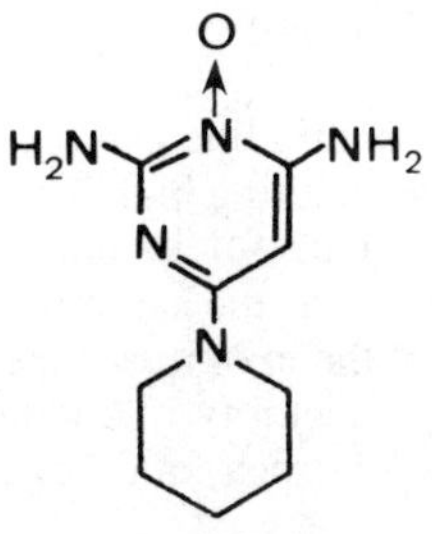

Minoxidil

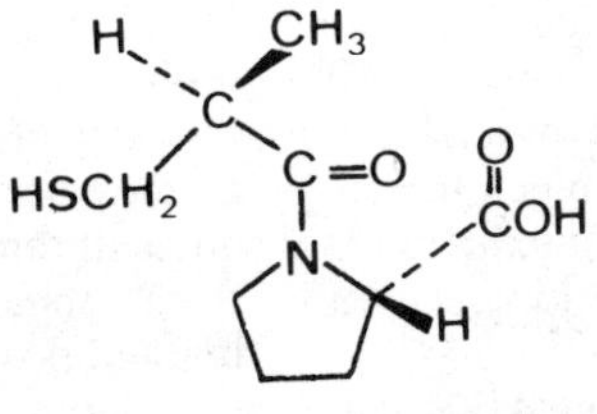

Captopril

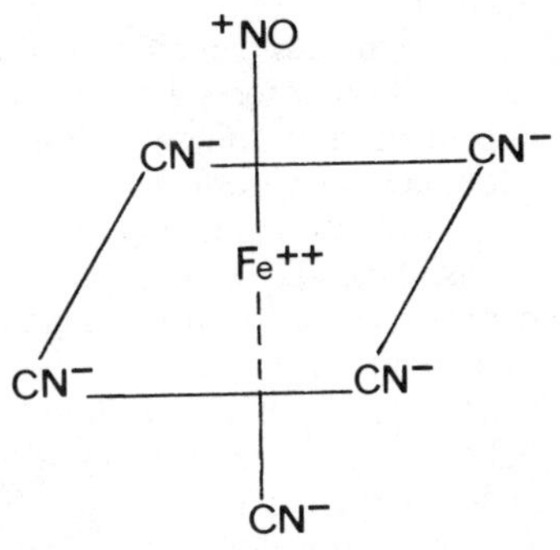

Nitroprusside

Figure 9–4. Chemical structures of antihypertensive drugs.

but are relatively infrequent. Lactation, associated with increased prolactin secretion, can occur in either men or women treated with methyldopa. This toxicity is probably mediated by actions on dopaminergic mechanisms in the hypothalamus.

Other important adverse effects of methyldopa are development of a positive Coombs test, which sometimes makes cross-matching blood for transfusion difficult and rarely is associated with hemolytic anemia, as well as hepatitis and drug fever.

CLONIDINE

Hemodynamic studies indicate that blood pressure lowering by clonidine results from reduction of cardiac output due to decreased heart rate and relaxation of capacitance vessels, with no consistent change in peripheral vascular resistance.

Reduction in arterial blood pressure by clonidine is accompanied by decreased renal vascular resistance and maintenance of renal blood flow. As with methyldopa, clonidine reduces blood pressure in the supine position and only rarely causes postural hypotension. Pressor effects of clonidine are not observed after ingestion of therapeutic doses of clonidine, but severe hypertension can complicate overdosage.

Pharmacokinetics & Dosage

In healthy individuals, the bioavailability of clonidine averages 75% and the half-life is 8–12 hours. About half of the drug is eliminated unchanged in the urine, suggesting that lower than usual doses may be effective in patients with renal insufficiency.

Because of its relatively short half-life and the fact that its antihypertensive effect is directly related to blood concentration, clonidine must be given twice a day to maintain smooth blood pressure control. Therapeutic doses are commonly between 0.2 and 1.2 mg/d. However, as is not the case with methyldopa, the dose-response curve of clonidine is such that increasing doses are more effective (but also more toxic). The maximal recommended dose is 2.4 mg/d.

Toxicity

Dry mouth and sedation are frequent and may be severe. Both effects are centrally mediated and dose-dependent and coincide temporally with the drug's antihypertensive effect.

The drug should not be given to patients who are at risk of mental depression and should be withdrawn if depression occurs during therapy. Concomitant treatment with tricyclic antidepressants may block the antihypertensive effect of clonidine. The interaction is believed to be due to α-adrenoceptor blocking actions of the tricyclics.

Withdrawal of clonidine after protracted use, particularly with high doses (greater than 1 mg/d), can result in life-threatening hypertensive crisis mediated by increased sympathetic nervous activity. Patients exhibit nervousness, tachycardia, headache, and sweating after omitting one or 2 doses of the drug. Although the incidence of severe hypertensive crisis is unknown, it is high enough to require that all patients who take clonidine be carefully warned of the possibility. If the drug must be stopped, this should be done gradually while other antihypertensive agents are being substituted. Treatment of the hypertensive crisis consists of reinstitution of clonidine therapy or administration of α- and β-adrenergic blocking agents.

Ganglionic Blocking Agents

Historically, drugs that block stimulation of postganglionic autonomic neurons by acetylcholine were among the first agents used in the treatment of hypertension. Most such drugs are no longer available clinically because of intolerable toxicities related to their primary action (see Chapter 4). Only one drug in this class (trimethaphan) is still used to treat hypertension.

TRIMETHAPHAN

Trimethaphan camsylate (Fig 9–4) is administered intravenously to take advantage of its rapid action in treating hypertensive crisis and to induce controlled hypotension for neurosurgery. The dependence of ganglionic blockade on blood level of the drug allows precise titration of blood pressure while other drugs are taking effect.

The antihypertensive effect of trimethaphan is to a large extent dependent upon pooling of blood in capacitance vessels. Patients must be tilted head up (usually with blocks under the head of the bed) for effective blood pressure lowering. Conversely, excessive hypotension can be rapidly treated by reverse tilting.

Adrenergic Neuron Blocking Agents

These drugs lower blood pressure by preventing normal physiologic release of norepinephrine from postganglionic sympathetic neurons (see Chapter 4).

GUANETHIDINE

In high enough doses, guanethidine can produce profound sympathoplegia. The resulting high maximal efficacy of this agent makes it useful in outpatient therapy of severe hypertension. For the same reason, guanethidine can produce all of the toxicities expected from "pharmacologic sympathectomy," including marked postural hypotension, diarrhea, and impaired ejaculation.

The structure of guanethidine includes a highly basic nitrogen (Fig 9–4) that prevents its entry into the central nervous system. As a result, this drug has none of the central effects seen with many of the other antihypertensive agents described in this chapter.

Bethanidine and **debrisoquin,** antihypertensive agents not yet released for clinical use in the USA, are similar in chemical structure and mechanism of antihypertensive action to guanethidine. **Bretylium,** an antiarrhythmia drug described in Chapter 12, is also structurally similar to guanethidine.

Mechanism & Sites of Action

Guanethidine inhibits the release of norepinephrine that occurs when a neuronal action potential reaches sympathetic nerve endings (Fig 9–5). This effect is probably responsible for most of the sympathoplegia that occurs in patients. Guanethidine is transported across the sympathetic nerve membrane by the same mechanism that transports norepinephrine itself, and uptake is essential for the drug's action. Once guanethidine has entered the nerve, it is concentrated in transmitter vesicles, where it replaces norepinephrine. Subsequently, the drug causes a gradual depletion of norepinephrine stores in the nerve ending.

Inhibition of norepinephrine release is probably related to guanethidine's local anesthetic properties. Although the drug does not impair axonal conduction in sympathetic fibers, local blockade of membrane electrical activity may occur in nerve endings, because the nerve endings specifically take up and concentrate the drug.

Because neuronal uptake is necessary for the hypotensive activity of guanethidine, drugs that block the catecholamine uptake process (see Chapter 4) block the uptake and subsequent effects of guanethidine. These include cocaine, tricyclic antidepressants, phenothiazines, phenoxybenzamine, and certain sympathomimetic amines.

When guanethidine first enters the neuron, norepinephrine is released. With usual doses, the amount of norepinephrine released is too small to have any significant effect; after rapid intravenous administration, however, sudden norepinephrine release can cause hypertension.

Guanethidine increases sensitivity to the hypertensive effects of exogenously administered sympathomimetic amines. This results from inhibition of neuronal uptake of such amines and, after long-term therapy with guanethidine, supersensitivity of effector smooth muscle cells, in a fashion analogous to the process that follows surgical sympathectomy (see Chapter 4).

The hypotensive action of guanethidine early in the course of therapy is associated with reduced cardiac output, due to bradycardia and relaxation of capacitance vessels, without consistent change in peripheral vascular resistance. With chronic therapy, cardiac output may return to normal, due in part to blood volume expansion, while peripheral vascular resistance decreases. Blood flow to splanchnic and renal beds is decreased relative to flow to heart, muscle, and brain. Renal hemodynamic effects may explain in part the marked tendency toward sodium and water retention during guanethidine therapy.

Pharmacokinetics & Dosage

The bioavailability of guanethidine is variable (3–50%). It is 50% cleared by the kidney. Retention of drug in nerve endings and uptake into other sites account for the very large volume of distribution and long half-life (5 days) of guanethidine. Thus, with constant

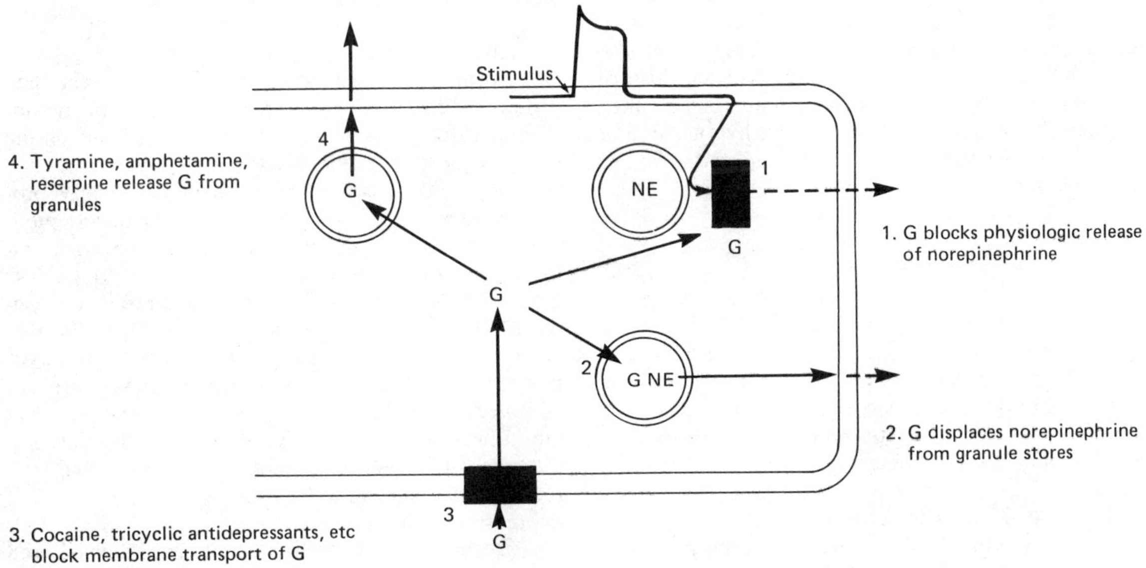

Figure 9–5. Guanethidine actions and drug interactions involving the adrenergic neuron. (G = guanethidine; NE = norepinephrine.)

daily dosing, the onset of sympathoplegia is gradual (maximal effect in 1–2 weeks), and sympathoplegia persists for a comparable period after cessation of therapy.

The daily dose required for a satisfactory hypotensive response varies greatly among individual patients. For this reason, therapy is usually initiated at a low dose, eg, 10 mg/d. As patients require 1–2 weeks for the hypotensive effect of a given daily dosage level to reach maximum, the dose should not ordinarily be increased at intervals shorter than 2 weeks. Because of the drug's long duration of action, maintenance doses need not be taken more than once a day.

Toxicity

Therapeutic use of guanethidine is often associated with symptomatic postural hypotension and hypotension following exercise, particularly when the drug is given in high doses. However, when it is used in lower doses (25–50 mg/d) for mild to moderate hypertension, orthostatic hypotension is not a significant problem. Injudicious treatment (excessive doses or too rapid escalation in dosage) may produce dangerously decreased blood flow to heart and brain or even overt shock. Guanethidine-induced sympathoplegia in men may be associated with delayed or retrograde ejaculation. Guanethidine commonly causes diarrhea, which results from increased gastrointestinal motility due to parasympathetic predominance in controlling the activity of intestinal smooth muscle.

Interactions with other drugs may complicate guanethidine therapy. Sympathomimetic agents at doses available in over-the-counter cold preparations can produce hypertension in patients taking guanethidine. Similarly, guanethidine can produce hypertensive crisis by releasing catecholamines in patients with pheochromocytoma. When tricyclic antidepressants are administered to patients taking guanethidine, the antihypertensive effect is attenuated, and severe hypertension may follow. A physician who is ignorant of this interaction may raise the dose of guanethidine; if the tricyclic antidepressant is then stopped, the patient may suffer severe hypotension or cardiovascular collapse from the unopposed action of guanethidine.

RESERPINE

Reserpine (Fig 9–4), an alkaloid extracted from the roots of an Indian plant, *Rauwolfia serpentina,* was one of the first effective drugs used on a large scale in the treatment of hypertension. At present, it is considered an effective and relatively safe drug for treating mild to moderate hypertension.

Mechanism & Sites of Action

Reserpine blocks the ability of adrenergic transmitter vesicles to take up and store biogenic amines, probably by interfering with an uptake mechanism that depends on Mg^{2+} and ATP. This effect occurs throughout the body, resulting in depletion of norepinephrine, dopamine, and serotonin in both central and peripheral neurons. Chromaffin granules of the adrenal medulla are also depleted of catecholamines, although to a lesser extent than are neurons elsewhere. Reserpine's effects on adrenergic vesicles appear irreversible; trace amounts of the drug remain bound to vesicular membranes for many days. Although sufficiently high doses of reserpine in animals can reduce catecholamine stores to zero, lower doses cause inhibition of neurotransmission that is roughly proportionate to the degree of amine depletion. Depletion of peripheral amines probably accounts for much of the beneficial antihypertensive effect, but a central component cannot be ruled out. The effects of low but clinically effective doses of reserpine resemble those of centrally acting agents (eg, methyldopa) in that sympathetic reflexes remain largely intact, blood pressure is reduced in supine as well as in standing patients, and postural hypotension is mild. Reserpine readily enters the brain, and depletion of cerebral amine stores causes sedation, mental depression, and parkinsonism symptoms.

At lower doses used for treatment of mild hypertension, reserpine lowers blood pressure by a combination of decreased cardiac output and decreased peripheral vascular resistance.

Pharmacokinetics & Dosage

Absorption, clearance, and metabolism have not been well defined. The drug disappears rapidly from the circulation, but its effects persist much longer, owing to irreversible inactivation of catecholamine storage granules, as described above.

The usual daily dose is less than 1 mg (typically, 0.25 mg), administered orally as a single dose. Although reserpine is available in injectable form, parenteral administration is rarely indicated.

Toxicity

At the low doses usually administered, reserpine produces little postural hypotension. Most of the unwanted effects of reserpine result from actions on the brain or gastrointestinal tract.

High doses of reserpine characteristically produce sedation, lassitude, nightmares, and severe mental depression; occasionally, these occur even in patients receiving low doses (0.25 mg/d). Much less frequently, ordinary doses of reserpine produce extrapyramidal effects resembling Parkinson's disease, probably as a result of dopamine depletion in the corpus striatum. Although these central effects are uncommon, it should be stressed that they may occur at any time, even after months of uneventful treatment. Patients with a history of mental depression should not receive reserpine, and the drug should be stopped if depression appears.

Reserpine rather often produces mild diarrhea and gastrointestinal cramps and increases gastric acid secretion. The drug should probably not be given to patients with a history of peptic ulcer.

Several retrospective studies have disclosed an apparent association between long-term treatment with reserpine and increased incidence of carcinoma of the breast. Most recent studies have failed to confirm this association.

PARGYLINE

Although pargyline and other inhibitors of monoamine oxidase have no place in the modern treatment of hypertension, their interesting mechanisms of action and their toxicity deserve mention. Pargyline is thought to lower blood pressure by increasing the concentration of an ineffective false transmitter in peripheral adrenergic nerve endings. Pargyline inhibits monoamine oxidase in gastrointestinal mucosa and thus allows unimpeded access of dietary tyramine to the systemic circulation. Tyramine is taken up into nerve endings and converted to octopamine, which replaces norepinephrine in catecholamine storage granules. Because octopamine is ineffective as a pressor agonist at postsynaptic α-adrenergic receptors, sympathoplegia results.

Depletion of endogenous norepinephrine is not complete enough, however, to prevent the severe toxicity that may result when pargyline-treated patients ingest the large quantities of tyramine found in certain wines and cheeses. In this situation, high concentrations of tyramine reach the nerve endings and release norepinephrine in large amounts onto sympathetic nerve endings, producing a hypertensive crisis. Pargyline is considered too dangerous for use in the treatment of hypertension because of the possibility of such hypertensive crises and because of its propensity to interact adversely with other drugs, including reserpine and opiates.

Adrenergic Receptor Antagonists

The pharmacology of drugs that antagonize catecholamines at α- and β-adrenergic receptors is presented in Chapter 8. Here we will concentrate on 2 drugs, propranolol and prazosin, primarily in relation to their use in treatment of hypertension. Other adrenergic antagonists will be considered only briefly.

PROPRANOLOL

Propranolol, a β-adrenergic blocking agent, is very useful for lowering blood pressure in mild to moderate hypertension. In severe hypertension, propranolol is especially useful in preventing the reflex tachycardia that often results from treatment with direct vasodilators.

Mechanism & Sites of Action

Propranolol antagonizes catecholamines at both β_1- and β_2-adrenergic receptors. Both its efficacy in treating hypertension as well as most of its toxic effects result from β-adrenergic blockade. When propranolol is first administered to a hypertensive patient, blood pressure decreases primarily as a result of a decrease in cardiac output associated with bradycardia. With continued treatment, however, cardiac output returns toward normal while blood pressure remains low, due to decreased peripheral vascular resistance.

Beta blockade in both brain and kidney has been proposed as contributing to the antihypertensive effect observed with β-adrenergic blockers. The brain appears unlikely to be the primary site of propranolol's action, because some beta-blockers that do not readily cross the blood-brain barrier (eg, nadolol, described below) are nonetheless effective antihypertensive agents.

Propranolol inhibits the stimulation of renin production by catecholamines (mediated by β_2 receptors) in animals and humans. It is likely that part of propranolol's effect is due to depression of the renin-angiotensin-aldosterone system, described above. Nonetheless, propranolol reduces blood pressure in hypertensive patients with normal or even low renin activity. In addition, beta-blockers relatively selective for β_1 receptors (such as metoprolol) are as effective in lowering blood pressure as is propranolol. Thus, depression of renin cannot in itself account for propranolol's usefulness in treating hypertension.

We are left with the idea that with chronic propranolol therapy, a long-term readjustment to the initial reduction in cardiac output leads to sustained reduction in peripheral vascular resistance and therefore blood pressure.

In mild to moderate hypertension, propranolol produces a significant reduction in blood pressure without prominent postural hypotension. As with many hypotensive drugs, propranolol may cause compensatory sodium retention and hypervolemia; many hypertensive patients receiving propranolol consequently require treatment with a diuretic.

Pharmacokinetics & Dosage

As described in Chapter 8, effective oral doses of propranolol are 10-fold (or more) greater than effective intravenous doses, owing to first-pass hepatic inactivation. The prominent first-pass effect partially accounts for the variability in doses required for clinically useful effects. The half-life is 3–6 hours.

Treatment of hypertension is usually started with 80 mg/d in divided doses. Effective antihypertensive doses range from 80 to 480 mg/d. Resting bradycardia and a reduction in the heart rate during exercise are indicators of propranolol's beta-blocking effect. Measures of these responses may be used as guides in regulating dosage. Propranolol can be administered once or twice daily.

Toxicity

The principal toxicities of propranolol result from blockade of cardiac, vascular, or bronchial beta receptors and are described in more detail in Chapter 8.

The most important of these predictable extensions of the beta-blocking action occur in patients with reduced myocardial reserve, asthma, peripheral vascular insufficiency, and diabetes.

When propranolol is discontinued after prolonged regular use, some patients experience an abstinence syndrome, including nervousness, tachycardia, increased intensity of angina, or increase of blood pressure. Myocardial infarction has been reported in a few patients. Although the incidence of these complications is probably low, propranolol should not be discontinued abruptly. The withdrawal syndrome may involve "up regulation" or supersensitivity of β-adrenergic receptors (see Chapter 2).

Finally, propranolol also produces a low incidence of effects not clearly attributable to β-adrenergic blockade, including diarrhea, constipation, nausea, and vomiting. Not infrequently, patients receiving propranolol complain of central nervous system effects reminiscent of those caused by methyldopa and clonidine, including nightmares, lassitude, mental depression, and insomnia.

OTHER BETA-ADRENERGIC BLOCKING AGENTS

Of the large number of beta-blockers tested, most have been shown to be effective in lowering blood pressure. The pharmacologic properties of 3 of these agents differ from those of propranolol in ways that may confer therapeutic benefit in certain clinical situations.

1. METOPROLOL

Metoprolol is approximately equipotent to propranolol in inhibiting stimulation of β_1-adrenergic receptors such as those in the heart but 50- to 100-fold less potent than propranolol in blocking β_2 receptors. Although metoprolol is in other respects very similar to propranolol, its relative cardioselectivity may be advantageous in treating hypertensive patients who also suffer from asthma, diabetes, or peripheral vascular disease. Studies of small numbers of asthmatic patients have shown that metoprolol causes less bronchial constriction than propranolol at doses that produce equal inhibition of β_1-adrenergic responses. The cardioselectivity is not complete, however, and asthmatic symptoms have been exacerbated by metroprolol. Usual antihypertensive doses of metoprolol range from 100 to 450 mg/d.

2. NADOLOL

Nadolol, a nonselective beta-antagonist, differs from propranolol chiefly in that it is not metabolized; it is almost entirely excreted in the urine. Nadolol can be administered once daily, owing to its relatively long half-life in plasma (up to 24 hours). Treatment with nadolol is usually begun with 40 mg/d. Upward adjustments in dosage to obtain a satisfactory therapeutic effect should take place no oftener than every 4 or 5 days, the period required to reach a steady-state plasma concentration at a given daily dose (see Chapter 3, Part I). Patients with reduced renal function should receive correspondingly reduced doses of nadolol.

3. LABETOLOL

Labetolol blocks both β- and α-adrenergic receptors. The block of beta receptors occurs at lower concentrations than are required for alpha blockade. Consequently, low doses of labetolol primarily result in beta blockade, while higher doses block alpha receptors as well and are effective in treating the hypertension of pheochromocytoma.

PRAZOSIN

Mechanism & Site of Action

Prazosin (Fig 9–4) produces most of its antihypertensive effect by blocking α_1-adrenergic receptors in arterioles and venules. Although this recently marketed agent is clearly effective in treating hypertension, its clinical advantages and disadvantages in comparison with older agents are not yet well defined.

Prazosin's selectivity for α_1 receptors is well established and may explain why this agent produces less reflex tachycardia than do nonselective alpha-antagonists such as phentolamine. This receptor selectivity allows norepinephrine to exert unopposed negative feedback (mediated by presynaptic α_2 receptors) on its own release (see Chapter 4); in contrast, phentolamine blocks both pre- and postsynaptic alpha receptors, with the result that reflex stimulation of sympathetic neurons produces greater release of transmitter onto beta receptors and correspondingly greater cardioacceleration.

Prazosin reduces arterial pressure by dilating both resistance and capacitance vessels. As expected, blood pressure is reduced more in the upright than in the supine position. Retention of salt and fluid occurs when prazosin is administered without a diuretic. The drug is clearly more effective when used in combination with other agents, such as propranolol and a diuretic, than when used alone.

Pharmacokinetics & Dosage

Prazosin is well absorbed but undergoes substantial first-pass metabolism in the liver. Prazosin is eliminated almost entirely by metabolism, with a plasma half-life of 3–4 hours, although the half-life of the antihypertensive effect is longer. Plasma concentrations are increased in patients with congestive heart failure, due primarily to reduced first-pass metabolism.

Treatment with prazosin should be initiated with a

low dose (1 mg 3 times daily) to prevent postural hypotension and syncope. Doses may be increased to 20 or 30 mg/d. Although long-term prazosin treatment causes relatively little postural hypotension, a number of patients develop bradycardia and a precipitous drop in standing blood pressure shortly after the first dose is absorbed. For this reason, the first dose should be administered at bedtime. While the mechanism of this first-dose phenomenon is not clear, it occurs more commonly in patients who are salt- and volume-depleted.

Aside from the first-dose phenomenon, the reported toxicities of prazosin are relatively infrequent and mild. These include dizziness, palpitations, headache, and lassitude. Some patients develop a positive test for antinuclear factor in serum while on prazosin therapy, but this has not been associated with rheumatic symptoms.

OTHER ALPHA-ADRENERGIC BLOCKING AGENTS

Phentolamine and **phenoxybenzamine** are useful in diagnosis and treatment of pheochromocytoma and in other clinical situations associated with exaggerated release of catecholamines (eg, phentolamine may be combined with propranolol to treat the clonidine withdrawal syndrome, described above). Their pharmacology is described in Chapter 8.

VASODILATORS

Mechanisms & Sites of Action

Within this class of drugs are the oral vasodilators, hydralazine and minoxidil, which are used for long-term outpatient therapy of hypertension; and the parenteral vasodilators, nitroprusside and diazoxide, which are used to treat hypertensive emergencies. These compounds act on the smooth muscle excitation-contraction coupling process.

All vasodilators relax smooth muscle of arterioles, thereby decreasing systemic vascular resistance. Sodium nitroprusside also relaxes veins. Decreased arterial resistance and decreased mean arterial blood pressure elicit compensatory responses, mediated by baroreceptors and the sympathetic nervous system (Fig 9–6), as well as renin, angiotensin, and aldosterone. These compensating responses counteract the hypotensive effect of the vasodilator. Because sympathetic reflexes are intact, vasodilator therapy does not cause orthostatic hypotension or sexual dysfunction.

Vasodilators work best in combination with other antihypertensive drugs that oppose the compensatory cardiovascular responses (Fig 9–6). Sympatholytic drugs are useful in blocking increases in heart rate, myocardial contractility, and plasma renin levels. Propranolol is particularly useful because cardiac sympathetic effects can be totally blocked without produc-

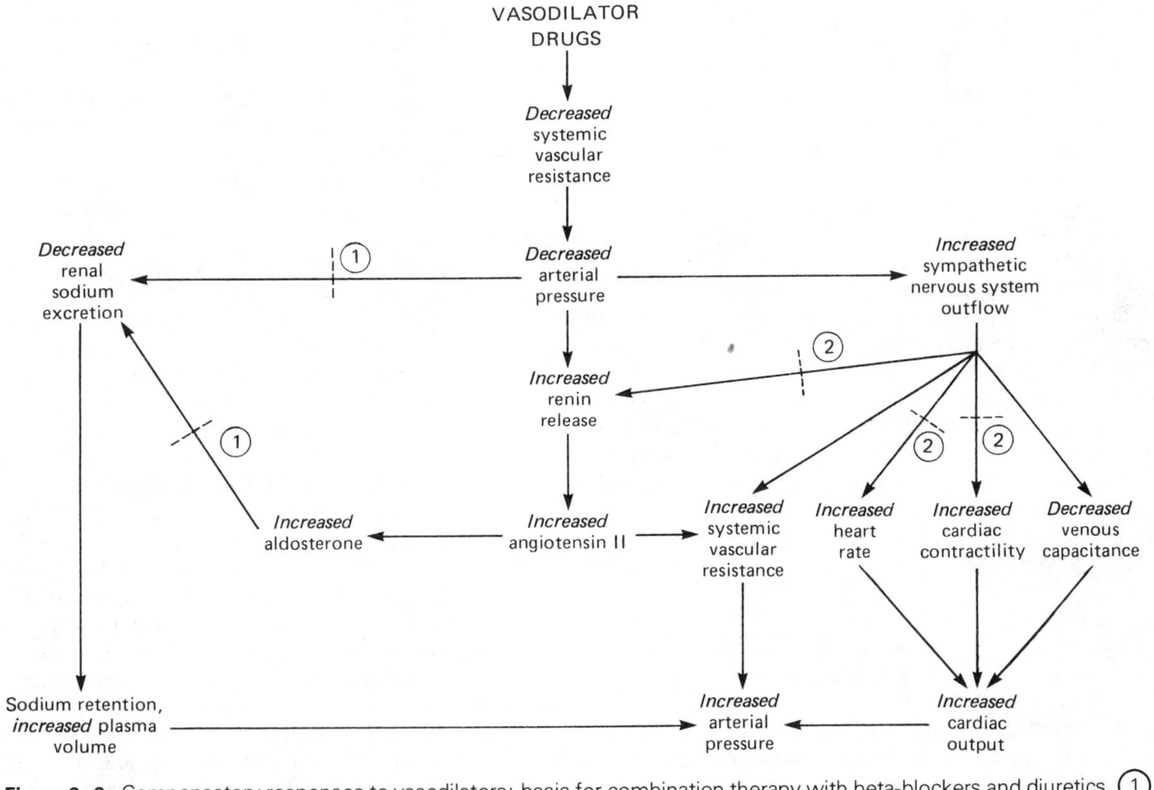

Figure 9–6. Compensatory responses to vasodilators; basis for combination therapy with beta-blockers and diuretics. (1) Effect blocked by diuretics. (2) Effect blocked by beta-blockers.

ing orthostatic hypotension. Diuretics are useful in preventing fluid retention and plasma volume expansion.

HYDRALAZINE

Hydralazine, a hydrazine derivative (Fig 9–4), dilates arterioles but not veins. It has been available for many years, although it was initially thought not to be particularly effective because tachyphylaxis to hypertensive effects developed rapidly. In the past 10 years, the benefits of combination therapy have been better appreciated, and hydralazine has had a resurgence in use.

Pharmacokinetics, Metabolism, & Dosage

Hydralazine is well absorbed and rapidly metabolized by the liver during the first pass, so that bioavailability is low (averaging 25%) and variable among individuals. It is metabolized in part by acetylation at a rate that appears to be bimodally distributed in the population. As a consequence, rapid acetylators have greater first-pass metabolism, lower bioavailability, and less antihypertensive benefit from a given dose than do slow acetylators. The half-life of hydralazine ranges from 2 to 4 hours, but vascular effects appear to persist longer than do blood concentrations—an observation that is consistent with experimental evidence of avid binding to vascular tissue.

Usual doses range from 40 to 200 mg/d. The higher dose was selected as the dose at which there is a small possibility of developing the lupus erythematosus-like syndrome described in the next section. However, higher doses result in greater vasodilatation and may be used if necessary. Dosing twice or 3 times daily provides smooth control of blood pressure.

Toxicity

The most common side-effects of hydralazine are headache, nausea, anorexia, palpitations, sweating, and flushing. In patients with ischemic heart disease, reflex tachycardia and sympathetic stimulation may provoke angina or ischemic arrhythmias. With doses of 400 mg/d or more, there is a 10–20% incidence—chiefly in persons who slowly acetylate the drug—of a syndrome characterized by arthralgia, myalgia, skin rashes, and fever that resembles lupus erythematosus. The syndrome is not associated with renal damage and is reversed by discontinuation of hydralazine. Peripheral neuropathy and drug fever are other serious but uncommon adverse effects.

MINOXIDIL

Minoxidil (Fig 9–4) is a very efficacious orally active vasodilator recently released for use in the USA. Like hydralazine, it dilates arterioles but not veins. Because of its greater potential antihypertensive effect, minoxidil should replace hydralazine when maximal doses of the latter are not effective or in patients with renal failure and severe hypertension, who do not respond well to hydralazine.

Pharmacokinetics, Metabolism, & Dosage

Minoxidil is well absorbed from the gastrointestinal tract and is metabolized, primarily by glucuronide conjugation, in the liver. Minoxidil is not protein-bound. Its half-life averages 4 hours, but its hypotensive effect after a single dose may persist for over 24 hours, probably as a result of avid binding to vascular smooth muscle.

Minoxidil is available only as an oral preparation. Generally, patients are started on 5 or 10 mg/d in 2 doses, and the daily dose is then gradually increased to 40 mg/d. Higher doses—up to 80 mg/d—have been used in treating severe hypertension, sometimes avoiding the requirement for nephrectomy.

Even more than with hydralazine, the use of minoxidil is associated with reflex sympathetic stimulation and sodium and fluid retention. Minoxidil must be used in combination with a beta-blocker and a loop diuretic.

Toxicity

Tachycardia, palpitations, angina, and edema are observed when doses of beta-blockers and diuretics are inadequate. Headache, sweating, and hypertrichosis, which is particularly bothersome in women, are relatively common.

SODIUM NITROPRUSSIDE

Sodium nitroprusside is a powerful parenterally administered vasodilator that is used in treating hypertensive emergencies as well as severe cardiac failure. Nitroprusside dilates both arterial and venous vessels, resulting in reduced peripheral vascular resistance and venous return.

In the absence of cardiac failure, blood pressure decreases, owing to decreased vascular resistance, while cardiac output does not change or decreases slightly. In patients with cardiac failure and low cardiac output, output increases due to afterload reduction. Heart rate typically increases, but less than is observed with other vasodilators.

Pharmacokinetics, Metabolism, & Dosage

Nitroprusside (Fig 9–4) is a complex of iron, cyanide groups, and a nitroso moiety. It is rapidly metabolized by uptake into red blood cells, where cyanide is liberated. Cyanide in turn is metabolized by the liver mitochondrial enzyme rhodanase, in the presence of a sulfur donor, to thiocyanate. Thiocyanate is distributed in extracellular fluid and slowly eliminated by the kidney.

Nitroprusside rapidly lowers blood pressure, and its effects disappear soon after discontinuation. The infusion rate is increased until blood pressure is controlled or until an administration rate likely to result in toxicity is achieved. Sodium nitroprusside is sensitive to light in aqueous solution and must therefore be made up fresh before each administration and covered with opaque foil. Infusion solutions should be changed after several hours. Doses typically begin at 0.5 μg/kg/min and may be increased up to 10 μg/kg/min as necessary to control blood pressure. Because of its efficacy and rapid onset of effect, the drug should be administered by infusion pump and arterial blood pressure continuously monitored via intra-arterial recording.

Toxicity

The most serious toxicity is related to accumulation of cyanide: metabolic acidosis, arrhythmias, excessive hypotension, and death have resulted. In a few cases, toxicity after relatively low doses of nitroprusside suggested a defect in cyanide metabolism. Administration of sodium thiosulfate as a sulfur donor facilitates metabolism of cyanide. Hydroxocobalamin combines with cyanide to form the nontoxic cyanocobalamin. Both have been advocated for prophylaxis or treatment of cyanide poisoning during nitroprusside infusion. Thiocyanate may accumulate over the course of prolonged administration, usually a week or more, particularly in patients with renal insufficiency who do not excrete thiocyanate at a normal rate. Thiocyanate toxicity is manifested as weakness, disorientation, psychosis, muscle spasms, and convulsions, and the diagnosis is confirmed by finding serum concentrations greater than 10 mg/dL. Rarely, delayed hypothyroidism occurs, owing to thiocyanate inhibition of iodide uptake by the thyroid. Methemoglobinemia during infusion of nitroprusside has also been reported.

DIAZOXIDE

Diazoxide is an effective and relatively long-acting parenterally administered arteriolar dilator that is used to treat hypertensive emergencies. Injection of diazoxide results in a sudden fall in systemic vascular resistance and mean arterial blood pressure associated with substantial tachycardia and increase in cardiac output.

Pharmacokinetics & Dosage

Diazoxide (Fig 9–4) is similar chemically to the thiazide diuretics but has no diuretic activity. It is bound extensively to serum albumin and to vascular tissue. Diazoxide is both metabolized and excreted unchanged; its metabolic pathways are not well characterized. Its half-life is approximately 24 hours, but the relationship between blood concentration and hypotensive action is not well established. The blood pressure-lowering effect after a rapid injection is established within 5 minutes and lasts for 4–12 hours. It was initially thought that rapid injection was mandatory to saturate plasma protein binding so that free drug could reach vascular tissue, but this idea is no longer generally accepted. Blood pressure is in fact lowered by constant infusion, although the extent of lowering for a given total dose is greater after rapid administration.

When diazoxide was first marketed, a dose of 300 mg by rapid injection was recommended. It appears, however, that excessive hypotension can be avoided by beginning with smaller doses (75–100 mg). If necessary, doses of 150 mg may be repeated every 5 minutes until blood pressure is lowered satisfactorily. Nearly all patients respond to a maximum of 3 or 4 doses. Because of reduced protein binding, hypotension occurs after smaller doses in persons with chronic renal failure, and smaller doses should be administered to these patients. The hypotensive effects of diazoxide are also greater if patients are pretreated with beta-blockers to prevent the reflex tachycardia and associated increase in cardiac output.

Toxicity

The most significant toxicity from diazoxide has been excessive hypotension, resulting from the recommendation to use a fixed dose of 300 mg in all patients. Such hypotension has resulted in stroke and myocardial infarction. The reflex sympathetic response can also provoke angina, electrocardiographic evidence of ischemia, and cardiac failure in patients with ischemic heart disease, and diazoxide should be avoided in this situation.

Diazoxide inhibits insulin release from the pancreas and is used to treat hypoglycemia secondary to insulinoma. Occasionally, hyperglycemia complicates diazoxide use, particularly in persons with renal insufficiency.

In contrast to the thiazide diuretics, diazoxide causes renal salt and water *retention*. However, because the drug is used for short periods only, this is rarely a problem.

CALCIUM ANTAGONISTS

Although primarily used thus far as antiarrhythmia and antiangina agents, calcium channel blockers also dilate peripheral arterioles and reduce blood pressure. The mechanism of action is believed to be inhibition of calcium influx in arterial smooth muscle. The pharmacology and toxicity of drugs used for this purpose are discussed in more detail in Chapter 10. **Nifedipine** and **verapamil** are currently being evaluated for treatment of hypertension in Europe; neither is approved for this use in the USA.

INHIBITORS OF ANGIOTENSIN

Although the causative roles of renin, angiotensin, and aldosterone in essential hypertension are still controversial, there do appear to be differences in the activity of this system among individuals. When controlled for daily sodium intake (assessed as 24-hour urinary sodium excretion) and serum potassium concentration, approximately 20% of patients with essential hypertension have inappropriately low and 20% have inappropriately high plasma renin activity. Blood pressure of patients with high-renin hypertension responds better to β-adrenergic blockers, which lower plasma renin activity, and to angiotensin inhibitors—supporting a role for excess renin and angiotensin in this population.

Mechanisms & Sites of Action

Renin release from the kidney cortex is stimulated by reduced renal arterial pressure, sympathetic neural stimulation, and reduced sodium delivery or increased sodium concentration at the distal renal tubule. Renin acts upon renin substrate, an α_2-globulin, to split off the inactive decapeptide angiotensin I that is then converted, primarily in the lung, to the arterial vasoconstrictor octapeptide angiotensin II that is in turn converted in the adrenal gland to angiotensin III (Fig 9–7). Angiotensin II has vasoconstrictor and sodium-retaining activity. Angiotensin II and III both stimulate aldosterone release. Angiotensin may contribute to maintaining high vascular resistance in hypertensive states associated with high plasma renin activity, such as renal arterial stenosis, some types of intrinsic renal disease, and malignant hypertension, as well as in essential hypertension after treatment with sodium restriction, diuretics, or vasodilators. Two compounds that inhibit the action of angiotensin have been extensively evaluated in humans.

SARALASIN

Saralasin (1-sar-8-ala-angiotensin II) is an analog and competitive inhibitor of angiotensin II. Saralasin blocks the pressor and aldosterone-releasing effects of infused angiotensin II and lowers blood pressure in high-renin states such as renal artery stenosis. Saralasin also has weak agonist activity, however, so that rapid injection or administration to persons without high circulating angiotensin II may increase rather than decrease blood pressure. This drug has proved to be a valuable research tool in determining the role of angiotensin II in experimental hypertension.

CAPTOPRIL

Captopril (Fig 9–4) inhibits the converting enzyme that hydrolyzes angiotensin I to angiotensin II and (under the name plasma kininase) inactivates bradykinin, a potent vasodilator. Unlike saralasin, captopril has no pressor activity. Thus, the hypotensive activity of captopril may result from an inhibitory action on the renin-angiotensin system and a stimulating action on the kallikrein-kinin system (Fig 9–7).

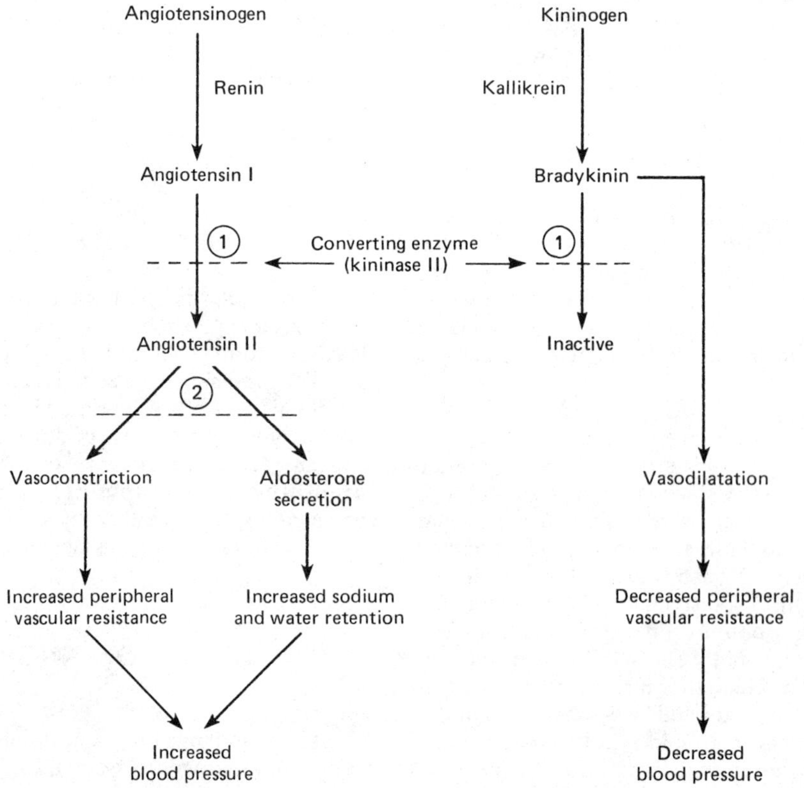

Figure 9–7. Sites of action of captopril and saralasin. (1) Site of captopril blockade. (2) Site of saralasin blockade.

Angiotensin II inhibitors lower blood pressure principally by decreasing peripheral vascular resistance. Cardiac output and heart rate are not significantly changed. Unlike direct vasodilators, captopril does not result in reflex sympathetic activation and can be used safely in persons with ischemic heart disease.

Although captopril is most effective in conditions associated with high plasma renin activity, there is no good correlation among subjects between plasma renin activity and hypotensive response. Accordingly, renin profiling is unnecessary. Captopril is usually reserved for patients who are unresponsive or intolerant to conventional drug therapy.

Pharmacokinetics & Dosage

Captopril is rapidly absorbed, with a bioavailability of about 70% after fasting; bioavailability is decreased by 30–40% if the drug is taken with food. It is metabolized chiefly to disulfide conjugates with other sulfhydryl-containing molecules. Less than half of an oral dose of captopril is excreted unchanged in the urine. Captopril is distributed to most body tissues, with the notable exception of the central nervous system. Although the half-life is not clearly established, most captopril is eliminated from the body within 6 hours.

Captopril is administered 2 or 3 times each day, taken 1–2 hours before meals. Maximal blood pressure response is seen 2–4 hours after the dose. At 1- to 2-week intervals, doses can be increased until blood pressure is controlled or to a maximum of 450 mg/d. Beyond this point, there probably is no further therapeutic benefit. Because captopril is partly eliminated by the kidney, less frequent dosing has been recommended for patients with renal insufficiency, but pharmacodynamic data to support this suggestion are lacking.

Toxicity

Toxicity from captopril is uncommon but may be serious, including bone marrow suppression and proteinuria. Neutropenia or pancytopenia usually occurs in the first month of therapy and resolves after the drug is discontinued, although fatal cases have been reported. Proteinuria is associated with minimal changes in kidney basal membranes and is reversible after stopping captopril in most, but not all, cases. It is recommended that blood counts and urinalyses be performed frequently (every 2 weeks) in the first few months of treatment. Minor toxic effects include altered sense of taste, allergic skin rashes, and drug fever, which may occur in as many as 10% of patients.

II. CLINICAL PHARMACOLOGY OF ANTIHYPERTENSIVE AGENTS

Hypertension presents a unique problem in therapeutics. It is usually a lifelong disease that causes few symptoms until the advanced stages. For effective treatment, medicines that are expensive and often produce adverse effects must be consumed daily. Thus, the physician must establish with certainty that hypertension is persistent and requires treatment and must exclude secondary causes of hypertension that might be treated by definitive surgical procedures. Persistence of hypertension, particularly in persons with mild elevation of blood pressure, should be established by finding an elevated blood pressure on at least 3 different office visits.

Once the presence of hypertension is established, the question of whether or not to treat and which drugs to use must be considered. The level of blood pressure, the age and sex of the patient, the severity of organ damage (if any) due to high blood pressure, and the presence of cardiovascular risk factors must all be considered. For example, an obese, apparently healthy middle-aged woman with mild hypertension and no cardiovascular risk factors might be treated with dietary caloric and sodium restriction and observation every 6 months. A young adult black man with mild hypertension but a strong family history of hypertension and coronary heart disease who has hyperlipidemia and is a heavy cigarette smoker should be treated more vigorously.

Once the decision is made to treat, a therapeutic regimen must be developed and the patient must be educated about the nature of hypertension and the importance of treatment. Selection of drugs is dictated by the level of blood pressure and the presence and severity of end organ damage. Severe high blood pressure with life-threatening complications requires more rapid treatment with more potent drugs. Most patients with essential hypertension, however, have had elevated blood pressure for months or years, and therapy is best initiated in a gradual fashion.

Successful treatment of hypertension requires that dietary instructions be followed and medications be taken as directed. Education about the natural history of hypertension and the importance of treatment as well as potential side-effects of drugs is essential. Follow-up visits should be frequent enough to convince the patient that the physician thinks the illness is serious. With each follow-up visit, the importance of treatment should be reinforced and questions—particularly concerning dosing or side-effects of medication—encouraged. Other factors that may improve compliance are simplifying dosing regimens and having the patient monitor blood pressure at home.

OUTPATIENT THERAPY OF HYPERTENSION

A general approach to outpatient management of hypertension has been presented by the Joint National Committee on Detection, Evaluation, and Treatment of High Blood Pressure. It consists of a number of sequential steps, combining drugs with different sites of action to maximize lowering of blood pressure while

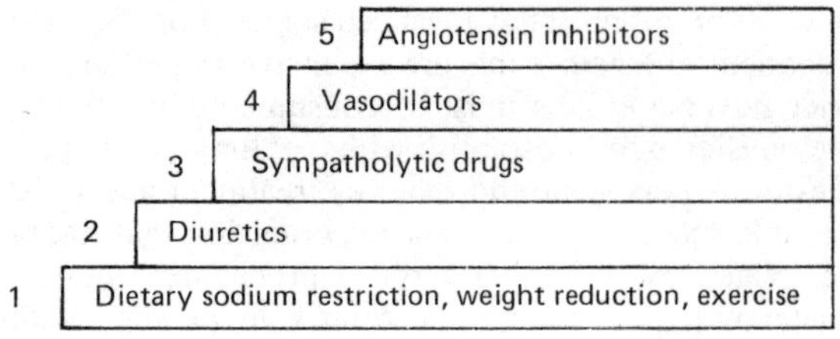

Figure 9–8. Stepped-care approach to treatment of hypertension.

minimizing side-effects. A modified version of the stepped-care approach is shown in Fig 9–8.

The initial step in treating hypertension may be nonpharmacologic. As discussed previously, sodium restriction may be effective treatment for as many as half of patients with mild hypertension. The average American diet contains about 200 mEq of sodium per day. A reasonable dietary goal in treating hypertension is 70–100 mEq of sodium per day, which can be achieved by not salting food during or after cooking and by avoiding processed foods that contain large amounts of sodium. Compliance with sodium restriction can be assessed by measuring 24-hour urinary excretion of sodium, which approximates sodium intake, before and after dietary instruction.

Weight reduction even without sodium restriction has been shown to normalize blood pressure in up to 75% of overweight patients with mild to moderate hypertension. Regular exercise has been shown in some but not all studies to lower blood pressure in hypertensive patients.

For most patients, diuretics are the first drug group used. Thiazide diuretics, combined with sodium restriction, are effective in normalizing blood pressure in most patients with mild hypertension and many with moderate hypertension. Loop diuretics are necessary in the presence of renal insufficiency with reduced glomerular filtration rate. Spironolactone may be used in the presence of hyperaldosteronism due to tumor, cardiac failure, or cirrhosis. At least 1 month should be allowed to evaluate the maximal antihypertensive effect of a particular diuretic.

Sympatholytic drugs are the next step, although propranolol can also be used as a first-step drug, particularly in persons with labile or high-renin essential hypertension or those unable to tolerate diuretics. All sympatholytic drugs are effective. Selection of a particular agent should be determined by anticipated side-effects, convenience of use, cost, and physician preference. Propranolol is often chosen for young active patients, because sedation is minimal and there is no orthostatic hypotension and less sexual dysfunction compared with other sympatholytic drugs. Centrally acting sympatholytics such as methyldopa and clonidine are more sedating—an effect that may be advantageous in the treatment of anxious patients. Because of its wide dose-response range, clonidine may be more effective than beta-blockers in treating severe hypertension. Peripheral-acting sympatholytic drugs such as reserpine and guanethidine are especially convenient, because they require only once-daily dosing and are less expensive than other sympatholytic agents. However, in larger doses required to treat more severe hypertension, reserpine causes excessive sedation and guanethidine causes orthostatic hypotension, diarrhea, and sexual dysfunction. Prazosin is effective in mild to moderate hypertension and is useful in patients who cannot tolerate beta-blockers (because of asthma, for example) or the sedating effects of centrally active drugs. In more severe hypertension, prazosin can be combined successfully with beta-blockers.

Vasodilators are added as the third drug class. Hydralazine is usually started first, and if maximal doses are reached without adequate control of blood pressure, minoxidil is substituted. Doses of diuretics or beta-blockers (or both) may have to be increased or, if other sympatholytic drugs are being used, beta-blockers are added to control the tendency toward sodium retention and reflex sympathetic stimulation due to vasodilators. Constant body weight and a heart rate of 80 or less are useful end points in adjusting doses of diuretics and beta-blockers, respectively.

There is no consensus about the next step to be taken if hypertension is still uncontrolled. Some authorities advise guanethidine, but this drug's unwanted effects may be incapacitating in severe hypertension, when large doses are required. Captopril is probably a better choice in that it acts by a different mechanism, may be additive or synergistic with actions of other drugs, and is usually well tolerated. More experience is necessary before firm recommendations about the role of captopril can be offered.

Assessment of blood pressure during office visits should include measurement of recumbent, sitting, and standing blood pressures. If a drug such as guanethidine that produces orthostatic hypotension is used, postexercise blood pressure should be measured as well. An attempt should be made to normalize blood pressure (mean blood pressure 100 mm Hg or less) in the posture or activity level that is customary for the patient. The extent of orthostatic hypotension and inhibition of reflex or exercise tachycardia are useful indicators of the effectiveness of or compliance with sympatholytic therapy. In addition to noncompliance with medication, causes of failure to respond to drug therapy include excessive sodium intake and inadequate diuretic therapy with excessive blood volume (this can be measured directly), and drugs such as antidepressants and over-the-counter sympathomimetics that can interfere with actions of some antihypertensive drugs or directly raise blood pressure.

MANAGEMENT OF HYPERTENSIVE EMERGENCIES

Despite the large number of patients with chronic hypertension, hypertensive emergencies are relatively rare. Marked or sudden elevation of blood pressure may be a serious threat to life, however, and prompt reduction of blood pressure is indicated. Most commonly, hypertensive emergencies occur in patients whose hypertension is severe and poorly controlled or in those who suddenly discontinue antihypertensive medications.

Clinical Presentation & Pathophysiology

Hypertensive emergencies include hypertension associated with vascular damage (termed malignant hypertension) and hypertension associated with hemodynamic complications such as cardiac failure, stroke, or dissecting aneurysm. The underlying pathologic process in malignant hypertension is a progressive arteriopathy with inflammation and necrosis of arterioles. Vascular lesions occur in the kidney, which releases renin, which in turn stimulates production of angiotensin and aldosterone, which further increases blood pressure.

Hypertensive encephalopathy is a classic feature of malignant hypertension. Its clinical presentation consists of severe headache, mental confusion, and apprehension. Blurred vision, nausea and vomiting, and focal neurologic deficits are common. If untreated, the syndrome may progress to convulsions, stupor, coma, and even death over a period of 12–48 hours.

Treatment of Hypertensive Emergencies

The general management of hypertensive emergencies requires monitoring the patient in an intensive care unit with continuous recording of arterial blood pressure. Rapid treatment is essential. Fluid intake and output must be monitored carefully and body weight measured daily as an indicator of total body fluid volume during the course of therapy. The first medication to be administered is usually a diuretic. Because it is likely that the patient will have compromised renal function, a drug that works in the presence of renal insufficiency, such as furosemide, should be selected. An appreciable diuresis should occur within 30 minutes and enhance the antihypertensive effects of other medications.

Dialysis may be an important alternative to the loop diuretics, particularly in patients with oliguric renal failure. Dialysis can remove excess fluid, correct electrolyte disturbances, and control symptoms of uremia. Uremic symptoms may be confusing in evaluating patients with hypertensive encephalopathy.

Additional parenteral antihypertensive medications are used to lower blood pressure rapidly; as soon as reasonable blood pressure control is achieved, oral antihypertensive therapy should be substituted, because this allows smoother long-term management of hypertension. The drugs most commonly used to treat hypertensive emergencies are the vasodilators sodium nitroprusside and diazoxide. Other drugs that may be effective include trimethaphan camsylate, hydralazine, reserpine, methyldopa, and angiotensin inhibitors.

Sodium nitroprusside is the most potent and predictably effective drug. Cardiac output may increase as a result of afterload reduction or decrease because of reduced venous return, depending on whether or not cardiac failure is present. Toxicity due to generation of cyanide is a major concern with high doses or during prolonged administration.

Diazoxide has the major advantage that once blood pressure is normalized, blood pressure remains low and returns only gradually over 4–10 hours to the pretreatment level. This means that once a patient is stabilized, monitoring can be less intensive compared with that required when a constant infusion of nitroprusside is given. The disadvantages of diazoxide are the possibility of excessive hypotension and reflex sympathetic stimulation, which is potentially detrimental to patients with coronary heart disease and dissecting aneurysm.

Trimethaphan's hypotensive effects are most pronounced when the patient is upright, and it is usually necessary to elevate the head of the bed to achieve a good hypotensive response. The drug is quite efficacious and acts immediately, and its hypotensive effects can be rapidly reversed by stopping the infusion and placing the patient in the head-down position. Trimethaphan is especially useful in treating patients with dissecting aneurysm, when venous pooling and decreased cardiac contractility are beneficial. Serious adverse consequences of ganglionic blockade include urinary retention and paralytic ileus.

Hydralazine lowers blood pressure after parenteral administration, but its effects are not predictable, and it rarely controls severe hypertension. **Reserpine** is quite effective in treating severe hypertension, but its onset of action is relatively slow, and high doses are required to lower blood pressure; these doses produce marked sedation and somnolence that complicate evaluation of hypertensive encephalopathy. **Methyldopa** infusions have been used to treat hypertensive emergencies, but the onset of antihypertensive effect is gradual, the degree of blood pressure lowering is unpredictable, and the effects are associated with somnolence.

Angiotensin II may play a significant role in maintaining the high vascular resistance observed in malignant hypertension. Although **captopril** and **saralasin** have been shown to decrease blood pressure dramatically in some patients with malignant hypertension, their role in the management of hypertensive emergencies has not been clearly defined. These drugs should be considered when other medications are not successful.

Phentolamine is an α-adrenoceptor blocker that has been used primarily in the diagnosis and management of pheochromocytoma. Both sympathetic neural activity and circulating catecholamines may contribute to maintenance of blood pressure in hypertensive emergencies, although this has not been well studied. If vasodilator therapy at maximally tolerated doses is inadequate in controlling blood pressure, added infusion of phentolamine should be considered.

• • •

References

Becker CE, Benowitz NL: Hypertensive emergencies. *Med Clin North Am* 1979;**63:**127.

Cohn JN, Burke LP: Nitroprusside. *Ann Intern Med* 1979; **91:**752.

Freis ED: Salt, volume and the prevention of hypertension. *Circulation* 1976;**53:**589.

Frohlich ED: Methyldopa: Mechanisms and treatment 25 years later. *Arch Intern Med* 1980;**140:**954.

Gifford RW Jr, Tarazi RC: Resistant hypertension: Diagnosis and management. *Ann Intern Med* 1978;**88:**661.

Graham RM, Pettinger WA: Prazosin. *N Engl J Med* 1979; **300:**232.

Haddy FJ: Mechanism, prevention and therapy of sodium-dependent hypertension. *Am J Med* 1980;**69:**746.

Heel RC et al: Captopril: A preliminary review of its pharmacological properties and therapeutic efficacy. *Drugs* 1980;**20:**409.

Helgeland A: Treatment of mild hypertension: A five year controlled drug trial. The Oslo study. *Am J Med* 1980;**69:**725.

Holland OB, Kaplan NM: Propranolol in the treatment of hypertension. *N Engl J Med* 1976;**294:**930.

Hypertension Detection and Follow-Up Program Cooperative Group: Five-year findings of the Hypertension Detection and Follow-Up Program. 1. Reduction in mortality of persons with high blood pressure, including mild hypertension. *JAMA* 1979;**242:**2562.

Koch-Weser J: Diazoxide. *N Engl J Med* 1976;**294:**1271.

Koch-Weser J: Drug therapy: Hydralazine. *N Engl J Med* 1976; **295:**320.

Koch-Weser J: Drug therapy: Metoprolol. *N Engl J Med* 1979; **301:**698.

Linas SL, Nies AS: Minoxidil. *Ann Intern Med* 1981;**94:**61.

Lowenstein J: Clonidine. *Ann Intern Med* 1980;**92:**74.

Pettinger WA: Clonidine, a new antihypertensive drug. *N Engl J Med* 1975;**293:**1179.

Reisin E et al: Effect of weight loss without salt restriction on the reduction of blood pressure in overweight hypertensive patients. *N Engl J Med* 1978;**298:**1.

Report of the Joint National Committee on Detection, Evaluation, and Treatment of High Blood Pressure: A cooperative study. *JAMA* 1977;**237:**255.

Report by the Management Committee: The Australian therapeutic trial in mild hypertension. *Lancet* 1980;**1:**1261.

The 1980 Report of the Joint National Committee on Detection, Evaluation, and Treatment of High Blood Pressure. *Arch Intern Med* 1980;**140:**1280.

Veterans Administration Cooperative Study Group on Antihypertensive Agents: Effects of treatment on morbidity in hypertension. 1. Results in patients with diastolic blood pressure averaging 115 through 129 mm Hg. *JAMA* 1967;**202:**1028.

Veterans Administration Cooperative Study Group on Antihypertensive Agents: Effects of treatment on morbidity in hypertension. 2. Results in patients with diastolic blood pressure averaging 90 through 114 mm Hg. *JAMA* 1970;**213:**1143.

Woosley RL, Nies AS: Guanethidine. *N Engl J Med* 1976; **295:**1053.

Vasodilators & the Treatment of Angina Pectoris | 10

Bertram G. Katzung, MD, PhD, & Kanu Chatterjee, MB, FRCP

Vasodilator drugs are used in several conditions involving tissue ischemia, but by far the most important one is angina pectoris. Angina is caused by the accumulation of metabolites in striated muscle; angina pectoris is the strangling chest pain that occurs when coronary blood flow is inadequate to supply the oxygen required by the heart.

Ischemic heart disease is the most common serious health problem in many western societies. By far the most frequent cause is atheromatous obstruction of the large coronary vessels. However, transient spasm of localized portions of these vessels can also cause significant myocardial ischemia and pain (variant or angiospastic angina).

The primary cause of angina pectoris is an imbalance between the oxygen requirement of the heart and the oxygen supplied to it via the coronary vessels. In classic angina, the imbalance occurs when the myocardial oxygen requirement increases, as during exercise. Classic angina is therefore "angina of effort." In variant angina, oxygen delivery decreases as a result of reversible coronary vasospasm. The primary objective of treatment in both forms of angina is to improve coronary blood flow. A secondary objective is reduction of the myocardial oxygen requirement. Both measures are used in clinical practice. Traditional treatment achieves the second goal through the use of organic nitrates—potent vasodilators—and several other classes of drugs. It is important to realize that the vasodilators useful in angina of effort do not act by dilating the obstructed coronary vessels but by dilating normal peripheral vessels and thus decreasing the work of the heart. Therefore, we will avoid the term "coronary vasodilator." Furthermore, careful study of newer agents has shown that not all vasodilators are effective in angina and, conversely, that some agents useful in angina (eg, propranolol) are not vasodilators.

This chapter is divided into 2 sections. The first describes the basic pharmacology of 2 important classes of vasodilators: the nitrates and the calcium influx inhibitors. The second section describes the clinical pathophysiology of angina pectoris and its management by means of the 2 classes of drugs and the β-adrenergic blocking agents.

History

Angina pectoris was first described as a distinct clinical entity by William Heberden in the latter half of the 18th century. In the second half of the 19th century, another English physician, T. Lauder Brunton, associated anginal attacks with events that raise blood pressure and experimented with amyl nitrite to lower blood pressure. Although transient relief was achieved, the compound was difficult to use properly, and it was not until the introduction of nitroglycerin in 1879 that effective relief of acute episodes of angina became possible. Subsequently, many other vasodilators were introduced for the treatment of angina. However, when careful double-blind clinical trials were done, most of these agents were found to be no better than placebo. In fact, several of the classic studies of the placebo effect were carried out in patients with angina. With the introduction of β-adrenergic blocking drugs, useful prophylactic therapy of angina became possible. More recently, the calcium influx blockers have been shown to be useful for prevention of anginal attacks, especially in variant angina.

I. BASIC PHARMACOLOGY OF VASODILATORS

NITRATES & NITRITES

Chemistry

These agents are simple nitric and nitrous acid esters of polyalcohols (Fig 10–1). They vary from extremely volatile liquids (amyl nitrite) through moderately volatile liquids (nitroglycerin) to solids (isosorbide dinitrate). Nitroglycerin may be considered the prototype of the group. Although it is used in the manufacture of dynamite, the formulations of nitroglycerin used in medicine are not explosive. The conventional sublingual tablet form of nitroglycerin may lose potency when stored as a result of volatilization and adsorption to plastic surfaces. Therefore, it should be kept in tightly closed glass containers. It is not sensitive to light.

Structure-activity studies indicate that all therapeutically active agents in this group are capable of releasing nitrite ion in vascular smooth muscle

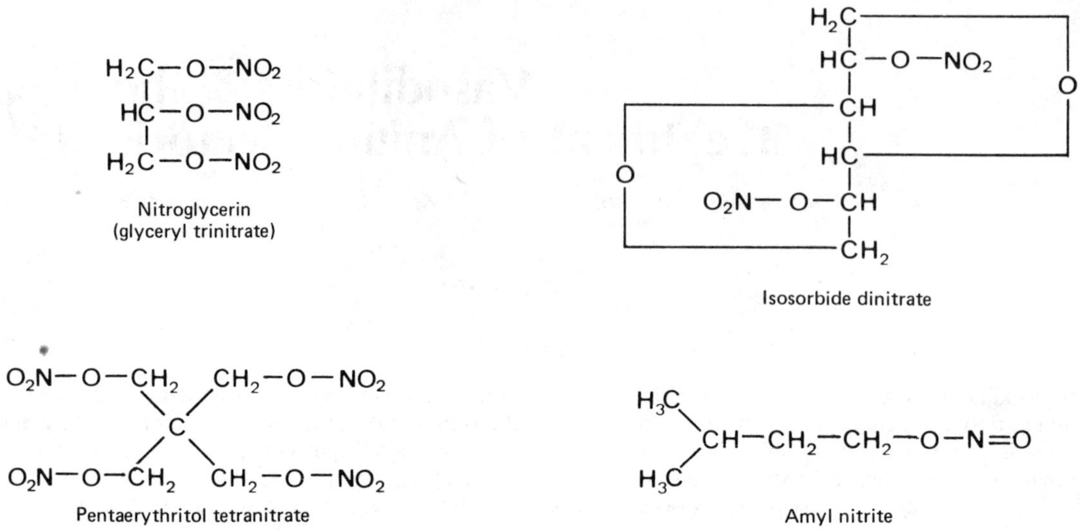

Figure 10–1. Chemical structures of 3 nitrates and amyl nitrite.

target tissues. Unfortunately, they all also appear to be capable of inducing cross-tolerance when given in large doses. Therefore, pharmacokinetic factors govern the choice of agent and mode of therapy when using the nitrates.

Pharmacokinetics

The use of organic nitrates is strongly influenced by the existence of a high-capacity hepatic organic nitrate reductase that inactivates the drug. Therefore, bioavailability of all orally administered organic nitrates is very low (typically less than 10%). Consequently, the sublingual route is preferred for achieving a therapeutic blood level rapidly. Nitroglycerin and isosorbide dinitrate are both absorbed efficiently by this route and reach therapeutic blood levels within a few minutes. However, the total dose administered by this route must be limited to avoid excessive effects; therefore, the total duration of effect is brief, typically 15–30 minutes. When much longer duration of action is needed, oral preparations are available that contain an amount of drug sufficient to result in sustained systemic blood levels in spite of first-pass hepatic inactivation. Other routes of administration available for nitroglycerin include transdermal absorption when applied to the skin as an ointment and buccal absorption from slow-release buccal preparations; these are described below.

Amyl nitrite and related nitrites are highly volatile liquids. Amyl nitrite is available in fragile glass ampules packaged in a protective cloth covering. The ampule can be crushed with the fingers, resulting in rapid release of inhalable vapors through the cloth covering. The inhalation route provides for very rapid absorption and, like the sublingual route, avoids the hepatic first-pass effect.

Once absorbed, the unchanged nitrate compounds have half-lives of only 2–8 minutes. The denitrated metabolites have much longer half-lives (1–3 hours) but are considerably less active as vasodilators.

Excretion, primarily in the form of glucuronide derivatives of the denitrated metabolites, is largely by way of the kidney.

Pharmacodynamics

Nitroglycerin and its analogs are unusually selective drugs: in therapeutic doses, their action is almost exclusively on smooth muscle cells.

A. Mechanism of Action: Nitroglycerin is probably denitrated in the smooth muscle cell. The resulting nitrite ion (NO_2^-) is thought to react with a specific receptor. The latter appears to include sulfhydryl (–SH) groups, since tolerance to nitrite involves a decrease in tissue sulfhydryl groups, and tolerance can be reversed with dithiothreitol, a sulfhydryl-regenerating agent. Little is known of the steps linking receptor binding of the nitrite ion and relaxation of smooth muscle. Some evidence suggests that an increase in cGMP is the first link. Other studies implicate the production of prostaglandin E or prostacyclin (PGI_2) as an important intermediate step. There is no evidence that autonomic receptors are involved in the primary nitrate response (although autonomic *reflex* responses are evoked when hypotensive doses are given).

B. Organ System Effects: Nitroglycerin relaxes all types of smooth muscle irrespective of the cause of the preexisting muscle tone (Fig 10–2). It has practically no direct effect on cardiac or skeletal muscle, and the reasons for this selectivity are unknown.

1. Vascular smooth muscle–All segments of the vascular system from large arteries through large veins relax in response to nitroglycerin (Fig 10–2). However, arterioles and precapillary sphincters are dilated less than other portions of the vascular tree, at least partly because of reflex responses. The primary

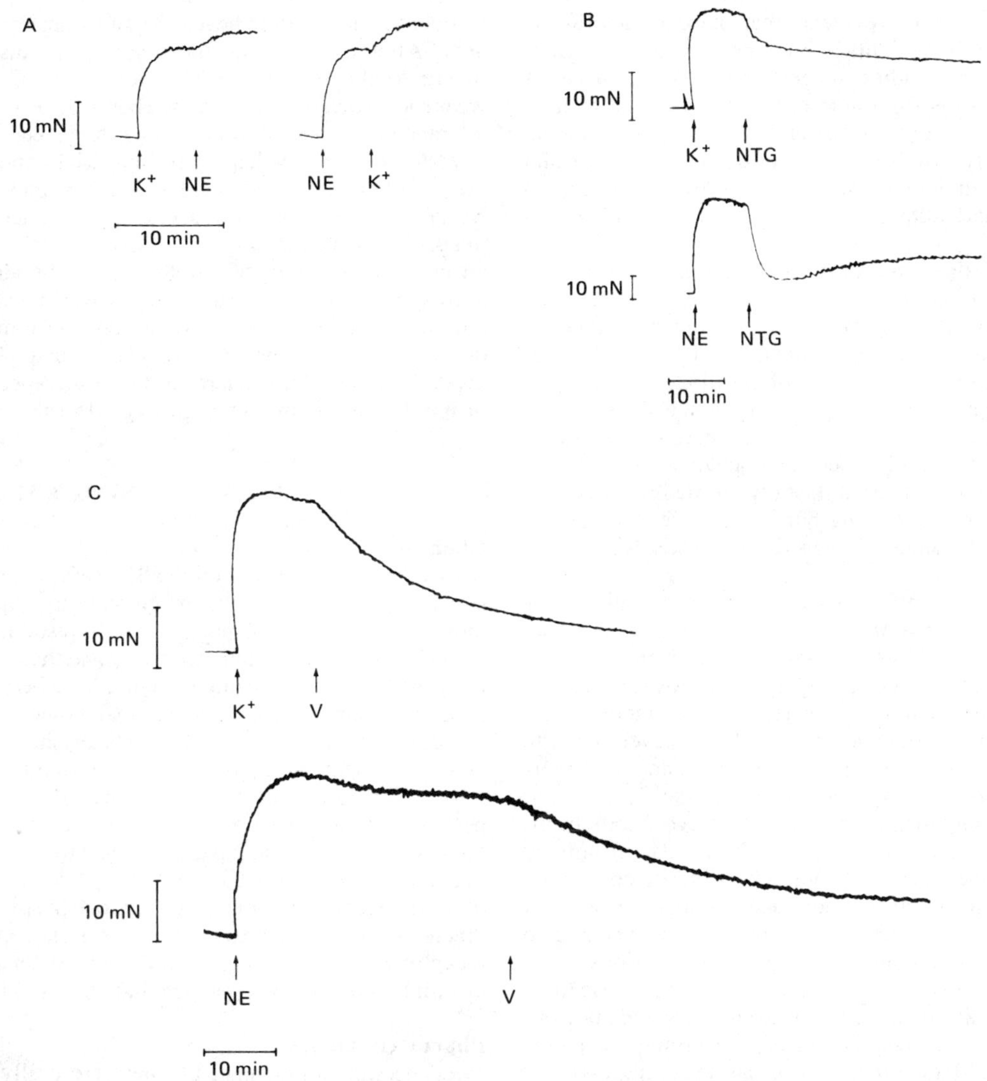

Figure 10–2. Effects of vasodilators on contractions of human vein segments studied in vitro. Panel *A* shows contractions induced by 2 vasoconstrictor agents, norepinephrine (NE) and potassium (K^+). Panel *B* shows the relaxation induced by nitroglycerin (NTG), 4 μM. The relaxation is prompt. Panel *C* shows the relaxation induced by verapamil (V), 2.2 μM. The relaxation is slower but more sustained. (Modified and reproduced, with permission, from Mikkelsen E, Andersson K-E, Bengtsson B: Effects of verapamil and nitroglycerin on contractile responses to potassium and noradrenaline in isolated human peripheral veins. *Acta Pharmacol Toxicol* 1978;**42**:14.)

direct result of an effective blood concentration is marked relaxation of the large veins with increased venous capacitance and decreased ventricular preload. Pulmonary vascular pressures and heart size are significantly reduced. In the absence of heart failure, cardiac output is reduced. Because venous capacitance is increased, orthostatic hypotension may be marked, and syncope can result. Dilatation of some large arteries may be significant: Temporal artery pulsations and a throbbing headache associated with meningial artery pulsations are frequent side-effects of nitroglycerin and amyl nitrite. In the presence of heart failure, preload is usually abnormally high; the nitrates and other vasodilators may have a beneficial effect on cardiac output in this condition (see Chapter 11).

The indirect effects of nitroglycerin consist of those reflexes evoked by baroreceptors responding to decreased arterial pressure (Fig 4–6). The primary mechanism of this reflex is sympathetic discharge; this consistently results in tachycardia and increased cardiac contractility. In the case of very rapidly acting agents (eg, inhaled amyl nitrite), arterial dilatation may be so marked as to cause a reflex venoconstriction.

In the isolated coronary-perfused heart (Langendorf preparation) and in normal subjects without coronary disease, nitroglycerin can induce a significant, if transient, increase in total coronary blood flow. In contrast, there is no evidence that total coronary flow is increased in patients with atherosclerotic angina. While some studies suggest that *redistribution* of coronary flow from normal to ischemic regions may play a role, most evidence suggests that relief of angina by nitroglycerin is the result of decreased myocardial oxygen requirement secondary to decreased preload and cardiac output (see Clinical Pharmacology, below).

2. Other smooth muscle organs–Relaxation of smooth muscle of the bronchi, gastrointestinal tract (including biliary system), and genitourinary tract has been demonstrated experimentally. Because of their brief duration, these actions of the nitrates are rarely of any clinical value. During recent years, the use of amyl nitrite and isobutyl nitrite as recreational (sex-enhancing) drugs has become popular with some segments of the population. Isobutyl nitrite is not licensed or advertised as a drug but is sold over-the-counter under such names as Rush, Bolt, Locker Room, and Dr. Bananas.

3. Other effects–Nitrite ion reacts with hemoglobin (which contains ferrous iron) to produce methemoglobin (which contains ferric iron). Because methemoglobin has a very low affinity for oxygen, large doses of nitrites can result in pseudocyanosis, tissue hypoxia, and death. The plasma level of nitrite resulting from even large doses of organic and inorganic nitrates is too low to cause significant methemoglobinemia in adults. However, sodium nitrite is used as a curing agent for meats. In nursing infants, the intestinal flora is capable of converting significant amounts of inorganic nitrate, eg, from well water, to nitrite ion. Thus, inadvertent exposure to large amounts of nitrite ion can produce serious toxicity. One therapeutic application of this otherwise toxic effect of nitrite has been discovered. Cyanide poisoning results from complexing of cytochrome iron by the CN^- ion. Methemoglobin iron has a very high affinity for CN^-; thus, administration of sodium nitrite ($NaNO_2$) soon after cyanide exposure will regenerate active cytochrome. The cyanmethemoglobin produced can be further detoxified by the intravenous administration of sodium thiosulfate ($Na_2S_2O_3$); this results in formation of thiocyanate ion (SCN^-), a less toxic ion that is readily excreted. Methemoglobinemia, if excessive, can be treated by giving methylene blue intravenously (Chapter 58).

Toxicity & Tachyphylaxis

The major acute toxicity of organic nitrates is a direct extension of therapeutic vasodilatation: orthostatic hypotension, tachycardia, and throbbing headache. With continuous exposure to nitrates, isolated smooth muscle may develop complete tolerance, and the intact human becomes at least partially tolerant. Continuous exposure to high levels of nitrates can occur in the chemical industry, especially where explosives are manufactured. When contamination of the workplace with volatile organic nitrate compounds is severe, workers find that upon starting their work week (Monday), they suffer headache and transient dizziness. After a day or so, these symptoms disappear owing to the development of tolerance. Over the weekend, when exposure to the chemicals is reduced, tolerance disappears, so symptoms recur each Monday. A more serious hazard of industrial exposure is the development of dependence. This may affect workers after months or years of exposure and manifests itself as variant angina occurring after 1–2 days away from the source of nitrates, eg, on Sunday of a normal work week. In the most seriously affected individuals, coronary vasospasm may cause myocardial infarction. There is no evidence that physical dependence develops as a result of the therapeutic use of nitrates for angina, even in large doses.

CALCIUM INFLUX–BLOCKING DRUGS

Chemistry

Verapamil, the first clinically useful member of this group, was the result of attempts to synthesize more active analogs of papaverine, a vasodilator alkaloid found in the opium poppy. Since then, dozens of agents of widely varying structure have been found to have the same fundamental pharmacologic action. A few of the clinically important agents are shown in Fig 10–3 along with papaverine, now of academic interest only. Two older compounds, prenylamine and perhexilene, are still available in many countries (not the USA) but appear to have significant disadvantages in comparison with the agents shown. A large number of newer agents are under investigation. In spite of the diverse structures represented in this group, the drug receptor is stereoselective: the R (+) isomer of verapamil has much lower potency than the S (–) isomer.

Pharmacokinetics

The calcium channel blockers are orally active agents that readily bind to plasma protein (80–90%). First-pass hepatic metabolism is extensive for verapamil and diltiazem. Elimination half-lives are 3–7 hours, with nifedipine and verapamil being excreted primarily in the urine and diltiazem in the feces. All 3 compounds are extensively metabolized (Table 10–1).

Pharmacodynamics

A. Mechanism of Action: Calcium channel blockers bind to membrane structures responsible for the "slow inward current"—structures thought to be channels much like the sodium channels of nerve but relatively selective for calcium. Tissues that require calcium influx for normal activity are therefore susceptible to block by these agents.

Calcium channel blockade by these drugs resembles sodium channel blockade by local anesthetics. The drugs act from the inner side of the membrane and bind more effectively to channels in depolarized membranes. The block is partially reversible by elevating the concentration of calcium, although the levels of calcium required are not clinically attainable. Partial

Table 10–1. Pharmacokinetics of some calcium influx-blocking drugs.

Drug	Absorption	Onset of Action	Plasma Half-Life	Disposition
Verapamil	> 90% after oral administration.	< 1½ min after intravenous, < 30 min after oral administration.	3–7 hours.	About 90% bound to plasma protein; 85% first-pass hepatic elimination after oral administration. About 70% eliminated by kidney; 15% by gastrointestinal tract.
Nifedipine	> 90% after oral or sublingual administration.	< 1 min after intravenous, < 3 min after sublingual, < 20 min after oral administration.	4 hours.	About 90% bound to plasma protein; metabolized to an acid lactate. Drug and metabolites excreted 80% in urine.
Diltiazem	> 90% after oral administration.	< 3 min after intravenous, < 3 min after oral administration.	4 hours.	Little bound to plasma protein but extensively deacetylated. Drug and metabolites excreted in feces.

reversal of block can also be obtained by the use of drugs that increase the transmembrane flux of calcium, such as adrenergic stimulants.

B. Organ System Effects:

1. Smooth muscle–Most types of smooth muscle are dependent on transmembrane calcium influx for normal resting tone and contractile responses. These cells are relaxed by the calcium influx inhibitors. Vascular smooth muscle appears to be the most sensitive (Fig 10–2), but similar relaxation can be shown for bronchiolar, gastrointestinal, and uterine smooth muscle. In the vascular system, arterioles appear to be more sensitive than veins; orthostatic hypotension is not a common side-effect. Blood pressure can be reduced, especially with nifedipine. The reduction in peripheral vascular resistance is one mechanism by

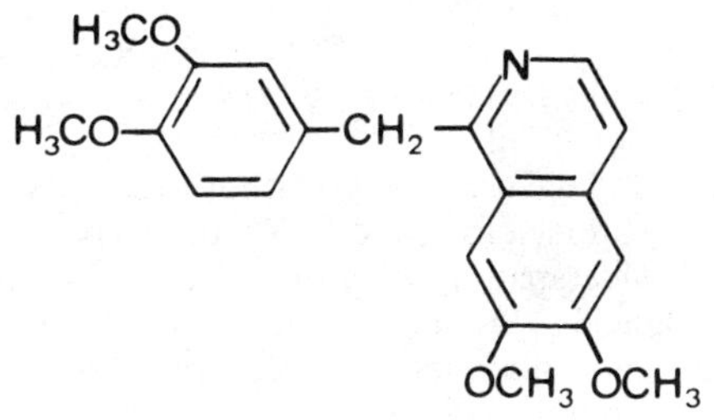

Papaverine

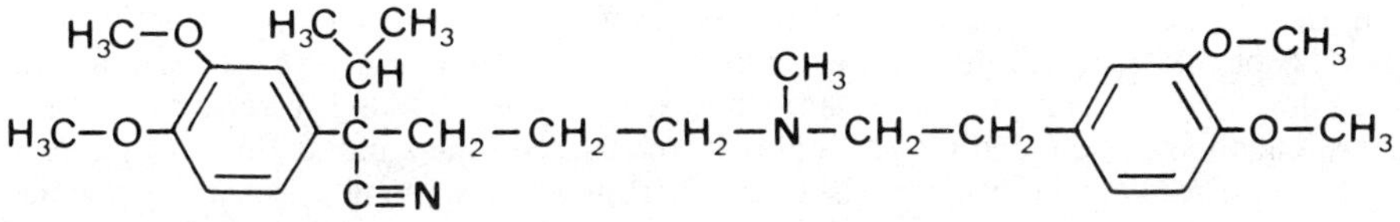

Verapamil

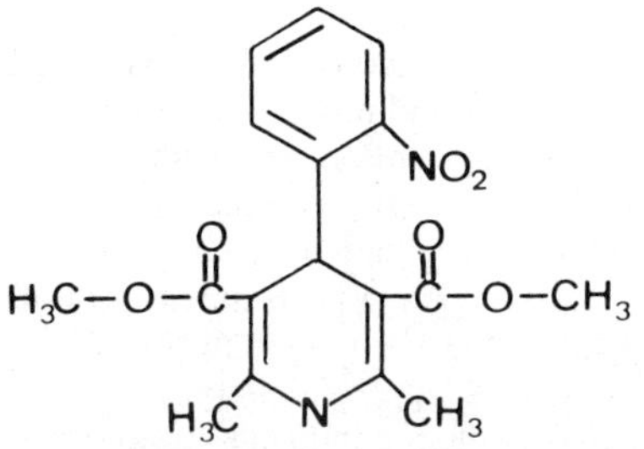

Nifedipine

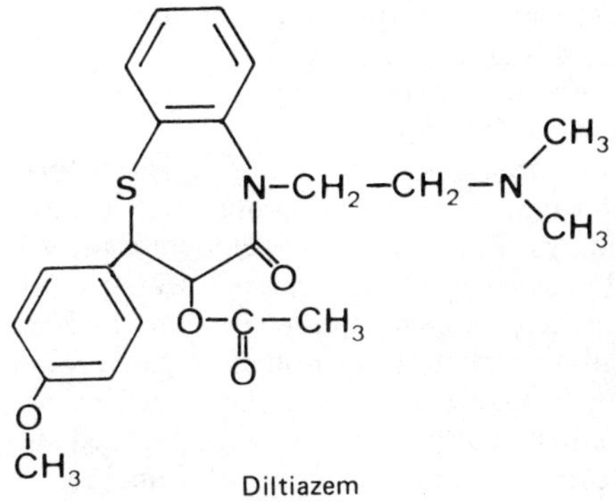

Diltiazem

Figure 10–3. Chemical structures of several calcium influx-blocking drugs.

which these agents may benefit the patient with angina of effort. Reduction of coronary arterial tone has been demonstrated in patients with variant angina.

2. Cardiac muscle–Cardiac muscle is highly dependent upon calcium influx for normal function. Impulse generation in the sinoatrial node and conduction in the atrioventricular node are blocked by all of the calcium influx inhibitors. Excitation-contraction coupling in all cardiac cells requires calcium influx, so these drugs reduce cardiac contractility and cardiac output in a dose-dependent fashion. This reduction in mechanical function is another mechanism by which the calcium influx inhibitors may reduce the oxygen requirement in patients with angina.

An additional benefit of calcium influx inhibition has been demonstrated in experimental myocardial infarction. Because ischemia causes membrane depolarization, calcium influx in ischemic cells is increased. Elevated intracellular calcium accelerates the activity of several ATP-consuming enzymes, which further depletes already marginal cellular energy stores, making the heart even more susceptible to ischemic damage. Protection by the calcium entry blockers against these damaging effects of calcium has been demonstrated by a reduction in the incidence of arrhythmias and in the ultimate size of developing infarctions in experimental animals.

Important differences between the available calcium influx inhibitors arise from the details of their interactions with cardiac ion channels and differences in their relative smooth muscle versus cardiac effects. Cardiac sodium channels are blocked by verapamil but less effectively than are calcium channels. Sodium block is less marked with diltiazem and nifedipine. Verapamil and diltiazem dissociate from the calcium channel receptor between action potentials relatively faster than does nifedipine; they therefore block tachycardias in calcium-dependent cells, eg, the atrioventricular node, more selectively than does nifedipine. (See Chapter 12 for additional details.) On the other hand, nifedipine appears to block smooth muscle calcium channels at concentrations below those required for significant cardiac effects; it is therefore less depressant on the heart than verapamil or diltiazem.

3. Skeletal muscle–Skeletal muscle is not depressed by the calcium influx inhibitors because it utilizes intracellular pools of calcium to support excitation-contraction coupling and does not require transmembrane calcium influx.

4. Other effects–Calcium influx inhibitors interfere with stimulus-secretion coupling in glands and nerve endings. The effect has been demonstrated experimentally in measurements of the secretion of pituitary and pancreatic polypeptide hormones and release of transmitters from synaptosomes prepared from brain tissue. Verapamil has been shown to inhibit insulin release in humans, but the dosages required are greater than those used in management of angina.

Preliminary evidence suggests that the calcium influx inhibitors may also interfere with platelet aggregation in vitro and the development of atheromatous lesions in rabbits fed a high-fat diet. These effects have not yet been reproduced in human studies.

In addition to angina pectoris, calcium influx inhibitors have been used in the therapy of hypertrophic cardiomyopathy, cardiac arrhythmias, migraine headache, hypertension, and premature labor.

Toxicity

The most important toxic effects reported for the calcium influx blockers are direct extensions of their therapeutic action. Excessive inhibition of calcium influx can cause serious cardiac depression, including cardiac arrest, bradycardia, atrioventricular block, and congestive heart failure. These effects have been rare in clinical use. Patients receiving β-adrenergic blocking drugs are more sensitive to the cardiodepressant effects of calcium influx inhibitors. Minor toxicity (not requiring discontinuation of therapy) includes flushing, edema, dizziness, and nausea.

II. CLINICAL PHARMACOLOGY OF DRUGS USED IN THE TREATMENT OF ANGINA

Pathophysiology of Angina

Angina pectoris is the symptomatic manifestation of myocardial ischemia, which is caused by an imbalance between myocardial oxygen supply and demand. Myocardial oxygen supply is primarily dependent on coronary blood flow; in most patients, arterial oxygen saturation and content are normal. An imbalance between myocardial oxygen supply and demand can occur either from a primary decrease in coronary blood flow, without an increase in myocardial oxygen demand, or from a disproportionate increase in myocardial oxygen demand in relation to the capacity to increase coronary blood flow. In patients with variant (Prinzmetal's) angina, a primary decrease in coronary blood flow is the principal mechanism. Effort angina (classic angina) is most frequently precipitated by an insufficient increase in coronary blood flow in response to an increase in myocardial oxygen demand.

Determinants of Myocardial Oxygen Demand

The major and minor determinants of myocardial oxygen requirement are set forth in Table 10–2. Unlike skeletal muscle, human cardiac muscle cannot develop an appreciable oxygen debt during stress and repay it later. As a consequence of its continuous activity, the heart's oxygen needs are relatively high, and it extracts approximately 75% of the available oxygen even under conditions of no stress. The oxygen is utilized to generate high-energy phosphates, and since oxidative metabolism is the primary source of cardiac energy, the rate of myocardial oxygen consumption parallels the cardiac energy requirements.

Table 10–2. Determinants of myocardial oxygen consumption.

Major	Minor
Heart rate	Fiber shortening
Contractility	Activation energy
Wall stress	Resting metabolism
Intraventricular pressure	
Ventricular radius (volume)	
Wall thickness	

The myocardial oxygen requirement increases when there is an increase in heart rate, contractility, arterial pressure, or ventricular volume. These hemodynamic alterations frequently occur during physical exercise, which often precipitates angina in patients with obstructive coronary artery disease. The relative contributions of basal metabolism, activation of contraction, and fiber shortening to the overall myocardial oxygen consumption appear to be small, but under pathologic conditions these apparently minor determinants of myocardial oxygen consumption may become relevant.

Because in the clinical setting it is not possible to measure all of the determinants listed in Table 10–2 directly, indirect measures are often used to assess changes in myocardial oxygen demand and consumption. One commonly used index is the "triple product" (heart rate × systolic blood pressure × ejection time), a measure closely related to the tension-time index. The tension-time index is calculated by multiplying the area (in mm Hg/s) under the systolic phase of the left ventricular pressure curve by the heart rate. The "double product" or rate-pressure product (systolic blood pressure × heart rate per minute) appears to be as reliable as the triple product as an indirect measure of myocardial oxygen consumption. These indices are limited, however, because they do not include left ventricular volume or contractile state.

Determinants of Coronary Blood Flow & Myocardial Oxygen Supply

Oxygen supply is a function of myocardial delivery and extraction. Since myocardial oxygen extraction is nearly maximal at rest, there is little reserve to meet increased demands; furthermore, the oxygen content of the blood cannot be significantly increased under normal atmospheric conditions. Thus, increased myocardial demands for oxygen in the normal heart are met by augmenting coronary blood flow.

Coronary blood flow is directly related to the perfusion pressure (aortic diastolic pressure) and the duration of diastole. Because coronary flow drops to negligible values during systole, the duration of diastole becomes a limiting factor for myocardial perfusion during tachycardia. Coronary blood flow is inversely proportionate to coronary vascular bed resistance. Resistance is determined by intrinsic factors, including metabolic products and autonomic activity; by various pharmacologic agents; and by the extravascular mechanical compression of the coronary arteries. The site of autoregulation appears to be the arteriolar resistance vessels.

A. Angina of Effort (Classic Angina): When the large coronary arteries are obstructed, as in atherosclerosis, their intraluminal resistance is added to the autoregulatory resistance of the arterioles and contributes significantly to the total coronary arterial resistance to blood flow. The relation between coronary artery stenosis and distal coronary artery bed resistance is thus important in the genesis of effort angina.

In most patients with classic angina, resting coronary blood flow is adequate and proportionate to myocardial oxygen demand at rest, indicating that resistance of the stenosis and resistance of the distal coronary vascular bed are below the limit for critical flow at rest. During exercise, as a result of autoregulatory vasodilatation, there is a 2- to 4-fold decrease in the resistance of the distal coronary vascular bed. Although such vasodilatation always increases flow, the increase in flow required for a given increase in demand becomes progressively curtailed as the degree of stenosis increases. Thus, despite an absolute increase in flow, relative myocardial ischemia develops, and angina is experienced that is proportionate to the increase in oxygen requirement.

B. Variant Angina: The pathogenesis of the variant form of angina pectoris is different from that of classic angina. Variant angina is characterized by cyclic recurrent chest pain at rest that is unrelated to effort but is associated with ST segment elevation on the ECG. Patients with this form of angina frequently have prolonged attacks of chest pain, which sometimes occur at the same time each day. Cardiac arrhythmias of various types occur during anginal attacks in about half of these patients. In some patients, prolonged anginal episodes may culminate in myocardial infarction and sudden death.

It has been noted that coronary sinus flow in these patients actually decreases during spontaneous rest angina. Thus, it seems highly probable that myocardial ischemia is precipitated in variant angina by spontaneous decrease in coronary blood flow unrelated to changes in myocardial oxygen demand.

The primary decrease in coronary blood flow during variant angina appears to be caused by a marked increase in tone of smooth muscle in the large epicardial coronary arteries (coronary artery spasm). Angiographic studies during spontaneous variant angina have documented coronary artery spasm and complete interruption of coronary blood flow. Localized spasm can also be provoked by intravenous injection of vasoconstrictors such as ergonovine; such spasm is usually accompanied by symptoms and electrocardiographic changes similar to those associated with the patient's spontaneous attacks. With relief of angina, restoration of flow and increase in luminal diameter of the arteries occur. The great majority of patients with variant angina also have fixed obstructive coronary artery disease; only a few have normal coronary arteries.

C. Unstable Angina: The term unstable angina

applies to angina of changing intensity. The patient population with unstable angina includes individuals with prolonged angina at rest who do not have evidence of myocardial necrosis at the time of initial presentation. In most patients, the syndrome of unstable angina consists of ischemic cardiac pain at rest that is severe enough to warrant hospitalization. Both coronary artery spasm and increased myocardial oxygen demand may be implicated in the pathogenesis of unstable angina.

Principles of Therapy of Angina

In addition to modification of the risk factors for coronary atherosclerosis (smoking, hypertension, hyperlipidemia), the treatment of angina and other manifestations of myocardial ischemia is based on reduction of myocardial oxygen demand and increase of coronary blood flow to the potentially ischemic myocardium to restore the balance between myocardial oxygen supply and demand. In classic angina, pharmacologic agents are effective mainly in reducing myocardial oxygen demand; surgical revascularization is the only method available that restores coronary blood flow and increases oxygen supply. In variant angina, some drugs are effective in preventing and reversing coronary spasm and therefore can increase oxygen supply.

Specific Therapeutic Interventions

NITRATES

Mechanisms of Clinical Effect

Nitroglycerin and other organic nitrates are direct smooth muscle relaxants and cause vasodilatation of the peripheral vascular bed. The beneficial and deleterious effects of nitrate-induced vasodilatation are summarized in Table 10–3.

A. Nitrate Effects in Angina of Effort: Decreased venous return to the heart as a result of peripheral venous pooling and the resulting reduction of intracardiac volume are the principal hemodynamic effects. Arterial pressure decreases because of modest reduction of systemic vascular resistance and decreased or unchanged cardiac output. Decreased intraventricular pressure and left ventricular volume are associated with decreased wall tension (Laplace relation) and resulting decreased myocardial oxygen requirement. In rare instances, a paradoxic increase in myocardial oxygen demand may occur as a result of excessive reflex tachycardia and increased contractility.

Nitrates also cause relaxation of smooth muscle of the large conductance arteries such as epicardial coronary arteries. Intracoronary or intravenous nitrate administration consistently increases the caliber of the epicardial coronary arteries. Coronary arteriolar resistance tends to decrease, though to a lesser extent. Since the collateral arteries respond in the same way as the larger coronary arteries and arterioles, nitrates can at least theoretically increase collateral blood flow. However, nitrates administered by the usual systemic routes consistently *decrease* overall coronary blood flow and myocardial oxygen consumption. Intracoronary injection of small doses of nitroglycerin, which increases total coronary blood flow but does not produce systemic hemodynamic effects, does not relieve angina. Yet systemic administration of nitroglycerin, which decreases arterial pressure and left ventricular volume, does relieve angina despite decreased coronary blood flow. These findings indicate that the relief of effort angina with nitrates is due primarily to decreased myocardial oxygen demand and not increased coronary blood flow. Collateral blood flow to the ischemic myocardium may increase, but the relative contribution of this beneficial effect in alleviating stress-induced myocardial ischemia remains uncertain.

B. Nitrate Effects in Variant Angina: In patients with variant angina, relaxation of smooth muscles of the epicardial coronary arteries and relief of coronary artery spasm is the principal mechanism by which nitrates exert their beneficial effects. These drugs cause an increase in regional coronary blood flow and myocardial perfusion associated with the relief of coronary artery spasm. Although intracoronary nitroglycerin injection appears to be the most effective method for relieving coronary artery spasm, this method of administration has little relevance in the clinical management of patients.

C. Nitrate Effects in Unstable Angina: Nitrates are also useful in the treatment of unstable angina, but the precise mechanism for their beneficial effects is not clear. Because both increased coronary vascular tone and increased myocardial oxygen demand can precipitate rest angina in these patients, nitrates may exert their beneficial effects both by dilating the epicardial coronary arteries and simultaneously reducing myocardial oxygen demand.

Table 10–3. Beneficial and deleterious effects of nitrates in the treatment of angina.

	Result
Potential beneficial effects	
Decreased ventricular volume	Decreased myocardial oxygen requirement.
Decreased arterial pressure	
Decreased ejection time	
Vasodilatation of epicardial coronary arteries	Relief of coronary artery spasm.
Increased collateral flow	Improved perfusion to ischemic myocardium.
Decreased left ventricular diastolic pressure	Improved subendocardial perfusion.
Potential deleterious effects	
Reflex tachycardia	Increased myocardial oxygen requirement.
Reflex increase in contractility	
Decreased diastolic perfusion time due to tachycardia	Decreased myocardial perfusion.

Clinical Use of Nitrates

Some of the forms of nitroglycerin and its congeners are listed in Table 10–4. Because of its rapid onset of action (1–3 minutes), sublingual nitroglycerin is the most frequently used agent for the immediate treatment of angina. Because its duration of action is short (not exceeding 20–30 minutes), it is not a suitable agent for maintenance therapy. The onset of action of intravenous nitroglycerin is also rapid (5 minutes), but its hemodynamic effects are quickly reversed with discontinuation of its infusion. Its clinical application, therefore, is restricted to the treatment of severe, recurrent rest angina. Slowly absorbed preparations of nitroglycerin include a buccal form, an oral preparation, and several transdermal forms. These formulations are claimed to provide effective blood concentrations for long periods.

The hemodynamic effects of sublingual or chewable isosorbide dinitrate, pentaerythritol tetranitrate, and erythrityl tetranitrate are achieved within 2–3 minutes after absorption; but their duration of action is relatively short, usually 90–120 minutes. Larger doses of these nitrates, like the long-acting preparations of nitroglycerin, are claimed to produce adequate plasma concentrations. Prolonged hemodynamic changes, including decreased left ventricular filling pressure and lower arterial pressure, have been documented. The recommended dosage schedules for commonly used long-acting nitrate preparations, along with their duration of action, are listed in Table 10–4.

Toxicity

The most common untoward effects of nitrate therapy are throbbing headache, which tends to decrease in intensity with continued therapy, and postural dizziness, weakness, or even frank syncope. Occasionally, excessive tachycardia occurs in response to hypotension, and angina may be worsened. Glaucoma, once thought to be a contraindication, does not worsen, and nitrates can be used safely in the presence of increased intraocular pressure. Nitrates, however, are contraindicated if intracranial pressure is elevated.

Whether tolerance and dependence develop to nitrates has remained controversial since nitroglycerin was first used for hypertension in the late 1880s. The tolerance and dependence that develops with chronic industrial exposure to organic nitrates is described above. Recent studies designed to evaluate this problem in patients receiving organic nitrates for angina for 4–40 weeks failed to yield any evidence of clinical tolerance. Furthermore, serial hemodynamic studies have documented sustained effects of nitrates in patients with chronic heart failure. However, because of the potential problem of nitrate withdrawal symptoms, nitrate therapy should be tapered rather than abruptly stopped if treatment is discontinued for any reason.

Table 10–4. Nitrate and nitrite drugs used in the treatment of angina.

Drug	Dose	Duration of Action
"Short-acting"		
Nitroglycerin, sublingual	0.15–1.2 mg	10–30 minutes
Isosorbide, sublingual	2.5–5 mg	10–60 minutes
Amyl nitrite, inhalant	0.18–0.3 mL	3–5 minutes
"Long-acting"		
Nitroglycerin, oral sustained-action	6.5–13 mg per 6–8 hours	6–8 hours
Nitroglycerin, 2% ointment	½–2 inches per 4 hours	3–6 hours
Nitroglycerin, slow-release buccal	1–2 mg per 4 hours	3–6 hours
Nitroglycerin, slow-release transcutaneous	10–25 mg per 24 hours	24 hours or longer
Isosorbide dinitrate, sublingual	2.5–10 mg per 2 hours	1½–2 hours
Isosorbide dinitrate, oral	10–60 mg per 4–6 hours	4–6 hours
Isosorbide dinitrate, chewable	5–10 mg per 2–4 hours	2–3 hours
Pentaerythritol tetranitrate	40 mg per 6–8 hours	6–8 hours
Erythrityl tetranitrate	10–40 mg per 6–8 hours	6–8 hours

BETA-ADRENERGIC RECEPTOR–BLOCKING AGENTS

Beta-blocking drugs (Chapter 8) are extremely useful in the management of stable and unstable angina pectoris. The beneficial effects of beta-blocking agents are related primarily to their hemodynamic effects—decreased heart rate, blood pressure, and contractility—which decrease myocardial oxygen requirements at rest and during exercise. Lower heart rate is also associated with an increase in diastolic perfusion time that may increase myocardial perfusion. It has been suggested that the beta-blocking agents can cause a favorable redistribution of coronary blood flow to the ischemic myocardium based on differential effects on the coronary vascular resistance in the relatively ischemic and nonischemic myocardial segments. However, reduction of heart rate and blood pressure—and consequently decreased myocardial oxygen consumption—appear to be the most important mechanisms for relief of angina and improved exercise tolerance.

Undesirable effects of beta-blocking agents include an increase in end-diastolic volume that accompanies slowing of the heart rate and an increase in ejection time. Increased myocardial oxygen requirements associated with increased left ventricular diastolic volume partially offset the beneficial effects of beta-blocking agents. These potentially deleterious effects of beta-blocking agents can be balanced by the concomitant use of nitrates. Indeed, combined therapy with beta-blockers and nitrates is an effective way to treat angina pectoris, since these 2 agents tend to offset each other's deleterious effects on myocardial oxygen requirements. The rationale for the use of combined nitrates and beta-blockers for treatment of angina is summarized in Table 10–5. Combined therapy re-

Table 10–5. Effects of β-adrenergic blocking drugs, nitrates, and combined beta-blocker–nitrate therapy in angina pectoris.

	Beta-Blockers	Nitrates	Combined Nitrates and Beta-Blocker
Heart rate	Decrease	Reflex increase	Decrease
Arterial pressure	Decrease	Decrease	Decrease
End-diastolic volume	Increase	Decrease	None or decrease
Contractility	Decrease	Reflex increase	None
Ejection time	Increase	Decrease	None
Diastolic perfusion time	Increase	Decrease	Increase

duces myocardial oxygen demand at rest and during exercise. The double rate-pressure product remains consistently lower during exercise with nitrate or beta-blocker therapy, and combination therapy produces synergistic effects. However, although exercise capacity increases, there is usually no change in the myocardial ischemia threshold, ie, the rate-pressure product at which symptoms occur.

There is no evidence that any particular beta-blocking agent is better than others in the management of angina. The undesirable cardiac effects of the different types of beta-blocking agents are also quite similar (Chapter 8).

The effective dose of any beta-blocker varies widely from patient to patient; individual titration against both rest and exercise heart rates is required along with monitoring blood pressure and evidence of cardiac function. In patients with severe effort angina, it may be necessary to decrease resting heart rate to 50–60 beats/min and maximal heart rate to 100–120 beats/min during exercise.

CALCIUM ENTRY-BLOCKING AGENTS

Drugs that block the calcium channel (often called the slow inward current channel) constitute an important family of agents for treatment of angina pectoris, especially the variant form. Nifedipine, verapamil, and diltiazem are presently available in the USA for prescription use. As mentioned previously, calcium influx inhibitors decrease myocardial contractile force, which in turn reduces myocardial oxygen requirements. Inhibition of calcium entry into arterial smooth muscle is associated with decreased arteriolar tone and systemic vascular resistance, resulting in decreased arterial and intraventricular pressure. Thus, left ventricular wall stress declines, which also reduces the myocardial oxygen requirements. Decreased heart rate with the use of some calcium entry-blocking agents (verapamil and diltiazem) causes a further decrease in myocardial oxygen demand. Calcium entry-blocking agents also relieve and prevent focal coronary artery spasm—the primary mechanism of variant angina. Use of these agents has thus emerged as the most effective treatment for this form of angina pectoris. As noted above, the calcium entry-blocking agents differ in their clinical cardiovascular effects. Sinoatrial and atrioventricular nodal tissue, which is mainly composed of "slow response" cells, is affected markedly by verapamil, moderately by diltiazem, and much less by nifedipine. Thus, verapamil and diltiazem decrease atrioventricular nodal conduction and are effective in the management of supraventricular reentry tachycardia and in decreasing ventricular responses in atrial fibrillation or flutter. Nifedipine does not affect atrioventricular conduction. Nifedipine appears to be a more potent arteriolar dilator than verapamil or diltiazem; thus, a fall in arterial pressure usually is more pronounced with nifedipine. Nonspecific sympathetic antagonism is most marked with diltiazem and much less with verapamil. Nifedipine does not appear to have this effect. Thus, significant reflex tachycardia in response to hypotension occurs most frequently with nifedipine and less so with verapamil. With diltiazem, decreased heart rate may accompany a fall in arterial pressure. These differences in pharmacologic effects should be considered in selecting calcium entry-blocking agents in the management of angina.

Calcium entry-blocking agents are effective in the long-term management of chronic stable angina. A number of studies have demonstrated an increase in exercise duration and a significant delay in the onset of effort angina. The comparative efficacy of calcium entry-blocking drugs, beta-blocking agents, and nitrates has not been established; preliminary studies suggest that there is little difference between these agents. However, calcium blockers, beta-blockers, and nitrates have all been shown to be more effective than placebo in reducing daily attacks of angina and in prolonging exercise tolerance. The combination of a beta-blocker and a calcium antagonist appears to be more effective than either drug alone in improving exercise duration and tolerance.

In studies of the mechanism of verapamil's beneficial effect in patients with effort angina, the rate-pressure product at the onset of angina remained unchanged. Thus, it appears that verapamil decreases myocardial oxygen demand in these patients. Nifedipine is an extremely potent peripheral vasodilator, and its hemodynamic actions suggest that it may produce its salutary effects in effort angina by reducing cardiac work because of the change in afterload. The antianginal effects of diltiazem have not been investigated extensively in patients with effort angina; however, the mechanisms of its beneficial effects are probably similar to those of verapamil and nifedipine.

Nifedipine, verapamil, and diltiazem are considerably more effective than the beta-adrenergic blocking drugs in relieving and preventing ischemic episodes in patients with variant angina. In approximately 70% of patients, angina attacks are completely abolished; in another 20%, marked reduction of frequency of anginal episodes is observed. Prevention of coronary artery spasm (in the presence or absence of fixed arteriosclerotic coronary artery lesions) is the principal mechanism for this beneficial response.

In patients with unstable angina with recurrent ischemic episodes at rest, the addition of nifedipine to beta-blocker and nitrate therapy can decrease the frequency of rest angina, the incidence of myocardial infarction, and the necessity for emergency myocardial revascularization.

Toxicity

The choice of a particular calcium entry-blocking agent should be made with knowledge of its specific potential adverse effects as well as of its pharmacologic properties. A combination of verapamil or diltiazem with beta-blockers may produce atrioventricular block. Nifedipine does not decrease atrioventricular conduction and therefore can be used more safely in the presence of atrioventricular conduction abnormalities. Combined beta-blocker and verapamil therapy may cause depression of ventricular function. In the presence of overt heart failure, all calcium entry-blocking agents can cause further worsening of heart failure as a result of their negative inotropic effect. However, nifedipine, a potent arteriolar dilator, decreases systemic vascular resistance and left ventricular ejection impedance, which may balance the detrimental negative inotropic effect. In patients with depressed left ventricular function, therefore, nifedipine might be the most appropriate choice. However, in the presence of relatively low blood pressure, nifedipine can cause further deleterious lowering of blood pressure. Verapamil and diltiazem appear to produce less hypotension and may be better tolerated in these circumstances. In patients with a history of atrial tachycardia, flutter, and fibrillation, verapamil provides a distinct advantage because of its antiarrhythmia effects. However, in the digitalized patient, verapamil should be used with caution, because it may increase digoxin blood levels through a pharmacokinetic interaction. Nifedipine has also been reported to increase digoxin blood levels.

Dosages and minor toxic effects of the calcium influx inhibitors are presented in Table 10–6.

Table 10–6. Dosage and toxicity of the calcium influx-blocking drugs.

Drug	Dose	Toxicity
Verapamil (Calan, Isoptin)	75–150 μg/kg intravenously; 80–160 mg every 8 hours orally.	Hypotension, myocardial depression, heart failure, dependent edema.
Nifedipine (Adalat, Procardia)	3–10 μg/kg intravenously; 10–40 mg every 8 hours orally.	Hypotension, dizziness, flushing, nausea, constipation, dependent edema.
Diltiazem (Cardiem, Herbesser)	75–150 μg/kg intravenously; 30–80 mg every 6 hours orally.	Hypotension, dizziness, flushing, bradycardia.

MYOCARDIAL REVASCULARIZATION & TRANSLUMINAL CORONARY ANGIOPLASTY

It is now well established that myocardial revascularization by coronary artery bypass surgery is extremely effective treatment for angina. About 70% of patients become asymptomatic, and another 20% have marked symptomatic relief. In patients with significant left main coronary lesions or with triple coronary vessel disease, better survival statistics have been obtained following coronary artery bypass surgery than with medical therapy. Transluminal coronary angioplasty (percutaneous transluminal coronary angioplasty, PTCA) also provides marked improvement in angina in patients with obstructive coronary artery disease. However, angioplasty can be performed only in a few selected patients with single- or double-vessel disease with proximal lesions. Nevertheless, following successful angioplasty (as with coronary artery bypass surgery), symptomatic relief along with improvement in angina threshold or regional myocardial function occurs in most patients.

In contrast to pharmacologic interventions, coronary artery bypass surgery and coronary artery angioplasty increase the heart rate × pressure product at the appearance of angina as well as exercise tolerance in patients with effort angina. The mechanism for the increased angina threshold is related to enhanced perfusion of the relatively ischemic myocardial segments

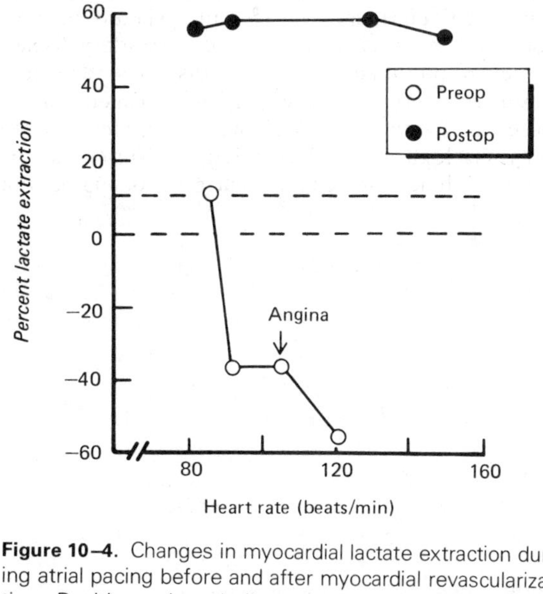

Figure 10–4. Changes in myocardial lactate extraction during atrial pacing before and after myocardial revascularization. Positive values indicate lactate extraction by the myocardium and adequate oxygen supply. Negative values indicate net lactate production by the heart and signify inadequate oxygen supply. Preoperatively, with increased heart rate and at the onset of angina, there was myocardial lactate production, indicating myocardial ischemia. Postoperatively, despite higher pacing rate, myocardial lactate extraction was normal and angina did not develop.

and improved regional myocardial metabolic function (Fig 10–4). Furthermore, increased regional perfusion has been documented by myocardial perfusion scintigraphy. Thus, the relief of effort-induced myocardial ischemia following revascularization balances the disparity between myocardial oxygen supply and demand by increasing the oxygen supply; in contrast, most pharmacologic agents do so by decreasing the myocardial oxygen demand.

GENERAL MANAGEMENT OF THE PATIENT WITH ANGINA

Both pharmacologic interventions and revascularization or angioplasty are effective for management of the angina syndromes. Therapy is aimed both at providing symptomatic relief and at prolonging life. The principal prognostic determinants are the degree of left ventricular dysfunction, the extent of coronary atherosclerosis, and the severity of myocardial ischemia. In patients with chronic stable angina, the degree of left ventricular dysfunction and the severity of the obstructive coronary artery disease should be determined before a therapeutic plan is offered. Noninvasive investigations such as echocardiography and angiography can provide significant information regarding the state of left ventricular function. Similarly, the severity and the extent of coronary atherosclerosis can be assessed in most instances by treadmill exercise tests with or without thallium 201 myocardial scintigraphy. When a high risk of myocardial infarction is suspected, coronary arteriography should be performed. If significant left main coronary artery disease or severe proximal triple-vessel disease is detected, coronary artery bypass surgery is indicated. In the absence of very high risk coronary artery lesions, the pharmacologic approach is preferable. Nitrates are the drugs of choice for the immediate relief of angina. For the long-term management of patients with chronic stable angina, a combination of nitrates and beta-blockers provides substantial benefit in most patients. The addition of calcium influx-blocking agents produces a synergistic effect and should be considered if nitrates and beta-blocker therapy fail to produce a satisfactory response. If the manifestations of myocardial ischemia continue despite combined drug therapy, surgical revascularization or angioplasty should be considered.

In patients with unstable angina, immediate therapy should be directed to the relief of rest angina, which can be achieved with aggressive nitrate and beta-blocker therapy in approximately 50% of patients. The addition of calcium entry-blocking agents to nitrates and beta-blockers will prevent recurrence of rest angina and myocardial ischemia in an even larger proportion of patients. In patients who continue to demonstrate manifestations of myocardial ischemia despite aggressive medical therapy, coronary arteriography should be undertaken with a view to revascularization or angioplasty. In patients who obtain complete relief of angina from pharmacologic interventions, elective coronary arteriography is desirable to determine whether revascularization or angioplasty is necessary or likely to be of benefit.

Because coronary artery spasm appears to be the principal mechanism of variant angina, nitrates and calcium entry-blocking agents should be considered first. In patients with additional obstructive coronary artery disease, beta-blockers may also be used concurrently. Patients who fail to respond to these pharmacologic interventions should undergo coronary arteriography to assess the presence and severity of obstructive coronary artery disease. In the absence of fixed obstructive coronary artery lesions, pharmacologic therapy should be continued. If severe fixed obstructive coronary artery lesions are present, revascularization or angioplasty should be considered.

• • •

References

Abrams J: Nitroglycerin tolerance: Fact or fancy. *Prac Cardiol* 1978;**4:**113.

Alterhog JH, Ekelund LG, Melin AL: Effect of nifedipine on exercise tolerance in patients with angina pectoris. *Eur J Cardiol* 1975;**8:**125.

Benson H, McCallie DP Jr: Angina pectoris and the placebo effect. *N Engl J Med* 1979;**300:**1424.

Bright GE: The effects of nitroglycerin on those engaged in its manufacture. *JAMA* 1914;**62:**201.

Carmichael P, Lieben J: Sudden death in explosives workers. *Arch Environ Health* 1963;**7:**50.

Chatterjee K et al: Improved angina threshold and coronary reserve following direct myocardial revascularization. *Circulation* 1975;**51:**1.

Cohn PF, Gorlin R: Physiologic and clinical actions of nitroglycerin. *Med Clin North Am* 1974;**58:**407.

Conti CR et al: Unstable angina pectoris: Randomized study of surgical vs. medical therapy. *Am J Cardiol* 1975;**35:**129.

Davidor ME, Mroczek WJ: The effect of sustained release nitroglycerin capsules on anginal frequency and exercise capacity. *Angiology* 1977;**28:**181.

Epstein SE et al: Angina pectoris: Pathophysiology, evaluation and treatment. *Ann Intern Med* 1971;**75:**263.

Ganz W, Marcus HS: Failure of intracoronary nitroglycerin to alleviate pacing-induced angina. *Circulation* 1972;**46:**880.

Gould KL, Lipscomb K: Effect of coronary stenosis on coronary flow reserve and resistance. *Am J Cardiol* 1974;**34:**48.

Grunzig A: Transluminal dilation of coronary artery stenosis. *Lancet* 1978;**1:**263.

Henry PD: Comparative pharmacology of calcium antagonists: Nifedipine, verapamil, and diltiazem. *Am J Cardiol* 1980;**46:**1047.

Hiller LD, Braunwald E: Coronary artery spasm. *N Engl J Med* 1978;**299:**695.

Hoffman JIE, Buckberg GD: The myocardial supply:demand ratio: A critical review. *Am J Cardiol* 1978;**41:**327.

Kukovetz WR et al: Evidence for cyclic GMP mediated relaxant effects of nitro-compounds in coronary smooth muscle. *Naunyn Schmiedebergs Arch Pharmacol* 1979;**310:**129.

Lawrie GM, Morris GC: Survival after coronary artery bypass surgery in specific patient groups. *Circulation* 1982;**65(Suppl 2):**43.

Levin RI et al: Nitroglycerin stimulates synthesis of prostacyclin by cultural human endothelial cells. *J Clin Invest* 1981;**67:**762.

Livesley B et al: Double blind evaluation of verapamil, propranolol, and isosorbide dinitrate against placebo in the treatment of angina pectoris. *Br Med J* 1973;**2:**375.

Mason DT, Braunwald E: The effects of nitroglycerin and amyl nitrite on arteriolar and venous tone in the human forearm. *Circulation* 1965;**32:**755.

Muller JE, Gunther SJ: Nifedipine therapy for Prinzmetal's angina. *Circulation* 1978;**57:**137.

Needleman P, Jakshik B, Johnson EM Jr: Sulfhydryl requirements for relaxation of vascular smooth muscle. *J Pharmacol Exp Ther* 1973;**187:**324.

Needleman P, Johnson EM Jr: Mechanism of tolerance development to organic nitrate. *J Pharmacol Exp Ther* 1973;**184:**709.

Plotnick GD et al: Rest angina with transient ST segment elevation: Correlation of clinical features with coronary anatomy. *Am J Med* 1978;**65:**257.

Prinzmetal M et al: Angina pectoris. 1. A variant form of angina pectoris. *Am J Med* 1959;**27:**375.

Reichek N et al: Sustained effects of nitroglycerin ointment in patients with angina pectoris. *Circulation* 1974;**50:**348.

Robinson BF: Relation of heart rate and systolic blood pressure to the onset of pain in angina pectoris. *Circulation* 1967;**35:**1073.

Rouleau J-L et al: Mechanism of relief of pacing-induced angina with oral verapamil: Reduced oxygen demand. *Circulation*, 1983. [In press.]

Russek HI: Propranolol and isosorbide dinitrate synergism in angina pectoris. *Am J Cardiol* 1968;**21:**45.

Takaro T et al: The Veterans Administration Cooperative Study of Stable Angina: Current status. *Circulation* 1982;**65(Suppl 2):**60.

Thadani U et al: Comparison of adrenergic beta-receptor antagonists in angina pectoris. *Br Med J* 1973;**1:**138.

Ulmsten U, Andersson K-E, Forman A: Relaxing effects of nifedipine on the nonpregnant human uterus in vitro and in vivo. *Obstet Gynecol* 1978;**52:**436.

Whitworth CG, Grant MM: Use of nitrate and vasodilators by glaucomatous patients. *Arch Ophthalmol* 1964;**71:**492.

Winbury MM, Howe BB, Hefner MA: Effect of nitrates and other coronary dilators on large and small coronary vessels: An hypothesis for the mechanism of action of nitrates. *J Pharmacol Exp Ther* 1969;**168:**70.

Wyatt HL et al: Effect of graded reductions in coronary perfusion on regional and total cardiac function. *Am J Cardiol* 1975;**36:**185.

11 | Cardiac Glycosides & Other Drugs Used in the Treatment of Congestive Heart Failure

Bertram G. Katzung, MD, PhD, & William W. Parmley, MD

Congestive heart failure occurs when the cardiac output is inadequate to provide the oxygen needs of the body. The cardiac glycosides comprise a group of steroid compounds that have complex primary effects on the mechanical and electrical functions of the heart. They also have effects on smooth muscle and other tissues. The principal therapeutic effect in congestive heart failure is an increase in cardiac contractility (positive inotropic action). Nevertheless, there is some doubt regarding the long-term efficacy of cardiac glycosides in patients with heart failure. On the other hand, there is general agreement that the commonly used glycosides have a narrow margin of safety and that less toxic compounds with positive inotropic actions are needed. Several experimental agents are candidates for this role, including **amrinone** and certain **β-adrenergic stimulants.** Furthermore, clinical research has shown that in some types of congestive failure, reduction of vascular tone by unloading the stressed myocardium gives effective relief. Thus, certain vasodilators have been used with considerable success. Such agents include **aminophylline** (which also has a positive inotropic action), **nitroprusside, nitroglycerin,** and **α-adrenergic antagonists.**

This chapter presents the basic pharmacology of the cardiac glycosides and amrinone, agents with primary cardiac inotropic effects. The clinical management of congestive heart failure with these agents and with vasodilators and diuretics is discussed in the second portion of the chapter.

I. BASIC PHARMACOLOGY OF DRUGS USED IN CONGESTIVE HEART FAILURE

DIGITALIS

Medicinal plants containing cardiac glycosides were known to the ancient Egyptians 3000 years ago, but these agents were used erratically and with variable success until the 18th century, when William Withering, an English physician and botanist, published a monograph describing the clinical effects of an extract of the foxglove plant (*Digitalis purpurea,* a major source of these agents). His book, *An Account of the Foxglove and Some of Its Medical Uses: With Practical Remarks on Dropsy and Other Diseases,* published in 1785, described in detail the indications for the use of cardiac glycosides and offered cautionary remarks about their toxicity. Unfortunately, many of Withering's recommendations were ignored in the subsequent enthusiastic use of these agents. It was not until about 60 years ago that the physiologic basis for the action of digitalis (the positive inotropic response) was clearly demonstrated and more rational use of the agents was reestablished.

Chemistry

All of the commonly used cardiac steroids, or cardenolides—of which **digoxin** may be considered the prototype—combine a steroid nucleus with an unsaturated lactone ring at the 17 position and a series of sugars linked to carbon 3 of the nucleus (Fig 11–1). Because they lack an easily ionizable group, their solubility is not pH-dependent.

Sources of these drugs include white and purple foxglove *(Digitalis lanata* and *D purpurea),* Mediterranean sea onion (squill), *Strophanthus gratus,* oleander, lily of the valley, milkweed, and numerous other tropical and temperate zone plants. During larval development, monarch butterflies concentrate cardenolides in their bodies from ingested milkweed—a factor that apparently protects adult butterflies from predation by birds, since the cardenolides are potent emetics in most birds. Certain toads have skin glands capable of elaborating **bufadienolides,** which differ from the cardenolides only in having a 6-membered lactone ring at the 17 position.

Structure-activity studies indicate that the lactone ring and the steroid nucleus are essential for activity. The other substituents—especially the sugar molecules in the 3 position—influence pharmacokinetic variables, including absorption, half-life, and metabolism. There is no clinical evidence that any of the natural cardenolides differs from the others in therapeutic index or maximal efficacy.

These agents are very stable if protected from strong light and low pH. Their shelf life is reported to be 1–5 years, depending on conditions of storage.

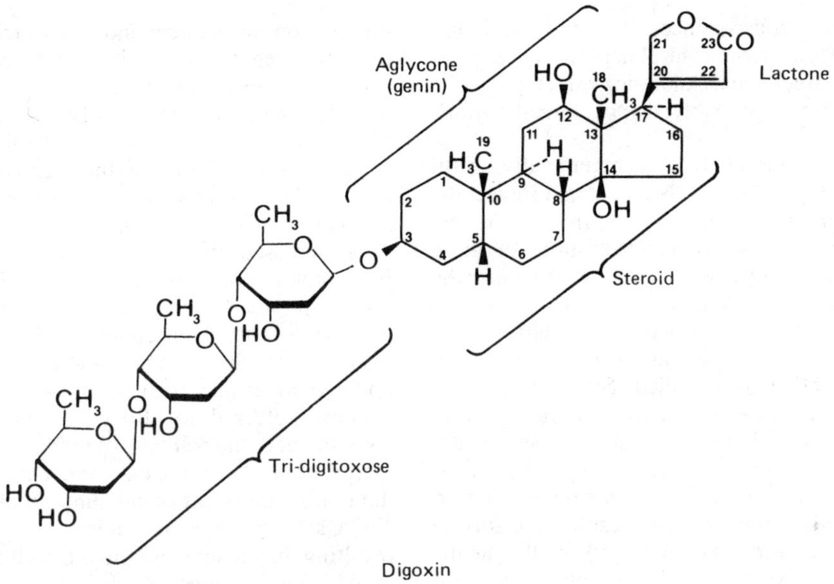

Figure 11–1. Structure of digoxin, a typical cardiac glycoside.

Pharmacokinetics

A. Absorption and Distribution: Cardenolides have both lipophilic (steroid nucleus) and hydrophilic (lactone ring, hydroxyl) groups. The balance of these 2 factors has an important effect on absorption, metabolism, and excretion, as shown by comparison (Table 11–1) of 3 of the most important agents: **digoxin, digitoxin,** and **ouabain.** As noted in the table, digoxin is fairly well absorbed after oral administration. However, because of its very narrow safety margin, even minor variations in bioavailability could cause serious toxicity or loss of effect. In fact, product formulation (factors in manufacture of the tablets) can modify the bioavailability of digoxin. As a result, digoxin tablets must pass dissolution tests before they can be marketed. Ouabain, because it is never used by the oral route, and digitoxin, because it is well absorbed under almost all circumstances, are not subject to this restriction. Digitalis leaf, a standardized preparation of the powdered plant material, contains chiefly digitoxin. Except for dosage, its properties are almost identical to those of digitoxin. Beta-methyldigoxin, a semisynthetic derivative of digoxin, is almost completely absorbed from the gut and is metabolized to digoxin in the body.

Once absorbed into the blood, all cardiac glycosides are widely distributed to tissues, including the central nervous system. The highest concentrations—for digoxin, 10–50 times higher than plasma—are found in heart, kidney, and liver.

B. Metabolism and Excretion: Digoxin is not extensively metabolized in humans but is largely excreted unchanged by the kidneys. Its elimination half-life is significantly prolonged in patients with renal impairment, and equations are available for adjusting digoxin dosage on the basis of creatinine clearance. In contrast, digitoxin is metabolized in the liver and excreted into the gut via the bile. Cardioactive metabolites as well as unchanged digitoxin can then be reabsorbed from the intestine, thus establishing an enterohepatic circulation that contributes to the very long half-life of this agent. Renal impairment does not significantly prolong the half-life of digitoxin, so this drug may occasionally be useful in patients with erratic or rapidly failing renal function. On the other hand, a variety of hepatic enzyme-inducing drugs (see Chapter 3) can reduce the blood level of digitoxin by accelerating its metabolism. Ouabain must be given parenterally and is therefore used only for acute therapy and rarely for more than a few doses. It is metabolized very little and excreted primarily by the kidney.

Table 11–1. Properties of 3 typical cardiac glycosides.

	Ouabain	Digoxin*	Digitoxin
Lipid solubility (oil/water coefficient)	Low	Medium	High
Oral availability (percentage absorbed)	0	75	>90
Half-life in body (hours)	21	40	168
Plasma protein binding (percentage bound)	0	20–40	>90
Percentage metabolized	0	<20	>80
Volume of distribution (L/kg)	18	6.3	0.6

*Beta-methyldigoxin is fully (100%) absorbed from the gut and is converted to digoxin in the body.

Pharmacodynamics

Digitalis has multiple direct and indirect cardiovascular effects, with both therapeutic and toxic (arrhythmogenic) consequences. In addition, it has undesirable effects on the central nervous system and gut. A small direct renal (diuretic) effect has been demonstrated but is probably of no clinical significance.

At the molecular level, all therapeutically useful cardiac glycosides *inhibit* **Na^+,K^+-ATPase,** the membrane-bound enzyme associated with the "sodium pump." Very low concentrations of these drugs have occasionally been observed to *stimulate* the enzyme, but this action is probably the result of catecholamine release. In contrast, inhibition over most of the dose range has been extensively documented in all tissues studied. Since the sodium pump is necessary for maintenance of normal resting potential in most excitable cells, it is generally believed that at least a portion of the toxicity of digitalis is caused by this enzyme-inhibiting action. It is also probable that this action is partly responsible for the therapeutic effect (positive inotropy) in the heart. Other molecular-level effects of digitalis have been studied in the heart and are discussed below.

A. Cardiac Effects: For clarity, the effects of digitalis on mechanical and on electrical function are discussed separately, but it must be realized that these changes occur simultaneously.

1. Mechanical effects–The therapeutic direct action of cardiac glycosides on mechanical function is to increase the intensity of the "active state" of the contractile apparatus—the interaction of the actin and myosin filaments of the cardiac sarcomere (Fig 11–2). This increased intensity is caused by increase in the free calcium concentration in the vicinity of the contractile proteins during systole, ie, by facilitation of excitation-contraction coupling. The precise mechanism by which this facilitation occurs is not fully understood. It may well be the result of inhibition of ATPase referred to above: Reduced transport of sodium out of the cell (at (1) in Fig 11–2) results in an increase in intracellular calcium. This increase reduces the normal transport of calcium out of the cell via the Na^+/Ca^{2+} exchange mechanism (at (1a) in Fig 11–2), resulting in an increase in intracellular calcium. A second possible mechanism is facilitation of calcium entry into the cell during the plateau of the action potential (at (2) in Fig 11–2). A third hypothesis is

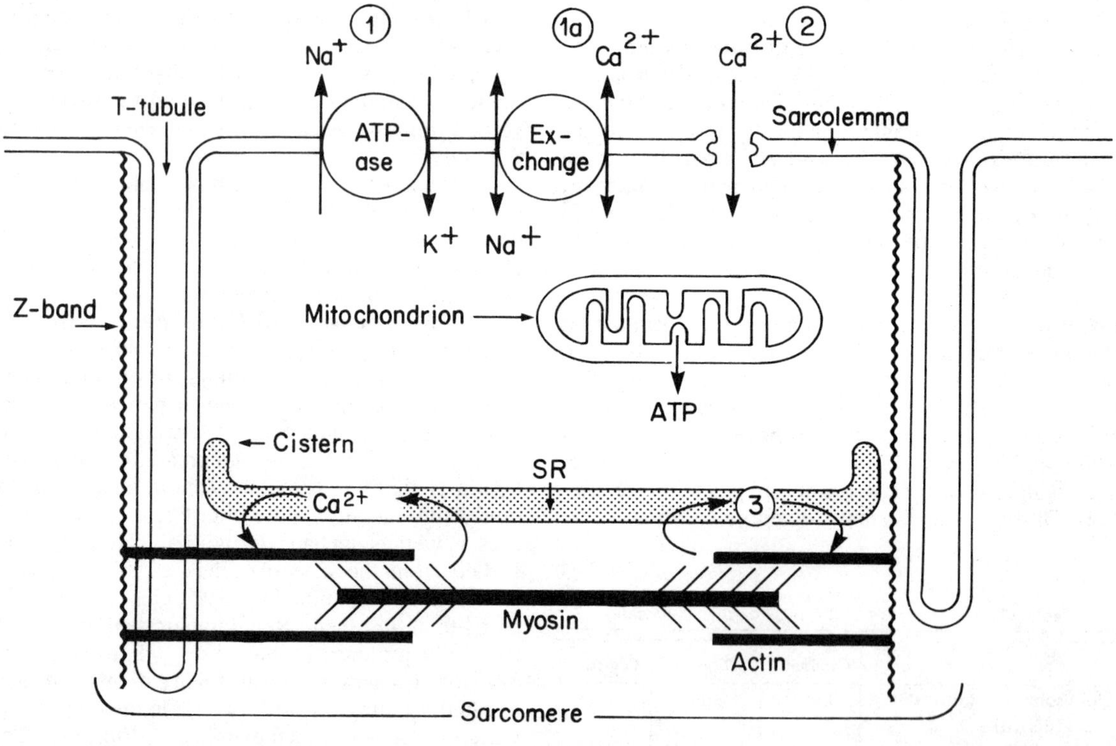

Figure 11–2. Schematic diagram of a sarcomere, the functional unit of a myocardial cell, with the possible sites of action of digitalis. Normal function involves the transduction of chemical energy (ATP, from the mitochondria) into mechanical shortening and tension development by the sliding of the thin actin filaments over the thicker myosin filaments. This reaction is brought about by an increase in free calcium ions in the vicinity of the actin strand. This calcium is released from the enlarged cisternae on the sarcoplasmic reticulum, the organelle that also sequesters calcium during relaxation. Release of the stored calcium is linked to membrane electrical activity (excitation) by "trigger calcium," which enters through membrane channels and thus couples excitation to contraction. Removal of excess calcium requires its exchange for sodium across the cell membrane and probably active pumping as well. Possible sites of digitalis action include (1) Na^+,K^+-ATPase (sodium pump), together with (1a), the Na^+/Ca^{2+} exchanger; (2) the ionic channel permeable to calcium; and (3) the sarcoplasmic reticulum (SR).

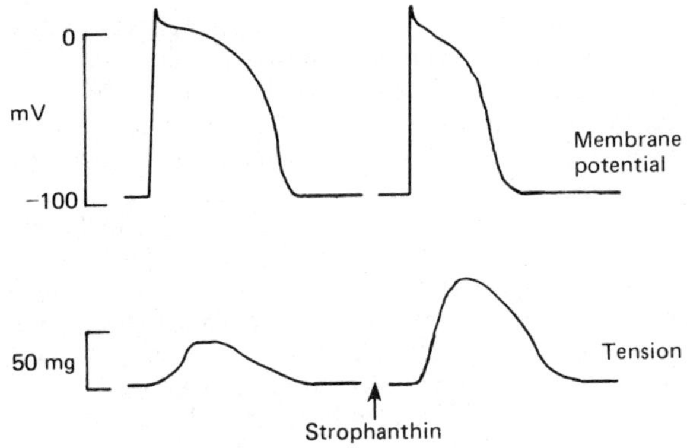

Figure 11–3. Typical effects of a nontoxic concentration of strophanthin, a rapidly acting cardiac glycoside, on the action potential and contractile response of isolated ventricular muscle. After 70 minutes of exposure to strophanthin, there is a marked increase in tension and a significant shortening of the action potential. There is little change in twitch duration or in action potential amplitude. (Redrawn, with permission, from Kassebaum DG: *J Pharmacol Exp Ther* 1963;**140**:331.)

that digitalis may increase the release of stored calcium from the sarcoplasmic reticulum (at ③ in Fig 11–2). It is possible that all 3 mechanisms participate in the action of digitalis.

The net result of the action of therapeutic concentrations of a cardiac glycoside is a distinctive increase in cardiac contractility (Fig 11–3). In isolated myocardial preparations, the rate of development of tension and of relaxation are both increased, with little or no change in time to peak tension. The duration of the contractile response is neither shortened (as in the case of β-adrenergic stimulation) nor prolonged (as in the case of methylxanthines such as theophylline). These effects occur in both normal and failing myocardium, but in the intact animal or patient the responses are modified by cardiovascular reflexes and the pathophysiology of congestive heart failure (see p 131).

2. Electrical effects–The effects of digitalis on the electrical properties of the heart in the intact organism are a complex mixture of indirect and direct actions. Direct actions on the membranes of cardiac cells follow a well-defined progression: an early, brief prolongation of the action potential with an increase in membrane resistance, followed by a protracted period of shortening of the action potential (especially the plateau phase) associated with a decrease in membrane resistance (Fig 11–3). This decrease in membrane resistance is probably the result of increased intracellular calcium, which is known to increase membrane potassium conductance. The latter change would result in action potential shortening. (See Chapter 12 for a discussion of the effects of ionic conductances on the action potential.) All of these effects can be observed in the absence of overt toxicity. Shortening of the action potential by direct drug action may contribute to the shortening of atrial and ventricular refractoriness (Table 11–2). With more toxic concentrations, resting membrane potential is reduced (made less negative) as a result of inhibition of the sodium pump and reduced intracellular potassium. As toxicity progresses, oscillatory depolarizing afterpotentials appear following normally evoked action potentials. When below threshold, these afterpotentials may interfere with normal conduction because of the further reduction of resting potential. Eventually, an afterpotential may reach threshold, eliciting an action potential (premature ventricular depolarization or "ectopic beat") that is coupled to the preceding normal one. If afterpotentials in the Purkinje conducting system regularly reach threshold in this way, bigeminy will be

Table 11–2. Actions of digitalis on cardiac electrical function. (Dominant effects in boldface.)

Effect	Atria	Atrioventricular Node	Ventricles, Purkinje System
Direct	Shortens refractory period.	Increases refractory period.	Shortens refractory period, or no significant effect.
	No significant effect on conduction velocity.	Decreases conduction velocity.	Decreases conduction velocity.
	Decreases normal automaticity; increases abnormal automaticity.	Increases or decreases normal automaticity; increases abnormal automaticity.	Increases or decreases normal automaticity; **increases abnormal automaticity.**
Indirect (ANS)			
1. Vagal	**Shortens refractory period (atria).**	**Increases refractory period.**	
	Decreases sinoatrial rate.	Decreases conduction velocity.	
2. Sympathetic (toxic doses)	Increases sinoatrial rate.	Shortens refractory period.	**Increases abnormal automaticity.**
		Junctional extrasystoles.	
Effect on ECG and rhythm			
Early	P wave changes.	**Lengthens P–R interval.**	**ST depression.**
Progressive toxicity	Premature atrial beats.	Second- or third-degree block.	**Ventricular premature depolarization.**
	Atrial fibrillation.	Junctional tachycardia.	Bigeminy.
			Ventricular tachycardia.
			Ventricular fibrillation.

recorded on the ECG. With further toxic deterioration, each afterpotential-evoked action potential will itself elicit a sizable afterpotential, and a self-sustaining arrhythmia (ventricular tachycardia) will be established. If allowed to progress, such a tachycardia may deteriorate into ventricular fibrillation.

Indirect actions of cardiac glycosides on the heart involve the autonomic nervous system and occur throughout the therapeutic and toxic dose ranges. In the lower portion of the dose range, cardioselective **parasympathomimetic** effects predominate. In fact, these atropine-blockable effects are probably responsible for a significant portion of all the electrical effects of digitalis (Table 11–2). This action involves sensitization of the baroreceptors, central vagal stimulation, and facilitation of muscarinic transmission at the cardiac muscle cell. Because cholinergic innervation is much richer in the atria, these actions affect atrial and atrioventricular nodal function more than Purkinje or ventricular function. Some of the cholinergic effects are useful in the treatment of certain arrhythmias (see p 132). At toxic levels, sympathetic outflow is increased by digitalis. This effect is not essential for typical cardenolide toxicity but sensitizes the myocardium and exaggerates all of the toxic effects of the drug.

The most common cardiac manifestations of glycoside **toxicity** include atrioventricular junctional rhythm, premature ventricular depolarizations, bigeminal rhythm, and second-degree atrioventricular blockade. However, it is claimed that digitalis can cause virtually every variety of arrhythmia. The membrane cardiotoxicity of digitalis was described above as involving resting depolarization (due to sodium pump inhibition) and oscillatory afterdepolarizations (caused by overload of intracellular calcium). The first effect may be responsible for a portion of the conduction abnormalities such as atrioventricular block. The second effect is probably responsible for most glycoside arrhythmias involving abnormal automaticity, including premature ventricular depolarizations, bigeminy, and ventricular tachycardia. These toxic effects are facilitated by hypokalemia and hypercalcemia. The former is especially important in the management of patients with digitalis-induced arrhythmias.

B. Effects on Other Organs: Cardiac glycosides affect all excitable tissues, including smooth muscle and the central nervous system. The mechanism of these effects has not been fully explored but probably involves the inhibition of Na^+,K^+-ATPase in these tissues. The depolarization resulting from depression of the sodium pump would be expected to increase spontaneous activity both in neurons and in smooth muscle cells. In addition, an increase in intracellular calcium could predictably increase smooth muscle tone. However, it should be remembered that in most cases of congestive heart failure treated with digitalis, a *decrease* in vascular tone is the net effect, resulting from a beneficial reduction of sympathetic tone (see below).

The gastrointestinal tract is the most common site of digitalis effects outside the heart. These actions include anorexia, nausea, vomiting, and diarrhea. This toxicity may be partially caused by direct effects on gastrointestinal smooth muscle but is also the result of central nervous system actions, including chemoreceptor trigger zone stimulation.

Central nervous system effects commonly include vagal and chemoreceptor zone stimulation, as noted above. Much less often, disorientation and hallucinations—especially in the elderly—and visual disturbances are noted. The last effect may include aberrations of color perception. Agitation and even convulsions are occasionally reported in patients taking digitalis.

Gynecomastia and galactorrhea are rare effects reported in men taking digitalis; it is not certain whether these effects represent a peripheral estrogenic action of these steroid drugs or a manifestation of hypothalamic stimulation.

ATPase-dependent transport processes such as aqueous humor and cerebrospinal fluid production, as well as sodium reabsorption in the kidney, can be shown experimentally to be inhibited by cardenolides. These effects are of no clinical significance.

Other Positive Inotropic Drugs Used in Heart Failure

Amrinone, an agent unrelated to digitalis or the catecholamines, and a group of β-adrenergic stimulants are under study as investigational agents. Aminophylline is sometimes used in the treatment of acute heart failure with pulmonary edema; it is of no value in the treatment of chronic congestive heart failure.

AMRINONE

Chemistry & Pharmacokinetics

Amrinone is a new bipyridine derivative that can be given orally or parenterally. It has an elimination half-life of about 2.6 hours, with 10–40% being excreted in the urine.

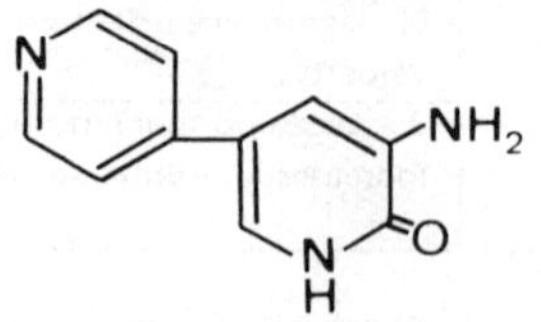

Amrinone

Pharmacodynamics

Amrinone directly increases myocardial contractility. The precise mechanism is unclear. In particular, it does not inhibit Na^+,K^+-ATPase, as does digitalis. It may increase levels of cAMP, as do the beta stimulants. The drug appears to increase inward calcium flux during the cardiac action potential. Amrinone's positive inotropic action is not affected by prior depletion of catecholamines with reserpine and therefore is not related to release of these amines. Similarly, the action of amrinone is not blocked by β-adrenergic blocking agents.

Amrinone also has some peripheral vasodilator effects that may be partly responsible for increased cardiac output in patients with heart failure. This combination of inotropic and vasodilator effects may be very desirable in achieving hemodynamic benefit. When given to patients with heart failure, amrinone increases output and reduces pulmonary capillary wedge pressure. There is little change in heart rate or arterial pressure. Although these acute effects are clearly beneficial, there are few long-term studies with amrinone. Some data suggest that it does produce sustained benefit in congestive heart failure.

The frequency of toxicity reported for amrinone is low, as would be expected for an agent so early in its investigational life. However, thrombocytopenia has been reported and may lead to bleeding. Since amrinone is a positive inotropic agent, it (like digitalis and other inotropic drugs) has the capacity to increase the myocardial oxygen requirement, which could be hazardous in patients with ischemic heart disease. Studies show, however, that the reduction in cardiac size produced by amrinone may offset the increase in contractility and cause a net decrease in oxygen demand. Nevertheless, ischemic side-effects are a potential complication with any positive inotropic agent.

BETA-ADRENERGIC STIMULANTS

The general pharmacology of these agents is discussed in Chapter 7. The search for positive inotropic drugs with less arrhythmogenic potential than digitalis and less tendency to increase heart rate than isoproterenol has led to the development of β_1-selective agents. At the same time, the successful use of vasodilators in congestive heart failure has resulted in an interest in selective β_2 agents for this condition.

Selective β_1-agonists that have been studied in patients with heart failure include **dobutamine** and **prenalterol.** These drugs produce an increase in cardiac output together with a decrease in ventricular filling pressure. Some tachycardia and increase in myocardial oxygen consumption have been reported. Thus, although these agents clearly increase cardiac contractility, it is unclear what net benefit they may have in patients with ischemic heart disease. The potential for producing angina or arrhythmias in such patients must be considered, as well as the tachyphylaxis that accompanies the chronic use of any β-adrenergic stimulant. No long-term studies are available for these drugs.

Beta$_2$-selective agonists such as **salbutamol** and **pirbuterol** have also been investigated in patients with congestive heart failure. These drugs act by relaxing smooth muscle and are effective vasodilators in some patients. They appear to be useful in increasing cardiac output and reducing pulmonary wedge pressure in such patients. How much of their effect is due to inotropic stimulation (an effect on the cardiac β_1 receptor) is unclear at present.

II. CLINICAL PHARMACOLOGY OF DRUGS USED IN CONGESTIVE HEART FAILURE

PATHOPHYSIOLOGY OF HEART FAILURE

Congestive heart failure is a syndrome with multiple causes that may involve the right ventricle, the left ventricle, or both. Its cardinal feature is that cardiac output falls short of what is required for normal tissue perfusion. Cardiac output in congestive heart failure is usually below the normal range. An intrinsic biochemical defect results in decreased cardiac contractility, which is usually responsive to positive inotropic drugs. This is typical of chronic failure resulting from coronary artery disease or hypertension or acute failure resulting from myocardial infarction. Rarely, "high-output" failure may occur. In this condition, the demands of the body are so great that even increased cardiac output is insufficient. High-output failure can result from hyperthyroidism, beriberi, anemia, and arteriovenous shunts. This form of failure responds poorly to positive inotropic agents.

The primary signs and symptoms of all types of congestive heart failure include tachycardia, decreased exercise tolerance and shortness of breath, peripheral and pulmonary edema, and cardiomegaly. Decreased exercise tolerance with rapid muscular fatigue is the major *direct* consequence of diminished cardiac output. The other manifestations result from attempts by the body to compensate for the intrinsic cardiac defect. Compensation involves 2 major mechanisms, as described in Chapter 4 and displayed in Fig 4–6). These are the sympathetic nervous system and the renin-angiotensin-aldosterone hormonal response (see also Fig 11–4). Increased sympathetic outflow causes tachycardia, increased cardiac contractility, and increased vascular tone—especially venous tone. Elevation of venous tone results in increased ventricular filling pressure, dilatation of the heart, and increased fiber stretch. Increased aldosterone secretion results in sodium and water retention with increased blood volume and, ultimately, edema.

Pathophysiology of Cardiac Performance

Cardiac performance is a function of 4 primary factors (Fig 11–4).

A. Preload: Preload refers to the diastolic loading conditions of the heart, eg, left atrial pressure (or pulmonary wedge pressure) for the left ventricle and right atrial pressure for the right. These are the "filling pressures" of their respective ventricles. The effect of

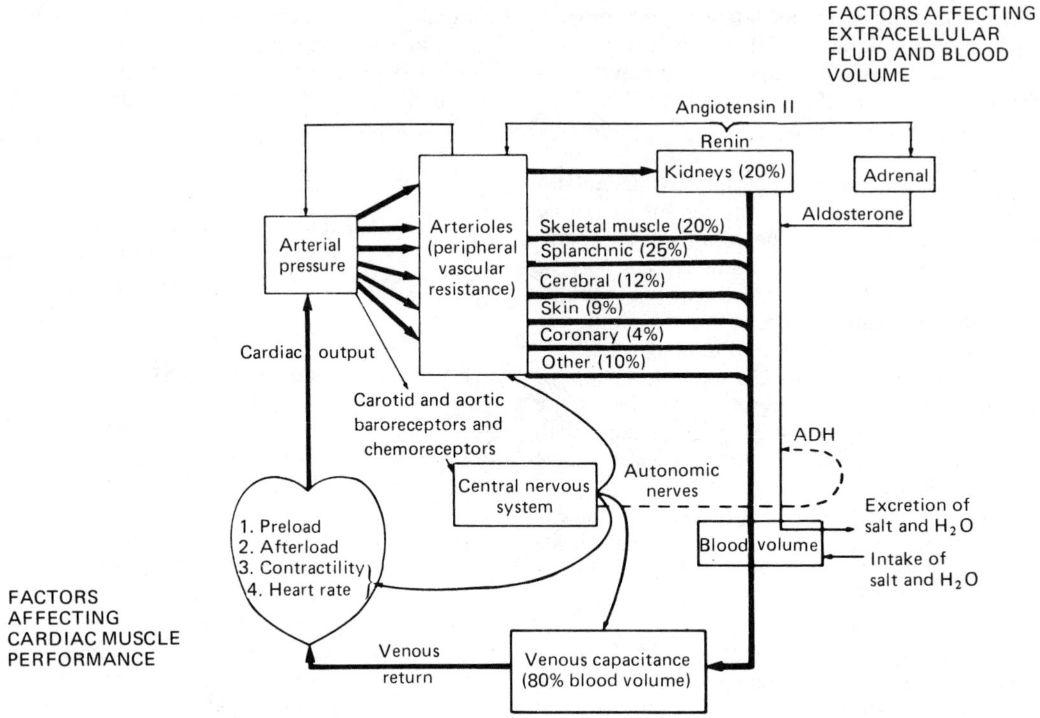

Figure 11–4. Schematic diagram of the cardiovascular system. (See text for details.) (Reproduced, with permission, from Parmley WW: Circulatory function and control. Page 1068 in: *Cecil Textbook of Medicine.* Saunders, 1979.)

altered preload on cardiovascular performance is illustrated in Fig 11–5. When some measure of left ventricular performance such as stroke volume or stroke work is plotted as a function of left ventricular filling pressure, the resulting curve is termed the **left ventricular function curve.** The ascending limb (below 15 mm Hg filling pressure) represents the classic Frank-Starling relation. Beyond approximately 15 mm Hg, there is a plateau of performance. Preloads greater than 20–25 mm Hg result in pulmonary congestion. As noted above, preload is usually increased in heart failure because of increased blood volume and venous tone. Reduction of high filling pressure is the goal of salt restriction and diuretic therapy in congestive heart failure.

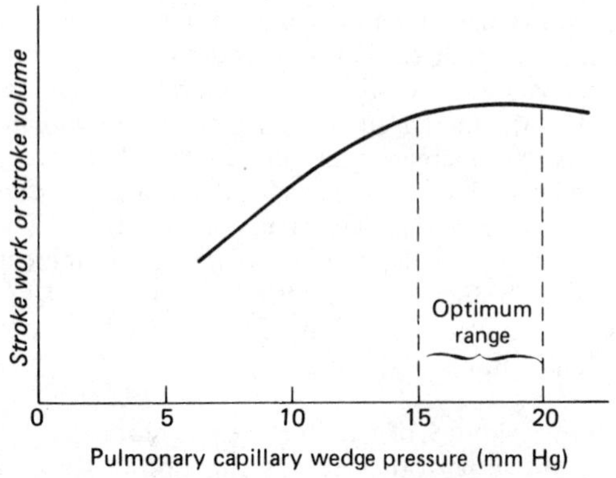

Figure 11–5. Ventricular function curve illustrating the relationship between stroke volume and left atrial (pulmonary capillary wedge) pressure. There is an increase in left ventricular performance up to a left ventricular filling pressure of 15–20 mm Hg. At higher filling pressures, pulmonary congestion and dyspnea ensue.

B. Afterload: Afterload is the resistance against which the heart must pump blood. Systemic vascular resistance is frequently increased in patients with congestive heart failure. The relationship between pressure, resistance, and cardiac output is expressed by the equation:

Arterial pressure = Cardiac output × Systemic vascular resistance

As cardiac output falls in chronic failure, there is a reflex increase in systemic vascular resistance, mediated in part by increased sympathetic outflow and circulating catecholamines (Fig 11–4). However, elevated vascular resistance may further reduce cardiac output by increasing resistance to ejection. This sets the stage for the use of drugs that reduce arteriolar tone in congestive heart failure.

C. Contractility: Contractility is the vigor of contraction of heart muscle. In patients with chronic low-output failure, the primary defect appears to be a reduction in the intrinsic contractility of the myocardium. As contractility decreases, there is a reduction in the velocity of muscle shortening and the rate of intraventricular pressure development (dp/dt). However, the heart is still capable of an increase in contractility in response to inotropic drugs. Thus, agents such as digitalis and amrinone may be helpful in improving the depressed cardiac output.

D. Heart Rate: The heart rate is an extremely important determinant of cardiac performance, as indicated by the following equation:

Cardiac output = Stroke volume × Heart rate

As the intrinsic function of the heart decreases in failure and stroke volume diminishes, an increase in heart rate is the first compensatory mechanism that comes into play to maintain cardiac output.

Pathophysiology of the Peripheral Vasculature in Congestive Heart Failure

The increase in systemic resistance that occurs at the arteriolar level is due to many factors. First, there is increased activity of the sympathetic nervous system, which increases resistance by α-adrenergic activation. Increase in plasma catecholamines is generally related to the severity of the heart failure. There is also an excessive increase in adrenergic tone during exercise, which frequently leads to a marked rise in vascular resistance. Although this helps maintain blood pressure in the face of an inadequate increase in cardiac output, it also increases the load against which the heart must work, which tends to further reduce cardiac output.

Activation of the renin-angiotensin-aldosterone system in heart failure has also been mentioned above. Angiotensin II is a potent arteriolar vasoconstrictor that directly increases vascular resistance. Furthermore, angiotensin II facilitates sympathetic outflow. As a result of these vasoconstrictor effects and retention of sodium, congestive heart failure is associated with increased wall stiffness in peripheral arteries.

The normal distribution of blood to various organs is schematically shown in Fig 11–4. As cardiac output is reduced in heart failure, renal blood flow and urine output are also decreased. On the other hand, regional circulations with powerful autoregulatory mechanisms (like the cerebral and coronary beds) tend to maintain their blood flow in spite of moderate reductions of arterial pressure and cardiac output. As output further diminishes, vascular regions such as the skin and splanchnic bed become vasoconstricted, and blood is thus preferentially shunted to vital organs.

The venous system holds 75–80% of the blood volume and thus serves as the major capacitance or storage system for the peripheral vascular system. In congestive heart failure, there is an increase in venous tone, caused by increased sympathetic tone and circulating catecholamines, as described above. This compensatory mechanism maintains venous return to the heart but may thereby further overload the right ventricle and the pulmonary circulation. For this reason, vasodilators that selectively dilate veins (eg, nitroglycerin) may be useful to redistribute blood in the vascular tree and reduce right and left atrial pressures. This effect may be particularly dramatic in patients with acute left heart failure in whom venodilators can promptly relieve the signs and symptoms of pulmonary congestion.

Important changes also occur in cardiovascular reflexes. Carotid, aortic, and left atrial pressure and stretch receptors are useful homeostatic mechanisms for maintaining an appropriate arterial pressure. In heart failure, reflex effects from these receptors may be blunted. This results in less tachycardia, for example, when arterial pressure is reduced with vasodilator drugs.

DIGITALIS IN CONGESTIVE HEART FAILURE

Because it has a moderate but persistent positive inotropic effect, digitalis can, in theory, reverse all the signs and symptoms of congestive heart failure. In an appropriate case, digitalis increases stroke work and cardiac output. This can be demonstrated by a shift of the ventricular function curve (Fig 11–6) from "depressed" to "adequate" or even "normal." The in-

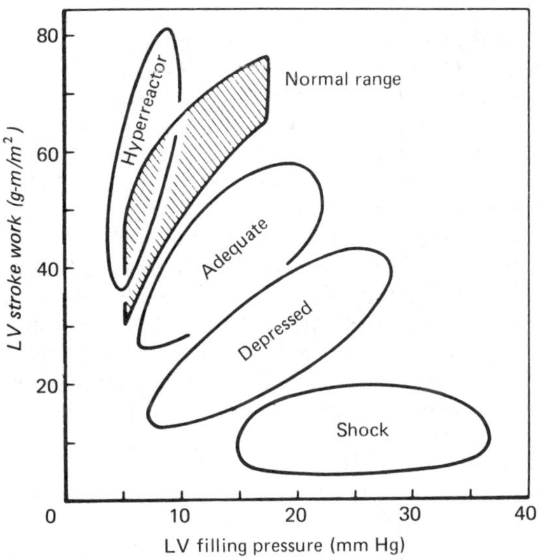

Figure 11–6. Relation of left ventricular performance to filling pressure in patients with acute myocardial infarction. The cross-hatched area is the range for normal, healthy individuals. Following infarction, there is a wide range of performance characteristics. In some patients, performance is in the normal or hypernormal range (hyperreactor). As the size of the infarct increases, however, function is shifted down and to the right. Similar depression is observed in patients with chronic congestive heart failure. (Reproduced, with permission, from: Swan HJC, Parmley WW: Congestive heart failure. Page 327 in: *Pathologic Physiology.* Sodeman WA, Sodeman WA Jr (editors). Saunders, 1979.)

creased output eliminates the stimuli evoking increased sympathetic outflow, and both heart rate and venous tone diminish. With decreased end-diastolic fiber tension (the result of increased systolic ejection and decreased filling pressure), heart size and oxygen demand decrease. Finally, increased renal blood flow improves glomerular filtration and reduces aldosterone-driven sodium reabsorption. Thus, edema fluid can be excreted, further reducing ventricular preload and the danger of pulmonary edema. It is important to note that the cardiac glycosides have the same effect on contractility in normal as in failing muscle, yet the actions of the drug in normal subjects and patients with congestive heart failure are quite different, owing to the very different reflex responses involved. In normal persons, digitalis increases cardiac contractility and ejection fraction, but homeostatic processes prevent any significant increase in cardiac output. Decreased heart rate and increased afterload are 2 contributing factors.

Administration & Dosage

Chronic treatment of a patient with digitalis requires careful attention to pharmacokinetics. Because of their long half-lives (Table 11–1), these agents accumulate in the body. According to the rules set forth in Chapter 3, it will take 3–4 half-lives to approach steady-state total body load when given at a constant dosing rate, ie, approximately 1 week for digoxin and 1 month for digitoxin. Since it is very important not to exceed the therapeutic range of plasma digitalis concentration, such a slow approach to "digitalization" is the safest dosing technique. If a more rapid effect is required, digitalization can be achieved quickly with a large loading dose (divided into 3 or 4 portions and given over 24–36 hours) followed by a maintenance dose. Typical doses used in adults are given in Table 11–3. It is essential that the patient be examined before each dose when using the rapid (3-dose) method of digitalization. Sensitive plasma digoxin radioimmunoassays are available at most medical centers and should be used when patient response is not as predicted from the dosing schedule.

Interactions

Important drug interactions must be considered in patients taking cardiac glycosides. All such patients are at risk of developing serious cardiac arrhythmias if hypokalemia develops, as in diuretic therapy or diarrhea. Furthermore, patients taking digoxin are at risk if given quinidine, which displaces digoxin from tissue binding sites, markedly decreasing its volume of distribution. Quinidine may also depress renal digoxin clearance. The plasma level of the glycoside may double within a few days after beginning quinidine therapy, and toxic effects may become manifest. A similar interaction with quinine, ibuprofen, and indomethacin has been reported in dogs, but it has not been demonstrated that these agents displace digoxin in humans. Quinidine does not alter volume of distribution or protein binding of digitoxin. However, it may prolong the half-life of this glycoside. Finally, agents that release catecholamines may sensitize the myocardium to digitalis-induced arrhythmias. Amantadine and many decongestants are among the clinically available drugs that have this potential toxicity.

Reduced responsiveness to cardiac glycosides may be due to intractably severe disease or patient noncompliance. In patients concurrently taking cholestyramine (Chapter 32), digitalis absorption is reduced. The digitalis dose required for therapeutic effect must usually be increased in hyperthyroid patients because of reduction in elimination half-life.

Table 11–3. Clinical use of cardiac glycosides. (These values are appropriate for adults with normal renal and hepatic function.)

	Digoxin	Digitoxin
Half-life	40 hours	168 hours
Therapeutic plasma concentration	0.5–2 ng/mL	10–25 ng/mL
Daily dose (slow loading or maintenance)	0.125–0.5 mg	0.05–0.2 mg
Rapid digitalizing dose	0.5–0.75 mg every 8 hours for 3 doses	0.2–0.4 mg every 12 hours for 3 doses
Time to peak effect	3–6 hours	6–12 hours

Other Clinical Uses of Digitalis

Digitalis is useful in the management of atrial arrhythmias because of its cardioselective parasympathomimetic effects. In atrial flutter, the depressant effect of the drug on atrioventricular conduction will help control an excessively high ventricular rate. The effects of the drug on the atrial musculature may convert flutter to fibrillation, with a further decrease in ventricular rate. In atrial fibrillation, the same "vagomimetic" action helps to control ventricular rate, thereby improving ventricular filling and increasing cardiac output indirectly as well as through its inotropic effect. Traditionally, digitalis was given prior to the administration of quinidine when quinidine was used to convert atrial fibrillation to normal sinus rhythm (see also Chapter 12). The atrioventricular depressant effect of the cardiac glycoside counteracts the antimuscarinic action of quinidine, which could otherwise lead to an undesirable increase in ventricular rate. Because quinidine increases the plasma concentration and toxicity of digoxin, this use of the latter drug requires caution. Digitalis is also valuable in the control of paroxysmal atrial and atrioventricular nodal tachycardia. Oral or, if necessary, cautious intravenous administration of digoxin may abruptly terminate such attacks, probably as the result of its vagomimetic action.

Toxicity

In spite of its recognized hazards, digitalis is still a widely and overused drug. In a large multicenter study, 17–27% of patients admitted for all medical conditions were taking digitalis on admission, and

5–25% of the identified group showed evidence of toxicity requiring at least temporary cessation of digitalis therapy.

Therapy of digitalis toxicity manifested as visual changes or gastrointestinal disturbances generally requires no more than withholding the drug. If cardiac arrhythmia is present and can definitely be ascribed to digitalis, more vigorous therapy may be necessary. For stable premature ventricular depolarizations or brief runs of bigeminy, oral potassium supplementation and withdrawal of the glycoside may be sufficient. If the arrhythmia is more serious, parenteral potassium and antiarrhythmia drugs may be required. Of the available antiarrhythmia agents, lidocaine, phenytoin, and propranolol are favored, although quinidine and verapamil can also be shown to be effective. Serum potassium levels and the ECG should be monitored during therapy of digitalis toxicity. In very severe digitalis intoxication (which usually involves suicidal overdose), serum potassium will already be elevated at the time of diagnosis. Furthermore, antiarrhythmia agents administered in this setting may lead to cardiac arrest. Such patients are best treated with digitalis antibodies or "Fab fragments" of such antibodies. Digoxin-specific antibody is available in many centers.

Digitalis-induced arrhythmias are frequently made worse by cardioversion; this therapy should be reserved for ventricular fibrillation if the arrhythmia is glycoside-induced.

CLINICAL MANAGEMENT OF CHRONIC HEART FAILURE

The major steps in the management of patients with chronic heart failure are outlined in Table 11–4. Reduction of cardiac work is a traditional form of therapy that is extremely helpful in most cases. It can be accomplished by reducing activity levels, weight reduction, and—especially important—control of hypertension. Sodium restriction is the next important step. Despite the availability of potent diuretics, one should advise patients about the necessity for salt restriction and encourage them to avoid excess salt through dietary restraint.

In patients without severe edema, some authorities recommend treatment with a positive inotropic agent (digitalis) as the next step. However, considerable evidence has accumulated against the universal efficacy of digitalis in patients with heart failure who are in normal sinus rhythm. Therefore, most clinicians prefer to start drug therapy with a diuretic, even in patients with minimal visible edema.

Table 11–4. Steps in the treatment of chronic heart failure.

1. Reduce workload of the heart.
   a. Limit activity level.
   b. Reduce weight.
   c. Control hypertension.
2. Restrict sodium.
3. Restrict water (rarely required).
4. Diuretics.
5. Digitalis.
6. Vasodilators.
7. Newer inotropic agents.

Diuretic therapy (Chapter 13) should be started with one of the thiazides, switching to more efficacious agents as required. The thiazides tend to increase excretion of sodium and chloride in approximately equivalent amounts. Sodium loss causes secondary loss of potassium, which is particularly hazardous if the patient is to be given digitalis. Therefore, serum electrolytes should be checked periodically in patients so treated. Hypokalemia can be treated with potassium supplementation or through the addition of potassium-sparing diuretics.

Furosemide and ethacrynic acid are very efficacious diuretics that should be reserved for patients with resistant edema. In some instances, diuresis may be so dramatic as to produce hypovolemia, hypotension, tachycardia, and severe electrolyte imbalance. When patients are given these drugs on a continuing basis, it is important to measure plasma electrolytes periodically to monitor possible volume depletion or electrolyte imbalance. Potassium supplementation may be required.

When a positive inotropic drug is to be used, a cardiac glycoside will be chosen; amrinone and the β-adrenergic stimulants are still investigational agents. It should be emphasized again that digitalis is a dangerous agent, and only about 50% of patients with normal sinus rhythm will have documentable relief of congestive failure. Better results are obtained in patients with atrial fibrillation. If the decision is made to use a cardiac glycoside, digoxin is the one chosen in the great majority of cases. (As noted in the first portion of this chapter, other glycosides are seldom needed.) When symptoms are mild, slow digitalization (Table 11–3) is safest and just as effective as the rapid method. If symptoms are moderately severe, the rapid oral method may be used, but the patient should be examined before each dose with particular attention to his cardiac rhythm. An ECG should be recorded if there is any doubt about the nature of the pretherapy rhythm or changes during digitalization. Intravenous digitalization is rarely required in chronic heart failure; it should be used only in hospitalized patients with careful monitoring.

Determining the optimal level of digitalis effect may be difficult. In patients with atrial fibrillation, reduction of ventricular rate is the best measure of glycoside effect. In patients in normal sinus rhythm, symptomatic improvement and reductions in heart size, heart rate during exercise, venous pressure, or edema may signify optimum drug levels in the myocardium. Unfortunately, toxic effects may occur before the therapeutic end point is detected. If slow digitalization is being employed, simple omission of one dose and halving of the maintenance dose will often bring the patient to the narrow range between suboptimal and toxic concentrations. Measurement of

Table 11–5. Vasodilators for use in chronic congestive heart failure.

Arteriolodilators	Combined Arteriolo- and Venodilators	Venodilators
Hydralazine Minoxidil	Prazosin Captopril Trimazosin Phenoxybenzamine Phentolamine	Nitrates

plasma digitalis levels is useful in patients who appear unusually resistant or sensitive; these assays are available for both digoxin and digitoxin.

If all of the above therapies are insufficient to maintain cardiovascular compensation, vasodilator drugs may be extremely helpful. A useful classification divides the drugs into selective venodilators, selective arteriolodilators, and drugs with nonselective vasodilatory effects (Table 11–5). Choice of agent should be based on the patient's signs and symptoms and hemodynamic measurements. Thus, in patients with high filling pressures in whom the principal symptom is dyspnea, the venodilators will be most helpful in reducing filling pressures and the symptoms of pulmonary congestion. In patients in whom fatigue due to low left ventricular output is a primary symptom, an arteriolodilator may be helpful in increasing forward cardiac output. In most patients with severe chronic failure that responds poorly to other therapy, the problem usually involves both elevated filling pressures and reduced cardiac output. In these circumstances, dilation of both arterioles and veins is required. To date, vasodilators have generally been used as supplements to standard therapy. Further study is required to determine whether or not vasodilator therapy may be considered as primary treatment, before digitalis or diuretics.

The predominant venodilator drugs comprise all forms of nitrates (Chapter 10). Although they chiefly dilate large veins, they may also dilate arterioles to some degree, particularly when given intravenously. Because of "first-pass" hepatic metabolism of orally administered nitrates, very high doses may be required to achieve effective venodilation in chronic therapy. An average oral dose of **isosorbide dinitrate** is approximately 40 mg 4 times daily, although doses considerably higher than this may be required in some patients. Because of the short duration of action of sublingually administered nitrates, only oral (nitroglycerin, isosorbide) or transdermal (nitroglycerin ointment) administration is suitable for chronic therapy.

The most commonly used arteriolar vasodilator is **hydralazine,** which causes direct relaxation of the arteriolar resistance bed (Chapter 9). Hydralazine is usually combined with nitrates to provide both venous and arteriolar dilatation. In general, one can begin at low doses (25–50 mg twice daily) and increase gradually to 150 mg twice daily. It is helpful to evaluate cardiac output directly in order to optimize the dose of hydralazine. In patients with chronic severe heart failure, hydralazine may produce a 50% increase in cardiac output and a 50% decrease in systemic vascular resistance. Hydralazine appears to be hemodynamically effective for long-term therapy, although it is not clear that this drug or any vasodilator combination prolongs survival. Side-effects are relatively frequent with hydralazine. Minoxidil is a powerful arteriolar vasodilator currently approved only for the treatment of resistant hypertension. Experimental studies in severe heart failure have demonstrated that its hemodynamic effects are similar to those of hydralazine. Sodium retention is a major unwanted effect.

Several drugs produce combined arteriolar and venous dilatation. Most of the useful agents are α-adrenergic blockers (Chapter 8). **Prazosin** has been extensively studied as a vasodilator for use in chronic heart failure. Prazosin produces an interesting first-dose effect, manifested by striking arteriolar and venous dilatation. This results in an increase in cardiac output along with a marked reduction in pulmonary capillary wedge pressure. Some degree of hypotension may also occur. Thus, the first dose of prazosin should be small (1 mg) and should be given under observation. After the first dose, there is frequently an attenuation of the effect on cardiac output, although pulmonary capillary wedge pressure may still be reduced. Several studies have demonstrated that despite this attenuated response, prazosin can be symptomatically beneficial in the long-term management of congestive heart failure. The usual dose is 3–5 mg 4 times daily. Development of tolerance may require decreasing or stopping prazosin for several days and then restarting it. If the patient needs vasodilator drugs, a combination of hydralazine and nitrates may be used in the interim.

Captopril, an angiotensin-converting enzyme inhibitor (Chapter 9), may be beneficial in some patients with congestive failure, although its only approved indication at present is hypertension. The reduction in aldosterone secretion, reduced angiotensin II levels, and elimination of sympathetic facilitation by angiotensin are all useful in reversing the compensatory mechanisms that contribute to the pathophysiology of congestive heart failure. In patients with severe congestive failure, captopril produces a modest increase in cardiac output, together with a reduction in left ventricular filling pressure. In contrast to hydralazine, captopril produces a modest reduction in arterial pressure. Despite this reduction in arterial pressure, there may be no change in heart rate or even a slight bradycardia. Thus, it may be difficult to use captopril in patients with low initial arterial pressure. Doses greater than 25 mg 4 times a day appear to be no more effective and may cause excessive hypotension. In studies to date, captopril appears to be most useful in patients whose congestive failure is associated with very high systemic vascular resistance.

In summary, therapy with vasodilator drugs confers immediate hemodynamic benefits, especially increased cardiac output and reduced pulmonary vascular pressure. Symptoms may also be significantly improved. However, it is not clear that these agents reduce the mortality rate in the seriously ill population studied so far.

MANAGEMENT OF ACUTE HEART FAILURE

Acute heart failure occurs frequently in patients with chronic failure. Such episodes are usually associated with increased exertion, emotion, salt in the diet, noncompliance with medical therapy, or increased metabolic demand occasioned by fever, anemia, etc. A particularly common and important cause of acute failure—with or without chronic failure—is acute myocardial infarction. Many of the signs and symptoms of acute and chronic failure are identical, but their therapies diverge because of the need for more rapid response and the relatively greater frequency and severity of pulmonary vascular congestion in the acute form.

Because of the need for rapid recognition and evaluation of changing hemodynamic status, it is much more important to obtain quantitative measurements in acute failure than in chronic failure. These measurements should include left ventricular filling pressure (pulmonary wedge pressure) and cardiac output in addition to heart rate, blood pressure, and heart size. The **stroke work index** (approximately stroke volume index times arterial pressure) is a useful derived variable that describes the external work performed by the heart.

Measurements of stroke work index and pulmonary capillary pressure from a large group of patients with acute myocardial infarction are illustrated in Fig 11–6. When filling pressure is greater than 15 mm Hg and stroke work index is less than 20 g-m/m^2, the mortality rate is high. It is apparent, therefore, that the effects of myocardial infarction on ventricular function are not uniform and that there can be no single standard therapy for the management of congestive failure in this condition.

Subsets of Patients Following Myocardial Infarction

Patients with acute congestive failure following myocardial infarction can be usefully characterized on the basis of 3 hemodynamic measurements: arterial pressure, left ventricular filling pressure, and cardiac index. One such classification is illustrated in Table 11–6.

(1) Hypovolemia: Subset 1 includes patients who are relatively hypovolemic following myocardial infarction. They usually have been taking diuretics or may have had inadequate fluid intake. The primary hemodynamic abnormality is low left ventricular filling pressure, which can be corrected by giving fluids. With an increase of filling pressure up to the optimal range of 15 mm Hg (Fig 11–5), hypotension disappears and cardiac output increases. This form of therapy is often all that is required to raise cardiac output and blood pressure to adequate levels. In patients with acute infarction, the amount of fluid required to increase filling pressure is often small—less than 500 mL.

(2) Pulmonary Congestion: The second subset—patients with pulmonary congestion—is a very large one and is also representative of other causes of acute heart failure. Such patients are characterized by a systolic blood pressure over 100 mm Hg and a filling pressure greater than 25 mm Hg, which leads to severe pulmonary congestion and dyspnea. Several pharmacologic agents may be helpful in the management of such patients. Diuretics are helpful because they reduce intravascular volume (Chapter 13). In addition, when given intravenously, powerful diuretics such as furosemide produce an immediate increase in compliance of systemic veins. This leads to peripheral pooling of blood, which reduces central blood volume and decreases right and left ventricular filling pressures. Morphine sulfate also is clinically effective in the management of acute pulmonary edema. Apart

Table 11–6. Therapeutic classification of subsets in acute myocardial infarction.*

Subset	Systolic Arterial Pressure (mm Hg)	Left Ventricular Filling Pressure (mm Hg)	Cardiac Index (L/min/m^2)	Therapy
1. Hypovolemia	< 100	< 10	< 2.5	Volume replacement.
2. Pulmonary congestion	100–150	> 20	> 2.5	Diuretics.
3. Peripheral vasodilatation	< 100	10–20	> 2.5	None, or vasoactive drugs.
4. Power failure	< 100	> 20	< 2.5	Vasodilators.
5. Severe shock	< 90	> 20	< 2.0	Vasoactive drugs, vasodilators, circulatory assist.
6. Right ventricular infarct	< 100	RVFP > 10 LVFP < 15	< 2.5	Provide volume replacement for low LVFP. Avoid diuretics.
7. Mitral regurgitation, ventricular septal defect	< 100	> 20	< 2.5	Vasodilators, circulatory assist, surgery.

*The numerical values are intended to serve as general guidelines and not as absolute cut-off points. Arterial pressures apply to patients who were previously normotensive and should be adjusted upward for patients who were previously hypertensive. (RVFP and LVFP = right and left ventricular filling pressure.)

from its ability to relieve the pain of infarction, the mechanisms by which it reduces pulmonary congestion are uncertain. Morphine produces some arteriolar dilatation, which may unload the ventricle and enhance its emptying. Morphine also has transient venodilating qualities that may help reduce right and left atrial pressures. Because morphine produces sedation, it may also reduce the work of breathing and be effective in part through this tranquilizing action. If bronchospasm is a prominent component of the pulmonary signs, aminophylline may also be helpful, since it combines bronchodilator, vasodilator, and positive inotropic actions (Chapter 17).

Mechanical interventions such as tourniquets on the limbs are also effective in pooling of blood in peripheral vessels and reducing right and left atrial pressures. Other measures infrequently required in pulmonary edema include rapid withdrawal of a unit of blood (if the patient has a normal hemoglobin) or positive pressure ventilation, which reduces venous return.

(3) Peripheral Vasodilatation: The third subset of patients following acute myocardial infarction is relatively small. These patients are hypotensive and yet have warm extremities because of peripheral vasodilatation. The usual response to the insult of myocardial infarction is a dramatic increase in peripheral vascular resistance in order to maintain arterial pressure. In some patients, however, this reflex is not operative, usually as a consequence of drug-induced autonomic blockade. These patients may not need any therapy, since pulmonary wedge pressure is usually normal and cardiac output satisfactory. If blood pressure is extremely low, however, a vasoactive drug such as dopamine should be considered to maintain arterial perfusion pressure at the desired level.

(4) "Power Failure": The fourth subset represents those patients who have moderate "power failure." Hemodynamic measurements show a reduction in arterial pressure, although not to shock levels, together with an elevation of left ventricular filling pressure and a reduction of cardiac index. The goal of therapy in these patients is to increase cardiac output and reduce ventricular filling pressure without further decrease in arterial pressure. Diuretics or nitrates are helpful in lowering filling pressures but will not increase cardiac output because the ventricle lacks sufficient power to pump against the systemic impedance. A combined venous and arteriolar dilator such as nitroprusside is extremely beneficial in such patients. Its venodilating effects reduce right and left atrial pressures by redistributing more blood into the periphery. Its arteriolodilating properties increase forward cardiac output by reducing systemic vascular resistance. The main limiting factor in the use of nitroprusside is the reduction in arterial pressure. If the dose is titrated carefully, however, this reduction in blood pressure may be minimized. A good rule of thumb is to consider giving nitroprusside if the systolic pressure is 90 mm Hg or higher. The effects of nitroprusside depend on the level of left ventricular filling pressure. This is

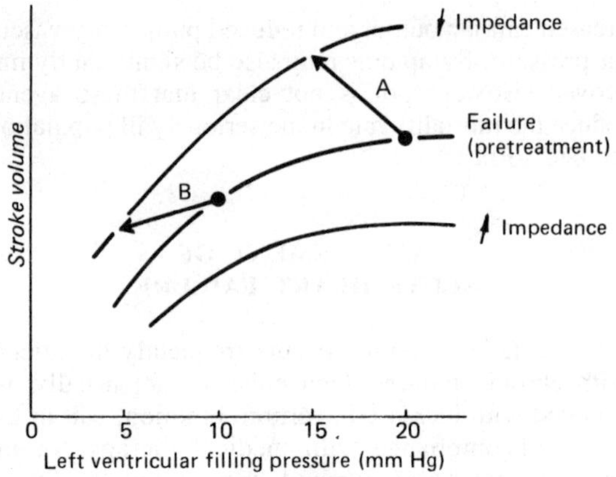

Figure 11–7. Effects of vasodilator therapy on left ventricular function. With the administration of a combined arteriolodilator and venodilator such as nitroprusside, function is shifted to a higher curve, reflecting the decreased impedance to ventricular ejection. A patient with heart failure on the pretreatment function curve with an initial filling pressure of 20 mm Hg will experience an increase in stroke volume along line *A,* up and to the left. If the patient was initially at a filling pressure of 10 mm Hg, nitroprusside would still shift performance to the upper curve, but this would result in a decrease of performance, along line ***B.*** (Reproduced, with permission, from Chatterjee K, Parmley WW: *Prog Cardiovasc Dis* 1977; **19**:305.)

illustrated diagrammatically in Fig 11–7. The middle curve in the figure represents a patient with moderately severe heart failure. If the patient has a high left ventricular filling pressure (20 mm Hg), the administration of sodium nitroprusside will shift ventricular function up and to the left, as illustrated by line *A*. If, however, the patient has been given large doses of diuretics and filling pressure has thereby been reduced to 10 mm Hg, nitroprusside will produce a different result. Although the patient moves to the upper curve with nitroprusside (line *B*), there is a reduction of stroke volume because the heart is on the steep ascending limb of the curve. This will worsen hypotension and tachycardia. If the patient is volume-loaded at this point, up to the optimal filling pressure of 15 mm Hg, the beneficial effect of nitroprusside will become evident. This example illustrates the importance of filling pressure: pulmonary wedge pressure should be maintained at about 15 mm Hg by either diuresis or volume administration, as required.

(5) Severe Shock: Subset 5 represents a group of patients with cardiogenic shock following myocardial infarction. These patients have very low arterial pressures, very high filling pressures, and low cardiac indices. Although diuretics may be helpful in lowering the elevated filling pressures, they will not increase cardiac output. Furthermore, the use of vasodilators in these patients is difficult, since the accompanying hypotension may be severe and may impair perfusion of vital organs. Since the mortality rate under these circumstances is high, it is often difficult to know whether any therapy is beneficial. Nevertheless, certain approaches may be helpful. If the arterial pressure is extremely low, it is useful to consider use of a catecholamine such as dopamine. By titrating the dose of this drug, one can produce an increase in arterial pressure that is adequate for peripheral tissue perfusion. At this point, one can cautiously add nitroprusside to lower pulmonary wedge pressure. The combined effects of these 2 agents on the heart tend to be additive, since they work through different mechanisms. Dopamine directly increases cardiac contractility, while nitroprusside produces venous and arteriolar dilatation. This therapy should be combined with an attempt to optimize left ventricular filling pressure. These patients are also candidates for circulatory assist measures (intra-aortic balloon) and consideration of cardiac catheterization and possible coronary bypass surgery.

(6) Right Ventricular Infarction: Group 6 comprises a subset of patients who have an inferior myocardial infarction that predominantly involves the right ventricle. The pattern shown in Table 11–6 occurs in approximately one-third of patients with inferior infarctions. In general, such patients are slightly hypotensive, with elevated central venous pressure and normal or low left ventricular filling pressure. Their hypotension is due to the fact that the right ventricle is unable to deliver sufficient blood to the left side of the heart to optimize left ventricular filling pressure and cardiac output. Therefore, the primary therapeutic goal is to optimize left ventricular filling pressure. This may require volume infusion despite elevated central venous pressure. One should avoid using diuretics, since reduction of volume may lead to further reduction of filling pressure with associated hypotension and tachycardia.

(7) Mitral Regurgitation and Ventricular Septal Defect: A seventh subset is mentioned for completeness, although these patients are also found in other subsets, particularly those with shock. These are patients with mechanical abnormalities such as acute severe mitral regurgitation or a ruptured interventricular septum. Vasodilator drugs such as nitroprusside are especially helpful in patients in this subset. Careful titration with the drug may be necessary to obtain optimal effect. The intra-aortic balloon is also helpful in management of these patients. Depending on the severity of the defect, cardiac surgery must be considered urgently as the most definitive form of therapy. However, vasodilator therapy may be necessary to stabilize the patient before surgery is possible.

• • •

References

Basic Pharmacology

Bigger JT Jr: The quinidine-digoxin interaction. *Mod Concepts Cardiovasc Dis* 1982;**51:**73.

Bodem G, Dengler HJ (editors): *Cardiac Glycosides*. International Boehringer-Mannheim Symposia. Springer-Verlag, 1978.

Jelliffe RW: An improved method of digoxin therapy. *Ann Intern Med* 1968;**69:**703.

Schwartz A, Lindenmayer GE, Allen JC: The sodium-potassium adenosine triphosphatase: Pharmacological, physiological, and biochemical aspects. *Pharmacol Rev* 1975;**27:**3.

Smith TW: Digitalis glycosides. (2 parts.) *N Engl J Med* 1973;**288:**719, 942.

Smith TW et al: Reversal of advanced digoxin intoxication with Fab fragments of digoxin-specific antibodies. *N Engl J Med* 1976;**294:**797.

Symposium: Newer aspects of cardiac glycoside action. *Fed Proc* 1977;**36:**2207.

Pathophysiology of Heart Failure

Abboud FM, Schmid PG: Circulatory adjustments to heart failure. Pages 249–260 in: *Heart Failure*. Fishman A (editor). Hemisphere Corp, 1978.

Braunwald E: Pathophysiology of heart failure. Pages 453–471 in: *Heart Disease*. Saunders, 1980.

Swan HJC, Parmley WW: Congestive heart failure. Pages 313–334 in: *Pathologic Physiology*, 6th ed. Sodeman WA, Sodeman WA Jr (editors). Saunders, 1979.

Zelis R et al: Autonomic adjustments to congestive heart failure and their consequences. Pages 237–247 in: *Heart Failure*. Fishman AP (editor). Hemisphere Corp, 1978.

Acute Myocardial Infarction

Chatterjee K et al: Hemodynamic and metabolic responses to vasodilator therapy in acute myocardial infarction. *Circulation* 1973;**48:**1183.

Forrester JS, Chatterjee K, Swan HJC: Medical therapy of acute myocardial infarction by application of hemodynamic subsets. *N Engl J Med* 1976;**295:**1356.

Parmley W, Chatterjee K: Evaluation of cardiac function in the coronary care unit. Chap 7, pp 86–98, in: *Acute Myocardial Infarction*. Vol 4. Donoso E, Lipski J (editors). Stratton Intercontinental, 1978.

Sobel BE, Braunwald E: The management of acute myocardial infarction. Pages 1353–1386 in: *Heart Disease*. Braunwald E (editor). Saunders, 1980.

Chronic Heart Failure

Chatterjee K, Parmley WW: The role of vasodilator therapy in heart failure. *Prog Cardiovasc Dis* 1977;**19:**301.

Chatterjee K, Parmley WW: Vasodilator therapy for chronic heart failure. Chap 22, pp 475–512, in: *Annual Review of Pharmacology and Toxicology*. Annual Reviews, 1980.

Colucci WS et al: Mechanisms and implications of vasodilator tolerance in the treatment of congestive heart failure. *Am J Med* 1981;**71:**89.

Lee DC-S et al: Heart failure in outpatients: A randomized trial of digoxin versus placebo. *N Engl J Med* 1982;**306:**699.

Smith TW, Braunwald E: The management of heart failure. Pages 509–570 in: *Heart Disease*. Braunwald E (editor). Saunders, 1980.

12 | Agents Used in Cardiac Arrhythmias

Luc M. Hondeghem, MD, PhD, & Jay W. Mason, MD

Cardiac arrhythmias are a frequent problem in clinical practice, occurring in up to 25% of patients treated with digitalis, 50% of anesthetized patients, and over 80% of patients with acute myocardial infarction. Arrhythmias may require treatment not only because too rapid, too slow, or asynchronous contractions reduce cardiac output but, more importantly, because some arrhythmias can precipitate more serious or even lethal rhythm disturbances—eg, early premature ventricular depolarization can precipitate ventricular fibrillation.

Arrhythmias can be treated with the drugs discussed in this chapter and with nonpharmacologic therapies, ie, pacemakers and cardioversion. This chapter describes the pharmacology of agents that suppress arrhythmias by a direct action on the cardiac cell membrane. Other modes of therapy are discussed briefly.

ELECTROPHYSIOLOGY OF NORMAL CARDIAC RHYTHM

The electrical impulse that triggers a normal cardiac contraction originates at regular intervals in the sinoatrial (SA) node (Fig 12–1), usually at a frequency of 60–100 beats per minute. This impulse spreads rapidly through the atria and enters the atrioventricular (AV) node, which is normally the only conduction pathway between the atria and ventricles. Conduction through the atrioventricular node is slow, requiring about 0.2 second. The impulse then propagates over the His-Purkinje system and invades all parts of the ventricles. Ventricular activation is complete in less than 0.1 second; therefore, contraction of all of the ventricular muscle is synchronous and hemodynamically effective.

Arrhythmias consist of cardiac depolarizations that deviate from the above description in one or more aspects; ie, there is an abnormality in the site of origin of the impulse, its rate or regularity, or its conduction.

Ionic Basis of Membrane Activity

The transmembrane potential of cardiac cells is determined by the concentrations of several ions—chiefly sodium (Na^+), potassium (K^+), and calcium (Ca^{2+})—on either side of the membrane and the permeability of the membrane to each ion. Ion channels—protein molecules that span the membranes—are the major routes by which ions diffuse through the membrane. These channels are relatively ion-specific, and the flux of ions through them is thought to be controlled by "gates" (probably flexible peptide chains). Each type of channel has its own type of gate (sodium and calcium channels are each thought to have 2 kinds of gates; potassium channels only one), and each kind of gate is opened and closed by specific transmembrane potential conditions.

Since movement of ions through these channels is passive and "downhill," other mechanisms must be present to maintain the average ionic concentrations inside the cell at appropriate levels. The most important of these active mechanisms is the sodium pump, Na^+,K^+-ATPase, described in Chapter 11. This pump and other active carriers of ions contribute indirectly to the transmembrane potential by maintaining the gradients necessary for diffusion through channels. In addition, they may contribute directly through electrogenic pumping.

At any given time, the potential across the cell membrane is a reflection of all of the processes just described. However, under certain conditions, a useful simplification can be applied to predict the transmembrane potential. These conditions require that the cell membrane be highly permeable to one ion and relatively impermeable to all others. When this is the case, the transmembrane potential, E_m, approximates the ionic equilibrium potential, E_{ion}. The equilibrium potential is given by the **Nernst equation,** which for sodium and potassium is (at body temperature):

$$E_{ion} = 61 \log (C_e/C_i)$$

where C_e and C_i are the extracellular and intracellular concentrations, respectively. The conditions required for application of the Nernst equation are approximated during rest (phase 4, Fig 12–1) and during the upstroke (phase 0) of most nonpacemaker cardiac cells.

The Resting Cell Membrane

During rest, the membrane of nonpacemaker cells is much more permeable to potassium than to other ions, so the membrane potential approaches the potas-

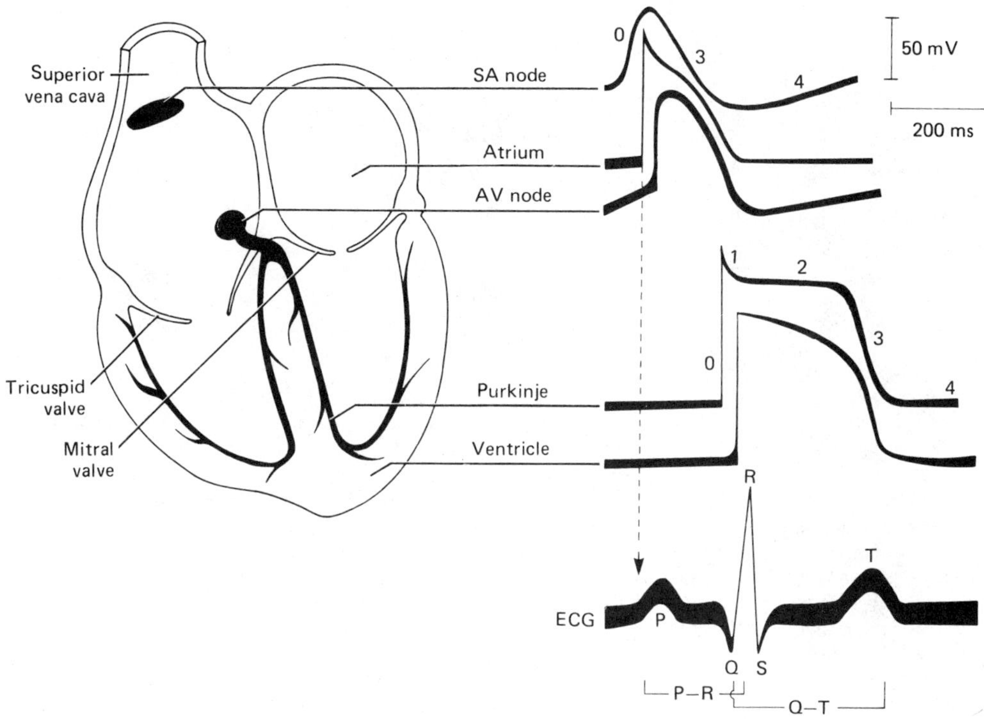

Figure 12–1. Schematic representation of the heart and normal cardiac electrical activity. Intracellular microelectrode recordings are shown for the 5 major cell types, along with an ECG recorded from the body surface. The cardiac action potential consists of 4 phases, demonstrated best in the Purkinje fiber action potential: phase 0 = upstroke, phase 1 = early fast repolarization, phase 2 = plateau, phase 3 = repolarization to the diastolic potential. Action potentials are separated by phase 4, the diastolic potential, which is stable in nonpacemaker cells such as atrial and ventricular fibers. In pacemaker cells, the membrane spontaneously depolarizes during phase 4, with the fastest depolarization occurring in the sinoatrial node, an intermediate rate in the atrioventricular node, and the slowest in Purkinje fibers. The sinoatrial and atrioventricular nodes have relatively less negative resting potentials, slower upstrokes, smaller amplitudes, and more rapid phase 4 depolarizations than other cardiac cells. Since the sinoatrial node is the fastest pacemaker, it resets latent pacemaker cells in the atrioventricular node and Purkinje system before they reach threshold. The ECG is the body surface manifestation of the depolarization and repolarization waves of the heart. The P wave reflects atrial activation; the QRS complex reflects ventricular activation; and the T wave coincides with ventricular repolarization. Thus, the P–R interval is a measure of atrioventricular conduction time and the Q–T interval reflects the duration of the ventricular action potential.

sium equilibrium potential. For typical values of K_e (4 mM) and K_i (150 mM), the potassium equilibrium potential, E_K, is −96 mV. The resting potential of ventricular muscle cells is −85 to −95 mV. Small variations in K_e can markedly alter E_K and, therefore, resting E_m. For example, when extracellular K^+ concentration is 2 mM, E_K is −114 mV; for K_e equal to 8 mM, E_K is −77 mV. Thus, changes in extracellular potassium ion concentration have dramatic and predictable effects on resting potential in nonpacemaker cells.

The situation in pacemaker cells is more complex, because during diastole these cells have a gradually increasing ratio of sodium (or calcium) permeability to potassium permeability. As a result, the diastolic potential is closer to E_K at the beginning of diastole than at its end, and a typical diastolic pacemaker depolarization is recorded during phase 4. Changes in extracellular potassium concentration have an effect on phase 4 depolarization in these cells in addition to that predicted by the Nernst relationship described above. Decreasing extracellular potassium decreases potassium permeability by an unknown mechanism; as a result, the membrane potential is more easily displaced from E_K toward E_{Na}, and pacemaker rate is enhanced. Conversely, increasing extracellular potassium causes an increase in potassium permeability, thus stabilizing the membrane potential close to E_K, and pacemaker rate is reduced.

Changes in resting potential occur in response to normal variations in extracellular potassium and also result from a number of pathologic conditions. The effects of these changes are described below.

The Active Cell Membrane

Normal atrial, Purkinje, and ventricular cells have sodium-dependent action potentials. Depolarization to the threshold voltage results in extremely rapid opening of the activation *(m)* gates of sodium channels (Fig 12–2). If the inactivation *(h)* gates of these chan-

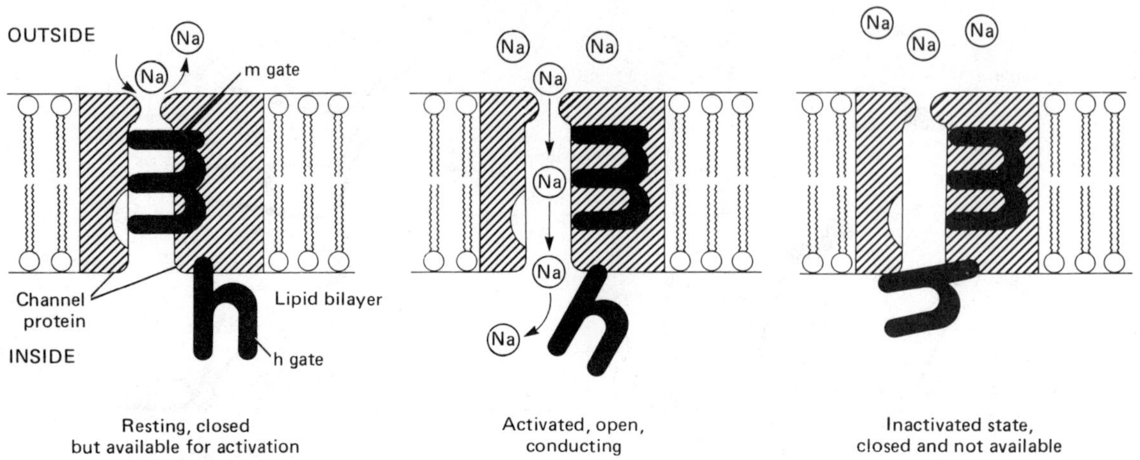

Figure 12–2. Schematic diagram of the cardiac sodium channel. The channel (shaded area) is a protein that spans the lipid bilayer membrane. In the resting, fully polarized membrane *(left),* the *h* gate is open and the *m* gate is closed, preventing any movement of sodium ions through the channel. With an appropriate stimulus, the *m* gate opens promptly, allowing a rapid influx of sodium ions *(middle).* After a few milliseconds, the more sluggish *h* gate closes, shutting off the sodium current *(right).* Additional stimuli applied to the inactivated channel cannot open it (the *m* gate is already open); therefore, it is "unavailable." The actual shapes of the channel and the gates are unknown, and those shown are purely symbolic. The light area at the lower left end of the channel is a possible location for a local anesthetic receptor.

nels have not already closed, the channels are now open or activated, and a very large increase in sodium permeability ensues. Sodium permeability now greatly exceeds permeability to any other ion. Extracellular sodium therefore diffuses down its electrochemical gradient, and the membrane potential approaches the sodium equilibrium potential, E_{Na} (about +50 mV when Na_e = 145 mM and Na_i = 20 mM). This intense sodium current is very brief, because depolarization, while opening the fast-moving *m* gates, also causes inactivation of sodium channels by closure of the slower *h* gates (Fig 12–2).

The depolarization caused by the sodium current produces phase 0 of the action potential (Fig 12–1) and leads to activation of calcium channels and, more slowly, of potassium channels. Calcium channels become activated and inactivated in what appears to be the same way as sodium channels, but in the case of calcium the transitions occur at more positive potentials and much more slowly. The plateau (phases 1 and 2) reflects the turning off of sodium current, the waxing and waning of calcium current, and the slow development of a repolarizing potassium current.

Final repolarization (phase 3) of the action potential results from completion of calcium channel inactivation and the growth of potassium permeability, so that the membrane potential once again approaches the potassium equilibrium potential.

The Effect of Resting Potential on Action Potentials

A key factor in the pathophysiology of arrhythmias and the actions of antiarrhythmia drugs is the relationship between the resting potential of a cell and the action potentials that can be evoked in it (Fig 12–3). Because the inactivation gates of sodium channels in the resting membrane close over the potential range –75 to –55 mV, fewer sodium channels are "available" for diffusion of sodium ions when an action potential is evoked from a resting potential of –60 mV than when it is evoked from a resting potential of –80 mV. Important consequences of the reduction in peak sodium permeability include reduced upstroke velocity (called $\dot{V}_{max}$, for maximum rate of change of membrane voltage), reduced action potential amplitude, reduced excitability, and reduced conduction velocity.

During the plateau of the action potential (phases 1 and 2), most sodium channels are inactivated. During the latter part of phase 3 and during the subsequent phase 4 resting potential, recovery from inactivation takes place (in the terminology of Fig 12–2, the *h* gates reopen), making the channels again available for excitation. Another important effect of less negative resting potential is prolongation of this recovery time, as shown in Fig 12–3. The prolongation of recovery time is reflected in an increase in the effective refractory period, ie, the time from the start of an action potential to the time when a second action potential can be evoked and propagated.

Reduction of the resting potential,* whether brought about by hyperkalemia, sodium pump block-

*The steady depolarization or reduction in resting potential referred to in this section should not be confused with the abrupt depolarization involved in a normal stimulus. A brief depolarizing stimulus, whether caused by a propagating action potential or by an external electrode arrangement, causes the opening of large numbers of activation gates, which are faster moving, before a significant number of inactivation gates can close.

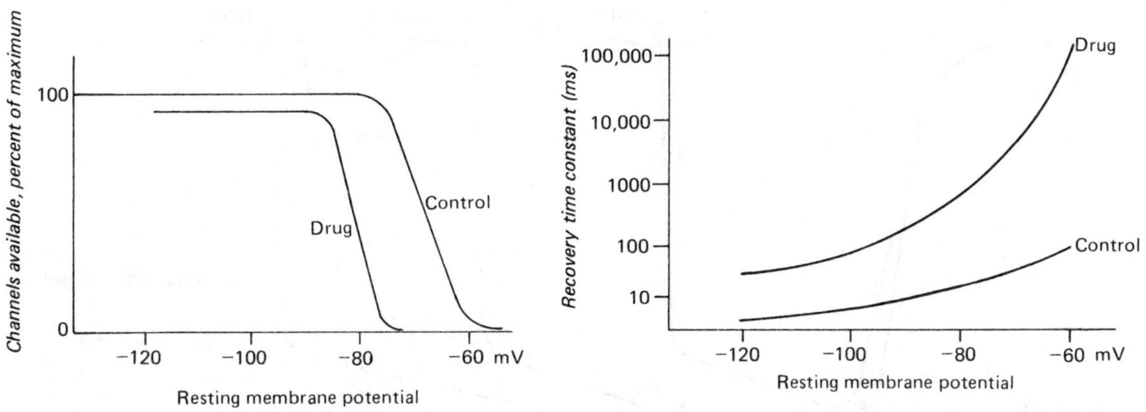

Figure 12–3. Dependence of sodium channel availability on membrane potential and time. As shown in the graph at *left,* the fraction of sodium channels "available" for opening in response to a stimulus is determined by the resting potential. The decrease in the fraction available when the resting potential is depolarized in the absence of drug (control curve) results from the closure of *h* gates in the channels. The shift in the curve illustrates the effect of a typical local anesthetic antiarrhythmia drug and may be caused by an interaction between the *h* gate and the drug molecule, or the drug may function like the *h* gate but at a more negative membrane potential. All sodium channels are inactivated during the plateau of the action potential. The time constant for recovery from inactivation after repolarization also depends on the resting potential. The graph at *right* shows that in the absence of drug, recovery occurs in less than 10 ms at normal resting potentials (–75 to –95 mV). Depolarized cells recover more slowly (note logarithmic scale). In the presence of sodium channel-blocking drugs, the time constant of recovery is increased, but the increase is far greater at depolarized potentials than at more negative ones.

ade, or ischemic cell damage, results in depressed sodium currents during the upstrokes of action potentials. Depolarization of the resting potential to levels positive to –55 mV abolishes sodium currents, since all sodium channels are inactivated. However, such severely depolarized cells have been found to support special action potentials under circumstances that increase calcium permeability or decrease potassium permeability. These "slow responses"—slow upstroke velocity and slow conduction—are important in some arrhythmias and probably constitute the normal electrical activity in the sinoatrial and atrioventricular nodes, since these tissues have a normal resting potential in the range of –50 to –70 mV.

MECHANISMS OF ARRHYTHMIAS

Many factors can precipitate or exacerbate arrhythmias: ischemia, hypoxia, acidosis or alkalosis, electrolyte abnormalities, excessive catecholamine exposure, autonomic influences, drug toxicity (eg, digitalis), overstretching of cardiac fibers, and the presence of scarred or otherwise diseased tissue. However, all arrhythmias result from (1) disturbances in impulse formation, (2) disturbances in impulse conduction, or (3) both.

Disturbances of Impulse Formation

The interval between depolarizations of a pacemaker cell is the sum of the duration of the action potential and the duration of the diastolic interval. Shortening of either duration results in an increase in pacemaker rate. The more important of the two, diastolic interval, is determined by 3 factors: maximum diastolic potential, slope of phase 4 depolarization, and threshold potential (Fig 12–4). Thus, vagal discharge slows pacemaker rate by making the maximum diastolic potential more negative and reducing the phase 4 slope; beta receptor-blocking drugs markedly reduce phase 4 slope. Acceleration of pacemaker discharge is often brought about by increased phase 4 depolarization slope, caused by hypokalemia, beta-adrenergic stimulation, fiber stretch, acidosis, and partial depolarization by currents of injury.

Latent pacemakers (cells that show slow phase 4 depolarization even under normal conditions, eg, some Purkinje fibers) are particularly prone to acceleration by the above mechanisms. However, all cardiac cells, including normally quiescent atrial and ventricular cells, may show repetitive pacemaker activity when depolarized under appropriate conditions, especially hypokalemia.

A special form of pacemakerlike activity results from digitalis toxicity (Chapter 11). Digitalis causes an increase in intracellular calcium, and this effect, if excessive, results in the triggering of oscillatory afterpotentials after each action potential (Fig 12–5). These oscillations (also called delayed afterdepolarizations) mimic phase 4 depolarization and can reach threshold, thereby evoking extrasystoles. In the severely intoxicated heart, the oscillation-extrasystole process becomes self-sustaining, and recordings show what appears to be a rapidly discharging ectopic pacemaker.

All pacemakers, normal and abnormal, are dependent upon phase 4 diastolic depolarization. Thus, for the reasons given above, hyperkalemia will tend to slow and hypokalemia to accelerate their rate of firing.

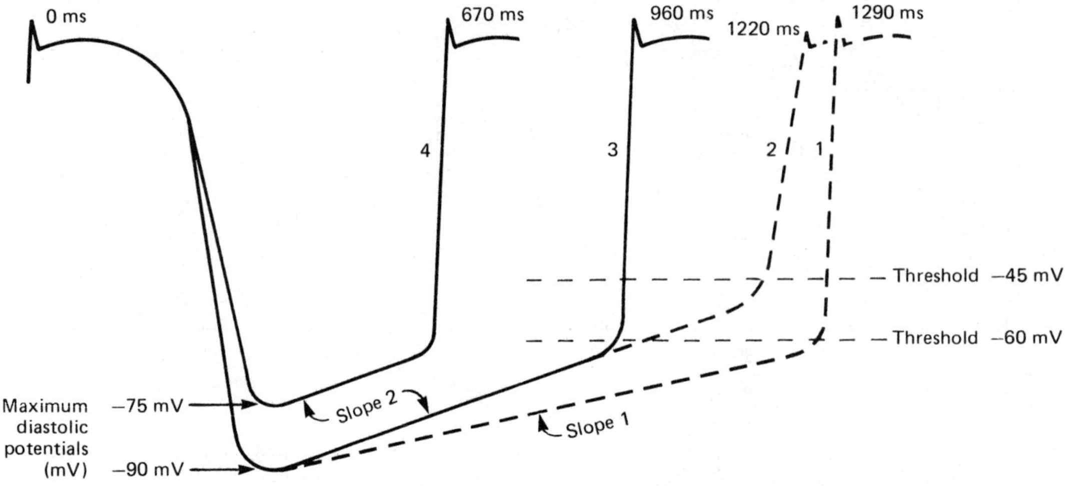

Figure 12–4. Determinants of pacemaker rate. The transmembrane potential from a Purkinje fiber pacemaker cell is shown schematically. The last action potential elicited by a normally conducted sinus impulse is shown at 0 ms, and the next sinus impulse originates 1000 ms later (not shown). An increase in phase 4 slope (from slope 1 to slope 2) would permit the cell to reach threshold and fire spontaneously as the action potential labeled 3. If there were also a depolarization of the maximum diastolic potential from –90 mV to –75 mV, the cell would reach threshold even sooner and fire spontaneously as action potential 4. Both changes would convert the cell from a latent to an overt pacemaker. Conversely, a change in threshold potential from –60 mV to –45 mV would delay the upstroke from 960 ms to 1220 ms and prevent this cell from becoming an overt pacemaker.

Disturbances of Impulse Conduction

Severely depressed conduction may result in several easily recognized arrhythmias, eg, atrioventricular nodal block, bundle branch block. A more subtle and more common abnormality of conduction is **reentry,** in which one impulse reenters and excites the heart more than once (Fig 12–6). In order for reentry to occur, 3 conditions must coexist: (1) There must be an obstacle (anatomic or physiologic) to homogeneous conduction, thus establishing a circuit around which the reentrant wavefront can propagate. (2) There must be unidirectional block at some point in the circuit. (3)

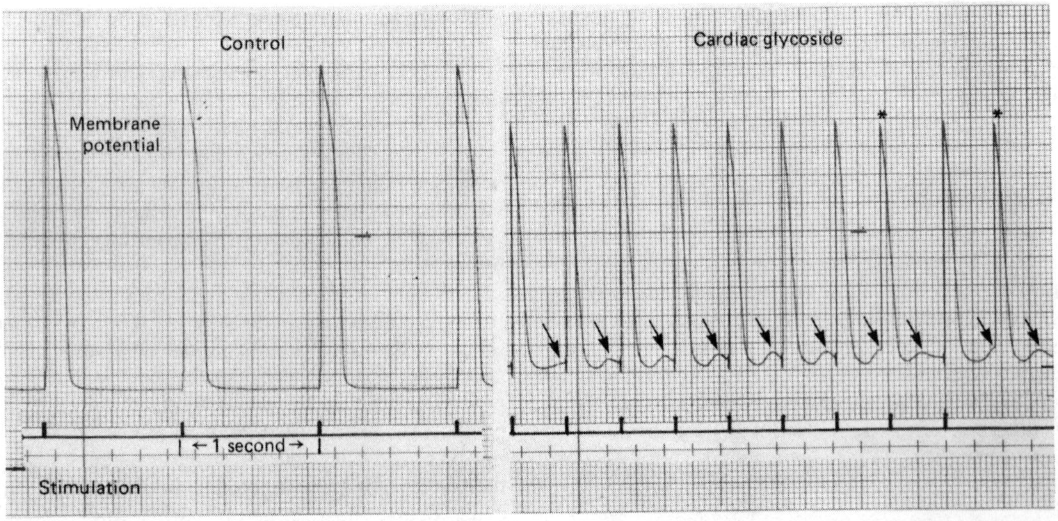

Figure 12–5. Induction of arrhythmia by a cardiac glycoside. The *left* side of the figure shows normal transmembrane action potentials in isolated cardiac muscle, produced by regular stimulation (lower tracing shows stimuli). After exposure to a toxic concentration of acetylstrophanthidin (*right* side), small oscillatory afterpotentials (arrows) occur after each action potential. Occasionally, such afterpotentials reach threshold during the regular sequence of stimuli and trigger an early action potential (first asterisk). Note that this action potential precedes the stimulus artifact (bottom tracing). After a pause in the regular driving stimulation, a second "extrasystole" (second asterisk) is evoked by an oscillatory afterpotential.

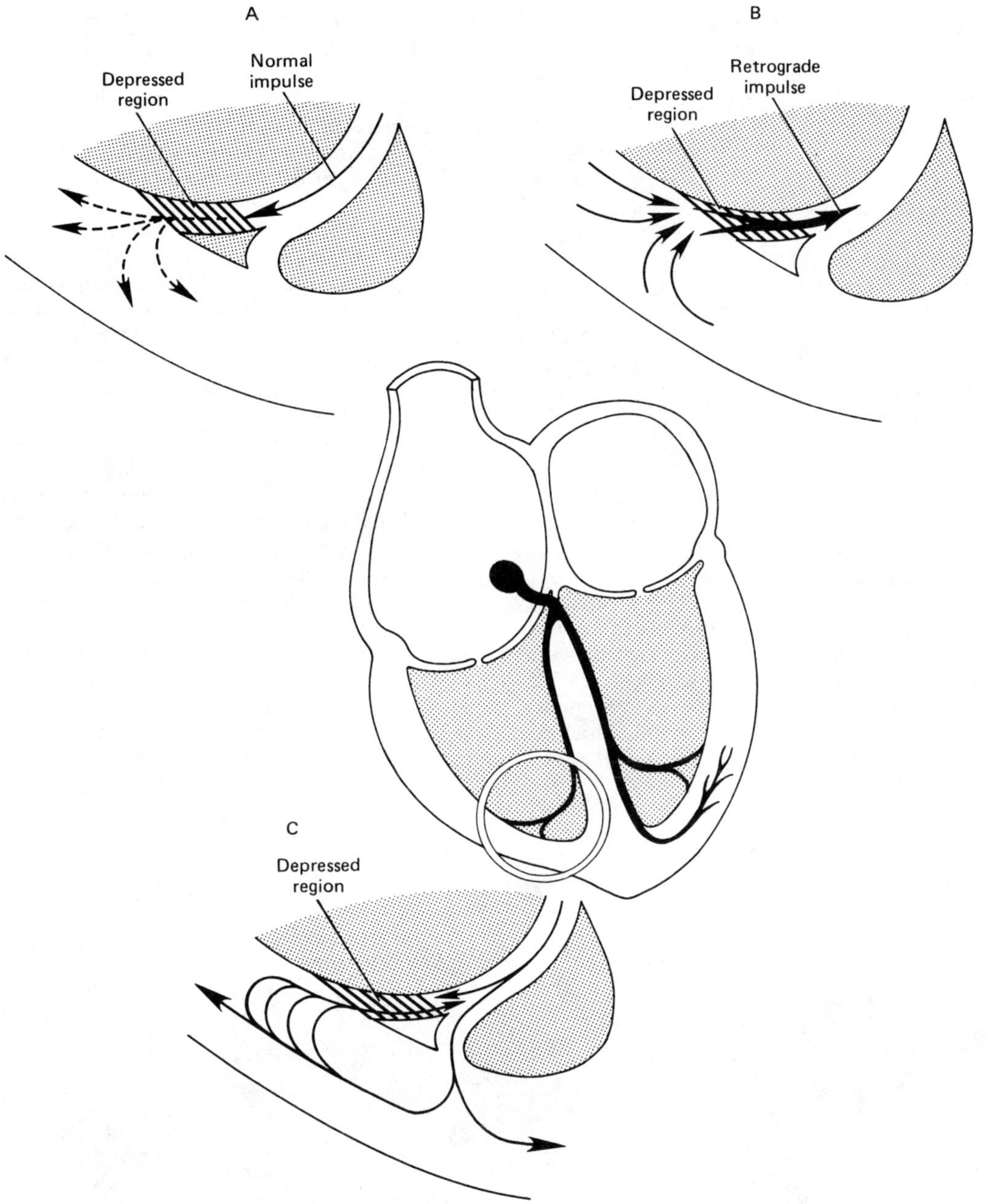

Figure 12–6. Unidirectional block and reentry. In panels *A* and *B*, a small free-running Purkinje fiber strand is shown traversing the ventricular cavity and entering a segment of the ventricular wall. Under normal circumstances, impulses can be conducted bidirectionally at the Purkinje-ventricular junction. However, under pathologic conditions, propagation of impulses may be blocked in one direction (unidirectional block). For example, if the terminal portion of the Purkinje strand is depolarized by excessive stretch (stippled area), the few depressed Purkinje cells (small current *source*) dilute their energy in a large number of healthy ventricular cells (large current *sink*) and may not be able to raise the ventricular membrane potential to threshold (panel *A*). In contrast, if the ventricle is excited first, a large number of healthy cells (large current source) may provide enough energy to excite Purkinje cells and conduct across the depressed area (panel *B*). This constitutes one of several ways by which unidirectional block may arise (panel *C*). If an area showing unidirectional block is part of a pathway around an obstacle, eg, part of the blood-filled ventricular cavity, an impulse traveling in the normal direction will not propagate but may approach the depressed segment from the ventricular side. As described above, the retrograde impulse may be propagated if the impulse conducts across the lesion (and if the conduction time is longer than the effective refractory period). The retrograde impulse will then reexcite tissue it had previously passed through, and a reentry arrhythmia will be established.

Conduction time around the circuit must be long enough so that the impulse does not enter refractory tissue as it travels around the obstacle—ie, the conduction time must exceed the effective refractory period.

Thus, reentry depends upon critically depressed conduction. If conduction is not sufficiently depressed, bidirectional conduction rather than unidirectional block will occur. In addition, even in the presence of unidirectional block, if the impulse travels around the obstacle too rapidly, it will enter tissue that is still refractory. If conduction is too depressed, bidirectional block rather than unidirectional block occurs; if the retrograde impulse is too weak, conduction may fail, or the impulse may arrive so late that it collides with the next regular impulse. Critically depressed conduction may be due to a depressed sodium current, a slow calcium current, or both. Drugs can abolish reentry either by improving critically depressed conduction (increasing the sodium or calcium current) or by further depressing it (blocking the sodium or calcium current).

Lengthening or shortening of the refractory period relative to a median value may also make reentry less likely. The longer the refractory period in tissue near the block, the greater the chance that the tissue will still be refractory when reentry is attempted. The shorter the refractory period near the block, the less likely it is that unidirectional block will occur.

I. BASIC PHARMACOLOGY OF THE ANTIARRHYTHMIA DRUGS

Mechanisms of Action

Arrhythmias are caused by abnormal pacemaker activity or abnormal impulse propagation. Thus, the aim of antiarrhythmia therapy is to reduce pacemaker activity and modify critically impaired conduction. The latter objective may involve improving conduction in the depressed region or suppressing it altogether. The major mechanisms for accomplishing these goals are (1) sodium channel blockade, (2) calcium channel blockade, (3) prolongation of the effective refractory period, and (4) blockade of sympathetic autonomic effects in the heart.

Antiarrhythmia drugs decrease automaticity, conduction, and excitability and increase the refractory period to a greater extent in depolarized tissue than in normally polarized tissue. This is accomplished chiefly by selectively blocking the sodium or calcium channels of depolarized cells (Fig 12–7). Therapeutically useful channel blocking drugs have a high affinity for open channels (ie, during phase 0) or inactivated channels (ie, during phase 2) but very low affinity for rested channels. Therefore, these drugs block electrical activity when there is a fast tachycardia (many channel openings per unit time) or if there is significant loss of resting potential (many inactivated channels).

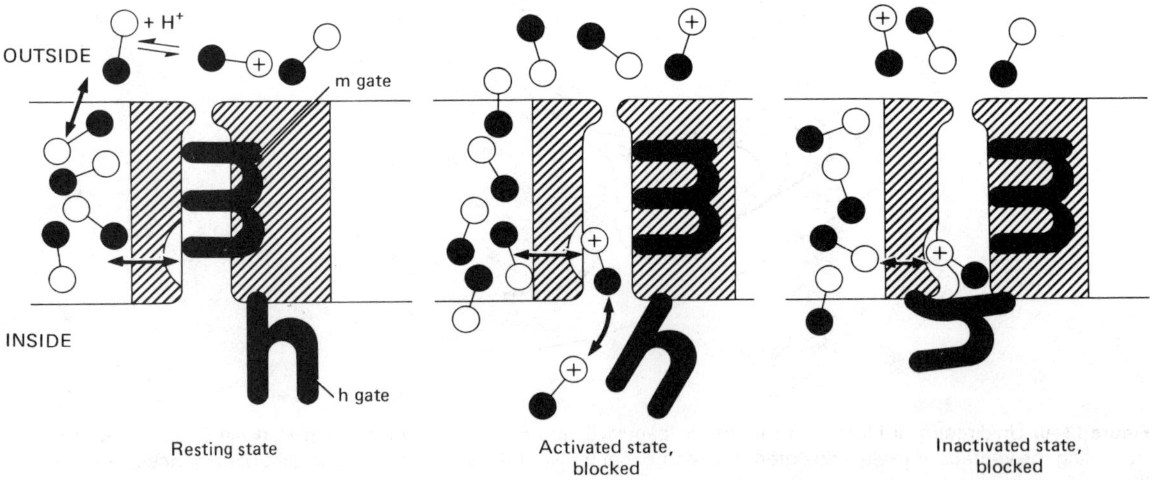

Figure 12–7. Interaction of antiarrhythmia drugs with the cardiac sodium channel. The diagram reproduces the schematic channel model shown in Fig 12–2. Local anesthetic antiarrhythmia molecules in solution in the extracellular fluid are divided into 2 forms: unchanged (lipid-soluble) and positively charged (less lipid-soluble) according to the pH and their pKas. Although the lipid membrane dissolves a large amount of uncharged drug, the drug cannot easily bind to the receptor site when the channel is in the rested state. The dissociation constant is very large. However, when the channel is open (*middle*, *m* gate withdrawn), drug molecules can reach the receptor site either from the lipid membrane side or from the intracellular space. The dissociation constant is now (for most antiarrhythmia drugs) relatively small. When drug is bound to the receptor, sodium ions cannot pass through the channel. When the channel is inactivated (*right*, *h* gate closed), drug molecules can still reach the receptor site, but only from the lipid membrane phase; access from the intracellular compartment is blocked. There may be some interaction between the *h* gate and drug that is bound to the receptor. The dissociation constant for this drug-receptor combination in the inactivated channel may be extremely small for certain drugs, eg, amiodarone.

Channels in normal cells that become blocked by a drug during normal activation-inactivation cycles will rapidly lose the drug from the receptors during the resting portion of the cycle. Channels in myocardium that is chronically depolarized, ie, has a resting potential less than −70 mV, will recover from block very slowly if at all.

In cells with abnormal automaticity, most of these drugs reduce the phase 4 slope (Fig 12–4) by blocking either sodium or calcium channels and thereby reducing the ratio of sodium (or calcium) permeability to potassium permeability. In addition, some agents may increase the threshold (make it more positive). Adrenergic receptor-blocking drugs indirectly reduce the phase 4 slope by blocking the positive chronotropic action of norepinephrine in the heart.

In critically depressed conduction with reentry, most of the antiarrhythmia agents slow conduction further by one or both of 2 mechanisms: (1) steady-state reduction in the number of available unblocked channels, which reduces the size of the action potential to a level below that required for propagation (Fig 12–3, left); and (2) prolongation of recovery time of the channels still able to reach the rested and available state, which increases the effective refractory period (Fig 12–3, right). As a result, early extrasystoles are unable to propagate at all; later impulses propagate more slowly and are subject to bidirectional conduction block. Several agents prolong the duration of the cardiac action potential, possibly through blockade of potassium channels. Such prolongation is usually directly reflected in an increase in effective refractory period, with the same beneficial results described above.

In one special case, reentry may result from *latent* pacemaker activity, especially in Purkinje fibers. Because phase 4 depolarization in latent pacemakers results in a less negative take-off potential for any subsequent action potential, the availability of sodium channels for the upstroke of that action potential may be reduced. As illustrated by the relationship in Fig 12–3 (left), this reduction in channel availability is very rapid in the potential range of −70 to −60 mV, and conduction velocity will be similarly reduced. This reduction may be sufficient to cause unidirectional block. Antiarrhythmia drugs can therefore (at least theoretically) *increase* conduction velocity in latent pacemaker cells by reduction of phase 4 depolarization in latent pacemaker cells.

By these mechanisms, antiarrhythmia drugs can suppress abnormal automaticity and conduction occurring in depolarized cells—rendering them electrically silent—while minimally affecting the electrical activity in normally polarized parts of the heart. However, as dosage is increased, these agents will also depress conduction in normal tissue, eventually resulting in *drug-induced* arrhythmias.

As noted above, extracellular potassium modulates the resting transmembrane potential. Therefore, hyperkalemia, by depolarizing the membrane and inactivating more channels, increases the depressant effects of antiarrhythmia drugs. When antiarrhythmia drug toxicity occurs, reduction of extracellular potassium levels (eg, by elevation of serum pH) may reverse the toxicity by hyperpolarizing the myocardium. This approach should only be considered if serum potassium is normal or high, since hypokalemia may also cause arrhythmias.

SPECIFIC ANTIARRHYTHMIA DRUGS

The antiarrhythmia agents can be divided into 4 distinct subgroups on the basis of mechanism of action: (1) Sodium channel blockers, all of which behave like local anesthetics. (In fact, the most popular parenteral antiarrhythmia drug, lidocaine, is also the most popular local anesthetic.) This is by far the most important group of antiarrhythmia drugs. (2) Calcium channel blockers, which seem to have some features in common with the local anesthetic group. (3) Drugs that prolong effective refractory period by some mechanism other than (or in addition to) blockade of sodium channels. (4) Drugs that reduce adrenergic activity in the heart.

Sodium Channel–Blocking Drugs

QUINIDINE

Although quinine was used sporadically as an antiarrhythmia drug during the 18th and 19th centuries, it was not until the early years of the 20th century that this isomer of quinine came into wide use. Quinidine is the most commonly used oral antiarrhythmia agent.

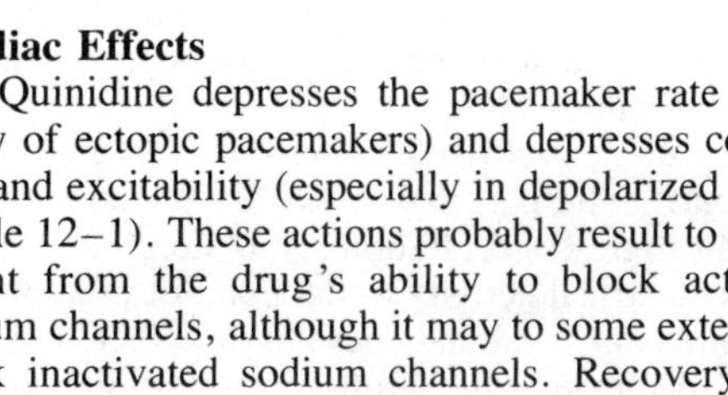

Quinidine

Cardiac Effects

Quinidine depresses the pacemaker rate (especially of ectopic pacemakers) and depresses conduction and excitability (especially in depolarized tissue) (Table 12–1). These actions probably result to a large extent from the drug's ability to block activated sodium channels, although it may to some extent also block inactivated sodium channels. Recovery from block proceeds more slowly in depolarized channels than in fully polarized channels. Thus, quinidine lengthens the refractory period and depresses excitabil-

Table 12–1. Membrane actions of antiarrhythmia drugs.

Drug	Block of Sodium Channels		Refractory Period		Calcium Channel Blockade	Effect on Pacemaker Activity	Adrenergic Blocking Action
	Normal Cells	Depolarized Cells	Normal Cells	Depolarized Cells			
Quinidine (many trade names)	+	++	↑	↑↑	0	↓↓	+
Procainamide (Pronestyl, others)	+	+++	↑	↑↑↑	0	↓	++
Disopyramide (Norpace)	+	+++	↑	↑↑	0	↓↓	0
Aprindine (investigational)	+	+++	0	↑↑	0	↓↓	0
Amiodarone (investigational)	+	+++	↑↑	↑↑↑	+	↓↓	+
Lidocaine (Xylocaine)	0	+++	↓	↑↑	0	↓↓	0
Tocainide (investigational)	0	+++	0	↑↑	0	↓↓	0
Mexiletine (investigational)	0	+++	0	↑↑	0	↓↓	0
Phenytoin (Dilantin)	0	+	↓	↑	+	↓	+
Verapamil (Calan, Isoptin)	0	+	0	↑↑	+++	↓↓	+
Propranolol (Inderal)	0	+	↓	↑↑	0	↓↓	+++
Bretylium (Bretylol)	0	0	↑↑↑	↑↑↑	0	↑↓*	++

*Bretylium may transiently increase pacemaker rate by causing catecholamine release.

ity and conduction in depolarized tissue more than in normal tissue.

Quinidine also lengthens the action potential duration, which is reflected in the ECG as a lengthening of the Q–T interval. Blockade of potassium channels with a reduction in repolarizing outward current may be responsible for this effect. It should be noted that lengthening of the action potential duration reduces the time spent at negative membrane potentials and will by itself therefore enhance the sodium-blocking efficacy of quinidine. This lengthening of the action potential duration and effective refractory period reduces the maximum reentry frequency.

Cardiac Toxicity

Quinidine has antimuscarinic actions in the heart that inhibit vagal effects. This can overcome its direct membrane effect and lead to increased sinus rate and increased atrioventricular conduction. In the presence of atrial fibrillation or flutter, the latter may result in an excessively high ventricular rate. However, this can be prevented by prior administration of digitalis (see Chapter 11).

A small percentage of patients given quinidine develop a syndrome called quinidine syncope, characterized by recurrent light-headedness and episodes of fainting. The symptoms are a result of a drug-induced rapid, disorganized ventricular tachycardia, resembling ventricular fibrillation, which usually terminates spontaneously but may recur incessantly or become sustained. It is associated with a striking prolongation of the Q–T interval.

In patients with sick sinus syndrome, quinidine may depress the pacemaker activity of the sinoatrial node. In toxic concentrations, this drug can depress cardiac electrical activity to the point of precipitating arrhythmias or asystole. These toxic effects are more likely to occur when the serum concentrations exceed 5 μg/mL and in the presence of high serum potassium levels (> 5 mEq/L). Widening of the QRS duration by 30% by quinidine administration is usually considered premonitory of serious toxicity. Toxic concentrations may depress contractility and lower blood pressure.

Extracardiac Effects

Quinidine possesses alpha-adrenergic receptor-blocking properties that can cause vasodilatation and a reflex increase in sinoatrial nodal rate. These effects are most prominent after intravenous administration (see below). Quinidine also has antimalarial, antipyretic, and oxytocic properties.

Extracardiac Toxicity

The most common side-effects are gastrointestinal: diarrhea, nausea and vomiting. The drug can also cause cinchonism (headache, dizziness, tinnitus). Rarely, quinidine can cause rashes, angioneurotic edema, fever, hepatitis, and thrombocytopenia. Quinidine increases digoxin plasma levels and may precipitate digitalis toxicity in patients taking that drug (see Chapter 11).

Pharmacokinetics & Dosage

Quinidine is usually administered orally and is rapidly absorbed from the gastrointestinal tract. It is 80% bound to plasma proteins. Quinidine is hydroxylated in the liver, but 20% is excreted unchanged in the urine. Its half-life is about 6 hours (Table 12–2) and may be longer in patients with congestive heart failure or hepatic or renal disease. Urinary excretion is enhanced in acid urine. Quinidine is usually administered orally as the sulfate, gluconate, or polygalacturonate salt. A test dose of 0.2 g is recommended to detect idiosyncrasies, and 0.2–0.6 g is then given 4–6 times daily. The therapeutic concentration in plasma is 3–5 μg/mL.

Parenteral administration of quinidine is occasionally necessary. Quinidine is absorbed after intramuscular injection of the sulfate in oil or the aqueous gluconate preparation. Intravenous administration of quinidine can be carried out successfully if proper precautions are observed. The intravenous dose should

Table 12–2. Clinical pharmacologic properties of antiarrhythmia drugs.

Drug	Effect on SA Nodal Rate	Effect on AV Nodal Refractory Period	Usefulness in Arrhythmias		Half-Life (hours)
			Supra-ventricular	Ventricular	
Quinidine (many trade names)	↑↓*	↑↓*	++	+++	6
Procainamide (Pronestyl, others)	↑↓*	↑↓*	++	+++	4
Disopyramide (Norpace)	↑↓*	↑↓*	++	+++	5
Aprindine (investigational)	↓	↑	++	+++	12
Amiodarone (investigational)	↓↓	↑↑	+++	+++	(weeks)
Lidocaine (Xylocaine)	None	None	None†	+++	1
Tocainide (investigational)	None	None	None†	+++	12
Mexiletine (investigational)	None	None	None†	+++	12
Phenytoin (Dilantin)	None	None	None†	+	24
Verapamil (Calan, Isoptin)	↑↓	↑↑	+++	+	6
Propranolol (Inderal)	↓↓	↑↑	++	++	8
Bretylium (Bretylol)	↑↓‡	↑↓‡	0	++	4

*Direct depressant action partly counteracted by anticholinergic effect.
†May be effective in atrial arrhythmias caused by digitalis.
‡Initial stimulation by release of endogenous norepinephrine followed by depression.

not exceed 10 mg/kg of quinidine gluconate and should not be given at a rate exceeding 0.5 mg/min. Intravenous administration of quinidine is usually associated with a decline in blood pressure as a result of its peripheral vasodilating action. Thus, when intravenous quinidine is used, blood pressure should be carefully monitored and supported when necessary with intravenous fluids.

Therapeutic Use

Quinidine is the most frequently prescribed oral antiarrhythmia agent. It has been found effective in nearly every form of arrhythmia: premature atrial contractions, paroxysmal atrial fibrillation and flutter, intra-atrial and atrioventricular nodal reentrant arrhythmias, Wolff-Parkinson-White tachycardias, premature ventricular contractions, and ventricular tachycardias.

PROCAINAMIDE

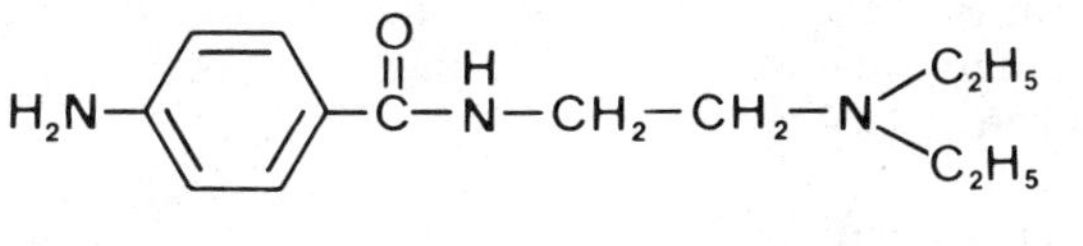

Procainamide

Cardiac Effects

The electrophysiologic effects of procainamide are similar to those of quinidine. It may be somewhat less effective in suppressing abnormal ectopic pacemaker activity but more effective in blocking sodium channels in depolarized cells.

Perhaps the most important difference between quinidine and procainamide is the less prominent anticholinergic action of procainamide. Therefore, the directly depressant actions of procainamide on sinoatrial and atrioventricular nodes are not as effectively counterbalanced by drug-induced vagolysis as in the case of quinidine. Procainamide also has ganglionic blocking properties and thus more potent negative inotropic effects than quinidine. In patients with preexisting ventricular dysfunction, procainamide may induce severe congestive heart failure.

Cardiac Toxicity

Procainamide's cardiotoxic effects are similar to those of quinidine. It is more likely than quinidine to produce severe or irreversible heart failure in toxic doses.

Extracardiac Effects

The ganglionic blocking effects of procainamide reduce peripheral vascular resistance and can cause hypotension. However, in therapeutic concentrations, its peripheral vascular effects are less prominent than those of quinidine. Hypotension is usually only seen during excessively rapid procainamide infusion.

Extracardiac Toxicity

The most troublesome side-effect of procainamide is a syndrome resembling lupus erythematosus and usually consisting of arthralgia and arthritis. In some patients, pleuritis, pericarditis, or parenchymal pulmonary disease also occur. Renal lupus is rarely induced by procainamide. During long-term therapy, serologic abnormalities (eg, increased antinuclear antibody titer) occur in nearly all patients. Approximately one-third of patients receiving long-term procainamide therapy develop lupus-related symptoms.

Other side-effects include nausea and diarrhea (about 10% of cases), rash, fever, hepatitis (less than 5%), and agranulocytosis (less than 0.1%).

Pharmacokinetics & Dosage

Procainamide can be administered safely by the

intravenous and intramuscular routes and is well absorbed orally, with 75% systemic bioavailability. It is metabolized to N-acetylprocainamide. The metabolic product has antiarrhythmia activity, but some patients respond differently to the 2 substances. Either or both may be the therapeutic form in a given patient. A few individuals rapidly acetylate procainamide and develop high levels of N-acetylprocainamide.

Procainamide's half-life is only 3–4 hours, which necessitates frequent dosing. Both procainamide and N-acetylprocainamide are eliminated chiefly by the kidneys. Thus, dosage must be reduced in patients with renal failure. The reduced volume of distribution and renal clearance associated with congestive heart failure also require reduction in dosage. The half-life of N-acetylprocainamide is considerably longer than that of procainamide, and it therefore accumulates more readily. Thus, it is important to measure plasma levels of both procainamide and N-acetylprocainamide, especially in patients with circulatory or renal impairment.

If rapid effect is needed, an intravenous loading dose of up to 12 mg/kg can be given safely at a rate of 0.4 mg/kg/min or less. This dose is followed by a maintenance dose of 2–5 mg/min, with careful monitoring of plasma levels.

Oral procainamide is frequently used improperly. If around-the-clock antiarrhythmia activity is required, the drug should be administered every 3 or 4 hours. In order to control ventricular arrhythmias, a total dose of 2–5 g daily is usually required. In an occasional patient who accumulates high levels of N-acetylprocainamide and in whom that compound is active, less frequent dosing may be possible.

Therapeutic Use

Like quinidine, procainamide is effective against most atrial and ventricular arrhythmias. However, many clinicians attempt to avoid long-term therapy because of the frequent dosing requirement and the common occurrence of lupus-related effects. Procainamide is the drug of second choice (after lidocaine) in most coronary care units for the treatment of ventricular arrhythmias associated with acute myocardial infarction.

DISOPYRAMIDE

Disopyramide phosphate is a relatively new drug closely related to an agent long used for its anticholinergic properties (isopropamide).

Cardiac Effects

The electrophysiologic effects of disopyramide are nearly indistinguishable from those of quinidine. Its cardiac anticholinergic effects are even more marked than those of quinidine. Therefore, digoxin should be administered with disopyramide in the treatment of atrial flutter or fibrillation.

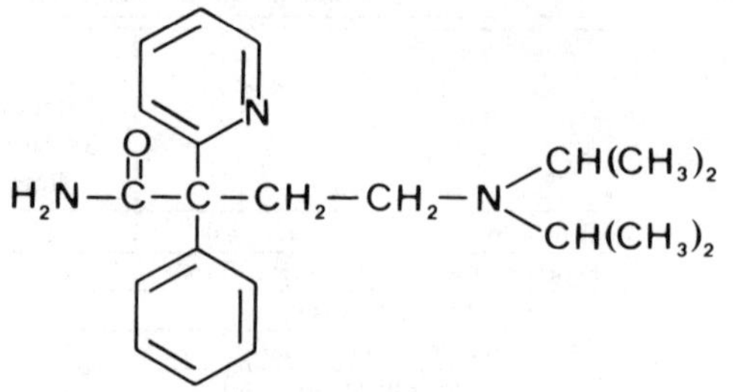

Disopyramide

Cardiac Toxicity

Toxic concentrations of disopyramide can precipitate all of the electrophysiologic disturbances described under quinidine. In addition, disopyramide's negative inotropic actions are frequently troublesome in patients with preexisting left ventricular dysfunction. Moreover, in rare instances, it may produce heart failure in subjects without prior myocardial dysfunction. Because of this adverse effect, disopyramide is not a first-line antiarrhythmia agent. It must be used with great caution in patients with congestive heart failure.

Extracardiac Effects & Toxicity

Disopyramide's anticholinergic activity accounts for most of its symptomatic side-effects: urinary retention in male patients with prostate hypertrophy, dry mouth, blurred vision, constipation, and worsening of preexisting glaucoma. These side-effects may require discontinuation of the drug.

Pharmacokinetics & Dosage

In the USA, disopyramide is only available for oral use. Bioavailability is about 50%. The drug is extensively protein-bound, but the extent of binding is variable and decreases with increasing dosage. As a result, measurements of plasma level are difficult to interpret. The drug is excreted by the kidneys and has a half-life of approximately 6–8 hours. The usual oral dose of disopyramide is 150 mg 3 times a day, but as much as 1 g daily may be required. In patients with renal impairment, this schedule must be reduced. Because of the danger of precipitating congestive heart failure, the use of large loading doses is not recommended.

Therapeutic Use

Although disopyramide has been shown to be effective in a variety of supraventricular arrhythmias, in the USA it is only approved for the treatment of ventricular arrhythmias. It is most commonly used when quinidine and procainamide have been poorly tolerated or ineffective.

APRINDINE

Aprindine is a sodium channel-blocking drug that resembles quinidine and disopyramide in its spectrum of action (Table 12–1) but has a higher affinity for inactivated sodium channels and a longer half-life.

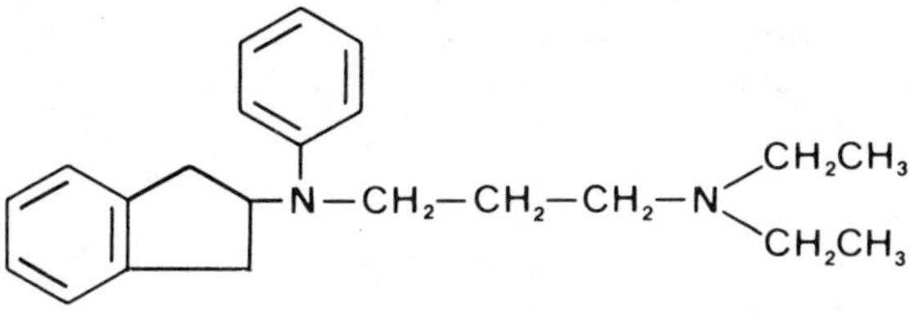

Aprindine

Aprindine is effective against a variety of ventricular and supraventricular arrhythmias. It is still in the clinical investigation stage of development in the USA. A therapeutic level (1–2 μg/mL) can be achieved by oral administration of 100–150 mg/d. In plasma concentrations above 2 μg/mL, it causes ataxia and other neurologic side-effects. Unfortunately, aprindine has also been implicated as a cause of agranulocytosis in as many as 1% of patients taking the drug for prolonged periods.

AMIODARONE

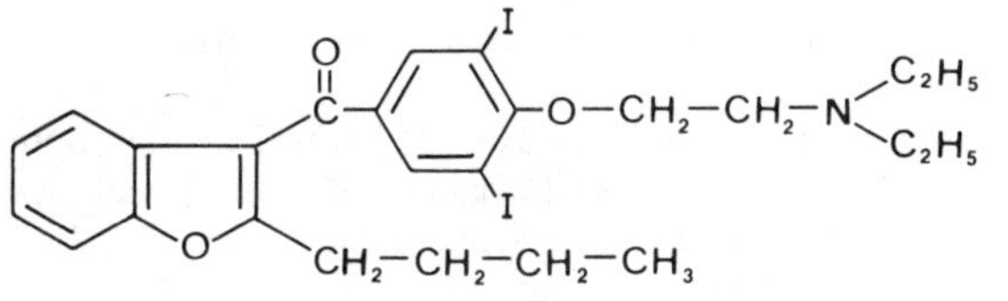

Amiodarone

Amiodarone has been widely used as an antiarrhythmia and antiangina agent in Europe but has only recently entered into clinical trials in the USA. It is very effective against a wide variety of arrhythmias, buut its prominent side-effects and unusual pharmacokinetics limit its use.

Cardiac Effects

Amiodarone has a broad spectrum of actions on the heart. It is a very effective blocker of sodium channels, but unlike quinidine it has a low affinity for activated channels, combining instead almost exclusively with channels in the inactivated state. Thus, the sodium-blocking action of amiodarone is most pronounced in tissues that have long action potentials, frequent action potentials, or less negative diastolic potentials. In therapeutic concentrations, amiodarone also markedly lengthens action potential duration by an unknown mechanism, perhaps involving blockade of potassium channels. Amiodarone is a weak calcium channel blocker as well as an inhibitor of beta-adrenergic receptors. Perhaps as a result of this combination of potentially antiarrhythmic effects, the drug can also be shown to be a powerful inhibitor of abnormal automaticity.

Amiodarone slows the sinus rate and atrioventricular conduction, markedly prolongs the Q–T interval, and slightly prolongs QRS duration. It increases atrial, atrioventricular nodal, and ventricular refractory periods. Induction of new ventricular arrhythmias or worsening of preexisting ones only rarely occurs during therapy with amiodarone. In patients with Wolff-Parkinson-White syndrome, the drug delays conduction, prolongs the effective refractory period, and may even totally abolish transmission through the accessory pathways.

Amiodarone also has antiangina effects. This may result from its weak noncompetitive alpha- and beta-adrenergic blocking properties as well as from its apparent ability to block calcium influx in coronary arterial smooth muscle.

Cardiac Toxicity

In patients with sinus or atrioventricular nodal disease, amiodarone may produce symptomatic bradycardia or heart block. It may also precipitate heart failure in susceptible patients.

Extracardiac Effects

Amiodarone causes peripheral vascular dilatation, presumably through its alpha-adrenergic blocking and calcium channel-inhibiting effects. In some patients, this may be beneficial; rarely, it may require discontinuation of the drug.

Extracardiac Toxicity

Amiodarone causes a remarkable variety of extracardiac side-effects. Few patients treated with 300 mg or less per day develop significant side-effects, but over one-third of patients receiving 1 g daily develop troublesome side-effects.

Amiodarone is deposited as microcrystals in tissue and can be found in virtually every organ. The most readily detected deposits are those in the cornea, which can be observed as yellowish-brown granules within a few weeks following initiation of therapy. These corneal deposits rarely cause visual symptoms except for an occasional halo in the peripheral visual fields, most prominent at night. Only infrequently does reduction of visual acuity occur that requires discontinuation or reduction of amiodarone dosage. Skin deposits of microcrystals can result in photodermatitis in about 25% of patients, requiring avoidance of sun exposure. In fewer than 1% of patients, a grayish-blue skin discoloration develops.

Thyroid dysfunction—both hypo- and hyperthyroidism—is the next most common side-effect (about 5% of patients). Thyroid function should be assessed prior to and throughout the duration of therapy with amiodarone.

Neurologic side-effects are unusual (< 5%) in low dosages but become very common (30–50%) in dosages above 600 mg/d. These effects include paresthesias, tremor, ataxia, and headaches.

In rare instances (< 1%), amiodarone may affect the gastrointestinal tract (eg, constipation), liver (eg, hepatocellular necrosis), or lung (eg, inflammation and fibrosis). Fatal lung fibrosis has been reported in 2 cases.

Despite this long list of adverse effects, amiodarone is a promising antiarrhythmia drug. Most of its common adverse effects resolve after discontinuation of therapy.

Pharmacokinetics & Dosage

Amiodarone has an extremely long half-life (a month or more). The effective plasma concentration is approximately 1 μg/mL, while the cardiac tissue concentration is about 30 times higher. It takes 15–30 days to load the body stores with sufficient amiodarone to estimate the drug's efficacy. Loading doses of 0.8–1.2 g daily for 2–4 weeks are used, after which the patient is maintained on 0.2–1 g daily. Because of the drug's long half-life, once-daily dosage is adequate.

Therapeutic Use

Amiodarone is very effective against both supraventricular and ventricular arrhythmias. In general, relatively low dosages (200–400 mg/d) can be used against paroxysmal atrial fibrillation and the circus movement associated with Wolff-Parkinson-White syndrome. Amiodarone appears to be especially effective against supraventricular arrhythmias in children. Furthermore, fewer side-effects are observed in pediatric patients than in adults.

LIDOCAINE

Lidocaine is the antiarrhythmia drug most commonly used by the intravenous route. It has an unusually low incidence of toxicity and a high degree of effectiveness in arrhythmia associated with acute myocardial infarction.

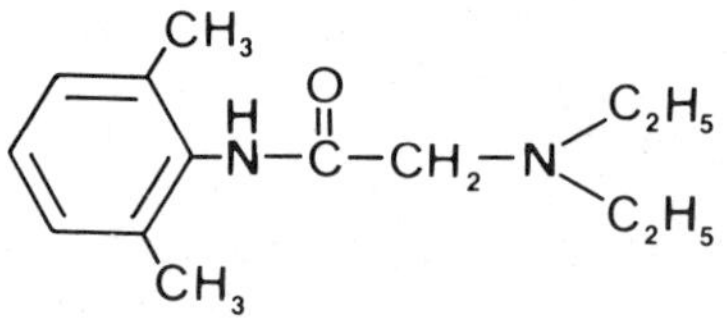

Lidocaine

Cardiac Effects

Lidocaine is a potent suppressor of abnormal cardiac activity, yet it appears to act exclusively on the sodium channel. Its interaction with this channel differs substantially from that of quinidine. Whereas quinidine mostly blocks sodium channels in the open state, lidocaine blocks primarily inactivated sodium channels. As a result, a large fraction (about 50%) of the unblocked sodium channels become blocked during each action potential plateau. During diastole, most of the sodium channels in normally polarized cells become drug-free. Since lidocaine usually shortens the action potential duration, diastole may be prolonged, thereby extending the time available for recovery. As a result, lidocaine has few electrophysiologic effects in *normal* cardiac tissue. In contrast, depolarized (inactivated) sodium channels remain largely blocked during diastole or actually become further blocked. Thus, lidocaine suppresses the electrical activity of the depolarized, arrhythmogenic tissues while minimally interfering with the electrical activity of normal tissues. These factors appear to be responsible for the fact that lidocaine is a very effective agent for suppressing arrhythmias associated with depolarization (eg, ischemia, digitalis toxicity), but it is relatively ineffective against arrhythmias occurring in normally polarized tissues (atrial flutter and fibrillation).

Cardiac Toxicity

Lidocaine is the least cardiotoxic of the currently used antiarrhythmia drugs. The drug exacerbates ventricular arrhythmias in fewer than 10% of patients (a good record). However, in diseased hearts, lidocaine does occasionally precipitate sinoatrial node standstill, change atrioventricular nodal block, or worsen impaired conduction (< 1%).

In large doses, especially in patients with preexisting heart failure, lidocaine may cause hypotension—partly by depressing myocardial contractility.

Extracardiac Toxicity

Lidocaine's most common side-effects—like those of other local anesthetics—are neurologic: paresthesias, tremor, nausea of central origin, lightheadedness, hearing disturbances, slurred speech, and convulsions. Convulsions occur mostly in elderly or otherwise vulnerable patients and are dose-related, usually short-lived, and respond to intravenous diazepam. In general, if plasma levels above 9 μg/mL are avoided, lidocaine is extremely well tolerated.

Pharmacokinetics & Dosage

Because of its very extensive first-pass hepatic metabolism, only 3% of orally administered lidocaine appears in the plasma. Thus, lidocaine must be given parenterally. When given by the intravenous route, lidocaine has a half life of 0.5–2 hours. In adults, a loading dose of 150–200 mg administered over about 4 minutes should be followed by a maintenance infusion of 2–4 mg/min to achieve a therapeutic plasma level of 2–6 μg/mL. Determination of lidocaine plasma levels is of great value in setting the infusion rate.

In patients with congestive heart failure, lidocaine's volume of distribution and total body clearance may both be decreased. However, since these effects counterbalance each other, the half-life may not be increased as much as predicted from clearance changes alone. In patients with liver disease, plasma clearance is markedly reduced and the volume of distribution is often increased; the elimination half-life in such cases may be increased 3-fold or more. The size of the initial bolus, the maintenance infusion, and the timing of plasma level determinations must be skillfully managed in patients with liver disease or heart failure.

Therapeutic Use

Lidocaine's major indication is suppression of ventricular tachycardia and prevention of fibrillation after acute myocardial infarction. Lidocaine is the agent of first choice in this setting. Impressive evidence has been obtained to justify the view that lidocaine actually reduces the incidence of ventricular fibrillation in the first few days after acute myocardial infarction. It remains controversial, however, whether lidocaine should be routinely administered to all patients after myocardial infarction.

Lidocaine is rarely effective in supraventricular arrhythmias except for those associated with Wolff-Parkinson-White syndrome or digitalis toxicity.

PHENYTOIN

Phenytoin (diphenylhydantoin) is an anticonvulsant agent with limited antiarrhythmia properties (Chapter 21). Because of its limited efficacy, it should only be considered as a last choice. It suppresses ectopic pacemaker activity, blocks the sodium current, and may interfere with the calcium current. It appears especially effective against digitalis-induced arrhythmias.

NEWER SODIUM CHANNEL-BLOCKING DRUGS

Tocainide and mexiletine are 2 lidocainelike drugs that are active by the oral route (Table 12–1). They have actions almost identical to those of lidocaine but much longer half-lives (Table 12–2). Other sodium channel-blocking agents currently under evaluation are encainide, lorcainide, flecainide, ethmozin, and propafenone.

Calcium Channel–Blocking Drugs

These drugs, of which verapamil is the prototype, were first introduced as antiangina agents and are discussed in some detail in Chapter 10. However, verapamil and several newer agents in this class are very effective antiarrhythmia drugs.

Only verapamil is discussed here. Other calcium channel-blocking agents in general use outside the USA and being investigated in the USA are diltiazem, nifedipine, lidoflazine, and flunarizine. Nifedipine appears to have little antiarrhythmia activity, whereas diltiazem may be as effective as verapamil.

VERAPAMIL

Cardiac Effects

Verapamil blocks both activated and inactivated calcium channels. Thus, its effect is more marked in tissues that fire frequently, are less completely polarized at rest, and in which activation depends exclusively on the calcium current. It is not surprising that verapamil has marked effects upon the sinoatrial and atrioventricular nodes. Atrioventricular nodal conduction and effective refractory period are invariably prolonged by therapeutic concentrations. Verapamil usually slows the sinoatrial node by its direct action, but its hypotensive action may occasionally result in a small reflex increase of sinoatrial nodal rate.

Verapamil can suppress oscillatory afterpotentials resulting from digitalis toxicity and may antagonize slow responses arising in severely depolarized tissue.

Cardiac Toxicity

Verapamil's cardiotoxic effects are dose-related and usually avoidable. Its negative inotropic effects may limit its clinical usefulness in damaged hearts (see Chapter 10). Verapamil can lead to atrioventricular block when used in large doses or in patients with partial atrioventricular block. This block can be treated with atropine, beta-adrenergic stimulants, or calcium. In patients with sinus node disease, verapamil can precipitate sinus arrest.

Extracardiac Effects & Toxicity

Verapamil causes peripheral vasodilatation, which may be beneficial in hypertension and peripheral vasospastic disorders. Its effects upon smooth muscle provide a number of therapeutic extracardiac effects (see Chapter 10).

Minor adverse effects include constipation, lassitude, nervousness, and peripheral edema.

Pharmacokinetics & Dosage

The half-life of verapamil is approximately 7 hours. Verapamil is extensively metabolized by the liver; after oral administration, its bioavailability is only about 20%. Therefore, verapamil must be administered with great caution in patients with hepatic dysfunction. Much smaller doses are required when the drug is administered intravenously.

In adult patients without heart failure or sinoatrial or atrioventricular nodal disease, an initial bolus of 5 mg is administered for treatment of supraventricular tachycardias, followed a few minutes later by a second 5-mg bolus if needed. Thereafter, 5- to 10-mg doses can be administered every 4–6 hours, or a constant infusion of 0.4 μg/kg/min may be used.

Effective oral dosage ranges from 120 to 600 mg daily, divided in 3 or 4 doses.

Therapeutic Use

Reentrant supraventricular tachycardia is the major indication for verapamil, and the drug is fast replacing previous treatments (propranolol, digoxin, edrophonium, vasoconstrictor agents, and cardioversion). Verapamil can also reduce the ventricular rate in atrial fibrillation and flutter. It may convert atrial flutter and fibrillation to sinus rhythm. In ventricular arrhythmias, verapamil appears to be only moderately effective.

Drugs That Prolong Effective Refractory Period by Prolonging Action Potential

At present, the only agents in this category are those which have additional effects that place them in one of the other subgroups. Quinidine and its congeners (especially amiodarone) effectively prolong action potential duration. However, as noted above, their actions on sodium channels also contribute to the measured increase in effective refractory period. Bretylium also prolongs action potential duration and refractory period but is better discussed with other adrenergic receptor-blocking drugs.

Drugs That Block Sympathetic Activity in the Heart

BETA-ADRENERGIC RECEPTOR–BLOCKING DRUGS

Cardiac Effects

Propranolol and similar drugs have antiarrhythmic properties by virtue of their adrenergic receptor-blocking action and direct membrane effects (Chapter 8). Of these drugs, some have selectivity for cardiac beta receptors (β_1-blockers); some have intrinsic sympathomimetic activity; some have marked direct membrane effects; and some prolong the cardiac action potential. The relative contributions of the beta-blocking and direct membrane effects to the antiarrhythmia effects of these drugs are not fully known. Although beta-blockers are fairly well tolerated, their efficacy for suppression of ventricular ectopic depolarizations is low. However, there is growing evidence that these agents can prevent recurrent infarction and sudden death in patients recovering from acute myocardial infarction (Chapter 8).

BRETYLIUM

Bretylium was first introduced as an antihypertension agent. It interferes with the neuronal release of catecholamines but also has direct antiarrhythmia properties.

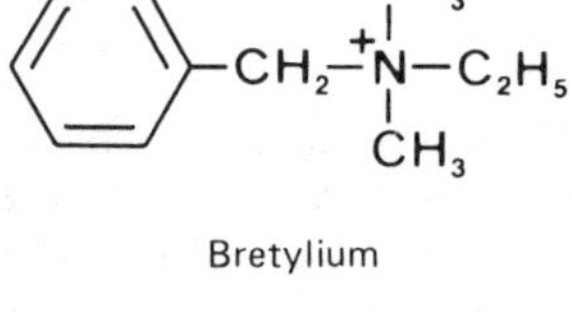

Bretylium

Cardiac Effects

Bretylium lengthens the ventricular (but not the atrial) action potential duration and effective refractory period. This effect is most pronounced in ischemic cells, which have shortened action potential durations. Thus, bretylium reverses the shortening in action potential duration precipitated by ischemia. Experimentally, it has been shown that bretylium markedly increases the strength of electrical stimulation needed to induce ventricular fibrillation (ventricular fibrillation threshold) and delays the onset of fibrillation after acute coronary ligation. This antifibrillatory action appears to be independent of its adrenergic blocking properties.

Since bretylium causes an initial release of catecholamines, it has some positive inotropic actions when first administered. This action may also *precipitate* ventricular arrhythmias and must be watched for at the onset of therapy with the drug.

Extracardiac Effects

These are predictable from the drug's sympathoplegic actions. The major side-effect is postural hypotension. This side-effect can be almost totally prevented by concomitant administration of a tricyclic antidepressant agent such as imipramine. Nausea and vomiting may occur after the intravenous administration of a bolus of bretylium.

Pharmacokinetics & Dosage

Bretylium is available only for intravenous use in the USA. In adults, an intravenous bolus of bretylium tosylate, 5 mg/kg, is administered over a 10-minute period. This dosage may be repeated after 30 minutes. Maintenance therapy is achieved by a similar bolus every 4–6 hours or by a constant infusion of 0.5–2 mg/min.

Therapeutic Use

Bretylium is usually used in an emergency setting, often during attempted resuscitation from ventricular fibrillation when lidocaine and cardioversion have failed. Its use in suppression of less severe ventricular arrhythmias is not established.

II. CLINICAL PHARMACOLOGY OF THE ANTIARRHYTHMIA AGENTS

PRINCIPLES OF ANTIARRHYTHMIA THERAPY

In addition to a thorough understanding of the pharmacokinetics and specific antiarrhythmia actions of the various antiarrhythmia agents, the clinician must employ certain basic principles and a growing number of technologic aids in treating patients with cardiac arrhythmias. The 3 main principles are (1) arrhythmia documentation, (2) drug efficacy assessment, and (3) plasma drug concentration determination. Antiarrhythmia drug therapy is rarely successful when any one of these principles is ignored.

Arrhythmia documentation has been greatly facilitated by recent technical advances, including in-hospital, computer-assisted ECG rhythm monitoring, ambulatory ECG monitoring, patient-initiated ECG event recording, and telephonic transmission of ECG signals. With these aids, it becomes inappropriate for assumptions to be made regarding the presence, absence, or nature of an arrhythmia.

The assessment of antiarrhythmia drug efficacy in individual patients has improved markedly in the past decade. The technical developments mentioned above make it possible to confirm, with statistical validation, the efficacy or inefficacy of an antiarrhythmia drug for a specific arrhythmia in a given individual. The physician's ability to choose the appropriate antiarrhythmia drug has also been expanded. Such a choice is based first upon the known spectrum of activity of any drug under consideration. Beyond that consideration, the choice must be empiric. The conventional approach to empiric drug selection in the past required that each drug be given a full therapeutic trial, usually requiring days or weeks of therapy with dose increments. This method relies upon frequent ambulatory monitoring and entails a certain risk in patients with life-threatening cardiac arrhythmias. A protracted trial-and-error testing period before settling on the most effective drug and the optimum dose may be dangerous. A newer technique, clinical cardiac electrophysiologic testing, now permits artificial induction of clinical arrhythmias and provides a basis for immediate and rapid antiarrhythmia drug efficacy assessment. By this new technique, the patient's arrhythmia can be repeatedly induced and terminated, using temporary pacing catheters to stimulate the heart. An antiarrhythmia drug is then administered intravenously, and arrhythmia induction is tried. Failure to induce the arrhythmia after drug administration is strongly predictive of long-term efficacy of the drug.

The third principle is antiarrhythmia drug concentration determination. Most antiarrhythmia drugs are variably absorbed and metabolized by patients, and this variability may be further exaggerated by congestive heart failure and impaired renal function. A drug cannot be considered ineffective unless plasma concentrations have been measured and found to be in the therapeutic range. In addition, since many antiarrhythmia drugs are characterized by a narrow therapeutic concentration range, patient safety often depends upon plasma level analysis.

WHEN SHOULD ARRHYTHMIAS BE TREATED?

Deciding when antiarrhythmia therapy is indicated is a complex matter. While the need to treat immediately life-threatening rhythm disturbances is usually obvious, other situations may be less so. Rhythms that produce significant symptoms should usually be treated, regardless of their risk to the patient, unless they present a small risk *and* the likelihood of successful therapy is small (as in certain instances of atrial fibrillation).

The area of greatest controversy concerns the therapy of premature ventricular contractions. Should all premature ventricular contractions be treated? Should the goal of therapy be to *totally* eliminate them? While there is no definite answer to either question, certain reasonable guidelines can be established:

(1) The simpler therapies should not be forgotten. Many patients benefit from reduction of excessive coffee intake, cigarette use, and alcohol consumption. Exercise, emotional stress, certain foods, and other avoidable environmental factors may trigger arrhythmias in susceptible patients. Identification and elimination of such factors should always be the first step after accurate diagnosis in the management of patients with cardiac rhythm disturbances.

(2) In patients without structural heart disease, ventricular arrhythmias generally do not have to be treated unless they are causing significant symptoms or are life-threatening (eg, ventricular tachycardia).

(3) Complex ventricular arrhythmias (eg, ventricular tachycardia) should be treated with the goal of eliminating them.

In some patients, the presence of heart disease may complicate the use of antiarrhythmia drugs. Heart failure and conduction system disease are the most important problems. Most antiarrhythmia drugs depress left ventricular function to a variable, dose-related extent. Disopyramide, verapamil, and beta-adrenergic blocking drugs are the most frequent offenders. In patients with atrioventricular nodal disease, verapamil, digitalis, and beta-blockers cause the most problems. In patients with conduction disease below the level of the atrioventricular node, therapy with disopyramide, quinidine, and procainamide and most of the experimental sodium channel-blocking drugs should only be started under careful continuous in-hospital monitoring.

Some arrhythmias do not respond to conventional or experimental drugs. In such cases, combinations of drugs may be tried. It is unwise to combine agents with similar electrophysiologic properties (eg, quinidine with procainamide, or verapamil with diltiazem). Overall, efficacy of combinations of 2 or more drugs that were ineffective when given singly in previous trials is low. If drug therapy fails, other measures may be considered (eg, pacing, cardioversion, and surgical procedures).

• • •

References

Coraboeuf E: Ionic basis of electrical activity in cardiac tissues. *Am J Physiol* 1978;**234:**101.

Grant AO et al: The influence of pH on the electrophysiological effects of licodaine in guinea pig ventricular myocardium. *Circ Res* 1980;**47:**542.

Grunblatt DJ, Koch-Weser J: Clinical pharmacokinetics. (2 parts.) *N Engl J Med* 1975;**293:**702, 964.

Harrison DC, Hefflin PJ, Winkle RA: Clinical pharmacology of antiarrhythmic drugs. *Prog Cardiovasc Dis* 1977;**20:**217.

Hoffman BF, Rosen MR: Cellular mechanisms of cardiac arrhythmias. *Circ Res* 1981;**49:**1.

Hoffman BF, Rosen MR, Wit AL: Electrophysiology and pharmacology of cardiac arrhythmias. 7. Cardiac effects of quinidine and procainamide. *Am Heart J* 1975;**89:**804.

Hondeghem LM, Katzung BG: Test of a model of antiarrhythmic drug action: Effects of quinidine and lidocaine on myocardial conduction. *Circulation* 1980;**61:**1217.

Lazzara R, Hope RR, El-Sherif BJ: Effects of lidocaine on hypoxic and ischemic cardiac cells. *Am J Cardiol* 1979;**41:**872.

Mason JW, Winkle RA: Accuracy of the ventricular tachycardia-induction study for predicting long-term efficacy and inefficacy of antiarrhythmic drugs. *N Engl J Med* 1980;**303:**1073.

McDonald TF, Pelser D, Trautwein W: On the mechanism of slow calcium channel block in heart. *Pfluegers Arch* 1980;**385:**175.

Mitchell LB, Schroeder JS, Mason JW: Comparative clinical electrophysiologic effects of diltiazem, verapamil and nifedipine: A review. *Am J Cardiol* 1982;**49:**629.

Oshita S et al: Effects of tocainide and lidocaine on the transmembrane action potentials as related to external potassium and calcium concentration in guinea pig papillary muscles. *Naunyn Schmiedebergs Arch Pharmacol* 1980;**314:**67.

Zipes DP, Troup PJ: New antiarrhythmic agents: Amiodarone, aprindine, disopyramide, ethmozin, mexiletine, tocainide and verapamil. *Am J Cardiol* 1978;**41:**1005.

Diuretics | 13

David G. Warnock, MD

Drugs acting on the renal tubules are useful in a variety of clinical conditions involving abnormal electrolyte or water metabolism. Because the anatomic segments of the nephron are highly specialized in function, the actions of each agent in this group can be best understood in relation to its site of action in the nephron and the normal physiology of that segment.

RENAL TUBULE TRANSPORT MECHANISMS

PROXIMAL TUBULES

Sodium bicarbonate, glucose, amino acids, and other organic solutes are preferentially reabsorbed in the early proximal tubule. As shown in Fig 13–1, the luminal concentrations of these solutes decrease along the length of the proximal tubule. Because of the high water permeability of the proximal tubule, the luminal fluid osmolality and sodium concentration remain relatively the same along the length of the proximal tubule. The luminal chloride concentration rises along the length of the proximal tubule—in contrast to the bicarbonate concentration, which falls. Therefore, bicarbonate is preferentially reabsorbed in the early proximal tubule, at least in comparison to chloride. Bicarbonate reabsorption by the proximal tubule is known to be critically dependent upon carbonic anhydrase activity. In the later portions of the proximal tubule, the luminal fluid closely resembles a simple NaCl solution (Fig 13–2). The reabsorptive process in the late proximal tubule therefore consists of isotonic NaCl reabsorption.

Organic acid secretory systems are located in the middle third of the proximal tubule (S_2 segment). These systems secrete a variety of organic acids (*p*-aminohippurate, diuretics, antibiotics, etc) into the luminal fluid from the bloodstream. Organic base secretory systems (creatinine, procainamide, choline, etc) are localized in the early (S_1) and middle (S_2) segments of the proximal tubules. These organic secretory systems are important determinants in delivery of diuretics to their active sites at the luminal aspects of tubule segments along the entire nephron. In

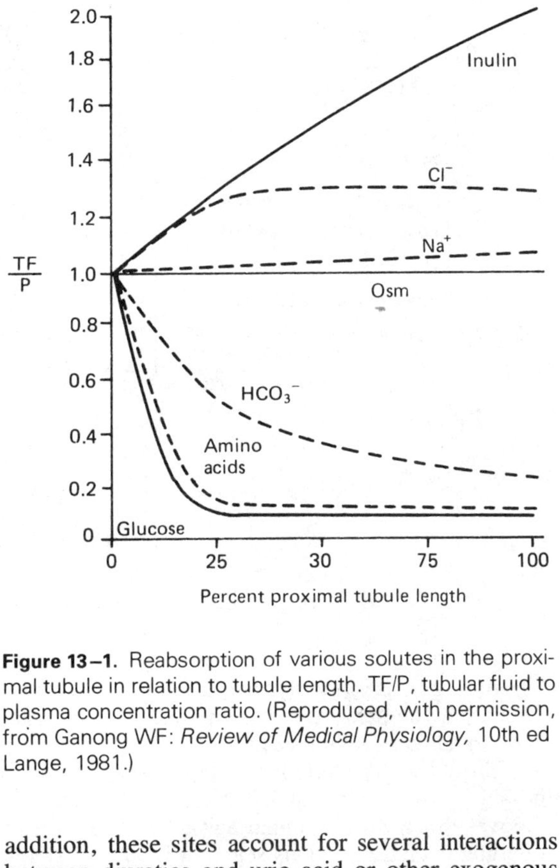

Figure 13–1. Reabsorption of various solutes in the proximal tubule in relation to tubule length. TF/P, tubular fluid to plasma concentration ratio. (Reproduced, with permission, from Ganong WF: *Review of Medical Physiology,* 10th ed Lange, 1981.)

addition, these sites account for several interactions between diuretics and uric acid or other exogenous organic compounds (eg, interactions between diuretics and probenecid).

LOOP OF HENLE

Water is abstracted from the thin descending limb of the loop of Henle by osmotic forces generated in the hypertonic medullary interstitium. Solute entry (eg, NaCl, urea) may occur in some species, but water abstraction appears to be the dominant process in most mammalian kidneys. Any impermeant solute in the lumen will oppose water abstraction and increase the delivery of salt and water to more distal sites. Important examples of impermeant solutes include osmotic

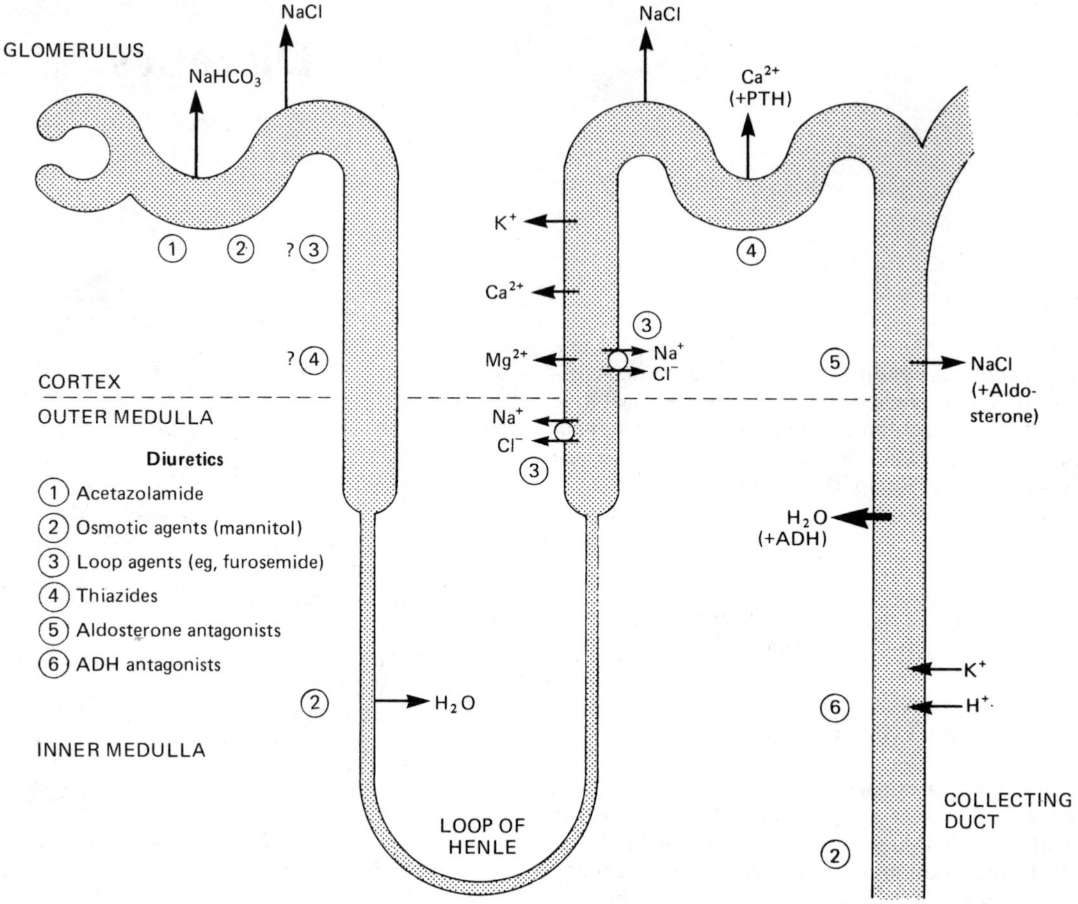

Figure 13–2. Tubule transport systems and sites of action of diuretics.

diuretics, glucose (in glycosuria), and bicarbonate (which may be present if proximal bicarbonate reabsorption has been inhibited).

The thick ascending limb of the loop of Henle is the site of an active NaCl reabsorptive system that removes salt from the lumen and adds it to the surrounding interstitium. This segment is extremely impermeable to water and therefore can be regarded as a diluting segment. Medullary portions of the thick ascending limb contribute to medullary hypertonicity and thereby also play an important role in concentration of urine. In contrast, NaCl reabsorbed from the cortical portions of the thick ascending limb does not provide a driving force for water abstraction from medullary structures and therefore does not participate in concentration of the urine. The NaCl transport system in the thick ascending limb is now regarded as a sodium chloride cotransport mechanism rather than an active "chloride" pump. A lumen-positive electrical potential present in this segment provides an important driving force for the reabsorption of divalent cations (Mg^{2+}, Ca^{2+}) and K^+. Inhibition of the thick ascending limb by "loop" diuretics causes an increase in urinary excretion of these cations in addition to NaCl.

DISTAL CONVOLUTED TUBULE

The distal convoluted tubule can be regarded as an example of a cortical diluting segment that reabsorbs NaCl and appears to be impermeable to water. In contrast to more distal sites, this segment does not appear to respond to aldosterone or antidiuretic hormone (ADH). This segment does have parathyroid hormone (PTH) receptors and is a site of active Ca^{2+} reabsorption.

COLLECTING TUBULES

NaCl is reabsorbed in the collecting tubules, and this transport system is regulated by mineralocorticoid hormones. In addition, K^+ and H^+ are secreted into the lumen, especially under conditions that enhance Na^+ reabsorption. The coupling between Na^+ reabsorption and K^+ (and H^+) secretion may involve several indirect mechanisms and can be completely dissociated in certain experimental settings, ie, it is not a simple "exchange." By whatever mechanism, there does appear to be a direct relation between Na^+ delivery to these sites and the resulting secretion of H^+ and K^+. These relations are accentuated during hypermineralocorticoid conditions and when distal Na^+ delivery is accompanied by an impermeant anion such as bicarbonate, phosphate, or sulfate.

In the presence of ADH, the collecting tubule (and duct) become very permeable to water. ADH levels are elevated during antidiuresis, and a concentrated urine is excreted. On the other hand, ADH secretion is suppressed during hypotonic volume expansion and by certain drugs, and relative large volumes of dilute urine are excreted.

1. BASIC PHARMACOLOGY OF DIURETICS

CARBONIC ANHYDRASE INHIBITORS

Carbonic anhydrase is present in many nephron sites, including the cytoplasm and the luminal and basolateral membranes, and in the red cells in the peritubular capillaries. The predominant site is in the proximal tubule, where this enzyme catalyzes the CO_2 hydration/dehydration reactions involved in bicarbonate reabsorption. Inhibitors of carbonic anhydrase cause sodium bicarbonate diuresis and a reduction in total body bicarbonate stores.

The carbonic anhydrase inhibitors were the forerunners of modern diuretics. They are unsubstituted sulfonamide derivatives and were developed when it was noted that bacteriostatic sulfonamides caused hyperchloremic metabolic acidosis with large volumes of alkaline urine. Subsequent sulfonamide diuretics (ie, thiazides) were developed to separate the natriuretic effect from the effects on bicarbonate handling.

Chemistry

The structure of acetazolamide is shown below. The $-SO_2NH_2$ (sulfamyl) group is essential for activity. Alkyl substitutions at this point completely block its effects on carbonic anhydrase activity.

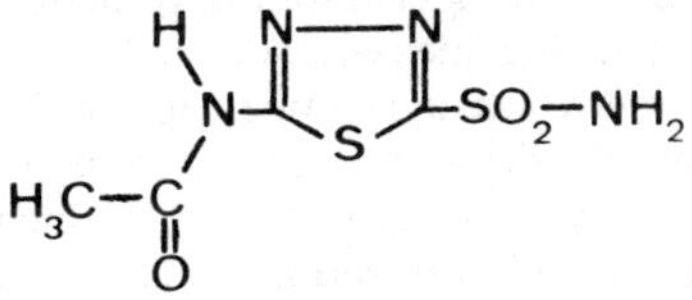

Acetazolamide

Pharmacokinetics

All of the carbonic anhydrase inhibitors are well absorbed after oral administration. Effects on urine pH are apparent within 30 minutes, are maximal at 2 hours, and persist for 12 hours after a single dose. Excretion is by tubular secretion in the S_2 segment of the proximal tubule.

Pharmacodynamics

Inhibition of carbonic anhydrase activity profoundly depresses bicarbonate reabsorption in the proximal tubule. Bicarbonate accumulates in the cells and in the luminal fluid. The discrepancy between luminal pH (which may become acid) and the elevation in the luminal bicarbonate concentration has been referred to as a "disequilibrium" pH. Nearly all of the bicarbonate-reabsorptive capacity of the superficial proximal tubule can be inhibited by acetazolamide, with an apparent I50 (concentration for 50% inhibition) of 4 μM. In contrast, substantial amounts of bicarbonate can still be absorbed at other nephron sites by one or more undefined carbonic anhydrase-independent mechanisms. The overall result of maximal acetazolamide administration is 85% inhibition of proximal bicarbonate reabsorption but only 45% inhibition of whole kidney bicarbonate reabsorption. The result is an acute bicarbonate-wasting condition. Depletion of the body stores of bicarbonate results in hyperchloremic metabolic acidosis and thereby reduces diuretic effectiveness of subsequent doses of the same drug.

An interesting effect of inhibition of proximal bicarbonate reabsorption is a parallel inhibition of chloride reabsorption in the proximal tubule. As a result, both $NaHCO_3$ and NaCl are delivered out of the proximal tubule during carbonic anhydrase inhibition. Most of the increased distal delivery of NaCl is picked up at downstream sites (ie, thick ascending limb), so the resulting natriuresis is accompanied by bicarbonate and not by chloride.

Many other secretory processes involve H^+ or HCO_3^- transport, which are mediated by carbonic anhydrase activity. Aqueous humor production is an important example, as noted below.

Clinical Indications & Dosage

A. Glaucoma: (See Table 13–1.) Aqueous humor contains a high concentration of bicarbonate ion. Inhibition of carbonic anhydrase decreases the rate of aqueous humor formation and thereby decreases intraocular pressure. This effect is of value in the chronic management of glaucoma, which is now the most common indication for use of carbonic anhydrase inhibitors.

Acetazolamide is also available in sustained-release capsules containing 500 mg and as the sodium salt in vials for parenteral administration.

Table 13–1. Carbonic anhydrase inhibitors used in treatment of glaucoma.

	Usual Oral Dose (1–4 Times Daily)
Acetazolamide (Diamox)	250 mg
Dichlorphenamide (Daranide, Oratrol)	50 mg
Ethoxzolamide (Cardrase, Ethamide)	125 mg
Methazolamide (Neptazane)	50 mg

B. Urinary Alkalinization: Uric acid and cystine are relatively insoluble in acid urines. Enhanced renal excretion can theoretically be achieved by increasing urinary bicarbonate excretion with carbonic anhydrase inhibitors. Similarly, renal excretion of weak acids (eg, aspirin) is increased by raising the urine pH. These effects are of relatively short duration and require bicarbonate infusion to maintain continuing bicarbonate diuresis.

C. Reduction of Total Body Bicarbonate Stores: Carbonic anhydrase inhibition will cause acute sodium bicarbonate diuresis as long as the filtered load of bicarbonate exceeds the renal capacity for bicarbonate absorption. This approach can be useful in chronic metabolic alkalosis associated with resistance to other diuretic agents. Another example is posthypercapnic metabolic alkalosis: Carbonic anhydrase inhibitors can be used to correct this condition if saline administration is ineffective or contraindicated because of elevated cardiac filling pressures.

D. Acute Mountain Sickness: Weakness, breathlessness, dizziness, and nausea can occur in mountain climbers who rapidly ascend above 3000 m and overexert themselves. The symptoms are usually mild and last for a few days. In some climbers, rapidly progressing pulmonary or cerebral edema can be life-threatening. Acetazolamide increases performance status and decreases overall symptomatology. A recent study (see Greene reference on p 168) proposed taking 500 mg (one sustained-release capsule) by mouth at night for 5 nights before a climb.

E. Other Uses: Carbonic anhydrase inhibitors have been used as adjuvants for the treatment of epilepsy, in some forms of hypokalemic periodic paralysis, and to increase urinary phosphate excretion during severe hyperphosphatemia.

Toxicity

A. Hyperchloremic Metabolic Acidosis: This is the predictable consequence of chronic reduction of body bicarbonate stores. Bicarbonate wasting will ultimately limit the diuretic efficacy of carbonic anhydrase inhibitors in direct proportion to the overall reduction in filtered load of bicarbonate.

B. Renal Stones: Phosphaturia and hypercalciuria occur during the bicarbonaturic response to carbonic anhydrase inhibition. Renal excretion of solubilizing factors (eg, citrate) may decline with chronic use. Calcium salts are relatively insoluble at alkaline pH, which means that renal stone formation can occur.

C. Renal K^+ Wasting: Potassium wasting can be severe, especially during the acute bicarbonate diuresis stage. This complication may limit the usefulness of carbonic anhydrase inhibitors in chronic metabolic alkalosis associated with prior diuretic administration.

D. Other Toxicities: Drowsiness and paresthesias are common following large doses. Hypersensitivity reactions (fever, rashes, bone marrow suppression, interstitial nephritis) can also occur.

Contraindications

Carbonic anhydrase inhibitors should be avoided in hepatic cirrhosis. Alkalinization of the urine will decrease urinary trapping of NH_4^+ and may contribute to the development of hepatic encephalopathy.

THIAZIDES

The thiazide diuretics emerged from efforts to synthesize more potent carbonic anhydrase inhibitors. Chemical modification of the parent compounds changed the anion composition of the diuresis. Increased chloride, rather than bicarbonate, accompanied by sodium appeared in the urine. Subsequent work has shown that the benzothiadiazides inhibit NaCl transport independently of any effect on carbonic anhydrase activity. Some members of this group retain significant carbonic anhydrase inhibitory activity, but this effect is not related to the primary mode of action.

Chemistry

The drugs in this group are called thiazides, benzothiadiazides, or simply sulfonamide diuretics. Substitutions and the nature of the heterocyclic rings vary between the different congeners, but all of them retain, in common with the carbonic anhydrase inhibitors, an unsubstituted sulfamyl group (Fig 13–3).

The structure-activity relations of the thiazides are complex. There is a wide range of potency with regard to carbonic anhydrase inhibition. On the other hand, the diuretic potency has clearly been dissociated from the ability to inhibit carbonic anhydrase activity. Some members of the group have hyperglycemic activity, but the structural requirements for this effect differ from those for diuresis. All of the members of this group have parallel dose-response curves and similar maximal effects on chloride excretion.

Pharmacokinetics

All of the thiazides are absorbed when given orally, but there are differences in their metabolism. Chlorothiazide, the prototype of the group, is less lipid-soluble and must be given in relatively large doses. Chlorthalidone is slowly absorbed and therefore appears to have a longer duration of action.

All of the thiazides are secreted by the organic acid secretory system and compete to some extent with the secretion of uric acid by that system. As a result, the uric acid secretory rate may be reduced, with a concomitant elevation in serum uric acid level. In the steady state, uric acid production and therefore renal excretion are not affected by the thiazides.

Pharmacodynamics

Thiazides inhibit NaCl reabsorption in the early segments of the distal tubule. Early clearance studies demonstrated an effect on NaCl reabsorption during excretion of diluted urine under water-loaded conditions. This finding suggested that the site of action was at a "cortical diluting segment," since there was no

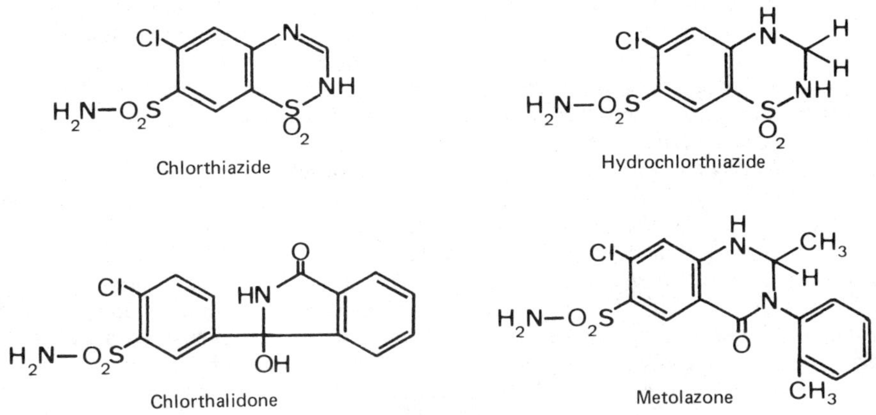

Figure 13–3. Thiazides and related agents.

appreciable effect on urinary concentration during elaboration of hypertonic urine. More recent studies have shown that the distal convoluted tubule is the site of action of thiazides and that there is no effect on thick ascending limb function. There may also be an effect on NaCl reabsorption in the late proximal tubule, but this is not observed in the usual clinical setting. Any increase in NaCl delivery out of the proximal tubule is picked up in the uninhibited thick ascending limb of the loop of Henle.

Very little is known about the NaCl transport system that is inhibited by thiazides. There is a lumen-negative electrical potential in the distal convoluted tubule, which is consistent with electrogenic Na^+ reabsorption. In contrast to the collecting tubule system, there does not appear to be any mineralocorticoid-dependent Na^+ transport in the distal convoluted tubule. There is an active reabsorptive process for Ca^{2+} in the distal convoluted tubule, which is modulated by parathyroid hormone (PTH). Thiazides do not inhibit Ca^{2+} reabsorption at this site. There may even be a relative stimulation of Ca^{2+} reabsorption when thiazides inhibit NaCl reabsorption. The overall effect is NaCl diuresis with a decrease in Ca^{2+} excretion. This effect may be hidden if volume expansion (eg, increased dietary salt intake) is superimposed upon chronic thiazide therapy.

Analogs

A large number of analogs are available. Three agents merit specific mention, because they differ from other thiazides with regard to the constituents of the heterocyclic ring structure: chlorthalidone, quinethazone, and metolazone. However, all 3 variants share with the thiazides an unsubstituted sulfonamide group.

Clinical Indications & Dosage

The general principles underlying the clinical use of thiazide diuretics are described later in this chapter. The usual therapeutic end point of diuretic therapy is mobilization of salt and water from interstitial compartments and reduction in "effective" circulating volume. Thiazide diuretics are often an appropriate choice because of the mild, sustained nature of their diuretic effect. More potent agents—or combinations of agents—may be required if the therapeutic response to thiazides is inadequate.

Table 13–2. Thiazides and related diuretics: Dosages.

	Daily Oral Dose	Frequency of Dosage
Bendroflumethiazide (Benuron, Naturetin)	2.5–10 mg	As single dose
Benzthiazide* (Aquatag, Exna)	25–100 mg	In 2 divided doses
Chlorothiazide* (Diuril)	0.5–1g	In 2 divided doses
Chlorthalidone† (Hygroton)	50–100 mg	As single dose
Cyclothiazide (Anhydron)	1–2 mg	As single dose
Hydrochlorothiazide* (Esidrix, Hydrodiuril, Oretic)	25–100 mg	As single dose
Hydroflumethiazide (Diucardin, Saluron)	25–100 mg	In 2 divided doses
Methyclothiazide (Aquatensen, Enduron)	2.5–10 mg	As single dose
Metolazone† (Diulo, Zaroxolyn)	2.5–10 mg	As single dose
Polythiazide (Renese)	1–4 mg	As single dose
Quinethazone† (Hydromox)	50–100 mg	As single dose
Trichlormethiazide* (Metahydrin, Naqua)	2–8 mg	As single dose

*Generic preparation available. Trade name included for identification only.
†Not a thiazide but a sulfonamide qualitatively similar to the thiazides.

A. Idiopathic Hypercalciuria: Thiazide therapy can reduce the urinary excretion of calcium and the degree to which urine is saturated with calcium salts. This effect is beneficial in calcium stone formers; a striking reduction in the incidence of new stone formation is generally seen. The reduction in urinary calcium excretion can be explained by the relative increase in calcium absorption induced by thiazides at the level of the distal convoluted tubule. This effect can be overcome by dietary salt excess, which may suppress proximal tubule reabsorption and increase urinary excretion of both Na^+ and Ca^{2+}.

B. Nephrogenic Diabetes Insipidus: Thiazide diuretics can reduce polyuria and polydipsia in patients who are not responsive to ADH. The beneficial effect is mediated through plasma volume reduction, with an attendant fall in glomerular filtration rate and enhanced proximal reabsorption of NaCl. Dietary sodium restriction can potentiate the beneficial effects of thiazides on urine volume in this setting. Lithium-induced nephrogenic diabetes insipidus may cause troublesome polyuria. Thiazides can be useful in this setting, but serum Li^+ levels must be carefully monitored, since these diuretics may *reduce* Li^+ clearance.

Toxicity

A. Weakness, Fatigability, Paresthesias: These dose-related toxic effects are similar to those of carbonic anhydrase inhibitors. Impotence has been reported as a side-effect of thiazide therapy.

B. Potassium Depletion and Metabolic Alkalosis: These effects accompany the volume contraction and secondary hyperaldosteronism that occur with diuretic therapy. These issues will be discussed with the K^+-sparing diuretics.

C. Impaired Carbohydrate Tolerance: Hyperglycemia and glycosuria may occur in susceptible patients who are overtly diabetic or have abnormal glucose tolerance tests. The effect is dose-related and is the result of impaired pancreatic release of insulin or a blockade of peripheral glucose utilization.

D. Hyperuricemia and Hyperlipidemia: Serum uric acid levels usually rise when patients are given thiazide diuretics. Most patients remain asymptomatic and do not require therapy to lower their uric acid levels. Gout may be precipitated or intensified in susceptible subjects. There is no convincing evidence that hyperuricemia is a cardiovascular risk factor at present. There are associations between hypertension, hyperuricemia, and hyperlipidemia, but it is not clear if diuretics modify or affect these associations. It is certain that effective antihypertensive therapy reduces the incidence of cardiovascular disease in hypertensive patients.

E. Hyponatremia: Life-threatening hyponatremia has occurred in a very small number of patients who had recently begun diuretic therapy. This effect may be related to reduction in the diluting capacity of the kidney or sustained release of ADH. Polydipsia and K^+ depletion may play important roles in the development of hyponatremia.

F. Allergic Reactions: Skin rashes occasionally occur. Serious allergic reactions are extremely rare but do include hemolytic anemia, thrombocytopenia, acute pancreatitis, cholestatic jaundice, and acute pulmonary edema.

Contraindications

Thiazides should be used cautiously in patients with hepatic cirrhosis to avoid K^+ depletion and hepatic encephalopathy. Renal insufficiency may be intensified by overzealous diuretic use in patients with established renal failure. Digitalis toxicity may become manifest or intensified as a result of diuretic-induced K^+ depletion.

LOOP AGENTS

These short-acting agents inhibit NaCl reabsorption in the thick ascending limb of the loop of Henle. Owing to the large NaCl absorptive capacity of this segment, agents that act at this site produce a diuretic effect much greater than that seen with any other diuretic group.

Chemistry

The 2 prototypical drugs of this group are furosemide and ethacrynic acid (Figs 13–4 and 13–5).

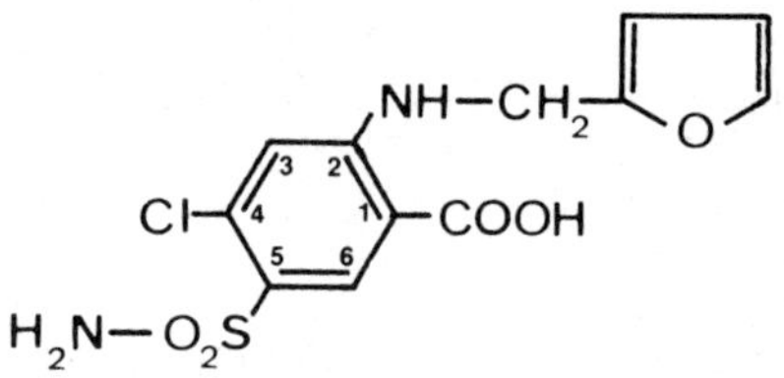

Furosemide

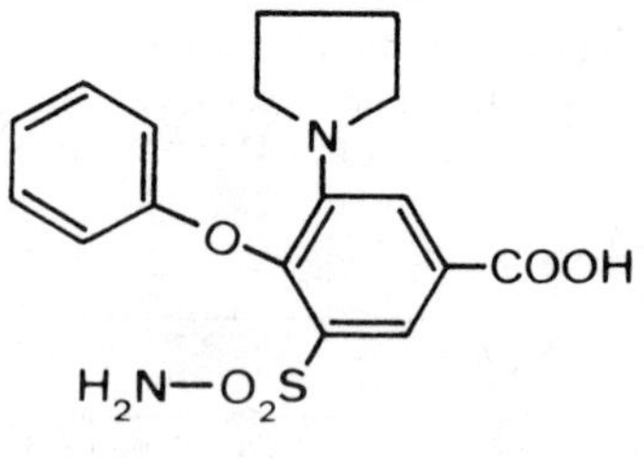

Piretanide

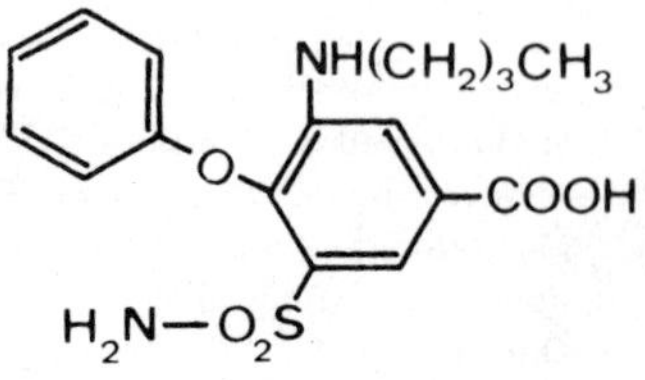

Bumetanide

Figure 13–4. Furosemide derivatives.

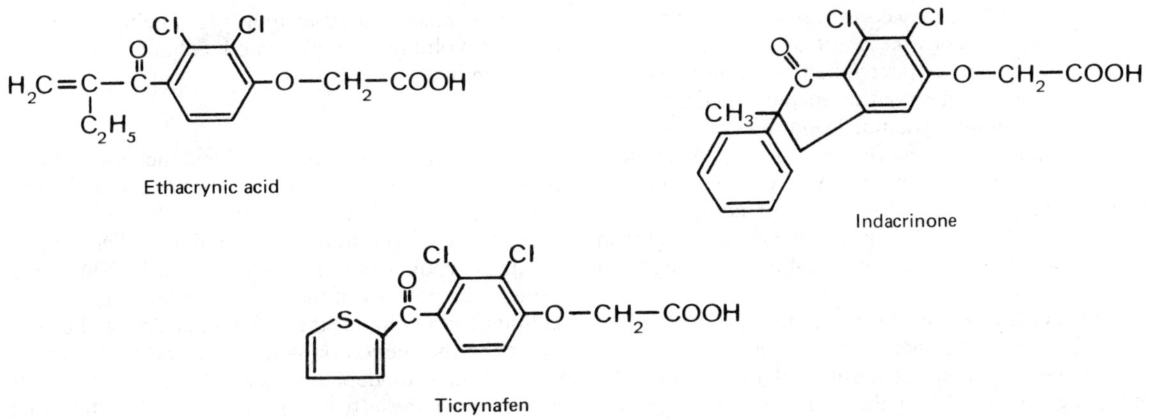

Figure 13–5. Ethacrynic acid derivatives.

The structures of **furosemide** and its analogs bumetanide and piretanide are shown in Fig 13–4. These agents have a carboxyl group with a sulfamyl moiety in the meta position (carbon number 5). A halide or phenoxy substitution is present at carbon 4, and a substituted amino group is present at carbon 2 or 3.

Ethacrynic acid is not a sulfonamide and therefore is chemically distinct from the thiazides and furosemide. Ethacrynic acid is a phenoxyacetic acid derivative that also contains an adjacent ketone and methylene group. The methylene group is fairly reactive and forms an adduct with the free sulfhydryl group of cysteine. The cysteine adduct appears to be the active form of the drug. Other members of this class (ie, phenoxyacetic acid derivatives, Fig 13–5) are currently being developed. The analogs reveal 2 interesting features: (1) the sulfhydryl reactivity is not a requirement for diuretic activity, and (2) all members of this class have uricosuric activity. In some instances, diuretic and uricosuric effects have been associated with separate stereoisomers.

Pharmacokinetics

The loop agents are rapidly absorbed and handled by renal secretion as well as filtration. Diuretic response is usually extremely rapid following intravenous injection. The duration of effect is usually 2–3 hours. The response to furosemide correlates positively with its urinary excretion rate. Defects in the secretory component of its clearance may result from simultaneous administration of agents such as indomethacin or probenecid. Metabolites of ethacrynic acid and furosemide have been identified, but it is not known if they have any diuretic activity.

Pharmacodynamics

These drugs inhibit NaCl transport in the thick ascending limb of the loop of Henle. The effect has been localized to a transport site at the luminal membrane and probably corresponds to a coupled entry mechanism for Na^+, Cl^-, and possibly K^+. It was formerly thought that an "active" chloride pump was present in the thick ascending limb. The current view favors a coupled NaCl transport system that is driven by a Na^+,K^+-ATPase-dependent pump in the basolateral membrane. The loop diuretics reduce the reabsorption of both Na^+ and Cl^- and diminish the normal lumen-positive potential across the tubule. These agents at high concentrations can be shown in vivo to inhibit various ATPases and mitochondrial transport systems. These metabolic effects are probably not related to the diuretic effects of these agents.

The thick ascending limb is thought to play an important role in divalent cation handling. Inhibition of active NaCl transport causes an associated increase in Mg^{2+} and Ca^{2+} excretion, perhaps because of the diminished positive potential across the tubule. Chronic use of loop agents has been associated with Mg^{2+} wasting and severe hypomagnesemia. Calcium excretion can be strikingly increased with loop agents and saline infusions, an effect of great usefulness in the acute management of hypercalcemia. This effect must be clearly distinguished from that of the thiazides, which *decrease* Ca^{2+} excretion.

Loop agents appear to have direct effects on blood flow through several vascular beds. Furosemide can be shown to increase renal blood flow and cause redistribution of blood flow within the renal cortex. The hemodynamic effects appear to involve the renin-angiotensin system and vasodilatory prostaglandins. However, the hemodynamic effects have not been directly linked to the diuretic response. Furosemide and ethacrynic acid have also been shown to improve pulmonary congestion and reduce left ventricular filling pressures as an acute hemodynamic effect before any measureable increase in urinary output occurs.

Clinical Indications & Dosage

A. Acute Pulmonary Edema: The therapeutic goal is rapid reduction of extracellular fluid volume and venous return so that right ventricular output and pulmonary vascular pressures are decreased. As described above, there may be an improvement in cardiac function that precedes the onset of diuresis. This response is due to an extrarenal hemodynamic response and may even be observed in anephric patients.

B. Refractory Edema: Loop diuretics are used when the patient does not respond to salt restriction or less potent diuretics. Diuresis will ensue as long as interstitial fluid is mobilized without compromising intravascular volume. Loop agents are also useful in patients who have diminished renal function and fluid overload.

C. Hypercalcemia: Loop agents can promote a striking increase in urinary excretion of calcium with a prompt reduction in the serum calcium level. The effect is very useful in the acute treatment of hypercalcemia. Inhibition of thick ascending limb function also causes marked excretion of NaCl, water, K^+, and Mg^{2+}. Extracellular fluid volume depletion must be prevented to ensure a continued diuretic response. The usual approach is to infuse normal saline and give furosemide (80–120 mg) intravenously. Once the diuresis begins, the rate of saline infusion can be matched with the urine flow rate to avoid volume depletion. Potassium may be added to the saline infusion if clinically indicated.

D. Anion and Cation Overdose: Various electrolyte disorders may respond to increases in urine flow rate. For example, halides seem to be reabsorbed in the thick ascending limb; loop diuretics are therefore useful in treating bromide, fluoride, and iodide poisoning. Saline solution must be administered to replace urinary losses of Na^+ and to provide Cl^-, so as to avoid extracellular fluid volume depletion. Hyperkalemia is another example where renal clearance of K^+ may be increased by the use of loop agents and saline infusion. These drugs are not useful in the treatment of lithium poisoning.

E. Acute Renal Failure: Loop agents can increase the rate of urine flow in acute renal failure in both clinical and experimental circumstances. This maneuver can convert oliguric renal failure to nonoliguric failure but seems not to have any beneficial effect on overall outcome, duration of renal failure, or survival. If it is known that a large pigment load has precipitated acute renal failure or threatens to do so, loop agents may "wash out" intratubular casts and ameliorate intratubular obstruction. Loop agents may be used to increase urine flow rates if hyperkalemia complicates the course of acute renal failure.

F. Hyperuricemia: Uricosuric congeners of ethacrynic acid include **indacrinone** (MK-196) and **ticrynafen** (tienilic acid). These agents inhibit proximal reabsorption of uric acid and are therefore uricosuric. Serum uric acid levels are diminished, but acute renal insufficiency can result if the urinary load of uric acid increases too rapidly. These agents may be useful in patients with symptomatic hyperuricemia who require diuretic therapy for management of hypertension or congestive heart failure. Cholestatic jaundice occurred with the use of ticrynafen, and the drug is no longer available in the USA. Loop agents also can *cause* hyperuricemia, presumably via extracellular volume depletion and enhanced proximal reabsorption.

Toxicity

Loop agents, like the thiazides, increase delivery of salt and water to more distal segments of the nephron. The predictable consequence of this effect is enhanced renal secretion of K^+ and H^+. The clinical result is hypokalemic metabolic alkalosis. This effect reflects the potency of the diuretic agent and the extracellular fluid volume status. These effects will be discussed in the section on potassium-sparing diuretics.

Magnesium depletion is another predictable consequence of the effects of loop agents on the thick ascending limb. Magnesium wasting can also occur with the thiazides, but clinically important hypomagnesemia seems to occur more commonly with chronic use of loop agents. Volume status is another factor that can influence divalent cation excretion. Loop agents are known for their hypercalciuric effect, but clinical instances of *hypercalcemia* have been noted. If chronic use of loop agents causes volume depletion, the proximal reabsorption of Ca^{2+} is apparently enhanced, resulting in volume contraction and hypercalcemia. Increased salt intake or use of less potent diuretics is indicated in this condition.

Ototoxicity is another well-described effect of loop agents. It is dose-related and usually (not always) reversible. This effect is seen with overzealous diuretic use in patients who have diminished renal function or are also receiving other ototoxic agents (ie, aminoglycoside antibiotics).

Contraindications

Idiosyncratic and hypersensitivity reactions occur with the use of loop agents. Acute allergic interstitial nephritis is well documented. It should be remembered that furosemide is a sulfonamide derivative and may demonstrate cross-reactivity in patients who are sensitive to other sulfonamides (ie, antimicrobial drugs used for urinary tract infections, carbonic anhydrase inhibitors, thiazides).

COMBINED USE OF LOOP AGENTS & THIAZIDES

Some patients are refractory to the usual doses of loop agents and are thus vulnerable to dose-related side-effects (eg, ototoxicity) if abnormally large amounts of the drugs are administered. Combinations can be used as an alternative approach if it is established that renal blood flow has not been compromised by prior volume depletion.

Thiazides and loop agents can be shown to inhibit NaCl absorption in the proximal tubule. This effect appears to be independent of any carbonic anhydrase activity of these agents but requires higher luminal concentrations of the drugs than is achieved with normal clinical use.

The proximal effect of thiazides is not usually appreciated, because any increase in NaCl delivery out of the proximal tubule is simply picked up in the next downstream segment; the thick ascending limb has a large capacity to reabsorb NaCl and probably masks any proximal effect of the thiazides. As a result, the usual clinical response to the thiazides is that associated with the inhibition of NaCl reabsorption in the distal convoluted tubule, as described previously. However, when thiazides and loop agents are administered together, a true synergy occurs. Both classes may then increase NaCl delivery out of the proximal tubule. With inhibition of the thick ascending limb by the loop agents and inhibition of the distal convoluted tubule by the thiazides, the overall result is a profound diuretic effect, which is greater than that achieved with either agent alone.

Metolazone seems to be the usual choice of thiazidelike drug in patients refractory to loop agents. If a patient has not responded to a reasonable dose of furosemide (eg, 200 mg), then 5–20 mg of metolazone can be administered along with furosemide. There is no reason to prefer metolazone over any of the other members of the thiazide group. Hydrochlorothiazide, 100 mg, should be as effective as a 20-mg dose of metolazone.

Clinical Indications

Combined use of loop diuretics and thiazides is useful in managing refractory edema or other forms of fluid overload where maximal diuretic efficacy is required. The combination does lessen the dose-dependent side-effects that accompany the use of loop agents alone. For this reason, the combination approach merits consideration. It can be encouraged if it decreases clinical reliance on inappropriately large doses of loop agents.

Toxicity

Very large amounts of fluid can be mobilized in patients who have been refractory to single agents. Routine outpatient use cannot be recommended because of the serious consequences of volume depletion. Potassium wasting is extremely common and requires parenteral K^+ administration with careful monitoring of the fluid and electrolyte status.

POTASSIUM-SPARING DIURETICS

The members of this group antagonize the effects of aldosterone at the cortical collecting tubule. Inhibition may occur by direct antagonism at the level of cytoplasmic mineralocorticoid receptors (spirolactones, including spironolactone and prorenone), by suppression of renin or angiotensin II generation (nonsteroidal anti-inflammatory agents, captopril), or by directly inhibiting Na^+ transport by the collecting tubule (triamterene, amiloride). These agents are used during states of mineralocorticoid excess, due either to primary hypersecretion (Cohn's syndrome, ectopic ACTH production) or to secondary hyperaldosteronism. Congestive heart failure, hepatic cirrhosis, and nephrotic syndrome are conditions associated with renal salt retention and diminished "effective" extracellular volume. Diuretic use contributes to further volume contraction and thereby intensifies secondary hyperaldosteronism. In the setting of enhanced

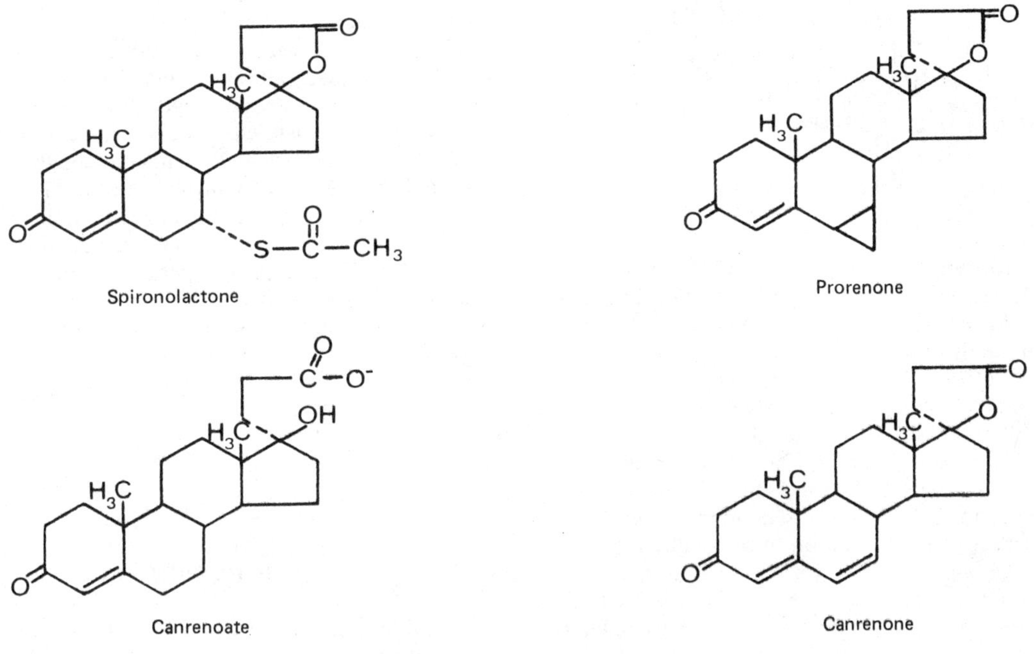

Figure 13–6. Spirolactones.

mineralocorticoid secretion and continuing delivery of Na^+ to distal nephron sites, renal K^+ wasting occurs owing to K^+ secretion at the level of the collecting tubule. Potassium-sparing diuretics, either direct or indirect antagonists of aldosterone, are used in this setting to blunt the K^+ secretory response and prevent depletion of the intracellular K^+ stores.

Pharmacokinetics

Spironolactone, prorenone, and the other spirolactones are synthetic steroids that bind to cytoplasmic mineralocorticoid receptors and prevent translocation of the receptor complex to the nucleus in the target cell. These agents act as competitive antagonists to aldosterone, and their structures are illustrated in Fig 13–6. Their onset and duration of action are therefore determined by the kinetics of aldosterone response in the target tissue. In addition, substantial inactivation of these agents occurs in the liver. The overall result is a rather slow onset of action, requiring several days before full therapeutic effect is achieved.

Triamterene is metabolized in the liver, but renal excretion is a major route of elimination for the active forms and the metabolites. Very little is known about the diuretic effects of the metabolites. **Amiloride** is excreted unchanged in the urine. The structures of triamterene and amiloride are shown in Fig 13–7.

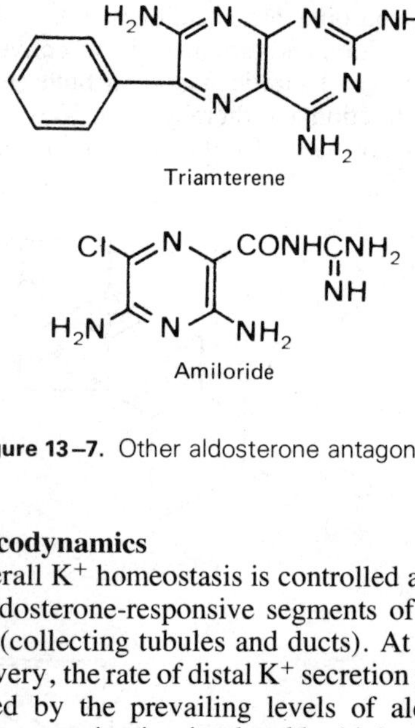

Figure 13–7. Other aldosterone antagonists.

Pharmacodynamics

Overall K^+ homeostasis is controlled at the level of the aldosterone-responsive segments of the distal nephron (collecting tubules and ducts). At any given Na^+ delivery, the rate of distal K^+ secretion is strongly influenced by the prevailing levels of aldosterone. Potassium secretion is stimulated by high aldosterone levels. There appears to be a direct effect of mineralocorticoids on K^+ secretion (or inhibition of K^+ absorption), as well as a secondary effect on Na^+ transport. Sodium absorption in the collecting tubule generates an electrical potential that is lumen-negative. This electrical force stimulates K^+ secretion into the lumen and in this way increases renal K^+ excretion. Aldosterone antagonists decrease the component of K^+ secretion coupled to Na^+ reabsorption and may also inhibit any direct effects of aldosterone on K^+ handling. Similar effects seem to pertain to H^+ handling by the collecting tubule. Aldosterone stimulates H^+ secretion by a direct effect as well as by a secondary effect resulting from the effects of aldosterone on Na^+ transport in this segment.

Analogs & Variants

Converting enzyme inhibitors are discussed in Chapters 9 and 15. Although not used therapeutically as K^+-sparing diuretics, these agents do antagonize the effects of aldosterone by interfering with its secretion. The renal side-effects of these agents can be understood in light of the clinical toxicities of the more traditional aldosterone antagonists.

Toxicity

These agents inhibit renal K^+ and H^+ secretory systems. Hyperkalemia and hyperchloremic metabolic acidosis are dose-related side-effects that occur when aldosterone antagonists are used as the sole diuretic agent. With fixed-dosage combinations of K^+-sparing and thiazide diuretics, there may be a fairly even balance, so that both the hypokalemia and the metabolic alkalosis due to the thiazide are ameliorated by the aldosterone antagonist. However, owing to variations in the bioavailability of the components of some of the fixed-dosage forms, the thiazide-associated side-effects may predominate (eg, metabolic alkalosis, hyponatremia). The clinical value of these combinations has never been adequately documented.

Synthetic steroidal agents may cause endocrine abnormalities by agonist effects on other steroid receptors. Gynecomastia and androgenlike side-effects have been reported with spironolactone.

Contraindications

These agents can cause severe, even fatal hyperkalemia in susceptible patients. Oral K^+ administration should be discontinued if aldosterone antagonists are administered. Patients with chronic renal insufficiency seem especially vulnerable in this regard and should not be treated with aldosterone antagonists. Patients with liver disease may have impaired metabolism of triamterene or spironolactone, and dosing must be carefully adjusted. Since triamterene and amiloride directly inhibit Na^+ transport in the collecting tubule, it follows that a diuretic response can be observed even in the absence of endogenous mineralocorticoid activity.

Dosages & Preparations

See Table 13–3.

AGENTS THAT AFFECT WATER EXCRETION

Antidiuretic hormone (ADH) acts at the collecting tubule to modulate the concentration of the final urine. ADH secretion is reduced during hypotonic

Table 13–3. Potassium-sparing diuretics and combination preparations.

Trade Name	Potassium-Sparing Agent	Hydrochlorothiazide	Frequency of Dosage
Aldactone	Spironolactone 25 mg	. . .	1–4 times daily
Aldactazide	Spironolactone 25 mg	25 mg	1–4 times daily
Dyrenium	Triamterene 100 mg	. . .	1–3 times daily
Diazide	Triamterene 50 mg	25 mg	1–4 times daily
Midamor	Amiloride 5 mg	. . .	Once daily
Moduretic	Amiloride 5 mg	50 mg	Once or twice daily

volume expansion, and large volumes of dilute urine are formed. During volume contraction and in hypertonic conditions, ADH is secreted and urine is concentrated by water abstraction.

It is important to appreciate the central role of the thick ascending limb during concentration as well as dilution of the urine. Urine concentration, modulated by ADH, is driven by the hypertonicity of the medullary interstitium that is generated by the salt transport out of the thick ascending limb and the countercurrent exchange system. Dilution of the urine is accomplished by the same salt transport systems in the thick ascending limb of the loop of Henle. Therefore, *both* concentration and dilution can be inhibited by loop agents, which inhibit salt transport in the thick ascending limb. Thiazides inhibit NaCl transport in segments that dilute the urine but do not contribute to the hypertonic medullary interstitium. Therefore, thiazides inhibit diluting ability but not the ability to maximally concentrate the urine.

Two additional groups that affect the excretion of water need to be specifically considered: osmotic diuretics and ADH antagonists.

Pharmacokinetics

Mannitol is an osmotic diuretic, ie, it obligates the renal excretion of water by virtue of its pharmacokinetic properties. This agent is not metabolized and is handled primarily by glomerular filtration, without any important tubular reabsorption or secretion. By definition, osmotic diuretics are poorly absorbed, which means that they must be given parenterally. If given by mouth, osmotic diarrhea can result. This effect can be used to potentiate the effects of K^+-binding resins or eliminate various toxic substances from the gastrointestinal tract in conjunction with activated charcoal.

ADH antagonists include Li^+ salts and tetracycline derivatives (demeclocycline). Lithium is reabsorbed to some extent in the proximal tubule and thereafter is neither secreted nor absorbed. Demeclocycline is metabolized in the liver.

Pharmacodynamics

Osmotic diuretics primarily limit water reabsorption in those segments of the nephron that are freely permeable to water: proximal tubule, descending limb of the loop, and collecting tubule. The presence of a nonreabsorbable solute such as mannitol prevents the normal absorption of H_2O by interposing a countervailing osmotic force. As a result, urine volume increases in conjunction with mannitol excretion, but natriuresis does not necessarily occur.

ADH antagonists inhibit the effects of ADH at the collecting tubule. This effect occurs at some step following cAMP generation by ADH, since the effects of cAMP itself can be antagonized by these drugs in various model systems.

Clinical Indications & Dosage

Osmotic diuretics are used to increase water excretion in preference to sodium excretion. This effect can be useful when renal hemodynamics are compromised or when avid Na^+ retention limits the response to conventional agents. It can be used to maintain urine volume and to prevent anuria that might otherwise result from presentation of large pigment loads to the kidney (eg, hemolysis or rhabdomyolysis). In oliguric patients, there may be no response to an osmotic diuretic. Therefore, a test dose of mannitol (12.5 g intravenously) is usually given first. Mannitol should not be continued unless there is an increase in urine flow rate to 50 mL/h during the next 3 hours. If there is a response, mannitol can then be given to maintain urine flow rates at about 100 mL/h.

Osmotic diuretics reduce total body water more than total body cation content and thus reduce intracellular volume. This effect is used to reduce intracranial pressure in neurologic conditions and to reduce intraocular pressure before ophthalmologic procedures. Other agents occasionally used include urea, glycerol, and sucrose.

ADH antagonists are clinically used to manage inappropriate ADH secretion syndrome when water restriction has failed to correct the abnormality. Serum levels can be monitored directly for Li^+ therapy, with a serum concentration of 1 mM as a desirable end point. Demeclocycline levels can be approximated by measurement of peak and trough levels using standard tetracycline determinations. In this way, the usual dose (900–1200 mg/d) can be adjusted to achieve a therapeutic serum level of 2 μg/mL.

Toxicity

Mannitol is rapidly distributed in the extracellular compartment and extracts water from the intracellular compartment. Hyponatremia and expansion of the extracellular fluid volume are the predictable consequences. This effect can be disastrous in patients with congestive heart failure and may produce florid pulmonary edema. Headache and nausea and vomiting are commonly observed in patients treated with osmotic diuretics.

The major complications of ADH antagonists relate to their pharmacologic effect. The syndrome of inappropriate ADH secretion is replaced by nephrogenic diabetes insipidus. Renal concentrating ability is abolished, and severe hypernatremia can result. Careful monitoring of the patient's fluid and electrolyte status is required. Side-effects associated with Li^+ therapy include tremulousness, mental obtundation, leukocytosis, and renal tubular acidosis.

II. CLINICAL PHARMACOLOGY OF DIURETICS

EDEMATOUS STATES

Salt and water retention with edema formation generally occurs in response to an "ineffective" arterial blood volume. Excessive diuretic therapy in this setting may lead to further compromise of the "effective" arterial blood volume and exacerbation of organ hypoperfusion. This sequence of events will intensify the homeostatic responses that caused salt retention in the first place. Judicious use of diuretics can mobilize interstitial edema fluid and restore plasma volume. Therefore, the use of diuretics to mobilize edema requires careful monitoring of the patient's hemodynamic status and an understanding of the pathophysiology of the underlying condition.

CONGESTIVE HEART FAILURE

The primary therapeutic goal in congestive heart failure is to improve cardiac function by increasing myocardial contractility. Reduction of pulmonary vascular congestion with diuretics may improve oxygenation and thereby improve myocardial function. On the other hand, if cardiac output is being maintained by high filling pressures, then diuretics may diminish venous return and thereby impair cardiac output. Reducing peripheral vascular resistance and improving cardiac function are more direct approaches to the underlying problem, but diuretic use in this setting should be regarded as an important part of therapy (see Chapter 11).

This issue is especially critical in right ventricular failure. Systemic rather than pulmonary vascular congestion is the hallmark of this disorder. Diuretic-induced volume contraction will predictably reduce venous return ("preload") and can severely compromise cardiac output. Furthermore, diuretic-induced metabolic alkalosis may complicate an underlying compensated respiratory acidosis and produce a mixed acid-base disturbance.

HEPATIC CIRRHOSIS

Liver disease is often associated with edema and with ascites in conjunction with elevated portal hydrostatic pressures and reduced plasma oncotic pressures. Ascites fluid is much more slowly mobilized than peripheral edema. Vigorous diuretic therapy in this setting can cause marked depletion of the "effective" arterial plasma volume, hypokalemia, and metabolic alkalosis. Hepatorenal syndrome and hepatic encephalopathy are particularly unfortunate consequences of overzealous diuretic use. Diuretic therapy can be useful in initiating and maintaining diuresis but must be viewed as an adjunct to the restriction of dietary salt intake and amelioration of the underlying cause of hepatic dysfunction.

NEPHROTIC SYNDROME

Reduction of the "effective" arterial plasma volume in conjunction with reduced plasma oncotic pressures may occur in the nephrotic syndrome. Diuretic use may cause further reductions in plasma volume that can impair glomerular filtration rate and may lead to hypotension and in some cases renal vein thrombosis. Patients with nephrotic syndrome may have expanded plasma volumes and usually present with diminished glomerular filtration rate and hypertension. Diuretic therapy may be beneficial in controlling the volume-dependent component of hypertension and reducing the contribution hypertension may make to their underlying renal disease.

NONEDEMATOUS STATES

HYPERTENSION

A thiazide diuretic is usually the first drug to be used for treating mild essential hypertension. Thiazides can produce adequate control in nearly two-thirds of patients with mild essential hypertension. Careful hemodynamic measurements have demonstrated a fall in peripheral vascular resistance and a sustained fall in plasma volume in patients who respond to chronic thiazide therapy. The importance of sustained plasma volume reduction is emphasized by the finding that liberalization of dietary salt intake can overcome the antihypertensive effects of thiazide therapy. Patients who do not respond to thiazides alone are often managed with one or more peripheral vasodilators. Salt and water retention is a predictable consequence of vasodilator therapy, so continued diuretic therapy is indicated.

Early studies suggested that diuretic therapy may directly reduce peripheral vascular resistance by an effect on vascular smooth muscle. These effects can be demonstrated most convincingly with parenteral administration of diuretics but are not necessarily related to the antihypertensive effect of thiazide diuretics. This issue will probably not be resolved until the cause of increased peripheral vascular resistance in essential hypertension is better understood.

It is worth reemphasizing that sustained reduction of plasma volume is a critical factor in the response to thiazide therapy. It is not practical to measure plasma volumes in all hypertensive patients. However, it may be useful to evaluate dietary salt intake and compliance in patients who do not respond to thiazides. Dietary history and urinary sodium excretion rates will identify patients who overcome the antihypertensive effects of thiazides by increasing salt intake. Patient compliance may be enhanced by once-a-day dosing with a thiazide that has a 12- to 18-hour duration of action (eg, hydrochlorothiazide). This approach matches the diuretic effect with the normal pattern of dietary salt intake.

RENAL POTASSIUM WASTING

Increased levels of aldosterone secretion cause marked renal K^+ secretion when distal Na^+ delivery is increased by diuretics or by high dietary salt intake. Distal H^+ secretion with generation of metabolic alkalosis occurs in the same setting. Recent studies suggest that total body K^+ depletion and hypokalemia may have severe cardiovascular consequences owing to left ventricular irritability. There is considerable controversy over the long-term effects of diuretic-induced K^+ depletion in patients not taking digitalis derivatives. Potassium depletion does cause a reduction in the number of Na^+,K^+-ATPase sites in skeletal muscle and may therefore alter the disposition of cardioactive glycosides. It is well recognized that diuretic-induced K^+ depletion can increase the incidence of digitalis toxicity.

Dietary K^+ supplementation is one approach to managing diuretic-induced K^+ depletion. Unfortunately, this approach is relatively expensive and requires faithful patient compliance, which is particularly hard to achieve in the case of oral KCl administration.

A recent approach emphasizes the importance of dietary Na^+ intake. In the steady state, dietary Na^+ intake will be reflected in the urinary excretion of Na^+. This relationship also pertains to patients chronically taking thiazides or loop diuretics. Once the initial diuresis is completed, the patient should then maintain normal salt balance. Therefore, even in the setting of chronic diuretic therapy, daily excretion of Na^+ is an accurate index of intake. If dietary salt intake is excessive, then distal delivery of Na^+ and urinary excretion of Na^+ will be high and distal K^+ (and H^+) excretion will be stimulated. Moderate restriction of dietary Na^+ intake (60–100 mEq/d) has been shown to potentiate the effects of diuretics in essential hypertension and to lessen renal K^+ wasting. Dietary Na^+ restriction is also indicated in states associated with avid renal Na^+ retention (congestive heart failure, cirrhosis, etc).

Potassium-sparing diuretics are indicated for the patient who has failed to respond to (or comply with) dietary Na^+ restriction or K^+ supplementation. Dietary counseling in the strongest terms should be tried before resorting to additional diuretic intervention.

• • •

References

General

Brenner BM, Rector FC Jr (editors): *The Kidney*, 2nd ed. Saunders, 1981.

Brooks BA, Lant AF: The use of the human erythrocyte as a model for studying the action of diuretics on sodium and chloride transport. *Clin Sci Mol Med* 1978;**54:**679.

Corvol P et al: Mechanism of the antimineralocorticoid effect of spirolactones. *Kidney Int* 1981;**20:**1.

Fries ED: Salt, volume, and hypertension. *Circulation* 1976; **53:**589.

Warnock DG, Eveloff J: NaCl entry mechanisms in the luminal membrane of the renal tubule. *Am J Physiol* 1982; **242:**F561.

Specific Agents

Araoye MA et al: Furosemide compared with hydrochlorothiazide: Long-term treatment of hypertension. *JAMA* 1978; **240:**1863.

Ashraf N, Locksley R, Arieff AI: Thiazide-induced hyponatremia associated with death or neurologic damage in outpatients. *Am J Med* 1981;**70:**1163.

Bear R et al: Effect of metabolic alkalosis on respiratory function in patients with chronic obstructive lung disease. *Can Med Assoc J* 1977;**22:**900.

Block WD, Shiner PT, Roman J: Severe electrolyte disturbances associated with metolazone and furosemide. *South Med J* 1978;**71:**380.

Case DB et al: Proteinuria during long-term captopril therapy. *JAMA* 1980;**244:**346.

DeTroyer A: Demeclocycline: Treatment for syndrome of inappropriate antidiuretic hormone secretion. *JAMA* 1977; **237:**2723.

Epstein M et al: Potentiation of furosemide by metolazone in refractory edema. *Curr Ther Res* 1977;**21:**656.

Greene MK et al: Acetazolamide in prevention of acute mountain sickness: A double-blind controlled cross-over study. *Br Med J* 1981;**283:**811.

Helgeland A et al: Serum triglycerides and serum uric acid in untreated and thiazide-treated patients with mild hypertension. *Am J Med* 1978;**64:**34.

Higashio T, Abe Y, Yamamoto K: Renal effects of bumetanide. *J Pharmacol Exp Ther* 1978;**207:**212.

Holland OB, Nixon JV, Kuhnert L: Diuretic-induced ventricular ectopic activity. *Am J Med* 1981;**70:**762.

Kleinknecht D et al: Furosemide in acute oliguric renal failure: A controlled trial. *Nephron* 1976;**17:**51.

Koechel DA: Ethacrynic acid and related diuretics: Relationship of structure to beneficial and detrimental actions. *Annu Rev Pharmacol Toxicol* 1981;**21:**265.

Levy ST, Forrest JM, Heninger GR: Lithium-induced diabetes insipidus: Manic symptoms, brain and electrolyte correlates, and chlorothiazide treatment. *Am J Psychiatry* 1973; **130:**1014.

MacLeod MD, Bell GM, Irvine WJ: Nephrogenic diabetes insipidus associated with dyazide (triamterene-hydrochlorothiazide). *Br Med J* 1981;**283:**1155.

Multicenter Diuretic Cooperative Study Group: Multiclinic comparison of amiloride, hydrochlorothiazide, and hydrochlorothiazide plus amiloride in essential hypertension. *Arch Intern Med* 1981;**141:**482.

Ram CVS, Garrett B, Kaplan NM: Moderate sodium restriction and various diuretics in the treatment of hypertension: Effects of potassium wastage and blood pressure control. *Arch Intern Med* 1981;**141:**1015.

Tan SY et al: Indomethacin-induced prostaglandin inhibition with hyperkalemia: A reversible cause of hyporeninemic hypoaldosteronism. *Ann Intern Med* 1979;**90:**783.

Tannenbaum PJ et al: The influence of dosage form on the activity of a diuretic agent. *Clin Pharmacol Exp Ther* 1968; **9:**598.

Tobert JA et al: Enhancement of uricosuric properties of indacrinone by manipulation of the enantiomer ratio. *Clin Pharmacol Ther* 1981;**29:**344.

Van Brummelen P, Woerlee M, Schalekamp MA: Long-term versus short-term effects of hydrochlorothiazide on renal haemodynamics in essential hypertension. *Clin Sci* 1979; **56:**463.

Warren SE, Blantz RC: Mannitol. *Arch Intern Med* 1981; **141:**493.

Histamine, Serotonin, & the Ergot Alkaloids | 14

Alan Burkhalter, PhD, & Oscar L. Frick, MD, PhD

Histamine and serotonin (5-hydroxytryptamine) are biologically active amines that are found in many tissues and have complex physiologic and pathologic effects. Together with endogenous polypeptides (Chapter 15) and prostaglandins (Chapter 16), they are sometimes called **autacoids** (Greek "self-remedy") or local hormones in recognition of these properties.

The roles of histamine and serotonin in normal physiology are not understood, and these compounds have no clinical application in the treatment of disease. However, compounds that selectively antagonize the actions of these amines are of considerable clinical usefulness. This chapter therefore emphasizes the basic pharmacology of the agonist amines and the clinical pharmacology of the antagonists. The ergot alkaloids, compounds with partial agonist activity at serotonin (and other) receptors, are discussed at the end of the chapter.

HISTAMINE

Histamine was synthesized in 1907 and later isolated from mammalian tissues. Early hypotheses concerning the possible physiologic roles of tissue histamine were based on similarities between histamine's actions and the symptoms of anaphylactic shock and tissue injury. Marked species variation has been observed, but in humans histamine is an important mediator of immediate allergic reactions, has an important role in gastric acid secretion, and, according to recent evidence, functions as a neurotransmitter in certain areas of the brain.

I. BASIC PHARMACOLOGY OF HISTAMINE

Chemistry & Pharmacokinetics

Histamine is 2-(4-imidazolyl)ethylamine (Fig 14–1). It occurs in plants as well as in animal tissues and is a component of many venoms and stinging secretions.

Histamine is formed by decarboxylation of the amino acid L-histidine, a reaction catalyzed in mammalian tissues by the enzyme histidine decarboxylase (Fig 14–1). Pyridoxal phosphate is required as cofactor. Once formed, histamine is either stored or rapidly inactivated by one of 2 amine oxidase enzymes and by methylation. Very little histamine is excreted unchanged. Certain tumors (systemic mastocytosis, urticaria pigmentosa, gastric carcinoid, and occasionally myelogenous leukemia) are associated with increased numbers of mast cells or basophils and with increased excretion of histamine and its metabolites.

Although histamine is found in most tissues, it is very unevenly distributed. Most tissue histamine exists in bound form in granules in mast cells or basophils; the histamine content of many tissues is directly related to their mast cell content. The bound form of histamine is biologically inactive, but many stimuli, as noted below, can trigger the release of mast cell histamine, allowing the free amine to exert its actions on surrounding tissues.

Non-mast cell histamine is found in several tissues including the brain. Both regional and intracellular distribution of brain histamine supports the possibility of transmitter or modulator function, especially in those parts of the brain concerned with temperature regulation.

Storage and release of histamine. In human mast cells and basophils, storage granules contain histamine complexed with the sulfated polysaccharide, heparin, and an acidic protein. The bound form of histamine can be released through several mechanisms. Certain amines, including drugs such as morphine and tubocurarine, can displace histamine from the heparin-protein complex. This type of release does not require energy and is not associated with mast cell injury or degranulation. Loss of granules from the mast cell will also release histamine, since sodium ions in the extracellular fluid rapidly displace the amine from the complex. Chemical and mechanical mast cell injury causes degranulation and histamine release.

More specific mechanisms also cause histamine release. Compound 48/80, a diamine polymer, specifically releases histamine from tissue mast cells by an exocytotic degranulation process requiring energy and calcium. The important pathophysiologic mechanism

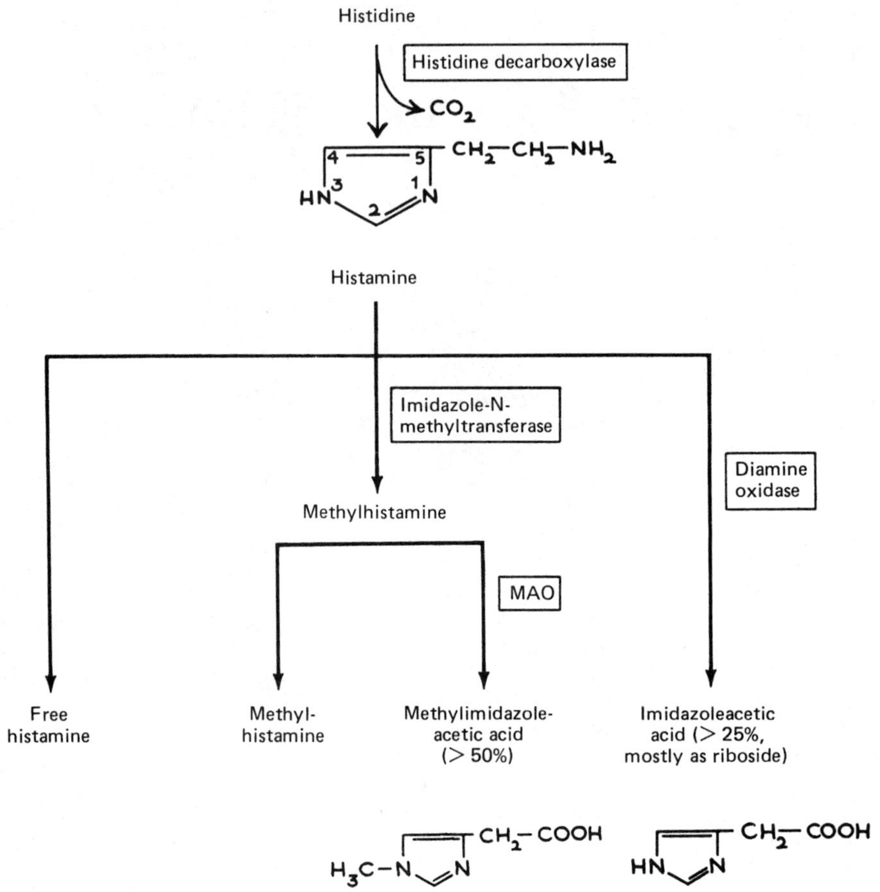

Figure 14–1. Synthesis, metabolism, and common urinary metabolites of histamine. (Modified and reproduced, with permission, from Meyers FH, Jawetz E, Goldfien A: *Review of Medical Pharmacology,* 7th ed. Lange, 1980.)

of histamine release is immunologic. Mast cells and basophils, if sensitized by IgE antibodies attached to their surface membranes, degranulate when exposed to the appropriate antigen. This type of release also requires energy and calcium. Degranulated mast cells will reaccumulate histamine over a period of days to weeks. Histamine released by this mechanism is a mediator in immediate (type I) allergic reactions. Substances released during IgG- or IgM-mediated immune reactions that activate the complement cascade also release histamine from mast cells and basophils.

By a negative feedback control mechanism, histamine appears to modulate the further release of histamine from sensitized mast cells. Thus, histamine may act to limit an allergic reaction by inhibiting the release of histamine and other mediators of the response (see Chapters 16 and 17).

Pharmacodynamics

A. Mechanism of Action: Histamine exerts its biologic actions by combining with specific cellular receptors located in or on the surface membrane. The actions of histamine antagonists indicate that there are at least 2 distinct types of receptors: $\mathbf{H_1}$ and $\mathbf{H_2}$. Responses at both types of receptors may involve alterations in membrane permeability to calcium or release of calcium from internal stores. Responses mediated by H_2 receptors have been convincingly shown to involve an elevation of intracellular cAMP. Less compelling evidence suggests an association of elevated cGMP with activation of H_1 receptors. It is not known whether these cyclic nucleotide alterations represent a cause or an effect of the changes in intracellular calcium concentration.

B. Tissue and Organ System Effects of Histamine: Histamine exerts powerful effects on smooth and cardiac muscle, on certain endothelial and nerve cells, and on the secretory cells of the stomach. However, sensitivity to histamine varies greatly among species. Humans, guinea pigs, dogs, and cats are quite sensitive, while mice and rats are much less so.

1. Cardiovascular system–In humans, injection or infusion of histamine causes a decrease in systolic and diastolic blood pressure and an increase in heart rate (Fig 14–2). The acute blood pressure changes are caused by the direct vasodilator action of histamine on

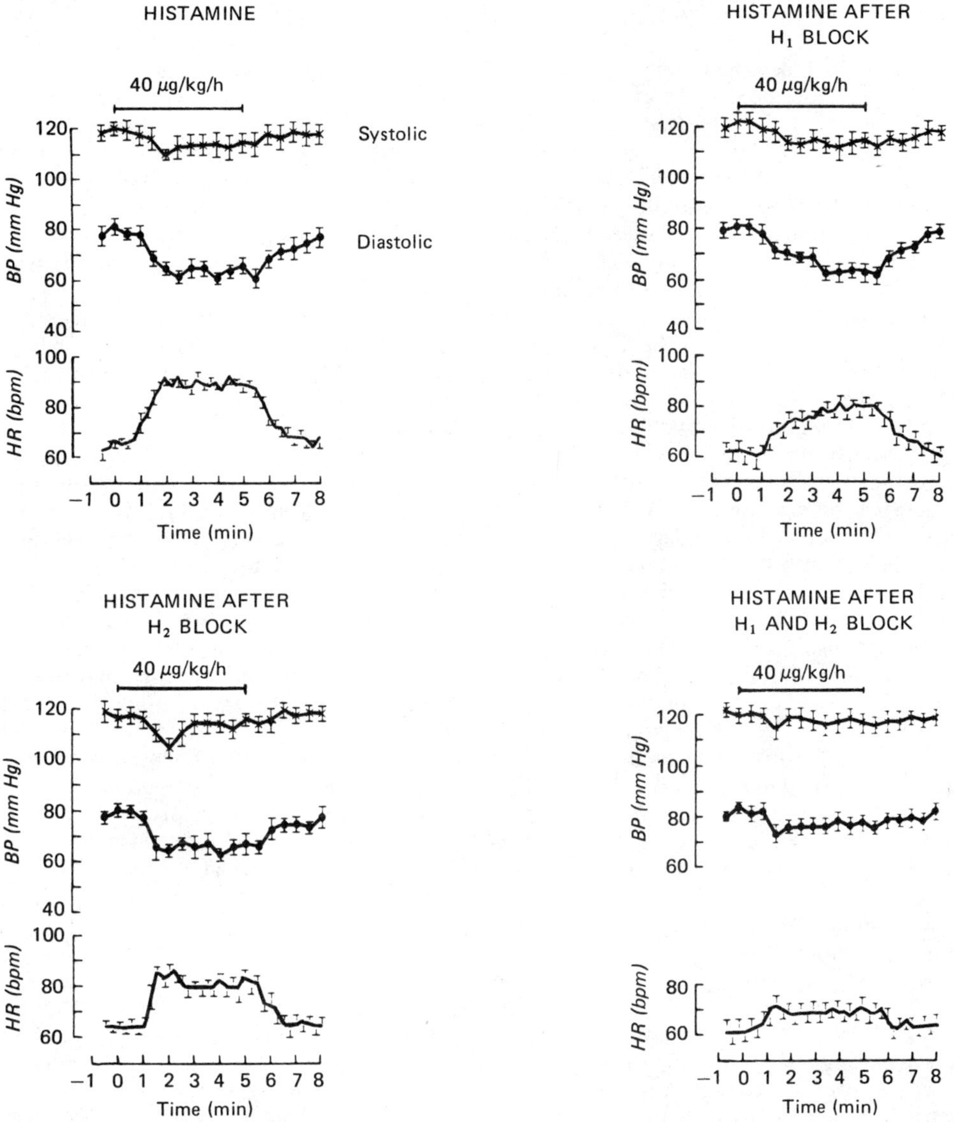

Figure 14–2. Effects of histamine and histamine antagonists on blood pressure and heart rate in humans. Histamine was infused at 40 µg/kg/h for 5 minutes as shown at the top of each panel. The H_1 antagonist was chlorpheniramine (10 mg intravenously). The H_2 antagonist was cimetidine (200 mg intravenously). (Modified and reproduced, with permission, from Torsoli A, Lucchelli PE, Brinblecombe RW [editors]: *H_2 Antagonists: H_2-Receptor Antagonists in Peptic Ulcer Disease and Progress in Histamine Research.* Excerpta Medica, 1980.)

arterioles and precapillary sphincters; the increase in heart rate involves both stimulatory actions of histamine on the heart and a reflex tachycardia. Flushing, a sense of warmth, and headache may also occur during histamine administration, consistent with the arteriolar dilating effect. Studies with histamine receptor antagonists show that both H_1 and H_2 receptors are involved in these cardiovascular responses to high doses, since a combination of H_1 and H_2 receptor-blocking agents is more effective in preventing the actions of histamine than either blocking agent alone (Fig 14–2). However, in humans, the cardiovascular effects of small doses of histamine can usually be antagonized by H_1 receptor antagonists alone.

Edema results from the action of histamine on H_1 receptors in the vessels of the microcirculation, especially the postcapillary vessels. The effect is associated with an increase in permeability of the vessel wall that has been ascribed to the separation of the endothelial cells, thus permitting the transudation of fluid and molecules as large as small proteins into the perivascular tissue. This effect is responsible for the urticaria (hives) that signals the intradermal release of histamine.

Direct cardiac effects of histamine include both increased contractility and increased pacemaker rate.

These effects are mediated chiefly by H_2 receptors. Their physiologic significance is unknown.

These cardiovascular effects may also be produced by the release of endogenous histamine from mast cells. Many of the cardiovascular signs and symptoms of anaphylaxis are due to released histamine, although other mediators are also involved.

2. Gastrointestinal tract smooth muscle–Histamine causes contraction of intestinal smooth muscle, and histamine-induced contraction of guinea pig ileum is a standard bioassay for histamine. The human gut is not as sensitive as that of the guinea pig, but large doses of histamine may cause diarrhea, partly as a result of this effect. This action of histamine is mediated by H_1 receptors.

3. Bronchiolar smooth muscle–Histamine causes bronchoconstriction. In the guinea pig, this effect is the cause of death from histamine toxicity, but in normal humans, bronchoconstriction following the usual doses of histamine is not marked. However, patients with bronchial asthma are very sensitive to histamine. The bronchoconstriction induced in these patients probably represents a hyperactive neural response, since they also respond excessively to many other stimuli, and the response can be blocked by autonomic blocking drugs such as ganglionic blocking agents as well as by H_1 receptor antagonists (Chapter 17). Inhalation provocation tests using increasing doses of histamine are of diagnostic value for bronchial hyperreactivity in patients with suspected asthma or cystic fibrosis. Such individuals may be 100- to 1000-fold more sensitive to histamine than normal individuals.

4. Other smooth muscle organs–In humans, histamine has insignificant effects on the smooth muscle of the eye and genitourinary tract, but in some species the effects on the uterus are of sufficient magnitude to form the basis for a bioassay.

5. Nerve endings–Histamine is a powerful stimulant of sensory nerve endings, especially those mediating pain and itching. This H_1-mediated effect is an important component of the urticarial response and reactions to insect and nettle stings. Some evidence suggests that local high concentrations can also depolarize efferent (axonal) nerve endings (see ¶ 7, below).

6. Secretory tissue–Histamine has long been recognized as a powerful stimulant of gastric acid secretion and, to a lesser extent, of gastric pepsin and intrinsic factor production. The effect is caused by activation of H_2 receptors on the parietal cells and is associated with increased adenylate cyclase activity and cAMP concentration. Other stimulants of gastric acid secretion such as acetylcholine and gastrin do not increase cAMP even though their maximal effects on acid output can be reduced—but not abolished—by H_2 receptor antagonists.

Histamine has insignificant effects on the activity of other glandular tissue at ordinary concentrations. Very high concentrations can cause adrenal medullary discharge.

7. The "triple response"–Intradermal injection of histamine causes a characteristic wheal-and-flare response first described over 50 years ago. The effect involves 3 separate cell types: microcirculatory smooth muscle, capillary or venular endothelium, and sensory nerve endings. At the site of injection, a reddening appears due to dilatation of small vessels, followed soon by an edematous wheal at the injection site and a red irregular flare surrounding the wheal. The flare is said to be caused by an axon reflex. As noted above, histamine stimulates nerve endings; the resulting impulses are thought to travel through other branches of the same axon, causing vasodilatation. The sensation of itch may also accompany the appearance of these effects. The wheal is due to local edema.

Similar local effects may be produced by injecting histamine liberators (compound 48/80, morphine, etc) intradermally or by applying the appropriate antigens to the skin of a sensitized person. Although most of these local effects can be blocked by prior administration of an H_1 receptor-blocking agent, H_2 receptors may also be involved.

Other Histamine Agonists

Small substitutions on the imidazole ring of histamine significantly modify the H_1 and H_2 selectivity of the compound. For example, 2-methylhistamine is relatively more specific for H_1 receptors, while 4-methylhistamine is a relatively specific H_2 agonist. The structures of two H_2-selective agents are shown below. **Betazole** is a drug used in testing gastric acid-secreting ability; **impromidine** is an experimental compound highly specific for H_2 receptors. **Clonidine,** an antihypertension drug, has selective H_2-activating effects; it has been proposed—thus far without convincing evidence—that its hypotensive effects result from selective activation of H_2 receptors in the brain (Chapter 9).

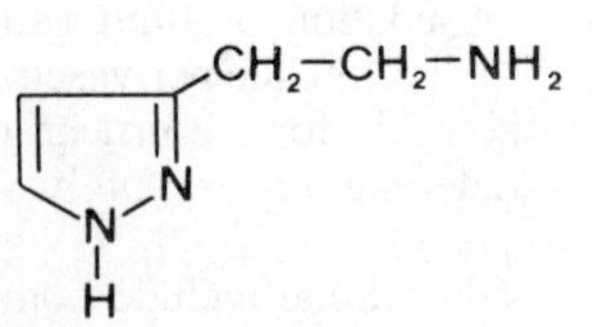

Betazole

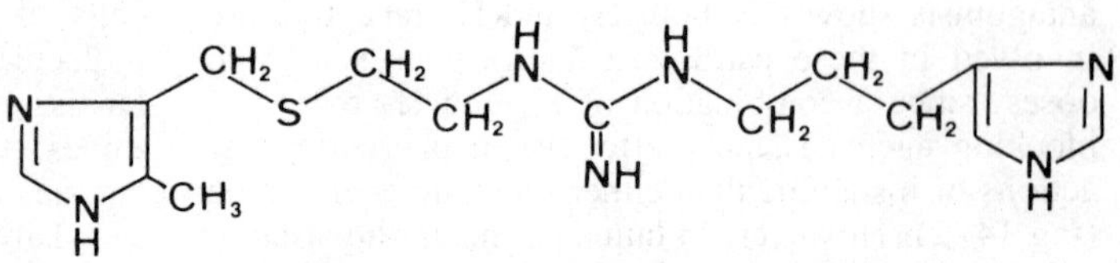

Impromidine

II. CLINICAL PHARMACOLOGY OF HISTAMINE

Clinical Uses

A. Testing Gastric Acid Secretion: The primary clinical use for histamine and its analogs is as a diagnostic agent in testing for gastric acid-secreting ability. Lack of an increase in acid secretion following histamine is consistent with a diagnosis of achlorhydria. Other possible diagnostic agents include gastrin or its analogs and the more selective H_2 agonists. Currently, betazole (Histalog) is the only alternative agonist available in the USA.

Use of histamine for this purpose involves injecting histamine phosphate, 2.75 mg subcutaneously, and measuring gastric acid secretion over the next 30–60 minutes. Other effects of histamine that are noted following this dose are flushing, hypotension, headache, and the appearance of wheals (hives, urticarial lesions) on the skin. These effects can be reduced by the simultaneous administration of an H_1 antagonist drug or (preferably) by substitution of betazole for histamine. Betazole hydrochloride, 0.5 mg/kg, or as a fixed dose of 50 mg, is given intramuscularly or subcutaneously. Though more selective than histamine as an H_2 agonist, it is not devoid of H_1 effects; use of an H_1 antagonist drug may be indicated.

B. Diagnosis of Pheochromocytoma: Histamine can cause release of catecholamines from adrenal medullary cells. Although this effect is not prominent in normal humans, massive release can occur in patients with pheochromocytoma. The response is caused partially by direct release of catecholamines and partly by an exaggerated overshoot in the homeostatic response to histamine-induced hypotension. This hazardous provocative test is now obsolete, since chemical assays are available for determination of the catecholamines and their metabolites in patients suspected of having this tumor.

Toxicity & Contraindications

Adverse effects following administration of histamine are dose-related. Flushing, hypotension, tachycardia, headache, wheals, bronchoconstriction, and gastrointestinal upset are noted.

Histamine should not be given to asthmatics or patients with active ulcer disease or gastrointestinal bleeding.

• • •

HISTAMINE ANTAGONISTS

The effects of histamine released in the body can be reduced in several ways. **Physiologic antagonists,** especially epinephrine, have smooth muscle actions opposite to those of histamine but act at different receptors. This is important clinically, because injection of epinephrine can be lifesaving in systemic anaphylaxis and in other conditions in which massive histamine release occurs.

Release inhibitors reduce the degranulation of mast cells and basophils that results from immunologic triggering of antigen-IgE interaction. Cromolyn appears to have this effect (Chapter 17) and is used in the treatment of asthma. $Beta_2$-adrenergic stimulant agents also appear capable of reducing histamine release.

Histamine **receptor antagonists** represent a third approach to the reduction of histamine-mediated responses. For over 40 years, compounds have been available that competitively antagonize many of the actions of histamine on smooth muscle. However, not until the H_2 receptor antagonist burimamide was described in 1972 was it possible to antagonize the gastric acid-stimulating activity of histamine. The development of selective H_2 receptor antagonists has led not only to more precise definition of histamine's actions in terms of receptors involved but also to more effective therapy of peptic ulcer.

H_1 Receptor Antagonists

When used without a modifying adjective, the word ''antihistamine'' refers to H_1 receptor antagonists. Compounds that competitively block histamine at H_1 receptor sites have been used clinically for many years, and over thirty H_1 antagonists are currently available in the USA. They are prescribed by physicians and are present in many nonprescription formulations such as ''cold pills'' and sleep aids (Chapter 64).

I. BASIC PHARMACOLOGY OF H_1 RECEPTOR ANTAGONISTS

Chemistry & Pharmacokinetics

The H_1 antagonists are stable lipid-soluble amines having the general structure illustrated in Fig 14–3. There are several chemical subgroups, and the structures of compounds representing different subgroups are shown in the figure. A listing of some of the available drugs is given in Table 14–1.

Most of these agents are similar with respect to absorption and distribution. They are rapidly absorbed following oral administration, with peak blood concentrations occurring in 1–2 hours. They are widely distributed throughout the body, including the central nervous system. They are extensively metabolized, primarily by microsomal systems in the liver. Most of the drugs have an effective duration of action of 4–6 hours following a single dose, but meclizine is longer-acting, with a duration of action of 12–24 hours.

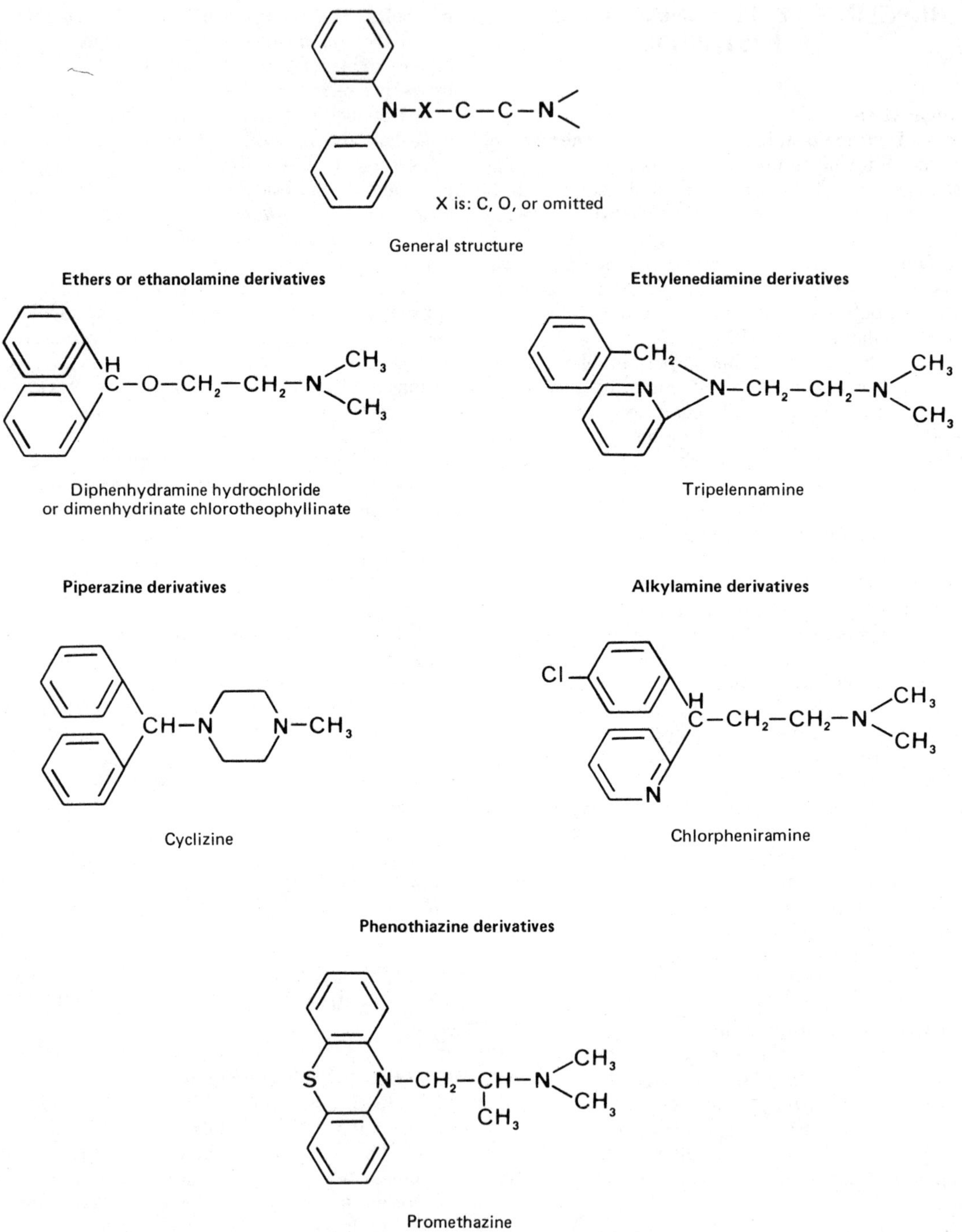

Figure 14–3. General structure of H_1 antagonist drugs and examples of the major subgroups.

Pharmacodynamics

A. Histamine Receptor Blockade: H_1 receptor antagonists block the actions of histamine by reversible, competitive antagonism at the H_1 receptor. They have negligible potency at the H_2 receptor. Therefore, the ability of these drugs to block a histamine action depends not only on the concentration of agonist and antagonist but also on the degree to which the action is mediated by H_1 receptors. For example, histamine-induced contraction of bronchiolar or gastrointestinal smooth muscle can be completely blocked by these agents, while the effects of histamine on the cardiovascular system are only partly blocked because of H_2 receptor-mediated actions (Fig 14–2). H_1 receptor

Table 14–1. Some H_1 antihistaminic drugs in clinical use.

Drug	Usual Adult Dose	Comments
Ethanolamines		
Carbinoxamine (Clistin)	4–8 mg	Slight to moderate sedation.
Dimenhydrinate (8-chlorotheophylline salt of diphenhydramine) (Dramamine, etc)	50 mg	Marked sedation; anti-motion sickness activity.
Diphenhydramine (Benadryl, etc)	25–50 mg	Marked sedation; anti-motion sickness activity.
Doxylamine (Decapryn)	1.25–25 mg	Marked sedation; anti-motion sickness activity.
Phenyltoloxamine (Histionex)	25–50 mg	Moderate sedation; component of OTC "sleep aids."
Ethylenediamines		
Antazoline (Vasocon-A)	1–2 drops	Ophthalmic solution.
Pyrilamine (Neo-Antergan)	25–50 mg	Moderate sedation; component of OTC "sleep aids."
Tripelennamine (PBZ)	25–50 mg	Moderate sedation.
Piperazine derivatives		
Chlorcyclizine (Perazil)	25–50 mg	Slight sedation; anti-motion sickness activity.
Cyclizine (Marezine)	25–50 mg	Slight sedation; anti-motion sickness activity.
Meclizine (Bonine, etc)	25–50 mg	Slight sedation; anti-motion sickness activity.
Alkylamines		
Brompheniramine (Dimetane)	4–8 mg	Slight sedation.
Chlorpheniramine (Chlortrimeton)	4–8 mg	Slight sedation; common component of OTC "cold" medication.
Dexbrompheniramine (Disomer)	2–4 mg	Slight sedation; active isomer of brompheniramine.
Dexchlorpheniramine (Polaramine)	2–4 mg	Slight sedation; active isomer of chlorpheniramine.
Pheniramine (Trimeton)	25–50 mg	Slight sedation.
Phenothiazine derivatives		
Promethazine (Phenergan)	10–25 mg	Marked sedation; antiemetic and antimuscarinic activity.
Miscellaneous		
Cyproheptadine (Periactin)	4 mg	Moderate sedation; also has antiserotonin activity.
Phenindamine (Thephorin)	25 mg	May cause stimulation.

antagonists block most of the local tissue effects, including the increase in capillary permeability and the axon reflex-mediated flare. H_2 receptor-mediated actions such as the increase in gastric acid secretion and inhibition of histamine release from mast cells are unaffected.

B. Actions Not Caused by Histamine Receptor Blockade: The H_1 receptor antagonists have many actions not ascribable to blockade of the actions of histamine. The large number of these actions probably results from the similarity of the H_1 antagonist general structure (Fig 14–3) to the structure of drugs that have effects at muscarinic cholinergic, alpha-adrenergic, serotonin, and local anesthetic receptor sites. Some of these actions are of therapeutic value and some are undesirable.

1. Sedation–The most common side-effect of H_1 antagonists is sedation, but the intensity of this action varies among chemical subgroups (Table 14–1) and among patients as well. The effect is sufficiently prominent with some agents to make them useful as "sleep aids" (Chapter 64) and unsuitable for daytime use. The effect resembles that of some antimuscarinic drugs and is considered very unlike the disinhibited sedation produced by sedative-hypnotic drugs. At ordinary dosages, children occasionally (and adults rarely) manifest excitation rather than sedation. At very high toxic dose levels, marked stimulation, agitation, and even convulsions may precede coma.

2. Nausea and vomiting–Several H_1 antagonists have significant activity in preventing motion sickness (Table 14–1). They are less effective against an episode of motion sickness already present. Certain H_1 antagonists, notably doxylamine (in Bendectin), have been used widely in the treatment of nausea and vomiting of pregnancy (see below).

3. Antiparkinsonism effects–Perhaps because of their anticholinergic effects (cf benztropine, Chapter 25), some of the H_1 antagonists have significant acute suppressant effects on the parkinsonismlike syndromes associated with certain antipsychotic drugs (Chapter 26).

4. Anticholinergic actions–Many of the H_1 antagonists, especially those of the ethanolamine and ethylenediamine subgroups, have significant atropinelike effects on peripheral muscarinic receptors. This action may be responsible for some of the (uncertain) benefits reported for nonallergic rhinorrhea but also may cause urinary retention and blurred vision.

5. Antiadrenergic actions–Weak alpha receptor-blocking effects can be demonstrated for many H_1 antagonists, especially those in the phenothiazine subgroup. This action may cause orthostatic hypotension in susceptible individuals.

6. Antiserotonin action–Strong blocking effects at serotonin receptors have been demonstrated for some H_1 antagonists, notably cyproheptadine. This drug is promoted as an antiserotonin agent and is discussed with that drug group. Nevertheless, it has a chemical structure that resembles the phenothiazine antihistamines and is a potent H_1 blocking agent.

7. Local anesthesia–Most of the H_1 antagonists are effective local anesthetics. They block sodium channels in excitable membranes in the same fashion as procaine and lidocaine. Diphenhydramine and promethazine are actually more potent as local anesthetics than is procaine. They are occasionally used to produce local anesthesia in patients allergic to the conventional local anesthetic drugs.

II. CLINICAL PHARMACOLOGY OF H_1 RECEPTOR ANTAGONISTS

Clinical Uses

A. Allergic Reactions: The H_1 antihistaminic agents are often the first drugs used to prevent allergic reactions or to treat their symptoms. In allergic rhinitis and urticaria, in which histamine is the primary mediator, the H_1 antagonists are the drugs of choice and are often quite effective. However, in bronchial asthma, which involves several mediators, the H_1 antagonists are largely ineffective (Chapter 17).

Angioedema may be precipitated by histamine-induced edema but appears to be maintained by bradykinins that are not affected by antihistaminic agents. For atopic dermatitis, antihistaminic drugs such as diphenhydramine are used mostly for their sedative side-effects and for some control of the itching.

The H_1 antihistamines used for treating allergic conditions are usually prescribed with the goal of minimizing sedative side-effects; the drugs in widest use are the alkylamines. However, this effect and the therapeutic efficacy of different agents vary widely among individuals, so it is common practice to give a patient samples from each major group to determine which is the most effective with the least side-effects. In addition, the clinical effectiveness of one group may diminish with continued use, and switching to another group may restore drug effectiveness for as yet unexplained reasons.

B. Motion Sickness and Vestibular Disturbances: Scopolamine and certain H_1 antagonists are the most effective agents available for the prevention of motion sickness. The antihistaminic drugs with the greatest effectiveness in this application are diphenhydramine and promethazine. The piperazines also have significant activity in preventing motion sickness and are less sedative in most patients. Dosage is the same as that recommended for allergic disorders (Table 14–1). Both scopolamine and the H_1 antagonists are more effective in preventing motion sickness when combined with ephedrine or amphetamine.

It is claimed that the antihistaminic agents effective in prophylaxis of motion sickness are also useful in Meniere's syndrome.

C. Nausea and Vomiting of Pregnancy: Several H_1 antagonist drugs have been studied for possible use in treating "morning sickness." The piperazine derivatives were withdrawn from such use when it was demonstrated that they have teratogenic effects in rodents. Doxylamine, an ethanolamine H_1 antagonist, is still promoted for this application as a component of Bendectin, a prescription medication that also contains pyridoxine. The question of fetal malformation resulting from this use of Bendectin is discussed below. In view of the weak evidence for the effectiveness of the drug in this condition, the use of Bendectin in vomiting of pregnancy should probably be discouraged.

Toxicity

The spectrum of side-effects of the H_1 antihistamines is described above. Several of these effects (sedation, anticholinergic action) have been used for therapeutic purposes, especially in OTC remedies (Chapter 64). Nevertheless, these 2 effects constitute the most common undesirable actions when these drugs are used to block histamine receptors. Appropriate selection of drugs with a lower incidence of these effects (Table 14–1) and trial of several drugs by the patient are the most effective methods for minimizing both toxicities.

Less common toxic effects of systemic use include excitation and convulsion in children, postural hypotension, and allergic responses. Drug allergy is relatively common, however, after topical use of H_1 antagonists. The effects of severe systemic overdosage resemble those of atropine overdosage and are treated in the same way (Chapters 6 and 58).

Possible teratogenic effects of doxylamine have been widely publicized in the lay press since 1978 as a result of case reports of fetal malformation associated with maternal ingestion of Bendectin. However, several large surveys, numbering over 60,000 pregnancies of which more than 3000 involved maternal Bendectin ingestion, detected no increase in the incidence of birth defects. In contrast, several case analysis studies of infants with malformations have suggested a weak correlation between Bendectin use and abnormalities. One clinical epidemiologic survey, supported by an experimental study in rodents, suggests that the incidence of congenital diaphragmatic hernia may be increased by maternal ingestion of doxylamine during the first trimester. Our inability to define the existence and extent of risk in this situation illustrates the difficulties involved in detecting small changes in the incidence of rare pathologic events.

H_2 Receptor Antagonists

The development of H_2 receptor antagonists, beginning in 1972, led to renewed interest in possible physiologic roles for histamine and to a classification of effects and both agonists and antagonists based upon histamine receptor subtypes. The frequency of peptic ulcer disease and related gastrointestinal complaints created great interest in the therapeutic potential of H_2 receptor antagonists. The ability to reduce gastric acid secretion has made cimetidine, the currently available member of this class, one of the most frequently prescribed drugs in the USA.

I. BASIC PHARMACOLOGY OF H_2 RECEPTOR ANTAGONISTS

Chemistry & Pharmacokinetics

The first two H_2 receptor antagonists, burimamide and metiamide, were imidazole com-

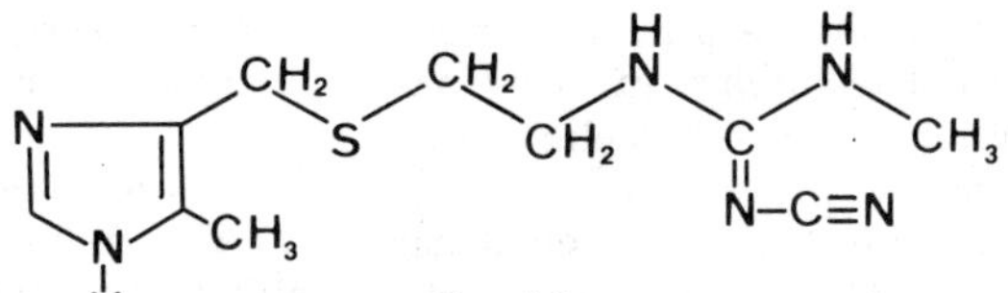

Cimetidine

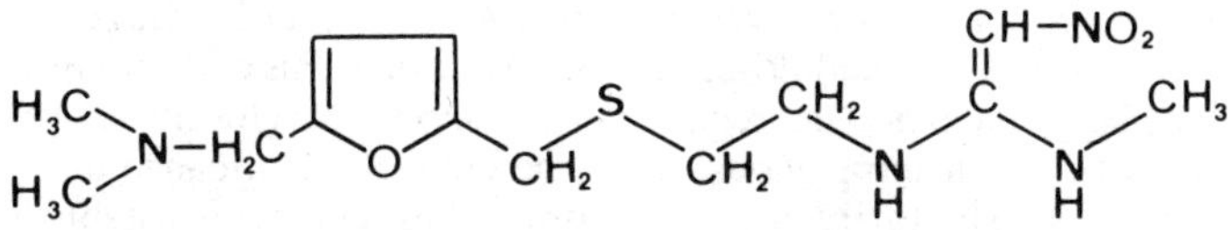

Ranitidine

pounds with long side chains containing a thiourea group. Burimamide was poorly absorbed after oral administration. Metiamide was well absorbed but, like many thiourea derivatives, caused blood dyscrasias (granulocytopenia) and was withdrawn from clinical use. Cimetidine, the third imidazole derivative of the series, lacks the thiourea moiety and appears to be relatively free of the granulocytopenic action of its predecessor. Ranitidine and tiotidine are potent experimental H_2 antagonists with neither imidazole nor thiourea moieties. Their long-term toxicity is not yet known (see below).

Cimetidine is well absorbed following oral administration, and peak plasma levels are observed 1–2 hours following each dose. The half-life of cimetidine in humans is approximately 2 hours, and the apparent volume of distribution is 2 L/kg. The drug is widely distributed, crosses the placenta, and has been detected in breast milk. Cimetidine is excreted mostly unchanged. Ranitidine has a slightly longer half-life and a slightly larger volume of distribution than cimetidine.

Pharmacodynamics

A. Mechanism of Action: Cimetidine and other known H_2 receptor antagonists reversibly compete with histamine at H_2 receptor sites. This action is quite selective in that the H_2 antagonists do not affect H_1 receptor-mediated actions. Conversely, the H_1 antagonists have no effect at H_2 receptors.

B. Organ System Effects:

1. Acid secretion and gastric motility–The most important action of H_2 receptor antagonists is to reduce the secretion of gastric acid. Cimetidine blocks the acid secretion stimulated by histamine, gastrin, cholinergic drugs, and vagal stimulation. The volume of gastric secretion and the concentration of pepsin are also reduced. While the ability of H_2 receptor antagonists to inhibit all phases of acid secretion has been interpreted as implicating histamine as a final common mediator of acid secretion, a more plausible hypothesis suggests that the full expression of stimuli such as gastrin and cholinergic impulses requires the participation of histamine in some manner.

Cimetidine has little effect on gastric smooth muscle function and on lower esophageal sphincter pressure. Other gastrointestinal secretions are not significantly reduced.

2. Other effects related to H_2 receptor blockade–In doses that suppress gastric acid secretion, cimetidine has little effect on the heart or on blood pressure. This observation is consistent with the idea that histamine has little role in the normal regulation of the cardiovascular system. However, as shown in Fig 14–2, cimetidine is effective in reducing the actions of administered histamine on the heart and vessels.

It has been predicted that H_2 receptor antagonists may enhance certain immune responses by blocking histamine's ability to decrease mediator release from mast cells and basophils; *experimentally,* increases in delayed hypersensitivity reactions can be shown in some patients receiving cimetidine. However, there is no evidence that clinical hypersensitivity reactions are increased in such patients.

II. CLINICAL PHARMACOLOGY OF H2 RECEPTOR ANTAGONISTS

Clinical Uses

A. Peptic Ulcer Disease: It is estimated that at least 10% of adults in the western world will suffer an active episode of peptic ulcer disease during their lifetimes. Although the mortality rate of this condition is low, the recurrence rate is high and the socioeconomic cost is great. It has long been known that "no acid = no ulcer," and medical therapy has focused on reducing acidity by the use of anticholinergic drugs and antacids. Anticholinergic drugs must be used in high doses that are associated with significant adverse effects. Antacids will relieve symptoms and, in high doses, can promote healing. However, very frequent dosing is required (Chapter 62), and compliance is poor except during the acute symptomatic phase of the disease. The effectiveness of cimetidine in reducing gastric acidity coupled with apparent low acute toxicity represents a significant advance in the treatment of this disease. Results of many clinical trials show that cimetidine is very effective in controlling symptoms during acute episodes and in promoting healing of duodenal ulcers. Prophylactic use at reduced dosage may prevent recurrence in many patients. Surgery for peptic ulcer patients is declining as a result of cimetidine therapy.

In the short-term treatment of active duodenal ulcer, cimetidine, 0.9–1.6 g/d, is given orally in divided doses. The dose should be less than this in elderly patients to minimize central nervous system toxicity. Following the acute phase, reduced dosage, eg, 400 mg at bedtime, may be given to prevent recurrence. Cimetidine may also be given intravenously. Almost all patients respond satisfactorily to oral cimetidine; the reasons for refractoriness in a few are unknown.

B. Zollinger-Ellison Syndrome: In this disorder, which may be rapidly fatal, hypersecretion of acid is due to a gastrin-secreting tumor. In many patients, cimetidine is effective in controlling symptoms related to excess acid secretion. The drug can be used in preparation for surgery or as primary treatment when surgery is not indicated.

C. Other Hypersecretion Conditions: In patients with systemic mastocytosis or basophilic leukemia associated with high blood histamine levels, cimetidine may be useful in controlling symptoms mediated by H_2 receptors. In other conditions in which the drug is used, such as reflux esophagitis, hiatal hernia, stress-induced ulcers, and iatrogenic ulcers, benefit is not clearly documented in the literature. In patients with *gastric* ulcer, cimetidine may relieve symptoms, possibly delaying the diagnosis of malignant disease. Nevertheless, the drug has been to an astonishing extent overprescribed. In recent surveys of several thousand patients receiving cimetidine, fewer than 50% had either indication for such therapy (duodenal ulcer or Zollinger-Ellison syndrome).

Toxicity

Cimetidine is well tolerated, and adverse effects are reported in only 1–2% of patients. The most commonly reported effects are diarrhea and nausea and vomiting. Rash, headache, dizziness, and constipation have been reported in fewer than 1% of patients. Less common and more serious toxic effects are as follows:

A. Central Nervous System Dysfunction: Slurred speech, delirium, and occasionally coma appear to be most common in elderly patients.

B. Endocrine Effects: Cimetidine may cause gynecomastia in men and galactorrhea in women. The incidence approaches 1% after 6 months of therapy. In addition, a reduction in sperm count has been reported in men taking cimetidine in large doses for Zollinger-Ellison syndrome. These antiandrogenic effects are rarely troublesome if therapy with the drug is limited to 8 weeks or less. Ranitidine may be free of these endocrine effects.

C. Blood Dyscrasias: Cimetidine therapy has been associated with granulocytopenia and even aplastic anemia in a very few instances. The incidence is clearly far below that associated with the use of metiamide. There are no studies of ranitidine given over long periods, but it too may induce reversible granulocytopenia when given for short periods.

Drug Interactions

Cimetidine can reduce liver blood flow and it inhibits the oxidative metabolism of other drugs, including warfarin-type anticoagulants, phenytoin, propranolol, chlordiazepoxide, diazepam, and theophylline. Patients taking warfarin-type anticoagulants should be closely monitored to avoid bleeding. The clinical significance of the interaction with other drugs has not been established. It is claimed that ranitidine does not cause these drug interactions.

• • •

SEROTONIN (5-HYDROXYTRYPTAMINE)

Before the identification of 5-hydroxytryptamine (5-HT), it was known that when blood is allowed to clot, a vasoconstrictor substance is released; this substance was called **serotonin.** Independent studies established the existence of a smooth muscle stimulant in intestinal mucosa; this was called **enteramine.** The synthesis of 5-hydroxytryptamine in 1951 permitted the identification of serotonin and enteramine as the same metabolite of 5-hydroxytryptophan.

I. BASIC PHARMACOLOGY OF SEROTONIN

Chemistry & Pharmacokinetics

Like histamine, serotonin is widely distributed in nature, being found in plant and animal tissues, venoms, and stings. It is an indoleethylamine formed in biologic systems from the amino acid L-tryptophan. The scheme shown in Fig 14–4 illustrates the hydroxylation of the indole ring followed by the decarboxylation of the amino acid. Hydroxylation at C5 is the rate-limiting step and can be blocked by *p*-chlorophenylalanine (PCPA, fenclonine) and by *p*-chloroamphetamine. These agents have been used experimentally to reduce serotonin synthesis in carcinoid tumor (see below).

After synthesis, the free amine is stored or is rapidly inactivated, usually by oxidation catalyzed by the enzyme monoamine oxidase. In the pineal gland, serotonin serves as a precursor of melatonin, a melanocyte-stimulating hormone. In mammals (including humans), over 90% of the serotonin in the body is found in enterochromaffin cells in the gastrointestinal tract. In the blood, serotonin is found in platelets, which lack the enzymes necessary for serotonin synthesis but are able to concentrate the

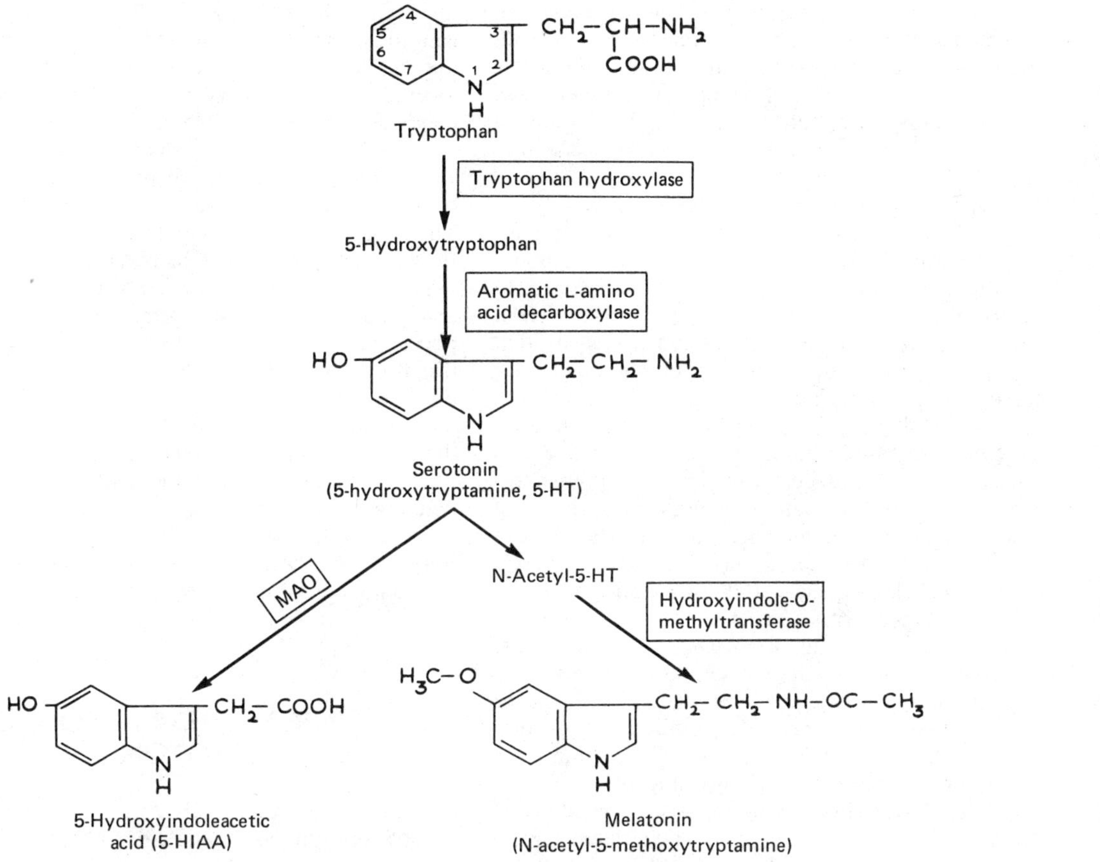

Figure 14–4. Synthesis and metabolism of serotonin. Note that the same enzyme catalyzes the decarboxylation of 5-hydroxytryptophan to serotonin and dopa to dopamine. (Modified and reproduced, with permission, from Meyers FH, Jawetz E, Goldfien A: *Review of Medical Pharmacology,* 7th ed. Lange, 1980.)

amine by means of an active carrier mechanism. Serotonin is also found in the raphe nuclei cell bodies of the brain stem, which contain cell bodies of tryptaminergic (serotoninergic) neurons that synthesize, store, and release serotonin as a transmitter. In rodents (but not in humans), serotonin is found in mast cells.

The function of serotonin in enterochromaffin cells is not clear. These cells synthesize serotonin, store the amine in a complex with ATP and with other substances in granules, and can release serotonin in response to mechanical and neuronal stimuli. Some of the released serotonin is taken up and stored in platelets.

Stored serotonin can be released by reserpine in much the same manner as this drug releases catecholamines from adrenergic vesicles (Chapter 9).

Serotonin is metabolized by monoamine oxidase, and the intermediate product, 5-hydroxyindoleacetaldehyde, is further oxidized by aldehyde dehydrogenase. When the latter enzyme is saturated, eg, by large amounts of acetaldehyde from ethanol metabolism, a significant fraction of the 5-hydroxyindoleacetaldehyde may be *reduced* in the liver to the alcohol 5-hydroxytryptophol. In humans consuming a normal diet, the excretion of 5-hydroxyindoleacetic acid is a measure of serotonin synthesis. Therefore, the 24-hour excretion of "5-HIAA" can be used as a diagnostic test for tumors that synthesize excessive quantities of serotonin, especially **carcinoid tumor.** A few foods (eg, bananas) contain large amounts of serotonin and must be prohibited during such diagnostic tests.

Pharmacodynamics

A. Mechanisms of Action: Serotonin exerts many actions, and, as in the case of histamine also, there are many species differences, making generalizations difficult. From studies with selective antagonists and results of tissue-binding experiments, it appears that the actions of serotonin are mediated through receptors located in or on the surface membranes of target cells. Two subsets of serotonin receptors have been identified and designated 5-HT_1 and 5-HT_2. Most peripheral serotonin receptors (in platelets, smooth muscle) appear to be of the 5-HT_2 variety. Both 5-HT_1 and 5-HT_2 types have been identified in brain.

The actions of serotonin on nerve and muscle cells are accompanied by changes in membrane permeability to ions such as sodium, potassium, and calcium, and stimulus-secretion coupling in enterochromaffin cells is associated with increased influx of calcium. The contraction or relaxation of smooth muscle caused by serotonin is often accompanied by elevated cGMP or cAMP, respectively, but the significance of the association between cyclic nucleotides and serotonin actions is not clear.

B. Tissue and Organ System Effects:

1. Cardiovascular system–A major direct effect of serotonin is to cause contraction of smooth muscle. In humans, serotonin is a powerful vasoconstrictor except in skeletal muscle and heart, where vessels are dilated. Serotonin can also elicit reflex bradycardia by activation of chemoreceptor nerve endings. A triphasic blood pressure response is often seen following injection of serotonin. Initially, there is a decrease in blood pressure and bradycardia caused by the chemoreceptor response. Following this decrease, blood pressure increases as a result of vasoconstriction. The third phase is again a decrease in blood pressure attributed to vasodilatation in vessels supplying skeletal muscle. Pulmonary and renal vessels seem especially sensitive to the vasoconstrictor action of serotonin. Serotonin also constricts veins, and venoconstriction with a resulting increased capillary filling appears responsible for the flush that is observed following serotonin administration. Serotonin has small direct positive chronotropic and inotropic effects on the heart that are probably of no clinical significance. However, continuously elevated blood levels of serotonin (which occur in carcinoid tumor) are associated with pathologic alterations in the endocardium (subendocardial fibroplasia) that may result in mechanical or electrical malfunction.

Serotonin causes aggregation of blood platelets by activating surface 5-HT_2 receptors. This response is not accompanied by release of the serotonin stored in the platelets, and its physiologic role is unclear.

2. Gastrointestinal tract–Serotonin causes contraction of gastrointestinal smooth muscle, increasing tone and facilitating peristalsis. This action is caused by the direct action of serotonin on smooth muscle plus a stimulating action on ganglion cells located in the intestinal wall. Serotonin has little direct effect on secretions, and what effects it has are generally inhibitory. It has been proposed that serotonin plays an important physiologic role as a local hormone controlling gastrointestinal motility. However, large doses of antagonists of serotonin are not associated with severe constipation. On the other hand, overproduction of serotonin—in carcinoid tumor—is associated with severe diarrhea.

3. Respiration–Serotonin has a small direct stimulant effect on bronchiolar smooth muscle in normal humans. In patients with carcinoid tumor, episodes of asthmatic bronchiolar obstruction occur in response to elevated levels of the amine. Serotonin also may cause marked hyperventilation, as a result of the chemoreceptor reflex response.

4. Nervous system–Like histamine, serotonin is a potent stimulant of pain and itch sensory nerve endings and is responsible for some of the symptoms caused by insect and plant stings. In addition, serotonin is a powerful activator of chemosensitive endings located in the coronary vascular bed. Activation of these afferent vagal nerve endings is associated with the chemoreceptor reflex (also known as the Bezold-Jarisch reflex). The reflex response is a triad consisting of bradycardia, hypotension, and hyperventilation. The bradycardia is mediated by vagal and motor outflow to the heart and can be blocked by atropine. The hypotension is a consequence of the decrease in cardiac output that results from bradycardia. The hyperventilation is mediated by a massive outflow of impulses from the respiratory center and is unaffected by atropine.

A variety of other agents are capable of activating the chemoreceptor reflex. These include nicotinic cholinergic stimulants and some cardiac glycosides, eg, ouabain.

Serotonin is present in a variety of sites in the brain. Its role as a neurotransmitter and its relation to the actions of drugs acting in the central nervous system are discussed in Chapters 18 and 26.

II. CLINICAL PHARMACOLOGY OF SEROTONIN

Serotonin has no clinical applications as a drug.

• • •

SEROTONIN ANTAGONISTS

The actions of serotonin, like those of histamine, can be antagonized in several different ways. Such antagonism is clearly desirable in those rare patients who have carcinoid tumor and may also be valuable in certain other conditions.

As noted above, serotonin synthesis can be inhibited by *p*-chlorophenylalanine and *p*-chloroamphetamine. However, these agents are too toxic for general use. Storage of serotonin can be inhibited by the use of reserpine, but the sympatholytic effects of this drug (Chapter 9) and the high levels of circulating serotonin that result from release prevent its use in carcinoid. Therefore, receptor blockade is the only available approach to therapeutic limitation of serotonin effects.

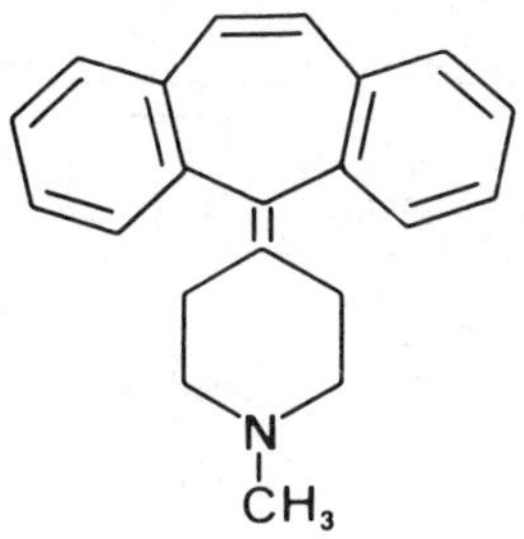

Cyproheptadine

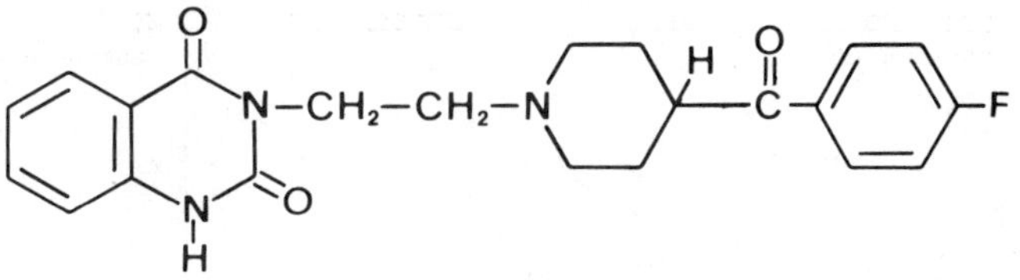

Ketanserin

SEROTONIN RECEPTOR ANTAGONISTS

Cyproheptadine and a number of experimental drugs have been identified as competitive serotonin receptor-blocking agents. In addition, the ergot alkaloids discussed in the last portion of the chapter are **partial agonists** at the serotonin receptor.

Cyproheptadine (Periactin) resembles the phenothiazine antihistaminic agents in chemical structure and has potent H_1 receptor-blocking actions. **Ketanserin** is an experimental agent with some selectivity for 5-HT_2 receptors and no reported H_1 blocking action.

The actions of cyproheptadine are predictable from its H_1 histamine and serotonin receptor affinities. It prevents the smooth muscle effects of both amines but has no effect on the gastric secretion stimulated by histamine. It has significant anticholinergic effects and causes sedation.

The major clinical applications of cyproheptadine are in the treatment of the smooth muscle manifestations of carcinoid tumor and in the postgastrectomy dumping syndrome. The usual dosage in adults is 12–16 mg/d in 3–4 divided doses.

• • •

THE ERGOT ALKALOIDS

Bertram G. Katzung, MD, PhD

Ergot alkaloids are produced by *Claviceps purpurea,* a fungus that infects grain—especially rye—under damp growing conditions. The ergot fungus has been called a "pharmaceutical factory," because this microorganism synthesizes histamine, acetylcholine, tyramine, and other biologically active products in addition to a score or more of ergot derivatives.

The accidental ingestion of ergot alkaloids in contaminated grain can be traced back more than 2000 years from descriptions of epidemics of the characteristic poisoning (ergotism). The most dramatic effects of poisoning are dementia with florid hallucinations; vasospasm, which may result in gangrene; and stimulation of uterine smooth muscle, which in pregnancy may result in abortion. The degree of each effect varies among reported epidemics and may represent a different mix of individual alkaloids in different crops of the fungus. In medieval times, ergot poisoning was called St. Anthony's fire after the saint whose help was sought in relieving the burning pain of vasospastic ischemia. Identifiable epidemics have occurred sporadically up to the present time (see References on p 185) and mandate continuous surveillance of all grains used for food.

In addition to the effects noted above, the ergot alkaloids produce a variety of other central nervous system and peripheral effects. Detailed structure-activity analysis and appropriate semisynthetic modifications have yielded a large number of agents with documented or potential clinical value.

I. BASIC PHARMACOLOGY OF ERGOT ALKALOIDS

Chemistry & Pharmacokinetics

Two major families of compounds that incorporate the tetracyclic **ergoline** nucleus may be identified: the amine alkaloids and the peptide alkaloids (Table

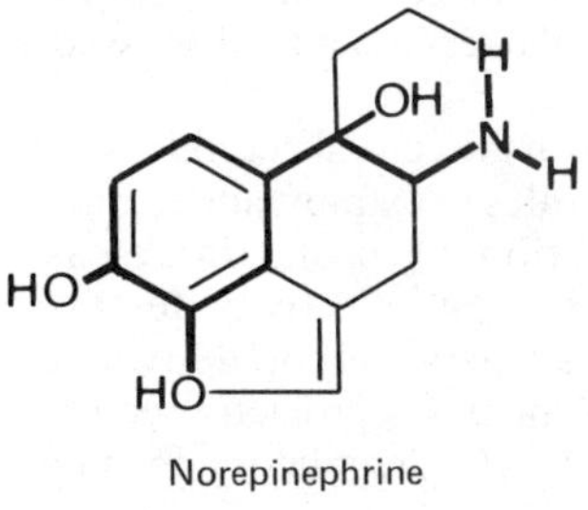

Norepinephrine

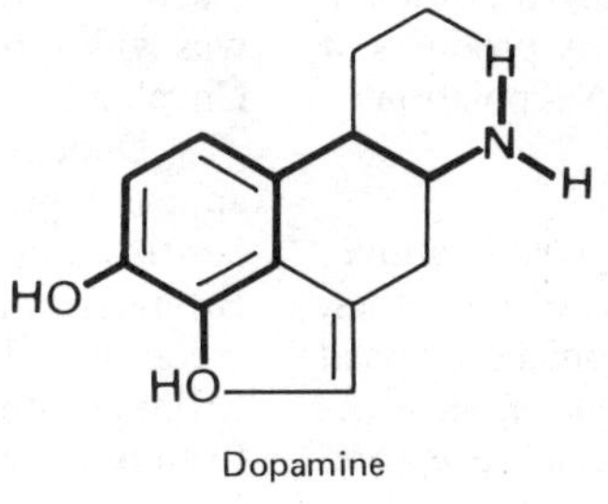

Dopamine

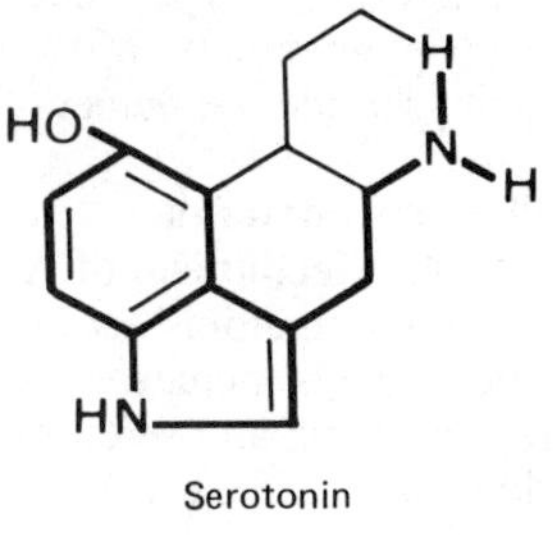

Serotonin

Table 14–2. Major ergoline derivatives (ergot alkaloids).

Amine alkaloids

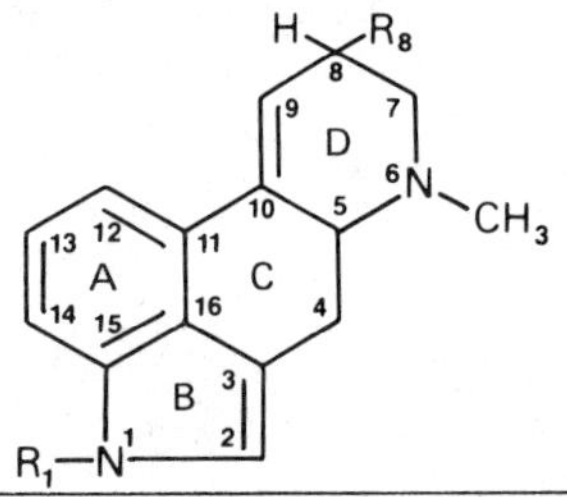

	R_1	R_8
6-Methylergoline	$-H$	$-H$
Lysergic acid	$-H$	$-COOH$
Lysergic acid diethylamide (LSD)	$-H$	$-C(=O)-N(CH_2-CH_3)_2$
Ergonovine (ergometrine)	$-H$	$-C(=O)-NH-CH(CH_2OH)-CH_3$
Methysergide	$-CH_3$	$-C(=O)-NH-CH(CH_2OH)-CH_2-CH_3$

Peptide alkaloids

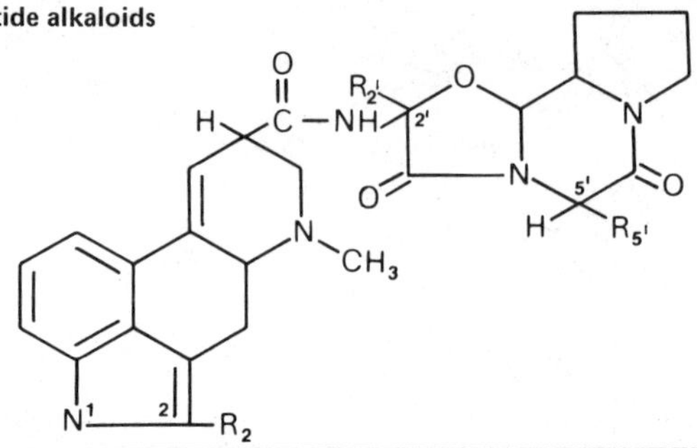

	R_2	R_2'	R_5'
Ergotamine	$-H$	$-CH_3$	$-CH_2-C_6H_5$
α-Ergokryptine	$-H$	$-CH(CH_3)_2$	$-CH_2-CH(CH_3)_2$
Bromocriptine	$-Br$	$-CH(CH_3)_2$	$-CH_2-CH(CH_3)_2$

14–2). Drugs of clinical importance are found in both classes. The structures shown on previous page compare norepinephrine, dopamine, and serotonin (heavy bonds) with the ergoline nucleus (light lines) and suggest one reason for the great pharmacologic versatility of the ergot alkaloids.

The ergot alkaloids are variably absorbed from the gastrointestinal tract. The oral dose of ergotamine is about 10 times larger than the intramuscular dose, but the speed of absorption and peak blood levels after oral administration can be improved by administration with caffeine (see below). The amine alkaloids are also absorbed from the rectum, the buccal cavity, and after administration by aerosol inhaler. Absorption after intramuscular injection is slow but usually reliable. Bromocriptine is more completely absorbed from the gastrointestinal tract than is ergotamine or the amine derivatives.

The ergot alkaloids are extensively metabolized in the body. The primary metabolites are hydroxylated in the A ring, and peptide alkaloids are also modified in the peptide moiety. Most of the excretory products of methysergide are demethylated at the N1 position.

Pharmacodynamics

A. Mechanism of Action: As suggested above, the ergot alkaloids act on several types of receptors. Their effects include agonist and antagonist actions at α-adrenergic and serotonin receptors and agonist action at central nervous system dopamine receptors. Furthermore, some members of the ergot family have a high affinity for presynaptic receptors, while others are more selective for postjunctional receptors. There is a powerful stimulant effect on the uterus and other smooth muscle that is not clearly associated with any of the preceding receptor types. Finally, an agonist effect at a putative tryptamine receptor on vascular smooth muscle has been proposed. Structural variations increase the selectivity of certain members of the family for specific receptor types (Table 14–3); clinical use of a given agent is not inevitably associated with all of the above actions.

B. Organ System Effects:

1. Central nervous system–As indicated by traditional descriptions of ergotism, certain of the naturally occurring alkaloids are powerful hallucinogens. Lysergic acid diethylamide (LSD_{25}, "acid") is the semisynthetic compound that most clearly demonstrates this action. In spite of extensive research, neither the mechanism nor any clinical value has been discovered for this dramatic effect. Abuse of this drug was widespread for several decades and is discussed in Chapter 29.

Dopamine receptors in the central nervous system appear to play important roles in extrapyramidal motor control and the regulation of prolactin release. Bromocriptine has the highest selectivity for these receptors of currently available ergot derivatives. Bromocriptine directly suppresses prolactin secretion from pituitary cells by activating regulatory dopamine

Table 14–3. Versatile actions of ergot alkaloids at several receptors.*

Ergot Alkaloid	Adrenergic Receptor		Dopamine Receptor	Serotonin Receptor		Smooth Muscle Stimulation
	Blockade	Activation	Activation	Blockade	Activation	
Lysergic acid diethylamide (LSD)	None	None	High	High	Low to none	Moderate
Ergonovine	None	Low	Low	Moderate	Low to none	High
Methysergide	None	Low to none	Low to none	High	Moderate	Low
Ergotamine	Moderate	Low	Low to none	Low	Moderate	High
Bromocriptine	Moderate	None	High	Low	None	None

*The reader is cautioned that receptor affinities cannot be equated with pharmacologic potency.

receptors. It competes for binding to these sites with dopamine itself and with other dopamine agonists such as apomorphine. The actions of bromocriptine on the extrapyramidal system are discussed in Chapter 25.

2. Vascular smooth muscle–The traditional view of ergot alkaloids as weak alpha-receptor antagonists and potent direct vasoconstrictor agents has given way in recent years to evidence of a much more complex pattern of vascular actions. As indicated in Table 14–3, this pattern includes agonist effects at alpha receptors, since some ergot-induced vasoconstriction is blocked by conventional alpha-receptor antagonists. Both agonist and antagonist effects probably occur at serotonin receptors as well. Activation of vasoconstrictor tryptamine receptors has also been proposed.

Despite the presence of alpha receptor-blocking activity in the alkaloids shown in Tables 14–2 and 14–3, their dominant effect on blood vessels is vasoconstriction. This action combines the agonist effects at alpha-adrenergic, serotonin, and, possibly, *separate* ergot (or tryptamine) receptors. The remarkably specific antimigraine action of certain ergot derivatives is thought to be related to their actions on the vascular serotonin receptor. Ergotamine and methysergide are the agents most widely used for the treatment of migraine.

After overdosage with ergotamine and similar agents, vasospasm is severe and prolonged (see Toxicity, below). This vasospasm is not reversed by alpha-antagonists, serotonin antagonists, or combinations of both. Only very powerful direct-acting vasodilators such as nitroprusside have been effective in this situation.

Ergotamine is typical of the ergot alkaloids with this spectrum of action (Table 14–3). The hydrogenation of ergot alkaloids at the 9 and 10 positions (Table 14–2) yields dihydro derivatives that have much lower direct smooth muscle and serotonin effects and more selective alpha receptor-blocking action.

3. Uterine smooth muscle–Like vascular smooth muscle, the action of ergot alkaloids on the uterus appears to combine adrenergic, serotonin, and other effects. However, the sensitivity of the uterus to the stimulant effects of ergot varies dramatically with hormonal status. As a result, the uterus at term is more sensitive than earlier in pregnancy and far more so than the nonpregnant organ.

In small doses, ergot preparations can evoke rhythmic contraction and relaxation of the uterus. At higher concentrations, these drugs induce powerful and prolonged contracture. Ergonovine (Table 14–3) is more selective than other ergot alkaloids in affecting the uterus and is the agent of choice in obstetric applications of these drugs.

4. Other smooth muscle organs–In most patients, the ergot alkaloids have no significant effect on bronchiolar smooth muscle. The gastrointestinal tract, on the other hand, varies dramatically in sensitivity among patients. Nausea, vomiting, and diarrhea may be induced by low doses in some patients but only by high doses in others. The effect is consistent with action on the central nervous system (emetic center) and on gastrointestinal serotonin receptors.

II. CLINICAL PHARMACOLOGY OF ERGOT ALKALOIDS

Clinical Uses

A. Migraine: Migraine headache in its classic form is characterized by a brief "aura" that may involve visual scotomas or even hemianopia and speech abnormalities, followed by a severe throbbing unilateral headache that lasts for a few hours to 1–2 days. The disease is familial in 60–80% of patients, more common in women, and usually has its onset in early adolescence through young adulthood, waning with advancing years. Attacks are usually precipitated by stress but often occur after rather than during the stressful episode. They vary in frequency from one attack a year to 2 or more a week.

Although the symptom pattern varies among patients, the severity of migraine headache justifies vigorous therapy in the great majority of cases.

The pathophysiology of migraine clearly involves some vasomotor mechanism, because the onset of headache is associated with a marked increase in amplitude of temporal artery pulsations, and relief of pain is accompanied by diminution in arterial pulsation. The chemical basis for these vascular changes is not clearly understood. Evidence strongly suggests that the onset of a migrainous aura is associated with an abnormal release of serotonin from platelets, while the arterial throbbing phase is associated with decrease of platelet and serum serotonin below normal concentrations. Other chemical triggers include falling levels of estrogen in women whose headache is linked to the menstrual cycle and elevated levels of prostaglandin E_1.

The efficacy of ergot derivatives in the therapy of migraine is so specific as to constitute a diagnostic test. Traditional therapy (ergotamine) is most effective when given during the prodrome of an attack and becomes progressively less effective if delayed. Ergotamine tartrate is available for oral, sublingual, rectal suppository, and inhaler use. It is often combined with caffeine (100 mg caffeine for 1 mg ergotamine tartrate) to facilitate absorption of the ergot alkaloid.

The vasoconstriction induced by ergotamine is long-lasting and cumulative when the drug is taken repeatedly, as in a severe attack. Therefore, patients must be carefully informed that no more than 6 mg of the oral preparation may be taken for each attack and no more than 10 mg per week. For very severe attacks, ergotamine tartrate, 0.25–0.5 mg, may be given intravenously or intramuscularly.

Because of the cumulative toxicity of ergotamine, safer agents useful for the prophylaxis of migraine have been sought. Methysergide, a derivative of the amine subgroup (Table 14–2), has been shown to be effective in this application in about 60% of patients. Unfortunately, significant toxicity (discussed below) occurs in almost 40%. As suggested in Table 14–3, there is some evidence of a difference in the agonist:antagonist ratios of methysergide and ergotamine when assayed on serotonin receptors. Regardless of the cause, methysergide is relatively *ineffective* in treatment of impending or active episodes of migraine. The dosage of methysergide maleate (Sansert) for prophylaxis of migraine is 4–8 mg/d.

Although relatively free of the rapidly cumulative vasospastic toxicity of ergotamine, chronic use of methysergide does induce important vascular disorders. Therefore, it is important that patients taking the drug have periodic drug holidays of 3–4 weeks every 6 months (see Toxicity).

Propranolol has also been found effective for the prophylaxis of migraine in some patients. Like methysergide, it is of no value in the treatment of acute migraine.

B. Hyperprolactinemia: Increased serum levels of the anterior pituitary hormone prolactin are associated with secreting tumors of the gland and also with the use of centrally acting dopamine antagonists, especially the antipsychotic drugs. Because of negative feedback effects, hyperprolactinemia is associated with amenorrhea and infertility in women as well as galactorrhea in both sexes.

Bromocriptine mesylate (Parlodel) is extremely effective in reducing the high levels of prolactin that result from pituitary tumors and has even been associated with regression of the tumor in some cases. The usual dosage of bromocriptine is 2.5 mg 2 or 3 times daily. Bromocriptine has also been used in the same dosage to suppress physiologic lactation.

C. Postpartum Hemorrhage: The introduction of ergot products into obstetrics in the latter part of the 18th century was accompanied by a dramatic increase in fetal and maternal mortality rates. It is now recognized that because the uterus at term is so sensitive to the stimulant action of ergot, even moderate doses produce a prolonged and powerful spasm of the muscle quite unlike natural labor. Therefore, ergot derivatives are useful only for control of late uterine bleeding and should never be given before delivery. Ergonovine maleate, 0.2 mg given usually intramuscularly, is effective within 1–5 minutes and is less toxic than other ergot derivatives for this application. It is given at the time of delivery of the placenta or immediately afterward if bleeding is significant.

D. Diagnosis of Variant Angina: Ergonovine produces prompt vasoconstriction in coronary vessels subject to spastic responses (Prinzmetal's or variant angina; see Chapter 10). Therefore, this ergot derivative may be administered via catheter into the coronary circulation during coronary angiography to diagnose variant angina.

E. Senile Cerebral Insufficiency: Dihydroergotoxine, a mixture of dihydro-α-ergokryptine and 3 similar dihydrogenated peptide ergot alkaloids,* has been promoted for many years for the relief of "senility." There is no evidence of significant benefit.

Toxicity & Contraindications

The most common toxic effects of the ergot derivatives are gastrointestinal disturbances, including diarrhea and nausea and vomiting. Activation of the medullary vomiting center and of the gastrointestinal serotonin receptors is involved. Since migraine attacks are often associated with these symptoms before therapy is begun, this side-effect is rarely a contraindication to therapy of acute migraine. However, in prophylactic management with methysergide, the effect is an important factor limiting use of the drug.

A more dangerous toxic effect of overdosage with agents like ergotamine and ergonovine is prolonged vasospasm. As described above, this sign of vascular smooth muscle stimulation may result in gangrene and require amputation. Most cases involve the circulation to the arms and legs. However, bowel infarction resulting from mesenteric artery vasospasm has also been reported. Peripheral vascular vasospasm caused by ergot is refractory to most vasodilators, but infusion of large doses of nitroprusside, a powerful direct-acting vasodilator, has been successful in some cases.

Chronic therapy with methysergide is associated with development of fibroplastic changes in the retroperitoneal space, the pleural cavity, and the endocardial tissue of the heart. These changes occur

*Available as ergoloid mesylates (many trade names).

insidiously over months and may present as hydronephrosis (from obstruction of the ureters) or a cardiac murmur (from distortion of the valves of the heart). Fortunately, most signs of toxicity appear to regress when administration of the drug is halted. However, the potential for injury is such that all patients taking methysergide should have periodic drug holidays and careful study if signs or symptoms of fibroplasia occur.

Other toxic effects of the ergot alkaloids include drowsiness and, in the case of methysergide, occasional instances of central stimulation and hallucinations. In fact, methysergide has been used as a substitute for LSD by members of the "drug culture."

Contraindications to the use of ergot derivatives consist of the obstructive vascular diseases and collagen disease.

There is no evidence that ordinary use of ergotamine or methysergide for migraine is hazardous in pregnancy. However, most clinicians counsel restraint in the use of these agents in pregnant patients.

• • •

References

Histamine

Beaven MA: *Histamine: Its Role in Physiological and Pathological Processes.* Monographs in Allergy, Vol 13, 1978.

Black JW et al: Definition and antagonism of histamine H_2-receptors. *Nature* 1972;**236:**385.

Cocco AE, Cocco DV: A survey of cimetidine prescribing. *N Engl J Med* 1981;**304:**1281.

Jick H et al: First-trimester drug use and congenital disorders. *JAMA* 1981;**246:**343.

Lebert PA et al: Ranitidine kinetics and dynamics. 1. Oral dose studies. 2. Intravenous dose studies and comparison with cimetidine. (2 parts.) *Clin Pharmacol Ther* 1981;**30:**539, 545.

Lomax P, Green MD: Histamine neurons in the hypothalamic thermoregulatory pathways. *Fed Proc* 1981;**40:**2741.

Milton-Thompson GJ et al: Intragastric acidity, bacteria, nitrite and nitroso compounds before, during, and after cimetidine treatment. *Lancet* 1982;**1:**1091.

Morelock S et al: Bendectin and fetal development: A study at Boston City Hospital. *Am J Obstet Gynecol* 1982;**142:**209.

Schade RR, Donaldson RMJ: How physicians use cimetidine: A survey of hospitalized patients and published cases. *N Engl J Med* 1981;**304:**1281.

Torsoli A, Lucchelli PE, Brinblecombe RW (editors): *H_2 Antagonists: H_2-Receptor Antagonists in Peptic Ulcer Disease and Progress in Histamine Research.* (Symposium.) International Congress Series 521. Excerpta Medica, 1980.

Serotonin

Cohen ML, Fuller RN, Wilkey KS: Evidence for 5-HT_2 receptors mediating contraction in vascular smooth muscle. *J Pharmacol Exp Ther* 1981;**218:**421.

Demoulin JC et al: 5-HT_2-receptor blockade in the treatment of heart failure. *Lancet* 1981;**1:**1186.

Essman WB (editor): *Serotonin in Health and Disease.* Vols 1–4. Spectrum, 1978.

Peroutka SJ, Lebovite RM, Snyder SH: Two distinct central serotonin receptors with different physiological functions. *Science* 1981;**212:**827.

Van Nueten JM et al: Vascular effects of ketanserin (R 41 468), a novel antagonist of 5-HT_2 serotonergic receptors. *J Pharmacol Exp Ther* 1981;**218:**217.

Ergot Alkaloids

Historical

Fuller JG: *The Day of St. Anthony's Fire.* MacMillan, 1968; Signet, 1969. [A narrative account of an epidemic of ergotism in France in 1951.]

Gabbai Dr, Lisbonne Dr, Pourquier Dr: Ergot poisoning at Pont St. Esprit. *Br Med J* (Sept 15) 1951;650.

King B: Outbreak of ergotism in Wollo, Ethiopia. (Letter.) *Lancet* 1979;**1:**1411.

Basic Pharmacology

Berde B: Ergot compounds: A synopsis. *Adv Biochem Psychopharmacol* 1980;**23:**3.

Muller-Schweinitzer E: Responsiveness of isolated canine cerebral and peripheral arteries to ergotamine. *Naunyn Schmiedebergs Arch Pharmacol* 1976;**292:**113.

Saxena PR: Selective vasoconstriction in carotid vascular bed by methysergide: Possible relevance to its anti-migraine effect. *Eur J Pharmacol* 1974;**27:**99.

Clinical Pharmacology

Anderson PK et al: Sodium nitroprusside and epidural blockade in the treatment of ergotism. *N Engl J Med* 1977;**296:**1271.

Anthony M, Hinterberger H, Lance JW: Plasma serotonin in migraine and stress. *Arch Neurol* 1967;**16:**544.

Harrington E et al: Migraine: A platelet disorder. *Lancet* 1981;**2:**720.

Thorner MO et al: Hyperprolactinemia: Current concepts of management including medical therapy with bromocriptine. *Adv Biochem Psychopharmacol* 1980;**23:**165.

15 | Polypeptides

Ian A. Reid, PhD

A variety of polypeptides exert important effects on vascular and other smooth muscles. These include the vasoconstrictors angiotensin II and vasopressin and several vasodilators, including bradykinin and other kinins, vasoactive intestinal peptide, and substance P.

ANGIOTENSIN

BIOSYNTHESIS OF ANGIOTENSIN

The pathway for the formation and metabolism of angiotensin II is summarized in Fig 15–1. The principal steps include enzymatic cleavage of angiotensin I from angiotensinogen by renin, conversion of angiotensin I to angiotensin II by converting enzyme, and degradation of angiotensin II by several peptidases.

Renin & Factors Controlling Renin Secretion

Renin specifically catalyzes hydrolytic release of the decapeptide angiotensin I from angiotensinogen. It has been classified as an acid protease and thus belongs to the same group of enzymes as pepsin and cathepsin D (which can also form angiotensin I from angiotensinogen under appropriate conditions). Renin has been purified to homogeneity and shown to be a glycoprotein with a molecular weight of 35,000–42,000. Inactive forms of renin, often referred to as "prorenins," are present in several body fluids and tissues. These can be activated by acidification, cold treatment, and various enzymes, including pepsin, cathepsin D, trypsin, and kallikrein, with or without a reduction in molecular weight. The extent to which inactive renin is converted to active renin in vivo is not known.

Most (probably all) of the renin in the circulation originates in the kidneys. Enzymes with reninlike activity are present in several extrarenal tissues, including blood vessels, uterus, salivary glands, and adrenal cortex, but no physiologic role for these enzymes has been established. Within the kidney, renin is synthesized and stored in a specialized area of the nephron, the juxtaglomerular apparatus. The juxtaglomerular apparatus is composed of vascular and tubular elements. Vascular elements include the afferent and efferent arterioles and a group of mesangial cells. The afferent arteriole and, to a lesser extent, the efferent arteriole and mesangial cells contain specialized granular cells called juxtaglomerular cells that serve as the site of synthesis, storage, and release of renin. The tubular component of the juxtaglomerular apparatus is the macula densa, a specialized tubular segment closely associated with the vascular components of the juxtaglomerular apparatus. The vascular and tubular components of the juxtaglomerular apparatus, including the juxtaglomerular cells, are innervated by adrenergic neurons.

The rate at which renin is secreted by the kidney is the primary determinant of activity of the renin-

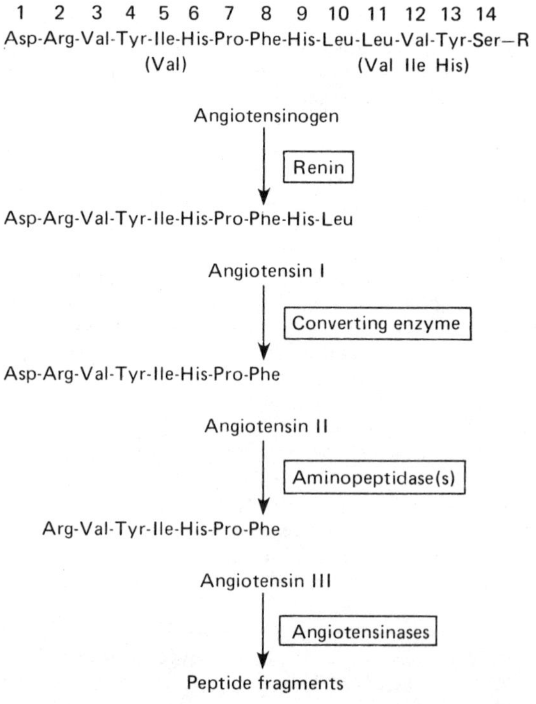

Figure 15–1. Chemistry of the renin-angiotensin system. The amino acid sequence of the amino terminal of equine and porcine angiotensinogen is shown. Bovine angiotensinogen contains Val in position 5, and human angiotensinogen contains Val-Ile-His in positions 11–13. R denotes the remainder of the protein molecule.

angiotensin system. Renin secretion is controlled by a variety of factors, including a renal vascular receptor, the macula densa, the sympathetic nervous system, angiotensin II, vasopressin, and potassium.

A. Renal Vascular Receptor: According to current concepts, the renal vascular receptor functions as a stretch receptor, decreased stretch leading to increased renin release and vice versa. The receptor is apparently located in the afferent arteriole, and it is possible that the juxtaglomerular cells themselves are sensitive to changes in stretch. Several stimuli to renin secretion, including alterations in renal perfusion pressure, are mediated via the renal vascular receptor.

B. Macula Densa: The macula densa contains a different type of receptor, apparently sensitive to changes in the rate of delivery of sodium or chloride to the distal tubule. Decreases in distal delivery result in stimulation of renin secretion, and vice versa, but the mechanisms involved are not well understood.

C. Sympathetic Nervous System: The sympathetic innervation of the juxtaglomerular apparatus plays an important role in the control of renin secretion. Maneuvers that increase renal neural activity cause stimulation of renin secretion, while renal denervation results in suppression of renin secretion. Norepinephrine released from the renal nerves has complex effects on renin secretion. It appears that norepinephrine can stimulate renin secretion by direct action on the juxtaglomerular cells. This effect is thought to be mediated by β-adrenergic receptors and may involve the activation of adenylate cyclase and the formation of cAMP. At present, it is not clear if these β-adrenergic receptors are of the β_1 or β_2 subtype. In some situations, norepinephrine stimulates renin secretion indirectly by way of α-adrenergic receptors. This stimulation apparently results from constriction of the afferent arteriole, with resultant activation of the renal vascular receptor and decreased delivery of sodium chloride to the macula densa. In other situations, α-adrenergic receptor stimulation may actually inhibit renin secretion, but the significance of this action is not understood.

The rate of renin secretion is also influenced by circulating epinephrine and norepinephrine. These catecholamines may act via the same mechanisms as the norepinephrine released locally from the renal sympathetic nerves. However, there is evidence that a major component of the renin secretory response to circulating catecholamines is mediated by way of extrarenal β-adrenergic receptors. The location of these receptors and the pathway by which they influence renin secretion remain to be determined.

D. Angiotensin, Vasopressin, and Potassium: Angiotensin II, vasopressin, and potassium all inhibit renin secretion. The inhibition of renin secretion by angiotensin II, which is thought to result from a direct action of the peptide on the juxtaglomerular cells, forms the basis of the short-loop negative feedback mechanism controlling renin secretion. Interruption of this feedback with antagonists of the renin-angiotensin system (see below) results in stimulation of renin secretion. Vasopressin may also inhibit renin secretion directly. It is effective at quite low concentrations and is probably an important modulator of the rate of renin secretion. Small changes in plasma potassium concentration lead to reciprocal changes in the rate of renin secretion. In contrast to angiotensin II and vasopressin, potassium appears to inhibit renin secretion indirectly by increasing the rate of delivery of sodium chloride to the macula densa.

Angiotensinogen

Angiotensinogen is the circulating protein substrate from which renin cleaves angiotensin I. Most of the angiotensinogen in the circulation originates in the liver. Angiotensinogen has been purified to homogeneity from the plasma of humans and several animal species and shown to be a glycoprotein with a molecular weight of 47,000–66,000. The amino acid sequence of the amino terminal of the molecule is known (Fig 15–1). In humans, the concentration of angiotensinogen in the circulation is less than the K_m (concentration for 50% of maximum reaction rate) for the renin-angiotensin reaction and is therefore an important determinant of the rate of formation of angiotensin. The production of angiotensinogen is regulated by corticosteroids, estrogens, and angiotensin II.

A. Corticosteroids: Angiotensinogen production is decreased following adrenalectomy or hypophysectomy and increased by administration of corticotropin or a variety of corticosteroids. The stimulation of angiotensinogen production by corticosteroids is related to their glucocorticoid activity rather than to their mineralocorticoid activity. As a consequence, plasma angiotensinogen concentration is increased in patients with Cushing's syndrome but not in those with primary aldosteronism.

B. Estrogens: Estrogens also increase angiotensinogen production, and elevations in plasma angiotensinogen concentration occur during pregnancy and in women taking estrogen-containing oral contraceptives. There is some evidence that stimulation of angiotensinogen production may be partly responsible for the hypertension occasionally associated with use of oral contraceptives.

C. Angiotensin II: Angiotensin II increases angiotensinogen production, apparently by direct action on the liver. This stimulatory effect may form the basis of a positive feedback mechanism that prevents angiotensinogen levels from falling when the utilization of angiotensinogen is increased during periods of hyperreninemia.

Angiotensin I

Although angiotensin I contains the peptide sequences necessary for all of the actions of the renin-angiotensin system, it has little or no biologic activity. Instead, it must be converted to angiotensin II by converting enzyme. Angiotensin I may also be acted on by plasma or tissue aminopeptidases to form [des-Asp^1]angiotensin I; this in turn is converted to [des-Asp[1]]angiotensin II (commonly known as angiotensin III) by converting enzyme.

Converting Enzyme (Peptidyl Dipeptidase, PDP, Kininase II)

Converting enzyme is a dipeptidyl carboxypeptidase that catalyzes the cleavage of dipeptides from the carboxyl terminal of certain peptides. Its most important substrates are angiotensin I, which it converts to angiotensin II; and bradykinin, which it inactivates (see below). It also cleaves enkephalins and substance P, but the physiologic significance of these effects has not been established. The action of converting enzyme is restricted by a penultimate prolyl residue, and angiotensin II is therefore not hydrolyzed by converting enzyme. Converting enzyme is distributed widely in the body, but its concentration is particularly high in the pulmonary circulation, and it is here that most conversion of angiotensin I to angiotensin II occurs. In most tissues, converting enzyme is located on the luminal surface of vascular endothelial cells and is thus in close contact with the circulation. The enzyme is a glycoprotein with a molecular weight of 130,000–140,000 and consists of a single polypeptide chain containing a molar equivalent of zinc. Its activity is dependent on the presence of chloride ion.

ACTIONS OF ANGIOTENSIN II

Angiotensin II exerts important actions at several sites in the body, including vascular smooth muscle, adrenal cortex, kidney, and brain. Through these actions, the renin-angiotensin system plays a key role in the regulation of fluid and electrolyte balance and arterial blood pressure. Overactivity of the renin-angiotensin system can result in hypertension and disorders of fluid and electrolyte homeostasis.

Effects on Blood Pressure

Angiotensin II is an extremely potent pressor agent—on a molar basis, approximately 40 times more potent than norepinephrine. The pressor response to intravenous angiotensin II is rapid in onset (10–15 seconds) and sustained during long-term infusions of the peptide. A large component of the pressor response to intravenous angiotensin II is due to direct contraction of vascular—especially arteriolar—smooth muscle. In addition, however, angiotensin II can also increase blood pressure through actions on the brain and autonomic nervous system. The central pressor effect of angiotensin II is mediated by the area postrema, a circumventricular organ located in the medulla oblongata. Like the other circumventricular organs, the area postrema lacks a blood-brain barrier and is therefore accessible to blood-borne angiotensin II. Infusion of angiotensin II into the vertebral arteries, which supply the area postrema, produces a prompt increase in blood pressure; this is abolished when a lesion is placed in the area postrema. Area postrema lesions have also been reported to decrease the pressor response to intravenous angiotensin II. The increase in blood pressure produced by intravertebral injection of angiotensin II is due to a combination of elevated total peripheral resistance resulting from increased sympathetic discharge and an increase in cardiac output secondary to withdrawal of vagal tone to the heart.

Angiotensin II also interacts with the peripheral autonomic nervous system. It facilitates sympathetic transmission by an action at adrenergic nerve terminals, increases the release of epinephrine and norepinephrine from the adrenal medulla, and stimulates autonomic ganglia. Of these actions, facilitation of adrenergic transmission is probably the most important. This effect results from both increased release and reduced reuptake of norepinephrine.

Angiotensin II also has a direct positive inotropic action on the heart. While this action may contribute to the increase in blood pressure, it is far less important than the vascular effects.

Effects on the Adrenal Cortex

Angiotensin II acts directly on the zona glomerulosa of the adrenal cortex to stimulate aldosterone biosynthesis and secretion. In high doses, angiotensin II may also stimulate glucocorticoid secretion. The stimulation of aldosterone secretion by angiotensin II results chiefly from increased conversion of cholesterol to pregnenolone, although, during long-term exposure to the peptide, the conversion of corticosterone to aldosterone may also be facilitated. Current evidence indicates that the renin-angiotensin system is one of the major regulators of aldosterone secretion, mediating, at least in part, the increases in aldosterone secretion that occur in sodium deficiency, renal hypertension, and congestive heart failure.

Effects on the Kidney

Angiotensin II acts directly on the kidney to cause renal vasoconstriction, increase proximal tubular sodium reabsorption, and, as mentioned above, inhibit the secretion of renin. The effects of angiotensin II on renal hemodynamics and sodium reabsorption can be produced by very low doses of angiotensin II and probably represent physiologic actions of the renin-angiotensin system.

Effects on the Central Nervous System

In addition to its central effects on blood pressure, angiotensin II also acts on the central nervous system to stimulate drinking and increase the secretion of vasopressin and ACTH. The most impressive responses are seen when the peptide is injected into the cerebral ventricles; the responses to intravenous angiotensin II are much less impressive. Dipsogenic responses to angiotensin II are apparently mediated by 2 circumventricular organs, the subfornical organ and the organum vasculosum of the lamina terminalis (OVLT). The relative importance of these 2 structures is not known at present. Proposed sites of angiotensin II effect on pituitary hormone secretion include the supraoptic nucleus and the posterior pituitary for vasopressin and the median eminence and anterior pituitary for ACTH. The physiologic significance of the effects of angiotensin II on drinking and pituitary hormone secretion is not known.

ANGIOTENSIN RECEPTORS & MECHANISM OF ACTION

The presence of specific angiotensin II receptors has been demonstrated in a variety of tissues, including vascular smooth muscle, adrenal cortex, kidney, uterus, and brain. Like the receptors for other polypeptide hormones, angiotensin II receptors are located on the plasma membrane of target cells, and this permits rapid onset of the various actions of angiotensin II.

The structure-activity relationships of angiotensin II have been studied extensively. Most studies have been based on the pressor action of the peptide, but the results probably apply to all of the actions. The amino terminal is not essential for activity, but it does influence receptor binding and duration of action (Fig 15–1). The amino acid at position 2 (arginine) also contributes to receptor affinity, but it does not influence the intrinsic activity of the peptide. The minimum structure of angiotensin II that has full intrinsic activity is the hexapeptide at positions 3–8 of the carboxyl terminal. The aliphatic side chains in residues 3, 5, and 7 are necessary to stabilize the secondary structure of the molecule, while the aromatic side chains in residues 4, 6, and 8 are essential for binding to receptors. Finally, the phenyl ring in position 8 is essential for intrinsic activity.

The nature of the intracellular signal generated in response to the binding of angiotensin II to its receptors has not been definitely identified. Possible second messengers for angiotensin II include potassium, cyclic nucleotides, and calcium. Further investigation is required, but it appears likely that many of the actions of angiotensin II involve changes in intracellular calcium concentration.

METABOLISM OF ANGIOTENSIN II

Angiotensin II is removed rapidly from the circulation, with a half-life of 15–60 seconds. It is metabolized during passage through most vascular beds (a notable exception being the lung) by a variety of peptidases collectively referred to as angiotensinases. Most of the metabolites of angiotensin II are biologically inactive, but the initial product of aminopeptidase action—[des-Asp^1]angiotensin II—retains considerable biologic activity.

ANTAGONISTS OF THE RENIN-ANGIOTENSIN SYSTEM

A wide variety of agents are now available that block the formation or actions of angiotensin II. These include drugs that block renin secretion; those that block the enzymatic action of renin; those that block the conversion of angiotensin I to angiotensin II; and those that block angiotensin II receptors.

Drugs That Block Renin Secretion

A number of drugs that interfere with the sympathetic nervous system inhibit the secretion of renin. Examples are clonidine, propranolol, and methyldopa. Clonidine inhibits renin secretion by causing a centrally mediated reduction in renal neural activity, but it may also exert a direct intrarenal action. Propranolol and other β-adrenergic blocking drugs act by blocking the intrarenal and extrarenal β-adrenergic receptors involved in the neural control of renin secretion. The mechanism by which methyldopa inhibits renin secretion has not been established.

Renin Inhibitors

The action of renin can be blocked by pepstatin, a pentapeptide that also inhibits the action of other proteases such as pepsin and cathepsin D. The use of pepstatin in vivo is restricted by its low solubility, but a more soluble form, N-acetylpepstatin, has been synthesized. Competitive inhibitors of renin based on the amino acid sequence around the cleavage site of angiotensinogen have been synthesized. The problem with most of these is low solubility. However, one of these peptides, Pro-His-Pro-Phe-His-Phe-Phe-Val-Tyr-Lys, is reasonably soluble and is an effective inhibitor of renin in vivo.

Converting Enzyme Inhibitors

A nonapeptide inhibitor of converting enzyme was originally isolated from the venom of the South American pit viper, *Bothrops jararaca*. The synthetic form of this peptide is (pyro)Glu-Trp-Pro-Arg-Pro-Gln-Ile-Pro-Pro, or **teprotide,** a highly effective inhibitor of converting enzyme used extensively in investigations of the role of the renin-angiotensin system in a variety of physiologic and pathologic situations. However, the use of teprotide is limited by the fact that it is active only when administered intravenously. A new class of converting enzyme inhibitors, directed against the active site of converting enzyme, has recently been synthesized. One such inhibitor is D-3-mercapto-methylpropanoyl-L-proline, or **captopril** (Fig 15–2). Like teprotide, captopril inhibits the conversion of angiotensin I to angiotensin II in vivo; unlike teprotide, captopril is effective when administered orally. Captopril is now used clinically as an antihypertensive agent (see Chapter 9). Other converting enzyme inhibitors are being studied. Like captopril, these inhibitors are orally active; unlike captopril, they are non-sulfhydryl-containing agents. One of the most effective of the new agents is N-[(S)-1-(ethoxycarbonyl)-3-phenylprolyl]-L-alanyl-L-proline, or MK-421 (see Fig 15–2). It should be noted that converting enzyme inhibitors not only block the conversion of angiotensin I to angiotensin II but also inhibit the degradation of bradykinin (see below). It is

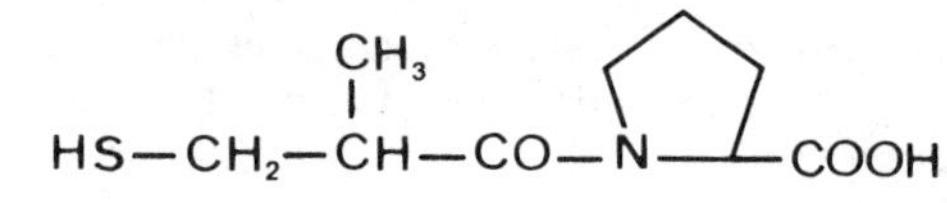

Captopril

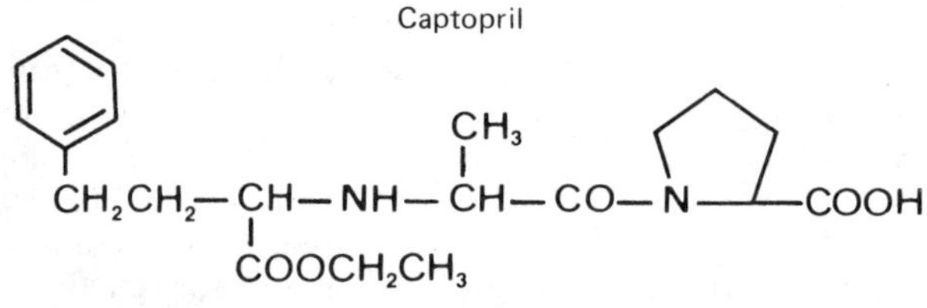

MK-421

Figure 15–2. Two orally active converting enzyme inhibitors: captopril and MK-421.

likely that this latter effect contributes significantly to the antihypertensive action of converting enzyme inhibitors.

Angiotensin Analogs

Substitution of aliphatic residues such as glycine, alanine, leucine, isoleucine, or threonine for the phenylalanine in position 8 of angiotensin II results in the formation of potent antagonists of the action of angiotensin II. Substitution of sarcosine (N-methylglycine) for the amino terminal aspartic acid prolongs the half-life of the peptides and thus enhances their potency. The best-known of these antagonists is [Sar^1,Val^5,Ala^8]angiotensin-(1–8)octapeptide, or **saralasin,** which has been used extensively in physiologic and clinical studies.

Asp-Arg-Val-Tyr-Ile-His-Pro-Phe

Angiotensin II

Sar-Arg-Val-Tyr-Val-His-Pro-Ala

Saralasin

Saralasin exhibits some agonist activity and may elicit pressor responses, particularly when circulating angiotensin II levels are low. This is true also of other angiotensin II antagonists, although some, eg, [Sar^1,Thr^8]angiotensin II, apparently have less agonist activity than saralasin. Saralasin and other angiotensin antagonists must be administered intravenously, and this severely restricts their use as antihypertensive agents. However, they can be used for the detection of renin-dependent hypertension and other hyperreninemic states. In general, angiotensin antagonists are less effective in lowering blood pressure than are converting enzyme inhibitors. This difference reflects both the agonist activity of angiotensin antagonists and the bradykinin-potentiating action of converting enzyme inhibitors.

Antibodies

Specific antibodies have been produced against renin, angiotensinogen, converting enzyme, angiotensin I, and angiotensin II. These are useful experimental tools but are not likely to have any clinical application.

KININS

BIOSYNTHESIS OF KININS

Kinins are a group of potent vasodilator peptides that are formed enzymatically by the action of enzymes known as kallikreins or kininogenases on protein substrates called kininogens. From the biochemical point of view, the kallikrein-kinin system has several features in common with the renin-angiotensin system.

Kallikreins

Kallikreins are present in plasma and in several tissues, including the kidneys, pancreas, intestine, sweat glands, and salivary glands. All kallikreins are serine proteases with active sites and catalytic properties very similar to those of enzymes such as trypsin, chymotrypsin, elastase, thrombin, plasmin, and other serine proteases. They are glycoproteins. Tissue kallikreins have molecular weights between 25,000 and 40,000; plasma kallikrein has a molecular weight of approximately 100,000.

Plasma kallikrein circulates in the blood as a precursor, prekallikrein, which is produced by the liver. Plasma kallikrein can be activated by trypsin, Hageman factor, and possibly kallikrein itself. Some glandular kallikreins exist as prekallikreins; others are present in active forms. In general, the biochemical properties of glandular kallikreins are quite different from those of plasma kallikreins. It has been shown that kallikreins can convert prorenin to active renin, but the physiologic significance of this action has not been established.

Kininogens

Kininogens—the precursors of kinins—are present in plasma, lymph, and interstitial fluid. At least 2 kininogens are present in plasma: a low-molecular-weight form (LMW kininogen) and a high-molecular-weight form (HMW kininogen). Both are acidic glycoproteins consisting of a single polypeptide chain. About 15–20% of the total plasma kininogen is in the high-molecular-weight form. It is thought that LMW kininogen crosses capillary walls and serves as the substrate for tissue kallikreins, while HMW kininogen is confined to the bloodstream and serves as the substrate for plasma kallikrein.

FORMATION OF KININS IN PLASMA & TISSUES

The pathway for the formation and metabolism of kinins is shown in Fig 15–3. Three kinins have been identified in mammals: bradykinin, lysylbradykinin (also known as kallidin), and methionyllysylbradykinin. They have the following structures:

Arg-Pro-Pro-Gly-Phe-Ser-Pro-Phe-Arg
1 2 3 4 5 6 7 8 9

Bradykinin

Lys-Arg-Pro-Pro-Gly-Phe-Ser-Pro-Phe-Arg

Lysylbradykinin (kallidin; Lys-bradykinin)

Met-Lys-Arg-Pro-Pro-Gly-Phe-Ser-Pro-Phe-Arg

Methionyllysylbradykinin (Met-Lys-bradykinin)

Note that each kinin contains bradykinin in its structure. Each kinin is formed from a kininogen by the action of a different enzyme. Bradykinin is released by plasma kallikrein, lysylbradykinin by glandular kallikrein, and methionyllysylbradykinin by pepsin and pepsinlike enzymes. The preferred substrate for plasma kallikrein is HMW kininogen, and the preferred substrate for tissue kallikrein is LMW kininogen. Some lysylbradykinin is converted to bradykinin by an aminopeptidase. The 3 kinins have been found in plasma, but bradykinin is the predominant type. All 3 kinins are also present in urine. Lysylbradykinin is the major urinary kinin and is probably formed by the action of renal kallikrein. Bradykinin is generated from lysylbradykinin by a renal aminopeptidase. Methionyllysylbradykinin occurs in acidified urine: acid activates uropepsinogen, which then catalyzes the release of methionyllysylbradykinin from urinary kininogens.

ACTIONS OF KININS

Effects on the Cardiovascular System

Kinins produce marked vasodilatation in several vascular beds, including the heart, kidney, intestine, skeletal muscle, and liver. In this respect, kinins are approximately 10 times more potent than histamine. The vasodilatation may result from a direct inhibitory effect of kinins on arteriolar smooth muscle or may be mediated by the release of vasodilator prostaglandins such as PGE_2 and PGI_2. In contrast, the predominant effect of kinins on veins is contraction; again, this may result from direct stimulation of venous smooth muscle or from the release of venoconstrictor prostaglandins such as $PGF_{2\alpha}$. Kinins also produce contraction of most visceral smooth muscle.

When injected intravenously, kinins produce a rapid fall in blood pressure that is due to the vasodilator action of the peptides. The hypotensive response to bradykinin is of very brief duration. Intravenous infusions of the peptide fail to produce a sustained decrease in blood pressure; prolonged hypotension can only be produced by progressively increasing the rate of infusion. The rapid reversibility of the hypotensive response to kinins is due primarily to reflex increases in heart rate, cardiac output, and myocardial contractility. In some species, bradykinin actually produces a biphasic change in blood pressure—an initial hypotensive response followed by an increase above the preinjection level. The increase in blood pressure appears to be due to a reflex activation of the sympathetic nervous system, although it is worth noting that under

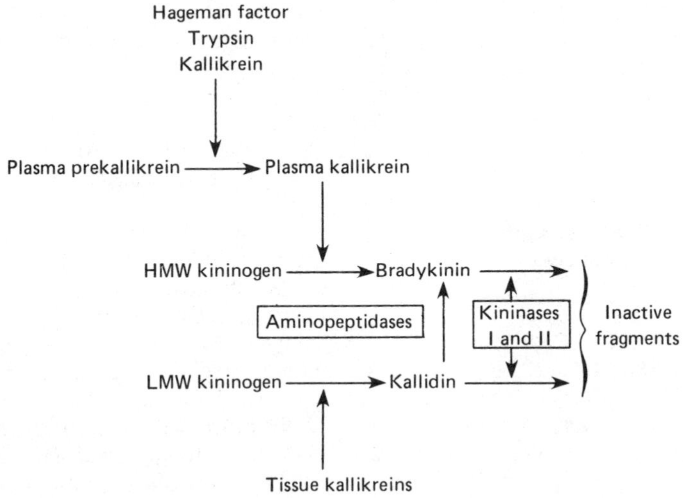

Figure 15–3. The kallikrein-kinin system. Kininase II is identical to peptidyl dipeptidase, converting enzyme.

some conditions, bradykinin can release catecholamines from the adrenal medulla and stimulate sympathetic ganglia. Bradykinin also increases blood pressure when injected into the central nervous system, but the significance of this effect is not clear, since it is unlikely that kinins cross the blood-brain barrier. Kinins have no consistent effect on sympathetic or parasympathetic nerve endings.

The arteriolar dilatation produced by kinins causes an increase in pressure and flow in the capillary bed, thus favoring efflux of fluid from blood to tissues. This effect may be facilitated by increased capillary permeability resulting from contraction of endothelial cells and widening of intercellular junctions and by increased venous pressure secondary to constriction of veins. As a result of these changes, water and solutes pass from the blood to the extracellular fluid; lymph flow increases; and edema may result.

Effects on Endocrine & Exocrine Glands

As noted earlier, prekallikreins and kallikreins are present in several glands, including the pancreas, kidney, intestine, salivary glands, and sweat glands, and can be released into the secretory fluids of these glands. The function of the enzymes in these tissues is not known. The enzymes (or active kinins) may diffuse from the organs to the blood and act as local modulators of blood flow. Since kinins have such marked effects on smooth muscle, they may also modulate the tone of salivary and pancreatic ducts and help to regulate gastrointestinal motility. Kinins also influence the transepithelial transport of water, electrolytes, glucose, and amino acids and may regulate the transport of these substances in the gastrointestinal tract and kidney. Finally, kallikreins may play a role in the physiologic activation of various prohormones, including proinsulin and prorenin.

Role in Inflammation

There is circumstantial evidence that kinins participate in the inflammatory process. Kallikreins and kinins can produce the basic symptoms of inflammation in animals, and the production of kinins is increased in inflammatory lesions produced by a variety of methods. Nevertheless, the extent to which kinins are involved in inflammatory process remains to be determined.

Effects on Sensory Nerves

The kinins are potent activators of sensory pain endings in the skin and the viscera.

KININ RECEPTORS & MECHANISMS OF ACTION

The biologic actions of kinins are thought to be mediated by specific receptors located on the membranes of the target tissues. There appear to be at least 2 types of receptors for bradykinin and the other kinins: B_1 receptors (eg, rabbit aorta) and B_2 receptors (eg, cat ileum and rat uterus). (Note that *B* here stands for bradykinin, not for beta-adrenergic.) Bioassay of B_1 receptor systems indicates that Lys-bradykinin and Met-Lys-bradykinin are approximately 10 and 76 times more potent than bradykinin, respectively. The octapeptide [des-Arg^9]bradykinin is 10 times more potent while the heptapeptide [des-Phe^8-des-Arg^9] bradykinin is inactive. Structure-activity studies have resulted in the discovery of specific, competitive inhibitors of the effects of kinins on B_1 receptors. An example of such an antagonist is [Leu^8-des-Arg^9]bradykinin. Bradykinin displays the highest affinity in most B_2 receptor systems, followed by Lys-bradykinin and then by Met-Lys-bradykinin. One exception is the B_2 receptor that mediates contraction of venous smooth muscle; this appears to be most sensitive to Lys-bradykinin. Pharmacologic inhibitors of the action of kinins on B_2 receptors are not yet available.

The mechanisms by which kinins produce their various effects are not well understood. As noted above, some of the actions may be mediated by generation of prostaglandins. Other responses may involve changes in the intracellular concentrations of calcium or cyclic nucleotides.

METABOLISM OF KININS

Kinins are metabolized rapidly (half-life less than 15 seconds) by nonspecific exo- or endopeptidases, commonly referred to as kininases. Two plasma kininases have been well characterized. **Kininase I,** apparently synthesized in the liver, is a carboxypeptidase that releases the carboxyl terminal lysine and arginine residues. It is a metalloprotease and is inhibited by edetate and *o*-phenanthroline. **Kininase II** is present in plasma and vascular endothelial cells throughout the body. It is identical to angiotensin-converting enzyme (peptidyl dipeptidase), discussed above. Kininase II inactivates kinins by cleaving the carboxyl terminal dipeptide phenylalanyl-arginine. Like angiotensin I, bradykinin is almost completely hydrolyzed during a single passage through the pulmonary vascular bed.

DRUGS AFFECTING THE KALLIKREIN-KININ SYSTEM

Relatively few drugs are available to modify the activity of the kallikrein-kinin system. Kinin synthesis can be inhibited with the kallikrein inhibitor **aprotinin (Trasylol).** Competitive antagonists of the B_1 receptor subtype have been synthesized (see above), but inhibitors of B_2 receptors are not yet available. The actions of kinins mediated by prostaglandin generation can be blocked nonspecifically by inhibitors of prostaglandin synthesis. Finally, the actions of kinins can be enhanced by agents that block the degradation of these peptides. Examples of such agents are teprotide and captopril, which inhibit kininase II (angiotensin-converting enzyme). However, it is difficult to determine if the effects of these agents result from accumulation of kinins or from reduced angiotensin II formation.

VASOPRESSIN

Vasopressin plays an important role in the long-term control of blood pressure through its action on the kidney to increase water reabsorption. This and other aspects of the physiology of vasopressin are discussed in detail elsewhere in this volume and will not be discussed here.

There is now considerable evidence that vasopressin also plays an important role in the short-term regulation of arterial pressure by its vasoconstrictor action. It has been shown, for example, that the peptide increases total peripheral resistance when infused in doses less than those required to produce maximum urine concentration. Such doses do not normally increase arterial pressure, because the vasopressor activity of the peptide is effectively buffered by reflex decreases in cardiac output. When the influence of these reflexes is removed by baroreceptor denervation or by other means, pressor sensitivity to vasopressin is greatly increased. Pressor sensitivity to vasopressin is also enhanced in patients with idiopathic orthostatic hypotension. Higher doses of vasopressin increase blood pressure even when baroreceptor reflexes are intact. These doses are generally higher than those required to produce maximum urine concentration; however, pressor responses can be elicited when plasma vasopressin concentration is increased to levels reached during nonhypotensive hemorrhage. Taken together, these observations indicate that at physiologic levels, vasopressin can exert important effects on cardiovascular regulation.

ANALOGS OF VASOPRESSIN

Since the molecular structures of vasopressin and oxytocin were first determined, many analogs of these neurohypophyseal peptides have been synthesized. Structure-activity studies have shown that the vascular receptors for vasopressin differ markedly from the renal receptors that mediate antidiuretic responses. Using this information, it has been possible to synthesize peptides with selective pressor or antidiuretic activity. The most specific vasopressor peptide synthesized to date is [Phe^2,Ile^3,Orn^8]vasotocin. Selective antidiuretic analogs include 1-deamino[D-Arg^8]arginine vasopressin (dDAVP) and 1-deamino[Val^4, D-Arg^8]arginine vasopressin (dVDAVP). Information on structure-activity relations has also made it possible to identify the molecular features required for binding to tissue receptors and for receptor activation. This has permitted the design of specific antagonists of the vasoconstrictor action of vasopressin. One of the most potent antagonists synthesized to date has the following structure: [1-(β-mercapto-β,β-cyclopentamethylene-propionic acid),2-(O-methyl)tyrosine]arginine vasopressin. This compound also has antioxytocic activity but does not antagonize the antidiuretic action of vasopressin. It does not interfere with the actions of other pressor agents such as angiotensin and norepinephrine.

These vasopressor antagonists have been particularly useful for investigating the role of endogenous vasopressin in cardiovascular regulation. The antagonists have no cardiovascular effects when administered to animals in which circulating vasopressin levels are within or below the normal range. However, when they are administered to water-deprived rats or dogs in which circulating vasopressin levels are elevated, prompt decreases in arterial pressure or total peripheral resistance occur. Vasopressin blockade also decreases blood pressure in adrenal-insufficient animals and markedly impairs blood pressure regulation during hemorrhage. Taken together, these and other observations demonstrate that, through its vasoconstrictor action, vasopressin plays an important role in cardiovascular regulation.

There is also some evidence that vasopressin plays a role in experimental hypertension in animals and may be involved in certain forms of human hypertension. Vasopressin antagonists of the type described above will be of value in the investigation of this important question.

VASOACTIVE INTESTINAL PEPTIDE

Vasoactive intestinal peptide (VIP) is a 28-amino-acid peptide closely related structurally to secretin and glucagon. Its structure is shown below:

VIP was originally extracted from porcine lung and was subsequently purified from porcine duodenum. It is now known that VIP is widely distributed in the central and peripheral nervous systems of humans and several animal species. It is also present in the circulation, but the weight of the evidence suggests that VIP functions as a neurotransmitter or neuromodulator rather than as a classic hormone.

VIP produces marked vasodilatation in most vascular beds, including peripheral systemic vessels, as well as the splanchnic, pulmonary, coronary, renal, and cerebral vessels. The vasodilator action of VIP is

His-Ser-Asp-Ala-Val-Phe-Thr-Asp-Asn-Tyr-Thr-Arg-Leu-Arg-Lys-Gln-Met-Ala-Val-Lys-Lys-Tyr-Leu-Asn-Ser-Ile-Leu-Asn-NH_2

Vasoactive intestinal peptide (VIP)

independent of adrenergic, cholinergic, serotinin, and histamine receptors and apparently results from a direct action of the peptide on vascular smooth muscle. As a result of this action, arterial pressure falls and cardiac output increases. The mechanism of the vasodilator action of VIP is not fully understood. However, it has been suggested that VIP binds to specific receptors in the blood vessels and stimulates cAMP production. This effect could be produced by VIP released from the VIP-containing nerve fibers that are associated with blood vessels or by VIP in the circulation.

In addition to dilating blood vessels, VIP relaxes tracheobronchial and gastrointestinal smooth muscle, stimulates intestinal water and electrolyte secretion, promotes hepatic glycogenolysis, causes neuronal excitation, and stimulates the release of several hormones including growth hormone, prolactin, and renin. The physiologic significance of these actions remains to be defined.

SUBSTANCE P

Substance P is an undecapeptide with the following structure:

Arg-Pro-Lys-Pro-Gln-Gln-Phe-Phe-Gly-Leu-Met

Substance P

It is present in the central nervous system, where it is thought to function as a neurotransmitter; and in the gastrointestinal tract, where it may play a role as a local hormone.

Substance P is a potent vasodilator and produces a marked hypotensive action in humans and in several animal species. The vasodilation apparently results from a direct inhibitory effect of the peptide on arteriolar smooth muscle. This action is mediated via specific receptors that differ from those mediating the actions of other vasodilators. In contrast to its effects on arteriolar smooth muscle, substance P stimulates contraction of venous, intestinal, and bronchial smooth muscle. It also causes secretion in the salivary glands, diuresis and natriuresis in the kidneys, and a variety of effects in the central and peripheral nervous systems.

The N-terminal region of substance P is not essential for activity, and several C-terminal fragments of the peptide, including the octa (4–11), hepta (5–11), and hexa (6–11) fragments, are also active. Indeed, depending on the preparation being studied, these peptides may be as potent as the intact undecapeptide or even more so.

• • •

References

Angiotensin

Fitzsimons JT: Angiotensin stimulation of the central nervous system. *Rev Physiol Biochem Pharmacol* 1980;**87:**117.

Ganten D, Hackenthal E, Vecsei P (editors): Renin-angiotensin-aldosterone system and hypertension. (Symposium.) *Klin Wochenschr* 1978;**56(Suppl 1).** [Entire issue.]

Genest J, Koiw E, Kuchel O (editors): *Hypertension: Physiopathology and Treatment.* McGraw-Hill, 1977.

Haber E: Specific inhibitors of renin. *Clin Sci* 1980;**59(Suppl 6):**7s.

Horovitz ZP (editor): *Angiotensin Converting Enzyme Inhibitors.* Urban & Schwarzenberg, 1981.

Johnson JA, Anderson RR: *The Renin-Angiotensin System.* Plenum Press, 1980.

Keeton TK, Campbell WB: The pharmacologic alteration of renin release. *Pharmacol Rev* 1980;**32:**81.

Laragh JH, Bühler FR, Seldin DW (editors): *Frontiers in Hypertension Research.* Springer-Verlag, 1981.

Page IH, Bumpus FM (editors): *Angiotensin.* Springer-Verlag, 1974.

Patchett AA et al: A new class of angiotensin-converting enzyme inhibitors. *Nature* 1980;**288:**280.

Peach MJ: Renin-angiotensin system: Biochemistry and mechanisms of action. *Physiol Rev* 1977;**57:**313.

Reid IA, Morris BJ, Ganong WF: The renin-angiotensin system. *Annu Rev Physiol* 1978;**40:**377.

Soffer L (editor): *Biochemical Regulation of Blood Pressure.* Wiley, 1981.

Stokes GS, Edwards KDG (editors): *Drugs Affecting the Renin-Angiotensin-Aldosterone System: Use of Angiotensin Inhibitors.* Vol 12 of: *Progress in Biochemical Pharmacology.* Karger, 1976.

Zimmerman BG: Adrenergic facilitation by angiotensin: Does it serve a physiological function? *Clin Sci* 1981;**60:**343. [Editorial review.]

Kinins

Regoli D, Barabé J: Pharmacology of bradykinin and related kinins. *Pharmacol Rev* 1980;**32:**1.

Schachter M: Kallikreins (kininogenases): A group of serine proteases with bioregulatory actions. *Pharmacol Rev* 1980;**31:**1.

Vasopressin

Möhring J et al: Greatly enhanced pressor response to antidiuretic hormone in patients with impaired cardiovascular reflexes due to idiopathic orthostatic hypotension. *J Cardiovasc Pharmacol* 1980;**2:**367.

Montani J-P et al: Hemodynamic effects of exogenous and endogenous vasopressin at low plasma concentrations in conscious dogs. *Circ Res* 1980;**47:**346.

Sawyer WH, Grzonka Z, Manning M: Neurohypophysial peptides: Design of tissue-specific agonists and antagonists. *Mol Cell Endocrinol* 1981;**22:**117. [Review article.]

Schwartz J, Reid IA: Effect of vasopressin blockade on blood pressure regulation during hemorrhage in conscious dogs. *Endocrinology* 1981;**109:**1778.

Vasoactive Intestinal Peptide

Said SI (editor): *Vasoactive Intestinal Peptide.* Raven Press, 1982.

Substance P

Couture R, Regoli D: Smooth muscle pharmacology of substance P. *Pharmacology* 1982;**24:**1.

16 | Prostaglandins & Other Eicosanoids

Marc E. Goldyne, MD, PhD

The therapeutic potential of prostaglandins stems from the increasing evidence of their profound physiologic effects as endogenously generated substances in animals and humans. Their biosynthesis has been demonstrated in every major organ of the human body, albeit to varying degrees. In addition to the prostaglandins, recent research has revealed the existence of other biologically active lipids and peptidolipids, biosynthesized from the same precursors as the prostaglandins through interrelated enzymatic pathways. These other lipids include the **thromboxanes, hydroperoxyeicosatetraenoic acids (HPETEs)** and **hydroxyeicosatetraenoic acids (HETEs),** and the **leukotrienes.** The expansion in the number of these interrelated compounds has led to the introduction of the all-inclusive term "eicosanoids," since they all derive from the same eicosaenoic (*eicosa* = 20-carbon; *enoic* = containing double bonds) acid precursors.

In the 1930s, 3 laboratories independently described a uterine smooth muscle-contracting activity deriving from semen. Von Euler named this active principle **prostaglandin** because of its assumed origin from the prostate gland. In the 1960s, Bergstrom et al showed that prostaglandin activity derived from several related compounds and named the first 2 prostaglandins E and F (PGE and PGF) because of their respective solvent partitioning into *e*ther and phosphate buffer (*f*osfat in swedish). Today, 9 prostaglandin groups are recognized.

In 1975, Hamberg et al described substances released by aggregating platelets (thrombocytes) that derived from the same precursors as the prostaglandins but differed in that they contained an oxane ring; thus the name **thromboxane** was coined. At the same time, Hamberg et al described another series of products synthesized from the prostaglandin precursor arachidonic acid. These substances lacked a cyclic structure and contained a hydroperoxy or hydroxyl substitution on the eicosatetraenoic (arachidonic) acid backbone and were accordingly labeled hydroperoxyeicosatetraenoic acids (HPETEs) and hydroxyeicosatetraenoic acids (HETEs).

In 1978, Parker et al demonstrated that the smooth muscle-contracting principle called **slow-reacting substance of anaphylaxis (SRS-A)** was a derivative of the prostaglandin precursor arachidonic acid. Subsequently, Borgeat et al isolated arachidonic acid derivatives from rabbit leukocytes that contained a conjugated triene bonding—hence the name **leukotrienes.** Subsequent work showed that SRS-A was in fact a combination of 2 of these leukotrienes.

Endogenously generated eicosanoids are synthesized at the cell membrane (Fig 16–1). The appropriate stimulus may vary, depending on the cell type. In response to this stimulus, phospholipase A_2 or a combination of phospholipase C and diglyceride lipase catalyzes the cleavage of an esterified eicosanoid precursor, such as arachidonic acid, from the 2 position of specific glycerophospholipids that constitute part of the lipid bilayer of the cell membrane. Once free, the arachidonic acid can activate several enzyme systems that are variably distributed among different cells. One enzyme, cyclooxygenase, converts arachidonic acid to unstable endoperoxide intermediates (PGG_2 and PGH_2). These can then be further metabolized through appropriate enzymatic activity to either the prostaglandins (PGD_2 through $PGF_{2\alpha}$ and PGI_2, also called prostacyclin) or to the thromboxanes. The E prostaglandins can be further metabolized to the B prostaglandins in vivo or to the A or B prostaglandins in vitro. Another group of enzymes collectively called lipoxygenases convert arachidonic acid to a series of HPETEs, which are then further metabolized to either a series of corresponding HETEs or to the leukotrienes.

The variety of prostaglandins or related lipids synthesized is cell type-specific. For example, epidermal cells produce D, E, and F group prostaglandins and 12-HETE but not thromboxanes. Vascular endothelium synthesizes primarily prostacyclin (PGI_2). Platelets, on the other hand, synthesize primarily thromboxanes.

Corticosteroids block all of the known pathways of eicosanoid metabolism by stimulating the synthesis of a protein called lipomodulin, which in turn inhibits the activity of phospholipases, thus preventing the initial release of arachidonic acid required to activate the subsequent enzymatic pathways. The nonsteroidal anti-inflammatory drugs (eg, aspirin, indomethacin, ibuprofen) block both prostaglandin and thromboxane synthesis by inhibiting cyclooxygenase activity. Aspirin specifically acetylates the enzyme, whereas the exact mechanism of inhibition by the other agents is

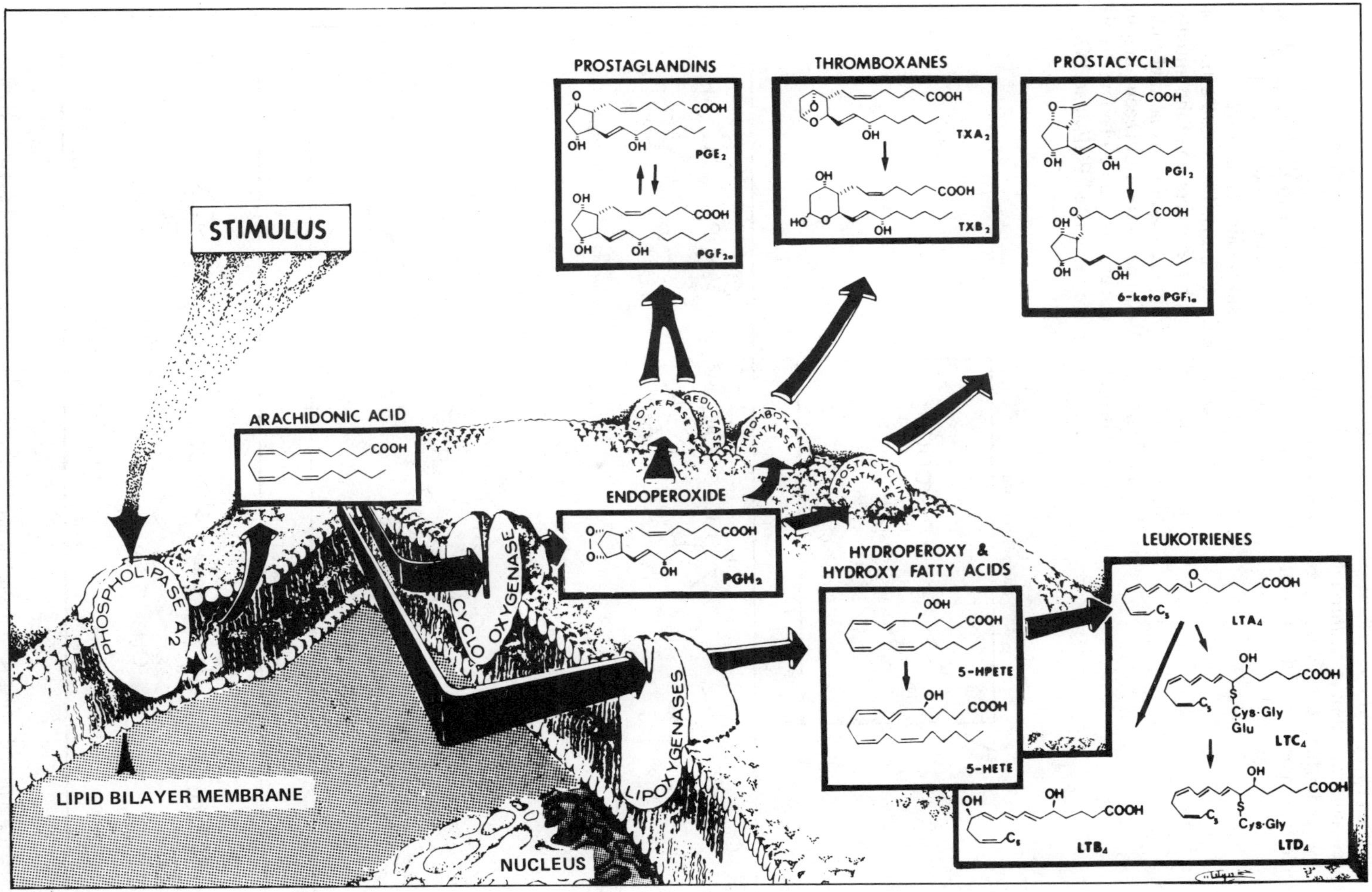

Figure 16–1. Biosynthesis of eicosanoids. The biosynthesis of prostaglandins and related lipids occurs for the most part at the cell membrane. However, the 5-lipoxygenase that catalyzes the generation of leukotrienes and 5-HETE may be a cytosolic enzyme. In response to an appropriate stimulus, a phospholipase is activated that cleaves arachidonic acid (a precursor of prostaglandins) from the phospholipids making up the lipid bilayer of the cell membranes. Free arachidonic acid activates several enzyme systems. One enzyme, cyclooxygenase, converts arachidonic acid into an unstable endoperoxide intermediate that can be further converted, through appropriate enzymatic activity, to prostaglandins (including prostacyclin) and thromboxanes. Another group of enzymes, the lipoxygenases, convert arachidonic acid to a series of hydroxy fatty acids (ie, HPETEs and HETEs) or, in conjunction with other enzymes, to the recently identified leukotrienes.

not fully understood. The nonsteroidal anti-inflammatory drugs do not, however, inhibit the lipoxygenase enzymes. In fact, by blocking utilization of the eicosanoid substrates by cyclooxygenase, they may cause an increased substrate utilization through the lipoxygenase pathways leading to increased production of (for example) the smooth muscle-stimulating leukotrienes.

I. BASIC PHARMACOLOGY OF PROSTAGLANDINS & OTHER EICOSANOIDS

Chemistry of Prostaglandins

The basic structure common to all prostaglandins, referred to as "prostanoic acid," consists of a pentane ring with 2 aliphatic side chains (Fig 16–2).

A. Prostaglandin Groups: There are 9 groups of prostaglandins that, with the exception of the initially discovered E and F groups, are arbitrarily assigned the letter designations A–I. They differ from each other in having substitutions at carbons 9 and 11. The 2 epimers of the F group are designated PGF_α and PGF_β.

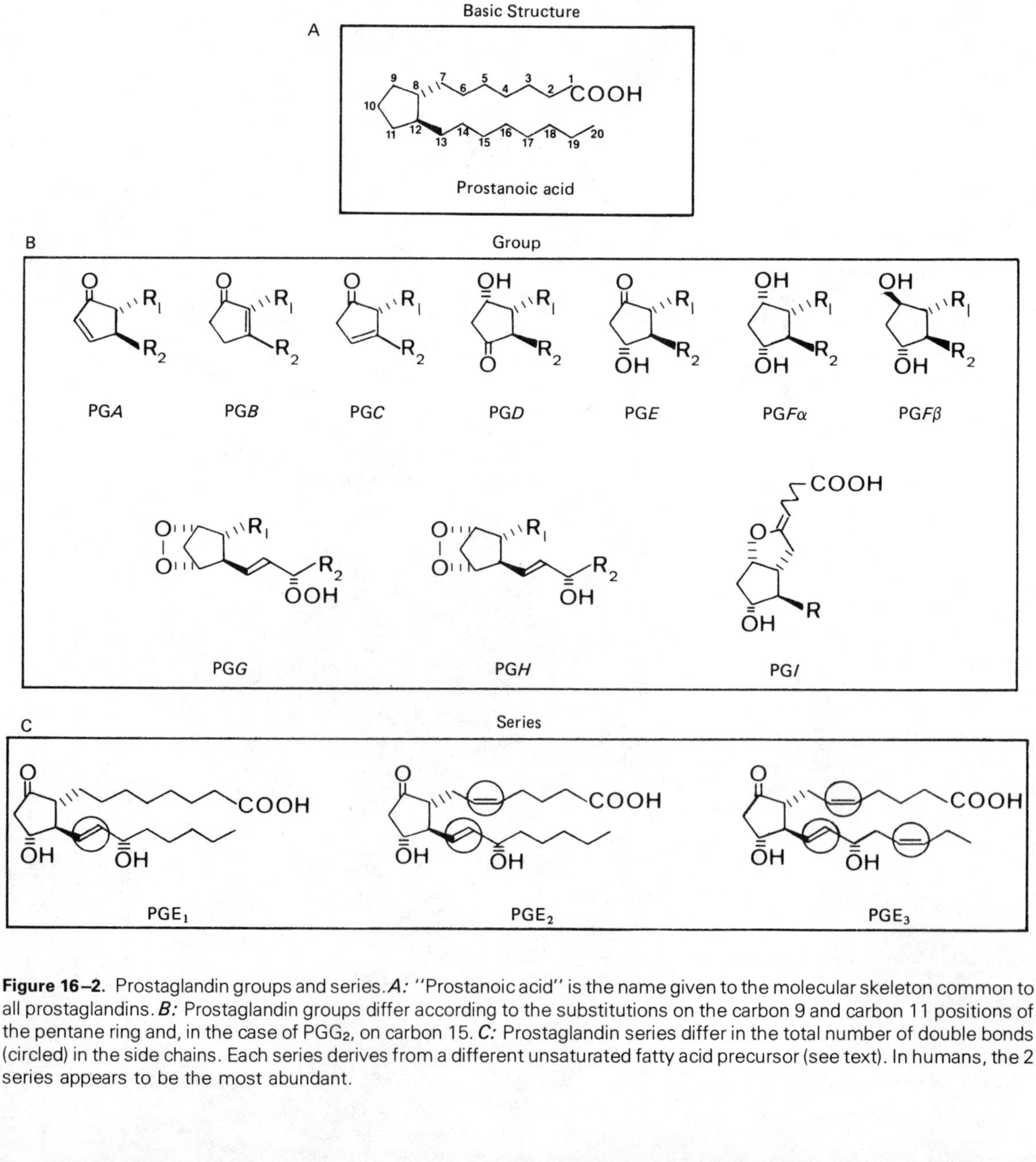

Figure 16–2. Prostaglandin groups and series. *A:* "Prostanoic acid" is the name given to the molecular skeleton common to all prostaglandins. *B:* Prostaglandin groups differ according to the substitutions on the carbon 9 and carbon 11 positions of the pentane ring and, in the case of PGG_2, on carbon 15. *C:* Prostaglandin series differ in the total number of double bonds (circled) in the side chains. Each series derives from a different unsaturated fatty acid precursor (see text). In humans, the 2 series appears to be the most abundant.

PGG and PGH are, as mentioned above, short-lived endoperoxide intermediates in the formation of all of the other prostaglandins. With the exception of PGG, which has a hydroperoxy substitution at carbon 15, all of the remaining prostaglandins possess a hydroxyl group at this position. In addition, all prostaglandins have a Δ^{13} double bond. The substitutions on the pentane ring appear responsible for the qualitative activities of the different groups, whereas the Δ^{13} bonding and carbon 15 hydroxyl group are required for full activity.

B. Prostaglandin Series: Each prostaglandin group except PGI can be classified in one of 3 series, designated by a subscript 1, 2, or 3 following the group designation. This subscript indicates the total number of double bonds in the 2 side chains of the prostaglandin molecule and reflects the fact that prostaglandins can be synthesized from 3 different eicosaenoic acids, which themselves differ in the total number of double bonds present. The 1 series derives from 8,11,14-eicosatrienoic acid (dihomo-γ-linolenic acid), the 2 series from 5,8,11,14-eicosatetraenoic acid, and the 3 series from 5,8,11,14,17-eicosapentaenoic acid. In humans, it appears that the 2 series is the most abundant. PGI exists only in the 2 and 3 series, since it requires the Δ^5 double bond for its synthesis.

Chemistry of Thromboxanes

The structure common to all thromboxanes is the presence of an oxane ring with the same 2 aliphatic side chains common to prostaglandins (Fig 16–1).

A. Thromboxane Groups: Two groups are recognized, designated TXA and TXB. TXA is a highly unstable oxane:oxetane compound with an aqueous half-life of 45 seconds. TXB is the stable spontaneous hydration derivative of TXA.

B. Thromboxane Series: Thromboxanes can also exist in any one of 3 series designated by a subscript 1, 2, or 3, depending, as with the prostaglandins, on the fatty acid precursor.

Chemistry of HPETEs & HETEs

The HPETEs derive from a different enzymatic pathway than the prostaglandins and thromboxanes and are not cyclic compounds (Fig 16–1). Their structure consists of the parent fatty acid with a hydroperoxy substituent. The position of this group is designated by a numerical prefix indicating the carbon position of the substitution (eg, 12-HPETE). The HPETEs are relatively unstable and are reduced enzymatically or nonenzymatically to the corresponding HETEs (eg, 12-HPETE → 12-HETE).

Chemistry of Leukotrienes

A. Leukotriene Groups: Five groups of leukotrienes have currently been identified, designated LTA through LTE (Fig 16–3). LTA is an unstable epoxide intermediate that interacts with glutathione S-transferase to produce LTC, which contains a carbon 5 hydroxyl group and a carbon 6 glutathione linked via the sulfur in the cysteinyl residue as a thioether. LTD results from the enzymatic removal of glutamic acid from glutathione. LTE is produced by the enzymatic removal of glycine from the LTD molecule. LTB is a dihydroxy derivative of 5-HPETE.

B. Leukotriene Series: As is the case with prostaglandins, 3 series of leukotrienes exist; they are designated by a subscript 3, 4, or 5 since, unlike the other eicosanoids, all of the double bonds in the parent trienoic, tetraenoic, and pentaenoic acids are retained.

Pharmacokinetics of Prostaglandins

The naturally occurring prostaglandins are rapidly degraded following their introduction into the systemic circulation. Whether endogenously generated or intravenously administered, PGE_2, for example, is quickly inactivated by the pulmonary, hepatic, and renal vascular beds. Such inactivation involves enzymatic oxidation of the carbon 15 hydroxyl group to a ketone (15-hydroxy prostaglandin dehydrogenase) and a reductive saturation of the Δ^{13} double bond (Δ^{13} prostaglandin reductase). In addition, there is beta and omega oxidation of the aliphatic side chains. These metabolites are excreted in the urine. Intravenous administration of labeled PGE_2 or $PGF_{2\alpha}$ in humans leads to rapid formation of the corresponding 15-keto-13,14-dihydro metabolites. Within 2 minutes, less than 3% of the initially administered compound remains in the blood; 40% is recovered as inactive metabolites. Within the blood, the half-life of most prostaglandins is less than 1 minute and of the metabolites about 8 minutes. Many tissues contain the enzymes necessary for prostaglandin degradation.

Pharmacokinetics of Thromboxanes

The biologically active TXA_2 is rapidly and spontaneously hydrated in the blood to TXB_2. Although the half-life of TXA_2 can be prolonged by the presence of albumin, this does not occur to a degree that would render the natural compound usable as a therapeutic agent. As with prostaglandins, thromboxane metabolites are excreted in the urine, and over 20 such metabolites have been described.

Pharmacokinetics of HPETEs & HETEs

Little is known about the metabolism of these hydroxy fatty acids, but both beta and omega oxidation probably occur.

Pharmacokinetics of Leukotrienes

The relatively recent isolation of the leukotrienes accounts for the scant information on their metabolism in humans. In porcine kidney, LTD_4, which has SRS-A activity, is converted to the less polar LTE_4, which is 8–12 times less potent as a smooth muscle stimulator. Local tissue breakdown of leukotrienes also occurs, and, as with other eicosanoids, the metabolites are probably excreted in the urine.

Mechanism of Action of Eicosanoids on Smooth Muscle

Prostaglandins as well as some of the other

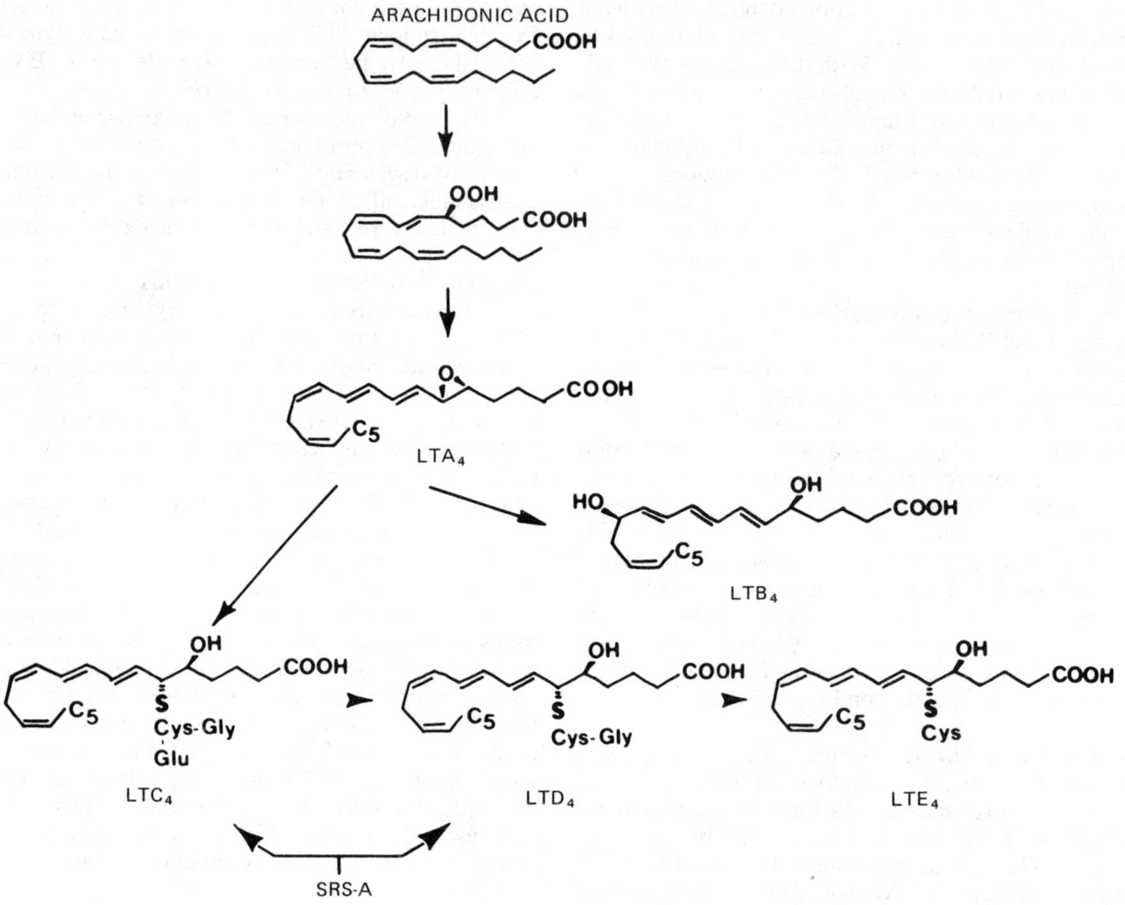

Figure 16–3. The leukotrienes synthesized from arachidonic acid. LTA_4 is an unstable epoxide intermediate in the synthesis of the remaining leukotrienes. LTC_4 and LTD_4 are the actual molecules that constitute the **slow-reacting substance of anaphylaxis (SRS-A)**. LTE_4 is an inactive metabolite of LTD_4. LTB_4 is a potent chemotactic substance for neutrophils and eosinophils.

eicosanoids appear to act in smooth muscle via specific receptors that are not blocked by conventional autonomic blocking agents (atropine, propranolol, phenoxybenzamine, hexamethonium) nor by antihistamine or antiserotonin drugs. Many of their actions appear to be associated with a change in the levels of one of the cyclic nucleotides, cAMP or cGMP, in the responding tissue. For example, venoconstriction in response to $PGF_{2\alpha}$ is associated with a rise in cGMP, whereas venodilatation induced by PGE_2 is associated with a rise in cAMP. This PGE_2-cAMP and $PGF_{2\alpha}$-cGMP association may change depending on the tissue. Nevertheless, an interaction between the prostaglandins or other eicosanoids and the cyclic nucleotides appears fairly well established for smooth muscle. The contraction of smooth muscle beds by various eicosanoids is associated with depolarization of the membrane potential, either alone or coupled with increased frequency and length of action potential bursts. Conversely, relaxation of smooth muscle by eicosanoids is associated with hyperpolarization.

Effects on Smooth Muscle

A. Vascular Smooth Muscle:

1. Prostaglandins–Prostaglandin activity is quite diverse among different vascular beds and different species. In animals, vascular smooth muscle itself synthesizes PGE_2, $PGF_{2\alpha}$, and PGI_2. In humans, PGE_2, PGI_2 (prostacyclin), and PGA_2 are generally regarded as arteriolar dilators, whereas $PGF_{2\alpha}$ is a weak arteriolar dilator but an effective venoconstrictor in some vascular beds. Intravenous administration of PGE_2 in humans induces facial flushing and vasodilatation in the systemic and pulmonary vascular beds. $PGF_{2\alpha}$ administered intravenously to humans (0.1–1 μg/kg/min) does not induce facial flushing and has no effect on systemic vascular resistance but increases local peripheral vascular resistance and pulmonary vascular resistance. In contrast to its general vasodilating effects, PGE_2 constricts human umbilical cord vessels, as does $PGF_{2\alpha}$. In the dog, prostaglandins of the E and A groups dilate the coronary vessels, whereas $PGF_{2\alpha}$ has no significant effect. The local synthesis of prostaglandins in various vascular beds may contribute to maintaining normal vascular tone.

2. Thromboxanes–The instability of TXA_2 makes its evaluation as a vasoactive agent difficult, although it has been shown in vitro to be a potent constrictor of umbilical vessels. TXB_2 has been shown in animals to have modest constrictor activity in the pulmonary vascular bed.

3. HPETEs and HETEs–These substances do not appear to significantly affect vascular smooth muscle tone.

4. Leukotrienes–There are few data regarding the effects of leukotrienes on vascular smooth muscle in humans. In vitro, LTC_4 and LTD_4 are weak constrictors of human pulmonary artery or vein smooth muscle. In other primates, intravenous injection of LTC_4 or LTD_4 (0.1 μg/kg) causes a decrease in peripheral vascular resistance; however, since LTC_4 and LTD_4 can induce PGE release from various tissues, the observed decrease may be an indirect effect. In animals, cutaneous arterioles appear to constrict initially and then relax in response to LTC_4 and LTD_4.

B. Respiratory Smooth Muscle:

1. Prostaglandins–In vitro, the E prostaglandins relax tracheal or bronchial smooth muscle and antagonize the contractile response induced by agents such as bradykinin, histamine, acetylcholine, and serotonin. PGI_2, also formed in lung tissue, relaxes bronchiolar smooth muscle. $PGF_{2\alpha}$ and PGD_2 are also produced by human lung. However, they are potent constrictors of human tracheal and bronchial smooth muscle. On a molar basis, $PGF_{2\alpha}$ inhaled as an aerosol mist is several times more potent than histamine. There is some evidence that these prostaglandins may participate in regulating bronchopulmonary tone.

2. Thromboxanes–TXA_2 is perhaps the most potent of the eicosanoids as a bronchoconstrictor. It can be released from human lung following immunologic stimulation and may also participate with the other eicosanoids in regulating physiologic and pathophysiologic aspects of respiratory smooth muscle response.

3. HPETEs and HETEs–Various HPETEs are synthesized in the lung, and rapidly reduced to their respective HETE derivatives. 5-HETE (0.001–1 μg/mL) produces slow contractions of isolated human bronchial smooth muscle, with a potency comparable to that of histamine. In addition, if given at subthreshold doses, 5-HETE will potentiate histamine-induced contractions. 15-HETE is somewhat less potent than either 5-HETE or histamine. 12-HETE is inactive.

4. Leukotrienes–In nanogram concentrations, LTB_4, LTC_4, and LTD_4 cause marked constriction of human peripheral lung segments and bronchial smooth muscle in vitro (Fig 16–4). Nebulized delivery of LTC_4 or LTD_4 induces bronchoconstriction, and comparison of FEV 1 values to expiratory flow at low lung volumes suggests that the major site of constriction is in the peripheral airways. Studies in animals show that

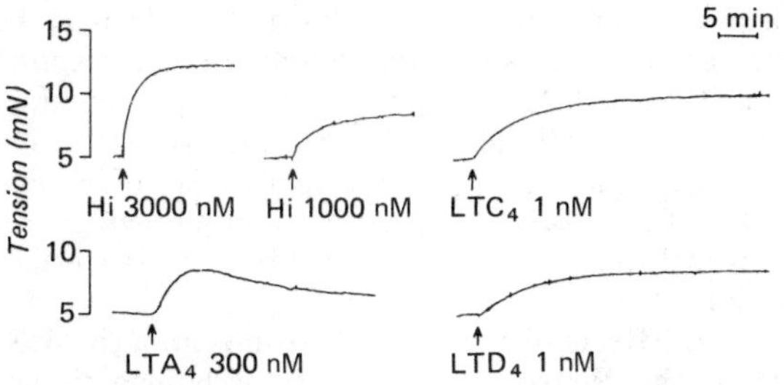

Figure 16–4. Contractions of isolated segments of human bronchi recorded after exposure to histamine (Hi) and the leukotrienes LTA_4, LTC_4, and LTD_4. LTC_4 and LTD_4, which together comprise SRS-A, are 300 times more potent than LTA_4 and 1000 times more potent than histamine. (Reproduced, with permission, from Dahlen S-E et al: *Nature* 1980;**288**:484.)

indomethacin, a potent inhibitor of prostaglandin and thromboxane synthesis, can block the effects of the leukotrienes on airway smooth muscle, suggesting that some of the actions of leukotrienes may be mediated by the prostaglandins or thromboxanes.

C. Gastrointestinal Smooth Muscle:

1. Prostaglandins–Various prostaglandins are produced throughout the gastrointestinal tract, the major ones being PGI_2, PGE_2, and $PGF_{2\alpha}$. In vitro studies with human gastrointestinal smooth muscle show that PGE_2 contracts longitudinal but relaxes circular smooth muscle. $PGF_{2\alpha}$ appears to contract both longitudinal and circular smooth muscle. However, in human gallbladder, $PGF_{2\alpha}$, while contracting longitudinal smooth muscle, was without effect on circular smooth muscle. PGI_2, in contrast to PGE_2, contracts circular smooth muscle. While these observations derive from in vitro studies, in vivo oral administration of E prostaglandins to humans increases bile concentration within aspirated gastric fluid. These results are compatible with PGE-induced relaxation of the pyloric sphincter. Furthermore, intravenous administration of PGE_2 or $PGF_{2\alpha}$ leads to colicky cramping, suggesting that these prostaglandins increase gastrointestinal smooth muscle activity in vivo. In animals, intravenous infusion of E prostaglandins decreases lower esophageal sphincter tone, again suggesting that in vivo, the E prostaglandins relax circular smooth muscle.

2. Thromboxanes–Although TXB_2 has been shown to be synthesized by gastric fundal and antral mucosal cells, the effects of thromboxanes on intestinal smooth muscle are not well established.

3. HPETEs and HETEs–The effects of these substances on gastrointestinal smooth muscle have not been well studied.

4. Leukotrienes–Before their structural elucidation, the SRS-A activity now known to be caused by LTC_4 and LTD_4 was determined on smooth muscle preparations from guinea pig ileum. This smooth muscle preparation demonstrates a slow onset but prolonged contractile response. However, this effect on gastrointestinal smooth muscle in animals may be species-specific, since rat ileum fails to respond to LTC_4 or LTD_4 at concentrations causing contraction of guinea pig ileum. However, the rat colon and stomach (fundus) are highly responsive to LTC_4 and LTD_4. The effects of leukotrienes on human gastrointestinal smooth muscle have not been clearly established.

D. Effects of Prostaglandins on Smooth Muscle of the Reproductive Tract: In human tissue, PGE_2 contracts the proximal quarter of the uterine tubes in vitro but relaxes the distal segments. In contrast, $PGF_{2\alpha}$ exerts a contractile effect on all segments. Intravenous injection of PGE_2 inhibits whereas $PGF_{2\alpha}$ increases tubal contractions, in keeping with the in vitro observations. Estrogens apparently enhance—whereas progesterone diminishes—the contractile response of the uterine tubes to the prostaglandins.

In the uterus, prostaglandins are synthesized primarily by the endometrium and act on myometrial smooth muscle. However, PGI_2 may be a product of the myometrium. Both PGE_2 and $PGF_{2\alpha}$ stimulate contractions of human myometrium in both pregnant and nonpregnant females. However, whereas intrauterine administration of PGE_2 in low doses (2–5 μg) produces contraction, higher doses (20–30 μg) cause relaxation. PGE_2 and PGI_2 cause relaxation of isolated human myometrium and can antagonize $PGF_{2\alpha}$-induced contractions. However, these in vitro effects may not always reflect in vivo action.

The effects of other eicosanoids on human reproductive tract smooth muscle are not well established.

E. Summary of Effects of Eicosanoids on Human Smooth Muscle: Table 16–1 summarizes the effects of the various eicosanoids on human smooth muscle beds. It is apparent that the responses elicited vary in different types of smooth muscle. Varying the dose of eicosanoid can also change the type of response observed.

Actions of Eicosanoids on Other Tissues

The endogenously synthesized eicosanoids probably serve a far broader array of regulatory functions than simple stimulation or inhibition of smooth muscle. In fact, they probably play a role as a fine-tuning system for a variety of basic cellular functions. The rapid inactivation of most eicosanoids within the organ in which they are synthesized or within the systemic circulation permits such cell-specific effects. Thus, no definition of the roles of eicosanoids is valid unless the responding tissue or cells under study are specifically identified. For example, for the platelet, thromboxane is a signal that induces aggregation, whereas to certain smooth muscle cells it is a signal that induces contraction. In the hypothalamus, PGE_2 activates the thermoregulatory center and induces fever, whereas to some smooth muscle cells it is a signal for relaxation and to others a signal for contraction. In the kidney, PGE_2 directly stimulates renin release as well as renal sodium loss. Local prostaglandins also seem to regulate distribution of renal blood flow. To thymic-derived lymphocytes, PGE_2 can be a signal that either enhances or suppresses proliferation depending on the subpopulation of lymphocytes. Such polyfunctional properties provide an explanation for the widespread and often confusing effects of eicosanoids when they are systemically administered at levels greater than can be achieved by normal endogenous metabolism. The same circumstance accounts for the difficulties inherent in using eicosanoids as therapeutic agents. Conversely, some of the side-effects of drugs that block synthesis of certain eicosanoids may stem from blockade of the physiologic functions of these endogenously generated compounds. For example, the ulcer-inducing effect of corticosteroids and aspirin or indomethacin may stem from their inhibition of prostaglandin generation by the gastric mucosa, since some prostaglandins have been shown to exert a cytoprotective effect on gastrointestinal mucosa.

Table 16–1. Effects of eicosanoids on smooth muscle in humans. (C = contraction; R = relaxation; 0 = no effect; ? = not determined.)

	Vascular System		Respiratory System		Gastrointestinal Tract		Reproductive Tract	
	Arterial	Venous	Tracheal	Bronchial	Longitudinal	Circular	Tubal	Uterine
PGE_2	R[1]	0	R	R	C	R	C[2]	C[3]
$PGF_{2\alpha}$	R[1]	C	C	C	C	C	C	C
PGI_2 (prostacyclin)	R	0	R	R	C	C	?	R
TXA_2	C	?	C	C	?	?	?	?
TXB_2	C	?	0	0	?	?	?	?
HETEs	0	0	C[4]	C[4]	?	?	?	?
LTC_4	C	C	C	C	?[5]	?[5]	?	?
LTD_4	C	C	C	C	?	?	?	?
LTE_4	0	0	0	0	?	?	?	?

[1] Both E and F prostaglandins constrict umbilical arteries.

[2] PGE_2 contracts proximal quarter but relaxes distal segment.

[3] Low dose range (2–5 μg) contracts; high dose range (20–30 μg) relaxes.

[4] 5-HETE > 15-HETE; 12-HETE is inactive.

[5] No reliable human studies.

II. CLINICAL PHARMACOLOGY OF PROSTAGLANDINS & OTHER EICOSANOIDS

The major clinical applications of agents in this group relate to their effects on smooth muscle. The effects of specific eicosanoids on various smooth muscle beds coupled with the knowledge of their endogenous synthesis have been used in 2 ways. The first involves direct use of prostaglandins or other eicosanoids as pharmacologic smooth muscle agonists; the second is concerned with the use of drugs that inhibit endogenous synthesis of eicosanoids and thereby modify smooth muscle activity.

EICOSANOIDS AS THERAPEUTIC AGENTS

In Gynecology

The ability of PGE_2 and $PGF_{2\alpha}$ to contract uterine smooth muscle—not only at term, as with oxytocin, but throughout pregnancy—has led to their use for inducing abortion as well as for the induction of term labor. However, since induction of term labor with these prostaglandins is accompanied by increased risks of uterine hypertonus and fetal bradycardia, their use in gynecologic practice has been primarily as abortifacients. When given intravenously, intramuscularly, or intravaginally, PGE_2 or $PGF_{2\alpha}$ is very effective in inducing second-trimester abortion. Intravaginal therapy is preferred, since this route reduces the stimulation of other smooth muscle beds that leads to side-effects of nausea, vomiting, abdominal cramping, diarrhea, hypotension or hypertension, headache, and asthmalike attacks. In addition, convulsions have been observed in susceptible individuals. Three preparations have been used: (1) dinoprost tromethamine ($PGF_{2\alpha}$, Prostin F2 alpha), for intra-amniotic administration; (2) carboprost tromethamine (15-methyl $PGF_{2\alpha}$, Prostin/15M), for intramuscular injection; and (3) dinoprostone (PGE_2, Prostin E2), as vaginal suppository. These agents appear to be preferable to intra-amniotic injection of hypertonic saline because of their more rapid onset of action and the lower incidence of major complications.

In Pulmonary Disease

The bronchodilator effect of PGE_2 has led to numerous studies of this prostaglandin as a possible agent to treat diseases associated with bronchoconstriction. However, inhalation of PGE compounds often causes severe irritation of the upper respiratory tract or induces paradoxic bronchoconstriction, thereby precluding its use as a therapeutically effective bronchodilator. Attempts to modify the structure of PGE_2 in order to diminish these untoward effects have so far led to a marked diminution in bronchodilator potency. This therapeutic area is still under investigation.

In Cardiovascular Disease

A significant therapeutic application of the E prostaglandins has been in the area of ductus-dependent cardiac malformations. The ability of alprostadil (PGE_1) to maintain patency of the ductus arteriosus has led to its evaluation as presurgical therapy for neonates suffering from transposition of the great arteries, pulmonary atresia, or pulmonary stenosis. Continuous infusion of 0.05–0.1 μg/kg/min intra-arterially or intravenously maintains ductal patency. FDA approval has been given for this use of PGE_1, and it is marketed as Prostin VR Pediatric.

PGE_1 and PGI_2 (prostacyclin) have been used investigationally as vasodilators for treatment of peripheral vascular diseases. At a dose of 2–4 μg/h, over a 10-minute period for each of 3 days, PGE_1 has in selected cases provided relief of pain and increase in skin temperature and is associated with healing of theretofore recalcitrant ulcers. PGI_2 infused intra-arterially or into the subclavian vein may produce a striking improvement in claudication. Muscle blood flow increased significantly in the affected extremities, and in some patients this effect lasted 4–6 weeks after treatment. Since generation of endogenous PGI_2 by vascular endothelium is decreased in atherosclerotic areas of vessel walls, it may be that PGI_2 infusion acts by reestablishing some mechanism essential for maintenance of vascular tone as well as by clearing platelet aggregations obstructing capillary beds in the affected extremities.

PGE_1 (6–10 ng/kg/min) has also been administered intravenously to patients suffering from systemic sclerosis with Raynaud's phenomenon. After administration of PGE_1 (but not of saline), increased skin temperature, improvement in cold tolerance, and reduced intensity of Raynaud attacks were reported. The improvement lasted for several weeks. Further evaluation of vasodilating prostaglandins in the treatment of occlusive vascular diseases is definitely warranted in light of these initial studies.

THERAPEUTIC INHIBITION OF ENDOGENOUS EICOSANOID SYNTHESIS

Several novel uses for the more potent nonsteroidal anti-inflammatory drugs (NSAIDs)—aspirin, indomethacin, mefanamic acid, ibuprofen, and naproxen—have been evaluated since the discovery that one of their pharmacologic effects is inhibition of prostaglandin and thromboxane synthesis.

NSAIDs & Dysmenorrhea

Current evidence strongly implicates excessive $PGF_{2\alpha}$ synthesis as an important factor in dysmenorrhea. High levels of $PGF_{2\alpha}$ are found in menstrual fluid of patients suffering from primary dysmenorrhea, and uterine cramping accompanies intravenous administration of sufficiently high doses of $PGF_{2\alpha}$. Clinical trials using indomethacin, ibuprofen, and naproxen have shown these drugs to be extremely effective in relieving the symptoms of dysmenorrhea. Aspirin is far less effective, perhaps because of the decreased sensitivity of uterine cyclooxygenase to aspirin when compared to the other NSAIDs. Typically, ibuprofen, 400 mg 4 times daily for 3 days prior to the expected menstrual period and continued for 3 days during menstruation, has produced significant relief of dysmenorrhea. Indomethacin has also been used with success when given in a dose of 50 mg at the first sign of an attack followed by no more than 2 repeat 50-mg doses over the ensuing 24 hours. While none of the NSAIDs have as yet been approved for use in management of primary dysmenorrhea, it is probable that one or several may in future be the treatment of choice for this disorder.

NSAIDs & Ductus Closure

Patency of the fetal ductus arteriosus is regarded as an active state caused by continual synthesis of either PGE_2 or PGI_2 by the ductal endothelium. This concept is supported by animal and human studies showing that PGE_1 and PGI_2 can maintain patency of the ductus and that agents which block prostaglandin synthesis cause closure of the ductus. Therapeutic advantage has been taken of this observation, and NSAIDs have been used to treat premature infants who develop respiratory distress due to failure of ductus closure. In such infants, administration of indomethacin (0.3–0.6 mg/kg/24 h) has succeeded in causing closure of the ductus, thereby precluding the need for surgical ligation (Chapter 33).

Current studies of a variety of diseases in which symptoms may derive from prostaglandin-induced smooth muscle activity offer promise of other uses for NSAIDs and other inhibitors of eicosanoid synthesis.

• • •

References

Benson LN et al: Role of prostaglandin E_1 infusion in the management of transposition of the great arteries. *Am J Cardiol* 1979;**44:**691.

Caldwell B, Behrman HR: Prostaglandins in reproductive processes. *Med Clin North Am* 1981;**65:**927.

Hirsh PD et al: Prostaglandins and ischemic heart disease. *Am J Med* 1981;**71:**1009.

Horton EW: Prostaglandins and smooth muscle. *Br Med Bull* 1979;**35:**295.

Hyman AL et al: Prostaglandins and the lung. *Med Clin North Am* 1981;**65:**789.

Metz SA: Anti-inflammatory agents as inhibitors of prostaglandin synthesis in man. *Med Clin North Am* 1981;**65:**713.

Olley PM et al: Clinical uses of prostaglandins and prostaglandin synthetase inhibitors in cardiac problems of the newborn. Page 913 in: *Advances in Prostaglandin and Thromboxane Research*. Vol 7. Samuelsson B, Ramwell P, Paoletti R (editors). Raven, 1980.

Piper PJ et al: Pharmacological studies on pure SRS-A, SRS, and synthetic leukotriene C_4 and D_4. Page 81 in: *SRS-A and Leukotrienes*. Piper PJ (editor). Research Studies Press, 1981.

Samuelsson B, Hammarstrom S: Nomenclature for leukotrienes. *Prostaglandins* 1980;**19:**645.

Samuelsson B et al: Prostaglandins and thromboxanes. *Annu Rev Biochem* 1978;**47:**997.

Bronchodilators & Other Agents Used in the Treatment of Asthma | 17

Homer A. Boushey, MD, & Michael J. Holtzman, MD

Asthma has been described as a disease characterized by increased responsiveness of the trachea and bronchi to various stimuli, manifested by widespread narrowing of the airways that changes in severity either spontaneously or as a result of therapy. The clinical hallmarks of asthma are recurrent, episodic bouts of coughing, shortness of breath, chest tightness, and wheezing. Its pathologic features are contraction of airway smooth muscle, mucosal thickening from edema and cellular infiltration, and inspissation in the airway lumen of abnormally thick, viscid plugs of mucus. Of these causes of airway obstruction, contraction of smooth muscle is most easily reversed by current therapy.

The most widely used bronchodilators are β-adrenergic stimulants (Chapter 7) and theophylline, a methylxanthine drug. Reversal of airway constriction can also be brought about by the use of antimuscarinic agents (Chapter 6). Two other types of drugs important in asthma are cromolyn, an inhibitor of mast cell degranulation, and corticosteroids.

This chapter presents the basic pharmacology of cromolyn and methylxanthines—agents whose medical use is almost exclusively for pulmonary disease. The other classes of drugs listed above are discussed in relation to the therapy of asthma.

A rational approach to the pharmacotherapy of asthma depends on an understanding of a conceptual model for the pathogenesis of the disease. In the classic immunologic model, asthma is a disease mediated by reaginic (IgE) antibodies bound to mast cells in the airway mucosa. On reexposure to an antigen, antigen-antibody interaction takes place on the surface of the mast cells, triggering both the release of mediators stored in the cells' granules and the synthesis and release of other mediators. The agents released include histamine, slow-reacting substance of anaphylaxis (SRS-A), eosinophil chemotactic factor (ECF), neutrophil chemotactic factor (NCF), and other compounds. In the traditional view, these agents diffuse throughout the airway wall and directly cause contraction of muscle, edema, cellular infiltration, and a change in mucus secretion that characterize the condition pathologically.

There are several features of asthma, however, that cannot be accounted for by this model. Most adults with asthma have no evidence of immediate hypersensitivity to antigens, and most attacks cannot be related to recent exposure to an unusual quantity of antigen. Even in patients with a history of asthma during the ragweed season and positive cutaneous and bronchial responses to ragweed antigen, the severity of asthma symptoms correlates poorly with the quantity of antigen in the atmosphere. Furthermore, bronchospasm can be provoked by nonantigenic stimuli, such as distilled water, exercise, cold air, sulfur dioxide, and rapid respiratory maneuvers.

In healthy nonasthmatic people, inhalation of small doses of mediators of anaphylaxis (eg, histamine) does not provoke bronchoconstriction. In people with asthma, however, inhalation of even smaller doses of the same mediator provokes intense symptomatic bronchospasm. This exaggerated sensitivity of the airways is sometimes called "nonspecific bronchial hyperreactivity" to distinguish it from the bronchospasm provoked by specific antigens. Bronchial hyperactivity appears to be fundamental to asthma's pathogenesis, for it is nearly ubiquitous in patients with asthma; its degree correlates positively with the symptomatic severity of the disease; and the events that increase bronchial reactivity (viral respiratory infections, exposure to oxidizing pollutants) have often been noted to cause symptomatic worsening of disease.

The mechanism underlying bronchial hyperreactivity is unknown, but it appears to involve parasympathetic reflex pathways (Fig 17–1). Thus, the bronchospasm provoked in dogs by histamine can be greatly reduced by pretreatment with an inhaled topical anesthetic agent, by blockade of the vagus nerves, and by pretreatment with atropine, a competitive antagonist of acetylcholine, in doses that have no effect on the responses of airway smooth muscle to histamine in vitro. Similar findings have been made in human studies. The abnormal, exaggerated bronchomotor response of asthmatic subjects to inhalation of histamine can be blocked by pretreatment with atropine or with aerosolized hexamethonium, a drug that inhibits transmission through parasympathetic ganglia (Chapter 6). Thus, the bronchoconstriction provoked by histamine appears in part to be due to a parasympathetic reflex response. The bronchial hyperreactivity of asthma may be due to an exaggeration of reflex responsiveness of the airways.

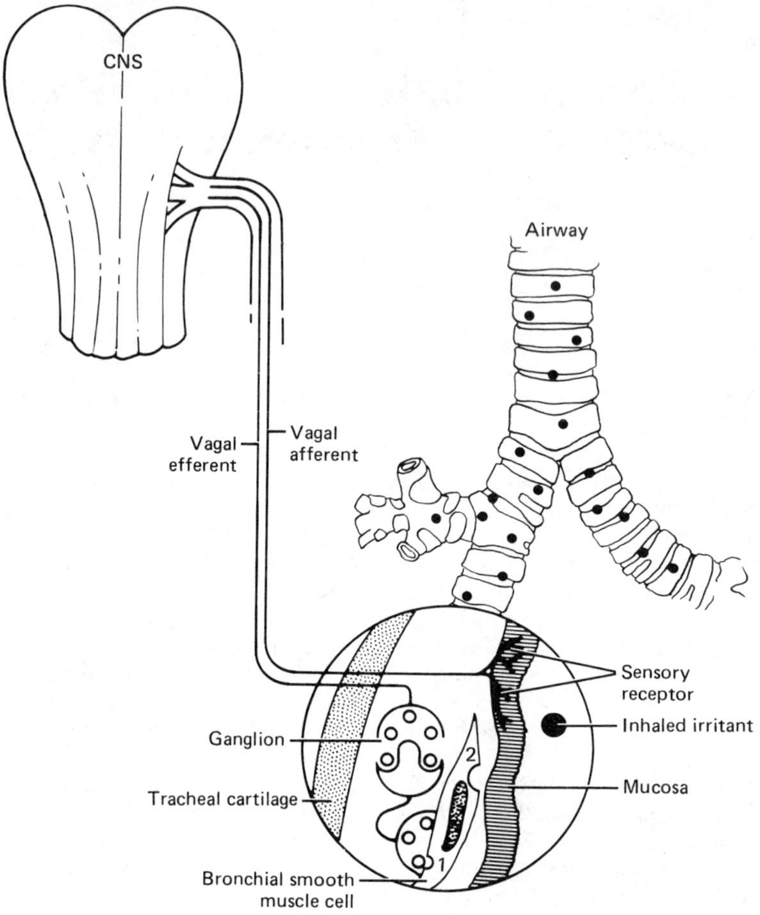

Figure 17–1. Mechanisms of response to inhaled irritants. The airway is represented microscopically by a cross section of the wall with branching vagal sensory endings lying adjacent to the lumen. Afferent pathways in the vagus nerves travel to the central nervous system; efferent pathways from the central nervous system travel to efferent ganglia. Postganglionic fibers release acetylcholine (○), which binds to muscarinic receptors (1) on airway smooth muscle. Released or inhaled stimulant (●) causes bronchoconstriction by 2 mechanisms: It diffuses across the airway epithelium and binds to receptors (2) on smooth muscle, provoking contraction; and it stimulates vagal sensory endings, causing reflex release of acetylcholine at the postganglionic nerve endings, further provoking muscle contraction.

The hypothesis suggested by these studies—that asthmatic bronchospasm results from a combination of release of mediators and an exaggeration of parasympathetic reflex responsiveness to their effects—suggests that asthma may be effectively treated by drugs with different modes of action. Asthmatic bronchospasm might be reversed or prevented, for example, by drugs that prevent mast cell degranulation (cromolyn, calcium channel antagonists), block the conduction along sensory or motor nerves to the airways (topical anesthetics), inhibit the effect of acetylcholine released from vagal motor nerves (muscarinic antagonists), or directly relax airway smooth muscle (adrenergic agents, theophylline). Some effective drugs, such as the corticosteroids, have an unknown mechanism of action and thus cannot be clearly related to this conceptual model.

I. BASIC PHARMACOLOGY OF BRONCHODILATORS & OTHER AGENTS USED IN THE TREATMENT OF ASTHMA

CROMOLYN

Cromolyn (disodium cromoglycate, Intal) is an unusual compound both chemically and in its mechanism of action. The drug is poorly soluble; for use in asthma, it must be applied topically by inhalation of the powder as described below. When given by inhalation or orally, less than 10% is absorbed, and most is excreted unchanged.

Mechanism of Action

Cromolyn has been shown to prevent antigen-

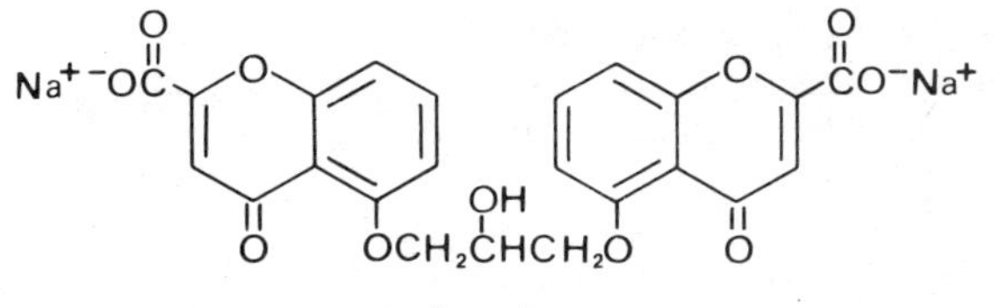

Cromolyn

induced degranulation from sensitized mast cells and lung fragments, apparently by preventing the transmembrane influx of calcium provoked by antigen-antibody interaction on the mast cell surface. From this mechanism of action, the drug can be predicted to be an effective prophylactic agent, interfering with the cascade of events that follows inhalation of antigen. Other experimental work, however, suggests that cromolyn may also inhibit phosphodiesterase, thus increasing intracellular cAMP, and that it may alter neural pathways that regulate smooth muscle tone.

Clinical Use of Cromolyn

In patients, the efficacy of cromolyn has been demonstrated in several circumstances. When used before exposure, the drug inhibits the immediate and, to a lesser extent, the late reactions to inhalation of antigen. Pretreatment with cromolyn blocks exercise-induced and aspirin-induced bronchoconstriction and protects against the bronchospasm provoked by a variety of industrial irritants, including toluene diisocyanate, wood dusts, soldering fluxes, piperazine hydrochloride, and certain enzymes. In controlled long-term studies of patients with intrinsic and extrinsic asthma, cromolyn was most effective in decreasing symptoms, but it also improved airway obstruction and decreased patient requirements for treatment with corticosteroids.

Cromolyn is absorbed poorly from the gastrointestinal tract and therefore is effective only when deposited directly into the airways. The current method of administration is via a Spinhaler apparatus that causes a capsule to be punctured and its powdered contents then carried by the inhaled air into the airways. The usual dose is 20 mg inhaled 4 times daily; the dose can be doubled if a response is not observed after 1–2 weeks of treatment. It may be useful to administer an inhaled adrenergic agonist just before the inhalation of cromolyn to dilate airways and thus obtain more widespread deposition of the drug. Because oral administration may increase patient compliance, several orally active compounds similar to cromolyn have been synthesized, but none are currently available.

METHYLXANTHINE DRUGS

The 3 important methylxanthines are theophylline, theobromine, and caffeine. Their major source is, of course, beverages (tea, cocoa, and coffee, respectively). Theophylline is important as a therapeutic agent in the treatment of asthma.

Chemistry

As shown below, theophylline is 1,3-dimethylxanthine; theobromine is 3,7-dimethylxanthine; and caffeine is 1,3,7-trimethylxanthine. The theophylline preparation most commonly used for therapeutic purposes is the theophylline-ethylenediamine complex **aminophylline.** A synthetic analog of theophylline (dyphylline) is both less potent and shorter-acting than theophylline. The pharmacokinetics of theophylline are discussed below. The metabolic products, partially demethylated xanthines (not uric acid), are excreted in the urine.

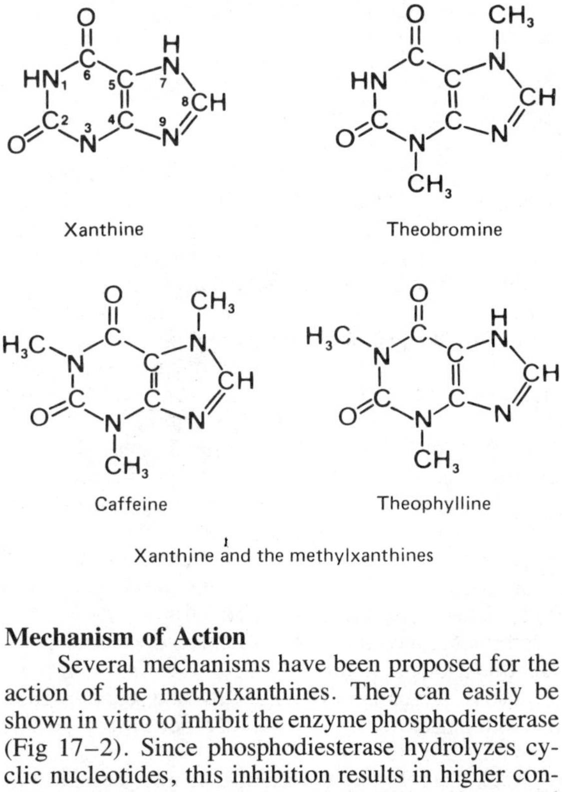

Xanthine and the methylxanthines

Mechanism of Action

Several mechanisms have been proposed for the action of the methylxanthines. They can easily be shown in vitro to inhibit the enzyme phosphodiesterase (Fig 17–2). Since phosphodiesterase hydrolyzes cyclic nucleotides, this inhibition results in higher concentrations of intracellular cAMP. This effect could explain the cardiac stimulation and smooth muscle relaxation produced by these drugs, but it is not certain that sufficiently high concentrations are achieved in all target tissues in vivo to bring about inhibition. A second mechanism that has recently been proposed involves inhibition of neural transmission at certain synapses, especially in the central nervous system, where adenosine, a structural analog, may be a neurotransmitter.

Pharmacodynamics of Methylxanthines

The methylxanthines have effects on the central nervous system, kidney, and cardiac and skeletal muscle as well as smooth muscle. Of the 3 agents, theophylline is most selective in its smooth muscle

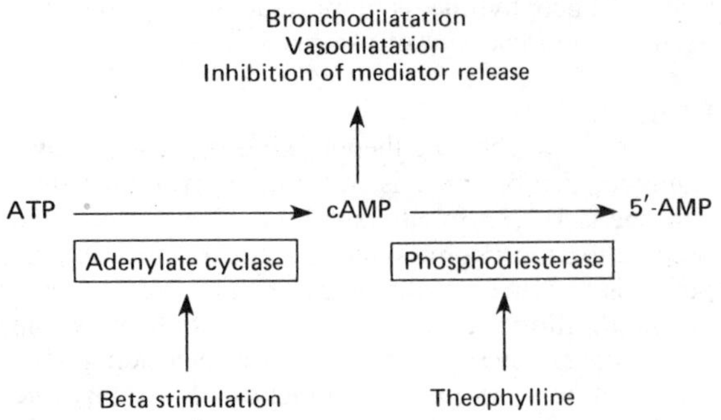

Figure 17–2. Intracellular levels of cAMP can be increased by beta-adrenergic agonists, which increase the rate of its synthesis by adenylate cyclase; or by phosphodiesterase inhibitors, such as theophylline, which slow the rate of its degradation.

effects, while caffeine has the most marked central nervous system effects.

A. Central Nervous System Effects: In low and moderate doses, the methylxanthines, especially caffeine, cause mild cortical arousal with increased alertness and deferral of fatigue. In unusually sensitive individuals, the caffeine contained in beverages, eg, 100 mg in a cup of coffee, is sufficient to cause nervousness and insomnia. At very high doses, medullary stimulation and convulsions may occur. Nervousness and tremor are primary side-effects in patients taking large doses of aminophylline for asthma.

B. Cardiovascular Effects: The methylxanthines have direct positive chronotropic and inotropic effects on the heart. In unusually sensitive individuals, consumption of a few cups of coffee may result in arrhythmias; but in most people, parenteral administration of higher doses of the methylxanthines produces only sinus tachycardia and increased cardiac output. Methylxanthines have occasionally been used in the treatment of pulmonary edema associated with heart failure (Chapter 11). These agents also relax vascular smooth muscle except in cerebral blood vessels, where they cause contraction.

C. Effects on Gastrointestinal Tract: The methylxanthines stimulate secretion of both gastric acid and digestive enzymes. However, even decaffeinated coffee has a potent stimulant effect on secretion, which means that the primary secretagogue in coffee is not caffeine.

D. Effects on Kidney: The methylxanthines—especially theophylline—are weak diuretics. This effect may involve both increased glomerular filtration and reduced tubular sodium reabsorption. The diuresis is not of sufficient magnitude to be therapeutically useful.

E. Effects on Smooth Muscle: The bronchodilatation produced by the methylxanthines is very useful in therapy. Tolerance does not develop, but side-effects, especially in the central nervous system, may limit the dose (see below). In addition to this direct effect on the airway smooth muscle, these agents inhibit antigen-induced release of histamine from lung tissue; their effect on mucociliary transport is unknown.

Clinical Use of Methylxanthines

Of the xanthines, theophylline is the most effective bronchodilator. Because it is only slightly soluble in water, it has been administered as a number of different salts containing varying amounts of theophylline base. The 2 commonly used theophylline salts are aminophylline, which contains 86% theophylline by weight; and oxtriphylline, which contains 64% theophylline by weight. Corrections must be made to ensure equivalent doses of theophylline for different preparations. Most preparations are well absorbed from the gastrointestinal tract; their absorption is not affected significantly by food. The absorption of rectal suppositories, however, is unreliable, and these preparations should be used only in special circumstances.

Improvements in theophylline preparations have come from alterations in the physical state of the drugs rather than from new chemical formulations. For example, several companies now provide anhydrous theophylline in a microcrystalline form in which the increased surface area allows solubilization for complete and rapid absorption after oral administration. In addition, several sustained-release preparations (eg, Slo-Phyllin, Theo-Dur) are now available and can produce therapeutic blood levels of theophylline for up to 12 hours. These preparations offer the advantages of less frequent drug administration, less fluctuation of theophylline blood levels, and, in many cases, more effective treatment of nocturnal bronchospasm.

An important advance in the use of theophylline is the availability of theophylline blood level measurements to monitor therapy. Therapeutic and toxic effects of theophylline are closely related to the plasma concentrations of the drug. Improvement in pulmonary function is well correlated with plasma concentration in the range of 5–20 mg/L. Anorexia, nausea, vomiting, abdominal discomfort, headache, and anxiety begin to occur at concentrations of 15 mg/L in some patients and become common at concentrations greater than 20 mg/L. Higher levels (generally greater than 40 mg/L) may cause seizures or arrhythmias; these may not be preceded by gastrointestinal or neurologic warning symptoms. Rational administration of theophylline, therefore, requires knowledge of its pharmacokinetics.

As described in Chapter 3, the initial or "loading" dose of a drug is determined by its volume of distribution (V_d) and the subsequent or "maintenance" dose by the rate of plasma clearance. The V_d for theophylline is proportionate to lean body weight but otherwise varies only slightly among individuals. On the average, $V_d = 0.5$ L/kg, so a plasma concentration of 10 mg/L will be achieved by a loading dose of 5 mg of theophylline per kilogram of body weight. Because aminophylline contains 86% theophylline by weight, this is approximately equivalent to 6 mg/kg of aminophylline. If administered intravenously, the loading dose should be given over 30 minutes, since rapid injection ("IV push") may result in transient toxic plasma levels with the risk of seizures or cardiac arrhythmias.

The plasma clearance of theophylline (often expressed as plasma half-life) has been shown to vary widely among healthy subjects and even more so among patients. Because theophylline is metabolized by the liver, changes in hepatic function can alter the drug's half-life. For example, a decrease in hepatic function from cirrhosis or decrease in hepatic blood flow from heart failure may decrease plasma clearance and lead to toxic concentrations of the drug. Induction of hepatic enzymes by cigarette smoking or by changes in diet may increase plasma clearance and cause inadequate concentrations of drug. In normal adults, the mean plasma clearance is 0.69 mL/kg/min. Children appear to clear theophylline faster than adults (1–1.5 mL/kg/min). Even when maintenance doses are altered to correct for the above factors, plasma concentrations vary widely.

For intravenous maintenance therapy, an infusion rate of 0.7 mg/kg/h may be used in stable patients; but in acutely ill patients, it should be decreased to approximately 0.6 mg/kg/h. In the presence of liver disease or heart failure, the dose should be decreased further (approximately 0.5 mg/kg/h). Theophylline levels should be measured 24 hours after starting treatment. For oral therapy, an initial dose equivalent to 3–4 mg/kg of theophylline every 6 hours is appropriate. Changes in dosage will result in a new steady-state concentration of theophylline in 1–2 days, so the dose may be increased at intervals of 2–3 days until therapeutic plasma concentrations are achieved (10–20 μg/mL) or until side-effects develop.

ADRENERGIC AGENTS

The adrenergic agonists, discussed in detail in Chapter 7, have several pharmacologic actions that are important in the treatment of asthma—ie, they relax airway smooth muscle and inhibit release of bronchoconstricting substances from mast cells. They may also increase mucociliary transport by increasing ciliary activity or by affecting the composition of mucous secretions. These effects may result from stimulation of adenylate cyclase, which catalyzes the formation of cAMP, although the exact role of increased intracellular concentrations of cAMP is still uncertain.

The best-characterized bronchodilator action of the adrenergic agonists on airways is relaxation of airway smooth muscle. Although there is no evidence for direct sympathetic innervation of human airway smooth muscle, there is evidence for the presence of adrenergic receptors on airway smooth muscle. In general, stimulation of β_2 receptors relaxes airway smooth muscle, inhibits mediator release, and causes skeletal muscle tremor as a toxic effect.

The adrenergic agents most widely used in the treatment of asthma include epinephrine, ephedrine, isoproterenol, and a number of β_2-selective agents (Fig 17–3). Because epinephrine and isoproterenol cause more cardiac stimulation (mediated by β_1 receptors), they should probably be reserved for special situations (see below). Ephedrine has no advantages over more selective agents except low cost, and it should be avoided if possible.

Epinephrine is an effective, rapidly acting bronchodilator when injected subcutaneously (0.4 mL of 1:1000 solution) or inhaled as a microaerosol from a pressurized canister (320 μg per puff). Maximal bronchodilatation is achieved 15 minutes after inhalation and lasts 60–90 minutes. Because epinephrine stimulates β_1 as well as β_2 receptors, tachycardia, arrhythmias, and worsening of angina pectoris are troublesome side-effects.

Ephedrine probably has the longest history of any drug used in treating asthma, for it was used in China for at least 2000 years before it was introduced into western medicine in 1924. Compared to epinephrine, ephedrine has a longer duration, oral activity, more pronounced central effects, and much lower potency. Because of the development of more efficacious and β_2-selective agonists, ephedrine is now used infrequently in treating asthma. It is available in 25- and 50-mg capsules and tablets but is most often prescribed in fixed-dose combination with theophylline and a sedative in commercial preparations. These fixed-dose combinations make rational adjustment of dosage of the individual agents impossible and should be avoided.

Isoproterenol is a potent bronchodilator; when inhaled as a microaerosol from a pressurized canister, 80–120 μg causes maximal bronchodilatation within 5 minutes. When the drug is given as an aerosolized solution from a nebulizer, the larger particle size generated results in a smaller quantity being delivered to the tracheobronchial tree, so larger doses must be given to achieve the same effect. Isoproterenol has a 60- to 90-minute duration of action. Cardiac side-effects (tachycardia, arrhythmias) can occur. Cardiac arrhythmias resulting from the use of high doses of inhaled isoproterenol may have caused the increase in mortality rate from asthma that occurred in Europe in the late 1960s. In the USA, where high-dose preparations were not available, this increase in mortality rate did not occur.

A new generation of adrenergic drugs, effective after oral administration, with a long duration of action and a significant degree of β_2 selectivity, has recently become available (Fig 17–3). These agents differ structurally from epinephrine in having a larger substitution on the amino group and in the position of the hydroxyl groups on the aromatic ring. **Metaproterenol (Alupent, Metaprel)** and **albuterol (Proventyl, Ventolin)** are available as metered dose inhalers; metaproterenol solution (5%) can be diluted in 0.3–1.5 mL of saline for delivery from a hand-held nebulizer. When given by inhalation, these agents cause bronchodilatation equivalent to that produced by

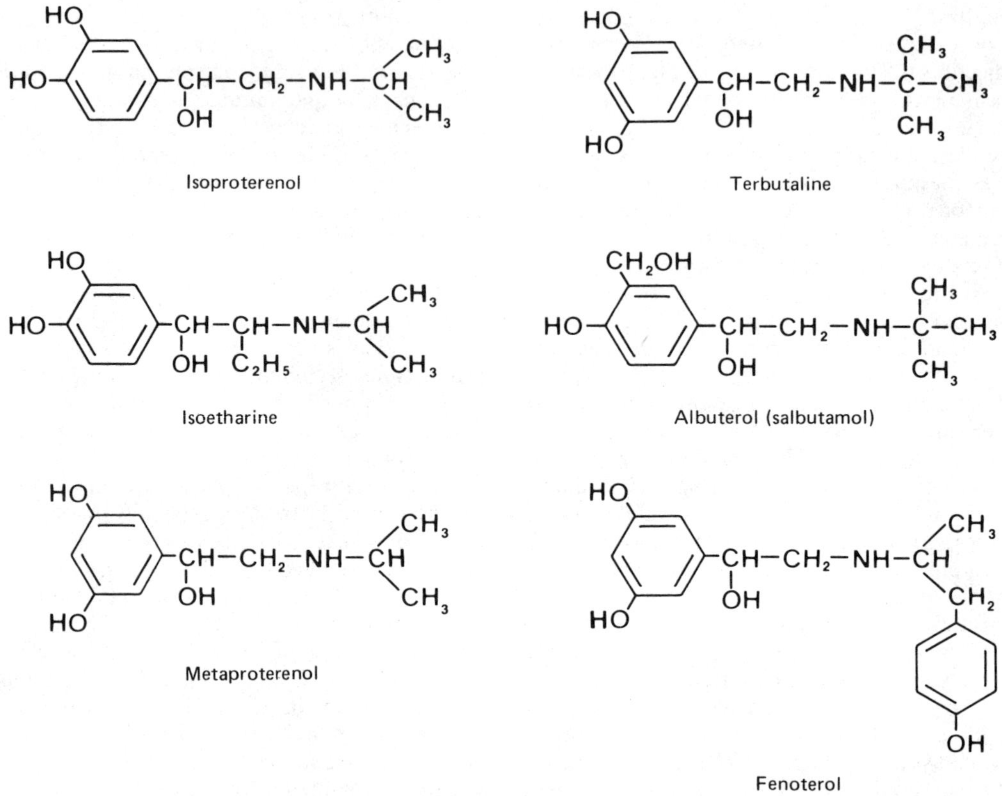

Figure 17–3. Structures of isoproterenol and several β_2-selective analogs.

isoproterenol. Bronchodilatation is maximal by 30 minutes and persists for 3–4 hours.

Metaproterenol and **terbutaline (Brethine, Bricanyl)** are prepared in tablet form (20 mg and 5 mg, respectively). One tablet 3 times daily is the usual regimen; the principal side-effects of skeletal muscle tremor, nervousness, and occasional weakness may be reduced by starting the patient on half-strength tablets for the first 2 weeks of therapy.

Only terbutaline is available for subcutaneous injection (0.25 mg). The indications for this route are similar to those for subcutaneous epinephrine—severe asthma requiring treatment in hospital—but it should be remembered that terbutaline's longer duration of action means that cumulative effects may be seen after repeated injections.

Although adrenergic agonists may be administered by inhalation or by the oral or parenteral routes, delivery by inhalation will result in the greatest local effect on airway smooth muscle with the least systemic toxicity. Aerosol deposition depends on the particle size, the pattern of breathing (tidal volume and rate of airflow), and the geometry of the airways. Even with particles in the optimal size range of 2–5 μm, 80–90% of the total dose of aerosol is deposited in the mouth or pharynx. Particles under 1–2 μm in size remain suspended and may be exhaled. Deposition can be increased by holding the breath in inspiration.

The preferred method for β_2-agonist inhalation is controversial. Available methods include dry aerosols (eg, metered-dose canisters) or wet aerosols (eg, compressed air-driven or hand bulb nebulizers, or intermittent positive-pressure breathing machines). Most studies have shown no significant differences in efficacy between the various methods of administration, although differences in cost are substantial. Metered-dose canisters are the most convenient but also depend most on proper delivery by the patient. It is therefore important to instruct patients carefully in how to achieve maximal aerosol deposition: delivering the aerosol during inspiration; breath-holding at full inspiration and only then exhaling slowly; then repeating the maneuver after a 5-minute pause. There is recent interest in combining different routes of administration to achieve greater bronchodilatation. For example, aerosols are deposited preferentially in the most dilated airways; drugs given intravenously or orally reach the lung via the circulation so their accessibility to the airways depends on the state of the blood vessels supplying the airways. Thus, combining routes of administration may allow a greater range of airways to be treated effectively.

Use of adrenergic agents by inhalation at first raised fears about possible tachyphylaxis or tolerance to β-adrenergic agonists, cardiac arrhythmias from β_1-adrenergic stimulation and hypoxemia, and arrhythmias from fluorinated hydrocarbons in Freon propellants. The concept that beta-agonist drugs cause worsening of clinical asthma by inducing tachyphylaxis to their own action remains unestablished. Most studies have shown only a small change in airway smooth muscle response to beta stimulation after prolonged treatment with beta-agonist drugs. Other experiments have demonstrated that arterial oxygen tension (Pa_{O_2}) may decrease after administration of beta-agonists if ventilation-perfusion ratios in the lung worsen. This effect may occur, however, with any class of bronchodilator drug, and the significance of such an effect will depend on the initial Pa_{O_2} of the patient. Supplemental oxygen may be necessary if the initial Pa_{O_2} is decreased markedly or if there is a large decrease in Pa_{O_2} during treatment with bronchodilators. Finally, there is concern over myocardial toxicity from Freon propellants contained in all of the commercially available metered-dose canisters. While fluorocarbons may sensitize the heart to toxic effects of catecholamines, such an effect occurs only at very high myocardial concentrations, which are not achieved if inhalers are used as recommended. In general, β_2-adrenergic agonists are safe and effective bronchodilators when given in doses that avoid systemic side-effects.

MUSCARINIC ANTAGONISTS

Leaves from *Datura stramonium* have probably been used for treating asthma for hundreds of years. Interest in the potential value of antimuscarinic agents has recently been increased by demonstration of the importance of the vagus nerves in the bronchospasm provoked by inhalation of allergen in allergic dogs and by the finding in humans with asthma that treatment with atropine aerosol can block the bronchoconstriction provoked by isocapnic hyperventilation with cold air, by histamine, and by antigen.

Mechanism of Action in Asthma

These drugs inhibit the effect of acetylcholine at the muscarinic receptors on airway smooth muscle and on mucus glands; they also block muscarinic receptors on cells lacking innervation, such as mast cells and basophils. Because the airways are innervated by the vagus nerves and because stimulation of these nerves causes contraction of airway smooth muscle and increased secretion of mucus, muscarinic antagonists effectively relax airway smooth muscle and decrease the secretion of mucus that occurs in response to vagal efferent activity. As described above, muscarinic antagonists therefore block vagal reflexes that may be responsible for airway narrowing in patients with asthma. By inhibiting the rise in intracellular cGMP stimulated by cholinergic agents, these drugs may also decrease mediator release from mast cells.

Clinical Use of Muscarinic Antagonists

Atropine is the prototypical muscarinic antagonist (Chapter 6). When atropine is given intravenously, bronchodilatation—caused by blockade of airway smooth muscle muscarinic receptors—is achieved at a much lower dose than increase in heart rate. The selectivity of atropine's effect can be increased further by administering the drug by inhalation. Dose-response studies of atropine sulfate aerosol show that a nebulized dose of 0.05–0.1 mg/kg causes maximal increases in baseline airway caliber—equivalent to what can be achieved with adrenergic agents—and that this effect persists for up to 5 hours. Although the dose varies among patients, the recommended dose is 0.05 mg/kg inhaled every 4–6 hours. Deposition of the aerosol in the mouth frequently causes a local drying effect. Side-effects due to systemic absorption include urinary retention, tachycardia, loss of visual accommodation, and agitation.

To achieve still greater selectivity of action, quaternary ammonium derivatives of atropine have been synthesized for increased bronchial effects. These compounds are poorly absorbed and do not enter the central nervous system readily; topical administration as an aerosol further enhances the ratio of bronchial to systemic effects. One of the drugs, **ipratropium bromide (Atrovent),** is undergoing clinical trials in the USA.

CORTICOSTEROIDS

Although corticosteroids have been used to treat asthma since 1950, their precise mechanism of action remains unknown. Like cromolyn, these drugs do not relax airway smooth muscle directly, but they may produce marked increases in airway caliber if administered for some time to patients with asthma. Corticosteroids may decrease airway obstruction by decreasing inflammation or by potentiating the effects of β-adrenergic agonists.

Clinical Use of Corticosteroids

In addition to uncertainty over their mechanism of action, there is controversy over the indications for corticosteroids in the treatment of asthma and their appropriate dosage schedule. Because of severe adverse effects when given chronically, corticosteroids are generally reserved for patients who do not improve adequately with other bronchodilators or who experience worsening symptoms despite maintenance bronchodilator therapy. Treatment is often begun with an oral dose of 30–60 mg of prednisone per day or an intravenous dose of 1 mg/kg of methylprednisolone every 6 hours; the daily dose is decreased gradually after airway obstruction has improved. In some patients, corticosteroid therapy can be discontinued in a week or 10 days, but in other patients symptoms may worsen as the dose is decreased to lower levels. Because adrenal suppression by corticosteroids is related to dose and because secretion of corticosteroids has a diurnal variation, low doses of corticosteroids may cause less adrenal suppression if taken early in the morning. Adrenal suppression can be better avoided by alternate-day treatment. This schedule is best achieved by gradually tapering 1 day's dose while increasing the alternate day's dose by the same amount.

Another effective method of decreasing systemic side-effects due to corticosteroid therapy is to administer the drug as an aerosol. The introduction of lipid-soluble corticosteroids such as beclomethasone (Beclovent, Vanceril) offers an effective method of delivering corticosteroids to the airways with minimal systemic absorption and reduced adverse effects. An average daily dose of 400 μg of the inhaled drug (2 puffs 4 times daily) is often as effective as oral corticosteroids in mild to moderate asthma and appears to be equivalent to about 10–15 mg/d of prednisone. Larger doses of inhaled steroid preparations may be more effective but may also cause a greater incidence of adrenal suppression. A special problem caused by inhaled topical corticosteroids is the occurrence of oropharyngeal candidiasis. Rinsing the mouth and gargling with water after each inhalation may prevent this complication. When it occurs, it responds to gargling with nystatin solution or to discontinuing the inhaled steroid. The drug is remarkably free of other complications, but when switching from chronic oral therapy to inhaled beclomethasone, the oral therapy must be tapered slowly to avoid precipitation of adrenal insufficiency.

II. CLINICAL PHARMACOLOGY OF DRUGS USED IN ASTHMA

Patients with mild asthma and only occasional symptoms generally require no more than an inhaled β-adrenergic agonist (eg, metaproterenol) on an "as needed" basis. If symptoms occur more frequently (more than 2 attacks a month) and the patient requires frequent aerosol inhalations or if nocturnal symptoms occur, maintenance treatment should include an oral theophylline compound and an inhaled β_2 agent taken at 4-hour intervals during waking hours. If symptoms remain poorly controlled or if side-effects become bothersome, it is important to check the plasma level of theophylline. If the level is in the therapeutic range (10–20 mg/L) and symptoms persist, an oral adrenergic agonist (eg, terbutaline, metaproterenol) may be added, although side-effects such as headache and tremor often limit the dose and usefulness of these agents. There may be a therapeutic advantage, however, in combining theophylline and adrenergic treatment in low doses in patients who develop side-effects from a high dose of either drug. Thus, the addition of an oral β_2-adrenergic agent will cause increased bronchodilatation in a patient with plasma levels of theophylline below 10 mg/L but will have little effect on airway caliber in a patient with plasma levels in the therapeutic range (10–20 mg/L). This observation does not imply that an aerosolized adrenergic agent is of no value in patients taking oral theophylline, for the inhaled drug has greater effect on large central airways, whereas the oral drug has greatest effect on smaller, more peripheral airways.

If airway obstruction remains severe despite bronchodilator therapy, corticosteroids may be started. After initial treatment with high doses of corticosteroids (eg, 30 mg/d of prednisone for 3 weeks), these drugs should be given in the lowest dose necessary to control symptoms. If possible, patients should then be converted to alternate-day corticosteroid therapy or therapy with inhaled beclomethasone.

Cromolyn is not usually beneficial in patients who require continuous steroid therapy. A therapeutic trial of cromolyn is warranted, however, in patients who require maintenance therapy with oral theophylline and an inhaled agent and in those whose symptoms occur seasonally or after clear-cut inciting stimuli such as exercise or exposure to animal dander or irritants. In a patient whose symptoms are continuous or occur without an obvious inciting stimulus, the value of cromolyn can only be established with a therapeutic trial of 40 mg inhaled 4 times a day for 4 weeks. If the patient responds to this therapy, the dose can be reduced to 20 mg 3 times daily.

The role of inhaled muscarinic antagonists in the treatment of asthma has not been defined. When adequate doses are given, their effect on airway resistance is as great as that of the adrenergic drugs, such as isoproterenol. The airway effects of antimuscarinic and adrenergic drugs given in full doses are not additive—ie, administration of an adrenergic drug does not cause further bronchodilatation in a person who has been treated with an antimuscarinic agent. The converse is also true: The addition of an antimuscarinic agent does not cause further bronchodilatation beyond that achieved with treatment with an inhaled adrenergic agent. Furthermore, no subgroup of patients with airflow obstruction has been identified who are more responsive to antimuscarinic than to adrenergic drugs.

When muscarinic antagonists are used for long-term treatment, they appear to be effective bronchodilators. Although it was predicted that muscarinic antagonists might "dry up" airway secretions, direct measurements of fluid volume secretion from single airway submucosal glands in animals show that atropine decreases secretory rates only slightly; however, the drug does prevent excessive secretion caused by vagal reflex stimulation. No cases of inspissation of mucus have been reported following administration of these drugs.

MANAGEMENT OF ACUTE ASTHMA

The treatment of acute attacks of asthma in patients reporting to the hospital requires more continuous assessment and objective measurement of lung function than is necessary for chronic outpatient therapy. Repeated measurements of arterial blood gas tensions and spirometry are generally necessary. Established treatment for severe attacks includes oxygen, bronchodilators, and corticosteroids. For example, the combination of β_2-adrenergic drugs given subcutaneously and by aerosol, aminophylline given by continuous intravenous infusion, and intravenous corticosteroids may all be necessary in severe attacks.

• • •

References

Austen KF, Orange RP: State of the art: Bronchial asthma. The possible role of the chemical mediators of immediate hypersensitivity in the pathogenesis of subacute chronic disease. *Am Rev Respir Dis* 1975;**112:**423.

Boushey HA et al: State of the art: Bronchial hyperreactivity. *Am Rev Respir Dis* 1980;**121:**389.

Cavanaugh MJ, Cooper DM: Inhaled atropine sulfate: Dose response characteristics. *Am Rev Respir Dis* 1976;**114:**517.

Gold WM, Kessler GF, Yu DYC: Role of vagus nerves in experimental asthma in allergic dogs. *J Appl Physiol* 1972;**33:**719.

Gross NJ: Sch 1000: A new anticholinergic bronchodilator. [Ipratropium.] *Am Rev Respir Dis* 1975;**112:**823.

Holtzman MJ et al: Effect of ganglionic blockade on bronchial reactivity in atopic subjects. *Am Rev Respir Dis* 1980;**122:**17.

Leifer KN, Wittig HJ: The beta-2 sympathomimetic aerosols in the treatment of asthma. *Ann Allergy* 1975;**35:**69.

McAllen MK, Kochanowski SJ, Shaw KM: Steroid aerosols in asthma: An assessment of betamethasone valerate. *Br Med J* 1974;**1:**171.

Paterson JW, Woolcock AJ, Shenfield GM: State of the art: Bronchodilator drugs. *Am Rev Respir Dis* 1979;**120:**1149.

Piafsky KM, Ogilvie RI: Dosage of theophylline in bronchial asthma. *N Engl J Med* 1975;**292:**1218.

Santa Cruz R et al: Tracheal mucous velocity in normal man and patients with obstructive lung disease: Effects of terbutaline. *Am Rev Respir Dis* 1974;**109:**458.

Sheppard D et al: Dose-dependent inhibition of cold air-induced broncho-constriction by atropine. *J Appl Physiol* 1982; **53:**169.

Van Arsdel PP, Paul GH: Drug therapy in the management of asthma. *Ann Intern Med* 1977;**87:**68.

Webb-Johnson JC, Webb-Johnson DC: Bronchodilator therapy. *N Engl J Med* 1977;**297:**476.

Yu DYC, Galant SP, Gold WM: Inhibition of antigen-induced broncho-constriction by atropine in asthmatic patients. *J Appl Physiol* 1972;**32:**823.

18 | Introduction to the Pharmacology of CNS Drugs

Roger Nicoll, MD

Drugs acting on the central nervous system (CNS) are the most widely used group of pharmacologically active agents and have extremely important medical uses. The practice of modern surgery, for example, would be impossible without general anesthetic agents. In addition to their use in therapy, drugs acting on the central nervous system are used on a daily basis without prescription to increase the sense of well-being. Caffeine, alcohol, and nicotine are socially accepted drugs in many countries, and their consumption is practiced worldwide. Because some of the drugs in this group cause pleasurable sensations when they are injected, ingested, or inhaled, societies have found it necessary to control their use and availability.

The mechanisms by which various drugs act on the central nervous system are not always clearly understood. Since the causes of many of the conditions for which these drugs are used (schizophrenia, anxiety, etc) are themselves poorly understood, it is not surprising that in the past much of CNS pharmacology has been purely descriptive. However, technologic advances over the past decade have led to greater understanding of how these drugs act. Studies on the mechanism of drug action have been useful not only for investigating the cellular and molecular basis of the condition for which a particular drug is given but also in providing clues about how the central nervous system normally operates. This chapter provides a broad outline of the functional organization of the central nervous system as a basis for understanding the actions of drugs on it.

THE SYNAPSE & SYNAPTIC POTENTIALS

It was not until the advent of glass microelectrodes that permit intracellular recording that a detailed description of synaptic transmission was possible. It is now well established that communication between neurons in the central nervous system occurs through chemical synapses in the vast majority of cases. A few instances of electrical coupling between neurons have been documented, and such coupling may play a role in synchronizing neuronal discharge. However, it is unlikely that these electrical synapses are an important site of drug action. The events involved in the release of transmitter from the presynaptic terminal have been studied most extensively at the vertebrate neuromuscular junction and at the giant synapse of the squid. An action potential in the presynaptic fiber propagates into the synaptic terminal and activates voltage-sensitive calcium channels in the membrane of the terminal. Calcium flows into the terminal, and the increase in intraterminal calcium concentration promotes the fusion of synaptic vesicles with the presynaptic membrane. The transmitter contained in the vesicles is released into the synaptic cleft and diffuses to the receptors on the postsynaptic membrane. Binding of the transmitter to its receptor causes a brief change in membrane conductance (permeability to ions) of the postsynaptic cell. The time delay from the arrival of the presynaptic action potential to the onset of the postsynaptic response is approximately 0.5 ms. Most of this delay is consumed by the release process, particularly the time required for calcium channels to open.

The first systematic analysis of synaptic potentials in the central nervous system was by Eccles et al, who recorded intracellularly from spinal motoneurons in the early 1950s. When a microelectrode enters a cell, there is a sudden change in the potential recorded by the electrode, which is typically about −70 mV (Fig 18–1). This is the resting membrane potential of the neuron. Two types of pathways, excitatory and inhibitory, impinge on the motoneuron. When an excitatory

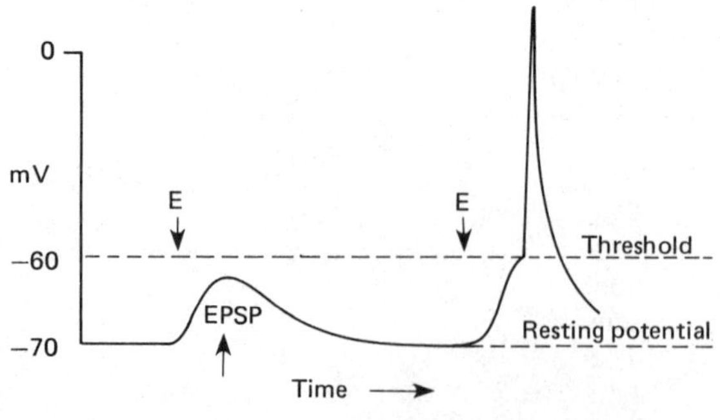

Figure 18–1. Excitatory synaptic potentials and spike generation. The figure shows a resting membrane potential of −70 mV in a postsynaptic cell. Stimulation of an excitatory pathway (E) generates transient depolarization. Increasing the stimulus strength increases the size of the depolarization, so that the threshold for spike generation is reached.

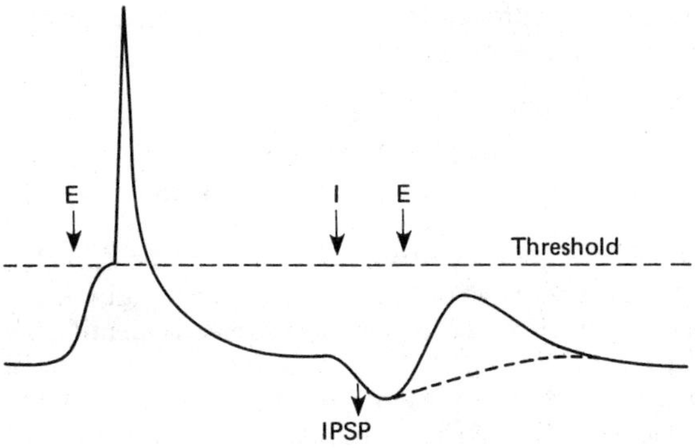

Figure 18–2. Interaction of excitatory and inhibitory synapses. On the left, a suprathreshold stimulus is given to an excitatory pathway (E). On the right, this same stimulus is given shortly after stimulating an inhibitory pathway (I), which prevents the excitatory potential from reaching threshold.

pathway is stimulated, a small depolarization or excitatory postsynaptic potential (EPSP) is recorded (Fig 18–1). This potential is due to the excitatory transmitter activating a large increase in sodium and potassium permeability. The duration of these potentials is quite brief, usually less than 20 ms. Changing the stimulus intensity to the pathway and therefore the number of presynaptic fibers activated results in a graded change in the size of the depolarization. This indicates that the contribution a single fiber makes to the EPSP is quite small. When a sufficient number of excitatory fibers are activated, the EPSP depolarizes the postsynaptic cell to threshold, and an all-or-none action potential is generated.

When an inhibitory pathway is stimulated, the postsynaptic membrane is hyperpolarized, producing an inhibitory postsynaptic potential (IPSP) (Fig 18–2). A number of inhibitory synapses must be activated together to appreciably alter the membrane potential. This hyperpolarization is due to a selective increase in membrane permeability to chloride ions that flow into the cell during the IPSP. If an EPSP that under resting conditions would evoke an action potential in the postsynaptic cell (Fig 18–2) is elicited during an IPSP, it no longer evokes an action potential, because the IPSP has moved the membrane potential farther away from the threshold for action potential generation. A second type of inhibition is termed presynaptic inhibition. In the central nervous system, this is limited to the sensory fibers entering the brain stem and spinal cord. The excitatory synaptic terminals of these sensory fibers receive synapses called axoaxonic synapses (Fig 18–4B). When activated, the axoaxonic synapses reduce the amount of transmitter released from the synapses of sensory fibers.

SITES OF DRUG ACTION

Virtually all of the drugs that act on the central nervous system produce their effects by modifying some step in chemical synaptic transmission. Fig 18–3 illustrates some of the steps that can be altered. These transmitter-dependent actions can be divided into presynaptic and postsynaptic categories.

Drugs acting on the synthesis, storage, metabolism, and release of neurotransmitters fall into the presynaptic category. Synaptic transmission can be depressed by blockade of transmitter synthesis or storage. For example, *p*-chlorophenylalanine blocks the synthesis of serotonin, and reserpine depletes the synapses of monoamines by interfering with intracellular storage. Blockade of transmitter catabolism can increase transmitter concentrations and has been reported to increase the amount of transmitter released per impulse. Drugs can also alter the release of transmitter. Capsaicin induces the release of the peptide substance P from sensory neurons, and tetanus toxin blocks the release of inhibitory amino acid transmitters. After the transmitter has been released into the synaptic cleft, its action is terminated either by uptake

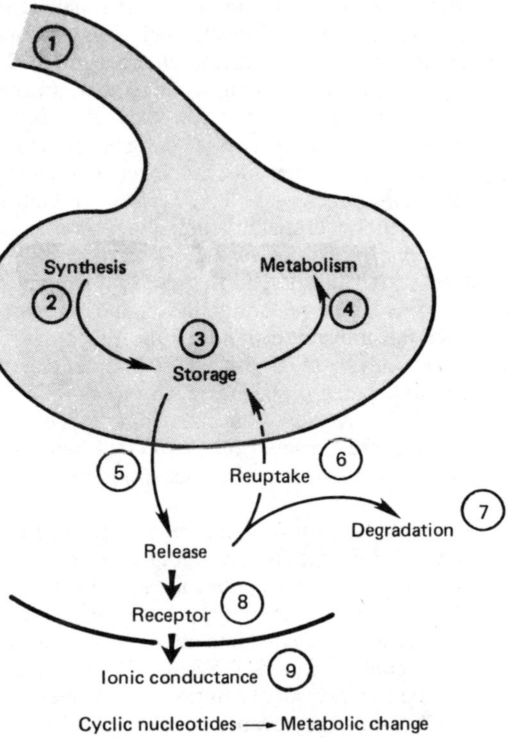

Figure 18–3. Sites of drug action. Schematic drawing of steps at which drugs can alter synaptic transmission. (1) Action potential in presynaptic fiber; (2) synthesis of transmitter; (3) storage; (4) metabolism; (5) release; (6) reuptake; (7) degradation; (8) receptor for the transmitter; (9) receptor-induced change in ionic conductance or level of cyclic nucleotides.

or degradation. For most neurotransmitters, there are uptake mechanisms into the synaptic terminal and also into surrounding neuroglia. Cocaine, for example, blocks the uptake of catecholamines at adrenergic synapses and thus potentiates the action of these amines. However, acetylcholine is inactivated by enzymatic degradation. Anticholinesterases block the degradation of acetylcholine and thereby prolong its action. No uptake mechanism has been found for any of the numerous recently discovered CNS peptides, and it has yet to be demonstrated whether specific enzymatic degradation terminates the action of peptide transmitters.

In the postsynaptic region, the transmitter receptor provides the primary site of drug action. Drugs can act either as neurotransmitter agonists, such as the opiates, which mimic the action of enkephalin, or they can block receptor function. Receptor antagonism is a common mechanism of action for CNS drugs. An example is strychnine's blockade of the receptor for the inhibitory transmitter glycine. This block is thought to be the mechanism underlying strychnine's convulsant action. Receptors are generally coupled to one of 2 transduction mechanisms. The receptors at most synapses in the central nervous system are coupled to ion channels, and receptor activation typically results in a brief opening of the channel. Drugs can act directly on the ion channel. For example, barbiturates enter and block the channel coupled to many excitatory neurotransmitter receptors. In other cases, receptors are coupled to enzymes, and receptor activation can lead to metabolic changes in the postsynaptic cell, most often as a consequence of elevations of cyclic nucleotide levels. Such metabolic changes can alter neuronal function either by changing the membrane properties of the cell or by changing neurotransmitter metabolism in the postsynaptic cell. These effects can be of long duration and can persist long after the transmitter has left the receptor. The methylxanthines are the best-known examples of drugs that can modify neurotransmitter responses mediated through cAMP. At high concentrations, the methylxanthines elevate the level of cAMP by blocking its metabolism and thereby prolong its action in the postsynaptic cell.

As should be clear from the above discussion, the selectivity of drug action is based almost entirely on the fact that different transmitters are used by different groups of neurons. Furthermore, these various transmitters are often segregated into neuronal systems that subserve broadly different CNS functions. Without such segregation, it would be impossible to selectively modify CNS function even if one had a drug that operated on a single neurotransmitter system. It is not entirely clear why the central nervous system has relied on so many neurotransmitters and segregated them into different neuronal systems, since the primary function of a transmitter is either excitation or inhibition; this could be accomplished with 2 transmitter substances or perhaps even one. That such segregation does occur has provided neuroscientists with a powerful pharmacologic approach for analyzing CNS function and treating pathologic conditions.

IDENTIFICATION OF CENTRAL TRANSMITTERS

Since drug selectivity is based on the fact that different pathways utilize different transmitters, it is a primary goal of neuropharmacologists to identify the transmitters in CNS pathways. Establishing that a chemical substance is a transmitter has been far more difficult for a given central synapse than for peripheral synapses. In theory, to identify a transmitter it is sufficient to show that stimulation of a pathway releases enough of the substance to produce the postsynaptic response. In practice, this experiment cannot be done satisfactorily for at least 2 reasons. First, the anatomic complexity of the central nervous system prevents the selective activation of a single set of synaptic terminals. Second, available techniques for measuring the released transmitter and applying the transmitter are not sufficiently precise to satisfy the quantitative requirements. Therefore, criteria have been established for transmitter identification.

Localization

A number of approaches have been used to prove that a suspected transmitter resides in the presynaptic terminal of the pathway under study. These include biochemical analysis of regional concentrations of suspected transmitters, often combined with interruption of specific pathways, and microcytochemical techniques. Immunocytochemical techniques have proved very useful in localizing peptides and synthetic enzymes for nonpeptide transmitters.

Release

To determine whether the substance can be released from a particular region, local collection (in vivo) of the extracellular fluid can sometimes be accomplished. In addition, in vitro slices of brain tissue can be stimulated electrically or chemically and the released substances measured. To determine if the release is relevant to synaptic transmission, it is important to establish that the release is calcium-dependent. As mentioned above, anatomic complexity often prevents identification of the synaptic terminals responsible for the release, and the amount collected in the perfusate is a small fraction of the amount actually released.

Synaptic Mimicry

Finally, application of the suspected substance should produce a response that mimics the action of the transmitter released by nerve stimulation. Microiontophoresis, which permits highly localized drug administration, has been a valuable technique in assessing the action of suspected transmitters. In practice, this criterion has 2 parts: physiologic and pharmacologic identity. To establish physiologic identity of action, the substance must be shown to initiate the same change in ionic conductance in the postsynaptic cell as synaptically released transmitter. This requires intracellular recording and determination of the reversal potential and ionic dependencies of the responses. However, since different transmitters can elicit identical ionic conductance changes, this finding is not sufficient. Thus, selective pharmacologic antagonism is used to further establish that the suspected transmitter is acting in a manner identical to synaptically released transmitter. Pharmacologic antagonism can be studied with extracellular recording and can therefore be used in those instances when it is technically impossible to obtain intracellular recordings.

CELLULAR ORGANIZATION OF THE BRAIN

Neuronal systems in the central nervous system can be divided in many instances into 2 broad categories: hierarchical systems and nonspecific or diffuse neuronal systems.

Hierarchical Systems

These systems include all of the pathways directly involved in sensory perception and motor control. The pathways are generally clearly delineated, being composed of large myelinated fibers that can often conduct action potentials in excess of 50 m/s. The information

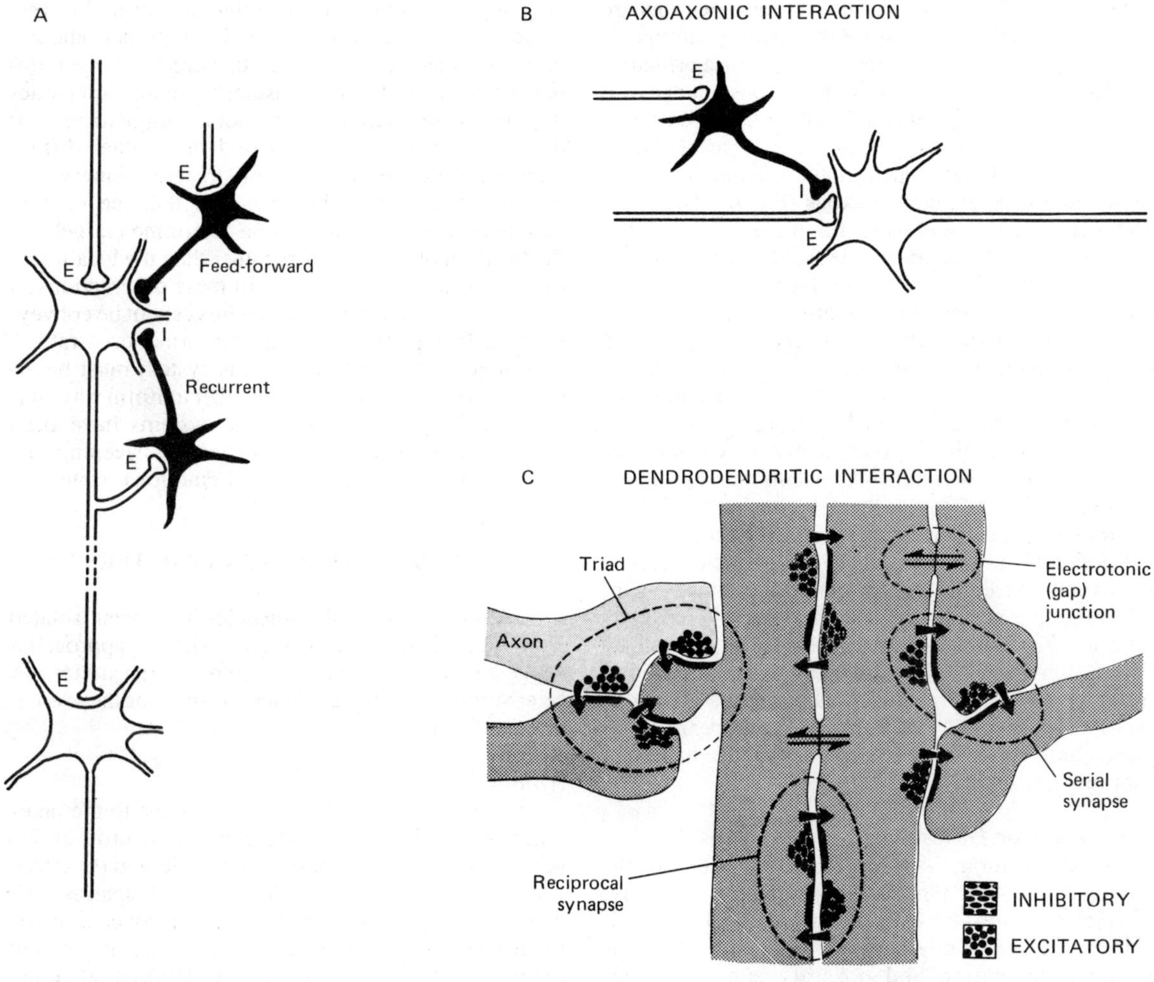

Figure 18–4. Pathways in the CNS. *A* shows 2 relay neurons and 2 types of inhibitory pathways, recurrent and feed-forward. The inhibitory neurons are shown in black. *B* shows the pathway responsible for presynaptic inhibition in which the axon of an inhibitory neuron synapses on the axon terminal of an excitatory fiber. *C:* Diagram illustrating that dendrites may be both pre- and postsynaptic to each other, forming reciprocal synapses, 2 of which are shown between the same dendrite pair. In triads, an axon synapses on 2 dendrites, and one of these dendrites synapses on the second. In serial synapses, a dendrite may be postsynaptic to one dendrite and presynaptic to another, thus connecting a series of dendrites. Dendrites also interact through low-resistance electrotonic ("gap") junctions (2 of which are shown). Except for one axon, all structures shown are dendrites. (Reproduced, with permission, from Schmitt FO, Dev P, Smith BH: *Science* 1976;**193**:114.)

is typically phasic, and in sensory systems the information is processed sequentially by successive integrations at each relay nucleus on its way to the cortex. A lesion at any link will incapacitate the system. Within each nucleus and in the cortex, there are 2 types of cells: relay or projection neurons and local circuit neurons (Fig 18–4A). The projection neurons that form the interconnecting pathways transmit signals over long distances. The cell bodies are relatively large, and their axons emit collaterals that arborize extensively in the vicinity of the neuron. These neurons are excitatory, and their synaptic influences are very short-lived. The excitatory transmitter released from these cells is not known, but aspartate and glutamate are leading candidates at many sites. Local circuit neurons are typically smaller than projection neurons, and their axons arborize in the immediate vicinity of the cell body. The vast majority of these neurons are inhibitory, and they release either gamma-aminobutyric acid (GABA) or glycine. They synapse primarily on the cell body of the projection neurons but can also synapse on the dendrites of projection neurons as well as with each other. A special class of local circuit neurons in the spinal cord forms axoaxonic synapses on the terminals of sensory axons (Fig 18–4B). Two common types of pathways for these neurons (Fig 18–4A) include recurrent feedback pathways and feed-forward pathways. In many sensory pathways, local circuit neurons may actually lack an axon and release neurotransmitter from dendritic synapses in a graded fashion in the absence of action potentials. Some pathways involving presynaptic dendrites of local circuit neurons are shown in Fig 18–4C.

Although there is a great variety of synaptic connections in these hierarchical systems, the fact that a limited number of transmitters are utilized by these neurons indicates that any major pharmacologic manipulation of this system will have a profound effect on the overall excitability of the central nervous system. For instance, selectively blocking GABA receptors with a drug such as picrotoxin results in generalized convulsions. Thus, while the mechanism of action of picrotoxin is quite specific in blocking the effects of GABA, the overall functional effect appears to be quite nonspecific, since GABA-mediated synaptic inhibition is so ubiquitous.

Nonspecific or Diffuse Neuronal Systems

Those neuronal systems that contain one of the monoamines—norepinephrine, dopamine, or 5-hydroxytryptamine—provide typical examples in this category. Certain other pathways emanating from the reticular formation and possibly some peptide-containing pathways also fall into this category. These systems differ in fundamental ways from the hierarchical systems, and the noradrenergic systems will serve to illustrate the differences.

Noradrenergic cell bodies are found primarily in a compact cell group called the locus ceruleus located in the caudal pontine central gray matter. The number of neurons in this cell group is quite small, approximately 1500 on each side of the brain in the rat. The axons of these neurons are very fine and unmyelinated. Indeed, they were entirely missed with classic anatomic techniques. It was not until the mid 1960s when the formaldehyde fluorescence histochemical technique was applied to the study of CNS tissues that the anatomy of the monoamine-containing systems was described. Because these axons are fine and unmyelinated, they conduct very slowly, in the range of 0.5 m/s. The axons branch repeatedly and are extraordinarily divergent. Branches from the same neuron can innervate several functionally different parts of the central nervous system. In the neocortex, these fibers have a tangential organization and therefore can monosynaptically influence large areas of cortex. The pattern of innervation in the cortex and nuclei of the hierarchical systems is diffuse, and the fibers form a very small percentage of the total number in the area. In addition, the axons are studded with periodic enlargements called varicosities that contain large numbers of vesicles. In many instances, these varicosities do not form synaptic contacts, suggesting that norepinephrine may be released in a rather diffuse manner, as occurs with the noradrenergic innervation of smooth muscle. This indicates that the cellular targets of these systems will be determined largely by the location of the receptors rather than the location of the release sites. Based on all of these observations, it is clear that the monoamine systems cannot be conveying specific topographic types of information—rather, vast areas of the central nervous system must be affected simultaneously and in a rather uniform way. It is not surprising, then, that these systems have been implicated in such global functions as sleeping and waking, attention, appetite, and emotional states.

CENTRAL NEUROTRANSMITTERS

A number of small molecules have been isolated from brain, and studies using a variety of approaches suggest that these agents may be neurotransmitters. A brief summary of the evidence for some of these compounds follows.

Amino Acids

The amino acids of primary interest to the pharmacologist fall into 2 categories: the neutral amino acids glycine and gamma-aminobutyric acid (GABA), and the acidic amino acids glutamate and aspartate. All of these compounds are present in high concentrations in the central nervous system and are extremely potent in modifying neuronal excitability. The neutral amino acids are inhibitory and selectively increase membrane permeability to chloride ions, thus mimicking the IPSP. Glycine concentrations are particularly high in the gray matter of the spinal cord, and destruction of the neurons in this area results in a marked fall in the concentration of glycine. In addition, strychnine, which is a potent spinal cord convulsant and has been used in some rat poisons, selectively antagonizes both the action of glycine and the IPSPs recorded in spinal cord neurons. Thus, it is generally agreed that glycine is released from spinal cord inhibitory local circuit neurons involved in postsynaptic inhibition. There is also good evidence that GABA is a widespread postsynaptic inhibitory transmitter in the brain. The IPSPs in most regions of the brain are blocked by the GABA antagonists picrotoxin and bicuculline, which both cause generalized convulsions. Immunohistochemical studies indicate that a large majority of the local circuit neurons synthesize GABA. A special class of local circuit neuron localized in the dorsal horn of the spinal cord also synthesizes GABA. These neurons form axoaxonic synapses with primary sensory nerve terminals and are responsible for presynaptic inhibition (Fig 18–4B).

Both glutamate and aspartate are also present in very high concentrations in the central nervous system. Virtually all neurons that have been tested are strongly excited by these 2 amino acids. However, the lack of selective antagonists has greatly limited research in this area. Thus, the evidence has come primarily from biochemical studies which have shown either (1) that glutamate or aspartate concentrations in a particular region fall when specific excitatory pathways to the region are cut, or (2) that the calcium-dependent release of either amino acid is reduced after such lesions.

Acetylcholine

Acetylcholine was the first compound to be identified pharmacologically as a transmitter in the central nervous system. Eccles showed in the early 1950s that excitation of Renshaw cells by motor axon collaterals was blocked by nicotinic antagonists. Furthermore, Renshaw cells were extremely sensitive to nicotinic agonists. These experiments were remarkable for 2 reasons. First, this early success at identifying a transmitter for a central synapse was followed by disappointment, because it remained the sole pathway for which the transmitter was known until the late 1960s, when comparable data became available for the neutral amino acids. Second, the motor axon collateral synapse remains the only clearly documented example of a cholinergic nicotinic synapse in the mammalian central nervous system. Most acetylcholine-sensitive neurons in the central nervous system appear to be excited primarily through a muscarinic receptor. The muscarinic effects have a much slower time course than either nicotinic effects on Renshaw cells or the effect of amino acids. Furthermore, this muscarinic excitation is unusual in that acetylcholine produces it by *decreasing* the membrane ion permeability, ie, the opposite of conventional transmitter action. A number of pathways are thought to contain acetylcholine, including neurons in the neostriatum, the medial septal nucleus, and the reticular formation, but progress in their investigation has been hampered by the lack of precise histochemical techniques.

Monoamines

These include the catecholamines (dopamine and norepinephrine) and 5-hydroxytryptamine (serotonin). Although these compounds are present in very small amounts in the central nervous system, extremely sensitive histochemical methods are available for localizing them. The methods include formaldehyde-induced fluorescence of the monoamines and immunohistochemical methods for localizing the individual synthetic enzymes.

A. Dopamine: The major pathways containing dopamine are the projection linking the substantia nigra to the neostriatum and the projection linking the ventral tegmental region to limbic structures, particularly the limbic cortex. The antiparkinsonism drug levodopa acts in the former area, and the antipsychotic drugs are thought to act in the latter. Dopamine-containing neurons are also present in the tuberobasal ventral hypothalamus and play an important role in regulating hypothalamohypophyseal function. Dopamine generally exerts a slow inhibitory action on CNS neurons, and this effect may be mediated through cAMP.

B. Norepinephrine: This system has already been discussed. Most noradrenergic neurons are located in the locus ceruleus or the lateral tegmental area of the reticular formation. Although the density of fibers innervating various sites differs considerably, most regions of the central nervous system receive diffuse noradrenergic input. When applied to neurons, norepinephrine produces a slow inhibition of spontaneous activity accompanied by hyperpolarization. In spite of this inhibitory effect, norepinephrine actually enhances excitatory inputs; this effect often predominates, so that the overall effect is to facilitate transmission. The mechanism for this enhancement of excitatory input is not entirely clear but may occur indirectly by disinhibition, ie, inhibition of inhibitory local circuit neurons. Facilitation of excitatory synaptic transmission is in accordance with many of the behavioral processes thought to involve noradrenergic pathways—attention, arousal, etc.

C. 5-Hydroxytryptamine (Serotonin): Most 5-HT pathways originate from neurons in the raphe or midline regions of the pons and upper brain stem. 5-Hydroxytryptamine is contained in unmyelinated fibers that diffusely innervate most regions of the central nervous system, but the density of the innervation varies. In most areas of the central nervous system, 5-hydroxytryptamine has a strong inhibitory action. This is associated with membrane hyperpolarization that may be due to an increase in potassium conductance. The overall effect of 5-hydroxytryptamine on impulse transmission is also generally inhibitory. Considerable speculation exists regarding the possible involvement of 5-hydroxytryptamine pathways in the hallucinations induced by LSD, since this compound can antagonize the peripheral actions of 5-hydroxytryptamine. However, LSD does not appear to be a 5-hydroxytryptamine antagonist in the central nervous system, and typical LSD-induced behavior is still seen in animals after destruction of raphe nuclei. Other proposed regulatory functions of 5-hydroxytryptamine-containing neurons include sleep, temperature, appetite, and neuroendocrine control.

D. Peptides: A great many CNS peptides have been discovered that produce dramatic effects both on animal behavior and on the activity of individual neurons. Some of the better known peptides have been mapped with immunohistochemical techniques and include enkephalin, endorphins, substance P, somatostatin, vasoactive intestinal polypeptide, and thyrotropin-releasing hormone. A particularly intriguing finding is that a peptide can coexist with a conventional nonpeptide transmitter in the same neuron. A good example of the approaches used to define the role of these peptides in the central nervous system comes from studies on substance P and its association with sensory fibers. Immunohistochemical studies have found substance P to be present in some of the small unmyelinated primary sensory neurons of the spinal cord and brain stem. In addition, stimulation of the sensory neurons releases substance P from the spinal cord. Application of substance P to neurons in the spinal cord excites neurons that are excited by painful stimuli. Painful stimuli are known to selectively activate unmyelinated sensory fibers. Finally, administration of the drug capsaicin to neonatal animals destroys unmyelinated sensory fibers that contain substance P and renders the animals insensitive to heat. Thus, it is believed that substance P may be an excitatory transmitter released from unmyelinated fibers that respond to painful thermal stimulation. Substance P is certainly involved in many other functions, since it is found in many areas of the central nervous system that are unrelated to pain pathways.

• • •

References

Bloom FE: Neurohumoral transmission and the central nervous system. Chap 12, pp 235–257, in: *Goodman and Gilman's The Pharmacological Basis of Therapeutics,* 6th ed. Gilman AG, Goodman LS, Gilman A (editors). Macmillan, 1980.

Cooper JR, Bloom FE, Roth RH: *The Biochemical Basis of Neuropharmacology,* 2nd ed. Oxford Univ Press, 1978.

Eccles JC: *The Physiology of Synapses.* Academic Press, 1964.

Hokfelt T et al: Peptidergic neurons. *Nature* 1980;**284:**515.

Iversen LL, Nicoll RA, Vale WW: Neurobiology of peptides. *Neurosci Res Program Bull* 1978;**16:**214.

Lipton ME, Killam KC, DiMascio A (editors): *Psychopharmacology: A Generation of Progress.* Raven Press, 1978.

McGreer PL, Eccles JC, McGreer EG: *Molecular Neurobiology of the Mammalian Brain.* Plenum Press, 1978.

Moore RY, Bloom FE: Central catecholamine neuron systems: Anatomy and physiology. *Annu Rev Neurosci* 1978;**2:**113.

Nicoll RA, Schenker C, Leeman SE: Substance P as a transmitter candidate. *Annu Rev Neurosci* 1980;**3:**227.

Rakic P: Local circuit neurons. *Neurosci Res Program Bull* 1975;**13:**293.

Shepherd GM: *The Synaptic Organization of the Brain.* Oxford Univ Press, 1974.

Sedative-Hypnotics | 19

Anthony J. Trevor, PhD, & Walter L. Way, MD

I. BASIC PHARMACOLOGY OF SEDATIVE-HYPNOTICS

Drug classifications are often based on clinical uses rather than on similarities in chemical structures or mechanisms of action. Assignment of a particular compound to the sedative-hypnotic class of drugs indicates that its major therapeutic use is to cause sedation (with concomitant relief of anxiety) or to encourage sleep. These clinical uses are of such magnitude that sedative-hypnotics have become the most frequently prescribed drugs worldwide.

An effective **sedative** should reduce anxiety and exert a calming effect with little or no effect on motor or mental functions. The degree of central nervous system depression caused by a sedative should be the minimum consistent with therapeutic efficacy. A **hypnotic** drug should produce drowsiness and encourage the onset and maintenance of a state of sleep that as far as possible resembles the natural sleep state. Hypnotic effects involve more pronounced depression of the central nervous system than sedation, and this can be achieved with most sedative drugs simply by increasing the dose.

Graded dose-dependent depression of central nervous system function is a characteristic of sedative-hypnotics. An increase in dose above that needed for hypnosis may lead to a state of general anesthesia, and certain sedative-hypnotic drugs can be used as adjunctive agents in anesthesia practice. At still higher doses, the sedative-hypnotics may depress respiratory and vasomotor centers in the medulla, leading to coma and death. Depression of a specific dysfunction also provides the basis for the use of certain drugs in this class as antiepileptic agents.

Individual sedative-hypnotic drugs may differ in terms of the relationship between the extent of central nervous system depression and dose. Examples of such dose-response relationships are shown in Fig 19–1. The steep slope for drug A indicates that clinically useful effects (eg, sedation) and undesirable central nervous system depression can occur over a relatively narrow dosage range. A flatter dose-response curve shown for drug B indicates a wider dosage range between sedative-hypnotic and toxic effects. In the case of deviations from linearity, as shown for drug C, even greater dosage increments would be needed to cause severe central nervous system depression. Obviously, sedative-hypnotics that can be shown to exhibit the dose-response relationships illustrated by drugs B or C offer a greater margin of safety in therapeutic use than those represented by drug A.

Chemical Classification of Sedative-Hypnotics

Drugs of the sedative-hypnotic class are of diverse chemical structure. In Table 19–1, representative examples of the different chemical groups are listed, and illustrative structures are shown. Based on extensive use since their introduction almost 80 years ago, the barbiturates can be regarded as prototypes of the class. Motivation to develop other sedative-hypnotics might be attributed to efforts to avoid certain undesirable features of the barbiturates, including their potential for habituation and physical dependence. Unfortunately, such efforts have not always been successful. For example, the piperidinediones such as glutethimide, introduced as "nonbarbiturates," are in fact chemically related and virtually indistinguishable from barbiturates in their pharmacologic properties. Because of the huge market for sedative-hypnotics, such "failed attempts" are often commercially successful.

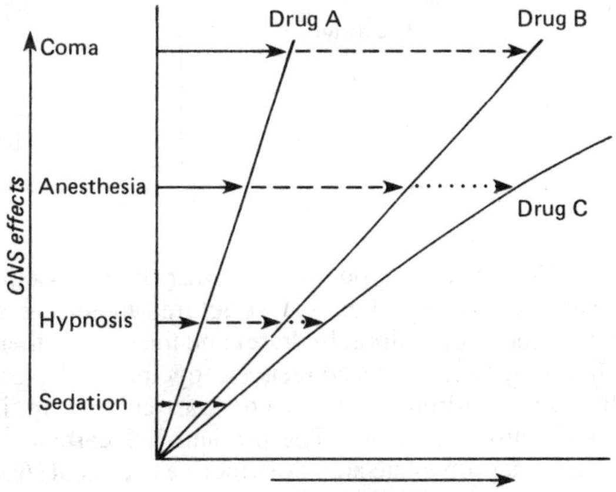

Figure 19–1. Theoretical dose-response curves for sedative-hypnotics.

Table 19–1. Chemical classes of sedative-hypnotics.

Class	Illustrative Structure	
Barbiturates Thiohexital Thiopental Hexobarbital Amobarbital Pentobarbital Phenobarbital	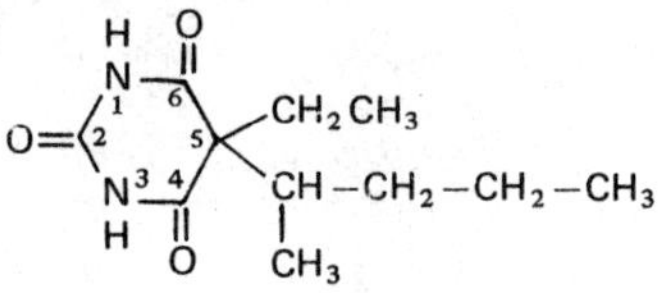	Pentobarbital
Piperidinediones Glutethimide Methyprylon	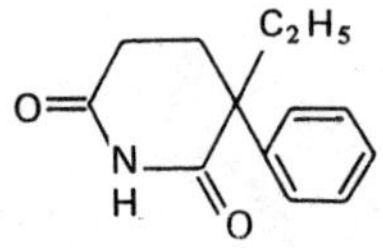	Glutethimide
Benzodiazepines Chlordiazepoxide Diazepam Flurazepam Lorazepam Oxazepam	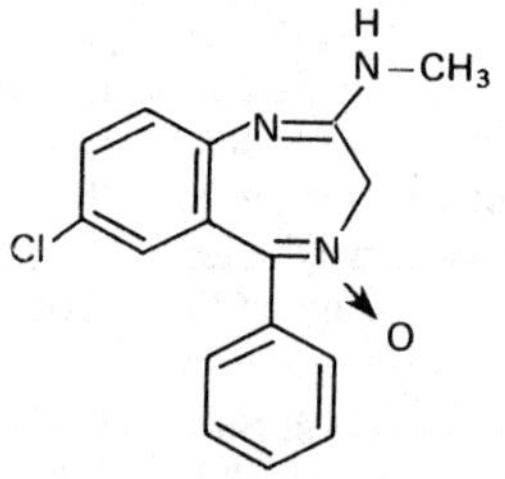	Chlordiazepoxide
Carbamates Meprobamate	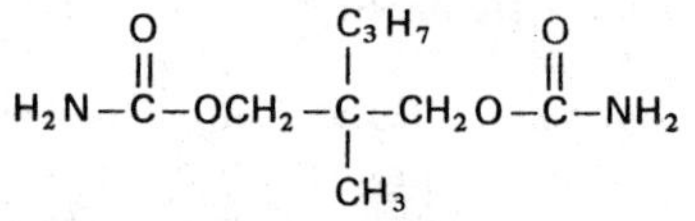	Meprobamate
Quinazolones Methaqualone	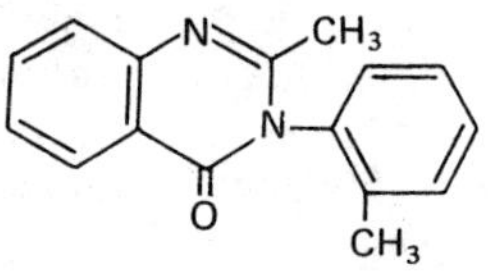	Methaqualone
Alcohols Ethanol Chloral hydrate Ethchlorvynol	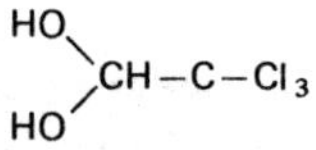	Chloral hydrate
Cyclic ethers Paraldehyde	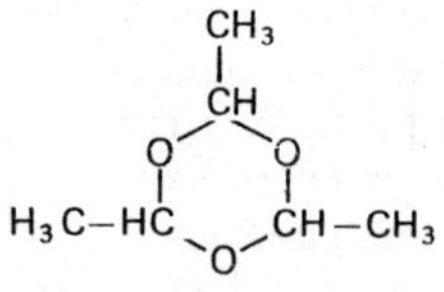	Paraldehyde

The sedative-hypnotic class also includes compounds of simple chemical structure, including alcohols (ethanol, chloral hydrate) and the cyclic ethers. Chloral hydrate and its congeners, together with paraldehyde, continue to be used, particularly in institutionalized patients. The propanediol carbamates such as meprobamate are of distinctive chemical structure but are practically equivalent to barbiturates in their pharmacologic effects, and their clinical use is declining. The benzodiazepines, introduced in 1961, have become the most frequently used sedative-hypnotics. Though more expensive, they appear to offer certain advantages over the barbiturates for sedation and hypnosis, as will be described below.

Other classes of drugs not included in Table 19–1 may exert sedative-hypnotic effects. For example, sedative and hypnotic effects can often be obtained with the antipsychotic tranquilizers, the tricyclic antidepressant drugs, and antihistaminic agents. As discussed in other chapters, these agents are different from conventional sedative-hypnotics in both their effects and their major therapeutic uses. Since they commonly exert marked effects on the peripheral autonomic nervous system, they are sometimes referred to as "sedative-autonomic" drugs. Compounds of this type are present in a number of over-the-counter sleep preparations, and their autonomic properties as well as their long duration of action can result in unwanted side-effects.

A. Absorption: When used to treat anxiety or sleep disorders, drugs of this class are usually given orally. The rates of oral absorption of sedative-hypnotics differ depending on a number of factors. In the stomach (pH 1–2), weakly acidic drugs such as the barbiturates and the piperidinediones are nonionized and, since they are lipid-soluble, are usually absorbed quite rapidly into the blood. One exception is glutethimide, which, because of its limited solubility in the aqueous gastric contents, may be absorbed slowly and erratically. Weakly basic drugs such as the benzodiazepines are absorbed most effectively at the higher pH found in the duodenum, which may explain their somewhat slower onset of effect than that of the barbiturates. One benzodiazepine, clorazepate, is converted to its active form, desmethyldiazepam, by acid hydrolysis in the stomach. Oral absorption of diazepam and the active metabolite of clorazepate is more rapid than that of the other commonly used benzodiazepines, whereas oxazepam is absorbed at the slowest rate. The bioavailability of several benzodiazepines, including chlordiazepoxide and diazepam, is unreliable after intramuscular injection.

B. Distribution: Transport of a sedative-hypnotic in the blood is a dynamic process in which drug molecules enter and leave tissues at rates dependent upon blood flow, concentration gradients, and permeabilities. Lipid solubility plays a major role in determining the rate at which a particular sedative-hypnotic enters the central nervous system. The thiobarbiturates (eg, thiopental), in which the oxygen on C2 is replaced by sulfur, are very lipid-soluble, and a high rate of entry into the central nervous system contributes to the rapid onset of their central effects. Diazepam is more lipid-soluble than chlordiazepoxide, and the central nervous system effects of the latter drug are slower in onset. Meprobamate has quite low solubility in lipids and penetrates the brain slowly even when given intravenously.

Redistribution of drug molecules from the central nervous system to other tissues is an important feature of the biodisposition of sedative-hypnotics. For example, thiobarbiturates are rapidly redistributed from the brain, first to highly perfused tissues such as skeletal muscle and subsequently to adipose tissue; these processes contribute to the termination of their major central nervous system effects. This may also be the case for other sedative-hypnotics, where the rate of metabolic transformation and elimination is much too slow in humans to account for the time required for dissipation of pharmacologic effects.

Administration of sedative-hypnotics during pregnancy should be done with the recognition that the placental barrier to lipid-soluble drugs is incomplete and that all of these agents are capable of reaching the fetus. The rate of achievement of equilibrium between maternal and fetal blood is slower than that for the maternal blood and central nervous system, partly because of lower blood flow to the placenta. Nonetheless, if sedative-hypnotics are given in the predelivery period, they may contribute to the depression of neonatal vital functions.

Many sedative-hypnotics bind to drug-binding sites on plasma proteins, and drug interactions between this class and other pharmacologic agents can occur. However, very few interactions appear to be based on competition for common binding sites on the plasma proteins. One exception is chloral hydrate, which increases the anticoagulant effects of warfarin by its displacement from such binding sites.

C. Biotransformation: As noted above, redistribution to tissues other than the brain may be as important as biotransformation in terminating the central nervous system effects of many sedative-hypnotics. However, metabolic transformation to more water-soluble metabolites is necessary for final clearance from the body of almost all drugs in this class. The microsomal drug-metabolizing enzyme systems of the liver are most important in this regard. Since few sedative-hypnotics are excreted from the body unchanged, the elimination half-life ($t_{1/2}$) of most drugs in this class depends mainly on the rate of their metabolic transformation.

With the exception of phenobarbital, only insignificant quantities of the barbiturates are excreted intact. The major metabolic pathways involve oxidation of chemical groups attached to C5, which are different for the individual barbiturates. The alcohols, acids, and ketones formed appear in the urine as glucuronide conjugates. Another type of metabolic reaction, glycosylation, involves direct attachment of glucose to N3 or N5 to form more water-soluble derivatives that can then be eliminated via the kidney. With very few exceptions, the metabolites of the barbiturates lack pharmacologic activity. The overall rate of hepatic metabolism in humans depends on the individual drug but (with the exception of the thiobarbiturates) is slow. The range of elimination half-life of thiopental and hexobarbital is a few hours, whereas that for most other barbiturates ranges from 18 to 48 hours. The elimination half-life of phenobarbital in humans may be as long as 4–5 days. Some biodispositional properties of representative barbiturates in humans are listed in Table 19–2. Secobarbital, pentobarbital, and amobarbital show few differences in the range of half-life or in plasma clearance rates. It would appear that the traditional classification of these barbiturates into short-acting, intermediate-acting, and long-acting drugs does not correlate well with these pharmacokinetic parameters. Multiple dosing with barbiturates with longer half-lives can lead to cumulative effects, though the development of tolerance may offset such problems to some extent.

All of the benzodiazepines undergo biotransformation via hepatic enzymes before excretion, but the

Table 19–2. Pharmacokinetic properties of barbiturates in humans.

Drug	Elimination Half-Life Range (hours)	Plasma Clearance (mL/min)	Metabolism Rate (percent per hour)	Comments
Methohexital	1–2	830	16–20	Given intravenously. Rapid onset and short duration.
Thiopental	3–6		12–15	
Hexobarbital	3–6	260	10–13	Given orally. Good bioavailability, slow tissue redistribution, slow biotransformation to inactive metabolites.
Secobarbital	18–36	53	2–6	
Pentobarbital	18–48	24	1–5	
Phenobarbital	24–96	6.5	< 1	Up to 30% excreted unchanged.

patterns and rates of metabolism depend on the individual drug. One important feature of benzodiazepine metabolism is formation of metabolites with central nervous system effects. Chlordiazepoxide and diazepam are both metabolized to several *active* compounds that contribute to their clinical and toxic effects. Desmethyldiazepam, the common active metabolite of both clorazepate and diazepam, has an elimination half-life of approximately 50 hours. Similarly, flurazepam, which is used mainly for hypnosis, is converted to an active metabolite with a half-life of 50–100 hours. This may account for unwanted central nervous system depression, including daytime sedation. The formation of active metabolites has complicated pharmacokinetic analyses of the benzodiazepines in humans, because the elimination half-life of the parent drug may have little relationship to the time course of pharmacologic effects. Those benzodiazepines for which either the parent drug or active metabolites have long half-lives are more likely to cause cumulative effects with multiple doses. Several drugs in this group, including oxazepam and lorazepam, which have a shorter half-life, are metabolized directly to inactive glucuronides. Cumulative and residual effects such as excessive drowsiness should be less of a problem with these agents. Some biodispositional properties of selected benzodiazepines are given in Table 19–3.

Most other sedative-hypnotics, including the piperidinediones and meprobamate, are biotransformed to more water-soluble compounds by hepatic enzymes. However, the metabolism of methaqualone is quite slow, which results in a long elimination half-life for the drug and the possibility of cumulative effects with continuous use. Trichloroethanol is the pharmacologically active metabolite of chloral hydrate and has a half-life of 6–10 hours. However, its toxic metabolite, trichloroacetic acid, is cleared very slowly and can accumulate with the nightly administration of chloral hydrate.

D. Excretion: The water-soluble metabolites of sedative-hypnotics are excreted mainly via the kidney. In most cases, changes in renal function do not have a marked effect on the elimination of parent drugs. Phenobarbital is excreted in the urine intact to a certain extent (20–30% in humans), and its elimination rate can be increased significantly by alkalinization of the urine. This is partly due to increased ionization at alkaline pH, since phenobarbital is a weak acid with a pK_a of 7.2. Only trace amounts of the benzodiazepines and less than 10% of a hypnotic dose of meprobamate appear in the urine unchanged.

E. Factors Affecting Biodisposition: The biodisposition of sedative-hypnotics can be influenced by various factors, particularly those that change rates of metabolic clearance. These include alterations in hepatic function resulting from disease, old age, or drug-induced increases in microsomal enzyme activities.

Table 19–3. Pharmacokinetic properties of benzodiazepines in humans.

Drug	Elimination Half-Life Range (hours)	Metabolites	Comments
Chlordiazepoxide	4–16	Active: desmethyl derivative, demoxepam, oxazepam.	Poor intramuscular bioavailability.
Clorazepate	50–100 (metabolites)	Active: desmethyldiazepam, oxazepam.	Hydrolyzed to active form in stomach.
Diazepam	50–150	Active: desmethyldiazepam, temazepam, oxazepam.	Poor intramuscular bioavailability.
Flurazepam	24–100 (metabolites)	Active: desalkyl derivative and others.	Long elimination half-lives of active metabolites.
Lorazepam	10–18	Inactive: glucuronides.	Elimination not much affected by age or liver disease.
Oxazepam	4–10	Inactive: glucuronides.	Slow oral absorption may delay onset of effects.
Temazepam	5–8	Possibly active.	Slow oral absorption.

Generally, decreased hepatic function results in reduction of the clearance rates of drugs metabolized via oxidative pathways. This group includes almost all of the barbiturates, the piperidinediones, meprobamate, and benzodiazepines such as chlordiazepoxide and diazepam. In very old patients or those with severe liver disease, the elimination half-lives of these drugs are usually increased significantly. If multiple normal doses of these sedative-hypnotics are given in such cases, one can anticipate the occurrence of cumulative or enhanced central nervous system effects.* Therefore, lower doses should be used in patients who may have limited hepatic function. Metabolism involving glucuronide conjugation appears to be less affected by old age or liver disease than oxidative metabolism.

The activity of hepatic microsomal drug-metabolizing enzymes may be increased in patients exposed to certain sedative-hypnotics on a chronic basis (enzyme induction; see Chapter 3). Drugs with longer elimination half-lives such as phenobarbital and meprobamate are most likely to cause this effect and result in an increase in the rate of their own hepatic metabolism as well as that of certain other drugs. Self-induction of metabolism is a possible mechanism contributing to the development of tolerance. Increased biotransformation of other pharmacologic agents by sedative-hypnotics is a potential mechanism underlying drug interactions. (See Appendix I.) The benzodiazepine group of sedative-hypnotics is somewhat less likely than the barbiturates to change hepatic drug-metabolizing enzyme activity with continuous use.

Pharmacodynamics

A. Sedation: Sedation can be defined as a decrease in responsiveness to a constant level of stimulation, with decrease in spontaneous activity and ideation. These behavioral changes occur at the lowest effective doses of the sedative-hypnotics. It is not yet clear whether antianxiety actions seen clinically are equivalent to or different from sedative effects. In experimental animal models, the sedative-hypnotic drugs are able to release punishment-suppressed behavior, and this disinhibition has been equated with antianxiety effects. However, the release of previously suppressed behavior may be more relevant to behavioral disinhibitory effects of these drugs, including euphoria, impaired judgment, and loss of self-control, which occur at doses slightly higher than those used to cause sedation. All sedative-hypnotic drugs are capable of releasing punishment-suppressed behavior in animals, but the benzodiazepines exert such effects at doses that do not cause general central nervous system depression. Phenothiazine antipsychotic drugs and tricyclic antidepressants are not effective in this experimental model.

B. Hypnosis: By definition, all of the sedative-hypnotics will induce sleep if high enough doses are given. Normal sleep is considered to consist of distinct stages, based on 3 physiologic measures: the electroencephalogram, the electromyogram, and the electro-oculogram (a measure of lateral movements of the eye). Based on the latter, 2 major categories can be distinguished: non-rapid eye movement (NREM) sleep, which represents approximately 70–75% of total sleep; and rapid eye movement (REM) sleep. REM and NREM sleep occur cyclically over an interval of about 90 minutes. The REM sleep stage is that in which most recallable dreams occur. NREM sleep progresses through 4 stages (1–4), with the greatest proportion (50%) of sleep being spent in stage 2. This is followed by delta or slow-wave sleep (stages 3 and 4), in which somnambulism and night terrors have been noted to occur.

The effects of drugs on the sleep stages have been studied extensively, although often with normal volunteer subjects rather than patients with sleep disorders. In the case of sedative-hypnotics, effects depend on several factors, including the specific drug, the dose, and the frequency of its administration. While some exceptions exist, the effects of sedative-hypnotics on patterns of normal sleep are as follows: (1) the latency of sleep onset is decreased (time to fall asleep); (2) the duration of stage 2 NREM sleep is increased; (3) the duration of REM sleep is decreased; and (4) the duration of slow-wave sleep is decreased.

More rapid onset of sleep and prolongation of stage 2 are presumably effects of clinical usefulness. However, the significance of effects on REM and slow-wave sleep is not clear. Use of sedative-hypnotics for more than a week or so leads to some tolerance to their effects on sleep patterns. Withdrawal after continued use can result in a "rebound" increase in the frequency of occurrence and duration of REM sleep. It is important to recognize that claims have often been made for superiority of one sedative-hypnotic over another based on differential actions on one stage of sleep or another. Since little is known about the function of any sleep stage, statements about the desirability of a particular drug based on its effects on sleep patterns can have no validity. Clearly, clinical criteria of efficacy in alleviating a particular sleeping problem are more useful. The ideal hypnotic—one that would promote sleep without any change in its natural pattern—has yet to be introduced.

C. Anesthesia: As shown in Fig 19–1, sedative-hypnotics in high doses will depress the central nervous system to a point known as stage III of general anesthesia (see Chapter 22). However, the suitability of a particular agent as an adjunct in anesthesia depends mainly on the physicochemical properties that determine its rapidity of onset and duration of effect. Among the barbiturates, thiopental and methohexital are very lipid-soluble, penetrating brain tissue rapidly following intravenous administration. Rapid tissue redistribution accounts for the short duration of action of these drugs, which are therefore useful in anesthesia practice. Certain of the benzodiazepines have been used intravenously in anesthesia, but most

*Surprisingly, there are only a few clinical studies that document this.

(eg, diazepam) have a relatively long half-life and form active metabolites that can lead to persistent postanesthetic depression when large doses are used. It is possible that new benzodiazepines that have much shorter half-lives will be more useful in anesthesia.

D. Anticonvulsant Effects: Most of the sedative-hypnotics are capable of inhibiting the development and spread of epileptiform activity in the central nervous system, but some selectivity exists in that certain drugs do so without marked central nervous system depression, so that normal mentation and activity are relatively unaffected. Of the barbiturates, phenobarbital and metharbital (converted to phenobarbital in the body) are effective in the treatment of grand mal and jacksonian epilepsy. Certain benzodiazepines also have selective actions: diazepam is used in status epilepticus and in the treatment of seizures induced by local anesthetics, and nitrazepam is used in certain infantile spasms and myoclonic seizures (see Chapter 21).

E. Muscle Relaxation: Some sedative-hypnotics, particularly members of the carbamate and benzodiazepine groups, exert inhibitory effects on polysynaptic reflexes and internuncial transmission, and at high doses may depress transmission at the skeletal myoneural junction. Selective actions of this type leading to muscle relaxation can be readily demonstrated in animals, and this has led to claims of usefulness for relaxing contracted voluntary muscle in joint disease or muscle spasm. Unfortunately, there is little clinical evidence to support such claims at dose levels that do not also cause significant depression of the central nervous system, leading to changes in mental or motor functions. What positive evidence does exist concerns specialized clinical situations such as the treatment with diazepam of spasticity in patients with cerebral palsy.

F. Effects on Respiration and Cardiovascular Function: At hypnotic doses in healthy patients, the effects of sedative-hypnotics on respiration are comparable to changes during natural sleep. However, sedative-hypnotics even at therapeutic doses can produce significant respiratory depression in patients with obstructive pulmonary disease. Effects on respiration are dose-related, and depression of the medullary respiratory center is the usual cause of death due to overdose of sedative-hypnotics.

At doses up to those causing hypnosis, no significant effects on the cardiovascular system are observed in healthy patients. However, in hypovolemic states, congestive heart failure, or other diseases impairing cardiovascular function, normal doses of sedative-hypnotics may cause cardiovascular depression, probably as a result of actions on the medullary vasomotor centers. At toxic levels, myocardial contractility and vascular tone may both be depressed by central and peripheral effects, leading to circulatory collapse. Respiratory and cardiovascular effects become more apparent when sedative-hypnotics are given intravenously.

Tolerance; Psychologic & Physical Dependence

Tolerance, a decrease in responsiveness to a drug following continuous exposure, is a common feature of the sedative-hypnotics. In some instances, it may result in a need to increase the dose to maintain symptomatic improvement or to promote sleep. It is important to recognize that **cross-tolerance** occurs between the sedative-hypnotics described here and also with ethanol (Chapter 20)—a feature of some clinical importance, as explained below. The mechanisms of development of tolerance to sedative-hypnotics are not well understood. An alteration in rates of metabolic inactivation with chronic administration may be partly responsible (metabolic tolerance), but changes in responsiveness of the central nervous system (pharmacodynamic tolerance) are more important.

The perceived desirable properties of relief of anxiety, euphoria, disinhibition, and promotion of sleep have led to the compulsive misuse of virtually all of the drugs classed as sedative-hypnotics. (See Chapter 29 for a detailed discussion of drug abuse.) The consequences of abuse of these agents can be defined in both psychologic and physiologic terms. The psychologic component may initially parallel simple neurotic behavior patterns hard to differentiate from those of the inveterate coffee drinker or cigarette smoker. When the pattern of sedative-hypnotic use becomes compulsive, more serious complications develop, including physical dependence and tolerance.

Physical dependence can be described as an altered physiologic state that requires continuous drug administration to prevent the appearance of an abstinence or withdrawal syndrome. As described more fully later, in the case of sedative-hypnotics this syndrome is characterized by states of increased excitability that may even progress to convulsions. All sedative-hypnotics are capable of causing physical dependence when used on a chronic basis. However, the severity of withdrawal symptoms differs between individual drugs and depends also on the magnitude of the dose used immediately prior to cessation of use. When higher doses of sedative-hypnotics are used, abrupt withdrawal will lead to more serious withdrawal signs. Differences in the severity of withdrawal symptoms between individual sedative-hypnotics relate in part to biodisposition properties, since drugs with long half-lives are eliminated slowly enough to accomplish gradual withdrawal with few physical symptoms.

Mechanisms of Action

Considering the multiple effects of sedative-hypnotics on central nervous system functions, together with the chemical heterogeneity of drugs in this class that can cause similar behavioral effects, it is not surprising that no unitary hypothesis exists regarding mechanisms of action. Consideration of the possible sites of action and the precise mechanisms underlying specific central nervous system effects has been aided by both neurophysiologic and neurochemical studies.

A. Neurophysiologic Actions: Neurophysiologic studies have revealed numerous sites in the central nervous system sensitive to actions of sedative-hypnotics. The midbrain reticular formation appears to be one site of barbiturate action, since these drugs increase the threshold for electrical stimulation and depress potentials evoked in the system by various stimuli at doses lower than those affecting conduction in sensory nerves. In addition, the barbiturates can depress neuronal activities in the posterior hypothalamus, the amygdaloid complex, and limbic structures, including the septal region and hippocampus.

Similar studies with various benzodiazepines suggest loci of actions in the limbic system as well as the thalamus and the midbrain reticular formation. The depression of evoked potentials in each of these anatomic regions can occur at doses of benzodiazepines that have little effect on the cortical electroencephalogram. Such selectivity can also be seen for other sedative-hypnotics. Meprobamate, for example, decreases the duration of electrical after-discharge evoked by stimulation of neurons in the septal region and amygdala at doses that have little effect on other neuronal activities.

Effects at the synaptic level have been studied extensively, especially for the barbiturates. At low dosage levels, these include reduced excitatory synaptic transmission with maintained synaptic inhibition, especially that involving glycine and GABA as chemical mediators. When used in anesthetic doses, the barbiturates may reduce sensitivity of postsynaptic membranes to excitatory neurotransmitters. Similar experiments with benzodiazepines have shown that these agents potentiate presynaptic inhibition at sites where GABA acts as an inhibitory neurotransmitter, including the cerebral cortex, substantia nigra, hippocampus, and cerebellum. These actions are relatively specific, since they occur at drug concentrations that have little direct effect on the actions of other chemical neurotransmitters such as glycine, norepinephrine, and serotonin.

B. Neurochemical Actions: Studies on the neurochemical actions of sedative-hypnotics have concentrated on effects on chemical neurotransmitters. For example, both barbiturates and benzodiazepines reduce stress-induced turnover of norepinephrine and serotonin in rat brain, particularly in cell bodies in the raphe nucleus. It has been difficult to establish whether such effects represent direct actions of the drugs or if they are metabolic sequelae of actions at other sites.

Recently, there have been demonstrations of high-affinity binding sites (receptors) for the benzodiazepines in various brain regions, including the cerebral cortex, midbrain, and hippocampus. These receptors appear to be located adjacent to—but are distinct from—GABA receptor sites. The interaction of benzodiazepines with these specific receptors leads to a facilitation of the inhibitory actions of GABA by mechanisms not fully understood. Current efforts are focused on the identification of endogenous substances (analogous to opioid peptides) that interact with benzodiazepine receptors.

II. CLINICAL PHARMACOLOGY OF SEDATIVE-HYPNOTIC DRUGS

TREATMENT OF ANXIETY STATES

Throughout history, the psychologic and behavioral responses to stress have been a significant part of human experience, and many ingenious approaches have been devised for relieving the various symptoms of anxiety. Before considering the clinical use of sedative-hypnotics, it is important to analyze the patient's symptoms carefully. If the patient presents with anxiety as a primary complaint, other psychiatric problems must be suspected. These may best be managed by psychotherapy or, when the situation warrants, by the use of pharmacologic agents such as the tricyclic antidepressants or antipsychotic drugs. Frequently, however, anxiety is secondary to organic disease states—acute myocardial infarction, angina pectoris, gastrointestinal ulcers, etc—which themselves require specific therapy. Another class of secondary anxiety states (situational anxiety) results from circumstances that may only have to be dealt with once or a few times, including anticipation of frightening medical or dental procedures and family illness or other tragedy. Even though situational anxiety tends to be self-limiting, the *short-term* use of sedative-hypnotics may be appropriate for the treatment of this and certain disease-associated anxiety states. Similarly, the acute use of a sedative-hypnotic as a premedicant prior to surgery or some unpleasant medical procedure is rational and proper (Table 19–4).

Historically, the rationale for the treatment of anxiety with sedative-hypnotics was quite empiric, since evidence for efficacy from well-controlled, blind clinical studies did not become available until the last decade. Difficulties in establishing efficacy can be related to many nonpharmacologic factors that influence the success of therapy, including personal expectations, personality of the therapist, environmental factors, and the placebo response. Although anxiety symptoms can now be ameliorated by drug therapy, it is difficult to demonstrate the superiority of one drug over another. Thus, a preference for a particular drug for a specific situation is based on factors other than pharmacologic effect.

Table 19–4. Clinical uses of sedative-hypnotics.

For relief of anxiety.
Hypnosis.
For sedation and amnesia before medical and surgical procedures.
Treatment of epilepsy and seizure states.
Premedication prior to anesthesia.
Intravenous administration, as a component of balanced anesthesia.
For control of ethanol or other sedative-hypnotic withdrawal states.
For muscle relaxation in specific neuromuscular disorders.
As diagnostic aids or for treatment in psychiatry.

Although phenobarbital, meprobamate, and certain sedative-autonomic drugs (hydroxyzine, diphenhydramine) continue to be used, the most commonly used drugs for treatment of anxiety are the benzodiazepines. The selection of benzodiazepines is based on several sound pharmacologic principles: (1) a relatively high therapeutic index (see drug B or C in Fig 19–1), since hypnotic and anesthetic doses are considerably higher than those causing sedation; (2) a low risk of drug interactions based on enzyme induction; (3) slow elimination rates, which may favor persistence of useful central nervous system effects; and (4) a low risk of physical dependence, with minor withdrawal symptoms.

Disadvantages of the benzodiazepines include the tendency to develop psychologic dependence, the formation of active metabolites, and their higher cost. As is true of all drugs of the sedative-hypnotic class, the benzodiazepines exert additive central nervous system depression when administered with other drugs, including ethanol. The patient should be warned of this possibility to avoid impairment of performance of any task requiring mental alertness and motor coordination.

Perhaps the most important guide to therapy is to use the drug selected with appropriate restraint to minimize adverse effects. A dose should be prescribed that does not impair mentation or motor functions during working hours. Some patients may tolerate the drug better if most of the daily dose is given at bedtime, with smaller doses during the day. Prescriptions should be written for short periods, since there is little justification for long-term therapy. The physician should make an effort to assess the efficacy of therapy from the patient's subjective responses. Plasma drug concentrations are too variable to be useful as a guide to dosage. Combinations of antianxiety agents should be avoided, and people taking sedatives should be cautioned about drinking and over-the-counter medications (see Chapter 64).

TREATMENT OF SLEEP PROBLEMS

The complaint of insomnia embraces a wide variety of sleep problems that include difficulty in falling asleep, frequent awakenings, short duration of sleep, and "unrefreshing" sleep. Insomnia is a serious complaint calling for careful evaluation to uncover possible causes (organic, psychologic, situational, etc) that can perhaps be managed without hypnotic drugs. Nonpharmacologic therapies sometimes useful include proper diet and exercise, avoiding stimulants before retiring, assuring a comfortable sleeping place, and retiring at a regular time each night. In some cases, however, the patient will need and should be given a sedative-hypnotic for a limited period. ***Note:*** *Long-term use of hypnotics is irrational and dangerous medical practice.*

The hypnotic drug selected should be one that provides sleep of fairly rapid onset (decreased sleep latency) and sufficient duration, with minimal "hangover" effects such as drowsiness, dysphoria, and mental or motor depression. Drugs with a favorable therapeutic index such as benzodiazepines are generally preferred. However, many benzodiazepines have slow elimination rates and are biotransformed to active metabolites—properties that are undesirable because they lead to cumulative and hangover effects. If hypnotics are used every night, tolerance can occur, leading to dose increases by the patient to produce the desired effect. It should be recalled that if physical dependence develops, the shorter-acting drugs are associated with more intense withdrawal signs when discontinued. The drugs commonly used for sedation and hypnosis are listed in Table 19–5 together with recommended doses.

OTHER THERAPEUTIC USES

Table 19–4 summarizes several other important clinical uses of drugs in the sedative-hypnotic class. Drugs used in the management of seizure disorders and for intravenous anesthesia are discussed in Chapters 21 and 22. For sedative and possible amnestic effects during medical or surgical procedures such as endoscopy and bronchoscopy, as well as premedication prior to anesthesia, oral formulations of shorter-acting drugs are preferred. When drug administration is under close supervision, the danger of accidental or intentional overdosage is less than in the outpatient situation, and a barbiturate may be as appropriate as any sedative-hypnotic. Meprobamate and, more recently, the benzodiazepines have frequently been used as central muscle relaxants, though evidence for general efficacy

Table 19–5. Dosages of drugs used commonly for sedation and hypnosis.

Sedation		Hypnosis	
Drug	Dosage	Drug	Dosage (at Bedtime)
Chlordiazepoxide (Librium)	10–20 mg 2–3 times daily	Chloral hydrate	500–1000 mg
Clorazepate (Tranxene)	5–7.5 mg twice daily	Flurazepam (Dalmane)	15–30 mg
Diazepam (Valium)	5 mg twice daily	Lorazepam (Ativan)	2–4 mg
Lorazepam (Ativan)	1–2 mg once or twice daily	Methaqualone (Quaalude)	150–250 mg
Oxazepam (Serax)	15–30 mg 3–4 times daily	Pentobarbital	100–200 mg
Phenobarbital	15–30 mg 2–3 times daily	Secobarbital	100–200 mg
		Temazepam (Restoril)	10–30 mg

without accompanying sedation is lacking. Sedative-hypnotics are occasionally used as diagnostic aids in neurology and psychiatry.

CLINICAL TOXICOLOGY OF SEDATIVE-HYPNOTICS

Direct Toxic Actions of Sedative-Hypnotics

Many of the common adverse effects of drugs in this class are those resulting from dose-related depression of central nervous system functions. In ambulatory patients, relatively low doses may lead to drowsiness, impaired judgment, and diminished motor skills, sometimes with a significant impact on personal relationships and job performance. Hangover effects are not uncommon following use of drugs with long half-lives for sleep problems in such patients. The most common reversible cause of confusional states in the elderly is overuse of sedative-hypnotics. At higher doses, toxicity may present as lethargy or a state of exhaustion or, alternatively, gross symptoms equivalent to those of ethanol intoxication. The titration of useful therapeutic effects against such side-effects is usually more difficult with sedative-hypnotics that exhibit steep dose-response relationships of the type shown in Fig 19–1 (drug A), including the barbiturates and piperidinediones. Unwanted depression of central nervous system functions also occurs more frequently when therapy is continued for longer periods and when drugs with long half-lives and active metabolites are used. The physician should be aware of variability among patients in terms of doses causing adverse effects. A relatively small dose in one individual may result in unwanted central nervous system depression that would require 2 or 3 times that dose in another patient. Variability is even more common in patients with cardiovascular or respiratory disease and hepatic impairment or in old age.

Sedative-hypnotics are the drugs most frequently involved in deliberate overdosage situations, in part because of their general availability as the most commonly prescribed pharmacologic agents. The benzodiazepines are generally considered to be "safer" drugs in this respect, since they have flatter dose-response curves. Epidemiologic studies on the incidence of drug-related deaths support this general assumption—eg, 0.3 deaths per million tablets of diazepam prescribed versus 11.6 deaths per million capsules of secobarbital in a recent study. Of course, many factors other than the specific sedative-hypnotic could influence such data—particularly the presence of other central nervous system depressants, including ethanol. In fact, most serious cases of drug overdosage, intentional or accidental, do involve polypharmacy; and when combinations of agents are taken, the practical "safety" of benzodiazepines may be less than the foregoing would imply.

The lethal dose of any sedative-hypnotic is variable (Chapter 58). If discovery of the ingestion is made early and a conservative treatment regimen is started, the outcome is rarely fatal, even following very high doses. On the other hand, for most sedative-hypnotics, with the exception of benzodiazepines, a dose as low as 10 times what is required for hypnosis may be fatal if the patient is not discovered or does not seek help in time. With severe toxicity, the respiratory depression from central actions of the drug may be complicated by aspiration of gastric contents in the unattended patient—an even more likely occurrence if ethanol is present. Loss of brain stem vasomotor control, together with direct myocardial depression, further complicates successful resuscitation. In such patients, treatment consists of mechanical respiration; maintenance of plasma volume, renal output, and cardiac function; and perhaps use of a positive inotropic drug such as dopamine, which preserves renal blood flow. Hemodialysis or hemoperfusion may be used to hasten elimination of some of these drugs (see Table 58–6).

Adverse effects of the sedative-hypnotic that are not referable to their central nervous system actions occur infrequently. Hypersensitivity reactions, including skin rashes, occur only occasionally with most drugs of this class. Reports of teratogenicity leading to fetal deformation following use of piperidinediones and certain benzodiazepines justify caution in the use of these drugs during pregnancy. Because barbiturates enhance porphyrin synthesis, they are absolutely contraindicated in patients with a history of acute intermittent porphyria.

Alterations in Drug Response

Depending on dosage and duration of use, tolerance may occur to many of the pharmacologic effects of sedative-hypnotics. This can be demonstrated experimentally in humans by changes in the effects of chronic use of these drugs on the electroencephalogram and other characteristics of the stages of sleep. Clearly, it must occur with respect to other effects, since it is known that chronic abusers sometimes ingest quantities of sedative-hypnotics many times the conventional dosage without experiencing severe toxicity. However, it should not be assumed that the degree of tolerance achieved is identical for all pharmacologic effects, and there is evidence that lethal dose ranges are not altered significantly with chronic use of sedative-hypnotics. Cross-tolerance between the different sedative-hypnotics, including ethanol, could lead to an unsatisfactory therapeutic response when standard doses of a drug are used in a patient with a recent history of abuse of these agents.

With chronic use of sedative-hypnotics, especially as doses are increased, a state of physical dependence can occur. This may develop to a degree unparalleled by chronic use of any other drug group, *including the opiates,* since withdrawal from a sedative-hypnotic can have severe and life-threatening manifestations. Withdrawal symptoms range from restlessness, anxiety, weakness, and orthostatic hypotension to hyperactive reflexes and generalized seizures. The severity of withdrawal symptoms depends to a large extent on the dosage range used immediately prior to discontinuance but also on the particular drug. For example, low doses of barbiturates such as secobarbital or pentobarbital (less than 400 mg/d) or diazepam (less than 40 mg/d) may produce only mild symptoms of withdrawal when discontinued. On the other hand, the use of more than 800 mg/d of barbiturates or 50–60 mg/d of diazepam for 60–90 days is likely to result in seizures if abrupt withdrawal is attempted. Symptoms of withdrawal are usually more severe following discontinuance of sedative-hypnotics with shorter half-lives. Symptoms are less pronounced with longer-acting drugs, which may partly accomplish their own withdrawal by virtue of their slow elimination. Cross-dependence, defined as the ability of one drug to suppress abstinence symptoms from discontinuance of another drug, is quite marked among sedative-hypnotics. This provides the rationale for therapeutic regimens in the management of withdrawal states. Thus, longer-acting drugs such as phenobarbital and diazepam can be used to alleviate withdrawal symptoms of shorter-acting drugs, including ethanol.

Drug Interactions

The most frequent drug interactions involving sedative-hypnotics are interactions with other central nervous system depressant drugs, leading to additive effects. These interactions have some therapeutic utility with respect to the use of these drugs as premedicants or anesthetic adjuvants. However, they can lead to serious adverse effects, including enhanced depression with concomitant use of many other drugs. Obvious additive effects can be predicted with use of alcoholic beverages, narcotic analgesics, anticonvulsants, phenothiazines, and other sedative-hypnotic drugs. Less obvious but just as important is enhanced central nervous system depression with a variety of antihistamines, antihypertensive agents, and antidepressant drugs of the tricyclic class.

Interactions involving changes in the activity of hepatic drug-metabolizing enzyme systems can occur, especially following continuous use of barbiturates and meprobamate. For example, in humans, barbiturates have been shown to increase metabolic degradation rates of dicumarol, phenytoin, digitalis compounds, and griseofulvin, effects that could lead to decrease in response to these agents. Cimetidine has recently been reported to double the elimination half-life of diazepam, presumably via inhibition of hepatic metabolism. As mentioned above, chloral hydrate may displace warfarin from plasma proteins to cause enhanced anticoagulant effects.

• • •

References

Allquander C: Dependence on sedative and hypnotic drugs. *Acta Psychiatr Scand* [*Suppl*] 1978;**270:**1.

Breimer DD: Clinical pharmacokinetics of hypnotics. *Clin Pharmacokinet* 1977;**2:**93.

Council on Scientific Affairs. Hypnotic drugs and treatment of insomnia report. *JAMA* 1981;**245:**749.

Greenblatt DJ et al: Benzodiazepines: A summary of pharmacokinetic properties. *Br J Clin Pharmacol* 1981;**11(Suppl 1):**11S.

Kay DC et al: Human pharmacology of sleep. Pages 83–210 in: *Pharmacology of Sleep.* Williams RL, Karacan I (editors). Wiley, 1976.

Mendelson WB: *The Use and Misuse of Sleeping Pills: A Clinical Guide.* Plenum Press, 1980.

Sepinwall J, Cook L: Behavioral pharmacology of antianxiety drugs. Chap 6, pp 345–393 in: *Biology of Mood and Antianxiety Drugs.* Vol 13 of: *Handbook of Psychopharmacology.* Iversen LL, Iversen SD, Snyder SH (editors). Plenum Press, 1978.

Skolnick P, Paul SM: The mechanism(s) of action of the benzodiazepines. *Med Res Rev* 1981;**1:**3.

Tallman JF et al: Receptors for the age of anxiety: Pharmacology of the benzodiazepines. *Science* 1980;**207:**274.

The Alcohols | 20

Nancy M. Lee, PhD, & Charles E. Becker, MD

Ethyl alcohol (ethanol) is a sedative-hypnotic consumed as a social drug. Alcohol abuse (alcoholism) is a complex disorder whose natural history and basic causes are not well-defined. It is a major medical and public health problem in many societies.

Many other alcohols with potentially toxic effects are used in chemical industries, some in enormous quantities. In spite of their potential toxicity, they are far less important because significant exposure to them is almost never deliberate. Methanol and ethylene glycol toxicity occur with sufficient frequency to warrant some discussion in this chapter.

I. BASIC PHARMACOLOGY OF ALCOHOLS

ETHANOL

Pharmacokinetics

Ethanol (CH_3CH_2OH) is a small water-soluble molecule that is absorbed rapidly and completely from the gastrointestinal tract. Ethanol vapor can also be readily absorbed in the lungs. After ingestion of alcohol in the fasting state, peak blood levels are reached within 40 minutes. The presence of food in the gut delays absorption. Distribution is rapid, with tissue levels rapidly approximating the blood concentration.

Over 90% of alcohol consumed is oxidized in the liver; the rest is excreted through the lungs and in urine. The rate of oxidation follows zero-order kinetics, ie, it is independent of time and concentration of the drug. The amount of alcohol oxidized per unit time is approximately proportionate to body weight or liver weight, and the rate of disappearance of alcohol from the body is markedly reduced or halted entirely by hepatectomy or liver damage. Two pathways of alcohol metabolism to acetaldehyde have been proposed. Acetaldehyde is then oxidized by a third metabolic process.

A. Alcohol Dehydrogenase Pathway: The main pathway for alcohol metabolism involves alcohol dehydrogenase, a cytosolic enzyme that contains zinc and catalyzes the conversion of alcohol to acetaldehyde, according to the following reaction:

$$CH_3CH_2OH + NAD^+ \xrightarrow{\text{Alcohol dehydrogenase}} CH_3CHO + NADH + H^+$$

This enzyme is located mainly in the liver; however, trace amounts can be found in other organs such as brain and testes.

In the reaction shown above, hydrogen ion is transferred from alcohol to the cofactor nicotinamide adenine dinucleotide (NAD) to form NADH. As a net result, alcohol oxidation generates an excess of reducing equivalents in the liver, chiefly as NADH. There is some controversy over whether chronic alcohol consumption affects the activities of hepatic alcohol dehydrogenase. Actually, alcohol dehydrogenase itself is not rate-limiting, but the velocity of oxidation may depend on the availability of the cofactor NAD; therefore, the increased rate of blood alcohol clearance in alcoholics is probably not due to increased alcohol dehydrogenase activity.

B. Microsomal Ethanol Oxidizing System (MEOS): This enzyme system, also known as the mixed function oxidase system (Chapter 3), uses NADPH instead of NAD as cofactor in the following reaction:

$$CH_3CH_2OH + NADPH + H^+ + O_2 \xrightarrow{\text{MEOS}} CH_3CHO + NADP^+ + H_2O$$

Since the K_m varies from 0.26 to 2 mM for alcohol dehydrogenase and from 8 to 10 mM for microsomal ethanol oxidizing system, it is thought that at low concentrations of alcohol, alcohol dehydrogenase is the main oxidizing system while at higher alcohol concentrations MEOS plays the more significant role. This may have important implications for the known interactions of alcohol (especially at high concentrations) with a host of other drugs also metabolized by this system. During chronic alcohol consumption, MEOS activity increases significantly. As described in Chapter 3, this induction of enzyme activity is associated with an increase in various constituents of the smooth fraction of the membranes involved in drug metabolism. Other "inducing" drugs such as barbiturates also enhance the rate of blood alcohol clearance.

C. Acetaldehyde Metabolism: It is now generally accepted that over 90% of the acetaldehyde formed from alcohol is also oxidized in the liver. While several enzyme systems may be responsible for this reaction, observations that acetaldehyde levels in the liver after ethanol administration are only 100–350 μmol have led to the conclusion that mitochondrial NAD-dependent **aldehyde dehydrogenase** (the apparent K_m for acetaldehyde is ~ 10 μM) is the main pathway for acetaldehyde oxidation. The product of this reaction is acetate, which can be further metabolized to CO_2 and water. Chronic alcohol consumption results in a decreased rate of acetaldehyde oxidation in intact mitochondria, although the enzyme activity is unaffected.

Tolerance & Physical Dependence

The consumption of alcohol over a long period may result in tolerance and physical dependence. Tolerance to the intoxicating effects of alcohol is a complex process involving changes in metabolism and poorly understood changes in the nervous system. Acute tolerance may occur after a few hours of drinking; this may occur in both alcoholics and social drinkers. Although minor degrees of metabolic tolerance after chronic alcohol use have been demonstrated in which the subject's capacity to metabolize the drug increases, the maximal increase in alcohol metabolism does not account for the magnitude of the observed clinical effect. Finally, as with other sedative-hypnotic drugs, there is a limit to tissue tolerance, so that only a relatively small increase in the lethal dose occurs with increasing doses.

Chronic alcohol drinkers, when forced to reduce or discontinue alcohol, experience a withdrawal syndrome, which indicates the existence of physical dependence. Although the mechanism of physical dependence to sedative-hypnotic drugs and alcohol is not known, it is recognized that both the rate of alcohol consumption and the duration determine the withdrawal syndrome. When consumption has been very high, merely reducing the rate of consumption may lead to signs of withdrawal.

Although tolerance and physical dependence are important components of alcohol abuse, the spectrum of illness associated with abuse of alcohol is so broad that it is difficult to contrive a simple definition of the phenomenon.

Pharmacodynamics of Acute Ethanol Abuse

A. Central Nervous System: The central nervous system is more markedly affected by acute alcohol consumption than any other organ system. Alcohol can lead to sedation and relief of anxiety, slurred speech, ataxia, impaired judgment, uninhibited behavior, or what is loosely called drunkenness.

Alcohol affects a variety of biochemical systems, including those concerned with energy metabolism, neurotransmitters, amino acids, proteins, ribonucleic acids, and neural membranes. However, little is known about the site of ethanol action in the brain. In view of the solvent properties of ethanol and its uniform distribution throughout the body, it is not surprising that it affects many systems. It has recently been shown that ethanol may affect the cell membrane by changing its fluidity (the membrane becomes more fluid in the presence of ethanol) and that tolerance may develop to this effect as a result of alteration in the ratio of saturated to unsaturated fatty acids and in the cholesterol content. The cell membrane is a fluid mosaic in which enzymes, receptors, and other components carry out their biologic activities. Thus, any system requiring a membrane component or membrane environment (eg, a neurotransmitter receptor) might be affected by alcohol.

Catecholamine, acetylcholine, and gamma-aminobutyric acid neurotransmitter systems have all been studied. Both central and peripheral noradrenergic neurons are affected by ethanol, with a transient decrease in norepinephrine levels and increase in its turnover; it has been shown that stimulation of the noradrenergic system can reverse some of alcohol's acute effects. On the other hand, pretreatment with levodopa prolongs ethanol narcosis. Ethanol inhibits the release of acetylcholine from cortical brain slices, presumably as a consequence of its reduction of passive Na^+ permeability. The studies of ethanol's action on the serotoninergic system have so far shown no consistent results. Ethanol also inhibits release of antidiuretic hormone from the pituitary, which accounts for its diuretic effect.

B. Heart: Significant depression of myocardial contractility has been observed in individuals who consume only moderate amounts of alcohol, ie, at a blood concentration of 100 mg/dL. Myocardial biopsies in humans before and after infusion of small amounts of alcohol have shown ultrastructural changes that may be associated with impaired myocardial function. Acetaldehyde is implicated as a cause of heart abnormalities by altering myocardial stores of catecholamines.

C. Smooth Muscle: Ethanol is a vasodilator, probably as a result of both central nervous system effects (depression of the vasomotor center) and direct smooth muscle relaxation caused by its metabolite, acetaldehyde. In cases of severe overdose, hypothermia consequent to vasodilatation may be marked. Ethanol also relaxes the uterus and has been used intravenously for the suppression of premature labor. However, the acute maternal toxicity of ethanol and the hazard to the fetus should relegate this therapeutic application to history, since other drugs (β_2-adrenergic stimulants and calcium influx inhibitors) appear to be more effective.

Consequences of Chronic Alcohol Consumption

The literature on alcoholism contains only limited data relating to precise dose-response relationships between chronic alcohol ingestion and injury of vital organ systems. The threshold for tissue and organ injury is an extremely unpredictable one in which the dose as well as various genetic and nutritional factors all may be critical.

A. Liver and Gastrointestinal Tract: Alcohol

in large doses creates a metabolic cascade effect, resulting in liver and gastrointestinal tract injury. The increased NADH/NAD ratio described above produces a change in the ratio of those metabolites that is dependent on the availability of NAD. It has been proposed that this altered ratio of NADH to NAD leads to a number of metabolic abnormalities in the liver, including reduced gluconeogenesis, hypoglycemia and ketoacidosis, and accumulation of fat in the liver parenchyma. Other factors such as heredity, associated disease, and the amount and duration of alcohol intake probably determine the severity of liver injury. Acetaldehyde also adversely affects liver function. Since metabolism of acetaldehyde via aldehyde dehydrogenase results in the generation of NADH, some of the acetaldehyde effects may be attributable to NADH excess. Acetaldehyde, however, is a very reactive compound that may have toxic effects of its own.

In some cases, nutritional factors are critical in alcohol-induced liver disease. It has been suggested that essential factors such as glutathione may be decreased in a malnourished alcoholic, thus removing a valuable scavenger of toxic free radicals that otherwise will injure the liver. Clinically significant alcoholic liver disease may be insidious in onset and progress without evidence of overt nutritional abnormalities. Alcoholic fatty liver may progress to alcoholic hepatitis and finally to cirrhosis. Hepatic failure may be the cause of death.

Other portions of the gastrointestinal tract may also be injured. Ingestion of alcohol increases gastric and pancreatic secretion and alters mucosal barriers that may enhance the risk of gastritis and pancreatitis. Acute gastrointestinal bleeding is often caused by alcoholic gastritis. The acute effects of alcohol on the stomach are related primarily to the toxic effect of ethanol on the mucosal membranes and have relatively little to do with increased production of gastric acid. Chronic alcoholics are prone to develop gastritis and increased susceptibility to blood and plasma protein loss during drinking, which may contribute to anemia and protein malnutrition. Alcohol also injures the small intestine, leading to diarrhea, weight loss, and multiple vitamin deficiencies. Malabsorption of vitamins, especially water-soluble ones, contributes to the clinical abnormalities. Thus, the statement sometimes made that malnutrition of alcoholic patients is due simply to dietary deficiency is probably not justified.

Although deficiencies in water-soluble vitamins were proposed in the past to account for most of the pathologic effects of alcohol, replacement doses of the vitamins do not protect against the injurious effects of alcohol. Thiamine deficiency, associated with Wernicke-Korsakoff syndrome, peripheral neuropathy, and beriberi heart disease, occurs in alcoholic patients, yet these nutritional deficiency syndromes are relatively rare in the alcoholic population.

B. Nervous System: As noted above, chronic ethanol consumption produces tolerance and physical dependence; when forced to reduce or discontinue the drug, the subject experiences withdrawal symptoms, which may consist of discomfort and hyperexcitability in mild cases and convulsions, toxic psychosis, and delirium tremens in severe ones. Consumption of large amounts of alcohol over extended periods (usually years) can also result in a number of neurologic deficits. The patient may have impairment of intellectual and motor functions, emotional lability, reduced perceptual acuity, and amnesia.

The most frequent neurologic abnormality in chronic alcoholism is a generalized symmetric peripheral nerve injury that begins with distal paresthesias of the hands and feet. While this is a diagnosis of exclusion requiring absence of other factors known to cause peripheral neuropathy, such neuropathies are commonly related to chronic alcohol use.

Wernicke-Korsakoff syndrome is a relatively uncommon but important entity characterized by paralysis of the external eye muscles, ataxia, and altered mentation, with amnesia and impairment of memory function. It is apparently associated with thiamine deficiency but is rarely seen in the absence of alcoholism. Wernicke-Korsakoff disease may be difficult to distinguish from the acute confusional state created by acute alcohol intoxication, which later blends in with the perceptual and behavioral problems associated with alcohol withdrawal. A distinguishing feature is the longer duration of the confusional state in Korsakoff's disease and the relative absence of the agitation that would be expected during withdrawal. Because of the importance of this pathologic condition, all patients suspected of Korsakoff's disease should receive thiamine therapy (50 mg intravenously once and 50 mg intramuscularly repeated daily until a normal diet is resumed).

Alcohol may also impair visual acuity, with painless bilateral blurring that occurs over several weeks of heavy alcohol consumption. Examination may reveal scotomas and reduced visual acuity for near and distant objects. Changes are usually bilateral and symmetric and may be followed by optic nerve degeneration. Ingestion of ethanol substitutes such as methanol (see below) causes severe visual disturbances.

C. Blood: Mild anemia resulting from alcohol-related folic acid deficiency is the most common hematologic disorder resulting from chronic alcohol abuse. Iron deficiency anemia may result from gastrointestinal bleeding, but sideroblastic anemia has also been described in alcoholic patients. Alcohol has also been implicated as a cause of several hemolytic syndromes some of which are associated with hyperlipidemia and severe liver disease. Alcohol directly inhibits the proliferation of all cellular elements in bone marrow.

Abnormalities in platelets and leukocytes have been described in alcoholics. These effects may account for some of the hemostatic impairment and increased frequency of infection in these individuals.

D. Cardiovascular System: The effect of alcohol on the cardiovascular system is now being given increasing attention. Alcohol can injure the cardiovascular system by producing severe nutritional abnormalities such as thiamine deficiency. Heart lesions have also been found to result from cobalt that was added to beer to stabilize the latter's foam.

Men and women who consume 3 or more drinks per day have higher systolic and diastolic blood pressures than abstainers independent of age, sex, race, smoking, coffee consumption, educational achievement, or weight. These findings suggest that the regular use of alcohol is a risk factor for hypertension. However, this conclusion is made less certain by the statistical manipulations required to exclude the effects of cigarette smoking and excessive coffee consumption, habits that are frequently associated with alcohol use.

Alcohol may affect the cardiovascular system by altering lipoprotein metabolism. Some individuals develop marked hyperlipidemia with moderate to heavy alcohol consumption, whereas others maintain normal levels. This variability suggests an underlying genetic heterogeneity. It has also been reported that one beneficial form of lipid—high-density lipoprotein (HDL)—increases with small amounts of alcohol consumption.

Patients undergoing alcohol withdrawal can develop severe arrhythmias that may reflect metabolic abnormalities of hypokalemia or alterations in magnesium metabolism. Seizures and syncope as well as sudden death during alcohol withdrawal may be due to these arrhythmias.

E. Endocrine System: Chronic alcohol use has important effects on the endocrine system and mineral and fluid electrolyte balance. Clinical reports of gynecomastia and testicular atrophy in alcoholics with cirrhosis suggest a derangement in steroid hormone balance. Gynecomastia and testicular atrophy have also been noted in alcoholics who have limited evidence of liver disease.

Alcoholics with chronic liver disease may have disorders of fluid and electrolyte balance, including ascites, edema, and effusions. These factors may be related to decreased protein synthesis and portal hypertension. Alterations of whole body potassium induced by vomiting and diarrhea, as well as severe secondary hyperaldosteronism, may contribute to muscle weakness and can be worsened by diuretic therapy. Abnormalities of trace metals such as zinc may also contribute to metabolic difficulties and infertility. Some alcoholic patients develop hypoglycemia, probably as a result of impaired hepatic gluconeogenesis. Some alcoholics also develop ketosis, caused by excessive lipolytic factors, especially increased cortisol and growth hormone.

F. Fetal Alcohol Syndrome: Chronic maternal alcohol abuse during pregnancy is associated with important teratogenic effects on the offspring. The abnormalities that have been characterized as fetal alcohol syndrome include multiple congenital abnormalities as set forth in Table 20–1. It is likely that heavy drinking in the first trimester of pregnancy has the greatest effect on fetal maldevelopment; heavy alcohol consumption near term may have a greater effect on fetal nutrition and birth weight. Although the extent to which alcohol alone causes these abnormalities is not clear, alcohol use during pregnancy appears to be a preventable cause of some fetal abnormalities.

Table 20–1. Most consistent features of the fetal alcohol syndrome.*

Growth and performance
Prenatal onset growth deficiency, more pronounced in length than in weight.
Concomitant microcephaly (small head circumference) even when corrected for small body weight and length.
Postnatal growth deficiency in weight and length, usually below third percentile.
Delay of intellectual development and/or mental deficiency (mean IQ from Seattle study = 64; range, 16–92).
Fine motor dysfunction (poor coordination).
Head and face
Microcephaly.
Short palpebral fissures (narrow eye slits).
Midfacial (maxillary) hypoplasia (underdevelopment of midfacial region).
Flattened, elongated philtrum (middle upper lip) associated with thin, narrow vermilion lip borders (highly specific to fetal alcohol syndrome).
Minor ear anomalies, including low-set ears.
Limbs
Abnormal creases in the palm of the hand.
Minor joint anomalies.
Syndactyly (fingers or toes joined together).
Clinodactyly (abnormal bending of fingers or toes).
Camptodactyly (one or more fingers constantly flexed at one or more phalangeal joints).
Heart
Ventricular and atrial septal defect (valve defects).
Brain
Absence of corpus callosum.
Hydrocephalus.
Brain cell migratory abnormalities.
Other
Minor genital anomalies.
Hemangiomas (benign tumors made up of blood vessels) in infancy.

*Data from Jones KL, Smith DW: The fetal alcohol syndrome. *Teratology* 1975;**12**:1.

G. Increased Risk of Cancer: Chronic alcohol ingestion has been shown to increase the risk for certain types of cancers, especially oropharyngeal, laryngeal, and esophageal cancers. Primary hepatocellular carcinoma is more likely to develop in patients with alcohol-related liver disease. There is also evidence of an increased incidence of prostatic and pancreatic cancer in alcoholics.

Alcohol-Drug Interactions

Interactions between ethanol and other drugs can have important clinical effects that result from alterations in the pharmacokinetics or pharmacodynamics of the second drug.

The most frequent pharmacokinetic alcohol-drug interactions occur as a result of alcohol-induced proliferation of the smooth endoplasmic reticulum of liver cells as described in Chapter 3. Thus, prolonged intake of alcohol without damage to the liver may enhance the metabolic biotransformation of other drugs. In contrast, *acute* alcohol use may *inhibit* metabolism of other drugs. This inhibition may be due to alteration of metabolism or alteration of liver blood flow. This acute alcohol effect may contribute to the commonly recognized danger of mixing alcohol with other drugs when performing activities requiring some skill, especially driving. Phenothiazines, tricyclic antidepressants, and sedative-hypnotic drugs are the most important drugs that may interact with alcohol by this mechanism.

Pharmacodynamic alcohol interactions are also of great clinical significance. Additive interaction with other sedative-hypnotics is most important. Alcohol also potentiates the pharmacologic effects of many nonsedative drugs including vasodilators and oral hypoglycemic agents. Alcohol also enhances the antiplatelet action of aspirin.

OTHER ALCOHOLS

Other alcohols related to ethanol have wide applications as industrial solvents and occasionally cause severe poisoning.

Methanol (methyl alcohol, wood alcohol; CH_3OH) is derived from the destructive distillation of wood. Methanol is used as a gasoline additive, as a home heating material, as an industrial solvent, and as a feedstock for bacterial synthesis of protein. Methanol is most frequently found in the home in the form of "canned heat" or in windshield washing materials. It can be absorbed through the skin or from the respiratory or gastrointestinal tracts. It is rapidly absorbed from the gastrointestinal tract and distributed in body water. The primary mechanism of elimination of methanol in humans is by oxidation to formaldehyde, formic acid, and CO_2:

$$CH_3OH \longrightarrow H\overset{O}{\overset{\|}{C}}H \longrightarrow H\overset{O}{\overset{\|}{C}}OH \longrightarrow CO_2 + H_2O$$

Methanol may also be removed by induced vomiting, and small amounts are excreted in the breath, sweat, and urine.

Various animal species show great variability in mean lethal doses of methanol. The special susceptibility of humans to methanol toxicity is probably due to the formate metabolite of methanol and not to methanol itself or to formaldehyde, the intermediate metabolite.

The enzyme chiefly responsible for methanol oxidation in the liver is alcohol dehydrogenase. Ethanol has a higher affinity than methanol for alcohol dehydrogenase; thus, saturation of alcohol dehydrogenase with ethanol can reduce formate production and is often used as treatment for acute methanol toxicity. Another agent known to inhibit alcohol dehydrogenase, 4-methylpyrazole, alone or in combination with ethanol, is probably of therapeutic value in methanol as well as ethylene glycol poisoning (see below).

Polyhydric alcohols such as **ethylene glycol** (CH_2OHCH_2OH) are used as heat exchangers, in antifreeze formulations, and as industrial solvents. Owing to the low volatility of the glycols, they produce little vapor hazard at ordinary temperatures. However, since they are used as antifreeze mixtures and as heat exchangers, they may be encountered in vapor or mist form, particularly if the temperature is high. Ethylene glycol appears to be considerably more toxic to humans than to many other animal species. As with other alcohols, ethylene glycol is metabolized by alcohol dehydrogenase to aldehydes, acids, and oxalate. The oxalate may be deposited in the renal tubules, causing acute renal failure. Prompt administration of ethanol or treatment with 4-methylpyrazole may prevent the development of metabolic acidosis.

II. CLINICAL PHARMACOLOGY OF ALCOHOLS

Ethanol is probably the least potent drug consumed by humans, yet it is the cause of more preventable morbidity and mortality than all other drugs combined, including the other drugs of abuse.

Although the disorder known as alcoholism is difficult to define, epidemiologic studies of alcohol consumption provide important information for predicting health-related factors that predispose to physical and psychologic problems. Approximately 80% of adults in the USA consume alcoholic beverages, with men and women probably consuming on an equal basis. It is estimated that 5–10% of the adult male population have alcohol-related problems at some time in their lives. Recent studies in almost 90,000 men and women who participated in multiphasic health examinations and were observed over a 10-year period disclosed a twice-normal mortality rate in persons who admitted to having 6 or more drinks a day; those taking 3–5 drinks a day had a rate 40–50% higher than normal. Cancer, hepatic cirrhosis, and accidents contributed significantly to the excessive mortality rate of heavy drinkers. Smoking, which is common in alcoholics, is also a possible mortality risk factor in heavy drinkers. The results of the study suggest that there is a threshold for increased mortality risk in the range of 3–5 drinks a day and that this risk rises sharply at a level of 6 or more drinks a day. There is also evidence that small amounts of alcohol (one beer a day) place patients at less risk of myocardial infarction than individuals who never consume alcohol.

The search for specific etiologic factors or the identification of significant predisposing variables for alcohol abuse has generally given disappointing results. Personality type, severe life stresses, psychiatric disorders, and parental role models are not reliable predictors of alcohol abuse. Comparisons of differences in alcohol metabolism are unreliable, and markers of disordered alcohol metabolism are not sufficiently predictive. It is clear that alcohol abuse is not equally distributed in all social groups, and its abuse appears to occur at a higher rate among relatives of alcoholics than in the general population. The rate of alcoholism in persons with an alcoholic biologic parent is almost 4 times that of a selected control group—a finding that has now been confirmed by several studies. It is difficult to distinguish between contributing factors of familial learning experiences and genetic variables, but current evidence suggests that genetic factors play a role in defining human alcohol use and medical complications. Genetic control of alcohol preference in animals has been clearly established. However, the nature of the genetic factors involved is still unknown.

MANAGEMENT OF ACUTE ALCOHOLIC INTOXICATION

Nontolerant individuals who consume alcohol in large quantities develop typical effects of acute sedative-hypnotic drug overdose, along with the cardiovascular effects described above (vasodilatation, tachycardia) and gastrointestinal irritation. Since tolerance is not absolute, even chronic alcoholics may become severely intoxicated. The degree of intoxication depends upon 3 factors: the blood ethanol concentration, the rapidity of the rise of the alcohol level, and the time during which the blood level is maintained. The pattern of drinking, the state of the absorptive surface of the gastrointestinal tract, and the presence in the body of other medications also affect the apparent degree of intoxication.

The most important goal in the treatment of acute alcohol intoxication is to prevent severe respiratory depression and aspiration of vomitus. Even with very high blood ethanol levels, survival is possible as long as the respiratory and cardiovascular systems can be supported. The lethal dose of alcohol varies widely because of varying degrees of tolerance. A normal nontolerant adult individual can metabolize 7–10 g of alcohol per hour (the ethanol content of 30 mL of 80-proof whiskey). The legal definition of intoxication in the USA varies in different states, but a blood level of 100 mg/dL or higher is often regarded as evidence of impaired judgment and performance sufficient for conviction of driving while impaired. The average blood alcohol concentration in fatal cases is about 400 mg/dL.

Metabolic alterations may require treatment of hypoglycemia and ketosis by administration of glucose. Alcoholic patients who are dehydrated and vomiting should also receive electrolyte solutions to enhance the excretion of ketone bodies. If vomiting is severe, large amounts of potassium may also be required as long as renal function is normal. Especially important is recognition of decreased phosphate stores, which may be aggravated by glucose administration. Low phosphate stores may contribute to poor wound healing, neurologic deficits, and increased risk of infection.

MANAGEMENT OF ALCOHOL WITHDRAWAL SYNDROME

When alcohol ingestion is abruptly discontinued, the characteristic syndrome of motor agitation, anxiety, insomnia, and reduction of seizure threshold occurs. The severity of the alcohol withdrawal syndrome is usually proportionate to the dose and the duration of alcohol abuse. However, this can be greatly modified by the use of other sedatives as well as by associated medical (eg, diabetes) or surgical factors (injury). In its mildest form, the alcohol withdrawal syndrome of tremor, anxiety, and insomnia occurs 6–8 hours after alcohol is stopped. These effects usually abate in 1–2 days. In some patients, more severe withdrawal reactions occur in which visual hallucinations, total disorientation, and marked abnormalities of vital signs occur. The more severe the withdrawal syndrome, the greater the need for meticulous investigation of possible underlying medical or surgical complications. The mortality risks of severe alcohol withdrawal have been overstated in the past. The prognosis is probably related chiefly to the underlying medical and surgical complications.

The major objective of drug therapy in the alcohol withdrawal period is prevention of seizures, delirium, and arrhythmias. Restoration of potassium, magnesium, and phosphate balance should be achieved rapidly if renal function is normal. Most persons in mild alcohol withdrawal do not need any other pharmacologic assistance.

Specific drug treatment for detoxification in severe cases involves 2 basic principles: substituting a long-acting sedative-hypnotic drug for alcohol and then gradually reducing ("tapering") the dose of the long-acting drug. Unfortunately, the most widely used "treatment" for alcohol withdrawal is renewed alcohol intake. Although alcohol can be slowly tapered, it is psychologically undesirable to maintain the patient on alcohol. Currently, benzodiazepines are preferred for this purpose. The benzodiazepines chlordiazepoxide and diazepam have pharmacologically active metabolites that may accumulate. Oxazepam is rapidly converted to inactive water-soluble metabolites that will not accumulate and is especially useful in alcoholic patients with liver disease. Benzodiazepines are poorly absorbed from intramuscular sites; when rapid clinical effects are required, the intravenous route is preferred.

Phenothiazine medications for alcohol withdrawal have potentially serious side-effects that probably outweigh their benefits. Antihistaminic medications have been used but with little justification.

Phenytoin (diphenylhydantoin) may be effective in preventing seizures in alcoholic patients with a history of seizures. Since phenytoin is poorly absorbed from intramuscular sites, the drug should be given by mouth or intravenously. A loading dose of 12–15 mg/kg is given, and the patient is maintained on 300 mg/d with monitoring of blood levels.

After the alcohol withdrawal syndrome has been treated acutely, sedative-hypnotic medications must be tapered slowly over several weeks. Complete detoxification is probably not achieved within a few days of sobering up. Several months may be required for restoration of normal nervous system function.

Disulfiram

Disulfiram (tetraethylthiuram), a widely used antioxidant in the rubber industry, has been shown to cause extreme discomfort to patients who drink alcoholic beverages. Disulfiram given by itself to nondrinkers has little effect; however, flushing, throbbing headache, nausea, vomiting, sweating, hypotension, and confusion occur within a few minutes after taking a drink. The effect may last 30 minutes in mild cases or several hours in severe ones. After the symptoms wear off, the patient is usually exhausted and may sleep for several hours.

Disulfiram acts by inhibiting **aldehyde dehydrogenase.** Thus, alcohol is metabolized as usual, but acetaldehyde is accumulated. The symptoms resulting from disulfiram plus alcohol are typical for acetaldehyde toxicity; the reaction is reproduced by acetaldehyde infusion in humans.

Disulfiram is rapidly and completely absorbed from the gastrointestinal tract; however, a period of 12 hours is required for its full action. Its elimination rate is very slow, so that the action may persist for several days after the last dose. The drug interacts with many other therapeutic agents.

Disulfiram should be considered as a pharmacologic adjunct in the treatment of alcoholism and should only be used in conjunction with behavioral therapies. When the drug is prescribed, the alcohol content of common nonprescription medications should be considered and communicated to the patient; some of these are listed in Table 64–2. Management with disulfiram should be initiated only when the patient has been free of alcohol for at least 24 hours. The safety of disulfiram in pregnancy has not been demonstrated. The duration of disulfiram treatment should be individualized and determined by the patient's responsiveness and clinical improvement. The usual oral dose is 250 mg daily taken at bedtime. Mandated use of disulfiram by court order is probably not efficacious.

MANAGEMENT OF INTOXICATION WITH OTHER ALCOHOLS

Methanol Intoxication

Severe methanol poisoning is usually encountered in chronic alcoholics and may not be recognized unless characteristic symptoms are noted in a group of patients. Because methanol is a much more potent toxin than ethanol, it is essential that patients with methanol poisoning be recognized and treated as soon as possible.

The most important initial symptom in methanol poisoning is a visual disturbance frequently described as "like being in a snowstorm." Visual disturbances are a universal complaint in epidemics of methanol poisoning. A complaint of blurred vision with a relatively clear sensorium should strongly suggest the diagnosis of methanol poisoning. In severe cases, the odor of formaldehyde may be present on the breath or in the urine. The development of bradycardia, prolonged coma, seizures, and resistant acidosis all indicate a poor prognosis.

Physical findings in methanol poisoning are generally nonspecific. Fixed dilated pupils have been described in severe cases. Optic atrophy is a late finding. The cause of death in fatal cases is sudden cessation of respiration.

It is critical that the blood methanol level be determined as soon as possible if the diagnosis is suspected. If the clinical suspicion of methanol poisoning is high, treatment should not be delayed. Methanol levels in excess of 50 mg/dL are probably an absolute indication for hemodialysis and ethanol treatment. Additional laboratory evidence includes metabolic acidosis with an elevated anion gap and osmolar gap (see Chapter 58). Ethylene glycol, paraldehyde, and salicylates may also cause an anion gap. A decrease in serum bicarbonate is a uniform feature of severe methanol poisoning. Ethylene glycol toxicity (see below) usually results in central nervous system excitation, increase in muscle enzymes, and hypocalcemia but not visual symptoms. Salicylate intoxication can be readily determined from salicylate levels in the blood.

The first treatment for methanol poisoning, as in all critical poisoning situations, is to establish respiration, with an artificial airway if necessary. Emesis can be induced if the patient is not comatose, is not having seizures, and has not lost the gag reflex. If any of these contraindications exists, the patient should be endotracheally intubated and gastric lavage carried out with a large-bore tube.

There are 3 "specific" modalities of treatment for severe methanol poisoning: suppression of metabolism by alcohol dehydrogenase to toxic products, dialysis to enhance removal of methanol and its toxic products, and alkalinization to counteract metabolic acidosis.

Because ethanol competes for alcohol dehydrogenase, which is responsible for metabolizing methanol to formic acid, it is essential to saturate this enzyme with the less toxic ethanol. The dose-dependent characteristics of ethanol metabolism and the variability induced by chronic ethanol intake require frequent monitoring of blood ethanol levels to ensure appropriate alcohol concentration. Ethanol may be given intravenously as a 10% solution.

With initiation of dialysis procedures, ethanol will also be eliminated in the dialysate, requiring alterations in the dose of ethanol. Hemodialysis is discussed in Chapter 57.

Because of profound metabolic acidosis in methanol poisoning, treatment with bicarbonate may be necessary. Quantities of bicarbonate to be administered should be based on estimated sodium intake, potassium balance, and cardiovascular status.

Since folate-dependent systems are probably responsible for the oxidation of formic acid to CO_2 in humans, it would probably be useful to administer folic acid to patients poisoned with methanol, although this has never been tested in clinical studies. 4-Methylpyrazole, by inhibiting alcohol dehydrogenase, may also be a useful adjunct in methanol poisoning when it becomes available for human use.

A special diagnostic problem occurs if a patient has a relatively low methanol level but visual symptoms are present. In this situation, laboratory tests for methanol itself should be repeated and confirmed with osmolality estimates. If visual impairment is present, hemodialysis should be started in spite of low methanol levels.

Ethylene Glycol Intoxication

Few clinical cases of ethylene glycol poisoning have been reported. As with methanol poisoning, there may be a delay in the onset of acidosis and renal insufficiency. Three stages of ethylene glycol overdose have been recognized. Initially, there is transient excitation followed by central nervous system depression. Severe acidosis then develops, and finally delayed renal insufficiency occurs. Ophthalmoscopic examination is usually normal, although occasional cases of papilledema have been described. Oxalate crystals are usually present in urine. Ethylene glycol-intoxicated patients have no detectable odor of alcohol on their breath. In severe cases, increased muscle enzyme and decreased calcium have been found in the plasma. The key to the diagnosis of ethylene glycol poisoning is the recognition of anion gap acidosis, osmolar gap, and oxalate crystals in the urine in a patient without visual symptoms. As with methanol poisoning, early alcohol infusion and dialysis are required. 4-Methylpyrazole therapy will also be of use in this situation when it becomes commercially available.

• • •

References

Becker CE: Acute methanol poisoning: The blind drunk. *West J Med* 1981;**135:**122.

Becker CE, Roe RL, Scott RA: *Alcohol as a Drug: A Curriculum on Pharmacology, Neurology and Toxicology.* R.E. Kreiger, 1979.

Goekas MC et al: Ethanol: The liver and the gastrointestinal tract. *Ann Intern Med* 1981;**95:**198.

Interactions of drugs with alcohol. *Med Lett Drugs Ther* (April 3) 1981;**23:**33.

Khama JM, Israel Y, Kalant H: Alcoholic liver pathology. Alcoholism and Drug Addiction Research Foundation of Ontario. 1973.

Klatsky AR, Friedman JD, Siegelaub AB: Alcohol and mortality: A ten year Kaiser Permanente experience. *Ann Intern Med* 1981;**95:**139.

Lieber CS: *Metabolic Aspects of Alcoholism.* University Park, 1977.

Neurobiological correlates of intoxication and physical dependence upon ethanol. (Symposium.) *Fed Proc* 1981;**40:**2048.

Rankin JG: Alcohol, drugs, and brain damage: Proceedings of a symposium: Effects of chronic use of alcohol and other psychoactive drugs on cerebral function. Alcoholism and Drug Addiction Research Foundation of Ontario. 1975.

Smith CM: *The Pharmacology of Sedative/Hypnotics, Alcohol and Anesthetic Sites and Mechanisms of Action in Drug Addiction, 1.* Martin WR (editor). Springer-Verlag, 1977.

Anticonvulsants | 21

Roger J. Porter, MD, & William H. Pitlick, PhD

Approximately 1% of the population of the USA has epilepsy, the second most common neurologic disorder after stroke. Epilepsy is a heterogeneous symptom complex—a chronic disorder characterized by recurrent seizures. Seizures are finite episodes of brain dysfunction resulting from abnormal discharge of cerebral neurons. The causes of seizures are many and include the gamut of neurologic diseases from infection to neoplasm to head injury. In only a few subgroups has heredity been proved to be a major contributing factor. The antiepileptic drugs described in this chapter are also used in patients with febrile seizures or with seizures occurring as part of an acute illness such as meningitis, even though the term epilepsy is not usually applied to such patients unless they later develop chronic seizures. Occasionally, seizures are caused by an acute underlying toxic or metabolic disorder, in which case appropriate therapy should be directed toward the specific abnormality, eg, hypocalcemia. In most cases of epilepsy, however, the choice of medication depends on the empirical seizure classification.

Before discovery of the antiepileptic drugs, treatment of epilepsy consisted of trephining, cupping, and the use of herbal medicines and animal extracts. In 1857, Sir Charles Locock reported the successful use of potassium bromide in the treatment of what is now known as catamenial epilepsy. In 1912, phenobarbital was first used for epilepsy, and in the next 25 years, 35 analogs of phenobarbital were studied as anticonvulsants. In 1938, phenytoin was found to be effective against experimental seizures in cats.

Between 1935 and 1960, tremendous strides were made both in the development of experimental models and in methods for screening and testing new antiepileptic drugs. During that period, 13 new antiepileptic drugs were developed and marketed. Following the enactment of requirements for proof of drug efficacy in 1962, antiepileptic drug development slowed dramatically. In the last 20 years, only 5 new antiepileptic drugs have reached the marketplace.

For a long time it was assumed that a single drug could be developed for treatment of all forms of epilepsy. It now appears unlikely that the wide variety of epileptic seizures can be managed successfully with just one drug. More than one mechanism may be responsible for the various seizures, and drugs useful for one seizure type may actually aggravate other types.

Table 21–1. Classification of seizure types.

Partial seizures
Elementary partial seizures.
Complex partial seizures.
Partial seizures secondarily generalized.
Generalized seizures
Generalized tonic-clonic (grand mal) seizures.
Absence (petit mal) seizures.
Atonic seizures.
Myoclonic (clonic) seizures.
Infantile spasms.*

*Infantile spasms is an epileptic syndrome rather than a specific seizure type; drugs useful in infantile spasms will be reviewed separately.

Drugs used in the treatment of the 2 major types of seizures (partial and generalized; Table 21–1) are quite distinct in their clinical effects and also fall into 2 pharmacologic classes, even though seizures may be induced experimentally by a wide variety of methods. The clinical aspects of generalized seizures, especially absence seizures, are highly correlated with experimental seizures produced in animals by subcutaneous administration of pentylenetetrazol (sometimes also called the Metrazol test). Likewise, partial seizures in humans correlate positively with experimental seizures elicited by the maximal electroshock (MES) test. In general, antiepileptic drugs effective against maximal electroshock seizures alter ionic transport across excitable membranes. Phenytoin, for example, is effective against partial seizures and maximal electroshock but with the exception of generalized tonic-clonic seizures is not effective against generalized seizures or those induced by subcutaneous pentylenetetrazol (scMet); it affects membrane potentials through its action on Ca^{2+} and Na^{+} fluxes. On the other hand, ethosuximide, which is active against certain generalized seizures and pentylenetetrazol, has little or no direct effect on ion fluxes across excitable membranes. The effectiveness of ethosuximide can be diminished by lipophilic substitution, in which more anti-maximal electroshock and less antipentylenetetrazol activity is observed. It is notable that the 2 distinct classes of antiepileptic drugs have apparently different mechanisms of action in spite of marked structural similarities between many of the drugs in the 2 groups. These differences in potency are indicated below in terms of ED50s for the 2 standard tests.

I. BASIC PHARMACOLOGY OF ANTICONVULSANTS

Chemistry

Approximately 16 major antiepileptic drugs are presently available. Thirteen of them can be classified into 5 very similar chemical groups: barbiturates, hydantoins, oxazolidinediones, succinimides, and acetylureas. These groups have in common a similar heterocyclic ring structure with a variety of substituents (Fig 21–1). The remaining 3 drugs are carbamazepine, valproic acid, and the benzodiazepines—all structurally dissimilar from each other.

For drugs with the basic structure shown in Fig 21–1, the substituents on the heterocyclic ring determine the pharmacologic class, either anti-maximal electroshock or antipentylenetetrazol. Very small changes in structure can alter the mechanism of action and clinical properties of a drug significantly. For example, the presence of a phenyl group at the R_1 position, as in phenytoin, produces activity against partial seizures; whereas an alkyl group, as in ethosuximide, produces activity against certain generalized seizures.

The development of new drugs involves structural modification based on knowledge of structure-activity relationships in the hope that a specific receptor exists for a drug with a particular spatial conformation. Even though a great many modifications and corresponding pharmacologic data exist, especially with such drugs as phenytoin and phenobarbital, only unproved hypotheses can be offered in an attempt to explain the nature of the drug receptors. Phenytoin, for example, has at least 3 major pharmacologic actions—it affects membrane conductance, alters reuptake of neurotransmitters, and changes hormonal balance—and it is not known which of these (if any) is

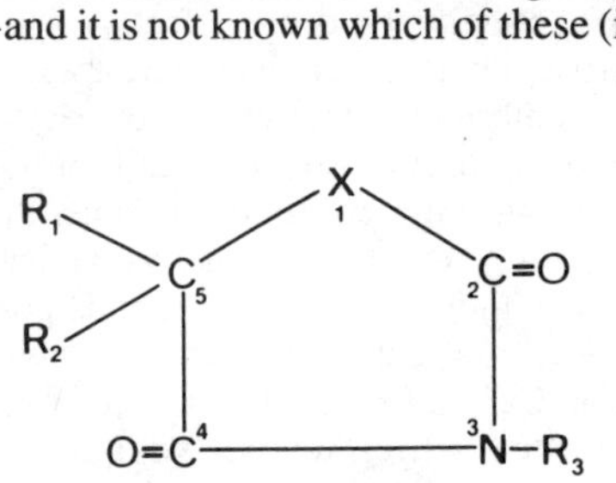

Figure 21–1. Antiepileptic heterocyclic ring structure. The "X" varies as follows: hydantoin derivatives, –N–; barbiturates, –C–N–; oxazolidinediones, –O–; succinimides, –C–; acetylureas, $-NH_2$ (N connected to C2). R_1, R_2, and R_3 vary within each subgroup.

responsible for the drug's anticonvulsant activity. In spite of these limitations, however, some generalizations regarding the structural requirements for anticonvulsant activity are possible. Common stereochemical features have been identified; most antiepileptic drugs possess 2 hydrophobic regions. When 2 antiepileptic drugs are compared and these regions are superimposed, 2 electron donor groups are found with similar orientation and position. The distances between these electron donor groups are critical for anticonvulsant activity. The 2,4-benzodiazepines, for example, which match the stereochemistry of known anticonvulsants, are more active than the 1,3-benzodiazepines. In general, to be active against partial seizures, the drug must have at least one phenyl ring as a hydrophobic region. Unfortunately, addition of hydrophobic groups reduces solubility, and diphenylbarbituric acid, which is effective against experimental seizures, is not useful clinically because of its very low solubility.

Pharmacokinetics

As a class, antiepileptic drugs exhibit many similar pharmacokinetic properties, even though their structural and chemical properties are often quite diverse. Although many of these compounds are only sparingly soluble, absorption is usually good, with 80–100% of the dose reaching the circulation. Bioavailability is a problem with phenytoin, in which both the rate and extent of absorption are highly dependent on the formulation.

Except for phenytoin, the benzodiazepines, and valproic acid, anticonvulsants are not highly bound to plasma proteins. Only the 3 named drugs are able to displace other highly bound drugs, and such drugs may also displace other anticonvulsants.

Antiepileptic drugs have low extraction ratios (see Chapter 3). An increase in the percentage of free drug will not change free concentrations but will reduce total drug concentrations and may lead the clinician to increase the dose; this increase in dose will result in higher free drug levels and possible drug toxicity. Sodium valproate is unique in that the fraction of drug bound is a function of the concentration of both the drug and the free fatty acids in plasma.

Antiepileptic drugs are cleared chiefly by hepatic mechanisms. Many, such as primidone and the benzodiazepines, are converted to active metabolites that are also cleared by the liver. The intrinsic ability of the liver to metabolize anticonvulsant drugs is generally low and, with the exception of phenytoin, independent of concentration. These drugs are predominantly distributed into total body water. Plasma clearance is relatively slow; many anticonvulsants are therefore considered to be medium- to long-acting. For most, half-lives are usually greater than 12 hours. The intrinsic clearance of antiepileptic drugs is sensitive both to those drugs and to other drugs. Phenobarbital and carbamazepine are potent inducers of hepatic microsomal enzyme activity.

DRUGS USED IN PARTIAL SEIZURES AND GENERALIZED TONIC-CLONIC SEIZURES

The major drugs for partial and generalized tonic-clonic seizures are phenytoin (and congeners), carbamazepine, and the barbiturates.

PHENYTOIN

Phenytoin (Dilantin) is the oldest nonsedative antiepileptic drug, introduced in 1938 following a systematic evaluation of compounds such as phenobarbital that altered electrically induced seizures in laboratory animals. It was known for decades as diphenylhydantoin (DPH).

Chemistry

Phenytoin is a diphenyl-substituted hydantoin with the structure shown below. Alkyl substituents at the 5 position result in sedative properties. The enantiomers of phenytoin are equipotent.

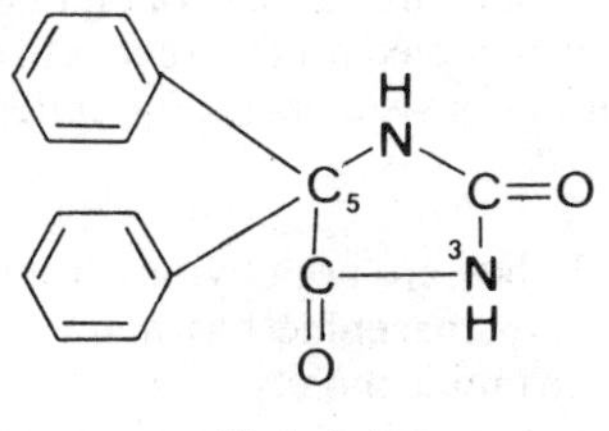

Phenytoin

Mechanism of Action

Phenytoin has major effects on several physiologic systems, but its most notable antiepileptic effects are those related to the movement of ions, particularly sodium, through cell membranes. Early studies indicated that phenytoin disrupted mechanisms involved in the experimental generation of repetitive action potentials; it does so in part by blocking sodium channels and decreasing the inward flux of sodium—similar to that observed with local anesthetics and tetrodotoxin. Phenytoin binds to both open and inactivated channels. This binding of phenytoin to sodium channels causes decreased sodium influx into nerve endings. A reduction of membrane permeability to Ca^{2+} is also observed. The inhibition of calcium influx across the cell membrane may explain the ability of phenytoin to inhibit a variety of calcium-induced secretory processes, including hormones and neurotransmitters. As a result, the drug inhibits the development and spread of seizure activity. Posttetanic potentiation is reduced. The ED50 of phenytoin against maximum electroshock in mice is 9.5 mg/kg; it has no activity against pentylenetetrazol seizures.

Clinical Use

Phenytoin is one of the most effective drugs against partial seizures and generalized tonic-clonic seizures. In the latter, it appears to be effective against attacks that are either primary or secondary to another seizure type.

Pharmacokinetics

Absorption of phenytoin is highly dependent on the formulation of the dosage form. Particle size and pharmaceutical additives affect both the rate and extent of absorption. Oral absorption of phenytoin sodium is nearly complete in most patients, although the time to peak may range from 3 hours to 12 hours. Absorption after intramuscular injection is unpredictable, and some drug precipitation in the muscle occurs; this route of administration is not recommended.

Phenytoin is highly bound to plasma proteins. It appears certain that the total plasma level decreases when the percentage that is bound decreases, as in uremia or hypoalbuminemia, but correlation of free levels with clinical states remains uncertain. Drug concentration in cerebrospinal fluid is proportionate to the free plasma level. Phenytoin is highly bound to brain proteins and is also reversibly stored in fat.

Phenytoin is metabolized primarily by parahydroxylation to 5-(*p*-hydroxyphenyl)-5-phenylhydantoin (HPPH), which is subsequently conjugated with glucuronic acid. The metabolites are clinically inactive and are excreted in the urine. Only a very small portion of phenytoin is excreted unchanged.

The pharmacokinetics of phenytoin are dose-dependent. At very low blood levels, phenytoin metabolism is proportionate to the rate at which the drug is presented to the liver, ie, first-order metabolism.

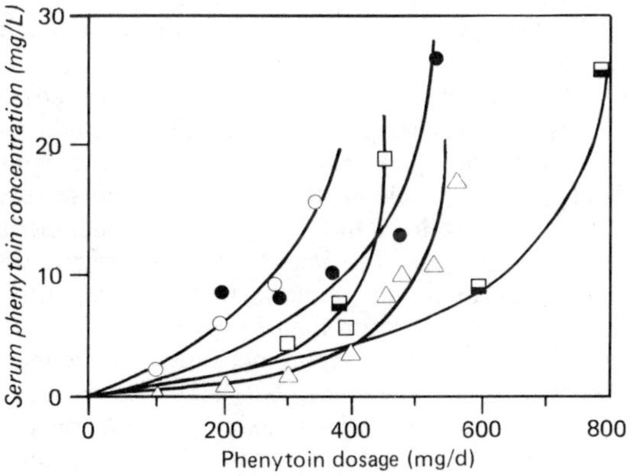

Figure 21–2. Nonlinear effect of phenytoin dosage on plasma concentration. Five different patients (identified by different symbols) received increasing dosages of phenytoin by mouth, and the steady-state serum concentration was measured at each dosage. The curves are not linear, since, as the dosage increases, the first-pass effect is proportionately less marked. Note also the marked variation among patients in the serum levels achieved at any dosage. (Modified, with permission, from Jusko WJ: Bioavailability and disposition kinetics of phenytoin in man. Pages 115–136 in: *Quantitative Analytic Studies in Epilepsy.* Kellaway P, Peterson I [editors]. Raven, 1977.)

However, as blood levels rise within the therapeutic range, the maximum capacity of the liver to metabolize phenytoin is reached (Fig 21–2). Further increases in dose, even though relatively small, may produce very large changes in phenytoin concentrations. In such cases, the half-life of the drug increases markedly, steady state is not achieved (since the plasma level continues to rise), and patients quickly develop symptoms of toxicity.

The half-life of phenytoin varies from 12 to 36 hours, with an average of 24 hours for most patients in the low to mid therapeutic range. Much longer half-lives are observed at higher concentrations. It takes 5–7 days to reach steady-state blood levels after every dosage change, and even longer at higher levels.

MEPHENYTOIN, ETHOTOIN, & PHENACEMIDE

Many congeners of phenytoin have been synthesized, but only 3 are marketed in the USA, and these are used to a limited extent. Mephenytoin (Mesantoin) has a methyl group at the 3 position of the heterocyclic ring, and one of the phenyl groups at the 5 position is replaced by an ethyl group (Fig 21–1). Ethotoin (Peganone) has an ethyl group at the 3 position of the heterocyclic ring and only one phenyl group at the 5 position. The third analog, phenacemide (Phenurone), is similar to phenytoin except that only one phenyl ring is present at carbon 5 and the heterocyclic ring has been opened to form a straight-chain phenylacetylurea compound. The ED50 of mephenytoin against maximal electroshock in mice is 61 mg/kg; its antipentylenetetrazol ED50 is 30 mg/kg. The anti-maximal electroshock ED50 of ethotoin is 86; its antipentylenetetrazol ED50 is 48.

In spite of their anti-maximal electroshock:antipentylenetetrazol ratios, mephenytoin and ethotoin, like phenytoin, appear to be most effective against generalized tonic-clonic seizures and partial seizures. No well-controlled clinical trials have documented their effectiveness. The incidence of severe reactions such as dermatitis, agranulocytosis, or hepatitis is higher for mephenytoin than for phenytoin.

Ethotoin may be recommended for patients hypersensitive to phenytoin, but larger doses are required. The side-effects and toxicity are generally less severe than those associated with phenytoin, but the drug appears to be less effective.

The pharmacokinetics of ethotoin and mephenytoin are not well established, but both drugs share with phenytoin the property of saturable metabolism within the therapeutic dosage range. Careful monitoring of the patient during dosage alterations with either drug is essential. Mephenytoin is metabolized to 5,5-ethylphenylhydantoin via demethylation. This metabolite, known as Nirvanol, is also active as an anticonvulsant. Both mephenytoin and Nirvanol are hydroxylated and undergo subsequent conjugation and excretion.

Therapeutic levels for mephenytoin range from 5 to 16 μg/mL, and levels above 20 μg/mL are considered toxic. Therapeutic blood levels of Nirvanol are between 25 and 40 μg/mL. A therapeutic range for ethotoin has not been established.

Phenacemide, the straight-chain analog of phenytoin, is a toxic drug of last resort for refractory partial seizures. It is active against both maximal electroshock and pentylenetetrazol seizures. Its mechanism of action is unknown. It is well absorbed and completely metabolized. The relationship between blood levels and effect has not been established. Serious and sometimes fatal side-effects have been reported in association with the use of phenacemide. Dose-related effects include behavioral changes, including psychosis and depressive reactions. Reactions of an idiosyncratic nature, including hepatitis, nephritis, and aplastic anemia, appear to be more frequent than with other antiepileptic drugs.

CARBAMAZEPINE

Closely related to imipramine and other antidepressants, carbamazepine (Tegretol) is a tricyclic compound effective in treatment of bipolar depression. It was initially marketed for the treatment of trigeminal neuralgia but has proved useful for epilepsy as well.

Chemistry

Although they are not obvious from its structure (Fig 21–3), carbamazepine has many similarities to phenytoin. The ureide moiety (–N–CO–NH_2) present in the heterocyclic ring of most antiepileptic drugs is also present in carbamazepine. Three-dimensional structural studies indicate that its spatial conformation is similar to that of phenytoin.

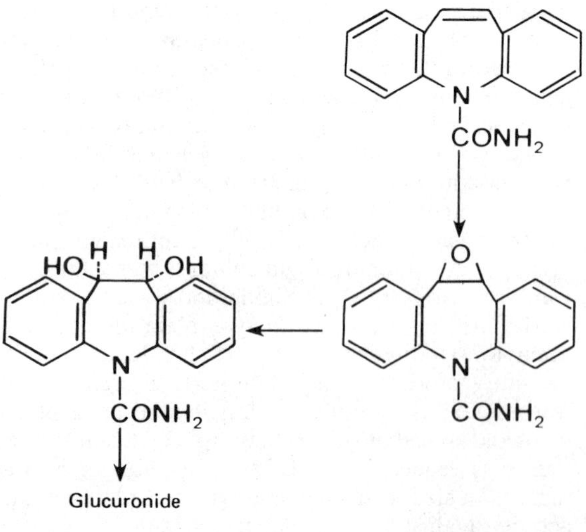

Figure 21–3. Carbamazepine and its metabolite. Carbamazepine (top) is oxidized to the epoxy intermediate, which opens to form the dihydroxy derivative.

Mechanism of Action

The mechanism of action of carbamazepine is unknown. Like phenytoin, carbamazepine shows activity against maximal electroshock seizures. Studies on membrane permeability indicate that carbamazepine, like phenytoin, diminishes sodium and, to a lesser degree, potassium conductance. Unlike phenytoin, however, carbamazepine has no significant effect on posttetanic potentiation. Carbamazepine also inhibits uptake and release of norepinephrine from brain synaptosomes but does not influence gamma-aminobutyric acid (GABA) uptake in brain slices, suggesting that its action is probably independent of the GABA-ergic system. Carbamazepine antagonizes ouabain-induced stimulation of adenylate cyclase by adenosine. The ED50 of carbamazepine against maximal electroshock in mice is 9 mg/kg; it has no antipentylenetetrazol activity.

Clinical Use

Carbamazepine is considered the drug of choice for partial seizures, and many physicians also use it first for generalized tonic-clonic seizures. It is used with phenytoin in many patients who are difficult to control. Carbamazepine is nonsedative in its usual therapeutic range. The drug is also very effective in some patients with **trigeminal neuralgia,** although older patients may tolerate higher doses poorly, with ataxia and unsteadiness. Some of these patients require specific surgical intervention.

Pharmacokinetics

The rate of absorption of carbamazepine varies widely among different patients, though almost complete absorption apparently occurs in all. Peak levels are usually achieved 6–8 hours after administration. Slowing absorption by giving the drug after meals helps the patient tolerate larger total daily doses.

Distribution is slow and generally limited to highly perfused tissues, and volume of distribution is roughly 1 L/kg of body weight. The drug is only 70% bound to plasma proteins; no displacement of other drugs from protein binding has been observed.

Carbamazepine has a very low systemic clearance of approximately 1 L/kg/d. The drug has a notable ability to induce microsomal enzymes. In several studies of epileptic patients or volunteers on dosage regimens exceeding 1 month, the clearance of carbamazepine increased 2-fold over initial treatment. Typically, the half-life of 36 hours observed in subjects following an initial single dose decreases to much less than 20 hours in subjects receiving continuous therapy. Considerable dosage adjustments are thus to be expected during the first weeks of therapy. These changes in dose may further alter the microsomal enzyme capacity. Carbamazepine also alters the clearance of other drugs. For example, carbamazepine has been shown to increase the clearance and decrease the half-life and steady-state blood levels of several other antiepileptic drugs such as phenytoin, primidone, valproic acid, or clonazepam.

Carbamazepine is completely metabolized in humans, in part to the 10,11-dihydro derivative, which is subsequently conjugated. The dihydro derivative is formed by way of a stable epoxide, carbamazepine-10,11-epoxide, which has been shown to have anticonvulsant activity (Fig 21–3). The contribution of this and other metabolites in the clinical activity of carbamazepine is unknown.

PHENOBARBITAL

Aside from the bromides, phenobarbital is the oldest of the currently available antiepileptic drugs. Although it has long been considered one of the safest of the antiepileptic agents, the use of other medications with lesser sedative effects has been urged.

Chemistry

The 4 derivatives of barbituric acid clinically useful as antiepileptic drugs are phenobarbital, mephobarbital, metharbital, and primidone. The first 3 are so similar that they will be considered together. Metharbital is methylated barbital, and mephobarbital is methylated phenobarbital; both are demethylated in vivo. The pK_as of these 3 compounds range from 7.3 to 7.9. Slight changes in the normal acid-base balance, therefore, can cause significant fluctuation in the ratio of the ionized/un-ionized species. This is particularly important for phenobarbital, the most commonly used barbiturate, whose pK_a of 7.3 is quite close to the plasma pH of 7.4.

X-ray crystallographic analysis of the structure of phenobarbital and its congeners indicates that the distance between the phenyl ring and the heterocyclic ring and the distance between ketonic oxygen atoms in the heterocyclic ring is critical for anticonvulsant activity. The 3-dimensional conformations of phenobarbital and N-methylphenobarbital are virtually identical to that of phenytoin. Both compounds possess a phenyl ring and are active against partial seizures.

Mechanism of Action

The exact mechanism of action of phenobarbital in preventing seizures is unknown. It seems clear that the drug elevates the seizure threshold and potentiates inhibitory pathways, but it has not been determined which, if any, of its known pharmacologic properties is responsible for its action. Direct activation of GABA receptors appears to correlate better with the hypnotic effects than with the anticonvulsant action of phenobarbital. The ED50 of phenobarbital against maximal electroshock in mice is 22 mg/kg; its antipentylenetetrazol ED50 is 13 mg/kg.

Clinical Use

Phenobarbital is useful in the treatment of partial seizures and generalized tonic-clonic seizures, although the drug is often tried for virtually every seizure type, especially when attacks are difficult to control. There is little evidence for its effectiveness in generalized seizures such as absence, atonic attacks, or infantile spasms; it may worsen certain patients with these seizure types.

Some physicians prefer either metharbital (Gemonil) or mephobarbital (Mebaral)—especially the latter—to phenobarbital because of supposed decreased side-effects. Only anecdotal data are available for such comparisons.

Pharmacokinetics

See Chapter 19.

PRIMIDONE

Primidone (Mysoline), or 2-desoxyphenobarbital (Fig 21–4), was marketed in the early 1950s. It was later reported that primidone was metabolized to phenobarbital and phenylethylmalonamide (PEMA). All 3 compounds are active anticonvulsants.

Mechanism of Action

Although primidone is converted to phenobarbital, the mechanism of action of primidone itself may be more like that of phenytoin, according to some recent studies. This may partially account for the increased use of primidone rather than phenobarbital in the treatment of complex partial seizures. The ED50 of primidone against maximal electroshock in mice is 11 mg/kg; the ED50 against pentylenetetrazol is 59 mg/kg.

Clinical Use

Primidone, like its metabolites, is effective against partial seizures and generalized tonic-clonic seizures and may be more effective than phenobarbital. It was previously considered to be the drug of choice for complex partial seizures, but most neurologists now prefer carbamazepine or phenytoin. Recent attempts to determine the relative potencies of the parent drug and its 2 metabolites have concentrated on newborn infants, in whom drug-metabolizing enzyme systems are very immature and in whom primidone is only slowly metabolized. Primidone has been shown to be effective in controlling seizures in this group, as well as in patients just beginning treatment with primidone; the latter show seizure control before phenobarbital concentrations reach the therapeutic range. Finally, animal studies suggest that greater protection against maximal electroshock seizures occurs with primidone than with phenobarbital alone, supporting the notion that primidone possesses independent activity. Nevertheless, the clinical use is similar to that of phenobarbital.

Pharmacokinetics

Primidone is absorbed slowly but completely. The time required to reach peak concentrations after oral administration is about 3 hours, but considerable variation has been reported.

Primidone is generally confined to total body water, with a volume of distribution of 0.6 L/kg of body weight. It is not highly bound to plasma proteins; approximately 70% circulates as unbound drug.

Primidone is metabolized by oxidation to phenobarbital, which accumulates very slowly, and by scission of the heterocyclic ring to form PEMA (Fig 21–4). Both primidone and phenobarbital are also hydroxylated at the para position of the phenyl ring and undergo subsequent conjugation and excretion.

Primidone has a larger clearance than other antiepileptic drugs (2 L/kg/d), corresponding to a half-life of 6–8 hours. PEMA clearance is approximately half that of primidone, but phenobarbital has a very low clearance. The appearance of phenobarbital corresponds to the disappearance of primidone. Phenobarbital therefore accumulates very slowly but eventually reaches therapeutic concentrations in most patients when therapeutic doses of primidone are administered. Phenobarbital levels derived from primidone are usually 2–3 times higher than primidone levels. PEMA has a half-life of 8–12 hours and therefore reaches steady state more rapidly than phenobarbital.

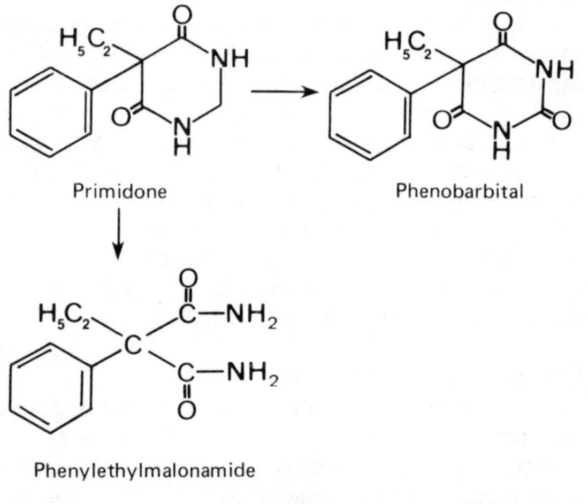

Figure 21–4. Primidone and its active metabolites.

DRUGS USED IN GENERALIZED SEIZURES

ETHOSUXIMIDE

Ethosuximide (Zarontin) was introduced in 1960 as the third of 3 marketed succinimides in the USA. Ethosuximide has very little activity against maximal electroshock but remarkable efficacy against pentylenetetrazol seizures and was introduced as a "pure petit mal" drug. Its popularity continues, based on its safety and efficacy; its role as the "first-choice" anti-absence drug remains undiminished, in part because of the idiosyncratic hepatotoxicity of the alternative drug, valproic acid.

Chemistry

Ethosuximide is the last antiepileptic drug to be marketed whose origin is in the antiepileptic heterocyclic ring structure. The 3 antiepileptic succinimides marketed in the USA are ethosuximide, phensuximide (Milontin), and methsuximide (Celontin). All 3 are substituted at the 2 position. (See structure below, and note difference in numbering relative to Fig 21–1). Methsuximide and phensuximide have phenyl substituents, while ethosuximide is 2-ethyl-2-methylsuccinimide. Many other substituted succinimides have antiepileptic activity, and several studies have demonstrated the optimal structural properties. Two substituents are optimal at the 2 position. If these substituents are small dialkyl groups, the compound will have antipentylenetetrazol activity. A phenyl group at the 2 position results in activity against maximal electroshock seizures but reduces activity against pentylenetetrazol seizures. Diphenyl compounds have no antipentylenetetrazol effects. Ethosuximide has an ED50 against maximal electroshock in mice of greater than 1000 mg/kg; its antipentylenetetrazol activity is 130 mg/kg.

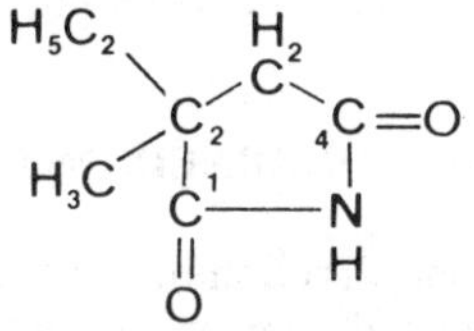

Ethosuximide

Mechanism of Action

The exact mechanism of action of the succinimides is undetermined. Ethosuximide does not inhibit the calcium influx into nervous tissue stimulated by maximal electroshock. Its lack of effect on membranes may be due to its hydrophilic nature. Addition of a phenyl group, which increases lipophilicity, results in increased anti-maximal electroshock activity. Other studies have shown that while ethosuximide can stimulate GABA release from presynaptic terminals, it does not elevate brain GABA levels.

Clinical Use

Ethosuximide is particularly effective against absence seizures, as might be expected from its activity in laboratory models. Documentation of its effectiveness required specific advances in quantitation of absence seizures; this was accomplished in the 1970s when the characteristic generalized 3/s spike-wave EEG abnormality was correlated with a decrement in consciousness, even when the abnormality occurs for only a few seconds. Long-term electroencephalographic recordings, therefore, provided the necessary quantitative method for determining the frequency of absence attacks and allowed rapid and effective evaluation of the efficacy of anti-absence drugs. Although ethosuximide was marketed in advance of the federal requirements for efficacy, these techniques were applied to later drugs such as clonazepam and valproic acid in documentation of their efficacy. This was accomplished by comparison with ethosuximide.

Pharmacokinetics

Absorption is complete following administration of the oral dosage forms. Peak levels are observed 3–7 hours after oral administration of the capsules. Animal studies indicate that chronic administration of the solution may prove irritating to the gastric mucosa.

Ethosuximide is uniformly distributed throughout perfused tissues and does not penetrate fat. Consequently, the volume of distribution approximates that of total body water, ie, 0.7 L/kg. It is not protein-bound, and spinal fluid concentrations are therefore equal to plasma concentrations.

Ethosuximide is completely metabolized, principally by hydroxylation. Four hydroxylated metabolites have been identified. These metabolites undergo subsequent conjugation and excretion. There is no evidence that these metabolites are pharmacologically active.

Ethosuximide has a very low total body clearance (0.5 L/kg/d). This corresponds to a half-life of approximately 40 hours, although values from 18 to 72 hours have been reported.

PHENSUXIMIDE & METHSUXIMIDE

Phensuximide (Milontin) and methsuximide (Celontin) are phenylsuccinimides that were developed and marketed before ethosuximide. They are used primarily as anti-absence drugs. Methsuximide is generally considered more toxic—and phensuximide less effective—than ethosuximide. Unlike ethosuximide, these 2 compounds have activity against maximal electroshock seizures, and methsuximide has been used for partial seizures by some investigators. The toxicity and lack of effectiveness of phensuximide when compared to methsuximide has been investigated, and the failure of the desmethyl metabolite to accumulate in the former probably explains its relatively weak effect. The desmethyl metabolite of methsuximide, however, has a half-life of 25 hours or more and exerts the major antiepileptic effect.

VALPROIC ACID & SODIUM VALPROATE

Valproic acid (Depakene), also available as the sodium salt, sodium valproate, was found to have antiepileptic properties when it was used as a solvent in the search for other drugs effective against seizures. It was marketed in France in 1969 but was not licensed in the USA until 1978.

Chemistry

Valproic acid is one of a series of fatty or carboxylic acids that have antiepileptic activity; this activity appears to be greatest for carbon chain lengths of 5–8 atoms. Branching and unsaturation do not significantly alter the drug's activity but may increase its lipophilicity, thereby increasing its duration of action. The amides and esters of valproic acid are also active antiepileptic agents.

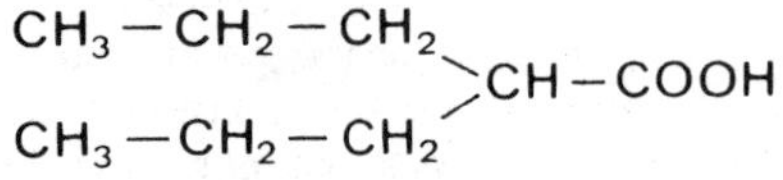

Valproic acid

Mechanism of Action

Valproic acid is active against both pentylenetetrazol and maximal electroshock seizures. Its ED50 in mice against pentylenetetrazol is 149 mg/kg; the ED50 against maximal electroshock is 272 mg/kg. As expected, it has little or no effect on sodium conductance, but at very high concentrations it increases potassium conductance. The greatest area of interest, however, has been the effect of valproic acid on GABA. Several studies have shown increased levels of GABA in brain after administration of valproic acid, though the mechanism for this increase remains unclear. If the effect is related to the enzymes necessary for either production or breakdown of GABA, it appears that valproic acid has a greater effect on inhibiting gamma transaminase (GABA-T) than on facilitating glutamic acid decarboxylase (GAD). At very high concentrations, valproic acid inhibits GABA-T in brain, thus increasing levels of GABA by blocking conversion of GABA to succinic semialdehyde. However, at the relatively low doses of valproic acid needed to abolish pentylenetetrazol seizures, brain GABA remains unchanged. Many investigators think that the changes in brain GABA do not represent a direct action of valproic acid but are instead due to an active metabolite or irreversible tissue binding. Another postulated model to explain the mechanism of action relates to the acidic properties of the drug. Valproic acid might cause a whole-body shift toward metabolic acidosis by stimulation of beta oxidation of fatty acids, resulting in an increase in circulating ketone bodies. These ketones could then be utilized to increase brain glycogen, which might protect against seizures induced by transient stimulation.

Clinical Use

Valproic acid is very effective against absence seizures and might be considered the drug of choice in this seizure type were it not for its hepatotoxicity. Because of this toxicity, ethosuximide is preferred. Valproic acid is unique in its ability to control certain types of myoclonic seizures; in some cases, the effect can be very dramatic. Its role in generalized tonic-clonic seizures is uncertain, but a few patients with atonic attacks may respond. There is no convincing evidence that the drug is effective in partial seizures or infantile spasms.

Pharmacokinetics

Valproic acid is well absorbed following an oral dose, with bioavailability greater than 80%. Peak blood levels are observed within 2 hours. Food may delay absorption, and decreased toxicity may result if the drug is given after meals.

Valproic acid has a pKa of 4.7 and is therefore completely ionized at physiologic plasma pH. The drug is also 90% bound to plasma proteins, though the fraction bound is somewhat reduced at blood levels greater than 150 μg/mL. Since it is both highly ionized and highly protein-bound, its distribution is essentially confined to extracellular water, with a volume of distribution of approximately 0.15 L/kg.

Approximately 20% of the drug is excreted as a direct conjugate of valproic acid. The remainder is metabolized by beta oxidation to a number of compounds; these are also subsequently conjugated and excreted.

Clearance for valproic acid is very low, corresponding to the small volume of distribution and accounting for a half-life of 9–18 hours. At very high blood levels, the clearance of valproic acid is dose-dependent. There appear to be offsetting changes in the intrinsic clearance and protein binding at higher doses.

OXAZOLIDINEDIONES

Trimethadione (Tridione), the first oxazolidinedione, was introduced as an antiepileptic drug in 1945 and remained the drug of choice for absence seizures until the introduction of succinimides in the 1950s. The use of the oxazolidinediones (trimethadione, paramethadione, and dimethadione) is now very limited.

Chemistry

The oxazolidinediones contain as a heterocyclic ring the oxazolidine ring (Fig 21–1) and are similar in structure to other antiepileptic drugs introduced before 1960. The structure includes only short-chain alkyl substituents on the heterocyclic ring, with no attached phenyl group.

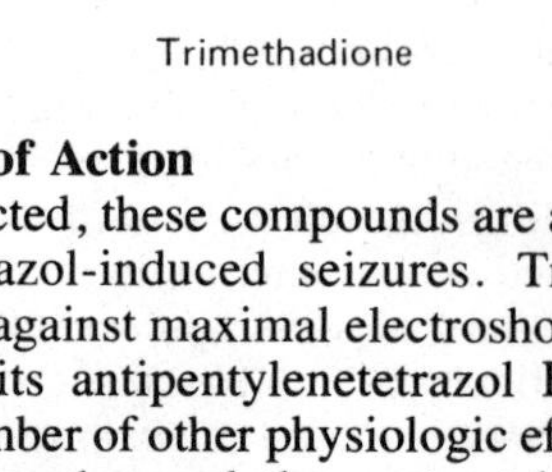

Trimethadione

Mechanism of Action

As expected, these compounds are active against pentylenetetrazol-induced seizures. Trimethadione has an ED50 against maximal electroshock in mice of 627 mg/kg; its antipentylenetetrazol ED50 is 301 mg/kg. A number of other physiologic effects of these drugs have been observed, the most notable of which is a reduction in synaptic transmission in the spinal cord during repetitive stimulation without affecting single-impulse transmission through monosynaptic pathways. In the brain, trimethadione increases the after-discharge threshold in the cortex. Some of these effects may be related to action of trimethadione on pre- and postsynaptic inhibition in synapses that utilize GABA as the neurotransmitter.

Pharmacokinetics

Trimethadione is rapidly absorbed, with peak levels reached within an hour after drug administration. It is distributed to all perfused tissues, with a volume of distribution that approximates that of total body water. It is not bound to plasma proteins. Trimethadione is completely metabolized in the liver by demethylation to 5,5-dimethyl-2,4-oxazolidinedione (dimethadione), which may exert the major antiepileptic activity. The drug has a relatively low clearance (1.6 L/kg/d), corresponding to a half-life of approximately 16 hours. The demethylated metabolite, however, is very slowly cleared and accumulates to a much greater extent than the parent drug. The clearance of dimethadione is 0.08 L/kg/d, reflected in a smaller volume of distribution and an extremely long half-life (240 hours).

OTHER DRUGS USED IN MANAGEMENT OF EPILEPSY

Some drugs are not classifiable by application to seizure type and will be discussed separately in this section.

BENZODIAZEPINES
(See also Chapter 19.)

Four benzodiazepines play prominent roles in the therapy of epilepsy, but their roles cannot be classified under a single seizure group. Although many benzodiazepines are quite similar chemically, subtle structural alterations result in differences in activity. Electronegative substituents in the 7 position are necessary for anticonvulsant activity; both Cl and NO_2 are effective. A phenyl group at the 5 position gives maximum anticonvulsant potency. Although they are quite different structurally from other antiepileptic drugs, the spatial conformation of the benzodiazepines is very similar to that of phenytoin. Possible mechanisms of action are discussed in Chapter 19.

Diazepam intravenously is the drug of choice for stopping continuous seizure activity, especially generalized tonic-clonic status epilepticus (see below). The drug is marketed as an adjunct to therapy and is occasionally given orally on a chronic basis, though it is not considered very effective in this application, probably because of the rapid development of tolerance, In mice, the anti-maximal electroshock ED50 for diazepam is 19 mg/kg, whereas the antipentylenetetrazol ED50 is 0.2 mg/kg.

Lorazepam is a newer benzodiazepine that, when given intravenously, appears in some studies to be more effective and longer-acting than diazepam in the treatment of status epilepticus.

Clonazepam (Clonopin) is a long-acting drug with documented efficacy against absence seizures and one of the most potent antiepileptic agents known. It is also effective in some cases of myoclonic seizures and has been tried in infantile spasms. Sedation is prominent, especially on initiation of therapy; starting doses should be small. Maximal tolerated doses are usually in the range of 0.1–0.2 mg/kg, but many weeks of gradually increasing daily dosage may be needed to achieve these doses in some patients. Therapeutic blood levels are usually less than 0.1 μg/mL and are not routinely measured in most laboratories. In mice, the ED50 against maximal electroshock is 87 mg/kg; the ED50 against pentylenetetrazol is 0.01 mg/kg.

Nitrazepam is not marketed in the USA but is used in many other countries, especially for infantile spasms and myoclonic seizures. It is less potent than clonazepam, and whether it has any clinical advantages over clonazepam remains unclear.

The pharmacokinetic properties of the benzodiazepines in part determine their clinical use. In general, the drugs are well absorbed, widely distributed, and extensively metabolized, with many active metabolites. The rate of distribution of benzodiazepines within the body is different from that of other antiepileptic drugs. Diazepam and lorazepam in particular are rapidly and extensively distributed to the tissues, with volumes of distribution between 1 and 3 L/kg. The onset of action, therefore, is also very rapid. Total body clearance of parent drug and metabolites, however, is very low, corresponding to half-lives of 40–50 hours.

Two prominent aspects of benzodiazepines limit their usefulness. The first is their pronounced sedative effect, which is unfortunate both in the treatment of status epilepticus and in chronic therapy. Children may manifest a paradoxic hyperactivity, as with barbiturates. The second problem is tolerance, in which seizures may initially respond, but within a few months the initial improvement may diminish. The remarkable antiepileptic potency of these compounds often cannot be realized because of these limiting factors.

ACETAZOLAMIDE

Acetazolamide (Diamox) is a diuretic whose main action is the inhibition of carbonic anhydrase (see Chapter 13). It has been proposed that the accumulation of carbon dioxide in the brain is the mechanism by which the drug exerts its antiepileptic activity. Acetazolamide has been used for all types of seizures but is severely limited by the rapid development of tolerance, with return of seizures usually within a few weeks. The drug may have a special role in epileptic women who experience seizure exacerbations at the time of menses; seizure control may be improved and tolerance may not develop, because the drug is not administered continuously. The usual dose is approximately 10 mg/kg up to a maximum of 1000 mg/d.

Another carbonic anhydrase inhibitor, **sulthiame,** was not found to be effective in clinical trials in the USA. It is marketed in some other countries.

BROMIDE

Bromide was introduced by Locock in 1857 and was the first antiepileptic drug with any measurable efficacy. Though largely discarded in favor of phenobarbital after the turn of the century, bromide is still occasionally useful, such as in management of epilepsy in patients with porphyria, in whom other drugs may be contraindicated. Its half-life is approximately 12 days, and it is given in doses of 3–6 g/d in adults to obtain plasma levels of 10–20 mEq/L. The mechanism of action of bromide as an antiepileptic agent is unknown. Major toxic problems are unfortunately frequent, including skin rashes, sedation, and behavioral changes.

II. CLINICAL PHARMACOLOGY OF ANTICONVULSANTS

SEIZURE CLASSIFICATION

The type of medication utilized for epilepsy is dependent upon the empirical nature of the seizure. For this reason, considerable effort has been made to classify seizures so that clinicians will be able to make a "seizure diagnosis" and thereby prescribe appropriate therapy. Errors in seizure diagnosis cause use of the wrong drugs, and an unpleasant cycle ensues in which poor seizure control is followed by increasing drug doses and medication toxicity. As noted above, seizures are divided into two groups: partial and generalized. Drugs used for partial seizures are more or less the same for the entire group, but drugs used for generalized seizures are determined by the individual seizure type. A shortened version of the International Classification of epileptic seizures is presented in Table 21–1.

Partial Seizures

Partial seizures are those in which a localized onset of the attack can be ascertained, either by clinical observation or by electroencephalographic recording; the attack begins in a specific locus in the brain. There are 3 types of partial seizures, determined to some extent by the degree of brain involvement by the abnormal discharge.

The least complicated partial seizure is the elementary or **simple partial seizure,** characterized by minimal spread of the abnormal discharge such that normal consciousness and awareness are preserved. For example, the patient may have a sudden onset of clonic jerking of an extremity lasting 60–90 seconds; residual weakness may last for 15–30 minutes after the attack. The patient is completely aware of the attack and can describe it in detail. The EEG may show an abnormal discharge highly localized to the involved portion of the brain.

The **complex partial seizure** also has a localized onset, but the discharge becomes more widespread (usually bilateral) and almost always involves the limbic system. Most (not all) complex partial seizures arise from one of the temporal lobes, possibly because of the susceptibility of this area of the brain to insults such as hypoxia or infection. Clinically, the patient may have a brief warning followed by an alteration of consciousness during which some patients may stare and others may stagger or even fall. Most, however, demonstrate fragments of integrated motor behavior called automatisms for which the patient has no memory. Typical automatisms are lip smacking, swallowing, fumbling, scratching, or even walking about. After 30–120 seconds, the patient makes a gradual recovery to normal consciousness but may feel tired or ill for several hours after the attack.

The last type of partial seizure is the **secondarily generalized attack,** in which a partial seizure immediately precedes a generalized tonic-clonic (grand mal) seizure. This seizure type is described below.

Generalized Seizures

Generalized seizures are those in which there is no evidence of localized onset. The group is quite heterogeneous.

Generalized tonic-clonic (grand mal) seizures are the most dramatic of all epileptic seizures and are characterized by tonic rigidity of all extremities, followed in 15–30 seconds by a tremor that is actually an interruption of the tonus by relaxation. As the relaxation phases become longer, the attack enters the clonic phase, with massive jerking of the body. The clonic jerking slows over 60–120 seconds, and the patient is usually left in a stuporous state. The tongue or cheek may be bitten, and urinary incontinence is common. Primary generalized tonic-clonic seizures begin without evidence of localized onset, whereas secondary generalized tonic-clonic seizures are preceded by another seizure type, usually a partial seizure. The medical treatment of both primary and secondary generalized tonic-clonic seizures is the same and utilizes drugs appropriate for partial seizures.

The **absence (petit mal) seizure** is characterized by both sudden onset and abrupt cessation. Its duration is usually less than 10 seconds and rarely more than 45 seconds. Consciousness is altered; the attack may also be associated with mild clonic jerking of the eyelids or extremities, with postural tone changes, autonomic phenomena, and automatisms. The occurrence of automatisms can complicate the clinical differentiation from complex partial seizures in some patients. Absence attacks begin in childhood or adolescence and may occur up to hundreds of times a day. The EEG during the seizure shows a highly characteristic 2.5–3.5 Hz spike-and-wave pattern. Atypical absence patients have seizures with postural changes that are more abrupt, and the patients are often mentally retarded; the EEG may show a slower spike-and-wave discharge, and the seizures may be more refractory to therapy.

Myoclonic jerking is seen, to a greater or lesser extent, in a wide variety of seizures, including generalized tonic-clonic seizures, partial seizures, absence seizures, and infantile spasms. Treatment of seizures that include myoclonic jerking should be directed at the primary seizure type rather than at the myoclonus. Some patients, however, have myoclonic jerking as the major seizure type, and some have frequent myoclonic jerking and occasional generalized tonic-clonic seizures without overt signs of neurologic deficit. In patients with the severe genetic syndrome of Unverricht-Lundborg, the myoclonus is progressive, severe, and associated with generalized tonic-clonic seizures and dementia. Many other kinds of myoclonus exist, and much effort has gone into the attempt to classify this entity. Further discussion is beyond the scope of this text.

Atonic seizures are those in which the patient has sudden loss of postural tone. If standing, the patient falls suddenly to the floor and may be injured. If seated, the head and torso may suddenly drop forward; the patient's face typically falls directly into a plate of food set on the table. Although most often seen in children, this seizure type is not unusual in adults. Many patients with atonic seizures wear helmets to prevent severe injury.

Infantile spasms is an epileptic syndrome and not a seizure type. The attacks, though sometimes fragmentary, are most often bilateral and are included for pragmatic purposes with the generalized seizures. These attacks are most often characterized clinically by brief, recurrent myoclonic jerks of the body with sudden flexion or extension of the body and limbs; the forms of infantile spasms are, however, quite heterogeneous. Ninety percent of affected patients have their first attack before the age of 1 year. Most patients are mentally retarded, presumably from the same origin as the spasms. The cause is unknown in many patients, but such widely disparate disorders as infection, kernicterus, tuberous sclerosis, and hypoglycemia have been implicated. In some cases, the EEG is characteristic. Drugs used to treat infantile spasms are effective only in some patients; there is no evidence that the mental retardation is alleviated by therapy, even when the attacks disappear.

THERAPEUTIC STRATEGY

For antiepileptic drugs, relationships between blood levels and therapeutic effects have been characterized to a particularly high degree. The same is true for the pharmacokinetics of these drugs. These relationships provide significant advantages in the development of therapeutic strategies for the treatment of epilepsy. Decisions on therapy are aided by blood level determinations, and decisions on dosage adjustments are based on pharmacokinetic data. The therapeutic index for most antiepileptic drugs is low, and toxicity is not uncommon. Thus, effective treatment of seizures requires an awareness of the therapeutic levels and pharmacokinetic properties as well as the characteristic toxicities of each agent. Measurements of antiepileptic drug plasma levels are extremely useful when combined with clinical observations and pharmacokinetic data.

MANAGEMENT OF EPILEPSY

Partial Seizures & Generalized Tonic-Clonic Seizures

The choice of drugs is usually limited to phenytoin, carbamazepine, or barbiturates. There has been a strong tendency in the past few years to limit the use of sedative antiepileptic drugs such as barbiturates and benzodiazepines to patients who cannot tolerate other medications. The trend in Europe has been to extend the use of carbamazepine, and North American physicians are gradually doing the same. In patients with resistant partial seizures, the combination of phenytoin and carbamazepine is preferred. Although the drugs described below are primarily used for either partial or generalized tonic-clonic seizures, their use in other seizure types is occasionally warranted.

PHENYTOIN

Therapeutic Levels & Dose

The therapeutic plasma level of phenytoin for most patients is between 10 and 20 μg/mL. A loading dose can be given either orally or intravenously; the latter is the method of choice for convulsive status epilepticus (discussed later). When oral therapy is started, it is common to begin adults at a dosage of 300 mg/d regardless of body weight. While this may be acceptable in some patients, it frequently yields steady-state blood levels below 10 μg/mL, the minimum therapeutic level for most patients. If seizures continue, higher doses are usually necessary to achieve plasma levels in the upper therapeutic range. Because of its dose-dependent kinetics, some toxicity may occur with only small increments in dose; the phenytoin dosage should be increased each time by only 25–30 mg in adults, and ample time should be allowed for the new steady state to be achieved before further increasing the dose. A common clinical error is to increase the dose directly from 300 mg/d to 400 mg/d; toxicity frequently occurs at a variable time thereafter. In children, a dose of 5 mg/kg/d should be followed by readjustment after steady-state plasma levels are obtained.

Two types of oral phenytoin sodium are currently available in the USA, differing in their respective rates of dissolution; one is absorbed rapidly and one more slowly. Only the latter can be given in a single daily dose, and care must be used when changing brands. Although rare patients being given phenytoin on a chronic basis have been proved to have low blood levels either from poor absorption or rapid metabolism, the most common cause of low levels is poor compliance.

Drug Interactions & Interference With Laboratory Tests

Drug interactions involving phenytoin are primarily related either to protein binding or to metabolism. Since phenytoin is highly bound, other highly bound drugs, such as phenylbutazone, sulfonamides, benzodiazepines, or anticoagulants can displace phenytoin from its binding site, causing an increase in free drug levels and intoxication when efforts are made to maintain total drug levels in the therapeutic range. The protein binding of phenytoin is markedly decreased in the presence of renal disease. A binding inhibitor, irreversible in the presence of uremia, may cause this displacement of phenytoin. The drug has an affinity for thyroid-binding globulin (TBG), which confuses some tests of thyroid function; the most reliable screening test of thyroid function in patients on phenytoin appears to be measurement of TSH.

Phenytoin has been shown to induce microsomal enzymes responsible for the metabolism of a number of drugs. Autostimulation of its own metabolism, however, appears to be insignificant. Other drugs, notably phenobarbital and carbamazepine, cause decreases in phenytoin steady-state concentrations through induction of hepatic microsomal enzymes. On the other hand, isoniazid inhibits the metabolism of phenytoin, resulting in increased steady-state concentrations when the 2 drugs are given together.

Toxicity

Dose-related side-effects caused by phenytoin are unfortunately similar to other antiepileptic drugs in this group, making differentiation difficult in patients receiving multiple drugs. Nystagmus occurs early, as does loss of smooth extraocular pursuit movements, but neither is an indication for decreasing the dose. Diplopia and ataxia are the most common dose-related side-effects requiring dose adjustment; sedation usually occurs only at considerably higher levels. Gingival hyperplasia and hirsutism occur to some degree in most patients; the latter can be especially unpleasant in females. Long-term chronic use is associated in some patients with coarsening of facial features and with peripheral neuropathy, usually manifested by diminished deep tendon reflexes in the lower extremities. Chronic use may also result in abnormalities of vitamin D metabolism leading to osteomalacia. Low folate levels and megaloblastic anemia have been reported, but the clinical importance of this observation is unknown.

Idiosyncratic reactions to phenytoin are relatively rare. Most commonly, a typical skin rash heralds the hypersensitivity of the patient to the drug, which is then appropriately discontinued. Fever may also occur, and in rare cases the skin lesions may be severe and exfoliative. Lymphadenopathy may be difficult to distinguish from malignant lymphoma, and although some studies suggest a causal relationship between phenytoin and Hodgkin's disease, the data are far from conclusive. Hematologic complications are exceedingly rare, although agranulocytosis has been reported in combination with fever and rash.

CARBAMAZEPINE

Therapeutic Levels & Dose

Carbamazepine is considered the drug of choice in partial seizures. It is available only in oral form. The drug is effective in children, in whom a dose of 15–25 mg/kg is appropriate. In adults, doses of 1 g or even 2 g are tolerated. Higher doses are achieved by giving multiple doses daily. In patients receiving 3 or 4 daily doses, in whom the blood is drawn just before the morning dose (trough level), the therapeutic level is usually 4–8 μg/mL; although most patients complain of diplopia above 7 μg/mL, others can tolerate levels above 10 μg/mL. When blood samples are drawn randomly, levels are frequently above 8 μg/mL, but fluctuations related to absorption make long-term comparisons difficult.

Drug Interactions

Drug interactions involving carbamazepine are almost exclusively related to the enzyme-inducing properties of this drug; as noted previously, the increased metabolic capacity of the hepatic enzymes may cause a reduction in steady-state carbamazepine concentrations, and an increased rate of metabolism of primidone, phenytoin, ethosuximide, valproic acid, and clonazepam. Other drugs such as propoxyphene, troleandomycin, and valproic acid may inhibit carbamazepine clearance and increase steady-state carbamazepine blood levels. Other anticonvulsants, however, such as phenytoin and phenobarbital, may decrease steady-state concentrations of carbamazepine through enzyme induction. No clinically significant protein binding interactions have been reported.

Toxicity

The most common dose-related side-effects of carbamazepine are diplopia and ataxia. The diplopia often occurs first and may last less than an hour during a particular time of day. Rearrangement of the divided daily dose can often remedy this complaint. Other dose-related complaints include mild gastrointestinal upsets, unsteadiness, and, at much higher doses, drowsiness. Hyponatremia and water intoxication have occasionally occurred and may be dose-related.

Considerable concern exists regarding the occurrence of idiosyncratic blood dyscrasias with carbamazepine, including fatal cases of aplastic anemia and agranulocytosis. Most of these have been in elderly patients with trigeminal neuralgia, and most have occurred within the first 4 months of treatment. A mild persistent leukopenia is also seen in some patients; this is not necessarily an indication to stop treatment but obviously requires careful monitoring. The most common idiosyncratic reaction is an erythematous skin rash; other idiosyncratic responses such as hepatic dysfunction are unusual.

BARBITURATES

Many consider the barbiturates (phenobarbital and primidone) the drugs of choice only for seizures in infants.

Therapeutic Levels & Dose

The therapeutic levels of phenobarbital in most patients range from 15 to 40 μg/mL. Documentation of effectiveness is best in febrile seizures, but levels below 15 μg/mL appear ineffective for prevention of febrile seizure recurrence. The upper end of the therapeutic range is more difficult to define, as many patients appear to tolerate chronic levels above 40 μg/mL.

Primidone is most efficacious when plasma levels are in the range of 8–12 μg/mL. Concomitant levels of its metabolite, phenobarbital, at steady state will usually vary from 15 to 30 μg/mL. Doses of 10–20 mg/kg/d are necessary to obtain these levels. It is very important, however, to start primidone at low doses and gradually increase over days to a few weeks to avoid prominent sedation and gastrointestinal complaints. When adjusting doses of the drug, it is important to remember that the parent drug will rapidly reach steady state (30–40 hours), but the active metabolites phenobarbital (20 days) and phenylethylmalonamide (3–4 days) will reach steady state much more slowly.

Toxicity

The toxic side-effects of primidone are similar to those of its metabolite, phenobarbital (see Chapter 19), except that drowsiness occurs early in treatment and may be prominent if the initial dose is too large; gradual increments are indicated when starting the drug in either children or adults.

Generalized Seizures

The drugs discussed below are used for treatment of most generalized seizures. The drugs used for generalized *tonic-clonic* seizures are the same as for *partial* seizures. Drugs used for infantile spasms will be reviewed separately.

Three drugs are effective against absence seizures. Two are nonsedative and therefore preferred: ethosuximide and valproic acid. Clonazepam is also highly effective but has disadvantages of dose-related side-effects and development of tolerance. The drug of choice is ethosuximide, even though valproic acid is effective in some ethosuximide-resistant patients. The major drawback in the use of valproic acid is its hepatotoxicity, discussed below.

Specific myoclonic syndromes are usually treated with valproic acid. It is nonsedative and can be dramatic in its effect. Other patients respond to clonazepam or other benzodiazepines, though high doses may be necessary, with accompanying sedation and drowsiness. A highly specific myoclonic syndrome, "intention myoclonus," which occurs after severe hypoxia, is characterized by myoclonus associated with volitional activity. Although further studies are needed, improvement in some patients with this unusual disorder has been reported using 5-hydroxytryptophan.

Atonic seizures are often refractory to all available medications, although some reports suggest that valproic acid may be beneficial. Benzodiazepines have been reported to improve seizure control in some patients but may worsen the attacks in others. If the loss of tone appears to be part of another seizure type (such as absence or complex partial seizures), every effort should be made to treat the other seizure type vigorously, hoping for simultaneous alleviation of the atonic component of the seizure.

ETHOSUXIMIDE

Therapeutic Levels & Dose

Therapeutic levels of 60–100 μg/mL can be achieved in adults with doses of 750–1500 mg/d, though lower or higher doses may be necessary. Some authors report that higher levels (up to 125 μg/mL) are needed in certain patients to achieve efficacy; such patients may tolerate the drug without apparent toxicity at these levels. Ethosuximide has a linear relationship between dose and steady-state plasma levels, and no change in pharmacokinetic parameters with age has been reported. The drug might be administered as a single daily dose were it not for its gastrointestinal side-effects; twice-a-day dosage is common. The time of day at which the level is measured is not particularly critical for ethosuximide, as its half-life is relatively long. No parenteral dosage form is available.

Drug Interactions

Administration of ethosuximide with valproic acid results in a decrease in ethosuximide clearance and higher steady-state concentrations due to inhibition of metabolism. No other drug interactions have been reported for the succinimides.

Toxicity

The most common dose-related side-effect of

ethosuximide is gastric distress, including pain, nausea, and vomiting. This can often be avoided by starting therapy at a low dose, with gradual increases into the therapeutic range. When the side-effect does occur, temporary dosage reductions may allow adaptation. Ethosuximide is a highly efficacious and safe drug for absence seizures; the appearance of relatively mild, dose-related side-effects should not immediately deter the physician from its use. Other dose-related side-effects include transient lethargy or fatigue and, much less commonly, headache, dizziness, hiccup, and euphoria. Behavioral changes are usually in the direction of improvement.

Non-dose-related or idiosyncratic side-effects of ethosuximide are extremely uncommon. Skin rashes have been reported, including at least one case of Stevens-Johnson syndrome. A few patients have had eosinophilia, thrombocytopenia, leukopenia, or pancytopenia; in none was it entirely certain that ethosuximide was the causal agent. The development of systemic lupus erythematosus has also been reported, but other drugs may have been involved.

VALPROIC ACID & SODIUM VALPROATE

The sodium salt of valproate is marketed in Europe as a tablet protected by aluminum foil, as it is quite hygroscopic. In Central and South America, the magnesium salt is available, which is considerably less hygroscopic. The free acid of valproate was first marketed in the USA in a capsule containing corn oil and is the predominant form of the drug available here, although the sodium salt is also used, in syrup, primarily for pediatric use. A calcium salt may also become available. There is little evidence that any of these various forms have any advantage over the other, with the possible exception of increased gastrointestinal side-effects of the capsules of valproic acid.

Therapeutic Levels & Dose

Doses of 25–30 mg/kg/d may be adequate in some patients, but others may require 60 mg/kg or even more. Therapeutic levels of valproic acid range from 50 to 100 μg/mL. The drug should not be abandoned until morning "trough" levels of at least 80 μg/mL have been attained; some patients may require and may tolerate levels in excess of 100 μg/mL.

Drug Interactions

As noted above, the clearance of valproic acid is dose-dependent, caused by changes in both the intrinsic clearance and protein binding. Valproic acid inhibits its own metabolism at low doses, thus decreasing intrinsic clearance. At higher doses, there is an increased free fraction of valproic acid, resulting in lower total drug levels than expected. It may be clinically useful, therefore, to measure both total and free drug levels. Valproic acid also displaces phenytoin from plasma proteins. In addition to binding interactions, valproic acid inhibits the metabolism of several drugs, including phenobarbital, phenytoin, and carbamazepine, leading to higher steady-state concentrations. The inhibition of phenobarbital metabolism may cause levels of the barbiturate to rise precipitously, causing stupor or coma. The inhibition of phenytoin metabolism may partially offset the reduction in total drug levels caused by displacement from plasma proteins.

Toxicity

The most common dose-related side-effects of valproic acid are nausea, vomiting, and other gastrointestinal complaints such as abdominal pain and "heartburn." The drug should be started gradually to avoid these symptoms; a temporary reduction in dose can usually alleviate the problems, and the patient will eventually tolerate higher doses. Sedation is uncommon with valproic acid alone but may be striking when valproate is added to phenobarbital. A fine tremor is frequently seen at higher levels. Other reversible side-effects, seen in a small number of patients, include weight gain, increased appetite, and hair loss.

The idiosyncratic toxicity of valproic acid is largely limited to hepatotoxicity, but this may be severe. Although most cases have been patients who are also taking other antiepileptic drugs, there seems little doubt that the hepatotoxicity of valproic acid has been responsible for 40 or 50 fatalities. The effect does not appear to be dose-related, nor is the age of the patient important, though most fatalities are pediatric because of the high utilization of the drug in this age group. Initial SGOT values may not be elevated in susceptible patients, though these levels do eventually become abnormal. Most fatalities have occurred within 4 months after initiation of therapy. Careful monitoring of liver function is obviously mandatory when starting the drug; the hepatotoxicity is reversible in some cases if the drug is withdrawn. It should be noted that valproic acid is an effective and popular antiepileptic drug and that only a very small number of patients have had severe toxic effects from its use.

The other observed idiosyncratic response with valproic acid is thrombocytopenia, though documented cases of abnormal bleeding are lacking.

OXAZOLIDINEDIONES

Therapeutic Levels & Dose

The therapeutic plasma level range for trimethadione has never been established, though trimethadione blood levels above 20 μg/mL and dimethadione levels above 700 μg/mL have been suggested. A dose of 30 mg/kg/d of trimethadione is necessary to achieve these levels in adults.

Drug Interactions

Relatively few drug interactions involving the methadione may competitively inhibit the demethylation of other drugs such as metharbital.

Toxicity

The most notable dose-related side-effect of the oxazolidinediones is sedation. An unusual side-effect is hemeralopia, a glare effect in which visual adaptation is impaired; it is reversible upon cessation of the drug. Accumulation of dimethadione has been reported to cause a very mild metabolic acidosis. Trimethadione has been associated with idiosyncratic dermatologic reactions, including rashes and exfoliative dermatitis, as well as toxic reactions involving the blood-forming organs; these have ranged from mild alterations in cell counts to fulminating pancytopenia. Other idiosyncratic reactions include reversible nephrotic syndrome, which may involve an immune reaction to the drug, as well as a myasthenic syndrome.

Drugs Used in Infantile Spasms

The treatment of infantile spasms is unfortunately limited to improvement of control of the seizures rather than other features of the disorder, such as retardation. Most patients receive a course of intramuscular corticotropin, though some clinicians note that prednisone may be equally effective and can be given orally. Clinical trials are under way to settle the matter. In either case, therapy must often be discontinued because of side-effects. If seizures recur, repeat courses of corticotropin or corticosteroids can be given, or other drugs may be tried. Other drugs widely used are the benzodiazepines such as clonazepam or nitrazepam, though their efficacy in this heterogeneous syndrome is unknown.

The rationale for the use of corticotropin or corticosteroids in the treatment of infantile spasms is based more on anecdotal evidence than on sound scientific studies. In some patients, corticotropin produces a dramatic improvement in seizure control with accompanying normalization of the EEG. Most studies, however, are poorly controlled and neglect the highly variable natural course of the disorder.

The basic mechanism of action of corticosteroids or corticotropin in the treatment of infantile spasms is unknown. It is known that glucocorticoids decrease septal-hippocampal excitability and thereby elevate convulsive thresholds of these limbic structures. It is not clear whether these agents interact directly with intracellular receptors involved in infantile spasms.

In spite of more than 20 years experience with corticosteroids and corticotropin for infantile spasms, the optimal dosage and duration of therapy have not been established. Initial studies suggested periods up to 12 weeks; most patients who responded showed improvement within 2–3 weeks and were continued on therapy for the full 12 weeks. With corticotropin, dosages were increased by 2–5 units daily until a level of 40–50 units daily was reached. Currently, a broad range of dosages are utilized, although most patients are treated with 25–40 units of corticotropin daily. A very few investigators recommend up to 240 units daily. In the 60% of patients who respond, seizure reduction is usually reported within 1–5 weeks. Corticotropin therapy may be continued for 3 months or more unless toxicity requires cessation. For corticosteroids, doses of 2 mg/kg of prednisolone or 0.3 mg/kg of dexamethasone have been utilized.

The toxic effects of corticotropin include hypertension, cushingoid obesity, gastrointestinal disturbances, skin changes, osteoporosis, and electrolyte imbalance. Neither corticotropin nor steroids affect the long-term prognosis for normal mental development.

Status Epilepticus

There are many forms of status epilepticus. The most common, generalized tonic-clonic status epilepticus, is a life-threatening emergency, requiring immediate cardiovascular, respiratory, and metabolic management as well as pharmacologic therapy. The latter virtually always requires intravenous administration of antiepileptic medications. Diazepam is the most effective drug in most patients for stopping the attacks and is given directly by intravenous push to a maximum total dose of 20 mg in adults. Intravenous diazepam may depress respiration (less frequently cardiovascular function), and facilities for resuscitation must be immediately at hand during its administration. The effect of diazepam is not lasting, but the 30- to 40-minute seizure-free interval allows more definitive therapy to be initiated. For patients who are not actually in the throes of a seizure, diazepam therapy can be omitted and the patient treated at once with a long-acting drug such as phenytoin.

The mainstay of continuing therapy for status epilepticus is intravenous phenytoin, which is effective and nonsedative. It should be given as a loading dose of 13–18 mg/kg in adults; the usual error is to give too little of the drug. Administration should be at a maximum rate of 50 mg/min. It is safest to give the drug directly by intravenous push, but it can also be diluted in saline; it precipitates rapidly in the presence of glucose. Especially in elderly people, careful monitoring of cardiac rhythm and blood pressure is necessary. At least part of the cardiotoxicity is from the diluent, propylene glycol, in which the phenytoin is dissolved.

In previously treated epileptic patients, the administration of a large loading dose of phenytoin may cause some dose-related toxicity such as ataxia. This is usually a relatively minor problem during the acute status episode and is easily alleviated by later adjustment of plasma levels.

For patients who do not respond to phenytoin, phenobarbital can be given in large doses: 100–200 mg intravenously to a total of 400–600 mg. Respiratory depression is a common complication, especially if diazepam has already been given, and there should be no hesitation in instituting intubation and ventilation.

Other drugs have been recommended for the treatment of generalized tonic-clonic status epilepticus, including intravenous lorazepam or lidocaine. General anesthesia may be necessary in highly resistant cases.

Special Aspects of the Toxicology of Antiepileptic Drugs

TERATOGENICITY

The potential teratogenicity of antiepileptic drugs is a controversial and important area. It is important because teratogenicity resulting from chronic drug treatment of millions of people throughout the world may have a profound effect even if the effect occurs in only a small percentage of cases. It is controversial because both epilepsy and antiepileptic drugs are heterogeneous and often inseparable in their effects. Furthermore, patients with severe epilepsy, in whom genetic factors rather than drug factors may be of greater importance in the occurrence of fetal malformations, are often receiving multiple antiepileptic drugs in high doses.

In spite of these limitations, it appears—from whatever cause—that children born to mothers taking antiepileptic drugs have an increased risk, perhaps 2-fold, of congenital malformations. It is noteworthy that one drug, phenytoin, has been implicated in a specific syndrome called **fetal hydantoin syndrome,** though not all investigators are convinced of its existence.

In dealing with the clinical problem of a pregnant woman with epilepsy, most students of epilepsy agree that while it is important to minimize antiepileptic drugs, both in numbers and doses, it is also important not to allow maternal seizures to go unchecked.

WITHDRAWAL

Withdrawal of antiepileptic drugs, whether by accident or by design, can cause increased seizure frequency and severity. There are 2 factors to consider: the effects of the withdrawal itself and the need for continued drug suppression of seizures in the individual patient. In many patients, both factors must be considered and dealt with. It is important to note, however, that the abrupt discontinuation of antiepileptic drugs ordinarily does not cause seizures in nonepileptic patients, provided that the drug levels are not above the usual therapeutic range when the drug is stopped.

Some drugs are more easily withdrawn than others. In general, withdrawal of anti-absence drugs is easier than withdrawal of drugs needed for partial or generalized tonic-clonic seizures. Barbiturates and benzodiazepines are the most difficult to discontinue; weeks or months may be required, with very gradual dosage decrements, to accomplish their complete removal, especially if the patient is not hospitalized.

OVERDOSE

Antiepileptic drugs are real or potential central nervous system depressants but are rarely lethal. Very high blood levels are usually necessary before overdoses can be considered life-threatening. The most dangerous effect of antiepileptic drugs after large overdoses is respiratory depression, which may be potentiated by other agents, such as alcohol. Treatment of antiepileptic drug overdose is supportive; stimulants should never be used. Efforts to hasten removal of antiepileptic drugs, such as urine alkalinization, are usually ineffective. Lipid dialysis has also been attempted; the data are too scanty to interpret its efficacy.

• • •

References

Browne TR, Penry JK: Benzodiazepines in the treatment of epilepsy. *Epilepsia* 1973;**14:**277.

Garretson LK: Pharmacology of anticonvulsants. *Pediatr Clin North Am* 1972;**19:**179.

Glaser GH, Penry JK, Woodbury DM (editors): *Antiepileptic Drugs: Mechanisms of Action*. Raven, 1980.

Glazko AJ: Antiepileptic drugs: Biotransformation, metabolism, and serum half-life. *Epilepsia* 1975;**16:**367.

Hooshmand H: Toxic effects of anticonvulsants: General principles. *Pediatrics* 1974;**53:**551.

Hvidberg EF, Dam M: Clinical pharmacokinetics of anticonvulsants. *Clin Pharmacokinet* 1976;**1:**161.

Kapetanovic IM et al: Mechanism of valproate-phenobarbital interaction in epileptic patients. *Clin Pharmacol Ther* 1981;**29:**480.

Penry JK, Newmark ME: The use of antiepileptic drugs. *Ann Intern Med* 1979;**90:**207.

Penry JK, Porter RJ: Epilepsy: Mechanisms and therapy. *Med Clin North Am* 1979;**63:**801.

Plaa GL: Acute toxicity of antiepileptic drugs. *Epilepsia* 1975;**16:**183.

Porter RJ, Penry JK, Lacy JR: Diagnostic and therapeutic reevaluation of patients with intractable epilepsy. *Neurology* 1977;**27:**1006.

Richens A: Interactions with antiepileptic drugs. *Drugs* 1977;**13:**266.

Theodore WH, Porter RJ: The removal of sedative-hypnotic antiepileptic drugs from the regimens of patients with intractable epilepsy. *Trans Am Neurol Assoc* 1980;**105:**1.

Woodbury DM, Penry JK, Schmidt RP (editors): *Antiepileptic Drugs*. Raven, 1972.

General Anesthetics | 22

Anthony J. Trevor, PhD, & Ronald D. Miller, MD

I. BASIC PHARMACOLOGY OF GENERAL ANESTHETICS

The attempted suppression of the pain of surgical procedures by the use of drugs dates from ancient times and includes the oral administration of ethanol and opiates. The first scientific demonstration of drug-induced anesthesia during surgery was in 1864, when William Morton used diethyl ether in Boston. Within a year, chloroform was introduced by James Simpson in Scotland, and this was followed almost 20 years later by the successful demonstration of the anesthetic properties of nitrous oxide, which had been first suggested by Priestley in 1776. Modern anesthesia dates from the 1930s, during which period the intravenous barbiturate thiopental was introduced. A decade later, curare was used in anesthesia to ensure adequate skeletal muscle relaxation. The first halogenated hydrocarbon, halothane, was introduced as an inhaled anesthetic in 1956 and has become the standard for comparison for several other more recently developed inhaled anesthetic drugs.

The state of "general anesthesia" usually includes analgesia, amnesia, loss of consciousness, inhibition of sensory and autonomic reflexes, and skeletal muscle relaxation. It can be produced by some but not all sedative-hypnotics (Chapter 19). The extent to which any individual anesthetic drug can exert these effects is variable. Also, it is desirable to be able to induce anesthesia smoothly and rapidly as well as to ensure rapid recovery from the effects of the anesthetic. An ideal anesthetic drug would also possess a wide margin of safety and be devoid of adverse effects. No *single* anesthetic agent is capable of achieving all of these desirable effects without some disadvantages when used alone. Thus, the modern practice of anesthesia involves the use of combinations of drugs, taking advantage of their individual desirable properties while attempting to minimize their potential for harmful actions. **Balanced anesthesia** includes the administration of medications preoperatively for sedation and analgesia, the use of neuromuscular blocking drugs intraoperatively, and the use of both intravenous and inhaled anesthetic drugs.

TYPES OF GENERAL ANESTHETICS

General anesthetics are usually given by inhalation or by intravenous injection.

Inhalational Agents

The chemical structures of the 5 most commonly used inhalational agents are shown in Fig 22–1. Nitrous oxide, a gas at ambient temperature and pressure, continues to be an important component of many anesthesia regimens. Halothane, enflurane, isoflurane, and methoxyflurane are volatile liquids. Other inhalational agents (not shown) include ether, cyclopropane, and chloroform, which have limited current use for reasons that include potential flammability (ether, cyclopropane) and organ toxicity (chloroform).

Intravenous Agents

Several drugs are used intravenously to achieve anesthesia:

(1) Thiobarbiturates (thiopental, methohexital).

(2) Neuroleptics in combination with narcotic analgesics (droperidol with fentanyl) to produce a state called neuroleptanesthesia.

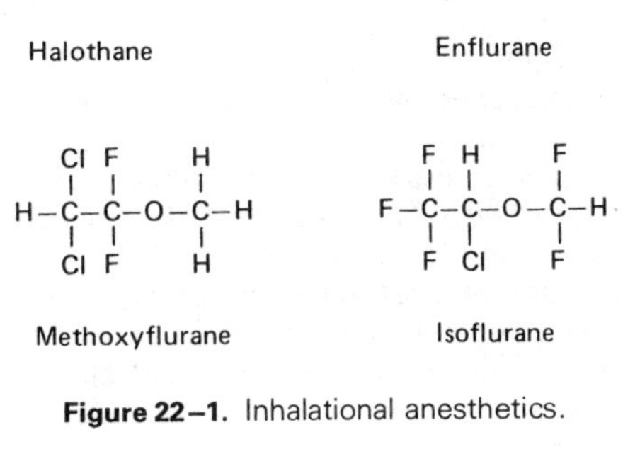

Figure 22–1. Inhalational anesthetics.

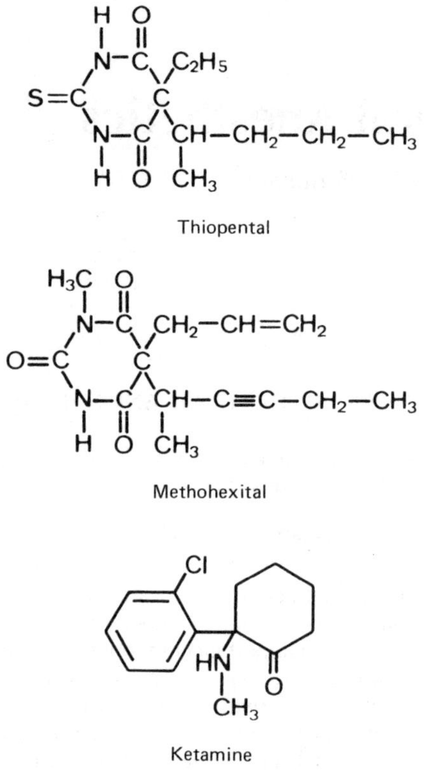

Figure 22–2. Intravenous anesthetics.

(3) Arylcyclohexylamines (ketamine), which produces a state called dissociative anesthesia.

(4) Miscellaneous drugs (propanidid, alfaxalone, etomidate), most of which are not currently available in the USA.

Fig 22–2 shows the structures of 2 commonly used barbiturates and ketamine.

SIGNS & STAGES OF ANESTHESIA

Since the introduction of general anesthetics, attempts have been made to correlate their observable effects or signs with the *depth* of anesthesia. Descriptions of the signs and stages of anesthesia (Guedel's signs) originate mainly from observations of the effects of diethyl ether, which has a slow onset of central action due to its high solubility in blood. These stages and signs may not occur so readily with the more rapidly acting modern inhaled anesthetics and are unusual with intravenous agents. Many of the signs refer to the effects of anesthetic agents on respiration, reflex activity, and muscle tone. Traditionally, anesthetic effects are divided into 4 stages of increasing depth of CNS depression.

I. Stage of analgesia: The patient initially experiences analgesia without amnesia. However, later in stage I, both analgesia and amnesia ensue.

II. Stage of excitement: During this stage, the patient often appears to be delirious and excited but definitely is amnesic. Respiration is irregular both in volume and rate, and retching and vomiting may occur. Incontinence and struggling sometimes occur. For these reasons, efforts are made to limit the duration and severity of this stage, which ends with the reestablishment of regular breathing.

III. Stage of surgical anesthesia: With the beginning of regular respiration, this stage extends to complete cessation of spontaneous respiration. Four planes of stage III have been described in terms of changes in ocular movements, eye reflexes, and pupil size, which under specified conditions may represent signs of increasing depth of anesthesia.

IV. Stage of medullary depression: When spontaneous respiration ceases, stage IV is present. This stage of anesthesia obviously includes severe depression of the respiratory center in the medulla and the vasomotor center as well. Without full circulatory support, coma and death rapidly ensue.

In modern anesthesia practice, the distinctive signs of each of the 4 stages described above are often obscured. Reasons for this include the relatively rapid onset of action of many inhaled anesthetics compared to that of diethyl ether and the fact that pulmonary ventilation is often controlled with the aid of a mechanical ventilator. In addition, the presence of other pharmacologic agents given pre- or intraoperatively can also influence the signs of anesthesia. Atropine, used to decrease secretions, also dilates pupils; drugs such as tubocurarine and succinylcholine affect muscle tone; and the narcotic analgesics exert depressant effects on respiration. The most reliable indications that stage III (surgical anesthesia) has been achieved are loss of the eyelash reflex and establishment of a respiratory pattern that is regular in rate and depth. The adequacy of ensuing depth of anesthesia for the particular surgical situation is assessed mainly by changes in respiratory and cardiovascular responses to stimulation.

MECHANISMS OF ACTION

The neuropharmacologic basis for the effects that characterize the stages of anesthesia appears to be a **differential sensitivity** to the anesthetics of specific neurons or neuronal pathways. Cells of the substantia gelatinosa in the dorsal horn of the spinal cord are very sensitive to relatively low anesthetic concentration in the central nervous system. A decrease in the activity of the dorsal horn interrupts sensory transmission in the spinothalamic tract, including that concerning nociceptive stimuli. These effects contribute to stage I, or analgesia. The disinhibitory effects of general anesthetics (stage II), which occur at higher brain concentrations, result from complex neuronal actions including blockade of many small inhibitory neurons such as Golgi type II cells, together with a paradoxic facilitation of excitatory neurotransmitters. A progressive depression of ascending pathways in the reticular activating system occurs during stage III, or surgical anesthesia, together with suppression of spinal reflex activity that contributes to muscle relaxation. Neurons in the respiratory and vasomotor centers of the medulla are relatively insensitive to the effects of the general anesthetics, but at high concentrations their activity is depressed, leading to cardiorespiratory collapse (stage IV).

Despite the apparent differences in sensitivity between various neurons in the central nervous system, the common neurophysiologic action of general anesthetics is to **increase the threshold** of cells to firing, resulting in decreased activity. Almost all anesthetics also **reduce the rate of rise of the action potential** by interfering with sodium influx. One interpretation of this effect is that the physical presence of anesthetic molecules blocks or distorts neuronal membrane channels involved in sodium conductance. Current theories of the possible mechanisms by which anesthetics interfere with the sodium channel include consideration of their molecular interactions with the lipid matrix of the membrane and with hydrophobic regions of specific membrane proteins. In experimental animals, general anesthesia can be reversed quite rapidly by high pressure (eg, 50–100 atm). This has led to suggestions that as the anesthetic molecule dissolves in the neuronal membrane, it causes a small expansion that distorts the sodium channel. High pressure restores the membrane to its former state to permit the normal influx of sodium that occurs during generation of the action potential.

PHARMACOKINETICS OF INHALED ANESTHETICS

Depth of anesthesia is determined by the concentrations of anesthetics in the central nervous system. The rate at which an effective brain concentration is reached (the rate of induction of anesthesia) depends on multiple pharmacokinetic factors that influence the uptake and distribution of the anesthetic. These factors determine the different rates of transfer of the inhaled anesthetic from the lung to the blood and from the blood to the brain and other tissues. These factors also influence the rate of recovery from anesthesia when inhalation of the anesthetic is terminated.

Uptake & Distribution

The **concentration** of an individual gas in a mixture of gases is proportionate to its **partial pressure** or **tension.** These terms are often used interchangeably in discussing the various transfer processes of anesthetic gases in the body. Achievement of a brain concentration of an anesthetic adequate to cause anesthesia requires transfer of that anesthetic from the alveolar air to blood and then to brain. The rate at which a given concentration of anesthetic in the brain is reached depends on the solubility properties of the anesthetic, its concentration in the inspired air, pulmonary ventilation rate, pulmonary blood flow, and the concentration gradient of the anesthetic between arterial and mixed venous blood.

Table 22–1. Properties of inhalational anesthetics.

Anesthetic	Blood:Gas Partition Coefficient	Brain:Blood Partition Coefficient	Minimum Alveolar Concentration (percent)
Nitrous oxide	0.47	1.1	>100
Isoflurane	1.40	2.6	1.40
Enflurane	1.80	1.4	1.68
Halothane	2.30	2.9	0.75
Methoxyflurane	12.00	2.0	0.16

Partition coefficients (at 37 °C) are from multiple literature sources. Minimum alveolar concentration (MAC) is the anesthetic concentration that produces immobility in 50% of patients exposed to a noxious stimulus.

A. Solubility: One of the most important factors influencing the transfer of an anesthetic from the lungs to the arterial blood is its solubility. The blood:gas partition coefficient is a useful index of solubility and defines the relative affinity of an anesthetic for the blood compared to air. This partition coefficient may be as low as 0.5 for anesthetics such as nitrous oxide or cyclopropane, which are quite insoluble in blood. Alternatively, the value may be higher than 10 for agents such as diethyl ether or methoxyflurane, which are very soluble in blood (Table 22–1). When an anesthetic with low blood solubility diffuses from the lung into the arterial blood, relatively few molecules are required to raise its partial pressure, and the arterial tension rises quickly. Conversely, for anesthetics with moderate to high solubility, more molecules dissolve before partial pressure is changed, and arterial tension of the gas will increase slowly. This inverse relationship between the blood solubility of an anesthetic and rate of rise of its tension in arterial blood is illustrated in Fig 22–3. The blood:gas partition coefficients for

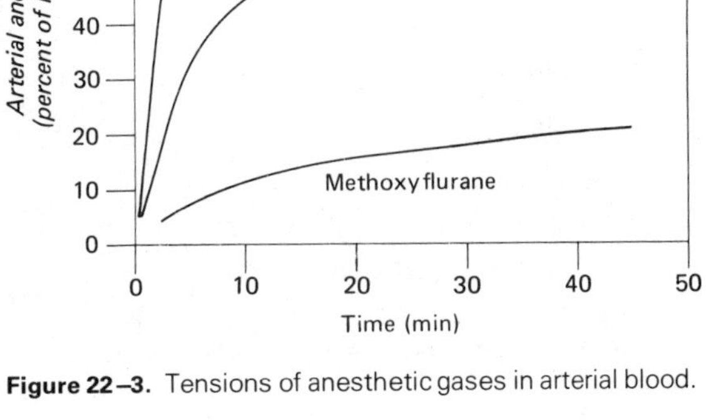

Figure 22–3. Tensions of anesthetic gases in arterial blood.

nitrous oxide, halothane, and methoxyflurane are 0.47, 2.3, and 12, respectively. Nitrous oxide, with low solubility in blood, reaches high arterial tensions rapidly, which in turn results in more rapid equilibrium with the brain and faster induction of anesthesia. In contrast, even after 40 minutes, methoxyflurane has reached only 20% of the equilibrium concentration.

B. Anesthetic Concentration in the Inspired Air: The concentration of an inhaled anesthetic in the inspired gas mixture has direct effects on both the maximum tension that can be achieved in the alveoli and the rate of increase in its tension in arterial blood. Increases in the inspired anesthetic concentration will increase the rate of induction of anesthesia by increasing the rate of transfer into the blood. Advantage is taken of this effect in anesthetic practice with inhaled anesthetics of moderate blood solubility such as enflurane or halothane, which have a relatively slow onset. For example, a 3–4% concentration of halothane may be inspired initially to increase rate of induction, and this is reduced to 1–2% for maintenance when adequate anesthesia is achieved.

C. Pulmonary Ventilation: The rate of rise of anesthetic gas tension in arterial blood is directly dependent on both the rate and depth of ventilation, ie, minute ventilation. The magnitude of the effect varies according to the blood:gas partition coefficient. An increase in pulmonary ventilation is accompanied by only a slight increase in arterial tension of an anesthetic with low blood solubility or low coefficient but can significantly increase tension of agents with moderate or high blood solubility (Fig 22–4). For example, a 4-fold increase in ventilation rate may double the arterial tension of halothane during the first 10 minutes of anesthesia, with little effect on the arterial tension of

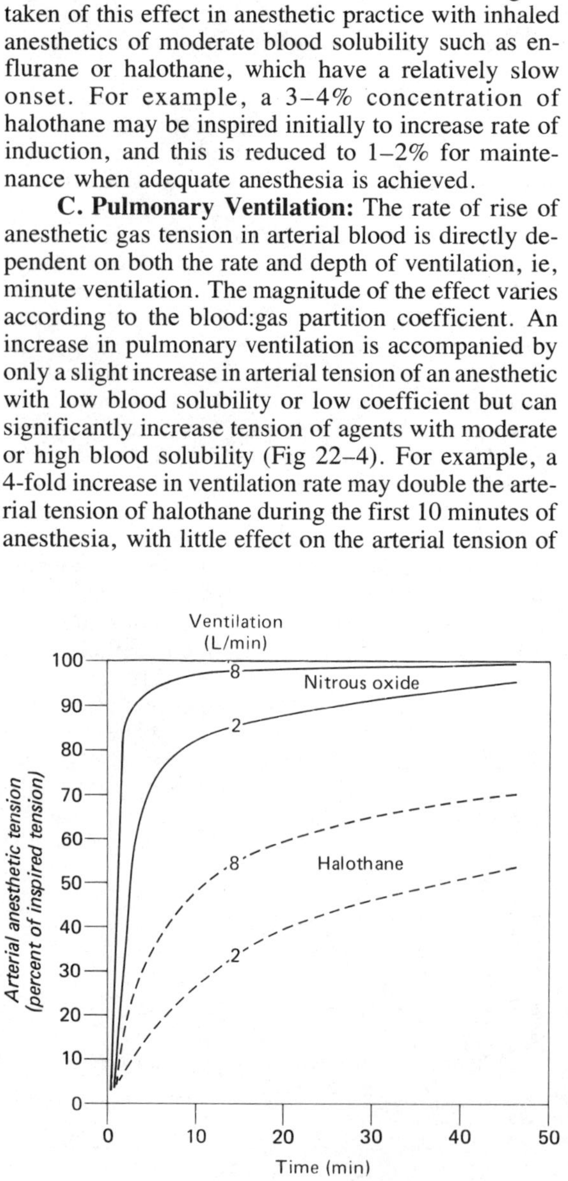

Figure 22–4. Ventilation rate and arterial anesthetic tensions.

nitrous oxide. Hyperventilation by mechanical control of respiration or by CO_2 stimulation increases the speed of induction of anesthesia with inhaled anesthetics that would normally have a slow onset. Depression of respiration by other pharmacologic agents, including narcotic analgesics, may slow the onset of anesthesia of some inhaled anesthetics if ventilation is not controlled.

D. Pulmonary Blood Flow: Changes in the rates of blood flow to and from the lungs influence transfer processes of the anesthetic gases. An increase in pulmonary blood flow (increased cardiac output) *lowers* the rate of rise in arterial tension, particularly for those anesthetics with moderate to high blood solubility. This is because increased pulmonary blood flow exposes a larger volume of blood to the anesthetic; thus, blood "capacity" increases and tension rises slowly. A decrease in pulmonary blood flow has the opposite effect and increases the rate of rise of arterial tension of inhaled anesthetics. In a patient with circulatory shock, the combined effects of decreased cardiac output (decreased pulmonary flow) and increased ventilation may accelerate the induction of anesthesia with some anesthetics. This is least likely to occur with nitrous oxide because of its low solubility.

E. Arterial-Venous Concentration Gradient: The anesthetic concentration gradient between arterial and mixed venous blood is dependent mainly on uptake of the anesthetic by the tissues; depending on the rate and extent of tissue uptake, venous blood returning to the lungs may contain significantly less anesthetic than that present in arterial blood. The greater this difference in tensions, the more time it takes to achieve equilibrium. Anesthetic entry into tissues is influenced by factors similar to those that determine transfer from lung to blood, including tissue:blood partition coefficient, rates of blood flow to the tissues, and concentration gradients.

During the induction phase of anesthesia, the tissues that exert greatest influence on the arterial-venous anesthetic concentration gradient are those which are highly perfused. These include the brain, heart, liver, kidneys, and splanchnic bed, which together receive over 75% of the resting cardiac output. In the case of anesthetics with relatively high solubility in these tissues, venous blood concentration will initially be very low, and equilibrium with arterial blood is achieved slowly.

During maintenance of anesthesia with inhaled anesthetics, there may continue to be transfer of these drugs between various tissues at rates dependent on solubility and blood flow. Muscle and skin, which together constitute 50% of body mass, accumulate anesthetics more slowly than the richly vascularized tissues, since they receive only one-fifth of the blood flow of the latter group. Although most anesthetic gases have high solubility in adipose tissues, low blood perfusion rates to these tissues delay accumulation, and equilibrium is unlikely to occur with anesthetics such as halothane and enflurane during the time anesthetics are usually required for surgery.

Elimination

The time to recovery from inhalational anesthesia depends on the rate of elimination of anesthetics from the brain after the inspired concentration of anesthetic has been decreased. Many of the processes of anesthetic transfer during recovery are similar to those that occur during induction of anesthesia. Factors controlling rate of recovery include the pulmonary blood flow and the magnitude of ventilation as well as solubility of the anesthetic in the tissues and the blood and in the gas phase in the lung. Two features of recovery, however, are quite different from what happens during induction of anesthesia. First, while transfer of an anesthetic from the lungs to blood can be enhanced by increasing its concentration in inspired air, the reverse transfer process cannot be enhanced, since the concentration in the lungs cannot be reduced below zero. Second, at the beginning of recovery, the anesthetic gas tension in different tissues may be quite variable, depending on the specific agent and the duration of anesthesia. With induction of anesthesia, the initial anesthetic tension in all tissues is zero.

Inhaled anesthetics that are relatively insoluble in blood and the brain are eliminated at faster rates than more soluble anesthetics. For example, the "washout" of nitrous oxide occurs at a fast rate, which leads to a rapid recovery from its anesthetic effects. Halothane is approximately twice as soluble in brain tissue and 5 times more soluble in blood than nitrous oxide; its elimination therefore takes place more slowly, and recovery from halothane anesthesia is less rapid. The duration of exposure to the anesthetic can have a marked effect on the time of recovery, especially in the case of more soluble anesthetics such as methoxyflurane. Accumulation of agents in tissues, including muscle, skin, and fat, increases with continuous inhalation; and blood tension may decline slowly during recovery as the anesthetic gradually leaves such tissues. Thus, if exposure to the anesthetic is short, recovery may be rapid. After prolonged anesthesia, recovery may be delayed even with anesthetics of modest solubility such as halothane.

Clearance of inhaled anesthetics by the lung into the expired air is the major route of their elimination from the body. However, metabolism by enzymes of the liver and other tissues may contribute to the elimination of anesthetics, usually to a lesser extent. For example, the washout of halothane during recovery is more rapid than that of enflurane, which would not be predicted from their respective solubilities. However, 15–20% of inspired halothane is metabolized during an average anesthetic procedure, while only 2–3% of enflurane is metabolized over the same period. Oxidative metabolism of halothane results in the formation of trifluoroacetic acid and release of bromide and chloride ions. Under conditions of low oxygen tension, halothane is metabolized to the chlorotrifluoroethyl free radical, which is capable of reacting with hepatic membrane components. The slow rate of metabolism of enflurane results in the formation of difluoromethoxydifluoroacetic acid and fluoride ion, which do not reach toxic levels. Methoxyflurane is metabolized by the liver at a faster rate than any other inhaled anesthetic and releases fluoride ions at levels that can be nephrotoxic. Nitrous oxide is metabolized to a very small extent.

MINIMUM ALVEOLAR ANESTHETIC CONCENTRATIONS

Inhaled anesthetics are delivered to the lungs in gas mixtures in which concentrations and flow rate are easy to measure and control. However, achievement of an anesthetic state depends on the concentration of the anesthetic in the brain, and that concentration is impossible to measure under clinical conditions. During general anesthesia, the partial pressure of the anesthetic in the brain equals that in the lung when steady state is reached. At this point, the measurement of the alveolar concentrations of different anesthetics provides a comparison of their relative potencies. The **minimum alveolar anesthetic concentration (MAC)** of an anesthetic is defined as that concentration which results in immobility in 50% of patients when exposed to a noxious stimulus such as surgical incision. Table 22–1 shows such concentrations for the common inhaled anesthetics, permitting comparison of their relative anesthetic potencies. The MAC value greater than 100% for nitrous oxide shows that it is the least potent, since not even 1 MAC can be reached at normal barometric pressures. Furthermore, the dose administered can be stated in multiples of MAC. While a dose of 1 MAC of any agent prevents movement in response to surgical incision in 50% of patients, individual patients may require from 0.5 to 1.5 MAC. In general, however, the dose-response relationship for inhaled anesthetics is steep; thus, over 95% of patients may fail to respond to a noxious stimulus at 1.1 MAC. The measurement of MAC values under controlled conditions has permitted quantitation of the effects of a number of variables on anesthetic requirements. For example, MAC values decrease in elderly patients but are not affected greatly by sex, height, and weight. Of particular importance is the presence of adjuvant drugs, which can change anesthetic requirement greatly. For example, when drugs such as the narcotic analgesics or sedative-hypnotics are present, MAC is decreased, which means that the inspired concentration of anesthetic should be decreased accordingly.

II. CLINICAL PHARMACOLOGY OF GENERAL ANESTHETICS

INHALED ANESTHETICS

General Overview of Clinical Use

Of the inhaled anesthetics available, nitrous oxide, halothane, enflurane, and isoflurane are most commonly used in the USA. As indicated previously, nitrous oxide lacks sufficient potency to produce surgical anesthesia by itself and therefore is usually used in combination with another inhaled or intravenous anesthetic to produce the total anesthetic state. Methoxyflurane is occasionally used, especially in obstetrical anesthesia, but not for prolonged procedures because of its nephrotoxicity, which is described below. Chloroform is not used because of its hepatotoxicity. Although cyclopropane and diethyl ether were the most commonly used anesthetics before 1960, they are rarely used now because of their flammable and explosive characteristics.

General Pharmacologic Effects

A. Effects on Cardiovascular System: Halothane, enflurane, and isoflurane all decrease mean arterial pressure in direct proportion to their alveolar concentration. With halothane and enflurane, the reduced arterial pressure appears to be caused by a reduction in cardiac output, since there is little change in systemic vascular resistance. In contrast, isoflurane has a depressant effect on arterial pressure as a result of a marked decrease in systemic vascular resistance; it has little effect on cardiac output.

Older anesthetics such as cyclopropane, diethyl ether, and fluroxene generally do not reduce arterial blood pressure or significantly change cardiac output. In fact, diethyl ether and cyclopropane often increase arterial blood pressure as a result of their ability to liberate catecholamines.

Inhaled anesthetics change heart rate either by altering the rate of sinus node depolarization directly or by shifting the balance of autonomic nervous system activity. Bradycardia is often seen with halothane and may be a result of direct depression of atrial rate. In contrast, methoxyflurane, enflurane, and isoflurane increase heart rate. All of these changes in heart rate have been determined in normal subjects undergoing surgery. The patient's excited state preoperatively or the stimulation of surgery intraoperatively will often alter the heart rate response to inhaled anesthetics.

All inhaled anesthetics tend to increase right atrial pressure in a dose-related fashion that reflects depression of myocardial function. In general, enflurane and halothane are very depressant to the myocardium, but cyclopropane, diethyl ether, and fluroxene are not. Inhaled anesthetics reduce myocardial oxygen consumption, primarily by decreasing those variables that control oxygen demand, such as arterial blood pressure and contractile force. Although certainly less depressant than the other inhaled anesthetics, nitrous oxide has also been found to depress the myocardium in a dose-dependent manner. However, nitrous oxide alone or in combination with potent inhaled anesthetics produces sympathetic stimulation that may obscure any cardiac depressant effects of the inhaled anesthetic. The combination of nitrous oxide plus halothane or enflurane, for example, appears to produce less depression at a given level of anesthesia than either more potent anesthetic given alone.

B. Effects on Respiratory System: With the exception of nitrous oxide and diethyl ether, all inhaled anesthetics cause a decrease in tidal volume and an increase in respiratory rate. However, the increase in rate is insufficient to compensate for the decrease in volume, resulting in a decrease in minute ventilation. All inhaled anesthetics are respiratory depressants, as gauged by the reduced response to various levels of carbon dioxide. The degree of ventilatory depression varies with anesthetic agents, with isoflurane and enflurane being the most depressant and diethyl ether the least depressant. All inhaled anesthetics except diethyl ether increase the resting level of P_{aCO_2} (the partial pressure of carbon dioxide in arterial blood). Because diethyl ether is a respiratory irritant, ventilation may remain sufficiently high to maintain normal P_{aCO_2}. However, if the patient is challenged with increasing inspired concentrations of carbon dioxide, the respiratory depressant effect of diethyl ether will become apparent. The ventilatory depressant effects of anesthetics are overcome by assisting or controlling ventilation via a mechanical ventilator during surgery. Inhaled anesthetics also depress mucociliary function in the airway. Thus, prolonged anesthesia may lead to pooling of mucus and then result in atelectasis and respiratory infections. On the other hand, inhaled anesthetics tend to be bronchodilators, with halothane probably one of the most potent. This effect has been utilized in the treatment of asthma.

C. Effects on Brain: Inhaled anesthetics decrease the metabolic rate of the brain. Nevertheless, most of them *increase* cerebral blood flow because they decrease cerebral vascular resistance. The increase in cerebral blood flow is often clinically undesirable. For example, in patients who have an elevated intracranial pressure because of brain tumor or head injury, the administration of an inhaled anesthetic may increase cerebral blood flow, which in turn will increase cerebral blood volume and further increase intracranial pressure.

Of the inhaled anesthetics, nitrous oxide increases cerebral blood flow the least, although when 60% nitrous oxide is added to halothane anesthesia, cerebral blood flow usually increases more than with halothane alone. Halothane, enflurane, and isoflurane in low doses have similar effects on cerebral blood flow. At higher doses, enflurane and isoflurane increase cerebral blood flow less than does halothane. If the patient is hyperventilated before the anesthetic is given, increase in intracranial pressure from inhaled anesthetics can be minimized.

Halothane, isoflurane, and enflurane have similar effects (eg, burst suppression) on the EEG up to doses of 1–1.5 MAC. At higher doses, the cerebral irritant effects of enflurane may lead to the development of a spike-and-wave pattern during which auditory stimuli can precipitate mild generalized muscle twitching that is augmented by hyperventilation. This seizure activity has never been shown to have any adverse clinical consequences. The effect is not seen clinically with the other inhaled anesthetics.

D. Effects on Kidney: To varying degrees, all inhaled anesthetics decrease glomerular filtration rate and effective renal plasma flow and increase filtration fraction. All the anesthetics tend to increase renal vascular resistance. Since renal blood flow decreases during general anesthesia in spite of well-maintained or even increased perfusion pressures, autoregulation of renal flow is probably impaired.

E. Effects on Liver: All inhaled anesthetics cause a decrease in hepatic blood flow, ranging from 15 to 45% of the preanesthetic flow. Despite transient changes in liver function tests intraoperatively, rarely does permanent change of liver function occur from the use of these agents. The possible hepatotoxicity of halothane is discussed below.

F. Effects on Uterine Smooth Muscle: Nitrous oxide appears to have little effect on uterine musculature. However, isoflurane, halothane, and enflurane are potent uterine muscle relaxants. This pharmacologic effect can be used to advantage when profound uterine relaxation is required for intrauterine fetal manipulation during delivery. In contrast, during dilatation and curettage for therapeutic abortion, these anesthetics may cause increased bleeding.

Toxicity

A. Hepatotoxicity (Halothane): Postoperative hepatitis is usually associated with factors such as blood transfusions, hypovolemic shock, and other surgical stresses rather than anesthetic toxicity. However, halocarbons can cause liver damage, and chloroform was identified as a hepatotoxin in the first decade of this century. Halothane was introduced into clinical practice in 1956; by 1963, several cases of postoperative jaundice and liver necrosis associated with halothane had been reported. However, several retrospective studies in which halothane was compared with other anesthetics showed no increased incidence in postoperative hepatic damage with halothane. In 1966, the United States National Halothane Study undertook a retrospective review of the incidence of fatal massive hepatic necrosis in a population of about 850,000 surgical patients. Results of the study were inconclusive and did not identify halothane clearly as a hepatotoxin. The incidence of massive necrosis associated with halothane was 7 out of 250,000 halothane administrations, or about 1 in 35,000 (not 1 in 10,000, as sometimes reported). Because halothane is such a valuable anesthetic, it is important to establish whether it is indeed a significant hepatotoxin before limiting its use. Unlike chloroform and fluroxene, which can produce fatty infiltration, centrilobular necrosis, and elevated transaminase concentrations, prolonged exposure of animals to halothane produces little evidence of liver damage. Several animal models have been developed to help define possible halothane-mediated hepatotoxicity. When rats are pretreated with phenobarbital and then exposed to hypoxic conditions with an inspired oxygen concentration of 7–14%, hepatotoxicity from halothane will occur. The mechanism underlying hepatotoxicity in the animals remains unclear, although these models suggest that it may depend on the production of a reactive metabolite (eg, a free radical) that either causes direct hepatocellular damage or initiates an immune-mediated response. Although this model is reproducible and well defined, its clinical applicability is uncertain because hypoxia is a necessary precondition for production of liver damage.

B. Nephrotoxicity (Methoxyflurane): In 1966, vasopressin-resistant polyuric renal insufficiency was first reported in 13 of 41 patients receiving methoxyflurane anesthesia for abdominal surgery. Subsequently, the causative agent was shown to be inorganic fluoride, an end product of the biotransformation of methoxyflurane.

C. Chronic Toxicity:

1. Mutagenicity–Under normal conditions, most modern and many previously used inhaled anesthetics are not mutagens and probably not carcinogens. On the other hand, anesthetics that contain the vinyl moiety (fluroxene and divinyl ether) may be mutagens.

2. Carcinogenicity–Several epidemiologic studies have suggested an increase in the cancer rate in operating room personnel who may be exposed to trace concentrations of anesthetic agents. However, no study has demonstrated the existence of a cause-and-effect relationship between anesthetics and cancer. Many other factors might account for the questionably positive results seen after a careful review of epidemiologic data. Most operating room theaters remove trace concentrations of anesthetics released from anesthetic machines via vents to the atmosphere.

3. Effects on reproduction–The most consistent finding reported from surveys conducted to determine the reproductive performance of female operating room personnel has been a higher than expected incidence of miscarriages. There are several problems in interpreting these studies, but in general it can be stated that the evidence is not strong.

On the other hand, the association of obstetric problems with surgery and anesthesia in pregnant patients is not open to question. In the USA, at least 50,000 pregnant women each year undergo anesthesia and surgery during pregnancy for indications unrelated to the pregnancy. The risk of abortion is clearly higher following this experience. It is not obvious whether the underlying disease, surgery, anesthesia, or a combination of these factors is the cause of the increased risk.

Another concern not yet substantiated is that anesthetics during pregnancy may lead to an increased incidence of congenital anomalies. If anesthetics are teratogenic, the risk must be very small.

INTRAVENOUS ANESTHETICS

ULTRA-SHORT-ACTING BARBITURATES

When sulfur is substituted for oxygen at carbon 2 on the parent barbiturate compound (Fig 22–2), the duration of barbiturate-induced narcosis is significantly shortened. Although there are several ultra-short-acting barbiturates, thiopental is the one most commonly used for induction of anesthesia, often in combination with inhaled anesthetics. The general pharmacology of the barbiturates is discussed in Chapter 19.

Following intravenous administration, thiopental crosses the blood-brain barrier and, if given in sufficient dosage, produces hypnosis in one circulation time. Similar effects occur with other ultra-short-acting barbiturates, eg, thiamylal and methohexital. With all of these barbiturates, plasma:brain equilibrium occurs rapidly (in approximately 1 minute) because of high lipid solubility. Thiopental rapidly diffuses out of the brain and other highly vascular tissues and is redistributed to muscle, fat, and eventually all body tissues (Fig 22–5). It is because of this rapid removal from brain tissue that a single dose of thiopental is so short-acting.

Metabolism following thiopental administration is much slower than redistribution and takes place primarily in the liver. Less than 1% of an administered dose of thiopental is excreted unchanged by the kidney. Thiopental is metabolized at the rate of 12–16% per hour in humans following a single dose.

With large doses, thiopental causes dose-dependent decreases in arterial blood pressure, stroke volume, and cardiac output. This is due primarily to its myocardial depressant effect; there is little change in total peripheral resistance. However, thiopental also markedly increases venous vessel compliance, resulting in pooling of blood and impaired venous return to the heart.

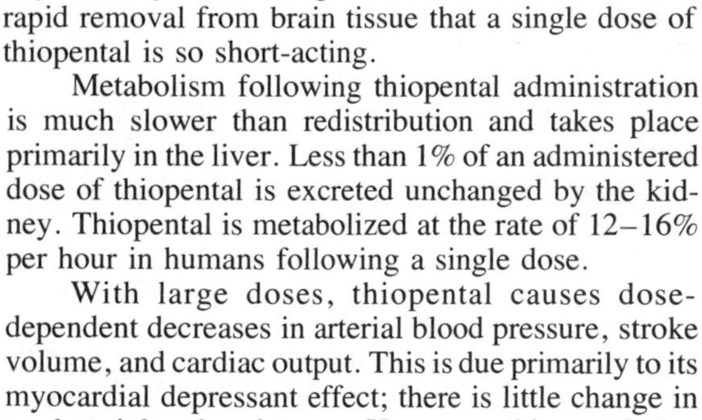

Figure 22–5. Redistribution of thiopental after an intravenous bolus administration.

Thiopental, like other barbiturates, is a potent respiratory depressant, lowering the sensitivity of the medullary respiratory center to carbon dioxide.

Cerebral metabolism and oxygen utilization are decreased after thiopental administration in proportion to the degree of cerebral depression. Cerebral blood flow is also decreased, but much less so than oxygen consumption. This makes thiopental a much more desirable drug for use in patients with cerebral swelling than the inhaled anesthetics, since intracranial pressure and blood volume are not increased.

Thiopental may reduce hepatic blood flow and glomerular filtration rate, but it produces no lasting effects on hepatic and renal function.

NEUROLEPTANESTHESIA

Neuroleptanesthesia is a term used to characterize a state in which the patient becomes completely disinterested and detached from the environment without loss of consciousness or the ability to obey commands or communicate with others. The desire to move or change body position is also lost. The most common drug combination used to produce this state is Innovar, which is a combination of droperidol, a butyrophenone, and fentanyl, a narcotic analgesic. This drug combination is usually used with nitrous oxide to produce complete general anesthesia.

KETAMINE

Ketamine—(±)-2-(*o*-chlorophenyl)-2-(methylamino)cyclohexanone; Fig 22–2—produces "dissociative anesthesia," characterized by catatonia, amnesia, and analgesia. Although it is a desirable anesthetic in many respects, ketamine has been associated with disorientation, sensory and perceptual illusions, and vivid dreams following anesthesia, effects that are termed "emergence phenomena." Diazepam, 0.2–0.3 mg/kg intravenously 5 minutes before administration of ketamine, reduces the incidence of these phenomena.

Ketamine, a lipophilic drug, is rapidly distributed into highly vascular organs, including the brain, and subsequently redistributed to less perfused tissues with concurrent hepatic metabolism and both urinary and biliary excretion.

Besides being a powerful analgesic, ketamine is the only intravenous anesthetic that routinely produces cardiovascular stimulation. Heart rate, arterial blood pressure, and cardiac output are usually significantly increased. The peak increases in these variables occur 2–4 minutes after intravenous injection and then slowly decline to normal over the next 10–20 minutes. Ketamine produces its cardiovascular stimulation by excitation of the central sympathetic nervous system.

Increases in plasma epinephrine and norepinephrine levels occur as early as 2 minutes after intravenous ketamine and return to control levels 15 minutes later.

Ketamine markedly increases blood flow, cerebral oxygen consumption, and intracranial pressure. Like most inhaled anesthetics, it is therefore a potentially dangerous drug when intracranial pressure is elevated.

In most patients, ketamine decreases the respiratory rate slightly for 2–3 minutes. Upper airway muscle tone is well maintained, and upper airway reflexes are usually (not always) active. Ketamine produces little other change in organ systems.

Because of the high incidence of postoperative psychic phenomena associated with its use, ketamine is not commonly used in general surgery in the USA, except for patients in shock and poor-risk geriatric patients, because of its cardiostimulatory properties. Because ketamine tends not to depress respiration and is short-acting, it is used quite often in outpatient anesthesia and in children undergoing dressing changes on burned tissue.

ETOMIDATE

Etomidate—(+)-ethyl 1-(α-methylbenzyl)-imidazole-5-carboxylate—is a carboxylated imidazole first synthesized in 1965. It causes rapid induction of anesthesia with minimal cardiovascular and respiratory changes. The compound has been studied extensively in Europe and is currently undergoing clinical trials in the USA. Distribution of etomidate is rapid, with a biphasic concentration curve showing distribution half-lives of 2.6 and 28.7 minutes. The drug is lipid-soluble and has a large volume of distribution (about 4.5 L/kg of body weight). Preliminary studies in humans indicate that almost 90% of the drug—of which only 2% is unchanged—eventually appears in the urine. This suggests that the total clearance of etomidate represents mostly metabolic clearance; the liver is the primary site of metabolism. Etomidate produces hypnosis within seconds, with no effect on heart rate, slight hypotension, and a low frequency of apnea. Unfortunately, it causes a high incidence of myoclonia and half of patients report pain during injection. The myoclonic movements are not associated with epileptiform discharges on the EEG.

ALTHESIN

Althesin is a proprietary mixture (also called Alfathesin) of 2 steroids: **alfaxalone** (3α-hydroxy-5α-pregnane-11,20-dione) and its 21-acetoxy ester, **alfadolone.** It induces sleep in less than 60 seconds, with a duration ranging from 2 to 13 minutes. The steroids are rapidly taken up by the liver, metabolized to more polar compounds possibly by conjugation, and then excreted in bile and urine. After 5 days, about 80% of the drug can be accounted for in the urine.

The drug causes hypotension to somewhat the same degree as thiopental and does not affect the heart rate.

Adverse reactions include skin rashes, hypotension, bronchospasm, and gastrointestinal distress (in that order of frequency).

PROPANIDID

Propanidid—4-[2-(diethylamino)-2-oxoethoxyl]3-methoxybenzeneacetic acid propyl ester—produces anesthesia with about the same rapidity as thiopental. Recovery is more complete and accumulation less likely with propanidid than with thiopental, since it is rapidly degraded by cholinesterase into inactive metabolites.

Propanidid causes hypotension, chiefly due to peripheral vasodilatation and a negative inotropic effect on the heart. Because of rapid recovery, an apparent lack of cumulative effect, and minimal cardiorespiratory effects, propanidid was at one time considered a promising anesthetic. However, numerous adverse reactions have been reported: Major epileptiform convulsions occur occasionally in patients with or without epilepsy, and severe hypotension with rash has occurred after injection.

• • •

References

Baden JM, Rice SA: Metabolism and toxicity of inhaled anesthetics. Page 383 in: *Anesthesia*. Miller RD (editor). Churchill Livingstone, 1981.

Cohen EN: Toxicity of inhalational anesthetic agents. *Br J Anaesth* 1978;**50:**665.

Eger EI II: *Anesthetic Uptake and Action*. Williams & Wilkins, 1974.

Eger EI II, Saidman LJ, Brandstater B: Minimum alveolar anesthetic concentration: A standard of anesthetic potency. *Anesthesiology* 1965;**26:**756.

Grogono AW, Seltzer JL: A guide to drug interactions in anesthetic practice. *Drugs* 1980;**19:**279.

Koblin DD, Eger EI II: Theories of narcosis. *N Engl J Med* 1979;**301:**1222.

Ngai SH: Effects of anesthetics on various organs. *N Engl J Med* 1980;**302:**564.

Sakai T, Takaori M: Biodegration of halothane, enflurane and methoxyflurane. *Br J Anaesth* 1978;**50:**785.

Trudell JR: Biophysical concepts in molecular mechanisms of anesthesia. Page 261 in: *Molecular Mechanisms of Anesthesia*. Fink BR (editor). Raven, 1980.

Vessey MP: Epidemiological studies of the occupational hazards of anaesthesia. *Anaesthesia* 1978;**33:**430.

White PF, Way WL, Trevor AJ: Ketamine: Its pharmacology and therapeutic uses. *Anesthesiology* 1982;**56:**119.

23 | Local Anesthetics

Luc M. Hondeghem, MD, PhD, & Ronald D. Miller, MD

Local anesthetics reversibly block impulse conduction along the axon. This action can be used to block pain sensation from—or sympathetic vasoconstrictor impulses to—specific areas of the body. Cocaine, the first such agent, was isolated by Niemann in 1860. It was introduced into clinical use by Koller in 1884 as an ophthalmic anesthetic. It was soon found to have strongly addicting central nervous system actions but was widely used, nevertheless, for 30 years, since it was the only local anesthetic drug available. In an attempt to improve the properties of cocaine, Einhorn in 1905 synthesized procaine, which became the dominant local anesthetic for the next 50 years. Since 1905, many local anesthetic agents have been synthesized. The goals of these efforts were reduction of local irritation and tissue damage, minimization of systemic toxicity, shorter onset of action, and longer duration of action. Lidocaine, currently the most popular agent, was synthesized in 1943 by Löfgren and may be considered the prototype local anesthetic agent.

I. BASIC PHARMACOLOGY OF LOCAL ANESTHETICS

Chemistry

Most local anesthetic agents consist of a lipophilic group (frequently an aromatic ring) connected by an intermediate chain (commonly including an ester or amide) to an ionizable group (usually a tertiary amine; Table 23–1). Optimal activity requires a delicate balance between the lipophilic and hydrophilic strengths of these groups. In addition to the general physical properties of the molecules, specific stereochemical configurations can also be important; ie, differences in the potency of stereoisomers have been documented for a few compounds. Since ester links (as in procaine) are more prone to hydrolysis than amide links, esters usually have a shorter duration of action.

Local anesthetics are weak bases. For therapeutic application, they are usually made available as salts for reasons of solubility and stability. In the body, they exist either as the uncharged base or as a cation. The relative proportions of these 2 forms is governed by their pK_a and the pH of the body fluids according to the Henderson-Hasselbalch equation:

$$\log \frac{\text{Cationic form}}{\text{Basic form}} = pK_a - pH$$

Since the pK_a of most local anesthetics is in the range of 8–9, the larger fraction in the body fluids at physiologic pH will be the charged, cationic form. The cationic form is thought to be the most active form at the receptor site, but the uncharged fraction is very important for rapid penetration of biologic membranes: the local anesthetic receptor is not accessible from the external side of the cell membrane (Fig 12–7). This partly explains why dentists and surgeons observe that local anesthetics are much less effective in infected tissues; these tissues have a low extracellular pH, so that a very low fraction of nonionized local anesthetic is available for diffusion into the cell.

Pharmacokinetics

Local anesthetics are usually administered by injection into the area of the nerve fibers to be blocked. Thus, absorption and distribution are not as important in controlling the onset of effect as in determining the rate of offset of anesthesia and the likelihood of central nervous system toxicity. Topical application of local anesthetics, on the other hand, requires drug diffusion for both onset and offset of anesthetic effect.

A. Absorption: Systemic absorption of injected local anesthetic from the site of administration is modified by several factors, including dosage, site of injection, drug-tissue binding, the presence of vasoconstricting substances, and the physicochemical and pharmacologic properties of the drug. Application of a local anesthetic to a highly vascular area such as the tracheal mucosa results in more rapid absorption and thus higher blood levels than if the local anesthetic had been injected into a poorly perfused area, such as tendon. For regional anesthesia involving block of large nerves, maximum blood levels of local anesthetic decrease according to site of administration in the following order: intercostal > caudal > epidural > brachial plexus > sciatic nerve.

Vasoconstrictor substances such as epinephrine reduce systemic absorption of local anesthetics from

Table 23–1. Structure and properties of some ester and amide local anesthetics.*

	Lipophilic Group	Intermediate Chain	Amine Substituents	Potency (Procaine = 1)	Duration of Action
Esters					
Cocaine	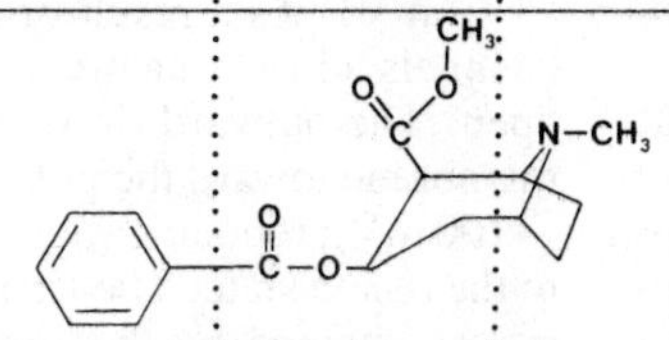			2	Medium
Procaine	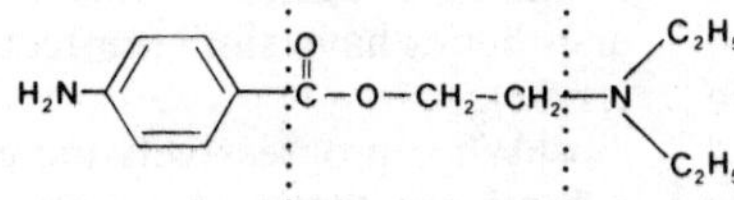			1	Short
Tetracaine	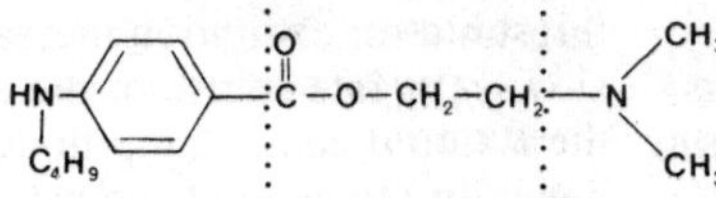			16	Long
Benzocaine	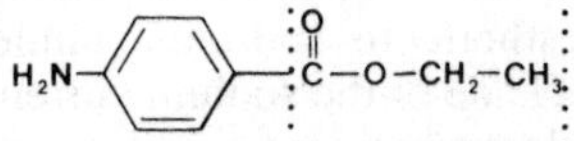			Surface use only	
Amides					
Lidocaine	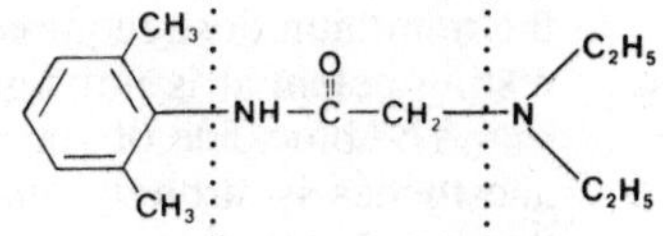			4	Medium
Mepivacaine	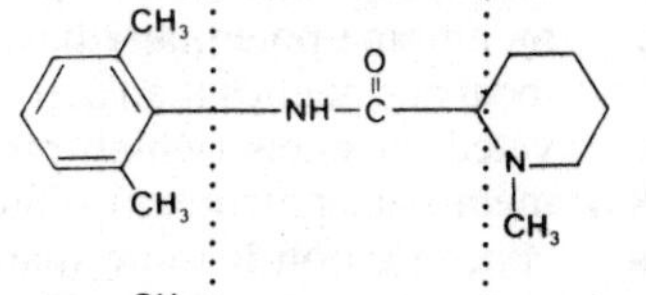			2	Medium
Bupivacaine	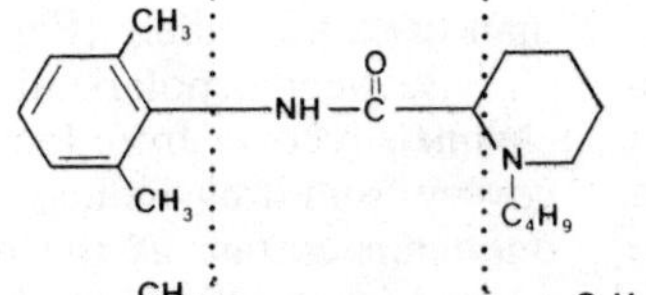			16	Long
Etidocaine	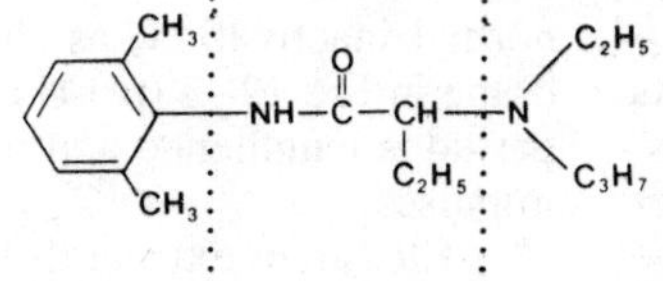			16	Long
Prilocaine	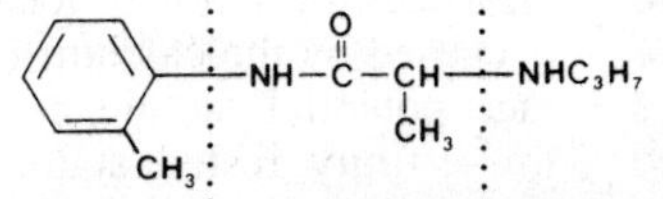			3	Medium

*Other chemical types are available including ethers (pramoxine), ketones (dyclonine), and phenetidin derivatives (phenacaine).

the depot site by decreasing regional blood flow in these areas. This is especially true for drugs with intermediate and short durations of action such as procaine, lidocaine, and mepivacaine (but not prilocaine). Neuronal uptake of the drug is presumably enhanced by the higher local drug concentration, and the systemic toxic effects of the drug are reduced, since blood levels are lowered by as much as one-third. The combination of reduced systemic absorption and enhanced uptake by the nerve is responsible for prolonging the local anesthetic effect by about 50%. Vasoconstrictors are less effective in prolonging anesthetic properties of the more lipid-soluble, long-acting drugs (bupivacaine, etidocaine), possibly because these molecules are highly tissue-bound.

B. Distribution: The amide local anesthetics are widely distributed after intravenous bolus administration. There is evidence that sequestration occurs in storage sites, possibly fat tissue. After an initial rapid distribution phase, which probably indicates uptake into highly perfused organs such as the brain, liver, kidney, and heart, a slower distribution phase occurs with uptake into moderately well perfused tissues, such as muscle and gut.

C. Metabolism and Excretion: Because of the extremely short plasma half-lives of the ester type agents (see below), their tissue distribution has not been studied. The local anesthetics are converted in the liver or in plasma to more water-soluble metabolites and then excreted in the urine. Since local anesthetics in the uncharged form diffuse readily through lipid, little or no urinary excretion of neutral form occurs. Acidification of urine will promote ionization of the tertiary base to the more water-soluble charged form, which is more readily excreted since it is not so easily reabsorbed by renal tubules.

Ester type local anesthetics are hydrolyzed very rapidly in the plasma by plasma cholinesterase. Therefore, they typically have very short half-lives, eg, less than 1 minute for procaine and chloroprocaine.

The amide linkage of amide local anesthetics is hydrolyzed by liver microsomal enzymes. There is considerable variation in the rate of liver metabolism of individual amide compounds, the approximate order being prilocaine (fastest) > etidocaine > lidocaine > mepivacaine > bupivacaine (slowest). As a result, toxicity from the amide type of local anesthetic is more likely to occur in patients with liver disease. For example, the average half-life of lidocaine may be increased from 1.8 hours in normal patients to over 6 hours in patients with liver disease.

Decreased hepatic removal of local anesthetics should also be anticipated in patients with reduced hepatic blood flow. For example, the hepatic elimination of lidocaine in animals anesthetized with halothane is slower than that measured in animals receiving nitrous oxide and curare. The reduced elimination may be related to decreased hepatic blood flow and to halothane-induced depression of hepatic microsomes. Propranolol may also prolong the half-life of amide local anesthetics such as lidocaine.

Pharmacodyamics

A. Mechanism of Action: The excitable membrane of nerve axons, like the membrane of cardiac muscle (Chapter 12) and neuronal cell bodies (Chapter 18), maintains a transmembrane potential of −90 to −60 mV. During excitation, the sodium channels open and a fast inward sodium current quickly depolarizes the membrane toward the sodium equilibrium potential (+40 mV). As a result of depolarization, the sodium channels close (inactivate) and potassium channels open. The outward flow of potassium repolarizes the membrane toward the potassium equilibrium potential (−100 mV); repolarization returns the sodium channels to the rested state. The transmembrane ionic gradients are maintained by the sodium pump. These characteristics are similar to those of heart muscle, and local anesthetics have similar effects in both tissues (Chapter 12).

When progressively increasing concentrations of a local anesthetic are applied to a nerve fiber, the threshold for excitation increases, impulse conduction slows, the rate of rise of the action potential declines, the action potential amplitude decreases, and, finally, the ability to generate an action potential is abolished. All of these effects result from the binding of the local anesthetic to sodium channels; binding results in blockade of the sodium current. If the sodium current is blocked over a critical length of the nerve, propagation across the blocked area is no longer possible. At the minimum dose required to block propagation, the resting potential is not significantly affected.

The blockade of sodium channels by most local anesthetics is strongly *state-dependent:* Channels in the rested state (which predominate at more negative membrane potentials) have a much lower affinity for local anesthetics than activated (open state) and inactivated channels (which predominate at more positive membrane potentials). Thus, the effect of a given drug concentration is more marked in rapidly firing axons than in resting fibers (Fig 23–1).

Between depolarizations of the axon, the sodium channels recover from local anesthetic block. The recovery from drug-induced block is one-thousandth to one-tenth as fast as the recovery of channels from normal inactivation, as shown for the cardiac membrane in Fig 12–3 (p 141). As a result, the refractory period is lengthened and the nerve can conduct fewer impulses.

Elevated extracellular calcium partially antagonizes the action of local anesthetics. This reversal is caused by the calcium-induced increase of the surface potential on the membrane, which favors the low-affinity rested state. Conversely, elevation of extracellular potassium depolarizes the membrane potential and favors the inactivated state. This enhances the effect of local anesthetics.

Structure-activity characteristics of local anesthetics. The smaller and more lipophilic the molecule, the faster the rate of interaction with the sodium channel receptor. Potency is positively correlated also with lipid solubility, as long as the agent

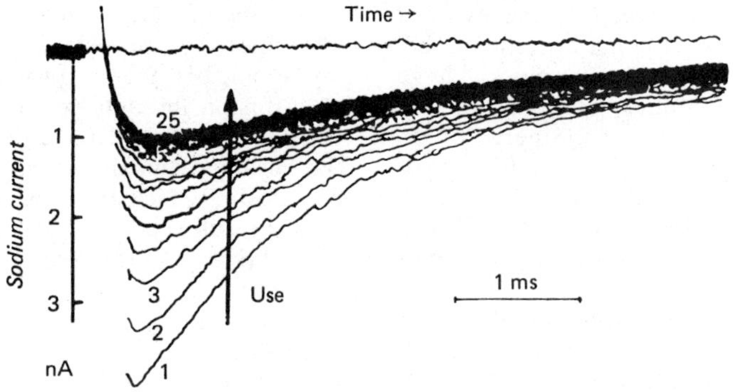

Figure 23–1. Effect of repetitive activity on the block of sodium current produced by a local anesthetic in a myelinated axon. A series of 25 pulses was applied, and the resulting sodium currents are superimposed. Note that the current produced by the pulses rapidly decreased from the first to the 25th pulse. A long rest period following the train resulted in recovery from block but the block could be reinstated by a subsequent train. nA = nanoamperes. (Modified slightly and reproduced, with permission, from Courtney KR: Mechanism of frequency-dependent inhibition of sodium currents in frog myelinated nerve by the lidocaine derivative GEA. *J Pharmacol Exp Ther* 1975;**195:**225.)

remains to some extent water-soluble, since water solubility is required for diffusion to the site of action. Lidocaine, procaine, and mepivacaine are more water-soluble than tetracaine, etidocaine, and bupivacaine. The latter agents are more potent and have longer durations of action. They also bind more extensively to proteins and will displace or be displaced from these binding sites by other drugs.

B. Actions:

1. Differential nerve block–Since local anesthetics are capable of blocking all nerves, their actions are not usually limited to the desired loss of sensation. Although motor paralysis may at times be desirable, it may also limit the ability of the patient to cooperate, eg, during obstetric delivery. During spinal anesthesia, motor paralysis may impair respiratory activity and autonomic nerve blockade may lead to hypotension. However, different types of nerve fibers differ significantly in their susceptibility to local anesthetic blockade on the basis of size and myelination (Table 23–2). Upon application of a local anesthetic to a nerve root, the smaller B and C fibers are blocked first. The small type A delta fibers are blocked next. Thus, pain fibers are blocked first; other sensations disappear next; and motor function is blocked last.

Local anesthetics preferentially block small fibers because the distance over which they can passively propagate an electrical impulse (related to the space constant) is shorter. During the onset of local anesthesia, when short sections of nerve are blocked, the small-diameter fibers are the first to fail to conduct. For the same reason, they will recover last upon washout of the drug. Myelinated nerves tend to become blocked before unmyelinated nerves of the same diameter. For this reason, the preganglionic beta fibers may be blocked before the smaller unmyelinated C fibers.

Another important reason for preferential blockade of sensory fibers follows directly from the state-dependent mechanism of action of local anesthetics and the fact that high-frequency discharge is blocked more readily than low-frequency discharge: Sensory fibers, especially pain fibers, have a high firing rate, whereas most motor fibers fire at a slower rate. As noted above, high rates of activity facilitate binding of local anesthetics to sodium channels.

An anatomic circumstance that sometimes creates exceptions to the above rules for differential nerve block is the location of the fiber in the peripheral bundle. In large nerve trunks, motor nerves are usually

Table 23–2. Relative size and susceptibility to block of types of nerve fibers.

Fiber Type	Function	Diameter (μm)	Myelination	Conduction Velocity (m/s)	Sensitivity to Block
Type A					
Alpha	Proprioception, motor	12–20	Heavy	70–120	+
Beta	Touch, pressure	5–12	Heavy	30–70	++
Gamma	Muscle spindles	3–6	Heavy	15–30	++
Delta	Pain, temperature	2–5	Heavy	12–30	+++
Type B	Preganglionic autonomic	<3	Light	3–15	++++
Type C					
Dorsal root	Pain	0.4–1.2	None	0.5–2.3	++++
Sympathetic	Postganglionic	0.3–1.3	None	0.7–2.3	++++

located circumferentially—hence, they are exposed first to the drug. Therefore, it is not uncommon that motor nerve block occurs before sensory block in large mixed nerves. In the extremities, proximal sensory fibers are located in the mantle of the nerve trunk, whereas the distal sensory innervation is in the core of the nerve. Thus, during infiltration block of a large nerve, anesthesia first develops proximally and then spreads distally as the drug penetrates into the core of the nerve.

2. Effects on other excitable membranes– Local anesthetics have weak neuromuscular blocking effects that are of little clinical importance. However, their effects on cardiac cell membranes are of major clinical significance. Some are useful antiarrhythmia agents (see Chapter 12) at concentrations lower than those required to produce nerve block.

II. CLINICAL PHARMACOLOGY OF LOCAL ANESTHETICS

Local anesthetics can provide temporary but complete analgesia of well-defined parts of the body after topical application, after injection in the vicinity of peripheral nerve endings and major nerve trunks, or after instillation within the epidural or subarachnoid spaces surrounding the spinal cord. In addition, block of autonomic sympathetic fibers can be used to evaluate the role of sympathetic tone in patients with peripheral vasospasm.

The choice of local anesthetic for a specific procedure is usually based on the duration of action required. Procaine (Novocain) and chloroprocaine (Nesacaine) are short-acting; lidocaine (Xylocaine, etc), mepivacaine (Carbocaine, Isocaine), and prilocaine (Citanest) have an intermediate duration of action; tetracaine (Pontocaine), bupivacaine (Marcaine), and etidocaine (Duranest) are long-acting drugs (Table 23–1).

As noted above, the anesthetic effect of the agents with short and intermediate durations of action can be prolonged by increasing the dose or by adding a vasoconstrictor agent, such as epinephrine or phenylephrine. The vasoconstrictor retards the removal of drug from the injection site. In addition, it decreases the blood level and hence the chance of toxicity.

The onset of local anesthesia is sometimes accelerated by the use of solutions saturated with carbon dioxide ("carbonated"). The high tissue level of CO_2 results in intracellular acidosis (CO_2 crosses membranes readily), which in turn results in intracellular accumulation of the cationic form of the local anesthetic.

Repeated injection of local anesthetics during epidural anesthesia results in loss of effectiveness (tachyphylaxis). This is probably a consequence of local extracellular acidosis. Local anesthetics are commonly marketed as hydrochloride salts (pH 4–6). After injection, the salts are buffered in the tissue to physiologic pH, thereby providing sufficient free base for diffusion through axonal membranes. However, repeated injections deplete the local available buffer. The ensuing acidosis increases the extracellular cationic form, which diffuses poorly into axons. The clinical result is apparent tachyphylaxis, especially in areas of limited buffer reserve, such as the cerebrospinal fluid.

Toxicity

Ultimately, local anesthetic agents are absorbed from the site of administration. If blood levels rise too high, effects on several organ systems may be observed.

A. Central Nervous System: Since prehistoric times, the natives of Peru have chewed the leaves of the indigenous plant *Erythroxylon coca,* the source of cocaine, to obtain a feeling of well-being and reduce fatigue. Intense central nervous system effects can be achieved by sniffing cocaine powder and smoking cocaine base. This abuse of the drug has recently gained in popularity (see Chapter 29). Other local anesthetics have been thought to lack the euphoriant effects of cocaine. However, recent studies indicate that some habitual cocaine users cannot differentiate between intranasal cocaine and lidocaine given by the same route.

Other central nervous system effects include sleepiness, light-headedness, visual and auditory disturbances, and restlessness. At higher concentrations, nystagmus and shivering may occur. Finally, overt tonic-clonic convulsions followed by central nervous system depression and death may occur with all local anesthetics, including cocaine. Local anesthetics apparently lead to depression of cortical inhibitory pathways, thereby allowing unopposed activity of excitatory components. This transitional stage of unbalanced excitation may be followed by generalized central nervous system depression if higher blood levels of local anesthetic are reached.

Over 90% of serious toxic reactions to local anesthetics are due to convulsions from excessive blood levels. These are best prevented by administering the smallest dose required for adequate anesthesia. When large doses must be administered, premedication with a benzodiazepine, eg, diazepam, 0.1–0.2 mg/kg parenterally, probably provides significant prophylaxis against seizures. If seizures do occur, it is essential to prevent hypoxemia. Although administration of oxygen is recommended in the treatment of convulsions from local anesthesia, oxygen inhalation does not prevent seizure activity. However, hyperoxemia after onset of seizures appears to be beneficial. Conversely, hypercapnia and acidosis appear to promote the occurrence of seizures. Thus, hyperventilation is recommended during treatment of seizures. Hyperventilation elevates blood pH, which in turn lowers extracellular potassium. This hyperpolarizes the transmembrane potential of axons, which favors the rested or low-affinity state of the sodium channels, resulting in decreased local anesthetic toxicity.

Seizures induced by local anesthetics can also be treated with small doses of short-acting barbiturates, eg, thiopental, 1–2 mg/kg intravenously, or diazepam, 0.1 mg/kg intravenously. The muscular manifestations can be suppressed by a short-acting neuromuscular blocking agent, eg, succinylcholine, 0.5–1 mg/kg intravenously. It should be emphasized that succinylcholine does not obliterate cortical manifestations on the electroencephalogram. In especially severe cases of convulsions, intubation of the trachea combined with succinylcholine administration and mechanical ventilation can prevent pulmonary aspiration of gastric contents and facilitate hyperventilation therapy.

B. Cardiovascular System: The cardiovascular effects of local anesthetics result partly from direct effects upon the cardiac and smooth muscle membranes and partly from indirect effects upon the autonomic nerves. As described in Chapter 12, local anesthetics block cardiac sodium channels and thus depress abnormal cardiac pacemaker activity, excitability, and conduction. They also depress the strength of cardiac contraction and cause arteriolar dilatation—except for cocaine, which causes vasoconstriction—both leading to hypotension. Although cardiovascular collapse and death usually occur only after large doses, they may result occasionally from the small amounts used for infiltration anesthesia.

As noted above, cocaine differs from the other local anesthetics in its cardiovascular effects. The blockade of norepinephrine reuptake results in vasoconstriction and hypertension. It may also precipitate cardiac arrhythmias. The vasoconstriction produced by cocaine can lead to ischemia of the nasal mucosa and, in chronic users, to ulceration of the mucous membrane and even damage to the septum. This vasoconstrictor property of cocaine can be used clinically to decrease bleeding from mucosal damage such as occurs with epistaxis.

C. Blood: The administration of large doses (> 10 mg/kg) of prilocaine during regional anesthesia may lead to accumulation of the metabolite *o*-toluidine, an oxidizing agent capable of converting hemoglobin to methemoglobin. When sufficient methemoglobin is present (3–5 mg/dL), the patient may appear cyanotic and the blood chocolate-colored. Such levels of methemoglobinemia are tolerated by healthy individuals but may cause decompensation in patients with cardiac or pulmonary disease and require immediate treatment. Reducing agents such as methylene blue or, less satisfactorily, ascorbic acid may be given intravenously to rapidly convert methemoglobin to hemoglobin.

D. Allergic Reactions: The ester type local anesthetics are metabolized to *p*-aminobenzoic acid derivatives. These metabolites are responsible for allergic reactions in a small percentage of the population. Amides are not metabolized to *p*-aminobenzoic acid, and allergic reactions to agents of the amide group are extremely rare.

• • •

References

Covino BG, Vassallo HG: *Local Anesthetics: Mechanisms of Action in Clinical Use*. Grune & Stratton, 1976.

Covino BG et al: Prolonged sensory/motor deficits following inadvertent spinal anesthesia. (Editorial.) *Anesth Analg (Cleve)* 1980;**59:**399.

Fink BR (editor): *Progress in Anesthesiology: Molecular Mechanisms of Anesthesia*. Vol 2. Raven Press, 1980.

Hille B: Local anesthetics: Hydrophilic and hydrophobic pathways for the drug-receptor reactions. *J Gen Physiol* 1977;**69:**497.

Mather LE, Cousins MJ: Local anesthetics and their current clinical use. *Drugs* 1979;**18:**185.

Savarese JJ, Covino BG: Pharmacology of local anesthetics. Page 563 in: *Anesthesia*. Miller RD (editor). Churchill Livingstone, 1981.

Tucker GT, Mather LE: The clinical pharmacokinetics of local anesthetics. *Clin Pharmacokinet* 1979;**4:**241.

24 | Skeletal Muscle Relaxants

Ronald D. Miller, MD

Drugs that affect skeletal muscle function fall into 2 major therapeutic groups: those used during surgical procedures to cause paralysis (neuromuscular blockers) and those used to reduce spasticity in a variety of neurologic conditions (spasmolytics). Members of the first group, as their name implies, interfere with transmission at the neuromuscular end-plate and are not CNS-active drugs. However, because they are used almost exclusively as an adjunct to general anesthesia, they are often discussed in connection with central nervous system agents. Drugs in the second group have traditionally been called "centrally acting" muscle relaxants. However, at least one of its important members (dantrolene) has no central effects, so the traditional name is somewhat inappropriate.

NEUROMUSCULAR BLOCKING DRUGS

History

During the 16th century, European explorers found that natives of the Amazon Basin of South America were using an arrow poison that produced death by skeletal muscle paralysis. This poison later became the subject of intense investigation. **Curare,** the active crude material, formed the basis for some of the earliest scientific studies in pharmacology. The active principle from curare, **tubocurarine (d-tubocurarine),** and its synthetic derivatives have had a tremendous influence on the practice of anesthesia and have been useful also in defining normal neuromuscular physiologic mechanisms.

Normal Neuromuscular Function

Theoretically, muscular relaxation and paralysis can occur from interruption of function at several sites, including the central nervous system, myelinated somatic nerves, unmyelinated motor nerve terminals, the cholinergic receptor, the motor end-plate, and the muscle membrane or contractile apparatus (Fig 24–1). The mechanism of neuromuscular transmission at the end-plate is similar to that described in Chapter 4, with arrival of an impulse at the motor nerve terminal, influx of calcium, and release of acetylcholine (Fig 24–1). Acetylcholine then diffuses across the synaptic cleft to the nicotinic cholinergic receptor located on the motor end-plate. When the receptor and acetylcholine interact, permeability of the membrane in the end-plate region increases to sodium primarily but also to potassium. Sodium moves from outside to inside the membrane, and the resting membrane potential depolarizes. This change in voltage is termed the end-plate potential. The magnitude of the end-plate potential is directly related to the amount of acetylcholine released. If the potential is small, the permeability and the end-plate potential return to normal without an impulse being propagated from the end-plate region to the rest of the muscle membrane. However, if the end-plate potential is large, the muscle membrane is depolarized, and the impulse will be propagated along the entire muscle fiber. Muscle contraction is then initiated by the process known as excitation-contraction coupling. The released acetylcholine is removed from the end-plate region by diffusion and rapid enzymatic destruction by acetylcholinesterase.

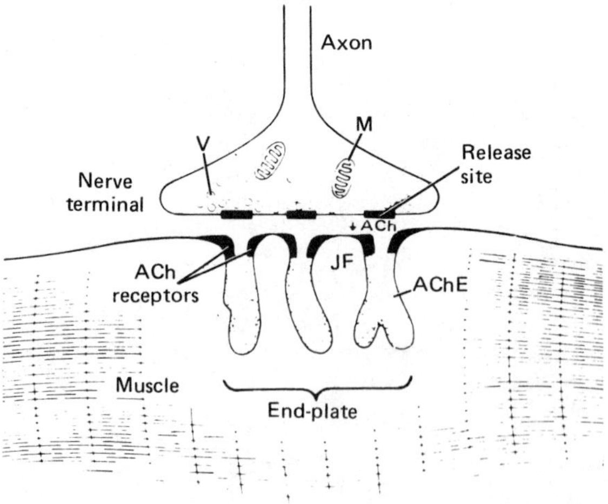

Figure 24–1. Schematic representation of the neuromuscular junction. V = transmitter vesicle; M = mitochondrion; ACh = acetylcholine; AChE = acetylcholinesterase; JF = junctional folds. (Reproduced with permission, from Drachman DB: Myasthenia gravis. *N Engl J Med* 1978;**298**:135.)

Blockade of normal end-plate function can occur by 2 mechanisms. Pharmacologic blockade of the agonist, acetylcholine, is characteristic of *antagonist* drugs like curare. Block of transmission can also be produced by an excess of depolarizing *agonist*. (This paradoxic effect also occurs at the ganglionic nicotinic cholinergic receptor.) The prototype depolarizing blocking drug is succinylcholine, although a similar depolarizing block can be produced by acetylcholine itself.

I. BASIC PHARMACOLOGY OF NEUROMUSCULAR BLOCKING DRUGS

Chemistry

All of the neuromuscular blocking drugs are structurally similar to acetylcholine. Often this resemblance is to 2 acetylcholine molecules linked end-to-end. In fact, succinylcholine is such a compound (Fig 24–2). In contrast to the single linear structure of depolarizing drugs such as succinylcholine, the nondepolarizing agents conceal the "double-acetylcholine" structure in a variety of bulky, relatively rigid ring systems (Figs 24–2 and 24–3). Another feature common to all useful drugs in this class is the quaternary nitrogen, which makes them poorly soluble in lipid. Agents currently available for use in the USA are shown in Figs 24–2 and 24–3. Two new agents currently in clinical trials are shown in Fig 24–4.

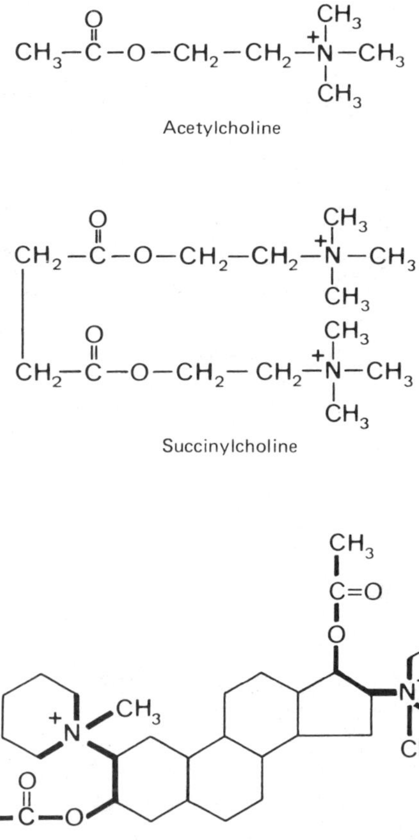

Figure 24–2. Structural relationship of succinylcholine, a depolarizing agent, and pancuronium, a nondepolarizing agent, to acetylcholine, the neuromuscular transmitter. Succinylcholine, originally called diacetylcholine, is simply 2 molecules of acetylcholine linked through the acetate methyl groups. Pancuronium may be viewed as 2 acetylcholinelike fragments *(outlined in dark print)* oriented on a steroid nucleus.

Pharmacokinetics of Neuromuscular Blocking Drugs

A. Nondepolarizing Drugs: The rate of disappearance of a nondepolarizing neuromuscular blocking drug from blood is characterized by a rapid initial disappearance followed by a slower decay (Fig 24–5). Distribution to tissues is the major cause of the initial decrease, whereas the slower decay is due to excretion. Because neuromuscular blocking drugs are highly ionized, they do not cross membranes well and have a limited volume of distribution—80–140 mL/kg, not much larger than blood volume.

Tubocurarine, metocurine (dimethyltubocurarine), and gallamine (Fig 24–3) are not metabolized. Gallamine is entirely dependent on the kidney for its elimination. In contrast, only about 50–60% of an injected dose of tubocurarine or metocurine is excreted in the urine over a 24-hour period in humans. The exact route of excretion of the remainder of these agents in humans is unclear, though it is presumed that biliary excretion accounts for most of it. Although the kidney is the major route of excretion for pancuronium, this drug is also metabolized (15–25%) to 3-hydroxy-, 17-hydroxy-, and 3,17-dihydroxypancuronium. Most of the remaining drug is excreted unchanged in the urine. 3-Hydroxypancuronium has about half the potency of its parent drug, pancuronium. Although the remaining metabolites also have neuromuscular blocking properties, they are very weak.

Vecuronium is a new short-acting neuromuscular blocking drug (Fig 24–4) that is not heavily dependent upon the kidney for its elimination. Only about 15% of an injected dose of this agent is eliminated by the kidney; presumably, the remainder is eliminated in the bile. It is not known whether it is metabolized. Atracurium (Fig 24–4) is another new, short-acting nondepolarizing muscle relaxant with many of the same characteristics as vecuronium; its metabolism has not been studied. It may undergo a form of spontaneous breakdown (Hofmann elimination) of the quaternary group. If this mechanism is proved for atracurium, it may be inferred that the drug does not depend on renal or hepatic mechanisms for inactivation.

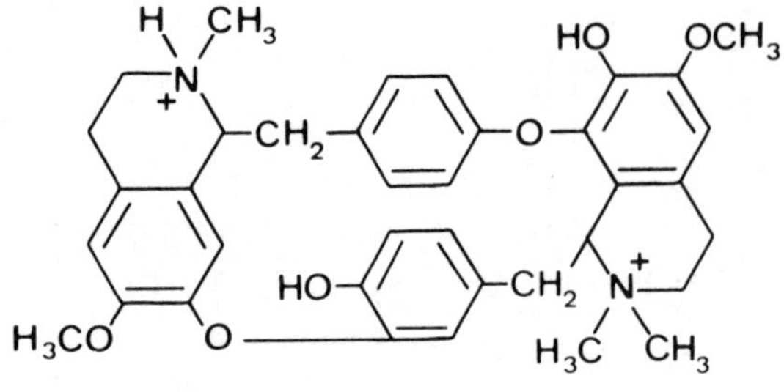

Tubocurarine

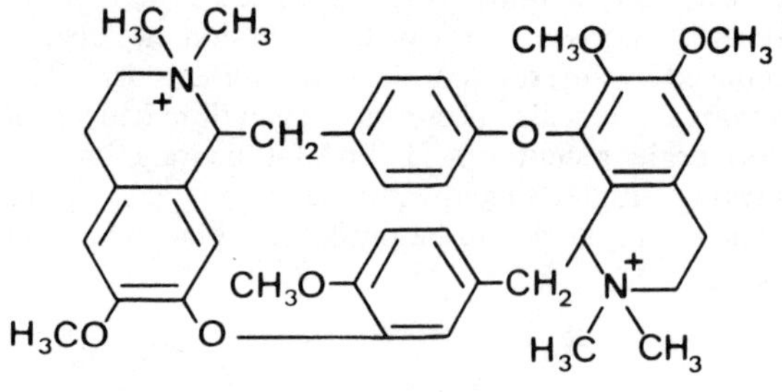

Dimethyltubocurarine

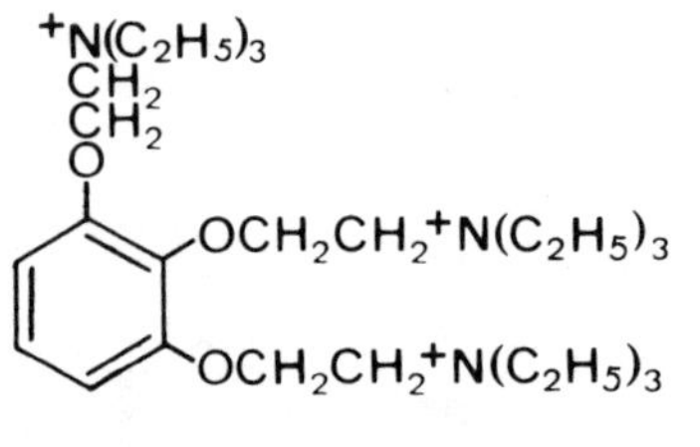

Gallamine

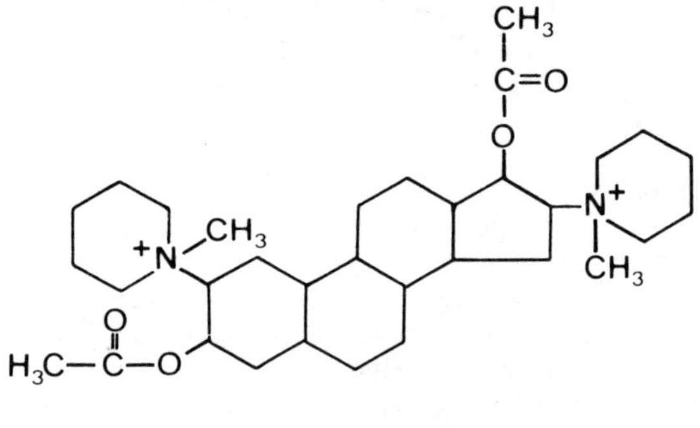

Pancuronium

Figure 24–3. Chemical formulas of nondepolarizing blocking drugs currently available in the USA.

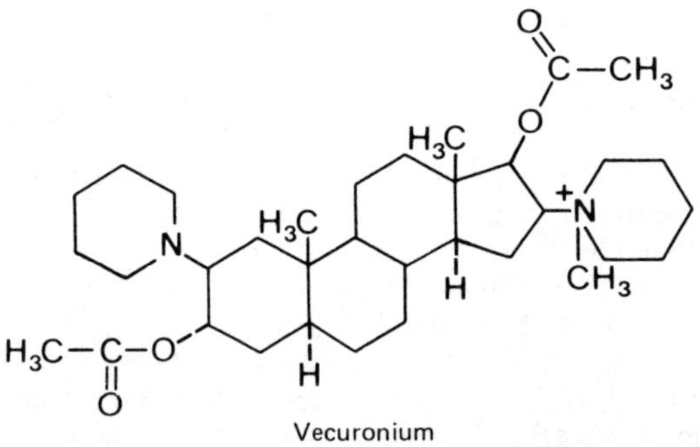

Vecuronium

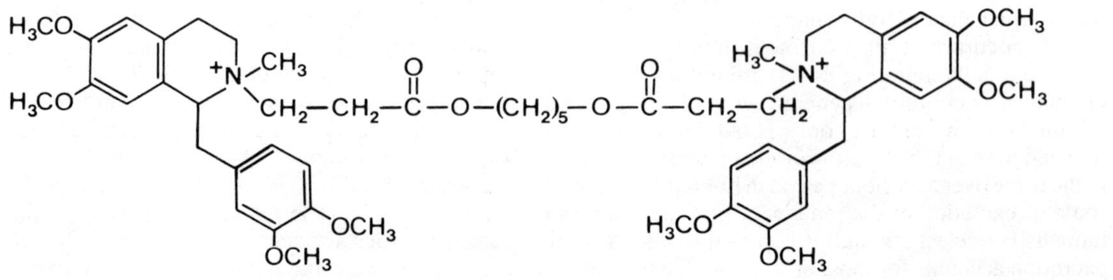

Atracurium

Figure 24–4. Chemical formulas of short-acting, nondepolarizing neuromuscular blocking drugs undergoing clinical trials in the USA and Europe.

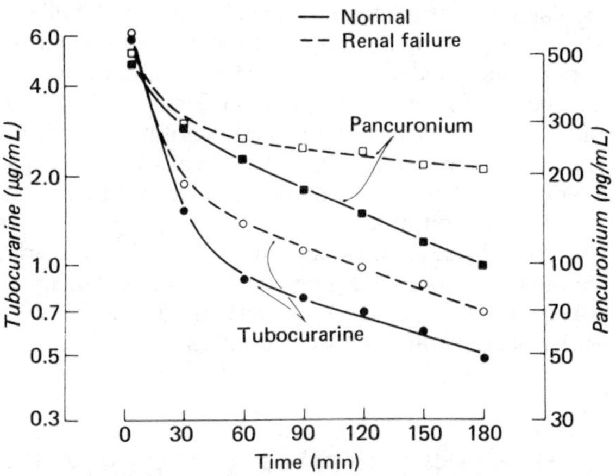

Figure 24–5. Rates at which the plasma concentrations of tubocurarine and pancuronium decrease in patients with and without renal failure. Note that the decay rates are about the same in patients with normal renal function. However, the decay rate is much slower in patients with renal failure receiving pancuronium than in those receiving tubocurarine. (Reprinted, with permission, from Miller RD, Savarese JJ: Pharmacology of muscle relaxants, their antagonists, and monitoring of neuromuscular function. In: *Anesthesia*. Miller RD [editor]. Churchill Livingstone, 1981.)

B. Depolarizing Drugs: The extremely brief duration of action of succinylcholine (5–10 minutes) is due chiefly to its rapid hydrolysis by pseudocholinesterase, an enzyme of the liver and plasma. The initial metabolite, succinylmonocholine, is a much weaker neuromuscular blocker. It in turn is metabolized to succinic acid and choline. Pseudocholinesterase has an enormous capacity to hydrolyze succinylcholine at a very rapid rate; as a result, only a small fraction of the original intravenous dose reaches the neuromuscular junction. Since there is little or no pseudocholinesterase at the motor end-plate, the neuromuscular blockade of succinylcholine is terminated by its diffusion away from the end-plate into extracellular fluid. Pseudocholinesterase, therefore, influences the duration of action of succinylcholine by controlling the rate at which the latter is hydrolyzed before it reaches the end-plate.

Neuromuscular blockade by succinylcholine may be prolonged in patients with an abnormal variant of pseudocholinesterase of genetic origin. The "dibucaine number"—a test for ability to metabolize succinylcholine—can be used to identify such patients. Under standardized test conditions, dibucaine inhibits the normal enzyme about 80% and an abnormal enzyme only 20%. Many genetic variants of pseudocholinesterase have been identified, although the dibucaine-related variants are the most important.

Mechanism of Action

A. Nondepolarizing Blocking Drugs: Neuromuscular blocking drugs classified as nondepolarizing antagonists—tubocurarine and metocurine (from curare), pancuronium, gallamine, vecuronium, and atracurium—produce a surmountable blockade. They are thought to combine with end-plate acetylcholine receptors but not to activate them. If sufficient receptors are occupied by a nondepolarizing neuromuscular blocking drug and are therefore unavailable to acetylcholine, neuromuscular transmission will fail. Since nondepolarizing blocking drugs prevent the postsynaptic membrane from depolarizing, they are also called stabilizing agents. This is the main mechanism by which these drugs act, but they may also have presynaptic effects; ie, they may decrease the amount of acetylcholine released in response to an impulse.

One consequence of the surmountable nature of the postsynaptic blockade produced by these agents is the fact that tetanic stimulation, by releasing a large quantity of acetylcholine, is followed by a transient posttetanic breakthrough or relief of the block (Fig 24–6). An important clinical consequence of the same

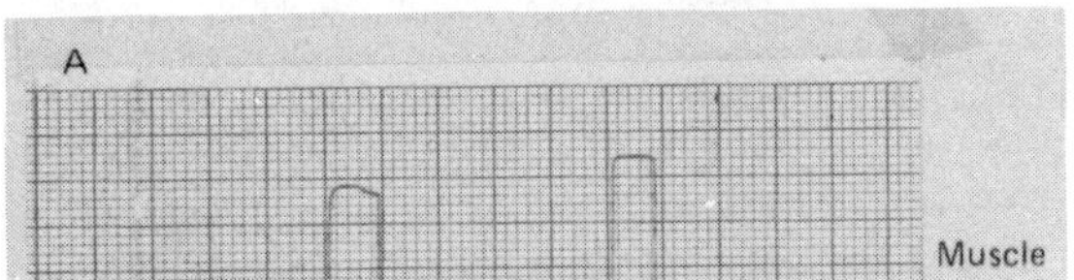

Figure 24–6. Effects of tubocurarine on neuromuscular transmission in humans. Panel *A* shows the twitch response induced by stimulation of the ulnar nerve in an anesthetized patient before curare was administered. The tetanic contractions (T) were evoked by stimulation at 50 pulses per second and were well maintained. A small increase (twitches marked by *) in twitch amplitude followed each tetanus. Panel *B* shows the effects of a small dose of tubocurarine in the same patient. The single stimulus twitch responses were reduced about 50%. The responses to tetanic stimulation showed a strong initial contraction followed by a rapid decline of tension ("fade"). The twitch responses following tetanic stimulation were increased by almost 80% (posttetanic potentiation).

Table 24–1. Comparison of a typical nondepolarizing muscle relaxant (tubocurarine) and a depolarizing muscle relaxant (succinylcholine).

	Tubocurarine	Succinylcholine Phase I	Succinylcholine Phase II
Administration of tubocurarine	Additive	Antagonistic	Augmented*
Administration of succinylcholine	Antagonistic	Additive	Augmented*
Effect of neostigmine	Antagonistic	Augmented*	Antagonistic
Initial excitatory effect on skeletal muscle	None	Fasciculations	None
Response to a tetanic stimulus	Unsustained	Sustained†	Unsustained
Posttetanic facilitation	Yes	No	Yes
Rate of recovery	30–60 min‡	4–8 min	> 20 min‡

*It is not known whether this interaction is additive or synergistic (superadditive).

†The amplitude is decreased, but the response is sustained.

‡The rate depends on the dose and on the completeness of neuromuscular blockade.

principle is the ability of cholinesterase inhibitors to reverse the blockade.

The characteristics of a nondepolarizing muscular blockade are summarized in Table 24–1.

B. Depolarizing Drugs:

1. Phase I block (depolarizing)–Succinylcholine is the only depolarizing neuromuscular blocking drug commonly used clinically. Its neuromuscular effects can be conveniently thought of as almost identical to those of acetylcholine, except that the former produces a longer effect. Succinylcholine reacts with a receptor to cause depolarization of the end-plate, and this in turn spreads to and depolarizes adjacent membranes, causing generalized disorganized contraction of muscle motor units. Because succinylcholine is not metabolized as rapidly as acetylcholine, the depolarized membranes remain depolarized and unresponsive to additional impulses. Because excitation-contraction coupling requires repolarization (''repriming'') and repetitive firing to maintain muscle tension, a flaccid paralysis results. Phase I block is potentiated, not reversed, by cholinesterase inhibitors.

Characteristics of a depolarizing blockade are summarized in Table 24–1.

2. Phase II block (desensitization)–With continued exposure to succinylcholine, the initial depolarization decreases; in other words, the membrane becomes repolarized. Despite this repolarization, the membrane cannot be depolarized again by acetylcholine as long as succinylcholine is present. The mechanism for the development of a phase II block is unknown. One hypothesis is that a nonexcitable area develops in the investing muscle membrane (immediately surrounding the end-plate) which becomes repolarized shortly after the arrival of succinylcholine. This area presumably impedes centrifugal spread of impulses initiated by the action of acetylcholine on the receptor. Because the end-plate is partially repolarized and still does not respond to acetylcholine, the membrane is said to be desensitized to the effects of acetylcholine. Therefore, this block has also been called a ''desensitization block.''

The characteristics of a phase II block are nearly identical to those of a nondepolarizing block, ie, a nonsustained response to a tetanic stimulus and reversal by acetylcholinesterase inhibitors.

II. CLINICAL PHARMACOLOGY OF NEUROMUSCULAR BLOCKING DRUGS

Skeletal Muscle Paralysis

Before the introduction of neuromuscular blocking drugs, adequate skeletal muscle relaxation could only be achieved by deep anesthesia that was often associated with hazardous depressant effects on various organ systems, especially the cardiorespiratory system. The drugs have made it possible to achieve adequate muscle relaxation for all surgical requirements without the depressant effects of deep anesthesia.

A. Nondepolarizing Drugs: During anesthesia, the intravenous administration of tubocurarine, 0.12–0.4 mg/kg, will first cause motor weakness; ultimately, skeletal muscles become totally flaccid and nonexcitable to stimulation (Fig 24–7). Muscles capable of rapid movement, such as those of the jaw and eye, are paralyzed before the larger muscles of the limbs and trunk. Lastly, the diaphragm is paralyzed and respiration ceases. If ventilation is controlled, no adverse effects occur. Recovery of muscles usually occurs in reverse order, with the diaphragm regaining function first. The above dose of tubocurarine usually lasts 30–60 minutes by gross evaluation; more subtle evidence of paralysis may last for another hour. Pancuronium and vecuronium are about 6 times more potent than tubocurarine, metocurine about 4 times more potent, and gallamine about one-fifth as potent. Atracurium is slightly more potent than tubocurarine.

B. Depolarizing Drugs: Following the intravenous administration of succinylcholine, 0.5–1 mg/kg, transient muscle fasciculations occur, especially over the cheeks and abdomen, although general anesthesia tends to attenuate them (Fig 24–8). As paralysis develops, the arm, neck, and leg muscles are involved at a time when there is only slight weakness of the facial and pharyngeal muscles. Respiratory muscle weakness follows. The onset of neuromuscular blockade from succinylcholine is very rapid, usually within 1 minute. Because of its rapid hydrolysis by pseudocholinesterase in the plasma and liver, the duration

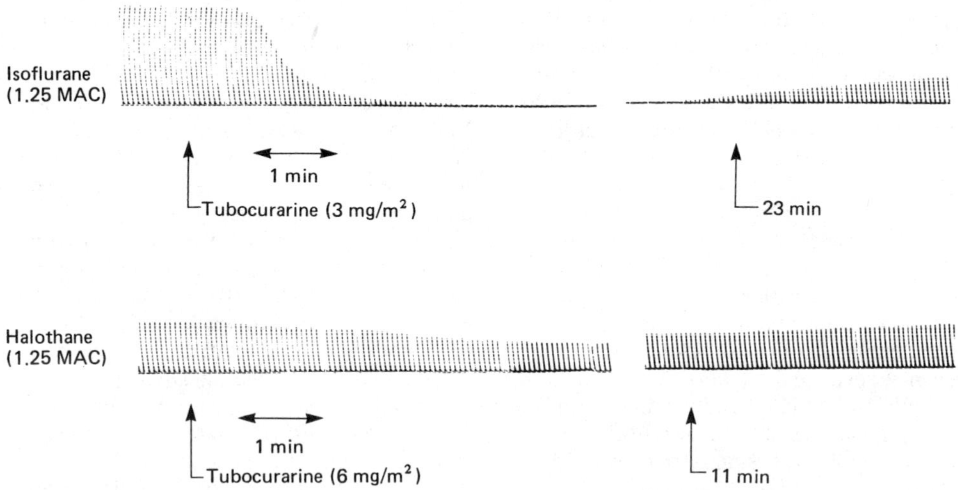

Figure 24–7. Neuromuscular blockade from tubocurarine during isoflurane and halothane anesthesia. Note that at equivalent levels of anesthesia, isoflurane augments the block far more than does halothane.

of neuromuscular block from this dose usually is 5–10 minutes.

Cardiovascular Effects

All of the currently used nondepolarizing muscle relaxants produce cardiovascular effects. Many of these effects are mediated by autonomic and histamine receptors (Table 24–2). Tubocurarine and, to a much lesser extent, metocurine produce hypotension. This hypotension probably results from the liberation of histamine and, in larger doses, from ganglionic blockade. Premedication with promethazine, an antihistamine drug, will attenuate tubocurarine-induced hypotension. Pancuronium causes a moderate increase in heart rate and to a lesser extent cardiac output, with little or no change in systemic vascular resistance. Although the tachycardia is primarily due to a vagolytic action, release of norepinephrine from adrenergic nerve endings and blockade of neuronal uptake of norepinephrine have been suggested as secondary mechanisms. Gallamine increases heart rate by both vagolytic action and sympathetic stimulation. The latter involves the release of norepinephrine from adrenergic nerve endings in the heart by an unknown mechanism.

Table 24–2. Autonomic effects of neuromuscular blocking drugs.

Drug	Effect on Autonomic Ganglia	Effect on Cardiac Muscarinic Receptors	Effect on Histamine Release
Succinylcholine	Stimulates	Stimulates	Slight
Tubocurarine	Blocks	None	Moderate
Metocurine	Blocks weakly	None	Slight
Gallamine	None	Blocks strongly	None
Pancuronium	None	Blocks moderately	None
Vecuronium	None	None	None
Atracurium	None	None	Slight

Succinylcholine-induced cardiac arrhythmias are many and varied. The drug stimulates all autonomic cholinergic receptors: nicotinic receptors in both sympathetic and parasympathetic ganglia and muscarinic receptors in the sinus node of the heart. In low doses, both negative inotropic and chronotropic responses occur that can be attenuated by administration of atropine. With large doses, positive inotropic and chronotropic effects may result. Bradycardia has been repeatedly observed when a second dose of the drug is

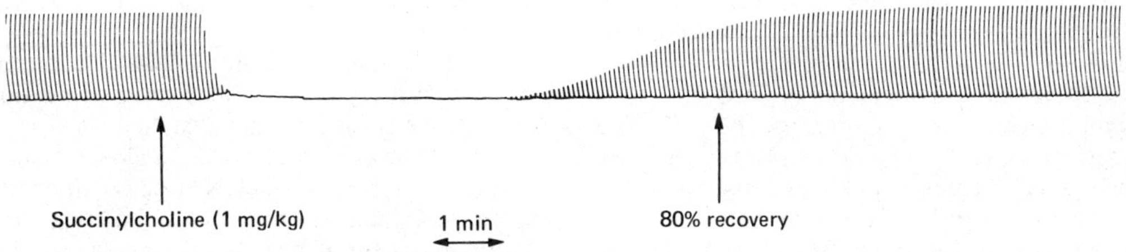

Figure 24–8. Neuromuscular blockade from succinylcholine during anesthesia. Fasciculations are not seen, because the anesthetic obliterated them.

given approximately 5 minutes after the first dose. This bradycardia can be prevented by thiopental, atropine, ganglionic blocking drugs, and nondepolarizing muscle relaxants. Direct myocardial effects, increased muscarinic stimulation, and ganglionic stimulation may all be involved in the bradycardia response.

Other Effects

A. Hyperkalemia: Some patients respond to succinylcholine by an exaggerated release of potassium into the blood, occasionally of such magnitude that cardiac arrest occurs. Patients with burns, nerve damage or neuromuscular disease, closed head injury and other trauma, peritoneal infections, and renal failure are especially susceptible. The mechanism of the hyperkalemic response has not been established, but it may be related to depolarization in association with the increased number of receptors that occur extrajunctionally in a denervated muscle or one that is not used.

B. Intraocular Pressure: Succinylcholine causes an increase in intraocular pressure. The increase is manifested 1 minute after injection, is maximal at 2–4 minutes, and subsides after 5 minutes. The mechanism for this effect has not been clearly defined, but it may involve contraction of tonic myofibrils or transient dilatation of choroidal blood vessels. Despite the increase in pressure, the use of succinylcholine for eye operations is not contraindicated unless the anterior chamber is to be opened.

C. Intragastric Pressure: In some patients, especially muscular ones, the fasciculations associated with succinylcholine will cause an increase in intragastric pressure ranging from 5 to 40 cm of water. This may make emesis more likely, with the potential hazard of aspiration of gastric contents.

D. Muscle Pain: The incidence of muscle pain following succinylcholine administration varies from 0.2 to 8.9%. It occurs more frequently in ambulatory than in bedridden patients. The pain is thought to be secondary to damage produced in muscle by the unsynchronized contractions of adjacent muscle fibers just before the onset of paralysis. Muscle damage has been verified by the occurrence of myoglobinuria following the use of succinylcholine.

Interactions With Other Drugs

A. Anesthetics: Inhaled anesthetics augment the neuromuscular block from nondepolarizing muscle relaxants in dose-dependent fashion. Of the drugs that have been studied, inhaled anesthetics augment the effects of muscle relaxants in the following order: Isoflurane and enflurane augment more than halothane, which in turn augments more than nitrous oxide-barbiturate-narcotic anesthesia (Fig 24–7). The most important factors involved in this interaction are the following: (1) Depression at sites proximal to the neuromuscular junction, ie, the central nervous system. (2) Increased muscle blood flow, which allows a larger fraction of the injected muscle relaxant to reach the neuromuscular junction. This is probably a factor only with isoflurane. (3) Decreased sensitivity of the postjunctional membrane to depolarization.

B. Antibiotics: Over 140 reports of enhancement of neuromuscular blockade by antibiotics, especially aminoglycosides, have appeared in the literature. Many of the antibiotics have been shown to cause a depression of evoked release of acetylcholine similar to that caused by magnesium. The same antibiotics also have postjunctional activity.

C. Local Anesthetics and Antiarrhythmia Drugs: In large doses, most local anesthetics block neuromuscular transmission; in smaller doses, they enhance the neuromuscular block from both nondepolarizing and depolarizing muscle relaxants.

In low doses, local anesthetics depress posttetanic potentiation, and this is thought to be a neural prejunctional effect. With higher doses, local anesthetics block acetylcholine-induced muscle contractions. This stabilizing effect is the result of blockade of the ionic channels linked to the nicotinic receptors.

Most antiarrhythmia drugs, including quinidine, enhance the block produced by nondepolarizing muscle relaxants. Quinidine appears to act at the prejunctional membrane, as judged by its lack of effect on acetylcholine-evoked twitch. However, large nonclinical doses of quinidine given intra-arterially produce a neuromuscular blockade of the depolarizing type that is augmented by edrophonium.

Reversal of Nondepolarizing Neuromuscular Blockade

The cholinesterase inhibitors effectively antagonize neuromuscular blockade by nondepolarizing drugs. Their general pharmacology is discussed in Chapter 5. Neostigmine and pyridostigmine antagonize nondepolarizing neuromuscular blockade by increasing the availability of acetylcholine at the muscle end-plate, mainly by inhibition of acetylcholinesterase. To a lesser extent, these agents also increase release of transmitter from the motor nerve terminal. In contrast, edrophonium antagonizes neuromuscular blockade purely by inhibiting acetylcholinesterase.

Other Uses of Neuromuscular Blocking Drugs

A. Control Of Ventilation: In patients who have ventilatory failure from various causes, such as obstructive airway disease, it is often desirable to control ventilation to provide adequate volumes and expansion of lungs. To eliminate chest wall resistance and ineffective spontaneous ventilation, paralysis is sometimes induced by administration of neuromuscular blocking drugs.

B. Treatment of Convulsions: Neuromuscular blocking drugs are sometimes used to attenuate or eliminate the peripheral manifestations of convulsions from such causes as epilepsy or local anesthetic toxicity. Although this approach is effective in eliminating the muscular manifestations of the conditions, it has no effect on the central processes involved, since neuromuscular blocking drugs do not cross the blood-brain barrier.

SPASMOLYTIC DRUGS

Bertram G. Katzung, MD, PhD

Spasticity is characterized by an increase in tonic stretch reflexes and flexor muscle spasms together with muscle weakness. It is often associated with cerebral palsy, multiple sclerosis, and stroke. The mechanisms underlying clinical spasticity appear to involve not the stretch reflex arc itself but higher centers, with damage to descending pathways that results in hyperexcitability of alpha motoneurons in the cord. Nevertheless, drug therapy may ameliorate some of the symptoms of spasticity by modifying the stretch reflex arc or by interfering directly with skeletal muscle excitation-contraction coupling. The components involved in these processes are shown in Fig 24–9.

Drugs modifying this reflex arc may modulate excitatory or inhibitory synapses (Chapter 18). Thus, to reduce the hyperactive stretch reflex, it is desirable to reduce the activity of the Ia fibers that excite the primary motoneuron or enhance the activity of the inhibitory internuncial neurons. These structures are shown in greater detail in Fig 24–10.

A variety of compounds used in the past can be loosely described as depressants of spinal "polysynaptic" reflex arcs (barbiturates: phenobarbital; glycerol ethers: mephenesin). However, it is clear from Fig 24–10 that nonspecific depression of synapses involved in the stretch reflex could reduce desirable inhibitory activity as well as excitatory transmission. In fact, in clinical use, phenobarbital and mephenesin have little specific spasmolytic effect, and such relief

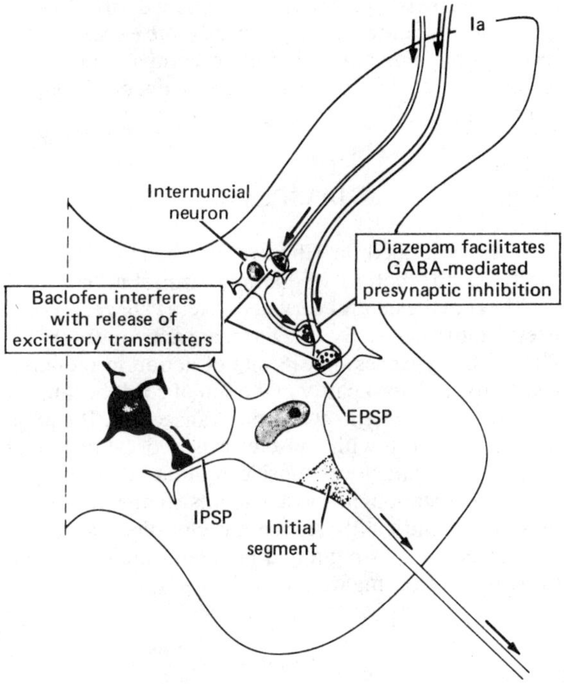

Figure 24–10. Postulated sites of spasmolytic action of diazepam and baclofen in the spinal cord. (Reproduced, with permission, from Young RR, Delwaide RJ: Drug therapy: Spasticity. *N Engl J Med* 1981;**304**:28.)

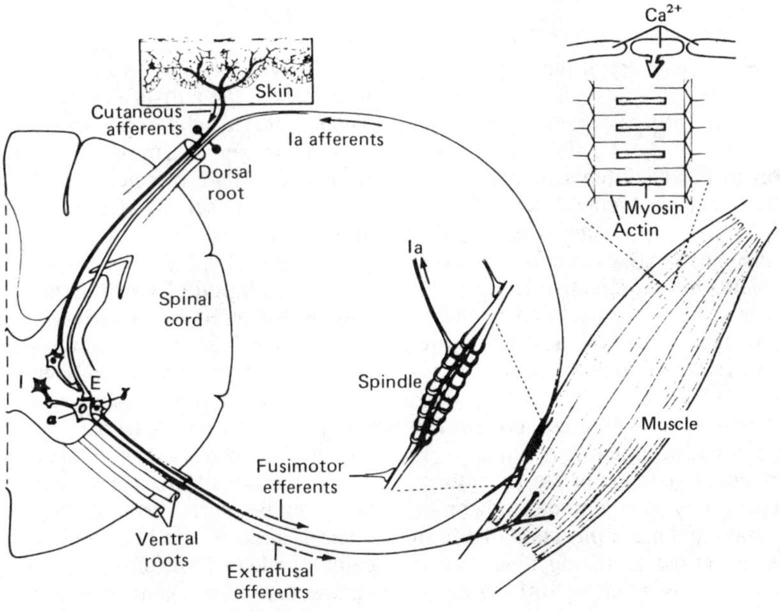

Figure 24–9. Diagram of the structures involved in the stretch reflex arc. I is an inhibitory interneuron; E indicates an excitatory presynaptic terminal, and Ca^{2+} denotes activator calcium stored in the sarcoplasmic reticulum of skeletal muscle. (Reproduced, with permission, from Young RR, Delwaide PJ: Drug therapy: Spasticity. *N Engl J Med* 1981;**304**:28.)

as may be produced appears to be the result of marked sedation. During the past decade, more specific therapy has become available. Unfortunately, the lack of a precisely quantifiable measure of clinical response—or, alternatively, an accurate experimental model—has prevented definitive comparison of the agents promoted for use in this heterogeneous group of conditions.

DIAZEPAM

As described in Chapter 19, benzodiazepines facilitate the action of gamma-aminobutyric acid (GABA) in the central nervous system. Diazepam has useful antispastic activity. Diazepam apparently acts at all GABA synapses, but its site of action in reducing spasticity is at least partly in the spinal cord, because it is effective in patients with cord transection. It can be used in patients with muscle spasm of almost any origin, including local muscle trauma. However, it produces sedation in most patients at the doses required to significantly reduce muscle tone. Dosage is usually begun at 4 mg/d and gradually increased to a maximum of 60 mg/d.

BACLOFEN
(Lioresal)

Baclofen (*p*-chlorophenyl GABA) was designed to be an orally active GABA-mimetic agent. The structure is shown below.

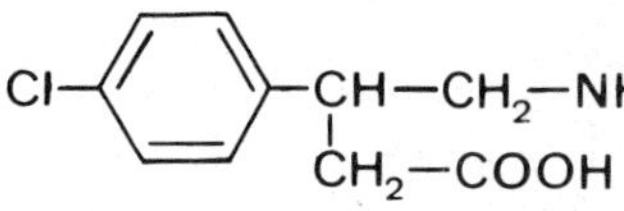

Baclofen

It is not clear, however, that baclofen acts in this way, since it is not antagonized by bicuculline, a GABA antagonist at many GABA-ergic sites (Chapter 18), nor does baclofen displace GABA from its receptors. On the other hand, bicuculline-insensitive GABA sites have recently been described, and baclofen might act at these synapses. In fact, baclofen may act at presynaptic inhibitory GABA receptors to reduce the release of excitatory transmitters.

Baclofen is at least as effective as diazepam in reducing spasticity but causes much less sedation. In addition, it does not reduce general muscle strength, as does dantrolene. It is rapidly and completely absorbed after oral administration and has a plasma half-life of 3–4 hours. Dosage is started at 15 mg twice daily, increasing, if tolerated, to as much as 100 mg daily. Toxicity of this drug includes drowsiness, to which the patient may become tolerant. Increased seizure activity has been reported in epileptic patients.

DANTROLENE
(Dantrium)

Dantrolene is a hydantoin derivative similar to phenytoin but with a unique mechanism of spasmolytic action outside the central nervous system. Its structure is shown below.

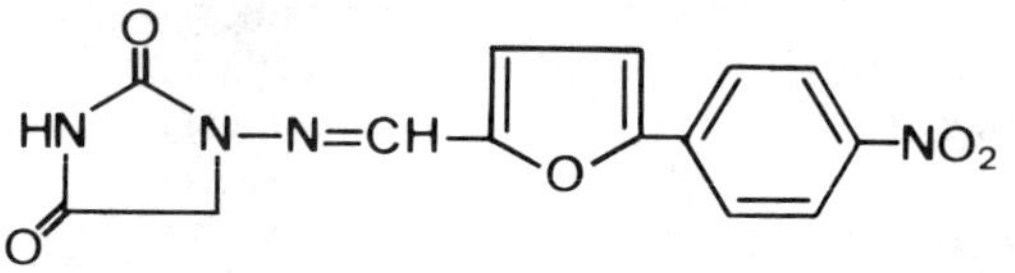

Dantrolene

Dantrolene reduces skeletal muscle strength by interfering with excitation-contraction coupling in the muscle fiber. The normal contractile response involves release of activator calcium from its stores in the sarcoplasmic reticulum of the sarcomere. This calcium brings about the tension-generating interaction of actin with myosin. Dantrolene interferes with the release of activator calcium from the sarcoplasmic reticulum. Thus, the action of this drug involves neither central synapses nor the neuromuscular junction; it is intracellular at the effector organ. Motor units that contract rapidly are more sensitive to the drug than are slow units. Cardiac muscle and smooth muscle are depressed only slightly, perhaps because the release of calcium from their sarcoplasmic reticulum (smooth muscle has very little) involves a somewhat different process.

Only about one-third of an oral dose of dantrolene is absorbed; the half-life of the drug is about 8 hours. Treatment is usually begun with 25 mg daily as a single dose, increasing to a maximum of 100 mg 4 times daily if necessary and tolerated. Major adverse effects are generalized muscle weakness, sedation, and occasionally hepatitis.

A special application of dantrolene is in the treatment of **malignant hyperthermia,** a rare disorder that can be triggered by a variety of stimuli, including general anesthesia and neuromuscular blocking drugs. Patients with this condition have a hereditary impairment of the ability of the sarcoplasmic reticulum to sequester calcium. A trigger event results in sudden and prolonged release of calcium, with massive muscle contraction, lactic acid production, and increased body temperature. Prompt treatment is essential to control acidosis and body temperature and to reduce calcium release. The latter is accomplished with intravenous dantrolene, starting with 1 mg/kg and repeating as necessary to a maximum of 10 mg/kg.

• • •

References

Neuromuscular Blockers

Kitz RJ: Molecular pharmacology of acetylcholinesterase. Page 333 in: *A Guide to Molecular Pharmacology and Toxicology*. Featherstone RM (editor). Marcel Dekker, 1977.

Miller RD, Savarese JJ: Pharmacology of muscle relaxants, their antagonists, and monitoring of neuromuscular function. Page 487 in: *Anesthesia*. Miller RD (editor). Churchill Livingstone, 1981.

Miller RD, Agoston S, Booij LDHJ: The comparative potency and pharmacokinetics of pancuronium and its metabolites in anesthetized man. *J Pharmacol Exp Ther* 1978;**207:**539.

Schoner PJ, Brown RL, Kirksey TD: Succinylcholine-induced hyperkalemia in burned patients. *Anesth Analg* 1969; **48:**764.

Waud BE, Waud DR: Physiology and pharmacology of neuromuscular blocking agents. Page 1 in: *Muscle Relaxants*. Katz RL (editor). Excerpta Medica, 1975.

Spasmolytics

Davidoff RA: Pharmacology of spasticity. *Neurology* 1980;**28:**46.

Young RR, Delwaide PJ: Drug therapy: Spasticity. (2 parts.) *N Engl J Med* 1981;**304:**28, 96.

25 | Pharmacologic Management of Parkinsonism & Other Movement Disorders

Michael J. Aminoff, MD

Many of the movement disorders have been attributed to disturbances of the basal ganglia, but the precise function of these anatomic structures is not yet clearly understood, and it is not possible to relate individual symptoms to involvement at specific sites.

Several different types of abnormal movement are recognized. **Tremor** consists of a rhythmic oscillatory movement around a joint and is best-characterized by its relation to activity. Tremor present at rest is characteristic of parkinsonism, when it is often associated with rigidity and an impairment of voluntary activity. Tremor may occur during maintenance of sustained posture (postural tremor) or during movement (intention tremor). A conspicuous postural tremor is the cardinal feature of benign essential or familial tremor. Intention tremor occurs in patients with a lesion of the brain stem or cerebellum, especially when the superior cerebellar peduncle is involved, and may also occur as a manifestation of toxicity from alcohol or certain other drugs.

Chorea consists of irregular, unpredictable, involuntary muscle jerks that may occur in different parts of the body and impair voluntary activity. In some instances, the proximal muscles of the limbs are most severely affected, and because the abnormal movements are then particularly violent, the term **ballismus** has been used to describe them. Chorea may be hereditary or may occur as a complication of a number of general medical disorders and of therapy with certain drugs.

Abnormal movements may be slow and writhing in character **(athetosis)** and in some instances are so sustained that they are more properly regarded as abnormal postures **(dystonia).** Athetosis or dystonia may occur with perinatal brain damage, with focal or generalized cerebral lesions, as an acute complication of certain drugs, as an accompaniment of diverse neurologic disorders, or as an isolated phenomenon of uncertain cause known as idiopathic torsion dystonia or dystonia musculorum deformans. Its pharmacologic basis is uncertain, and treatment is unsatisfactory.

Tics are sudden coordinated abnormal movements that tend to occur repetitively, particularly about the face and head, especially in children, and can be suppressed voluntarily for short periods of time. Common tics include, for example, repetitive sniffing or shoulder shrugging. Tics may be single or multiple and transient or chronic. Gilles de la Tourette's syndrome is characterized by chronic multiple tics; its pharmacologic management is discussed at the end of this chapter.

PARKINSONISM
(Paralysis Agitans)

Parkinsonism is characterized by a combination of rigidity, bradykinesia, tremor, and postural instability that can occur for a wide variety of reasons but is usually idiopathic. The course is generally progressive, leading to increasing disability unless effective treatment is provided. The normally high concentration of dopamine in the basal ganglia of the brain is reduced in parkinsonism, and pharmacologic attempts to restore dopaminergic activity with levodopa and dopamine agonists have been successful in alleviating many of the clinical features of the disorder. An alternative but complementary approach has been to restore the normal balance of cholinergic and dopaminergic influences on the basal ganglia with anticholinergic drugs.

LEVODOPA
(Larodopa)

Dopamine does not cross the blood-brain barrier and therefore has no therapeutic effect in parkinsonism. However, (−)-3-(3,4-dihydroxyphenyl)-L-alanine (levodopa), the immediate metabolic precursor of dopamine, does penetrate the brain, where it is decarboxylated to dopamine. Several dopamine agonists have also been developed and may lead to clinical benefit, as discussed below.

Dopamine receptors can be classified according to various biochemical and pharmacologic features. They have, for example, been subdivided according to whether they are linked to an adenylate cyclase. Cyclic adenosine monophosphate (cAMP) is formed with activation of this cyclase and may well be responsible for mediating certain tissue-specific responses to dopamine. Other responses to dopamine apparently do not involve the stimulation of an adenylate cyclase or accumulation of cAMP. The designation D_1 has been proposed for those receptors linked to adenylate cyclase and D_2 for those that are not.

Dopamine receptors of the D_1 type are located in the zona compacta of the substantia nigra and presynaptically on striatal axons coming from cortical neurons and from dopaminergic cells in the substantia nigra. The D_2 receptors are located postsynaptically on striatal neurons and presynaptically on axons in the substantia nigra belonging to neurons in the basal ganglia. The benefits of dopaminergic antiparkinsonism drugs appear to depend on stimulation of the D_2 receptors. Dopaminergic ergot derivatives such as lergotrile or bromocriptine that are powerful stimulators of the D_2 receptors have antiparkinsonism properties, whereas certain dopaminergic blockers that are selective D_2 antagonists can induce parkinsonism.

Chemistry

As discussed in Chapter 4, dopa is the precursor of dopamine and norepinephrine. Its structure is shown in Fig 25–1. Levodopa is the levorotatory stereoisomer of dopa.

Pharmacokinetics

Levodopa is rapidly absorbed from the small intestine, but its absorption depends on the rate of gastric emptying and the pH of the gastric contents. Plasma concentrations usually peak between 1 and 2 hours after an oral dose, and the plasma half-life is usually between 1 and 3 hours, though it varies considerably between individuals. About two-thirds of the dose appears in the urine as metabolites within 8 hours of an oral dose, the main metabolic products being

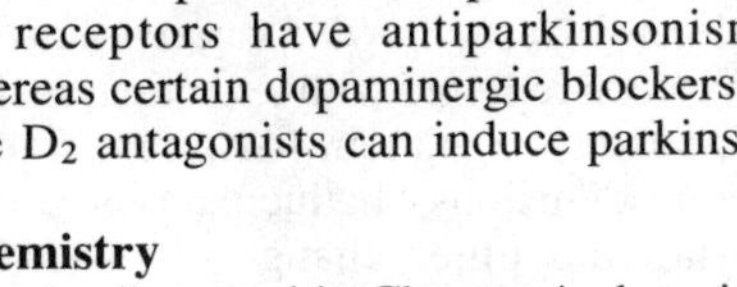

Dihydroxyphenylalanine (dopa)

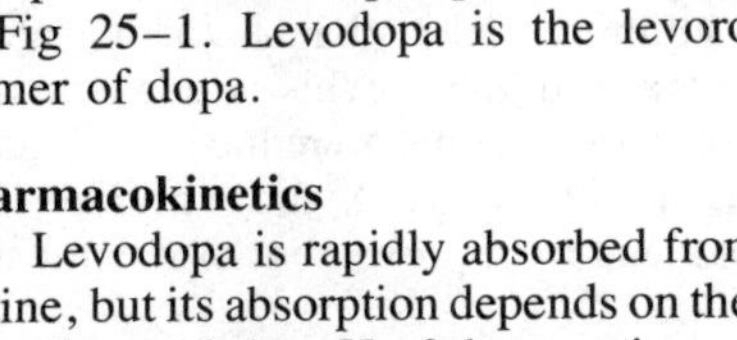

Carbidopa

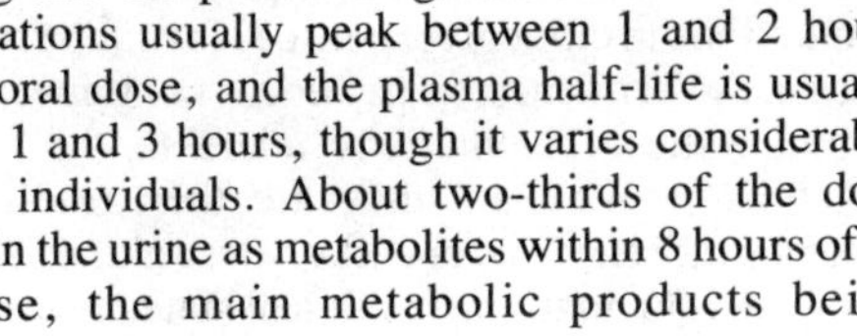

Deprenyl

Figure 25–1. Some drugs used in the treatment of parkinsonism.

3-methoxy-4-hydroxyphenylacetic acid (homovanillic acid, HVA) and dihydroxyphenylacetic acid (DOPAC). Unfortunately, only about 1–3% of administered levodopa actually enters the brain unaltered, the remainder being metabolized extracerebrally, predominantly by decarboxylation to dopamine, which does not penetrate the blood-brain barrier. This means that levodopa must be given in large amounts when it is used alone. However, when it is given in combination with a dopa decarboxylase inhibitor that does not penetrate the blood-brain barrier, the peripheral metabolism of levodopa is reduced, plasma levels of levodopa are higher, plasma half-life is longer, and more dopa is available for entry into the brain. Indeed, concomitant administration of a peripheral dopa decarboxylase inhibitor may reduce the daily requirements of levodopa by approximately 75%.

Clinical Use

In considering the use of levodopa in patients with parkinsonism, it is important to appreciate that the best results are obtained in the first few years of treatment. This is sometimes because the daily dose of levodopa must be reduced with time in order to avoid side-effects at doses that were well tolerated at the outset. The reason that side-effects develop in this way is unclear, but selective denervation or drug-induced supersensitivity may be responsible. Some patients also become less responsive to levodopa, so that previously effective doses eventually fail to produce any therapeutic benefit. Responsiveness to levodopa may ultimately be lost completely, perhaps because of the disappearance of dopaminergic nigrostriatal nerve terminals or some pathologic process directly involving the striatal dopamine receptors. For such reasons, the benefits of levodopa treatment usually begin to diminish after about 3 or 4 years of therapy irrespective of the severity of the original disorder or the initial therapeutic response. Moreover, levodopa therapy does not stop the progression of parkinsonism, and long-term therapy may lead to a number of problems in management such as development of the on-off phenomenon discussed below. It may therefore be better practice to reserve levodopa therapy until the parkinsonism is advanced or there is significant functional disability and to use other drugs for early management.

When levodopa is used, it is generally given in combination with carbidopa (Fig 25–1), a peripheral decarboxylase inhibitor, for the reasons set forth above. **Sinemet** is a preparation containing carbidopa and levodopa in fixed proportion (1:10 or 1:4). Treatment is started with a small dose, eg, Sinemet-10/100 (carbidopa 10 mg, levodopa 100 mg) 3 times daily and gradually increased depending upon the therapeutic response and development of side-effects. Most patients ultimately require Sinemet-25/250 (carbidopa 25 mg, levodopa 250 mg) 3 or 4 times daily.

Levodopa can ameliorate all of the clinical features of parkinsonism, but it is particularly effective in relieving bradykinesia and any disabilities resulting from it. When it is first introduced, about one-third of patients respond very well and one-third less well. Most of the remainder either are unable to tolerate the medication or simply fail to respond at all.

Side-Effects

A. Gastrointestinal Effects: When levodopa is given without a peripheral decarboxylase inhibitor, anorexia and nausea and vomiting occur in about 80% of patients. These side-effects can be minimized by taking the drug in divided doses, with or immediately after meals, and by increasing the total daily dose very slowly; antacids taken 30–60 minutes before levodopa may also be beneficial. The vomiting has been attributed to stimulation of an emetic center located in the brain stem but outside the blood-brain barrier to dopamine and to peripheral decarboxylase inhibitors. Fortunately, tolerance to this emetic effect develops in many patients after several months. Antiemetics such as phenothiazines are sometimes given but may reduce the antiparkinsonism effects of levodopa.

When levodopa is given in combination with carbidopa to reduce its extracerebral metabolism, gastrointestinal side-effects are much less frequent and troublesome, occurring in fewer than 20% of cases, so that patients can tolerate proportionately higher doses.

B. Cardiovascular Effects: A variety of cardiac arrhythmias have been described in patients receiving levodopa, including tachycardia, ventricular extrasystoles, and, rarely, atrial fibrillation. This effect has been attributed to increased catecholamine formation peripherally. The incidence of such arrhythmias is low, even in the presence of established cardiac disease, and may be reduced still further if the levodopa is taken in combination with a peripheral decarboxylase inhibitor. In parkinsonism patients who also have heart disease, the anticipated benefits of levodopa, especially when combined with carbidopa, generally outweigh the slight risk of inducing a cardiac arrhythmia.

Postural hypotension is common, often asymptomatic, and tends to diminish with continuing treatment. Hypertension may also occur, especially in the presence of monoamine oxidase inhibitors or other sympathomimetics or when massive doses of levodopa are being taken.

C. Dyskinesias: Dyskinesias occur in about 80% of patients receiving levodopa therapy for long periods. The development of dyskinesias is dose-related, but there is considerable individual variation in the dose required to produce them. Dyskinesias seem to occur more commonly in patients receiving levodopa combined with a peripheral decarboxylase inhibitor than in those receiving levodopa alone. Moreover, with continuing treatment, dyskinesias may develop at a dose of levodopa that previously was well tolerated. They can be alleviated or reversed by lowering the daily dose of levodopa, but usually at the expense of reduced antiparkinsonism benefit; many patients are therefore willing to tolerate even a marked dyskinesia, because their mobility is so greatly improved by the medication. In some instances, dyskinesias are less marked if levodopa is prescribed alone rather than in combination with carbidopa; in other instances, a drug holiday (see below) may help control the problem. Pharmacologic attempts to counteract the dyskinesia with drugs used to treat chorea have generally not been successful or require the use of drugs that tend to worsen the parkinsonism.

The form and nature of dopa dyskinesias vary widely in different patients but tend to remain constant in character in individual patients. Chorea, ballismus, athetosis, dystonia, myoclonus, tics, and tremor may occur individually or in any combination in the face, trunk, or limbs. Choreoathetosis of the face and distal extremities is the most common presentation.

D. Behavioral Effects: A wide variety of mental side-effects have been reported with levodopa, including depression, anxiety, agitation, insomnia, somnolence, confusion, delusions, hallucinations, nightmares, euphoria, and other changes in mood or personality. Such side-effects are more common in patients taking levodopa in combination with a decarboxylase inhibitor rather than levodopa alone, presumably because higher levels are reached in the brain. The only treatment is to reduce or withdraw the medication if necessary. A drug holiday (see below) may also lead to improvement of mental side-effects.

E. Fluctuations in Response: Unpredictable fluctuations in clinical response to levodopa occur with increasing frequency as treatment continues. In some patients, these fluctuations relate to the timing of levodopa intake, and they are then referred to as wearing-off reactions or end-of-dose akinesia. In other instances, fluctuations in clinical state are unrelated to the timing of doses (on-off phenomenon). In the on-off phenomenon, off-periods of marked akinesia alternate over the course of a few hours with on-periods of improved mobility but often marked dyskinesia. The phenomenon is most likely to occur in patients who responded well to treatment initially. The exact mechanism is unknown, but the off-period can sometimes be shown to relate to falling plasma levels of levodopa. Patients may benefit from taking their medication at more frequent intervals in smaller doses during the day or from the addition of dopamine agonists such as bromocriptine (see below) to the drug regimen. Alternatively, a brief holiday from levodopa under careful medical supervision may help in restoring its effectiveness.

F. Miscellaneous Side-Effects: Mydriasis may occur and may precipitate an attack of acute glaucoma in some patients. Other reported but rare side-effects include various blood dyscrasias; a positive Coombs test with evidence of hemolysis; hot flushes; aggravation or precipitation of gout; abnormalities of smell or taste; brownish discoloration of saliva, urine, or vaginal secretions; priapism; and mild—usually transient—elevations of blood urea nitrogen and of serum transaminases, alkaline phosphatase, and bilirubin.

Drug Holidays

A drug holiday may help in alleviating some of the neurologic and behavioral side-effects of levodopa and in the management of the on-off phenomenon. Patients must be under close medical supervision. The optimal duration of such a break in treatment with levodopa is unclear, but it has varied from 3 to 21 days in different studies. Up to about two-thirds of patients show improved responsiveness to levodopa when the drug is reinstituted, and, because they can be managed on lower doses than before, mental side-effects and dyskinesias are less troublesome. Fluctuations in response (on-off phenomenon) are reduced in many instances. Unfortunately, there is no way of predicting which patients will respond satisfactorily to the holiday.

Drug Interactions

Pharmacologic doses of pyridoxine (vitamin B_6) enhance the extracerebral metabolism of levodopa and may therefore prevent its therapeutic effect unless a peripheral decarboxylase inhibitor is also taken. Levodopa should not be given to patients taking monoamine oxidase A inhibitors or within 2 weeks of their discontinuation, because such a combination can lead to hypertensive crises.

Contraindications

Levodopa should not be given to psychotic patients, as it may exacerbate the mental disturbance. It is also contraindicated in patients with closed-angle glaucoma, but those with chronic open-angle glaucoma may be given levodopa if intraocular pressure is well controlled and can be monitored. It is best given combined with carbidopa to patients with cardiac disease, but even so there is a slight risk of cardiac dysrhythmia. Patients with active peptic ulcer must also be managed carefully, since gastrointestinal bleeding has occasionally occurred with levodopa. Because it may activate malignant melanoma, its use should be avoided in patients with a history of melanoma or with suspicious undiagnosed skin lesions.

BROMOCRIPTINE
(Parlodel)

The enzymes responsible for synthesizing dopamine are depleted in the brains of parkinsonism patients, and drugs acting directly on dopamine receptors may therefore have a beneficial effect additional to that of levodopa. Moreover, drugs specifically affecting certain (but not all) dopamine receptors may have more limited side-effects than levodopa. There are a number of dopamine agonists with antiparkinsonism activity. Some, such as apomorphine, piribedil, and lergotrile, have such serious side-effects that they cannot be used clinically, but others may have a role in treatment of parkinsonism.

The most promising group of dopaminergic agonists currently being evaluated are ergot derivatives. Several ergot derivatives have been used experimentally in the treatment of parkinsonism, but **bromocriptine** (structure shown in Chapter 14) is the most promising drug and currently the only one in widespread use. It has also been used to treat certain endocrinologic disorders, especially hyperprolactinemia (see Chapters 14 and 35), but in lower doses than those required to counteract parkinsonism. The drug is absorbed to a variable extent from the gastrointestinal tract, peak plasma levels being reached within 1–2 hours after an oral dose. It is excreted in the bile and feces.

Bromocriptine is an expensive drug best reserved for parkinsonism patients taking levodopa who have end-of-dose akinesia or on-off phenomena or who are becoming refractory to treatment with levodopa. Partial replacement of levodopa with bromocriptine may then be valuable. Optimal results are obtained by a combination of levodopa and bromocriptine in doses less than the maximum tolerable doses of each. The results of bromocriptine treatment are generally disappointing in patients totally unresponsive to levodopa, and addition of bromocriptine to patients receiving optimal levodopa therapy may cause intolerable side-effects. Bromocriptine does not complicate treatment with anticholinergic drugs or amantadine, and these drugs can be continued without change in dosage in patients who are to be given bromocriptine as well.

Clinical Use

The usual daily dose of bromocriptine in parkinsonism is between 10 and 60 mg, but in about one-fourth to one-half of cases therapeutic doses either fail to provide sustained benefit or cannot be tolerated. In order to minimize unwanted side-effects, the dose of bromocriptine should be built up slowly over about 2 or 3 months from a starting level of 2.5 mg twice daily after meals; the dose of levodopa taken concurrently may have to be gradually lowered to about half of that previously required. However, because occasional patients are very sensitive to the hypotensive effect of bromocriptine and may even collapse within an hour of the first dose, a test dose of 1 mg should be given initially, with food and with the patient in bed. If vascular collapse occurs, recovery is usually rapid and spontaneous, and patients often tolerate subsequent doses well. Treatment with bromocriptine should be stopped if it leads to psychiatric disturbances, cardiac dysrhythmia, erythromelalgia, ergotism, or other intolerable side-effects.

Side-Effects

A. Gastrointestinal Effects: Anorexia and nausea and vomiting are especially common when bromocriptine therapy is introduced and can be minimized by taking the medication with meals. Other gastrointestinal side-effects include constipation, dyspepsia, and symptoms suggestive of reflux esophagitis. Bleeding from peptic ulceration has also been reported.

B. Cardiovascular Effects: Postural hypotension is fairly common, especially at the initiation of therapy. Painless digital vasospasm is a complication of long-term treatment that can be reversed by lowering the dose. Cardiac arrhythmias may also occur with bromocriptine and are an indication for discontinuing treatment.

C. Dyskinesias: Abnormal movements similar to those induced by levodopa can also be produced by bromocriptine. Treatment consists of reducing the total dose of dopaminergic drugs being taken.

D. Mental Disturbances: Confusion, hallucinations, delusions, and other psychiatric reactions are established complications of dopaminergic treatment of parkinsonism. They are more common and severe with bromocriptine than with levodopa itself. Such side-effects clear on withdrawal of the offending medication.

E. Miscellaneous Side-Effects: Headache, nasal congestion, increased arousal, pulmonary infiltrates, and erythromelalgia are other reported side-effects of bromocriptine. Erythromelalgia consists of red, tender, painful, swollen feet and, occasionally, hands, at times associated with arthralgia; symptoms and signs clear within a few days of withdrawal of bromocriptine.

Contraindications

Bromocriptine treatment is contraindicated in patients with a history of psychiatric illness or recent myocardial infarction. It is best avoided in patients with peripheral vascular disease or peptic ulceration.

MONOAMINE OXIDASE INHIBITORS

Two types of monoamine oxidase have been distinguished. Monoamine oxidase A metabolizes norepinephrine and serotonin; monoamine oxidase B metabolizes dopamine. **Deprenyl** (Fig 25–1), a selective inhibitor of monoamine oxidase B, retards the breakdown of dopamine; in consequence, it enhances and prolongs the antiparkinsonism effect of levodopa and may reduce mild on-off or wearing-off phenomena. Its use for this purpose is experimental at present. Deprenyl has no useful therapeutic effect on parkinsonism when given alone.

The combined administration of levodopa and an inhibitor of both forms of monoamine oxidase must be avoided, since it may lead to hypertensive crises, probably because of the peripheral accumulation of norepinephrine.

AMANTADINE
(Symmetrel)

Amantadine, an antiviral agent, was by chance found to have antiparkinsonism properties. Its mode of action in parkinsonism is unclear, but it may potentiate dopaminergic function by influencing the synthesis, release, or reuptake of dopamine. Release of catecholamines from peripheral stores has been documented.

Pharmacokinetics

Peak plasma concentrations of amantadine are reached 1–4 hours after an oral dose. The plasma half-life is between 2 and 4 hours, most of the drug being excreted unchanged in the urine.

Clinical Use

Amantadine is less potent than levodopa, and its benefits may be short-lived, often disappearing after only a few weeks of treatment. Nevertheless, during that time it may favorably influence the bradykinesia, rigidity, and tremor of parkinsonism. The standard dose is 100 mg orally twice daily.

Side-Effects

Amantadine has a number of central nervous system side-effects that can be reversed by stopping the drug. These include restlessness, depression, irritability, insomnia, agitation, excitement, hallucinations, and confusion. Overdosage may produce an acute toxic psychosis. With doses several times higher than recommended, convulsions have occurred.

Livedo reticularis sometimes occurs in patients taking amantadine and usually clears within a month after the drug is withdrawn. Other dermatologic reactions have also been described. Peripheral edema, another well-recognized complication, is not accompanied by signs of cardiac, hepatic, or renal disease and responds to diuretics. Other adverse reactions include headache, congestive heart disease, postural hypotension, urinary retention, and gastrointestinal disturbances (eg, anorexia, nausea, constipation, and dry mouth).

Contraindications

The drug should be used with caution in patients with a history of seizures or congestive heart failure.

ANTICHOLINERGIC DRUGS

A number of centrally acting anticholinergic preparations are available that differ in their potency and in their efficacy in different patients.

Clinical Use

Treatment is started with a low dose of one of the drugs in this category, the level of medication gradually being increased until benefit occurs or side-effects limit further increments. Anticholinergic drugs may improve the tremor and rigidity of parkinsonism but have little effect on bradykinesia. If patients fail to respond to one anticholinergic drug, a trial with another is certainly warranted and may be successful. Some of the more commonly used drugs are listed in Table 25–1.

Table 25–1. Some drugs with anticholinergic properties used in parkinsonism.

Drug	Usual Daily Dose (mg)
Benztropine mesylate (Cogentin)	1–6
Biperiden (Akineton)	2–12
Chlorphenoxamine (Phenoxene)	150–400
Cycrimine (Pagitane)	5–20
Ethopropazine (Parsidol)	150–300
Orphenadrine (Disipal, Norflex)	150–400
Procyclidine (Kemadrin)	7.5–30
Trihexyphenidyl (Artane)	6–20

Side-Effects

Anticholinergic drugs have a number of central nervous system side-effects, including drowsiness, mental slowness, inattention, restlessness, confusion, agitation, delusions, hallucinations, and mood changes. Such side-effects are sometimes precipitated by intercurrent infections and usually subside within a few days after withdrawal of the offending substance. Other common side-effects include dryness of the mouth, blurring of vision, mydriasis, urinary retention, nausea and vomiting, constipation, tachycardia, tachypnea, increased intraocular pressure, palpitations, and cardiac arrhythmias. Acute suppurative parotitis sometimes occurs as a complication of dryness of the mouth.

If anticholinergic medication is to be withdrawn, this should be accomplished gradually rather than abruptly in order to prevent acute exacerbation of parkinsonism.

Contraindications

Anticholinergic drugs should be avoided in patients with prostatic hypertrophy, obstructive gastrointestinal disease (eg, pyloric stenosis or paralytic ileus), or closed-angle glaucoma. In parkinsonism patients receiving anticholinergic medication, concomitant administration of other drugs with anticholinergic properties—eg, tricyclic antidepressants or antihistamines—may precipitate some of the complications mentioned above.

GENERAL COMMENTS ON DRUG MANAGEMENT OF PATIENTS WITH PARKINSONISM

There is no means of influencing the course of idiopathic parkinsonism, and the benefits of levodopa therapy often diminish with time. In view of this, pharmacologic treatment of mild parkinsonism may initially be unnecessary and is probably best avoided until there is some degree of disability or until symptoms begin to have a significant impact on the patient's life-style. When treatment becomes necessary, it is best to start with amantadine or an anticholinergic drug, reserving levodopa until there is definite incapacity. In patients with more severe parkinsonism, levodopa is usually prescribed in combination with carbidopa as Sinemet, and amantadine or an anticholinergic drug (or both) may be necessary as well for optimal benefit. Physical therapy is also helpful in improving mobility. In patients with severe parkinsonism and long-term complications of levodopa therapy, such as the on-off phenomenon, a trial of treatment with bromocriptine may be worthwhile. All patients require continual support and encouragement to maintain an independent existence.

DRUG-INDUCED PARKINSONISM

Reserpine and the related drug tetrabenazine deplete biogenic monoamines from their storage sites, while haloperidol and the phenothiazines block dopaminergic receptors. These drugs may therefore produce a parkinsonian syndrome, usually within 3 months after introduction, which is related to high dosage and clears over a few weeks or months after withdrawal. If treatment is necessary, anticholinergic drugs are preferred. Levodopa is of no help if neuroleptic drugs are continued and may in fact aggravate the mental disorder for which antipsychotic drugs were prescribed originally.

OTHER MOVEMENT DISORDERS

Tremor

Tremor consists of rhythmic oscillatory movements. Physiologic postural tremor is enhanced in amplitude by anxiety, fatigue, thyrotoxicosis, and intravenous epinephrine or isoproterenol. Propranolol reduces its amplitude, and, if administered intra-arterially, prevents the response to isoproterenol in the perfused limb, presumably through some peripheral action. Certain drugs—especially the bronchodilators, tricyclic antidepressants, and lithium—may produce a dose-dependent exaggeration of the normal physiologic tremor that is readily reversed by discontinuing the drug. Although the tremor produced by sympathomimetics such as terbutaline (a bronchodilator) is blocked by propranolol, which antagonizes both β_1- and β_2-adrenergic receptors, it is not blocked by metoprolol, a β_1-selective antagonist, suggesting that such tremor is mediated mainly by the β_2 receptors.

Essential tremor is a postural tremor, sometimes familial, that is clinically similar to physiologic tremor. Dysfunction of β_1 receptors has been implicated in some instances, since the tremor may respond dramatically to standard doses of metoprolol as well as to propranolol. The most useful approach is with propranolol, but whether the response depends on a central or peripheral action is unclear. The pharmacokinetics, pharmacologic effects, and adverse reactions of propranolol are discussed in Chapter 8. Daily doses of propranolol on the order of 120 mg (60–240 mg) are usually required, and reported side-effects have been few. Propranolol should be used with caution in patients with congestive cardiac failure, heart block, asthma, or hypoglycemia. Patients can be instructed to take their own pulse and call the physician if significant bradycardia develops. Metoprolol, a relatively selective β_1-blocker, is sometimes useful in treating tremor when patients have concomitant pulmonary disease that contraindicates use of propranolol. Small quantities of alcohol may also suppress essential tremor, but only for a short time and by an unknown mechanism. Diazepam, chlordiazepoxide, mephenesin, and antiparkinsonism agents have been advocated in the past but are generally worthless.

Intention tremor—tremor present during movement but not at rest—sometimes occurs as a toxic manifestation of alcohol or drugs such as phenytoin. Withdrawal or reduction in dosage provides dramatic relief. There is no satisfactory pharmacologic treatment for intention tremor due to other neurologic disorders.

Rest tremor is usually due to parkinsonism.

Huntington's Disease

This dominantly inherited disorder is characterized by progressive dementia and chorea that usually begin in adulthood. The development of chorea seems to be related to an imbalance of dopamine, acetylcholine, gamma-aminobutyric acid (GABA), and perhaps other neurotransmitters in the basal ganglia. Pharmacologic studies indicate that chorea results from functional overactivity in dopaminergic nigrostriatal pathways, perhaps because of increased responsiveness of postsynaptic dopamine receptors or deficiency of a neurotransmitter that normally antagonizes dopamine. Drugs that impair dopaminergic neurotransmission, either by depleting central monoamines (eg, reserpine, tetrabenazine) or by blocking dopamine receptors (eg, phenothiazines, butyrophenones), often alleviate chorea, whereas dopaminergic drugs such as levodopa tend to exacerbate it.

Both GABA and the enzyme (glutamic acid decarboxylase) concerned with its synthesis are markedly reduced in the basal ganglia of patients with Huntington's disease, and GABA receptors are usually implicated in inhibitory pathways. There is also a significant decline in concentration of choline acetyltransferase, the enzyme responsible for synthesizing acetylcholine, in the basal ganglia of these patients. These findings may be of pathophysiologic significance and have led to attempts to alleviate chorea by enhancing central GABA or cholinergic activity. Unfortunately, such pharmacologic manipulations have been disappointing, yielding no consistently beneficial response, and as a consequence the most commonly used drugs for controlling dyskinesia in patients with Huntington's disease are still those that interfere with dopaminergic activity. With all of the latter drugs, however, reduction of abnormal movements may be associated with iatrogenic parkinsonism.

Reserpine depletes cerebral dopamine by preventing intraneuronal storage; it is introduced in low doses (eg, 0.25 mg daily), and the daily dose is then built up gradually (eg, by 0.25 mg every week) until benefit occurs or side-effects become troublesome. A daily dose of 2–5 mg is often effective in suppressing abnormal movements, but side-effects may include hypotension, depression, sedation, diarrhea, and nasal congestion. Tetrabenazine resembles reserpine in depleting cerebral dopamine and has less troublesome side-effects, but it is available in the USA only on an experimental basis. Treatment with postsynaptic dopamine receptor blockers such as phenothiazines and butyrophenones may also be helpful. Haloperidol is started in a small dose, eg, 1 mg twice daily, and increased every 4 days depending upon the response. If haloperidol is not helpful, treatment with increasing doses of perphenazine up to a total of about 20 mg daily sometimes helps. The pharmacokinetics and clinical properties of these drugs are considered in greater detail elsewhere in this book.

It has recently been reported that low doses of a dopamine agonist may reduce the choreiform movements of patients with Huntington's disease, perhaps because of activation of presynaptic or self-inhibitory dopamine receptors whose stimulation results in inhibition of the activity of dopaminergic neurons. Such an approach remains experimental at this time but may prove to have some useful therapeutic application in the future.

Other Forms of Chorea

Treatment is directed at the underlying cause when chorea occurs as a complication of general medical disorders such as thyrotoxicosis, polycythemia vera rubra, systemic lupus erythematosus, hypocalcemia, and hepatic cirrhosis. Drug-induced chorea is managed by withdrawal of the offending substance, which may be levodopa, an anticholinergic drug, amphetamine, lithium, phenytoin, or an oral contraceptive. Neuroleptic drugs may also produce an acute or tardive dyskinesia (discussed below). Sydenham's chorea is temporary and usually so mild that pharmacologic management of the dyskinesia is unnecessary, but dopamine blocking drugs are effective in suppressing it.

Ballismus

The biochemical basis of ballismus is unknown, but the pharmacologic approach to management is the same as for chorea. Treatment with haloperidol, perphenazine, or other dopaminergic blocking drugs may be helpful.

Athetosis & Dystonia

The pharmacologic basis of these disorders is unknown, and there is no satisfactory medical treatment for them. Occasional patients with dystonia may respond to diazepam, amantadine, anticholinergic drugs, levodopa, carbamazepine, baclofen, haloperidol, or phenothiazines. A trial of these pharmacologic approaches is worthwhile even though often not successful.

Tics

The pathophysiologic basis of tics is unknown. Chronic multiple tics (Gilles de la Tourette's syndrome) may require treatment if the disorder is severe or is having a significant impact on the patient's life. The most effective pharmacologic approach is with haloperidol, and patients are better able to tolerate this drug if treatment is started with a small dose (eg, 0.25 or 0.5 mg daily) and then increased very gradually over the following weeks, most patients ultimately requiring a total daily dose of 3–8 mg. If haloperidol is not helpful, fluphenazine, clonazepam, clonidine, or carbamazepine should be tried. The pharmacologic properties of these drugs are discussed elsewhere in this book.

Drug-Induced Dyskinesias

The pharmacologic basis of the acute dyskinesia or dystonia sometimes precipitated by the first few doses of a phenothiazine is not clear. In most instances, parenteral administration of an anticholinergic drug such as benztropine (2 mg intravenously) or biperiden (2–5 mg intravenously or intramuscularly) is helpful, while in other instances diazepam (10 mg intravenously) alleviates the abnormal movements.

Tardive dyskinesia is a disorder characterized by a variety of abnormal movements that develop after long-term neuroleptic drug treatment. A reduction in dose of the offending medication, a dopaminergic receptor blocker, commonly worsens the dyskinesia, while an increase in dose may suppress it. These clinical observations, and the exacerbation in the movement disorder that is produced by levodopa, suggest that tardive dyskinesia relates to increased dopaminergic function, but its precise pharmacologic basis is unclear. It would seem, therefore, that phenothiazines cause a short-term reversible blockade of dopaminergic receptors but that over the long term they increase dopaminergic function. Whether this latter effect depends upon the development of denervation supersensitivity, increased dopamine synthesis, or diminished reuptake of dopamine at central synapses is not known.

There is some evidence that GABA is involved in a striatonigral feedback loop modulating the activity of dopaminergic cells in the substantia nigra, and GABA efferents also pass from the striatum to the globus pallidus and thalamus. GABA-mediated activity may diminish the activity of nigrostriatal dopaminergic cells and thereby decrease involuntary movements. **Muscimol** (3-hydroxy-5-aminomethylisoxazole), a semirigid structural analog of GABA, has been given to a small number of patients with tardive dyskinesia, and at oral doses of 5–9 mg daily consistently attenuated their involuntary movements in one study. However, muscimol has behavioral side-effects that limit any role for it in the treatment of tardive dyskinesia. Other attempts to increase central GABA activity (eg, with benzodiazepines or sodium valproate) have not yielded consistent benefit. Attempts to restore the balance between dopaminergic and cholinergic activity by increasing the latter with oral choline or lecithin have been helpful in some instances but not in others, and the same is true of treatment with deanol acetamidobenzoate, a drug related to acetylcholine. The drugs most likely to provide immediate symptomatic benefit are those interfering with dopaminergic function, either by depletion (eg, reserpine, tetrabenazine) or receptor blockade (eg, phenothiazines, butyrophenones). Paradoxically, the receptor blocking drugs are the very ones that also cause the dyskinesia, and they are probably best avoided to prevent the development of a spiral phenomenon in which continuing aggravation of the dyskinesia by the drugs used to control it necessitates increasingly higher doses for its temporary suppression.

Because tardive dyskinesia developing in adults is usually irreversible and has no satisfactory treatment, care must be taken to reduce the likelihood of its occurrence. Antipsychotic medication should be prescribed only when necessary and should be withheld periodically to assess the need for continued treatment and to unmask incipient dyskinesia. Thioridazine, a phenothiazine with a piperidine side chain, is an effective antipsychotic that seems less likely than most to cause extrapyramidal reactions, perhaps because it has little effect on dopamine receptors in the striatal system. Finally, anticholinergic drugs should not be prescribed routinely in patients receiving neuroleptics, since the combination may increase the likelihood of dyskinesia.

Wilson's Disease

Wilson's disease, a recessively inherited disorder of copper metabolism, is characterized biochemically by reduced serum copper and ceruloplasmin concentrations, pathologically by markedly increased concentration of copper in the brain and viscera, and clinically by signs of hepatic and neurologic dysfunction. Treatment involves the removal of excess copper, followed by maintenance of copper balance. The most satisfactory agent currently available for this purpose is **penicillamine** (dimethylcysteine), a chelating agent that forms a ring complex with copper. It is readily absorbed from the gastrointestinal tract and rapidly excreted in the urine. A common starting dose in adults is 500 mg 3 or 4 times daily. After remission occurs, it may be possible to lower the maintenance dose, generally to not less than 1 g daily, which must thereafter be continued indefinitely. Side-effects include nausea and vomiting, nephrotic syndrome, a lupuslike syndrome, pemphigus, myasthenia, arthropathy, optic neuropathy, and various blood dyscrasias. Treatment should be monitored by frequent urinalysis and complete blood counts. Dietary copper should also be kept below 2 mg daily by the exclusion of chocolate, nuts, shellfish, liver, mushrooms, broccoli, and cereals; and distilled or demineralized water may have to be provided if tap water contains more than 0.1 mg of copper per liter. Potassium disulfide, 20 mg 3 times daily with meals, reduces the intestinal absorption of copper and should also be prescribed.

• • •

References

Bianchine JR: Drug therapy of parkinsonism. *N Engl J Med* 1976;**295:**814.

Calne DB et al: Advances in the neuropharmacology of parkinsonism. *Ann Intern Med* 1979;**90:**219.

Fahn S, Calne DB: Considerations in the management of parkinsonism. *Neurology* 1978;**28:**5.

Lieberman A et al: Long-term efficacy of bromocriptine in Parkinson disease. *Neurology* 1980;**30:**518.

Marsden CD, Parkes JD: Success and problems of long-term levodopa therapy in Parkinson's disease. *Lancet* 1977;**1:**345.

Parkes JD: Adverse effects of antiparkinsonian drugs. *Drugs* 1981;**21:**341.

Seeman P: Brain dopamine receptors. *Pharmacol Rev* 1981;**32:**229.

Antipsychotics & Lithium | 26

Leo Hollister, MD

ANTIPSYCHOTICS

The term **antipsychotics** is one of several applied to a group of drugs that have been used mainly for treating schizophrenia but are effective in some other psychoses as well. The preferred term in Europe is **neuroleptics,** connoting the capacity of these drugs to affect several integrating systems of the brain, including the ability to cause movement disorders. The term **major tranquilizers** has fortunately fallen into disuse, since it confounds these drugs with **minor tranquilizers** (actually sedative-hypnotics), which they resemble only superficially.

History

No acceptable forms of drug treatment were available for treating schizophrenia until the early 1950s, when both reserpine and chlorpromazine appeared almost simultaneously. Chlorpromazine had been developed as an antihistamine and reserpine as an antihypertensive agent. Fortuitous observations of their calming properties led to trials in psychiatric patients. Initial clinical trials were enthusiastically reported. Over the years, reserpine became obsolete as an antipsychotic drug, since it was not believed to be as effective as chlorpromazine and was more likely to produce mental depression. The success of chlorpromazine led to the introduction of numerous phenothiazine derivatives. During the past 30 years, many different chemical structures have been shown to share the spectrum of pharmacologic activities associated with antipsychotic activity.

Nature of Psychosis & Schizophrenia

The term "psychosis" denotes a variety of mental disorders. Schizophrenia is a particular kind of psychosis characterized mainly by a clear sensorium but a marked thinking disturbance. The pathogenesis is unknown.

Largely as a result of research stimulated by the discovery of antipsychotic drugs, it has been proposed that genetic predisposition is a necessary but not always sufficient condition underlying the psychotic disorders. The ensuing abnormality is thought to reside primarily, but not exclusively, in overactivity of dopaminergic pathways of the brain, particularly in the mesolimbic-frontal dopaminergic system (Fig 26–1). Whether the overactivity is due to excessive synthesis and release of dopamine presynaptically or impaired metabolism or enhanced postsynaptic receptor sensitivity is uncertain. The "dopamine hypothesis" of schizophrenia is based on 3 circumstantial lines of evidence: (1) virtually all antipsychotic drugs block postsynaptic dopamine receptors; (2) increasing dopaminergic activity by administering levodopa sometimes produces a schizophreniform psychosis; and (3) abuse of sympathomimetic stimulants, which increase release of dopamine, produces a paranoid state resembling paranoid schizophrenia.

More recently, evidence has been adduced that some schizophrenic patients show brain atrophy as measured by CT scan and that these patients are generally refractory to treatment with drugs, following a deteriorating course. On the other hand, patients without this structural abnormality may have a functional

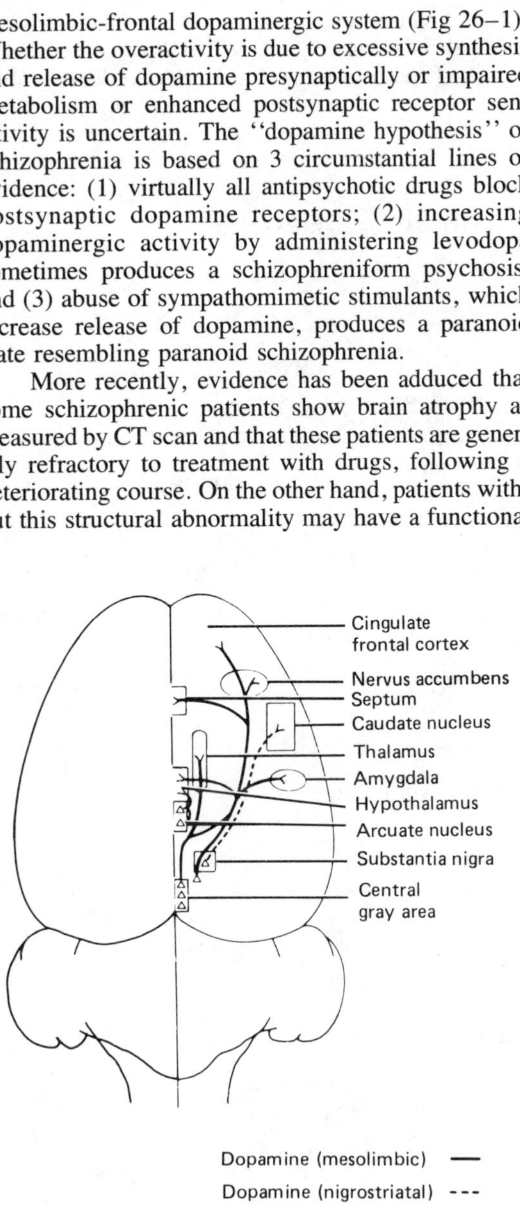

Figure 26–1. Diagrammatic section of brain showing the 2 principal dopaminergic tracts of the mesolimbic-frontal system and the nigrostriatal system.

abnormality of the dopamine system that is corrected by antipsychotic drugs. Even in the latter instance, the amelioration of schizophrenia is at best partial, manifested by clearer thinking, more acceptable behavior, and some degree of social and vocational rehabilitation.

I. BASIC PHARMACOLOGY OF ANTIPSYCHOTIC DRUGS

Chemical Types

A number of chemical structures have been associated with antipsychotic properties. The drugs can be classified into 4 major groups as shown in Fig 26–2.

A. Phenothiazine Derivatives: Three subfamilies of phenothiazines, based primarily on the side chain of the molecule, are in use. Aliphatic derivatives, exemplified by chlorpromazine, are the least potent. Piperidine derivatives (eg, thioridazine) and piperazine derivatives are more potent in the sense that they are effective in lower milligram doses. However, the piperazine derivatives are also more specific in their pharmacologic effects.

B. Thioxanthene Derivatives: This group of drugs is exemplified primarily by thiothixene. In general, this group of compounds is slightly less potent than their phenothiazine homologs.

C. Butyrophenone Derivatives: This rapidly growing group, of which haloperidol is the most widely used, has a somewhat different structure than the other 2 groups. Diphenylbutylpiperidines are closely related compounds.

ANTIPSYCHOTIC DRUGS

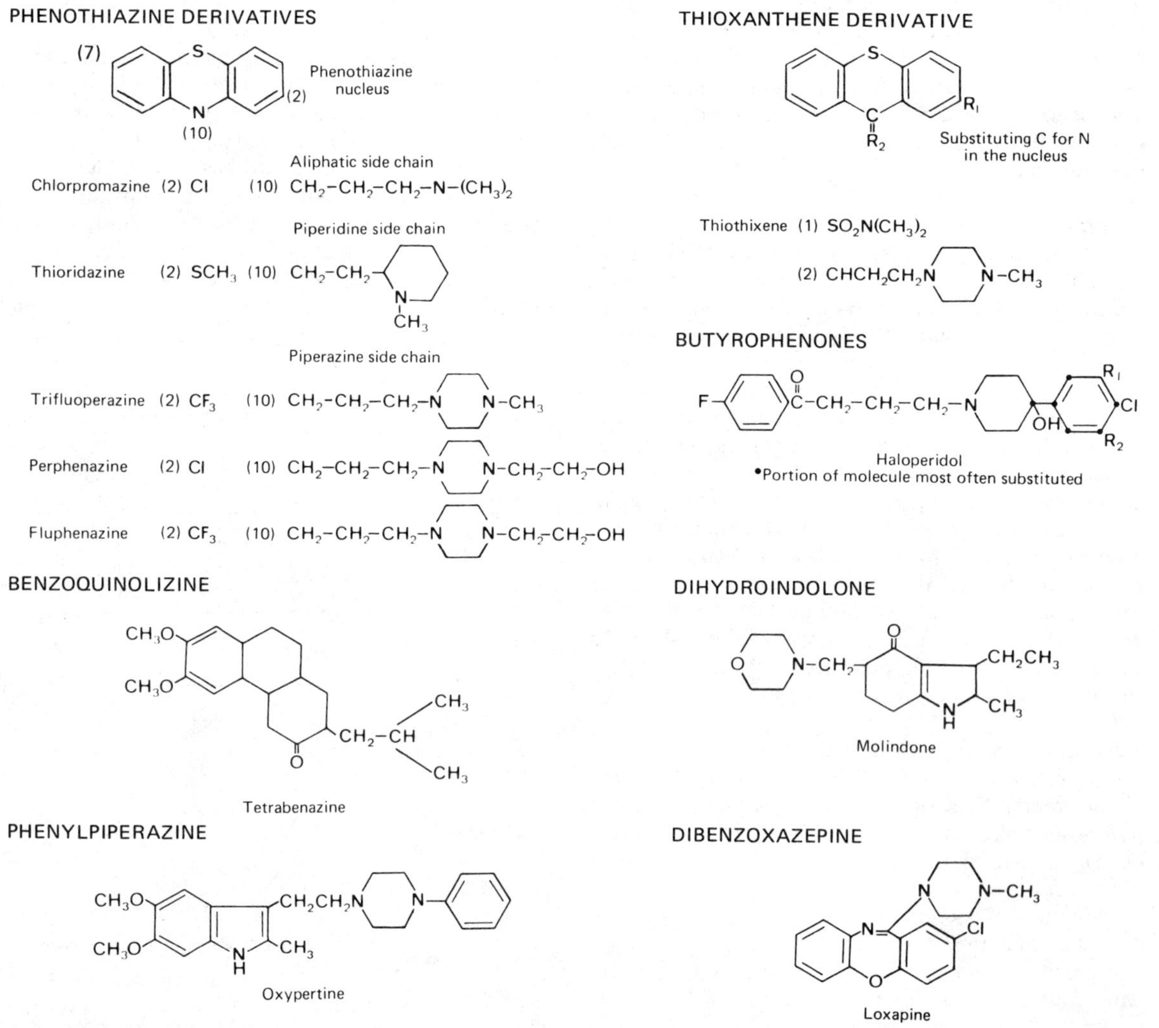

Figure 26–2. Structural formulas, of phenothiazines, thioxanthenes, butyrophenones, and a miscellaneous group of antipsychotics. Only representative members of each type are shown.

D. Miscellaneous Structures: These include benzoquinolizines (tetrabenazine), dihydroindolone derivatives (molindone), phenylpiperazine derivatives (oxypertine), and some tricyclic structures with a 6–7–6 ring structure (loxapine).

Pharmacokinetics

A. Metabolism: Chlorpromazine may have one of the most complicated routes of metabolism of any drug, with 60 or so identified metabolites. Various routes include nuclear transformations of the tricyclic portion (hydroxylations with subsequent conjugation as well as sulfoxidation of the sulfur atom) and transformations of the aliphatic side chain (demethylations, N-oxidation, and deamination). Some of the metabolites may be active, especially the 7-hydroxy metabolite.

Thioridazine produces 2 active metabolites, mesoridazine and sulforidazine, both from sulfoxidations on the thiomethyl ring substituent. Ring sulfoxidation results in an inactive metabolite. Trifluoperazine has metabolic pathways similar to those of chlorpromazine, with the addition of opening of the piperazine moiety and formation of a free amine. The thioxanthenes are metabolized like the phenothiazines. Metabolism of haloperidol involves N-dealkylation, oxidation, and conjugation. Although an active hydroxy metabolite is formed, its concentrations are inconsequential.

B. Distribution and Excretion: Most antipsychotics are highly lipid-soluble and protein-bound (92–99%). Thus, they tend to have large volumes of distribution (usually more than 7 L/kg). Bioavailability following oral administration is quite variable, tending to be low (25–35%) with drugs such as chlorpromazine that are extensively metabolized and higher with drugs such as haloperidol that have simpler metabolic pathways. The plasma half-lives tend to be short, ranging from 10 to 20 hours, but the clinical duration of the antipsychotic action is much longer than the short plasma half-life would indicate. Urinary metabolites of chlorpromazine may be found weeks after the last dose of chronically administered drug, suggesting that a large amount of the drug is sequestered in tissues. The importance of active metabolites in determining the clinical effects of these drugs is not known.

Pharmacologic Effects

A. Effects on Dopaminergic Synapses: A number of pharmacologic and biochemical actions of these drugs suggest that they should be called **dopamine antagonists.** Blockade of postsynaptic dopamine receptors in the mesolimbic system of the brain probably accounts for their ability to ameliorate schizophrenia, while the same action in the nigrostriatal pathway may account for the unwanted parkinsonism symptoms that result from prolonged administration. These 2 actions of antipsychotic drugs, apparently so disparate, have similar mechanisms of action. Blockade of dopamine receptors in the tuberoinfundibular dopamine pathway releases prolactin from the tonic inhibitory control of dopamine, resulting in hyperprolactinemia. Thus, the same pharmacodynamic action may have psychiatric, neurologic, and endocrine consequences.

Despite their ability to block postsynaptic dopamine receptors, these drugs are only partially effective in schizophrenia. Furthermore, their effects can be easily antagonized by administering dopamine precursors, such as levodopa, or dopamine receptor agonists, such as apomorphine. These findings suggest either that dopamine receptor blockade is incomplete or that the antipsychotic action is due to some other mechanism, possibly in conjunction with the effect at dopamine synapses.

With continued use of antipsychotics, some patients develop supersensitivity of dopamine receptors, especially in the nigrostriatal system, that leads to the clinical manifestation called **tardive dyskinesia,** characterized by choreoathetoid movements resembling those associated with Huntington's disease. This change apparently occurs as a compensatory mechanism against the blockade of dopamine receptors (Fig 26–3). Whether such supersensitivity of receptors in

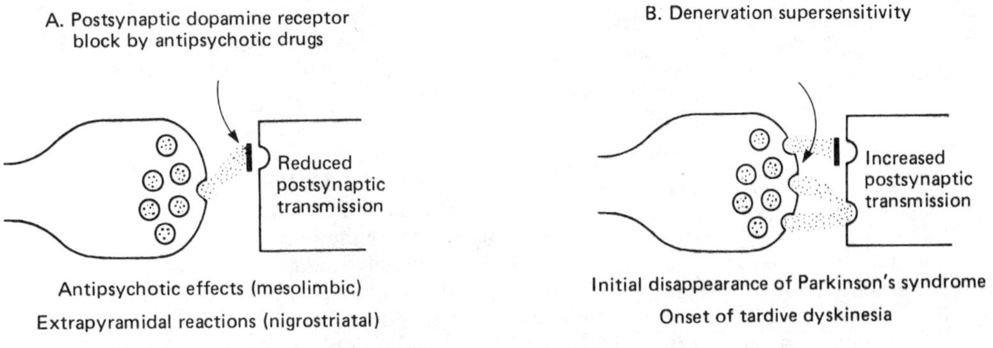

Figure 26–3. *A:* Postsynaptic dopamine receptor blockade by antipsychotic drugs produces 2 actions: antipsychotic effects and extrapyramidal reactions. *B:* Continued treatment is thought to lead to increased dopamine stores presynaptically and new and supersensitive receptors postsynaptically. Compensatory mechanisms may eliminate initial parkinsonism, but if overcompensation occurs, the symptoms may be replaced by those of tardive dyskinesia.

the mesolimbic system leads to tolerance to the antipsychotic effects of these drugs is currently under investigation.

B. Effects on Other Neurotransmitters: Although some antipsychotics have antiserotonin or antinoradrenergic actions, it is uncertain how these contribute to the therapeutic effects. Some investigators have suggested that the antinoradrenergic action may be related to their ability to control excitement as well as their peripheral effects such as orthostatic hypotension. Many antipsychotics also show evidence of central blockade of histamine H_1 receptors, an action that may relate to their sedative effects. All have varying degrees of antimuscarinic action, thioridazine being most potent. This action may reduce the intensity of parkinsonism, but it is also manifested peripherally by many common side-effects, such as dry mouth, blurred vision, constipation, and difficulty in urination. Some of these effects are summarized in Table 26–1.

C. Psychologic Effects: Most antipsychotic drugs cause unpleasant reactions in nonpsychotic individuals; the combination of sleepiness, restlessness, and autonomic effects create experiences unlike those associated with more familiar sedatives or hypnotics. Performance is impaired as judged by a number of psychomotor and psychometric tests. In general, the more active the drug or the larger the dose, the greater the impairment as shown by psychomotor tests. The crucial clinical question of the effects of such impairment on various potentially hazardous functions, such as driving, during therapeutic administration is still unsettled.

D. Neurophysiologic Effects: Antipsychotic drugs produce shifts in the pattern of electroencephalographic frequencies, chiefly in the direction of slowing and increased synchronization. The slowing (hypersynchrony) is sometimes focal or unilateral, which may lead to erroneous diagnostic interpretations. Both the frequency and the amplitude changes induced by psychotropic drugs are readily apparent and can be confirmed by sophisticated electronic techniques.

Table 26–1. Unwanted pharmacologic effects of antipsychotic drugs.

Type	Manifestations	Mechanism
Autonomic nervous system	Cycloplegia, dry mouth, difficulty urinating, constipation.	Muscarinic cholinergic blockade.
	Orthostatic hypotension, impotence, failure to ejaculate.	Alpha-adrenergic blockade.
Central nervous system	Parkinson's syndrome, akathisia, dystonias.	Dopamine receptor blockade.
	Tardive dyskinesia.	Supersensitivity of dopamine receptors.
	Toxic-confusional state.	Muscarinic cholinergic blockade.
Endocrine system	Amenorrhea-galactorrhea, infertility, impotence.	Dopamine receptor blockade resulting in hyperprolactinemia.

Electroencephalographic changes associated with antipsychotic drugs appear first in subcortical electrodes, supporting the view that their chief action is exerted at subcortical sites. The hypersynchrony produced by these drugs may account for their activating effect on the EEG in epileptic patients, as well as their occasional elicitation of seizures in patients with no history of seizure disorders.

E. Endocrine Effects: Antipsychotic drugs produce striking side-effects on the reproductive system. Amenorrhea-galactorrhea, false-positive pregnancy tests, and increased libido have been reported in women, whereas men have been troubled by decreased libido and gynecomastia. Some of these effects are secondary to loss of the tonic inhibition of prolactin secretion by dopamine; others may be due to increased peripheral conversion of androgens to estrogens.

F. Cardiovascular Effects: Orthostatic hypotension and high resting pulse rates frequently result from use of the "high-dose" phenothiazines. Mean arterial pressure, peripheral resistance, and stroke volume are decreased, and pulse rate is increased.

Abnormal ECGs have been observed, especially with thioridazine. Changes include prolongation of the Q–T interval and abnormal configurations of the ST segment and T waves, the latter being rounded, flattened, or notched. These changes are readily reversible upon withdrawal of the drug.

G. Animal Screening Tests: Inhibition of conditioned (but not unconditioned) avoidance behavior is one of the tests most predictive of antipsychotic action. Another is the inhibition of amphetamine- or apomorphine-induced stereotyped behavior. This inhibition no doubt is related to the dopamine receptor-blocking action of the drugs, countering these 2 dopamine agonists. Other tests that may predict antipsychotic action are reduction of exploratory behavior without undue sedation, induction of a cataleptic state, inhibition of intracranial stimulation of reward areas, and prevention of apomorphine-induced vomiting. It is difficult to see the pertinence of many of these tests to any model of clinical psychosis.

II. CLINICAL PHARMACOLOGY OF ANTIPSYCHOTIC DRUGS

Indications

A. Psychiatric Indications: Schizophrenia is the primary indication for these drugs, which presently constitute the only clearly efficacious treatment. Unfortunately, some patients do not respond at all, and virtually none show a complete response. Because some schizophrenics have a favorable course with prolonged remission after an initial episode, most physicians recommend discontinuing drug therapy after remission has been achieved following the first episode.

Schizo-affective schizophrenic disorders may be more similar to affective disorders than to schizophrenia. Nonetheless, the psychotic aspects of the illness require treatment with antipsychotics, which may be used in combination with other drugs, such as antidepressants or lithium. Mania during manic-depressive disorder is most effectively treated with antipsychotics, although lithium alone may suffice in milder cases. As mania subsides, the antipsychotic drug may be withdrawn. Nonmanic excited states may also be managed by antipsychotics, but attempts to define the diagnosis should not be abandoned.

Psychoses associated with old age, notably Alzheimer's disease, may show some symptomatic improvement with antipsychotics. Disturbed behavior, emotional lability, and abnormal sleep-wake cycles may be improved, but the basic disorder is untouched.

Gilles de la Tourette's syndrome, characterized by unpredictable barking tics and outbursts of foul language, has been successfully managed with haloperidol and may also be responsive to other antipsychotics.

The use of antipsychotics as primary treatment for depression is controversial. Because of the danger of tardive dyskinesia, most clinicians would use them only adjunctively in patients with agitated or psychotic depressions.

Acute brain syndromes following withdrawal from alcohol or other drugs should not be treated with antipsychotics. Substitution of a pharmacologically equivalent drug, stabilization on that drug, and subsequent gradual withdrawal are the time-honored principles of management. Acute adverse reactions associated with the use of other social drugs may be aggravated by antipsychotics but can be managed with simple sedatives. Overdoses of amphetamine and related stimulants are best managed with haloperidol, which is also likely to help the delirium of medically or surgically ill patients.

Antipsychotics in small doses have been promoted for relief of anxiety associated with minor emotional disorders. The antianxiety sedatives (Chapter 19) are far better in every respect, including safety and acceptability to patients.

B. Nonpsychiatric Indications: Most antipsychotic drugs, with the exception of thioridazine, have a strong antiemetic effect. This action is due to dopamine receptor blockade, both centrally (in the chemoreceptor trigger zone of the medulla) and peripherally (on receptors in the stomach). Some drugs, such as prochlorperazine and benzquinamide, are promoted solely as antiemetics. Phenothiazines with shorter side chains have considerable H_1 receptor-blocking action and have been used for relief of pruritus or, in the case of promethazine, as preoperative sedatives. The butyrophenone droperidol is used in combination with a meperidinelike drug, fentanyl, in "neuroleptanesthesia." The use of these drugs for nonpsychiatric indications is described in Chapter 22.

Choice of Drug

A rational choice of antipsychotic drugs may be based on differences between chemical structures and the attendant pharmacologic differences, since the differences between groups are greater than the differences within groups. Thus, one might select one member of each of the 3 subfamilies of phenothiazines, a member of the thioxanthene and butyrophenone group, and perhaps 2 members of the miscellaneous group. A possible selection is shown in Table 26–2.

No basis exists for choosing drugs for use against "target symptoms," as there is no evidence of specificity in their effects. The physician whose practice often or sometimes requires prescribing drugs for long-term management of psychotic disorders does not need to know all of the drugs but should become familiar with the effects—including the side-effects—of one or two drugs in each class. The best guide for selecting a drug for individual patients is their past responses to drugs. The trend in recent years has been away from the "low-potency" agents such as

Table 26–2. Some representative antipsychotic drugs.

Drug Class	Drug	Advantages	Disadvantages
Phenothiazines			
Aliphatic	Chlorpromazine[1]	Generic	Many side-effects; probably should not be used (obsolete).
Piperidine	Thioridazine[2] (Mellaril)	Slight extrapyramidal syndrome.	800 mg/d limit; no parenteral form; (?) cardiotoxicity.
Piperazine	Fluphenazine[3] (Permitil, Prolixin)	Depot form also available (enanthate, decanoate).	(?) Increased tardive dyskinesia.
Thioxanthene	Thiothixene[4] (Navane)	Parenteral form also available; (?) decreased tardive dyskinesia.	Uncertain.
Butyrophenone	Haloperidol (Haldol)	Parenteral form also available.	Severe extrapyramidal syndrome.
Dibenzoxazepine	Loxapine (Loxitane)	(?) No weight gain.	Uncertain.
Dihydroindolone	Molindone (Moban)	(?) No weight gain.	Uncertain.

[1] Other aliphatic phenothiazines: Promazine (Sparine, generic), triflupromazine (Vesprin).
[2] Other piperidine phenothiazines: Piperacetazine (Quide), mesoridazine (Lidanar, Serentil).
[3] Other piperazine phenothiazines: Acetophenazine (Tindal), perphenazine (Trilafon), carphenazine (Proketazine), prochlorperazine (Compazine, generic), trifluoperazine (Stelazine).
[4] Other thioxanthenes: Chlorprothixene (Taractan).

chlorpromazine and thioridazine to the "high-potency" drugs such as thiothixene, haloperidol, and fluphenazine. Chlorpromazine, in fact, should probably now be considered obsolete in view of its high incidence of side-effects (see below).

Doses

The range of effective doses among various antipsychotics is quite broad. Even with individual drugs in each class, a wide range of doses may be used, since therapeutic margins are substantial. Assuming that doses are equivalent, there is no evidence that any antipsychotic drug is superior in overall efficacy to any other. However, some patients who fail to respond to one drug may respond to another, and for this reason, several drugs may have to be tried to find the one most effective for an individual patient.

Some dose relationships between various antipsychotic drugs, as well as possible therapeutic ranges, are shown in Table 26–3.

Plasma Concentrations & Clinical Effects

Attempts to define a therapeutic range of plasma concentrations of antipsychotic agents are beset by many difficulties. A range of 150–300 ng/mL has been suggested for chlorpromazine, but the evidence is tenuous. Ranges of 7–20 ng/mL have been suggested for haloperidol, although some very refractory patients may benefit from levels up to 50 ng/mL. Clinical monitoring of plasma concentrations of these drugs, although technically feasible, is not warranted at this time.

Pharmaceutical Preparations

Well-tolerated parenteral forms of the high-potency drugs are available for rapid initiation of treatment as well as for maintenance treatment in noncompliant patients. Since the parenterally administered drugs may have much greater bioavailability than the oral forms, doses should be only a fraction of what might be given orally. Fluphenazine decanoate is the drug most widely used for parenteral maintenance therapy. A single intramuscular dose of this drug may be adequate for long periods (1–4 weeks). However, the release characteristics of such preparations are somewhat uncertain. While their value in maintenance treatment is established for noncompliant patients, these preparations offer no advantage over oral doses in compliant patients. Thus, they should not be used routinely.

Table 26–3. Dose relationships of antipsychotics.

	Minimum Effective Therapeutic Dose (mg)	Usual Range of Daily Doses (mg)
Chlorpromazine (Thorazine)	100	100–1000
Thioridazine (Mellaril)	100	100–800
Mesoridazine (Lidanar, Serentil)	50	50–400
Piperacetazine (Quide)	10	20–160
Trifluoperazine (Vesprin)	5	5–60
Perphenazine (Trilafon)	10	8–64
Fluphenazine (Permitil, Prolixin)	2	2–60
Thiothixene (Navane)	2	2–120
Haloperidol (Haldol)	2	2–100
Loxapine (Loxitane)	10	20–160
Molindone (Lidone, Moban)	10	20–200

Dosage Schedules

Antipsychotics may be given in divided daily doses initially while an effective dose level is being sought. They need not always be equally divided doses, even when given orally. After an effective daily dose has been defined for an individual patient, doses can be given less frequently. Once-daily doses are feasible for many patients during chronic maintenance treatment. Simplification of dosage schedules leads to better compliance. Maximum dose units of many drugs are being increased by manufacturers to meet the needs of once-daily dosing.

Maintenance Treatment

A small minority of schizophrenic patients may remit from an acute episode and require no further drug therapy for prolonged periods. In most cases, however, schizophrenia is a chronic disorder that only partially remits, so that drug therapy must be continued indefinitely.

The issue is whether treatment should be continuous or intermittent. Advocates of "drug holidays" maintain that many patients do not relapse for substantial periods after treatment is stopped once remission has been achieved with drugs, and that such interruptions in treatment diminish the total amount of exposure to drugs and lessen the likelihood of tardive dyskinesia. The contrary view is that there is no way of predicting who will relapse early; that it is better to keep maintenance doses at minimal levels to reduce total exposure to drugs; that some evidence suggests tardive dyskinesia may be more likely to occur with interrupted maintenance dose schedules; and that rapid and unexpected relapse may undo much of the hard-won rehabilitative gains afforded by a good treatment program. The issue is not decided.

Drug Combinations

Combining antipsychotic drugs confounds evaluation of the efficacy of the drugs being used. Tricyclic antidepressants may be used with antipsychotics, but only for clear symptoms of depression complicating schizophrenia. They are of no proved efficacy for alleviating the social withdrawal and blunted affect of the psychotic. Lithium is sometimes added with benefit to antipsychotic agents when patients fail to respond to the latter drugs alone. It is uncertain whether such instances represent misdiagnosed cases of mania. Sedative drugs may be added for relief of anxiety or insomnia not controlled by antipsychotics.

The drugs most frequently combined with antipsychotics are antiparkinsonism agents. Although it has been claimed that concurrent use of these drugs reduces the bioavailability of chlorpromazine, the evidence is uncertain, and the effect is probably of little clinical consequence in any case. It has also been suggested that these drugs undo the therapeutic action of antipsychotics; but when the choice is between this theoretical possibility and the real problem of treating parkinsonism, most clinicians prefer to treat with antiparkinsonism drugs.

Adverse Reactions

Most of the unwanted effects of antipsychotics are extensions of their known pharmacologic actions, but a few are allergic and some are idiosyncratic.

A. Behavioral Effects: Antipsychotic drugs are unpleasant to take—the more so the less psychotic the patient. Many patients stop taking their drug because of the unpleasant side-effects, which may be mitigated by giving small doses during the day and the major portion at bedtime. A "pseudodepression" that may be due to akinesia from these drugs usually responds to treatment with antiparkinsonism drugs. Other "pseudodepressions" may be due to using higher doses than needed in a partially remitted patient, in which case decreasing the dose may relieve the symptom. Toxic-confusional states may occur with very high doses of drugs that have prominent anticholinergic actions. The development of supersensitivity of receptors that are blocked by the antipsychotic agents could result in tolerance to the drugs or even a drug-resistant form of psychosis. This is a matter of current concern.

B. Neurologic Effects: Parkinson's syndrome, including akathisia and acute dystonias (spastic torticollis or retrocollis), may occur at any time during antipsychotic therapy and is usually responsive to conventional antiparkinsonism drugs of the anticholinergic type. Such drugs may not have to be used throughout treatment; attempts to discontinue their use should be made every 3–4 months. Prophylactic use of antiparkinsonism drugs may be useful in patients at high risk of developing extrapyramidal reactions, such as children or young adults being treated with substantial doses of high-potency drugs. Otherwise, it seems better to await the development of symptoms severe enough to warrant treatment.

Tardive dyskinesia, a late-appearing syndrome of abnormal choreoathetoid movements, is the most important unwanted effect of antipsychotics. It has been proposed that it is caused by a relative cholinergic deficiency secondary to supersensitivity of dopamine receptors in the caudate-putamen. Older women treated for long periods are most susceptible to the disorder, although it can occur at any age and in either sex. The prevalence varies enormously, but tardive dyskinesia is estimated to occur in 20–40% of chronically treated patients. Early recognition is important, since advanced cases may be difficult to reverse. Decreasing the dosage of antipsychotic drug, eliminating anticholinergic drugs such as antiparkinsonism agents and tricyclic antidepressants, and adding diazepam or reserpine have been tried in an attempt to mitigate this complication. The most promising treatment may be oral administration of acetylcholine precursors: choline or lecithin. Lecithin is hydrolyzed to yield choline in the liver and has fewer side-effects.

C. Autonomic Nervous System Effects: Most patients become tolerant to the anticholinergic side-effects of antipsychotic drugs. Those who are made too uncomfortable or who are impaired, as with urinary retention, should be given bethanechol, a peripherally acting cholinomimetic. Orthostatic hypotension or impaired ejaculation, common complications of chlorpromazine therapy, should be managed by switching to drugs with less marked adrenergic blocking actions.

D. Metabolic and Endocrine Effects: Weight gain is common and requires monitoring of food intake. Hyperprolactinemia in women results in the amenorrhea-galactorrhea syndrome and infertility; in men, loss of libido, impotence, and infertility may result. Chlorpromazine also increases serum cholesterol levels.

E. Toxic or Allergic Reactions: Agranulocytosis is no longer a major risk except with low-potency drugs, eg, chlorpromazine. Clozapine, a promising drug several years ago, produced the greatest epidemic of drug-induced agranulocytosis in medical history and is now seldom used. Cholestatic jaundice is now rare, even with chlorpromazine.

F. Ocular Complications: Deposits in the anterior portion of the eye (cornea and lens) are a common complication of chlorpromazine therapy. They may accentuate the normal processes of aging of the lens. Thioridazine is the only antipsychotic drug that causes retinal deposits, which in advanced cases may resemble retinitis pigmentosa. The deposits are usually associated with "browning" of vision. The maximum daily dose of thioridazine has been limited to 800 mg/d to reduce the possibility of this complication.

G. Cardiac Toxicity: Thioridazine in doses exceeding 300 mg daily is almost always associated with minor abnormalities of T waves that are easily reversible. Overdoses of thioridazine are associated with major ventricular arrhythmias, cardiac conduction block, and sudden death; it is not certain whether thioridazine can cause these same disorders when used in therapeutic doses. In view of possible additive anticholinergic and quinidinelike actions with various tricyclic antidepressants, thioridazine should not be combined with the latter drugs.

H. Use in Pregnancy; Dysmorphogenesis: Although the antipsychotic drugs appear to be relatively safe in pregnancy, a small increase in risk could be missed. Questions about whether to use these drugs during pregnancy and whether to abort a pregnancy in which the fetus has already been exposed must be decided individually.

I. Malignant Neuroleptic Syndrome: This early complication of treatment appears to be an idiosyncratic response. It often follows an initial large dose of antipsychotic drug. High fever, mutism, extrapyramidal disturbances, and autonomic signs are characteristic. Death occurs unless cooling and rehydration are prompt and vigorous. This syndrome is somewhat different from the "heat stroke" that may occur during chronic treatment with these drugs during periods of high ambient temperature.

Drug Interactions

Pharmacodynamic interactions are more frequent than pharmacokinetic ones and are of greater importance clinically. The most important pharmacodynamic interaction of the antipsychotics is an additive depressant effect when they are used along with various other central nervous system depressants. Such drugs include conventional sedative-hypnotics, antihistamines, opiates, and alcohol. Neuroleptics have relatively little respiratory depressant action when taken by themselves, but they may have a modest additive effect when taken with other drugs that also depress respiration.

The anticholinergic effects of various antipsychotics vary in intensity, but they are often used with other drugs, such as antiparkinsonism agents or tricyclic antidepressants, that are strongly anticholinergic. The onset of anticholinergic delirium in the presence of psychosis may be deceiving, so that more drug is mistakenly added. Peripheral anticholinergic effects are more easily recognized.

The alpha-adrenergic receptor-blocking actions of some neuroleptics, especially chlorpromazine and thioridazine, are quite strong and may produce additive orthostatic hypotensive effects when combined with monoamine oxidase inhibitors or tricyclic antidepressants. On the other hand, chlorpromazine may reverse the antihypertensive effects of drugs that work on alpha receptors, such as guanethidine, clonidine, bethanidine, debrisoquin, and possibly methyldopa.

Thioridazine has quinidinelike effects perhaps related to its cardiotoxicity. Other drugs with such actions include quinidine and procainamide, tricyclic antidepressants, and hydroxyzine. The use of thioridazine with any of these classes of drugs should be avoided, since the arrhythmogenic potential of the drug may be increased.

Pharmacokinetic interactions are of less importance. Colloidal antacids, kaolin, and activated charcoal adsorb chlorpromazine and probably also other phenothiazines and tricyclic antidepressants as well as other drugs concurrently administered. It would seem desirable to separate by at least 1–2 hours the ingestion of such antacids and the subsequent administration of any drug.

Chlorpromazine, perphenazine, haloperidol, chlorprothixene, and thioridazine inhibit the hydroxylation of imipramine and nortriptyline, and the reverse is true to some extent. Thus, concurrent administration of both types of drugs may lead to elevated plasma concentrations of both. This interaction—at least between nortriptyline and perphenazine—seems to occur only with large doses of either drug.

A possible interaction between phenothiazines (specifically thioridazine) and phenytoin might be of greater consequence. Inhibition of metabolism of phenytoin, which has a narrow therapeutic range, has led to serious clinical toxicity.

Overdoses

Poisonings with antipsychotics are rarely fatal, with the exception of those due to mesoridazine and thioridazine. In general, drowsiness proceeds to coma, with an intervening period of agitation. Neuromuscular excitability may proceed to convulsions. Pupils are miotic, and deep tendon reflexes are decreased. Hypotension and hypothermia are the rule, although fever may be present later in the course. The lethal effects of mesoridazine and thioridazine are related to their actions on the heart.

Patients should be monitored in an intensive care setting for the usual vital signs, venous pressure, arterial blood gases, and electrolytes. Attempts at gastric lavage should be made even if several hours have elapsed since the drug was taken, since gastrointestinal motility is decreased. Activated charcoal effectively binds most of these drugs, following which a saline cathartic may be given. Hypotension often responds to fluid replacement. If a pressor agent is to be used, norepinephrine or dopamine is preferred to epinephrine, whose unopposed β-adrenergic receptor-stimulant action in the presence of alpha blockade may cause vasodilatation. Seizures may be treated with either diazepam or phenytoin, the latter being given with an initial loading dose. Management of overdoses of thioridazine and mesoridazine, which are complicated by cardiac arrhythmias, is similar to that for tricyclic antidepressants (Chapter 27).

LITHIUM

Lithium is often referred to as an "antimanic" drug, but some cases of depression also seem to respond. In many parts of the world, lithium is referred to as a "mood-stabilizing" agent because of its primary action of preventing mood swings in patients with manic-depressive (bipolar) disorder. Other drugs possibly effective in preventing mood swings include carbamazepine, clonidine, and spironolactone, but lithium is the only one clearly established as useful.

Nature of Manic-Depressive Disorder

Manic-depressive illness is a frequently diagnosed and very serious emotional disorder. Patients with cyclic attacks of mania have many symptoms of paranoid schizophrenia (grandiosity, bellicosity, paranoid thoughts, and overactivity). The gratifying response to lithium therapy of patients with manic-depressive disorder has made such diagnostic distinctions important.

Bipolar disorder has a strong genetic component and seems to be biologically determined. The episodes of mood swings are generally unrelated to life events.

The exact biologic disturbance has not been identified, but a preponderance of catecholaminergic activity is thought to be present. Drugs that increase this activity tend to exacerbate mania, whereas those that reduce activity of dopamine or norepinephrine relieve mania. Acetylcholine may also be involved. The nature of the abrupt switch from mania to depression experienced by some patients is uncertain.

Drugs for Manic-Depressive Disorder

When mania is mild, lithium alone may be effective treatment. In more severe cases, it is almost always necessary to give one of the antipsychotic drugs also. After mania is controlled, the antipsychotic drug may be stopped and lithium continued as maintenance therapy.

Unlike antipsychotic or antidepressant drugs, which exert several actions on the central or autonomic nervous system, lithium ion produces only mild sedation and is devoid of adrenergic blocking or anticholinergic effects. Since it is a small inorganic ion, lithium is easily measured in body fluids such as plasma, urine, or saliva, is distributed in body water, and is not metabolized. Thus, its kinetics can be studied much more easily, and plasma or tissue concentrations can be correlated with clinical effects. A third attribute of considerable interest has been the prophylactic use of lithium in preventing both mania and depression. It is indeed remarkable that a so-called functional psychosis can be controlled so easily by such a simple chemical as lithium carbonate.

Lithium may be combined with antipsychotics when mania breaks through a prophylactic treatment program, or with antidepressants when depression becomes apparent. Although haloperidol was alleged to be a poor drug to combine with lithium, it seems in retrospect to be no different from other neuroleptics. All neuroleptics may produce more severe extrapyramidal syndromes when combined with lithium.

I. BASIC PHARMACOLOGY OF LITHIUM

No single mechanism accounts for the therapeutic effect of lithium. Its effects on neurotransmitters, cell membranes, cations, and water have been the major avenues of inquiry.

Lithium is thought to accelerate the presynaptic destruction of catecholamines, to inhibit release of transmitters at the synapse, and to decrease the sensitivity of the postsynaptic receptor. All of these actions would tend to correct the overactivity of catecholaminergic systems presumed to occur in mania. Many of these actions of lithium are acute and have not been demonstrated to be sustained during chronic treatment.

Presynaptic and postsynaptic regulation of neurotransmission is intimately involved with various cations of physiologic importance, eg, sodium, potassium, magnesium, and calcium. Neurotransmitter release is probably calcium-dependent, while the configuration of postsynaptic receptors may be altered by sodium. The passage of lithium into cells, where it exerts its major action, is intimately concerned with these ions as well.

Both calcium and magnesium are required for stabilization of cell membranes, tending to make them less fluid. Displacement by lithium of either calcium or magnesium might increase membrane permeability.

In extracellular fluid, lithium acts similarly to potassium and stimulates sodium efflux from cells, both by cation exchange and by stimulation of the Na^+-K^+ pump mechanism. Lithium also enhances the entry of choline into cells, but the significance of this action is uncertain.

The rather simple pharmacokinetic properties of lithium are summarized in Table 26–4.

II. CLINICAL PHARMACOLOGY OF LITHIUM

Manic-Depressive (Bipolar) Disorder

Agreement is almost universal that lithium carbonate is the preferred treatment for bipolar disorder, especially in the manic phase. Because its onset of action is slow, concurrent use of antipsychotic drugs may be required for severely manic patients. The overall success rate for attaining remission from the manic phase of bipolar disorder is about 60–80%. Maintenance (prophylactic) therapy in patients with classic manic-depressive disorder is now well accepted. In general, control with maintenance lithium is about 60–70% effective.

Some clinicians find that depressive episodes during typical bipolar illness may respond better when a tricyclic antidepressant is added to lithium maintenance during this period. Rapidly cycling manic-depressive episodes have been linked to treatment with tricyclic antidepressants. Carbamazepine may be useful in such situations.

Table 26–4. Pharmacokinetics of lithium.

Absorption	Rapid. Virtually complete within 6–8 hours; peak plasma levels in 30 minutes to 2 hours.
Distribution	In total body water; slow entry into intracellular compartment. Apparent volumes of distribution of 0.5–0.9 L/kg body weight; some sequestration in bone. No protein binding.
Metabolism	None.
Excretion	Virtually entirely in urine. Lithium clearance about 20% of creatinine. Plasma half-life about 20 hours.

Other Applications

Acute endogenous depression is not generally considered to be an indication for treatment with lithium. On the other hand, recurrent endogenous depressions with a cyclic pattern are controlled by lithium and imipramine, both of which are superior to a placebo.

Schizo-affective disorders are characterized by a mixture of schizophrenic symptoms and altered affect in the form of depression or excitement. Antipsychotic drugs alone or combined with lithium are used in the excited phase; tricyclic antidepressants are used if depression is present.

Alcoholism is commonly believed to have a high association with depression and mania. When the 2 conditions exist, lithium may be useful in reducing drinking. Lithium has no established efficacy in the absence of affective symptoms.

Lithium is not regarded as useful for schizophrenia. Whether lithium added to antipsychotic drugs can enhance their efficacy in ordinary schizophrenia is an unsettled question.

An interesting application of lithium currently being investigated is the management of aggressive, violent behavior in prisoners. These men, both in and out of prison, have explosive responses to minimal provocation, possible brain damage with nonspecific abnormal EEGs, and long histories of violent criminal behavior. Sufficient studies are available to suggest that this may be an important indication for the use of lithium.

Doses & Dosage Schedules

Before treatment is started, one should obtain recent laboratory data such as a complete blood count, urinalysis, common biochemical tests, tests of thyroid function, and an ECG. Patients over 50 years of age should also have a creatinine clearance test. These tests serve as baseline measurements in assessing possible complications of treatment.

The patient's age and body weight and renal function should be considered in determining initial appropriate doses of lithium carbonate. The initial volume of distribution of lithium will be the same as body water, or about 0.5 L/kg body weight for women and 0.55 L/kg for men. The proportion of body water may decrease slightly in older individuals. What is more important in older patients is a subtle decrease in renal function. Any patient over 50 years of age is likely to have a decreased creatinine clearance, which may reach 50% or less of the usual normal values without abnormal elevation of serum creatinine.

A daily lithium dose of 0.5 mEq/L body water will produce the desired serum lithium concentration in the range of 0.9–1.4 mEq/L after a week of treatment if renal function is normal. If this level is not precisely reached, the dose can then be altered in arithmetic fashion to achieve the desired concentration in serum. Each 300-mg dose unit of lithium carbonate contains approximately 8 mEq of lithium.

It is almost always necessary to give lithium in divided doses to avoid gastric distress. Two to 4 divided doses may be needed, depending on the total daily dose. Medication is best taken with or shortly after meals.

Monitoring Treatment

Clinicians have relied heavily on measurements of plasma concentrations for assessing both the dose required for satisfactory treatment of acute mania and the adequacy of maintenance treatment. These measurements are customarily taken 10–12 hours after the last dose, so all data in the literature pertaining to these concentrations reflect this interval.

Maintenance Treatment

The decision to use lithium as prophylactic treatment depends on many factors: the frequency and severity of previous episodes, a crescendo pattern of appearance, and the degree to which the patient is willing to follow a program of indefinite maintenance therapy. If the present attack was the patient's first, one might prefer to terminate treatment after it has subsided. Patients who have one or more episodes of illness per year are candidates for maintenance treatment. However, if the patient is unreliable, it may be better to alert the family to the initial signs of recurrence and be prepared to provide prompt treatment when needed. Some patients with mania discontinue treatment voluntarily, feeling that their spirits and initiative are suppressed by lithium.

Drug Interactions

Renal clearance of lithium is reduced about 25% in the presence of oral diuretics, and doses may have to be reduced by a similar amount. A similar reduction in lithium clearance has been noted with several newer nonsteroidal anti-inflammatory drugs that block synthesis of prostaglandins. It is not known whether this interaction extends to aspirin and acetaminophen.

Side-Effects & Complications

Many side-effects associated with lithium treatment occur at varying times after treatment is started. Some are harmless, while others may presage the onset of toxicity. It is important to be alert to side-effects that may signify impending serious toxic reactions.

A. Neurologic and Psychiatric Side-Effects: Tremor is one of the most frequent side-effects of lithium treatment, occurring at therapeutic dose levels. Propranolol, which has been reported to be effective in essential tremor, also alleviates lithium-induced tremor. Other neurologic abnormalities that have been reported include choreoathetosis, motor hyperactivity, ataxia, dysarthria, and aphasia. Psychiatric disturbances are generally marked by mental confusion and withdrawal or bizarre motor movements.

B. Effects on Thyroid Function: Lithium probably decreases thyroid function in most patients exposed to the drug, but the effect is reversible or nonprogressive. Some patients develop frank thyroid enlargement, but only about 15% show symptoms of hypothyroidism.

C. Nephrogenic Diabetes Insipidus: Polydipsia and polyuria are often associated with lithium treatment, occurring at therapeutic plasma concentrations. The principal physiologic lesion involved is loss of the ability of the distal tubule to conserve water under the influence of antidiuretic hormone (ADH, vasopressin). Resistance of lithium-induced nephrogenic diabetes insipidus to vasopressin has led to other attempts at therapy. Chlorothiazide is moderately successful (see Chapter 13). Such treatment is not without risk, for sodium depletion may augment lithium toxicity.

D. Edema: Edema is a frequent side-effect of lithium treatment and may be related to some effect of lithium on sodium retention. Although weight gain may be expected in patients who become edematous, water retention alone probably does not account for all of it.

E. Cardiac Side-Effects: Reduced amplitude of T waves is a frequent finding during lithium treatment if the ECG tracing is examined carefully. No evidence of myocardial damage can be found when enzyme tests are done during periods of T wave abnormality, and the effect seems to be readily reversible. The sinus node may also be susceptible to toxic effects of lithium, with depression of its normal pacemaker function. The drug is definitely contraindicated in the "sick sinus" syndrome.

F. Use During Pregnancy: Renal clearance of lithium increases during pregnancy and reverts to lower levels immediately after delivery. A patient whose serum lithium concentration is in a good therapeutic range during pregnancy may develop toxic levels following delivery. Special care in monitoring lithium levels is needed at these times. Lithium is transferred to nursing children through breast milk, in which it has a concentration about one-third to one-half that of serum. Lithium toxicity in newborns is manifested by lethargy, cyanosis, poor suck and Moro reflexes, and possibly hepatomegaly.

The issue of dysmorphogenesis is not settled. One report suggests an alarming increase in the frequency of cardiac anomalies, especially Ebstein's anomaly, in lithium babies. At present one must observe the old rule that says no drug should be used during pregnancy unless the need for it outweighs the possible risk to the fetus.

G. Miscellaneous Side-Effects: Transient acneiform eruptions have been noted early in lithium treatment. Some of them subside with temporary discontinuation of treatment and do not recur with its resumption. Folliculitis is less dramatic and probably occurs more frequently. Leukocytosis is always present during lithium treatment, probably reflecting a direct effect on leukopoiesis rather than mobilization from the marginal pool. This "side-effect" has now become a therapeutic effect in patients with low leukocyte counts. Disturbed sexual function has been reported in men treated with lithium.

Overdoses

Therapeutic overdoses are more common than those due to deliberate or accidental ingestion of the drug. Therapeutic overdoses are usually due to accumulation of lithium resulting from some change in the patient's status, such as diminished serum sodium, use of diuretics, fluctuating renal function, or pregnancy. Since the tissues will have already equilibrated with the blood, the plasma concentrations of drugs may not be excessively high in proportion to the degree of toxicity; any value over 2 mEq/L must be considered as indicating potential toxicity.

A primary consideration is to rid the patient of the drug. Because of the physically large amounts of drug involved in cases of acute deliberate overdosage (one may be dealing with 30–60 g), absorption is slow. Lavage should be done with a wide-bore tube, as the material tends to clump and may be difficult to remove through smaller tubes. Saline cathartics should follow lavage. Charcoal is not an effective adsorbent in this instance. As lithium is a simple ion, it is dialyzed readily. Both peritoneal dialysis and hemodialysis are effective, though the latter is preferred. Dialysis should be continued until the plasma concentrations fall below the usual therapeutic range.

• • •

References

Antipsychotics

Branchey MH et al: High- and low-potency neuroleptics in elderly psychiatric patients. *JAMA* 1978;**239:**1860.

Carlsson A: Antipsychotic drugs, neurotransmitters and schizophrenia. *Am J Psychiatry* 1978;**135:**164.

Chouinard G, Jones BD: Neuroleptic-induced supersensitivity psychosis: Clinical and pharmacologic characteristics. *Am J Psychiatry* 1980;**137:**16.

Donlon PT, Tupin JP: Successful suicides with thioridazine and mesoridazine. *Arch Gen Psychiatry* 1977;**34:**955.

Donlon PT et al: High versus standard dosage fluphenazine hydrochloric acid in acute schizophrenia. *J Clin Psychiatry* 1978;**39:**800.

Itoh H et al: Malignant neuroleptic syndrome: Its present status in Japan and clinical problems. *Psychiatr Neurol Jpn* 1977;**31:**565.

Johnstone EC et al: Mechanism of the antipsychotic effect in the treatment of acute schizophrenia. *Lancet* 1978;**1:**848.

Kobayashi RM: Drug therapy of tardive dyskinesia. *N Engl J Med* 1977;**296:**257.

Rivera-Calimlim L et al: Correlation between plasma concentrations of chlorpromazine and clinical response. *Commun Psychopharmacol* 1978;**2:**215.

Rome HP: The classification of schizophrenia: A historical review. *Psychiatr Ann* 1979;**9:**12.

Schooler NR et al: Prevention of relapse in schizophrenia. *Arch Gen Psychiatry* 1980;**37:**16.

Stevens JR: Schizophrenia and dopamine regulation in the mesolimbic system. *Trends Neurosci* 1979;**1:**102.

Tarsy D, Baldessarini RJ: The pathophysiologic basis of tardive dyskinesia. *Biol Psychiatry* 1977;**12:**431.

Tuma AH, May PRA: And if that doesn't work, what next? A study of treatment failures in schizophrenia. *J Nerv Ment Dis* 1978;**167:**566.

Lithium

Albrecht J, Kampf D, Müller-Oerlinghausen B: Renal function and biopsy in patients on lithium therapy. *Pharmakopsychiatr Neuropsychopharmakol* 1980;**13:**228.

Amdisen A: Serum lithium monitoring and clinical pharmacokinetics of lithium. *Clin Pharmacokinet* 1977;**2:**73.

Bunney WE Jr et al: Mode of action of lithium: Some biological considerations. *Arch Gen Psychiatry* 1979;**36:**898.

Goodwin FW (editor): Lithium ion. *Arch Gen Psychiatry* 1979;**36:**833.

Greil W et al: Interindividual differences in the Na^+-dependent Li^+ countertransport system and in the Li^+ distribution ratio across the red cell membrane among Li^+-treated patients. *Psychopharmacology* 1977;**53:**19.

Hansen HE, Amdisen A: Lithium intoxication: Report of 23 cases and review of 100 cases from the literature. *Q J Med* 1978;**186:**123.

Jefferson JW, Greist JH: *Primer of Lithium Therapy.* Williams & Wilkins, 1977.

Quitkin F, Rifkin A, Klein DF: Prophylaxis of affective disorders. *Arch Gen Psychiatry* 1976;**33:**337.

Report of the APA Task Force: The current status of lithium therapy. *Am J Psychiatry* 1975;**132:**997.

Vestergaard P, Amdisen A, Schou M: Clinically significant side effects of lithium treatment: A survey of 237 patients in long-term treatment. *Acta Psychiatr Scand* 1980;**62:**193.

Antidepressants | 27

Leo Hollister, MD

Nature of Depression

Depression is readily diagnosed when it is the chief complaint, but unfortunately it rarely is; a host of complaints may mask the true underlying disorder. Patients with vague complaints that resist explanation as manifestations of somatic disorders and those who may be called "neurotics" or "crocks" should be suspected of being depressed.

Depression and anxiety are symptoms that usually occur together. The initial complaints of depressed patients are often physical; and some manifestations, such as fatigue, headache, insomnia, and gastrointestinal disturbances, resemble those of simple anxiety. Other complaints may be more distinctive: anorexia and weight loss, bad taste in the mouth, chronic pain, loss of interest, inactivity, loss of sexual desire, and a general feeling of despondency. The constellation of fatigue, musculoskeletal complaints, sleep disorder, and loss of joy in living is characteristic of depression. Guilt as a symptom is almost unique to depression; if anger is directed outward rather than inward, hostility rather than depression may dominate the clinical picture. The core depressive syndrome consists of somatic complaints, anxiety and tension, guilt, and various manifestations of depressed mood.

Depression is a heterogeneous disorder that has been characterized and classified in a variety of ways. A simplified classification based on presumed origin is as follows: (1) "reactive" or "secondary" depression (most common; over 60%), occurring in response to real stimuli such as grief, illness, etc; (2) "endogenous" depression, a genetically determined biochemical disorder manifested by inability to cope with ordinary stress (about 25%); and (3) depression associated with manic-depressive disorder (about 10–15%). Drugs discussed in this chapter are used chiefly in management of the second type. Table 27–1 indicates how the 3 types may be differentiated.

I. BASIC PHARMACOLOGY OF ANTIDEPRESSANTS

Chemistry

A variety of different chemical structures have been found to have antidepressant activity. The number is constantly growing, but as yet no group has been found to have a clear therapeutic advantage over the others. Table 27–4 lists clinically used antidepressants and their trade names.

A. Tricyclics: (Fig 27–1.) Tricyclic antidepressants—so called because of the characteristic 3-ring nucleus—have been used clinically for over 2 decades. They closely resemble the phenothiazines chemically and, to a lesser extent, pharmacologically. Like the latter drugs, they were first thought to be

Table 27–1. Differentiation of types of depression.

Type	Diagnostic Features	Comments
Reactive	Loss (adverse life events). Physical illness (myocardial infarct, cancer). Drugs (antihypertensives, alcohol, hormones). Other psychiatric disorders (senility).	More than 60% of all depression. Core depressive syndrome: depression, anxiety, bodily complaints, tension, guilt. May respond spontaneously or to a variety of ministrations.
Endogenous	Precipitating life event not adequate for degree of depression. Autonomous (unresponsive to changes in life). May occur at any age (childhood to old age). Biologically determined (family history).	About 25% of all depressions. Core depressive syndrome plus "vital" signs: abnormal rhythms of sleep, motor activity, libido, appetite. Usually respond specifically to antidepressants or ECT. Tend to recur throughout life.
Manic-depressive	Characterized by episodes of mania. Cyclic; mania alone, rare; depression alone, occasional; mania-depression, usual.	About 10–15% of all depressions. May be misdiagnosed as endogenous if hypomanic episodes are missed. Lithium carbonate stabilizes mood. Mania may require antipsychotic drugs as well; depression managed with antidepressants.

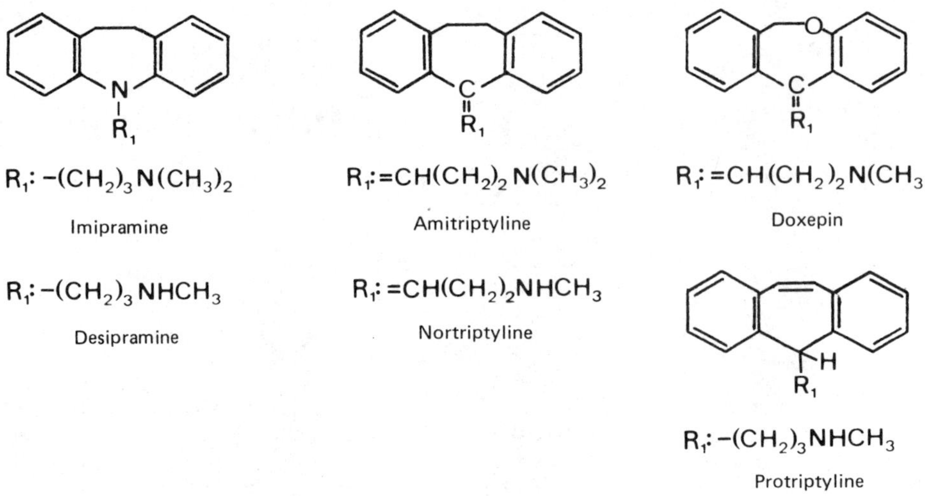

Figure 27–1. Structural relationships between various tricyclic antidepressants.

useful as antihistamines and later as antipsychotics. The discovery of their antidepressant properties was a fortuitous clinical observation. Imipramine and amitriptyline are the prototypical drugs of the class and the most commonly used.

B. Monoamine Oxidase (MAO) Inhibitors: (Fig 27–2.) MAO inhibitors may be classified as hydrazides, exemplified by the C–N–N moiety, as in phenelzine and isocarboxazid; or nonhydrazides, which lack such a moiety, as in tranylcypromine. Tranylcypromine bears a close resemblance to dextroamphetamine, which is itself a weak inhibitor of MAO. It retains some of the sympathomimetic characteristics of the amphetamines.

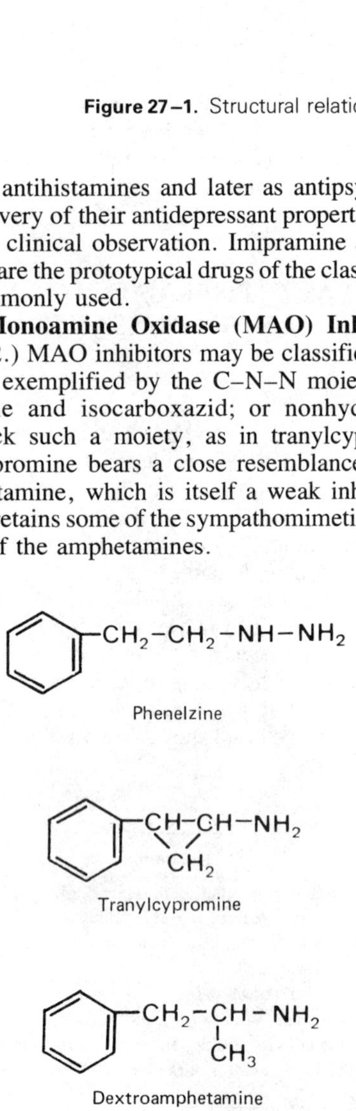

Figure 27–2. Some monoamine oxidase inhibitors. Phenelzine has a hydrazide configuration, while tranylcypromine has a cyclopropyl amine side chain compared with the isopropyl amine side chain of dextroamphetamine.

C. Sympathomimetic Stimulants: Dextroamphetamine, other amphetamines, and amphetamine surrogates such as pipradrol and methylphenidate are occasionally used as antidepressants. Although the action of amphetamines in blocking MAO has generally been regarded as too weak to confer significant antidepressant action, it may contribute to an antidepressant action in some people.

D. "Second-Generation" Drugs: (Fig 27–3.) A number of new antidepressant drugs with different chemical structures have been introduced into clinical practice in recent years. Not only do some of these drugs have unconventional structures, but some also differ considerably in their pharmacologic effects from tricyclics, especially in their actions on biogenic amine neurotransmitters. None of these drugs are more effective than the older tricyclic agents in treating depression, but to varying degrees they may have less anticholinergic side-effects, less cardiotoxicity, and a faster onset of action.

Pharmacodynamics

Drugs used to treat mental depression are not central nervous system stimulants and are actually contraindicated in organic or drug-induced central nervous system depression. Studies of the mode of action of antidepressants have largely focused on the effects on various aminergic neurotransmitters in the brain.

A. Amine Hypothesis: Soon after the introduction of reserpine in the early 1950s, it became apparent that the drug could induce depression in patients being treated for hypertension and schizophrenia as well as in normal subjects. Within the next few years, pharmacologic studies revealed that the principal mechanism of action of reserpine was to inhibit the storage of amine neurotransmitters such as serotonin and norepinephrine in the vesicles of presynaptic nerve endings. Reserpine induced depression and depleted stores of

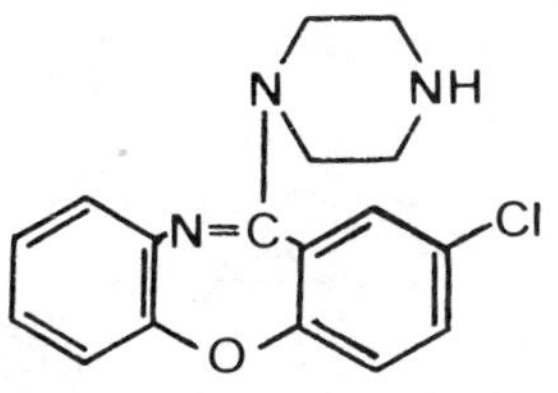

Amoxapine

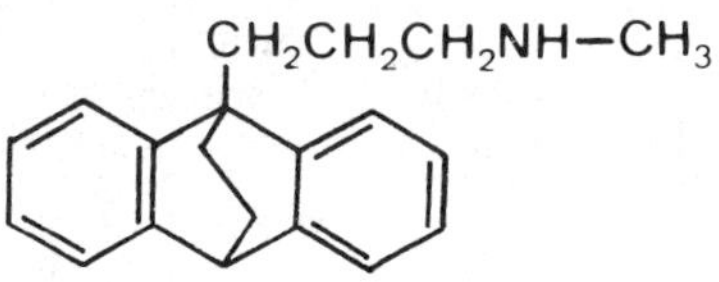

Maprotiline

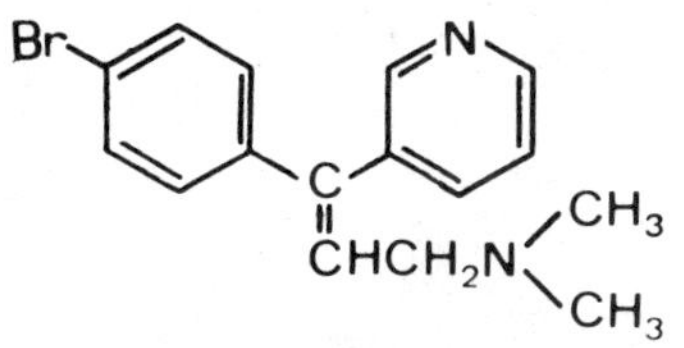

Zimelidine

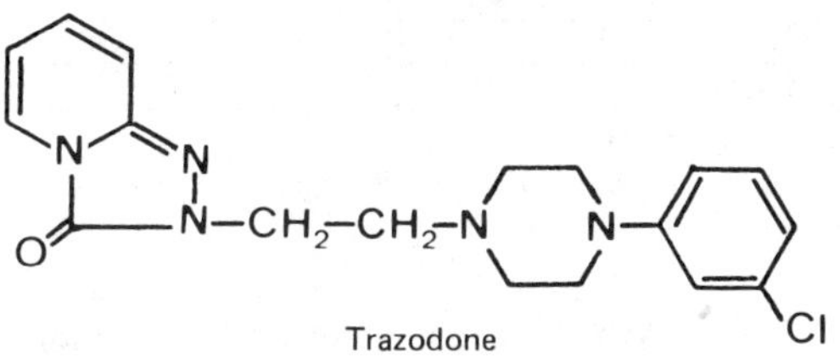

Trazodone

Figure 27–3. Some "second-generation" antidepressants.

aminergic neurotransmitters; therefore, it was reasoned, depression must be associated with decreased functional aminergic transmission. This simple syllogism provided the basis for what became known as the amine hypothesis of depression.

B. Action of Antidepressants on Biogenic Amine Neurotransmitters: The amine hypothesis was buttressed by studies on the mechanism of action of various types of antidepressant drugs. Tricyclics block the amine reuptake pump, the "off switch" of aminergic neurotransmission (see Table 27–2 and Chapter 4). Such an action presumably permits a longer sojourn of neurotransmitter at the receptor site. MAO inhibitors block a major degradative pathway for the amine neurotransmitters, which presumably permits more amines to accumulate presynaptically and more to be released. Amphetaminelike sympathomimetics also block the amine pump but are thought to act chiefly by increasing the release of catecholaminergic neurotransmitters. Thus, these 3 classes of antidepressant drugs might remedy a deficiency in aminergic neurotransmission, although by somewhat different mechanisms. Some of the "second-generation" antidepressants have similar effects on aminergic neurotransmitters, while others have mild or minimal effects.

Table 27–2. Pharmacologic differences among several tricyclic antidepressants. (0 = none, + = slight, ++ = moderate, +++ = high).

Drug	Sedation	Anticholinergic Effects	Block of Amine Pump	
			For Serotonin	For Norepinephrine
Imipramine	++	++	++	++
Amitriptyline	+++	+++	+++	+
Desipramine	+	+	0	+++
Nortriptyline	++	++	+	++
Doxepin	+++	+++	Weak	
Protriptyline	0	++	Not known	

C. Consequences of Increased Aminergic Neurotransmission: Increased aminergic neurotransmitters in the synapse were long thought to *increase* postsynaptic responses in a deficient system. Such conclusions were based on observations of the results of acute dosage. Clinically, however, drugs are given chronically for their antidepressant action. When they are administered chronically to animals and the postsynaptic consequences are measured by the generation of cAMP, *subsensitivity* of the postsynaptic receptor is observed. Thus, the evidence now strongly suggests that downstream neurotransmission is *decreased* rather than increased.

D. Peripheral Effects: See Adverse Effects, below.

Pharmacokinetics

A. Tricyclics: Absorption of most tricyclics is incomplete, and there is significant first-pass metabolism. As a result of high protein binding and relatively high lipid solubility, volumes of distribution tend to be very large. Tricyclics are metabolized by 2 major routes: transformation of the tricyclic nucleus and alteration of the aliphatic side chain. The former route involves ring hydroxylation and conjugation to form glucuronides; the latter, primarily demethylation of the nitrogen. Monodemethylation of tertiary amines leads to active metabolites, such as desipramine and nortriptyline (Fig 27–1). The proportion of monodemethylated metabolites formed varies from one patient to another. In general, the proportion of amitriptyline to its metabolite nortriptyline favors the parent drug. The converse is the case with imipramine and its metabolite desipramine. The pharmacokinetic parameters of various antidepressants are summarized in Table 27–3.

B. Monoamine Oxidase Inhibitors: These drugs produce an "irreversible" inhibition of MAO that persists even after the drug is no longer detectable in plasma. In following the effectiveness of a dosage

Table 27–3. Pharmacokinetic parameters of various antidepressants.

Drug	Bioavailability (percent)	Protein Binding (percent)	Plasma $t_{1/2}$ (hours)	Active Metabolites	Volume of Distribution (L/kg)	Therapeutic Plasma Concentrations (ng/mL)
Imipramine	29–77	76–95	9–24	Desipramine	15–30	> 180 total
Amitriptyline	31–61	82–96	31–46	Nortriptyline	5–10	80–200 total
Nortriptyline	32–79	93–95	18–93	10-Hydroxy	21–57	50–150
Desipramine	60–70	73–90	14–62	*	22–59	145†
Protriptyline	*	90–95	54–198	*	19–57	70–170
Doxepin	13–45	*	8–24	Desmethyl	9–33	30–150
Clomipramine	*	*	22–84	Desmethyl	7–20	240–700
Maprotiline	37–67	*	36–108	*	*	200–300

*No data available.
†Lower concentrations may be effective, but no data are available.

regimen, it has been more useful to measure the inhibition of MAO activity in platelets than to measure the plasma levels of the drug directly. Present feeling is that optimal antidepressant effect from these drugs requires about 60–80% inhibition of the enzyme—a degree achieved with doses of approximately 1 mg/kg/d of phenelzine.

C. Second-Generation Drugs: The pharmacokinetics of these drugs and of the tricyclics are similar. Although the claim for many second-generation drugs is faster onset of clinical action, neither a pharmacokinetic nor a pharmacodynamic explanation for this clinical effect is apparent. Some of these drugs are said to have less cardiotoxicity than tricyclics when taken in overdose quantities.

Clinical Indications

The major indication for these drugs is to treat depression, but a number of other uses have been established by clinical experience.

A. Depression: This indication has been kept broad deliberately, even though evidence from clinical studies strongly suggests that the drugs are specifically useful only in endogenous depressions. Endogenous depressions are diagnosed not so much by their severity as by their quality. Formerly, they were referred to as "vital" or "vegetative"—reflecting the characteristic disturbances of major body rhythms of sleep, hunger and appetite, sexual drive, and motor activity. The diagnosis of endogenous depression may be uncertain in individual patients, so that on balance it is probably better to treat too many patients with tricyclics than to miss treating those who might benefit. Many of the other types of depression respond to nonspecific treatment. Thus, when heterogeneous groups of depressed patients are treated with tricyclics, it is difficult to demonstrate the efficacy of tricyclics as compared with placebo treatment.

B. Enuresis: Enuresis is an established indication for tricyclics. Proof of efficacy for this indication is substantial, but drug therapy is not the preferred approach. The beneficial effect of drug treatment lasts only as long as drug treatment is continued.

C. Chronic Pain: Clinicians in pain clinics have found tricyclics to be especially useful for treating a variety of chronically painful states that often cannot be definitely diagnosed. Whether such painful states represent depressive equivalents or whether such patients become secondarily depressed after some initial pain-producing insult is not clear. It is even possible that the tricyclics (sometimes phenothiazines are also used in combination) work directly on pain pathways.

D. Other Indications: Less frequent and less well documented indications include obsessive-compulsive-phobic states, cataplexy associated with narcolepsy, acute panic attacks, and school phobia, minimal brain damage, and hyperkinesis in children.

II. CLINICAL PHARMACOLOGY OF ANTIDEPRESSANTS

Choice of Drug

Controlled comparisons of the available antidepressants have usually led to the conclusion that they are roughly equivalent drugs. Although this may be true for groups of patients, individual patients may for uncertain reasons fare better on one drug than on another. Thus, finding the right drug for the individual patient must be accomplished empirically at present. The past history of the patient's drug experience, if available, is the most valuable guide. At times such a history may lead to the exclusion of tricyclics, as in the case of patients who have responded well in the past to MAO inhibitors.

Tricyclic antidepressant drugs are apt to be most successful in patients with clearly "endogenous" characteristics, including psychomotor retardation, poor appetite and weight loss, and loss of libido. MAO inhibitors in adequate doses may also be useful for such patients.

Tricyclics differ mainly in the degree of sedation (amitriptyline and doxepin cause the most, protriptyline the least) and the amount of anticholinergic effects (amitriptyline and doxepin have the largest, desipramine the least) (Table 27–2). Although it is often argued that more sedative drugs are preferable for markedly anxious or agitated depressives while the least sedative drugs are preferable for patients with psychomotor withdrawal, this hypothesis has not been tested.

MAO inhibitors are helpful in patients described as having "atypical" depressions—a nonspecific designation scarcely helpful in their identification. Depressed patients with considerable attendant anxiety, phobic features, and hypochondriasis are the ones who respond best to these drugs. Either phenelzine or tranylcypromine may be used.

A claim made for some "second-generation" antidepressants is that they act more quickly. For patients in whom a rapid response is especially desirable, a drug such as amoxapine might be tried. Another claim is that some of the drugs such as maprotiline, trazodone, or mianserin have less anticholinergic side-effects than most tricyclics. These effects can be a limiting factor for many patients—limiting either the dose of drug tolerated or the patient's willingness to take the drug. One of the newer agents might be considered for such patients. Finally, some of the newer drugs seem not to have the cardiotoxic effects of the tricyclics when they are taken in overdose quantities. Accordingly, patients with major heart problems might best be treated with a less hazardous drug.

Doses

The usual dose ranges of antidepressants are shown in Table 27–4. Doses are almost always determined empirically; the patient's acceptance of side-effects is the usual limiting factor. Tolerance to some of the objectionable side-effects may develop, so that

Table 27–4. Usual daily doses of antidepressant drugs.

Drug	Dose (mg)
Tricyclics	
Amitriptyline (Elavil, etc)	75–200
Clomipramine	75–300
Desipramine (Norpramin, Pertofrane)	75–200
Doxepin (Adapin, Sinequan)	75–300
Imipramine (Tofranil, etc)	75–200
Nortriptyline (Aventyl, Pamelor)	75–150
Protriptyline (Triptil, Vivactil)	20–40
Trimipramine (Surmontil)	75–200
Monoamine oxidase inhibitors	
Isocarboxazid (Marplan)	20–50
Phenelzine (Nardil)	45–75
Tranylcypromine (Parnate)	10–30
Tetracyclics	
Maprotiline (Ludiomil)	75–300
Mianserin	30–120
Bicyclics	
Viloxazine	100–300
Zimelidine	50–300
Dibenazepines	
Amoxapine (Asendin)	150–300
Miscellaneous	
Nomifensine (Merital)	75–200
Trazodone (Desyrel)	50–600

the usual pattern of treatment has been to start with small doses, increasing either to a predetermined daily dose, or to one that produces relief of depression, or to the maximum tolerated dose. The effective dose of an antidepressant varies widely depending upon many factors. Undertreatment has been thought to be a frequent cause of apparent failure of drug therapy to relieve depression.

Dosage Schedules for Treating the Acute Episode

The plasma half-lives of many antidepressants are long enough so that single daily doses in the early evening hours can be used (Table 27–4). The sedative and anticholinergic actions of these drugs are less bothersome when the drug is taken in the evening. However, the patient should be warned of these side-effects and should construe them as evidence of the action of the drug. Patients should be warned also that noticeable improvement may be slow, perhaps taking 3 weeks or more. Inability to tolerate side-effects and discouragement with treatment are 2 major causes for noncompliance and for failure of tricyclics to relieve depression.

Maintenance Treatment

Whether or not to undertake long-term maintenance treatment of a depressed patient depends entirely on the natural history of the disorder. If the depressive episode was the patient's first and if it responded quickly and satisfactorily to drug therapy, it is rational to gradually withdraw treatment over a period of a few months. If relapse does not occur, drug treatment can be stopped until the next attack occurs, which is unpredictable but nearly certain. On the other hand, a patient who has had several previous attacks of depression, especially if each succeeding attack was more severe and more difficult to treat, is a prime candidate for maintenance therapy.

Drug treatment of endogenous depression should be continued for at least 2 months. Doses for maintenance treatment may be one-half to two-thirds lower than what is required for management of the acute episode. Some patients have been on maintenance treatment for years with apparent good control of their illness and no long-term adverse effects. Members of the household should be instructed in how to detect early signs of relapse; the patients themselves may be poor judges of that.

Monitoring Plasma Concentrations

Routine monitoring of plasma concentrations of antidepressants, while technically feasible for most drugs, is still of uncertain value. Experience with monitoring of plasma concentrations of tricyclics suggests that about 20% of patients become noncompliant at some time or other. Thus, a "poor response" in a patient for whom an adequate dosage of drug has been prescribed may be shown by measurement of the plasma drug concentration to be due merely to failure to take the drug. Blood for plasma drug level determinations should be obtained in the postabsorptive state, about 10–12 hours after the last dose. Even when sampling time is constant, the same patient may show variation in both the total plasma concentration and the proportion of parent drug versus metabolites while on a constant dose at steady-state conditions. Under no circumstances should the laboratory test results be permitted to overrule the physician's clinical judgment.

Adverse Effects

Adverse effects of various antidepressants are summarized in Table 27–5. Most common unwanted effects are minor, but they may seriously affect the acceptance of drug treatment by the patient; the more seriously depressed the patient is, the more likely it is that unwanted effects will be tolerated. Most normal persons find that even moderate doses of these drugs cause disagreeable symptoms.

A. Sedation: Although we think of antidepressants as "activators," tricyclics—with the possible exception of protriptyline—are strongly sedative. Complaints of lassitude, fatigue, and loss of energy are common, especially early in treatment. If doses are too high, the patient may sleep at inappropriate times. Sedative effects are less bothersome when a single daily dose is taken at night. MAO inhibitors, especially those with sympathomimetic actions such as tranylcypromine, may produce mild degrees of stimulation.

B. Sympathomimetic Actions: These effects of various antidepressants may be obscured by other more prominent actions on the autonomic nervous system, but they are explainable on the basis of known pharmacologic actions of most of these drugs. Tremor is extremely common; treatment with a beta-blocking drug such as propranolol or nadolol may be helpful. Some patients may become agitated and manic with tricyclics, but one should always consider the possibility that they are really manic-depressive.

C. Anticholinergic Effects: Dry mouth, constipation, urinary hesitancy, and loss of visual accommodation are the most frequent anticholinergic side-effects. More extensive anticholinergic action may result in paralytic ileus or urinary retention, especially in elderly patients. Treatment with bethanechol, a peripherally acting cholinomimetic, may counter the peripheral anticholinergic action of the tricyclics.

D. Cardiovascular Effects: Palpitation, tachycardia, and orthostatic hypotension were recognized early as unwanted effects of these drugs. Later, arrhythmias and electrocardiographic abnormalities were described. Congestive heart failure and sudden death are rare complications.

E. Psychiatric Effects: Confusional reactions are most often seen in patients over 40 years of age. The situation may be made worse if the patient is also receiving other drugs with anticholinergic action, such as antipsychotics or antiparkinsonism drugs.

A central anticholinergic syndrome consisting of delirium, anxiety, hyperactivity, hallucinations, disorientation, and seizures has been described for many drugs with anticholinergic action, especially when they are taken in combination. A good general rule is that any patient showing new or bizarre mental symptoms while receiving antidepressant medication should have the drug discontinued until the situation can be appraised. Some writers have recommended treatment with physostigmine, but most cases respond quickly enough to simple discontinuation of the drug.

F. Neurologic Effects: Tremor is common and is more similar to essential tremor than to the tremor of Parkinson's disease. Paresthesias are less common and may herald the rare development of peripheral neuropathy. Other neurologic abnormalities are usually signs of therapeutic overdoses. Although Parkinson's syndrome has been reported, it is extremely rare. Tardive dyskinesia has not occurred.

G. Allergic or Toxic Reactions: Skin rashes are uncommon. Cholestatic jaundice and agranulocytosis have been reported but are now so rare as to hardly merit consideration.

H. Metabolic and Endocrine Effects: Weight gain is frequent with these drugs, just as it is with the phenothiazines. It may be due in part to increased appetite with remission of depression, but a central action is probably responsible also. Some patients have complained of a craving for sweets, and beverages containing sugar are often used to relieve dry mouth.

The syndrome of inappropriate secretion of antidiuretic hormone has been reported with various tricyclics.

I. Birth Defects: As is the case with so many drugs, it is not clear whether or not the antidepressant

Table 27–5. Side-effects of antidepressants.

Type	Minor, Early	Major
Sedation	Lassitude, fatigue.	Sleepiness; impaired consciousness with alcohol and other drugs.
Sympathomimetic	Tachycardia, tremor, sweating.	Agitation, insomnia, aggravation of psychosis.
Anticholinergic	Blurred vision, constipation, urinary hesitancy, fuzzy thinking.	Aggravation of glaucoma, paralytic ileus, urinary retention, delirium.
Cardiovascular	Orthostatic hypotension, electrocardiographic abnormalities.	Delayed cardiac conduction, arrhythmias, cardiomyopathy, sudden death.
Psychiatric	Confusion.	Central anticholinergic syndrome, withdrawal.
Neurologic	Paresthesias, electroencephalographic alterations.	Seizures, neuropathy.
Allergic/toxic		Cholestatic jaundice, agranulocytosis.
Metabolic/endocrine	Weight gain, sexual disturbances.	Gynecomastia, amenorrhea.
Birth defects		Uncertain.

drugs have been responsible for birth defects in infants born to mothers taking the drugs early in pregnancy. The evidence is not very persuasive, and the results of national surveys are equivocal. Even so, it is still good practice to accept the conventional wisdom that unless a drug is necessary for preserving life or maintaining adequate function, it should not be used in pregnancy.

Drug Interactions

A. Pharmacodynamic Interactions: Many of the pharmacodynamic interactions of antidepressants with other drugs have already been discussed. Sedative effects may be additive with other sedatives, especially alcohol. Patients taking tricyclics should be warned that use of alcohol may lead to greater than usual impairment of driving ability. MAO inhibitors, by increasing stores of catecholamines, sensitize the patient to indirectly acting sympathomimetics such as tyramine, which is found in many fermented foods and beverages, and to sympathomimetic drugs that may be administered therapeutically, such as diethylpropion or phenylpropanolamine.

B. Pharmacokinetic Interactions: Reversal of the antihypertensive action of guanethidine is a dramatic interaction (see Chapter 9). The blood pressure not only returns quickly to high levels but may overshoot to dangerously high levels. Guanethidine is concentrated in sympathetic nerve endings by the same amine pump that is blocked by tricyclics. Thus, it is prevented from reaching its site of action. A similar reversal of action of other antihypertensives, such as methyldopa and clonidine, has been described. Although doxepin is less likely than other tricyclics to produce this interaction, because it is considerably less potent in blocking the amine pump, interaction can occur with high doses of the drug. MAO inhibitors predictably prolong the half-lives of the many drugs that are oxidatively deaminated.

Overdoses

Tricyclics are extremely dangerous when taken in overdose quantities, and depressed patients are more likely than others to be suicidal. Prescriptions should therefore be limited to amounts less than 1.25 g, or 50 dose units of 25 mg, on a "no refill" basis. If suicide is a serious possibility, the tablets should be entrusted to a family member. The drugs must be kept away from children.

Both accidental and deliberate overdoses are frequent and are a serious medical emergency. Major symptoms include (1) coma with shock and sometimes metabolic acidosis; (2) respiratory depression with a tendency to sudden apnea; (3) agitation or delirium both before and after consciousness is obtunded; (4) neuromuscular irritability and seizures; (5) hyperpyrexia; (6) bowel and bladder paralysis; and (7) a great variety of cardiac manifestations, including conduction defects and arrhythmias. Cardiac problems are the principal distinguishing features.

Management of cardiac problems is difficult. Antiarrhythmia drugs having the least depressant effect on cardiac conduction should be used. Lidocaine, propranolol, and phenytoin have been used successfully, but quinidine and procainamide are contraindicated. Physostigmine given in small (0.5-mg) intravenous boluses to a total dose of 3–4 mg may awaken the patient and reverse the cardiac arrhythmia. It is more likely to be effective for supraventricular than for ventricular arrhythmias. Continual cardiac monitoring is essential, and facilities must be at hand for resuscitation if needed. Arterial blood gases and pH should be measured frequently, since both hypoxia and metabolic acidosis predispose to arrhythmias. Sodium bicarbonate and intravenous potassium chloride may be required to restore acid-base balance and to correct hypokalemia. Electrical pacing must be used in refractory cases.

Other treatment is entirely supportive. After placement of a cuffed endotracheal tube, attempts should be made to remove residual drug from the gastrointestinal tract. Absorption may be slow because of the strong anticholinergic effects. Activated charcoal may be used to bind the drug, which may subsequently be removed by catharsis. Ventilatory assistance is of prime importance. Shock is best treated with fluids or plasma expanders, since adrenergic receptors may be blocked. Hyperpyrexia is treated by cooling. Seizures may be treated with intravenous phenytoin (which may also double as an antiarrhythmia agent) or diazepam. Patients should not be discharged until they have been conscious for a day or 2 and most abnormal signs have disappeared. Measurement of plasma concentrations of the drug may be helpful in deciding about the safety of discharge. Virtually all patients who survive recover completely with no permanent sequelae.

Intoxication with MAO inhibitors is unusual. Agitation, delirium, and neuromuscular excitability are followed by obtunded consciousness, seizures, shock, and hyperthermia. Supportive treatment is usually all that is required, although sedative phenothiazines with alpha-adrenergic receptor-blocking action, such as chlorpromazine, may be useful.

• • •

References

Davis JM: Overview: Maintenance therapy in psychiatry. 2. Affective disorders. *Am J Psychiatry* 1976;**133:**1.

Garver DL, Davis JM: Biogenic amine hypothesis of affective disorders. *Life Sci* 1979;**24:**383.

Hekimian LJ, Friefhoff AJ, Deever E: A comparison of the onset of action and therapeutic efficacy of amoxapine and amitriptyline. *J Clin Psychiatry* 1978;**39:**633.

Hollister LE: Monitoring tricyclic antidepressant plasma concentrations. *JAMA* 1979;**241:**2530.

Hollister LE: Treatment of depression with drugs. *Ann Intern Med* 1978;**89:**78.

Kiloh LG et al: The relationship of the syndromes called endogenous and neurotic depression. *Br J Psychiatry* 1972;**121:**183.

Montgomery SA et al: Amitriptyline plasma concentration and clinical response. *Br Med J* 1979;**1:**230.

Morris JB, Beck AT: The efficacy of antidepressant drugs. *Arch Gen Psychiatry* 1974;**30:**667.

Pinder RM et al: Maprotiline: A review of its pharmacological properties and therapeutic efficacy in mental depressive states. *Drugs* 1977;**13:**321.

Shaw DM: The practical management of affective disorders. *Br J Psychiatry* 1977;**130:**432.

Sorensen B et al: The practical significance of nortriptyline plasma control: A prospective evaluation under routine conditions in endogenous depression. *Psychopharmacology* 1978;**59:**35.

Narcotic Analgesics & Antagonists | 28

Walter L. Way, MD, & E. Leong Way, PhD

The black bag carried by physicians in general practice today would almost certainly contain a narcotic analgesic, probably morphine sulfate. One hundred years ago, morphine would without question have been the most important drug in the bag; since there were no antibiotics, hormonal agents, or antipsychotic drugs, the practitioner depended heavily on drugs that would at least provide symptomatic relief. Not only could opium and its derivatives be counted upon to allay severe pain of different origins, it would also control diarrhea, cough, anxiety, and insomnia. For these reasons, Sir William Osler called morphine "God's own medicine."

Compounds similar to morphine that produce pain relief and sedation have traditionally been called narcotic analgesics to distinguish them from the antipyretic analgesics such as aspirin and acetaminophen (Chapter 33). However, the term "narcotic" is an imprecise one, since narcosis signifies a stuporous state whereas the opiates produce analgesia without loss of consciousness. The terms "opiate" and "opioid analgesic" are more precise, but established usage of a word is always difficult to extinguish. Consequently, "narcotic analgesics" are now understood to include natural and semisynthetic alkaloid derivatives from opium as well as their synthetic surrogates with actions that mimic those of morphine. In the 1950s, it was found that nalorphine, an antagonist of morphine, itself had analgesic effects. In recent years, more potent analgesics that also possess morphine antagonist properties have found extensive applications in clinical situations where morphine might be used. The recent discovery of endogenous peptides with analgesic properties suggests that synthetic peptides with opioid characteristics may in the future also be included in this group. In this chapter, "narcotic analgesic" and "opiate" will be used interchangeably as general terms for compounds of the narcotic analgesic class. Morphine is considered the prototypic agonist.

History

The source of opium, the crude substance, and morphine, one of its purified constituents, is the opium poppy, *Papaver somniferum*. The plant was used at least 6000 years ago, and there are accounts of it in ancient Egyptian, Greek, Roman, and Chinese documents. It was not until the 18th century that the addiction liability of opium began to cause concern. Until quite recently, opiates were used indiscriminately for analgesia and sedation and to control diarrhea and cough.

The modern basis of pharmacology was established by Sertürner, a German pharmacist, who described the isolation of a pure active alkaline substance from opium in 1803. This first isolation in chemically pure form of an active principle from a plant was a landmark event in that it made it possible to derive a standardized potency for a natural product. Sertürner ingested the substance himself and gave it to his friends to produce a deep narcotic state. He proposed the name "morphine" for the compound—after Morpheus, the Greek god of dreams.

I. BASIC PHARMACOLOGY OF THE NARCOTIC ANALGESICS

Source

Opium is obtained from the opium poppy by incision of the seed pod after the petals of the flower have dropped. The white latex that oozes out turns brown and hardens on standing. This sticky brown gum is opium. It is scraped off and kneaded into a homogeneous mass that contains about 20 alkaloids, including morphine, codeine, thebaine, and papaverine. Thebaine and papaverine are not narcotic analgesics, but thebaine is the precursor of several semisynthetic opiate agonists (eg, etorphine, an experimental agent 500–1000 times as potent as morphine) and antagonists (naloxone). Papaverine is a vasodilator with no established clinical applications that nevertheless inspired the development of verapamil, an important calcium channel-blocking drug (Chapter 12). The principal alkaloid in opium is morphine, present in a concentration of about 10%. Codeine is present in less than 0.5% concentration; it is synthesized commercially from morphine. Cultivation of the opium poppy is now restricted by international agreement, but illicit production of opium is difficult to control.

Table 28–1. Chemical structures of narcotic analgesics and antagonists.

Basic Structure	Strong Agonists	Mild to Moderate Agonists	Mixed Agonist-Antagonists	Antagonists
Phenanthrenes	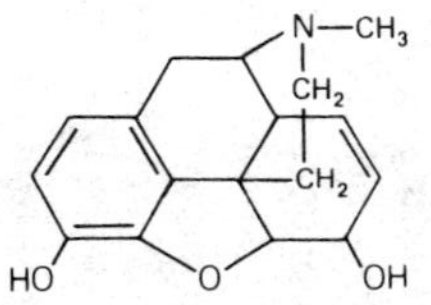 Morphine	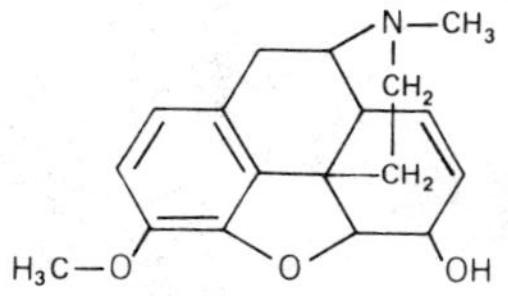 Codeine	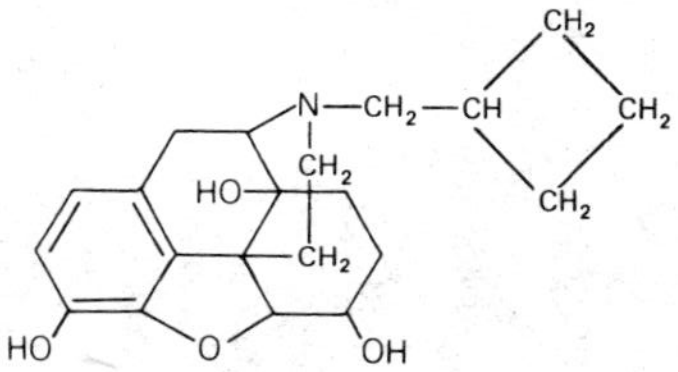 Nalbuphine (Nubain)	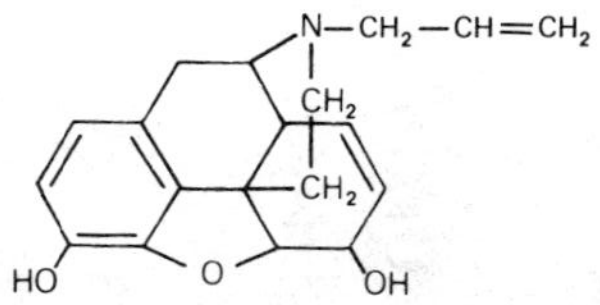 Nalorphine (Nalline)*
	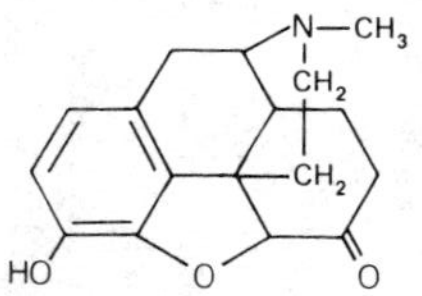 Hydromorphone (Dilaudid)	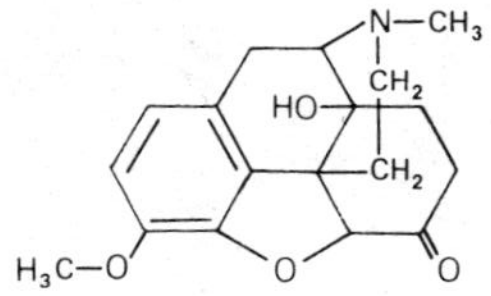 Oxycodone (Percodan)	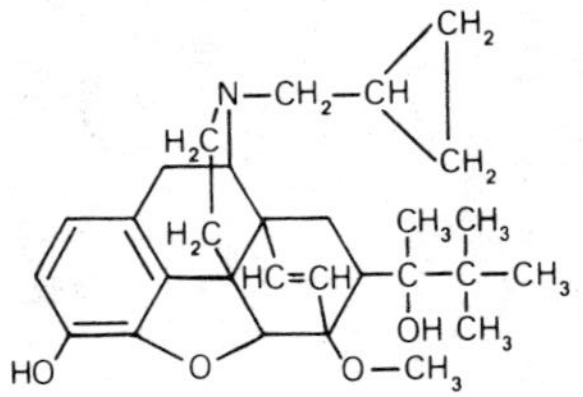 Buprenorphine (Temgesic)	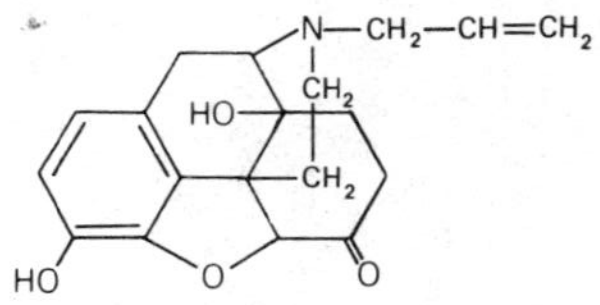 Naloxone (Narcan)
	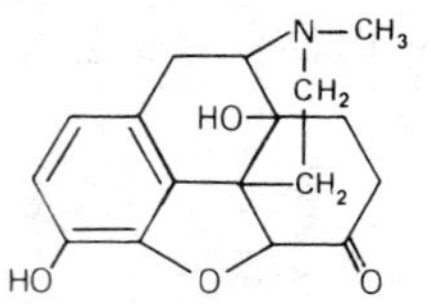 Oxymorphone (Numorphan)	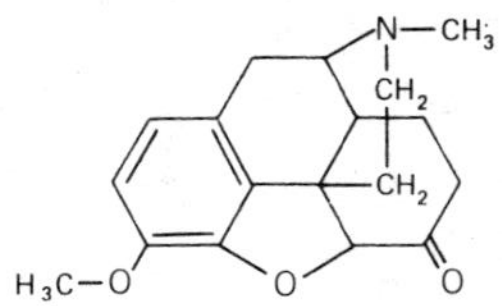 Hydrocodone (Hycodan)		
Phenylheptylamines	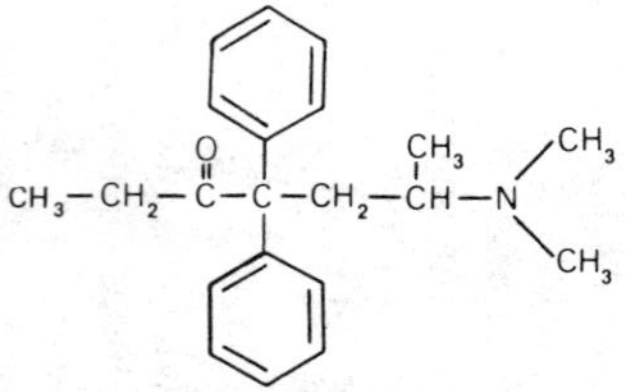 Methadone	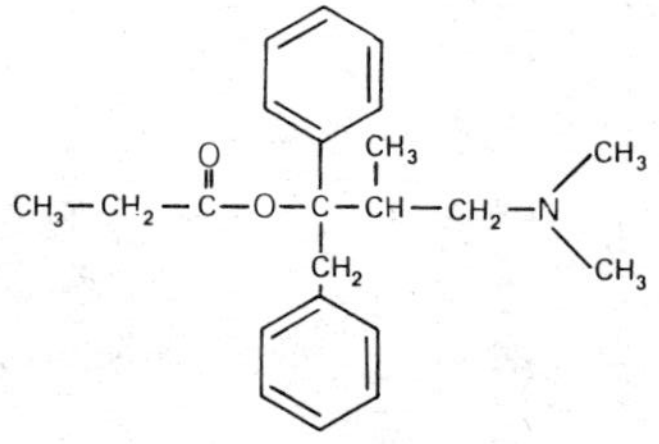 Propoxyphene (Darvon)		

Phenylpiperidines	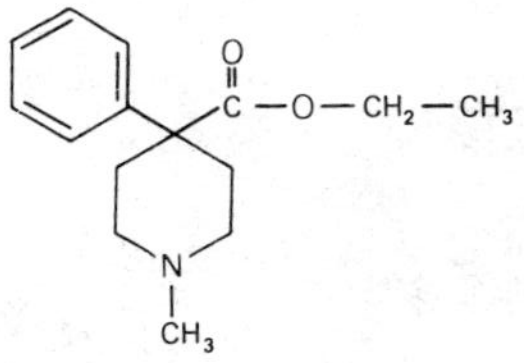 Meperidine (Demerol) 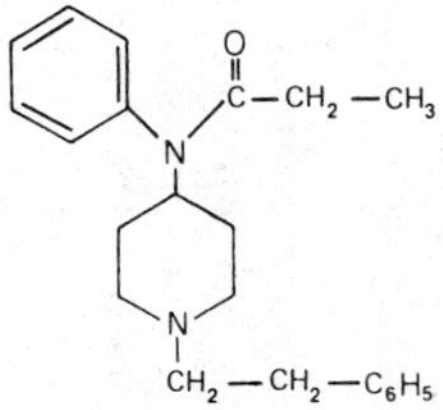 Fentanyl (Sublimaze)	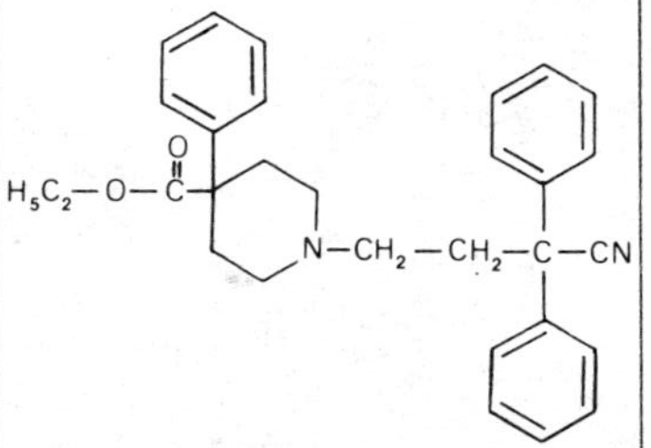 Diphenoxylate		
Morphinans	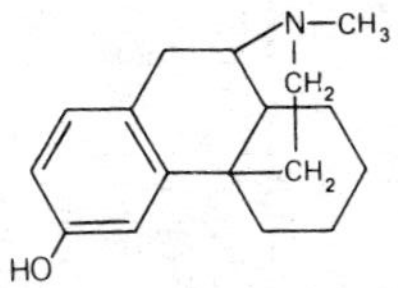 Levorphanol (Levo-Dromoran)		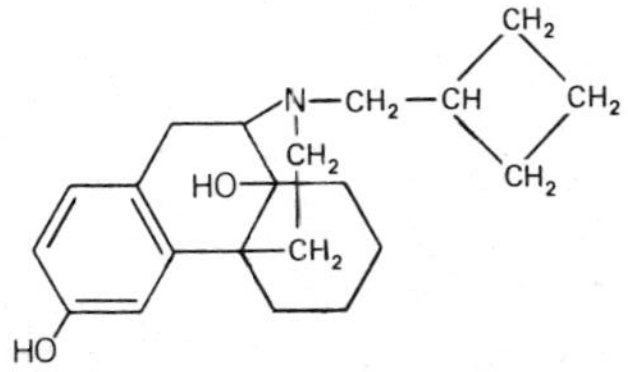 Butorphanol (Stadol)	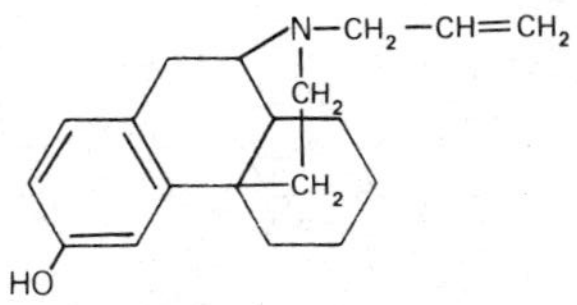 Levallorphan (Lorfan)*
Benzomorphans			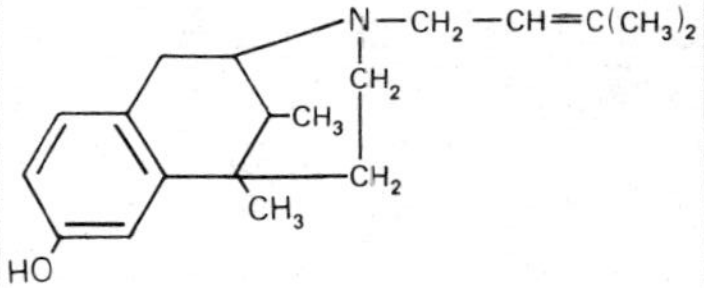 Pentazocine (Talwin)	

*Not a pure antagonist. See text for explanation.

Chemistry

Since the early discoveries in alkaloid chemistry, many compounds with opiate agonist activity have been synthesized. Several different families may be identified, all bearing a common "backbone" as shown in Fig 28–1. Several important members of these families are shown in Table 28–1, and some of their properties are summarized in Table 28–2. Relatively small molecular alterations may drastically change the action of these compounds, converting an agonist to an antagonist or to a compound with both agonist and antagonist effects—a "mixed agonist-antagonist."

Antagonist properties are associated with replacement of the methyl substituent on the nitrogen atom with larger groups—allyl in the case of nalorphine and naloxone; methylcyclopropane or methylcyclobutane for several other agents.

Substitutions at the C3 and C6 hydroxyl groups of morphine significantly alter pharmacokinetic properties. Methyl substitution at the phenolic hydroxyl at C3 reduces susceptibility to first-pass hepatic inactivation of the molecule by glucuronide conjugation. Therefore, drugs such as codeine and oxycodone have a higher ratio of oral:parenteral potency. Acetylation of both hydroxyl groups of morphine yields heroin, which penetrates the blood-brain barrier much more rapidly than morphine. It is rapidly hydrolyzed in the tissues to monoacetylmorphine and morphine. In Table 28–1, compounds are listed according to their agonist, mixed agonist-antagonist, or antagonist properties. The pharmacologic basis for their different properties is discussed below.

Pharmacokinetics

A. Absorption: Most narcotic analgesics are well absorbed from subcutaneous and intramuscular sites as well as from the mucosal surfaces of the nose and gastrointestinal tract. However, although absorption from the gastrointestinal tract may be rapid, the pharmacologic potency of some compounds taken by this route may be considerably less than after parenteral administration, because of significant first-pass metabolism in the liver after absorption. Therefore, the oral dose required to elicit a therapeutic effect for such compounds may be considerably higher than that required when parenteral administration is used (Chapter 3). Narcotic analgesics with a free hydroxyl group (eg, morphine) are usually metabolized by conjugation with glucuronic acid. Since the amount of β-glucuronidase, the enzyme responsible for this reaction, varies considerably in different individuals, the effect of a specified oral dose of a compound that will be metabolized by conjugation is difficult to predict.

Examples of compounds that have high oral: parenteral potency ratios are codeine and oxycodone. Their greater effectiveness by the oral route is thought to result from a decrease in first-pass metabolism, because their conjugation is prevented by a methyl group on the aromatic hydroxyl group.

B. Distribution: The uptake of opiates by various organs and tissues is a function of both physiologic and chemical factors. Although all narcotic analgesics bind to plasma proteins with varying degrees of affinity after absorption, the compounds rapidly leave the blood and localize in highest concentrations in parenchymatous tissues such as lungs, liver, kidneys, and spleen. Although drug concentrations in skeletal muscle may be much lower, this tissue serves as the main reservoir for the drug because of its greater bulk. However, accumulation in fatty tissue can also become important, particularly after frequent high-dose administration of highly lipophilic opiates that are slowly metabolized, eg, fentanyl. Brain concentrations of narcotic analgesics are usually relatively low in comparison to most other organs, although the blood-brain barrier is traversed readily by compounds in which the aromatic hydroxyl at C3 is substituted, as in heroin and codeine. Difficulty in gaining access to the brain appears to be greater with ampholytic agents such as morphine. However, this barrier is lacking in the infant. Since the narcotic analgesics also traverse the placenta, their use for obstetric analgesia can result in the delivery of an infant with depressed respiration.

C. Metabolism: The opiates are converted mostly to polar metabolites, which are then readily excreted by the kidneys. Compounds that have free hydroxyl groups are readily conjugated with glucuronic acid; examples are morphine and levorphanol. Esters (eg, meperidine, heroin) are rapidly hydrolyzed by common tissue esterases. Heroin is hydrolyzed to monoacetylmorphine and finally to morphine, which is then conjugated with glucuronic acid. The narcotic analgesics are also N-demethylated by the liver, but this is a minor pathway. In the presence of liver disease, therapeutic blood levels can probably be achieved with lower than usual doses of these compounds.

D. Excretion: The polar metabolites of the opiates are excreted mainly in the urine. Small amounts of the unchanged drug may also be excreted in the urine. Glucuronide conjugates are also excreted in the bile, but enterohepatic circulation represents only a small portion of the excretory process.

Pharmacodynamics

A. Mechanism of Action: Brain loci involved in the transmission of pain and in the alteration of reactivity to nociceptive (painful) stimuli appear to be the primary but not the only sites at which opiates act. In general, sites that display a high affinity for exogenous ligands such as morphine also contain high concentrations of endogenous peptides having opioid properties. The generic term for this class of substances is **endorphin,** a blend of the words "endogenous" and "morphine." Several types of endorphins have been isolated and identified. The **enkephalins** are pentapeptides: met-enkephalin (Tyr-Gly-Gly-Phe-Met) and leu-enkephalin (Tyr-Gly-Gly-Phe-Leu). Beta-endorphin is the 31-residue carboxyl terminus of the pituitary protein β-lipotropin. It is a highly potent endogenous opioid peptide with pharmacologic

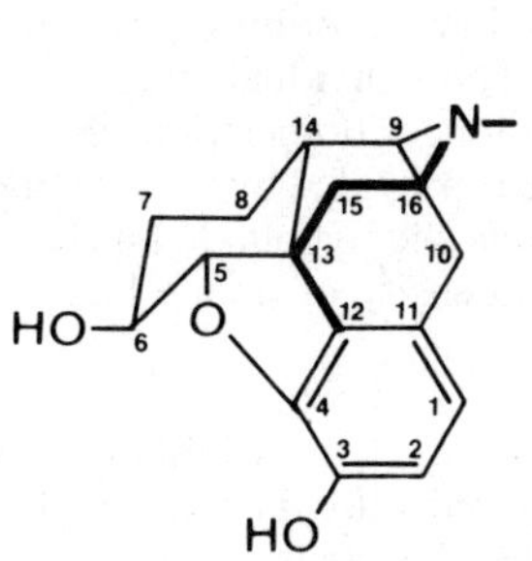

Morphine
(phenanthrene
alkaloid)

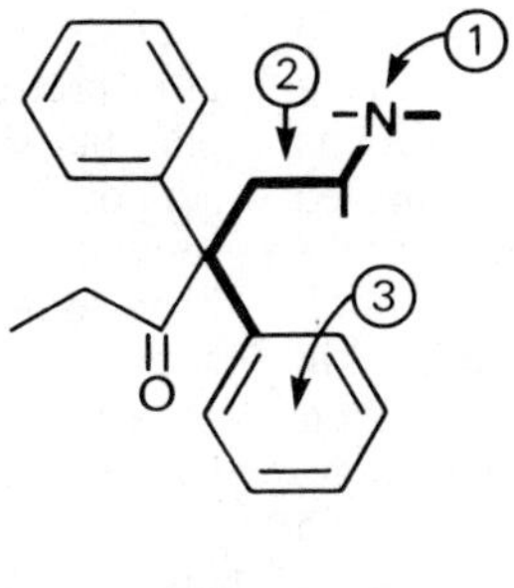

Methadone
(phenylheptylamine)

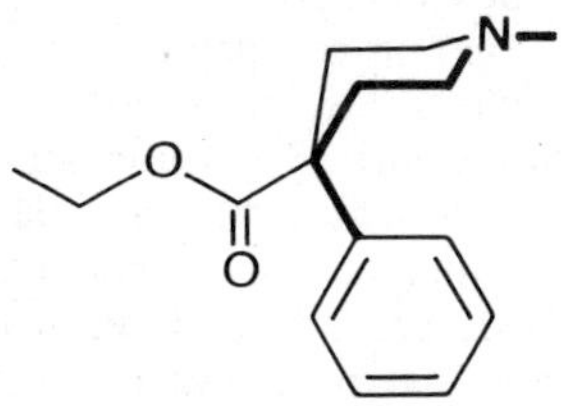

Meperidine
(phenylpiperidine)

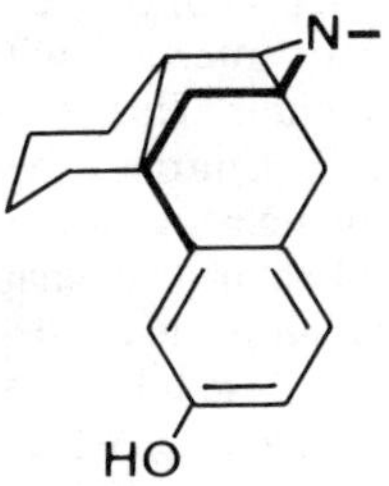

Levorphanol
(morphinan)

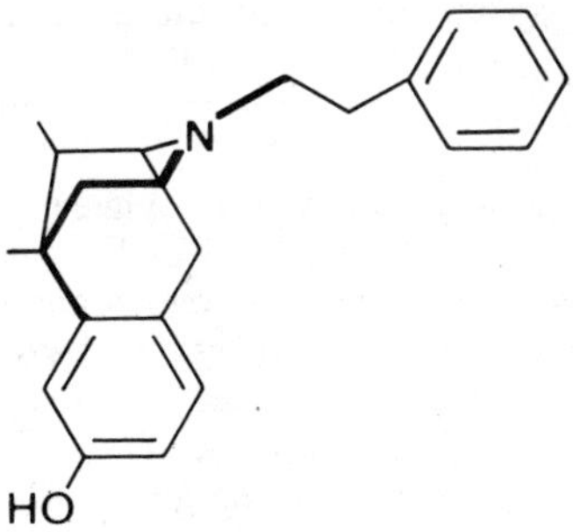

Phenazocine
(benzomorphan)

Figure 28–1. The chemical structures of an opium alkaloid and 4 examples of synthetic narcotic analgesics written to emphasize the structure common to all: (1) a tertiary nitrogen; (2) a short hydrocarbon chain held in a plane perpendicular to the page; (3) a flat aryl group held in the plane of the page. (Modified and reproduced, with permission, from Meyers FH, Jawetz E, Goldfien A: *Review of Medical Pharmacology,* 7th ed. Lange, 1980.)

Table 28–2. Useful narcotic analgesics.

Generic Name	Proprietary Name	Approximate Dose (mg)	Oral:Parenteral Potency Ratio	Duration of Analgesia (hours)	Maximum Efficacy	Addiction/Abuse Liability
Morphine		10	Low	4–5	High	High
Hydromorphone	Dilaudid	1.5	Low	4–5	High	High
Oxymorphone	Numorphan	1.5	Low	3–4	High	High
Methadone	Dolophine	10	High	4–6	High	High
Meperidine	Demerol	60–100	Medium	2–4	High	High
Alphaprodine	Nisentil	30–50	Parenteral use only	1–2	High	High
Fentanyl	Sublimaze	0.2	Parenteral use only	1–1½	High	High
Levorphanol	Levo-Dromoran	1.5–1.2	High	4–5	High	High
Codeine		30–60†	High	3–4	Low	Medium
Oxycodone*	Percodan	4.5†	Medium	3–4	Moderate	Medium
Dihydrocodeine*	Drocode	16†	Medium	3–4	Moderate	Medium
Propoxyphene	Darvon	60–120†	Oral use only	4–5	Very low	Low
Pentazocine	Talwin	30–50†	Medium	3–4	Moderate	Low
Nalbuphine	Nubain	0.5–1	Parenteral use only	3–6	High	Low
Buprenorphine	Temgesic	0.3	Parenteral use only	4–8	High	Low
Butorphanol	Stadol	2	Parenteral use only	3–4	High	Low

*Available only in tablets containing aspirin, etc.
†Analgesic efficacy at this dose not equivalent to 10 mg of morphine. See text for explanation.

properties very similar to those of morphine and 5–10 times more potent on a molar basis. Neo-endorphin is a 17-amino-acid peptide containing leu-enkephalin in its sequence. Potent endorphins have also been identified in the adrenal medulla and the posterior pituitary; the one from the latter organ has been named dynorphin. It is anticipated that other endorphins will be isolated in the future, and it will be an enormous task to map their neuronal pathways and determine their physiologic roles. Thus, a natural system appears to be present in the body that can release endorphins in response to pain and perhaps other stimuli; these opioid peptides may then bind to opiate receptors to modify transmission along pain pathways. Morphine and the other narcotic analgesics apparently mimic the actions of these endogenous ligands by binding with the opiate receptors located throughout the body; this interaction gives rise to pharmacologic effects.

1. Receptor types–Several types of opiate receptors have been identified at various sites in the central and peripheral nervous systems. Exogenous and endogenous ligands bind at these loci to varying degrees, and the predominance and nature of the combination between a particular substance and a specific receptor give rise to a characteristic pharmacologic profile.

Analgesia at the supraspinal level as well as the euphoriant, respiratory depressant, and physical dependence properties of morphine (typical agonistlike effects) result principally from combination with μ receptors. The κ receptors are responsible primarily for the expression of analgesia at the spinal level, miosis, and sedation. The σ receptor seems related to the dysphoric, hallucinogenic, and cardiac stimulant effects. Other receptors have been postulated based on in vitro experiments, but their significance in vivo is unclear.

2. Receptor distribution–Opiate binding or recognition sites have been identified by radioligand binding, autoradiographic, and immunohistochemical techniques. A high density of narcotic analgesic binding sites is present in the dorsal horn of the spinal cord and certain subcortical regions of the brain. Some of the brain opiate binding sites that are concerned with pain transmission include the nucleus raphe magnus and locus ceruleus of the brain stem, the midbrain periaqueductal gray area, and several hypothalamic and thalamic nuclei. Binding of an opiate at these supraspinal sites greatly augments the effect at the spinal level to reduce nociceptive input and thereby raise the pain threshold. Certain spinal cord cells containing narcotic analgesic binding sites have been identified as short interneurons terminating on pain-transmitting primary central sensory afferents containing the peptide transmitter substance P (Chapter 18). Substance P neurons have been hypothesized to transmit pain, and opiates and endorphins have been shown to inhibit the release of substance P.

The brain sites involved in altering reactivity to pain are less well identified. It has been suggested that pathways between the diencephalon and the frontal cortex are involved, since the effects of narcotic analgesics bear some resemblance to those occurring after prefrontal lobotomy. The individual is aware of pain but states that it is no longer bothersome. Some support for such a postulate is provided by the fact that several nuclei of the thalamus and hypothalamus have been found to have a high density of opiate binding sites.

3. Neurochemical effects–Electrical activity in specific areas of the nervous system is inhibited by narcotic analgesics, and the reduction in neuronal firing is accompanied by a general decrease in the release of certain neurotransmitters. Since the release of transmitter substances is known to be coupled with the entry of calcium into the neuron, it has been suggested that the action of opiates depends upon their ability to selectively interfere with calcium influx and lower brain calcium. This reduction in intracellular calcium in specific neurons where opiates act causes a deficiency in neurotransmitter release with decreased activation of their postsynaptic sites.

In contrast to the depression of calcium entry into neurons caused by a single exposure to opiates, chronic exposure, which is associated with tolerance and dependence, causes an elevation of intracellular calcium content in neurons.

Another recent hypothesis attempts to relate narcotic analgesic effects to an inhibitory action on adenylate cyclase. The postulate is based principally on the effects of opiates on hybrid neuroblastoma cells in culture and has not been validated by experiments in the intact animal. Opiate effects on calcium and adenylate cyclase may be closely related, but definitive experiments to establish this relationship have not been carried out.

The release of several neurotransmitters is inhibited by narcotic analgesics; these transmitters include acetylcholine, norepinephrine, dopamine, 5-hydroxytryptamine, and substance P. Earlier attempts to explain opiate action by linking certain effects with a single neurotransmitter have not been successful, mainly because no one neurotransmitter can account for all of the varied effects of the narcotic analgesics.

4. Tolerance and physical dependence–With frequently repeated administration of therapeutic doses of morphine or its surrogates, there is a gradual loss in effectiveness, called **tolerance.** To reproduce the original response, a larger dose must be administered. With the development of tolerance, **physical dependence** occurs, so that continued administration of the drug becomes necessary to prevent a characteristic withdrawal or abstinence syndrome (Chapter 29).

The mechanism of development of tolerance and physical dependence is not related to pharmacokinetic factors but is a true cellular adaptive response. It has been suggested that the accumulation of neuronal calcium following frequent opiate administration may be partially responsible, since the ability to sequester calcium increases with chronic opiate administration and calcium readily antagonizes opiate effects. Discontinuing the narcotic would then result in loss of the ability to sequester calcium and in enhanced release of a number of neurotransmitters. The increased transmitter release may be the immediate cause of the abstinence syndrome.

The clinical aspects of tolerance and physical dependence are discussed below.

B. Organ System Effects of Morphine and Its Surrogates: The actions given below for morphine, the prototype agonist opiate, are also observed with all of the other agonists (Table 28–1). The agonist-antagonist agents, when given to a patient who has not recently received an agonist agent, also produce analgesia, but with minor variations in effects as noted below. Characteristics of specific members of these 2 groups are discussed below.

The pure antagonists and the agonist-antagonists, when given to a subject who has received an agonist, will have very different effects, as noted at the end of this chapter.

1. Central nervous system effects–The principal effects of the narcotic analgesics are on the central nervous system; the more important ones include analgesia, euphoria, sedation, and respiratory depression. With repeated use, a high degree of tolerance occurs to all of these effects (Table 28–3).

a. Analgesia–A painful sensation, no matter what its origin, consists of the noxious input plus the reaction of the organism to the stimulus. The analgesic properties of the opiates are related to their ability to change both pain *perception* and the *reaction* of the patient to pain. Experimental and clinical studies indicate that narcotic analgesics can effectively raise the threshold for pain, but their effects on the reactive component can only be inferred from subjective effects on the patient. In the presence of effective analgesia, pain may still be noted or perceived by the patient, but even very severe pain is no longer an all-consuming and destructive sensory input.

b. Euphoria–After a dose of morphine, a patient in pain or an addict experiences a pleasant floating sensation and freedom from anxiety and distress. However, other patients and some normal subjects (not in pain) experience dysphoric rather than pleasant effects after a dose of narcotic analgesic. Dysphoria is a disquieted state accompanied by both restlessness and a feeling of malaise. In general, if a real indication exists for administration of a narcotic analgesic, the most common affective response is euphoria.

Table 28–3. Extent of tolerance developed to some of the effects of the opiates.

High Degree of Tolerance	Moderate Degree of Tolerance	Minimal or No Tolerance
Analgesia	Bradycardia	Miosis
Euphoria, dysphoria		Constipation
Mental clouding		Convulsions
Sedation		
Respiratory depression		Antagonist actions
Antidiuresis		
Nausea and vomiting		
Cough suppression		

c. Sedation–Drowsiness and clouding of mentation are frequent concomitants of opiate action, and there may be some impairment of reasoning ability. There is little or no amnesia. Sleep is induced by opiates more frequently in the elderly than in young, healthy individuals. Ordinarily, the patient can be easily aroused from sleep. However, the combination of morphine with other central depressant drugs, such as the sedative-hypnotics, may result in profound depression. Marked sedation occurs more frequently with compounds closely related to the phenanthrene derivatives and less frequently with the synthetic agents such as meperidine and fentanyl. In contrast to humans, a number of species (cats, horses, cows, pigs) manifest excitation rather than sedation when given opiates. The reason for this difference is unknown.

d. Respiratory depression–All of the narcotic analgesics can produce significant respiratory depression by inhibiting brain stem respiratory mechanisms. Alveolar P_{CO_2} may increase, but the most significant aspect of this depression is decreased responsiveness to carbon dioxide. Many well-designed studies have demonstrated this effect, chiefly as a depressed response to a carbon dioxide challenge. The respiratory depression is dose-related and is influenced significantly by the degree of other sensory input occurring at the same time. For example, it is possible to partially overcome the opiate-induced respiratory depression by stimulation of various sorts. When strongly painful stimuli that have prevented the depressant action of a large dose of an opiate are relieved, respiratory depression may suddenly become marked. A small to moderate decrease in respiratory function, as measured by P_{CO_2} elevation, may be well tolerated in the patient without prior respiratory impairment. However, in individuals with increased intracranial pressure, asthma, chronic obstructive pulmonary disease, or cor pulmonale, this decrease may not be tolerated.

e. Cough suppression–Suppression of the cough reflex is a well-recognized action of narcotic analgesics. Codeine in particular has been used to good advantage in persons suffering from pathologic cough and in patients in whom it is necessary to maintain ventilation via an endotracheal tube. However, cough suppression by opiates may allow accumulation of secretions and thus lead to airway obstruction and atelectasis. Tolerance develops to the cough suppressant action of narcotic analgesics (Table 28–3).

f. Miosis–Constriction of the pupils is seen with virtually all of the narcotic agonists. Miosis is also a pharmacologic action to which little or no tolerance develops; thus, it is valuable in the diagnosis of opiate overdose, since even highly tolerant addicts will have miosis. The action can be blocked by atropine and by narcotic antagonists.

g. Truncal rigidity–An intensification of tone in the large trunk muscles has been noted with a number of opiates. It is believed that this is the result of an action of the narcotics at the spinal cord level. Truncal rigidity reduces thoracic compliance and thus interferes with ventilation. This action may be overcome by administration of a narcotic antagonist.

h. Emesis–The narcotic analgesics can activate the brain stem chemoreceptor trigger zone to produce nausea and vomiting. There may be another component to these effects in that ambulation seems to increase the incidence of nausea and vomiting, perhaps by an action on the vestibular apparatus.

2. Peripheral effects–

a. Cardiovascular system–Most narcotic analgesics have no significant direct effects on the heart and no major effects on cardiac rate or rhythm or on blood pressure. Exceptions to this generalization will be noted below as the specific drugs are discussed. Blood pressure is usually well maintained in subjects receiving opiates unless the cardiovascular system is stressed, in which case hypotension may occur. This hypotensive effect is probably due to peripheral arterial and venous dilatation, which has been attributed to a number of mechanisms including release of histamine and central depression of vasomotor-stabilizing mechanisms. No consistent effect on cardiac output is seen, and the ECG is not significantly altered. However, caution should be exercised in patients with decreased blood volume, since the above mechanisms make these patients quite susceptible to blood pressure decreases. Narcotic analgesics affect cerebral circulation minimally except when P_{CO_2} rises as a consequence of respiratory depression. Increased P_{CO_2} leads to cerebral vascular dilatation and a concomitant decrease in cerebral vascular resistance, increase in cerebral blood flow, and increase in cerebrospinal fluid pressure (intracranial pressure).

b. Gastrointestinal tract–Constipation has long been recognized as an effect of narcotic analgesics, although the effects of the narcotics on smooth muscle of the gut are generally stimulatory. There is considerable variation in the response at different levels of the gut. The effects may be mediated through an action on the central nervous system as well as a local one. In the stomach, motility may be decreased but tone may increase—particularly in the central portion; gastric secretion of hydrochloric acid is decreased. Small intestine resting tone is increased, with periodic spasms, but the amplitude of nonpropulsive contractions is markedly decreased. In the large intestine, propulsive peristaltic waves are diminished and tone is increased; this delays passage of the fecal mass and allows increased absorption of water, which leads to constipation. The large bowel actions are the basis for the use of narcotics in management of diarrhea. There is a clinical impression that the benzomorphans (eg, pentazocine) cause less constipation than other opiates.

c. Biliary tract–The narcotics constrict biliary smooth muscle, which may result in biliary colic. The sphincter of Oddi may constrict, resulting in reflux of biliary and pancreatic secretions and elevated plasma amylase and lipase levels.

d. Genitourinary tract–Renal function is depressed by opiates. It is believed that in humans this is chiefly due to decreased renal plasma flow. This contrasts with animal studies, in which reduced urine output seems to result from increased secretion of antidiuretic hormone as well as reduced renal perfusion. Ureteral and bladder tone is increased by therapeutic doses of the narcotic analgesics. Increased urethral sphincter tone may precipitate urinary retention, especially in postoperative patients. Occasionally, ureteral colic caused by a renal calculus is made worse by the increase in ureteral tone.

e. Uterus–The narcotic analgesics may prolong labor. The mechanism for this action is unclear, but both direct smooth muscle depressant effects of the opiates and their central nervous system effects may reduce uterine tone.

f. Neuroendocrine–Narcotic analgesics stimulate the release of antidiuretic hormone, prolactin, and somatotropin but inhibit the release of luteinizing hormone. These effects are of importance in that they may reflect regulatory roles in these systems by endogenous opioid peptides and are probably mediated by effects in the hypothalamus.

g. Miscellaneous–Therapeutic doses of the narcotic analgesics will produce flushing and warming of the skin accompanied sometimes by sweating and itching; central effects and histamine release may be responsible for these reactions.

C. Effects of Agonist-Antagonists: Pentazocine and other agonist-antagonist drugs usually produce sedation in addition to analgesia when given in therapeutic doses. At higher doses, sweating, dizziness, and nausea are common, but severe respiratory depression may be less common than with pure agonists. When it does occur, respiratory depression may be reversed by naloxone but not by other agonist-antagonists such as nalorphine. Psychotomimetic effects, with hallucinations, nightmares, and anxiety, have been reported following the use of agonist-antagonist agents.

II. CLINICAL PHARMACOLOGY OF THE NARCOTIC ANALGESICS

Management of pain is essential to good medical practice and requires careful consideration of proper dose, type of drug, and the disease being treated. There are many situations in which analgesia must be provided before a definitive diagnosis can be reached. Indeed, in some acute situations relief of pain may actually facilitate history-taking and physical examination and thus speed the diagnostic process.

Use of these drugs in acute situations may be contrasted to their use in chronic pain management, where other factors must be considered—particularly tolerance and physical dependence. In all instances, the factors that should enter into the decision about choice of drug include the following: (1) Is analgesia needed? (2) Will the narcotic analgesic obscure or alter the signs and symptoms of the underlying disorder? (3) Are the pharmacologic effects of the opiate liable to worsen the condition for which they are being used, eg, by increasing cerebrospinal fluid pressure or producing respiratory depression? (4) Do the narcotic agent's adverse effects impose a significant hazard? (See Table 28–4.) (5) Is there a possibility of significant drug interaction between the narcotic agent and other drugs the patient is receiving? (See Table 28–5.) (6) Are tolerance and drug dependence likely to develop?

Table 28–2 shows the variability in agonist efficacy of different narcotic drugs. It is therefore necessary to select a drug appropriate to the type and severity of pain being treated to make certain that adequate analgesia is provided. The level of pain associated with various disease states also varies; thus, the postoperative pain of a forearm fracture may be adequately treated with codeine; the severe pain of a kidney stone may not. Each drug has a therapeutic ceiling, and to attempt to raise the ceiling with higher doses creates a risk of significant drug side-effects and therapeutic failure.

Clinical Use of Narcotic Analgesics

A. Analgesia: Severe, *constant* pain is usually relieved with the more efficacious narcotics, but sharp, intermittent pain does not appear to be as amenable to relief. An attempt should be made to quantify the pain; this information should be used to select the proper agent and to monitor its effects. In this evaluation and selection process, such considerations as route of administration (oral versus parenteral administration), duration of action, ceiling effect (maximal efficacy), duration of therapy, and past experience with narcotics are of obvious importance.

The pain associated with cancer and other terminal illnesses must be treated adequately, and concerns about tolerance and dependence should be set aside in favor of making the patient as comfortable as possible. Research by workers in the hospice movement has demonstrated that fixed-interval administration of narcotic medication (a regular dose at a regular time) is more effective in achieving pain relief than dosing on demand. In addition, drugs such as the amphetamines have been shown to enhance the actions of the narcotics and thus may be very useful adjuncts in the patient with chronic pain.

Narcotic analgesics are often employed during obstetric labor. Because all of the narcotics cross the placental barrier and reach the fetus, care must be taken to minimize neonatal narcotic depression. If this occurs, immediate injection of naloxone will reverse the depression. The phenylpiperidine drugs (eg, meperidine) appear to produce less depression in newborn infants than does morphine; this may justify their use in obstetric practice.

The acute, severe pain of renal and biliary colic often requires a strong agonist opiate for adequate relief. However, the increase in smooth muscle tone may cause a paradoxic *increase* in pain secondary to increased spasm around the stone. An increase in the dose of opiate is usually successful in providing analgesia. Other measures such as anticholinergic drugs and nitrates are rarely useful in this situation.

B. Acute Pulmonary Edema: The relief produced by intravenous morphine in dyspnea from pulmonary edema associated with left ventricular failure is truly remarkable. The mechanism is not clear but probably involves a reduction in *perception* of shortness of breath and the anxiety associated with it as well as a reduction in cardiac preload (reduced venous tone) and afterload (decreased peripheral resistance). (See also Chapter 11.)

C. Cough: Suppression of cough can be obtained at doses lower than those needed for analgesia. However, in recent years the use of narcotic analgesics to allay cough has diminished largely because a number of effective synthetic compounds have been developed that are neither analgesic nor addictive. These agents are discussed in the section on antitussives.

D. Diarrhea: Diarrhea from almost any cause can be controlled with the narcotic analgesics, but if diarrhea is associated with infection such use must not substitute for appropriate chemotherapy. Opium preparations (eg, paregoric) have long been used to control diarrhea, but in recent years opiates with more selective gastrointestinal effects have been developed, eg, diphenoxylate. Formulations are cited below that have been prepared specifically for this purpose.

E. Applications in Anesthesia: The narcotics are frequently used as premedicant drugs before anesthesia and surgery because of their sedative, anxiolytic, and analgesic properties. The narcotics are also used intraoperatively both as adjuncts to other anesthetic agents and, in high doses (eg, 1–3 mg/kg of morphine, or 0.02–0.075 mg/kg of fentanyl), as the primary anesthetic agent (see Chapter 22), most commonly in cardiovascular surgery and other types of high-risk surgery where a primary goal is to minimize cardiovascular depression. In such situations, mechanical respiratory assistance must be provided.

Recently, there has been great interest in the use of opiates as regional analgesics by administration into the epidural or subarachnoid spaces of the spinal cord. This interest is based on the laboratory finding that there is a spinal component of opiate action and that there are a great many opiate receptors in the dorsolateral horn of the spinal cord. Theoretically, therefore, the epidural application of opiates might selectively produce analgesia without impairment of motor, autonomic, or sensory functions other than pain. A number of studies have, in the main, confirmed these expectations. Long-lasting analgesia (6–30 hours) with minimal side-effects can be achieved by epidural administration of 3–5 mg of morphine. However, it has been noted that respiratory depression may occur hours after the drug is injected.

Toxicity & Undesired Effects

Direct toxic effects of the narcotic analgesics that are extensions of their acute pharmacologic actions

Table 28–4. Toxic effects of the opiates.

Behavioral restlessness, tremulousness, hyperactivity (in dysphoric reaction).
Respiratory depression.
Nausea and vomiting.
Increased intracranial pressure.
Postural hypotension accentuated by hypovolemia.
Constipation.
Urinary retention.
Itching around nose, urticaria (more frequent with parenteral administration).

include the adverse effects of nausea, vomiting, constipation, and respiratory depression (Table 28–4). In addition, the following must be considered.

A. Tolerance and Dependence: Drug dependence of the opiate type is marked by tolerance, a relatively specific withdrawal or abstinence syndrome, and pronounced craving or psychologic dependence. Just as there are pharmacologic differences between the various narcotics, there are also differences in abuse potential and the severity of withdrawal effects. For instance, administration of a narcotic antagonist to a methadone-dependent person is followed by severe withdrawal symptoms. Propoxyphene, a related compound, causes less marked dependence, and the withdrawal syndrome appears to be milder although qualitatively similar to that of other narcotics. The addiction liabilities of the mixed agonist-antagonist opiates appear to be considerably less than those of the agonist drugs. Heroin addicts usually resort to pentazocine only when agonists are not available.

1. Tolerance–As mentioned above, repeated administration of therapeutic doses of any opiate results in a gradual loss of effectiveness. Although development of tolerance begins with the first dose of an opiate, tolerance generally does not become clinically manifest until after 2–3 weeks of frequent experience with ordinary therapeutic doses. Tolerance develops most readily when large doses are given at short intervals and is minimized by giving small amounts of drug with larger intervals between doses. Thus, compulsive abusers of opiates may develop tolerance very rapidly.

Depending on the compound and the effect measured, the degree of tolerance may be as great as 35-fold. Marked tolerance usually develops to the analgesic, euphoriant, and respiratory depressant effects. It is possible to produce respiratory arrest in a nontolerant person with a dose of 60 mg of morphine, whereas in addicts maximally tolerant to opiates as much as 2000 mg of morphine taken over a 2- or 3-hour period may not produce significant respiratory depression. Tolerance also develops to the antidiuretic, emetic, and hypotensive effect but not to the miotic, convulsant, and constipating actions (Table 28–3).

Tolerance to the euphoriant and respiratory effects of the narcotics dissipates within a few days after the drugs are discontinued. Tolerance to the emetic effects may persist for several months after withdrawal of the drug. The rates at which tolerance appears and disappears, as well as the degree of tolerance, may also differ considerably among the different narcotic analgesics. For instance, tolerance to methadone develops more slowly and to a lesser degree than to morphine.

Cross-tolerance is an extremely important characteristic of the narcotics, ie, patients tolerant to morphine are also tolerant to all other agonist opiates. Morphine, meperidine, methadone, and their congeners exhibit cross-tolerance not only with respect to their analgesic actions but also to their euphoriant, sedative, and respiratory effects.

Tolerance develops also to the agonist-antagonist analgesics but to a much lesser extent than to the agonists. Such effects as hallucinations, sedation, hypothermia, and respiratory depression are reduced after repeated administration of the agonist-antagonist drugs. However, tolerance to agonist-antagonist agents does not generally include cross-tolerance to the agonist opiates. It is also important to note that tolerance does not develop to the antagonist actions of the mixed agonist-antagonists nor to those of the pure antagonists.

2. Physical dependence–The development of physical dependence on an opiate after its repeated administration is an invariable accompaniment of tolerance. Failure to continue administering the drug results in a characteristic withdrawal or abstinence syndrome that reflects an exaggerated rebound from the acute pharmacologic effects of the opiate. The signs and symptoms of withdrawal include rhinorrhea, lacrimation, yawning, chills, goose pimples, hyperventilation, hyperthermia, mydriasis, muscular aches, vomiting, diarrhea, anxiety, and hostility (see also Chapter 29). The number and intensity of the signs and symptoms are largely dependent on the degree of physical dependence that has developed. Administration of an opiate suppresses abstinence signs and symptoms almost immediately. The time of onset, the intensity, and the duration of the abstinence effects depend on the drug used and may be related to its biologic half-life. With morphine or heroin, withdrawal signs usually start within 6–10 hours after the last dose. Peak effects are seen at 36–48 hours, after which most of the signs and symptoms gradually subside. By 5 days, most of the effects have disappeared, but some may persist for months. In the case of meperidine, the withdrawal syndrome largely subsides within 24 hours, whereas with methadone several days are required to reach the peak of the abstinence syndrome, and it may last as long as 2 weeks. The slower subsidence of methadone effects is associated with a less intense syndrome, and this is the basis for its use in the detoxification of heroin addicts.

A transient, explosive abstinence syndrome—antagonist-precipitated withdrawal—can be induced in a subject physically dependent on opiates by administering naloxone or other antagonist. Within 5 minutes after injection of the antagonist, signs and symptoms similar to those seen after abrupt discontinuance appear, peaking in 10–20 minutes and largely subsiding after 1 hour. In contrast to the relatively mild abstinence syndrome that results from methadone withdrawal (cessation of drug administration), antagonist-precipitated methadone abstinence syndrome may be very severe.

In the case of the agonist-antagonist agents, withdrawal signs and symptoms can be induced after repeated administration followed by abrupt discontinuance of pentazocine, cyclazocine, or nalorphine, but the syndrome appears to be quite different from that produced by morphine and other agonists. Anxiety, loss of appetite and body weight, tachycardia, chills, increase in body temperature, and abdominal cramps have been noted. The syndrome can be precipitated by naloxone in dependent subjects, but high doses are required.

3. Psychologic dependence–The euphoria, indifference to stimuli, and sedation usually caused by the narcotic analgesics, especially when injected intravenously, tend to promote their compulsive use. In addition, the addict experiences abdominal effects that have been likened to an intense sexual orgasm. These factors constitute the primary reasons for opiate abuse liability and are strongly reinforced by the development of physical dependence, since the drug user rationalizes continued use of the drug as the means of preventing abstinence symptoms, ie, to remain "normal."

Under no circumstances should adequate pain relief be denied simply because a narcotic exhibits potential for abuse or because laws complicate the process of prescribing narcotics. However, there are certain principles that can be followed by the clinician to avoid the problems presented by tolerance and dependence when using narcotic analgesics: (1) Establish therapeutic goals before starting opiate therapy. This tends to limit the potential for physical dependence. (2) When drugs equivalent to morphine must be used, attempt to limit both the dosage and duration of administration. (3) Instead of narcotic analgesics, especially in chronic management, consider using less efficacious agents or compounds exhibiting less pronounced withdrawal symptoms on discontinuance.

B. Diagnosis and Treatment of Opiate Overdosage: The diagnosis of narcotic overdosage may be very simple (known addict, needle marks, brought to hospital by friends who appear to be using drugs), or it may be very difficult—as in any comatose patient for whom no past history is available. Intravenous injection of naloxone, 0.1–0.2 mg, can provide quick information about whether coma is due to opiate overdose. Treatment is with the same drug, 0.4–0.8 mg given intravenously, and repeated every 2–3 minutes for 2–3 doses. In using naloxone in the severely depressed newborn, it is important to start with doses of 5–10 μg/kg and to consider a second dose of up to a total of 25 μg/kg if no response is noted. Use of the antagonist should not, of course, delay the institution of other therapeutic measures, especially respiratory support.

C. Contraindications and Cautions in Therapy:

1. Use of pure agonists with mixed agonist-antagonists–When a mixed agonist-antagonist agent such as pentazocine is given to a patient also receiving an agonist (eg, morphine or meperidine), the possibility of diminishing analgesia or perhaps inducing a state of withdrawal is present; combining agonist with agonist-antagonist opiates should be done cautiously, if at all.

2. Use during pregnancy–In pregnant women who are chronically using opiates, the fetus may become addicted in utero and may manifest withdrawal symptoms in the early postpartum period. A daily dose as small as 6 mg of heroin (or equivalent) will result in mild withdrawal symptoms in the infant, and twice that much may result in severe signs and symptoms, including irritability, shrill crying, diarrhea, or even seizures. Recognition of the problem is aided by a careful history and physical examination. Initial treatment of the neonate may consist of giving paregoric, 0.12–0.24 mL/kg orally (1 mL of paregoric is equivalent to 0.4 mg of morphine) or methadone, 0.1–0.5 mg/kg orally. Large intravenous doses of the piperidine derivatives (meperidine, fentanyl, etc) should be avoided, since they cause central nervous system stimulation, particularly in infants and children. More recently, diazepam, 0.1 mg/kg intravenously, has been used in the treatment of neonatal withdrawal syndrome. The pharmacologic basis for this is unclear.

3. Use in patients with impaired pulmonary function–In patients with borderline respiratory reserve, the depressant properties of the narcotic analgesics may lead to acute respiratory failure. In addition, carbon dioxide retention caused by respiratory depression results in cerebral vasodilatation; in patients with elevated intracranial pressure, this may lead to lethal alterations in brain function.

4. Use in patients with impaired hepatic function–Morphine and its congeners are metabolized primarily by conjugation to glucuronides in the liver; their use in patients in prehepatic coma may thus be questioned.

5. Use in patients with endocrine disease–Patients with adrenal insufficiency (Addison's disease) and those with hypothyroidism (myxedema) have prolonged and exaggerated responses to opiates.

Drug Interactions

Because seriously ill or hospitalized patients may

Table 28–5. Narcotic drug interactions.

Sedative-hypnotics: Increased central nervous system depression, particularly respiratory depression.
Antipsychotic tranquilizers: Increased sedation. Variable effects on respiratory depression. Accentuation of cardiovascular effects (anticholinergic and α-blocking actions).
MAO inhibitors: Absolute contraindication to all narcotic analgesics because of the high incidence of hyperpyrexic coma; hypertension has also been reported.

require a large number of drugs, there is always a possibility of drug interactions when the narcotic analgesics are administered. Table 28–5 lists some of these drug interactions and the reasons for not combining the named drugs with opiates.

SPECIFIC AGENTS

The following section describes the most important widely used narcotic analgesics, along with features peculiar to specific agents. Data about doses approximately equivalent to 10 mg of intramuscular morphine, oral:parenteral efficacy, duration of analgesia, maximum efficacy, and addiction and abuse liability are presented in Table 28–2.

Strong Agonists

PHENANTHRENES

Morphine, hydromorphone, and **oxymorphone** are strong agonists useful in treating severe pain. These prototypic agents have been described in detail above. **Heroin** is a potent and fast-acting narcotic, but its use is prohibited by legislation in the USA. Double-blind studies have not supported the claim that heroin is more effective than morphine in severe chronic pain.

PHENYLHEPTYLAMINES

Methadone has a pharmacodynamic profile very similar to that of morphine but is somewhat longer-acting. Acutely, its analgesic potency and efficacy are at least equal to those of morphine. Methadone gives reliable effects when administered orally. Tolerance and physical dependence develop more slowly with methadone than with morphine. As noted above, the withdrawal signs and symptoms occurring after abrupt discontinuance of methadone are milder, although more prolonged, than those of morphine. These properties make methadone a useful drug for detoxification and for maintenance of the chronic relapsing heroin addict. For detoxification of a heroin-dependent addict, low doses of methadone (5–10 mg orally) are given twice or 3 times daily for 2 or 3 days. Upon discontinuing methadone, the addict experiences a mild but endurable withdrawal syndrome. For maintenance therapy of the narcotic recidivist, tolerance to 50–100 mg/d of oral methadone is deliberately produced; in this state, the addict exhibits cross-tolerance to heroin that prevents most of the addiction-reinforcing effects of heroin. The rationale of maintenance programs is that blocking the reinforcement obtained from abuse of illicit opiates removes the motive for criminal activity and makes the addict more amenable to psychiatric and rehabilitative therapy. The pharmacologic basis for the use of methadone in maintenance programs is sound and the sociologic basis is rational, but some methadone programs fail because nonpharmacologic management is inadequate.

PHENYLPIPERIDINES

Meperidine and **fentanyl** are the most widely used agents in this family. Fentanyl is used chiefly as part of the anesthesia regimen during surgery. Meperidine has significant anticholinergic effects, which may be a contraindication if tachycardia would be a problem. It is also reported to have a negative inotropic action on the heart.

MORPHINANS

Levorphanol is a synthetically prepared narcotic analgesic closely resembling morphine in its action.

Mild to Moderate Agonists

PHENANTHRENES

Codeine, oxycodone, dihydrocodeine, and **hydrocodone** are all somewhat less potent than morphine or have side-effects that limit the maximum tolerated dose when one attempts to achieve analgesia comparable to that of morphine. These compounds are rarely used alone but are combined in formulations containing aspirin or acetaminophen and other drugs.

PHENYLHEPTYLAMINES

Propoxyphene is chemically related to methadone but has low analgesic activity. Various studies have reported its potency at levels ranging from no better than placebo to half as potent as codeine, ie, 120 mg propoxyphene = 60 mg codeine. Its true potency probably lies somewhere between these extremes, and its analgesic effect is additive to that of an optimal dose of aspirin. However, its low efficacy makes it unsuitable, even in combination with aspirin, for severe pain. Although propoxyphene has a low abuse liability, the increasing incidence of deaths associated with its misuse in recent years has caused it to be scheduled as a controlled substance with low potential for abuse.

PHENYLPIPERIDINES

Diphenoxylate is not used for analgesia but for the treatment of diarrhea. It is not scheduled for control because the likelihood of its abuse is remote. The poor solubility of the compound limits its use for parenteral injection. As an antidiarrheal drug, it is usually used in combination with atropine (Lomotil, other names).

Loperamide (Imodium) is another phenylpiperidine derivative used to control diarrhea. Its potential for abuse is low because of its limited ability to gain access to the brain. The usual dose is 4 mg to start and then 2 mg after each diarrheal stool.

Mixed Agonist-Antagonists

PHENANTHRENES

Nalbuphine and **buprenorphine** are potent members of this class and are given parenterally. At doses higher than usual, there seems to be a definite ceiling—not noted with morphine—to the respiratory depressant effect. Unfortunately, when respiratory depression from these agents does occur, it may be relatively resistant to naloxone reversal.

MORPHINANS

Butorphanol is similar to nalbuphine and buprenorphine but appears to produce more sedation at equianalgesic dose.

BENZOMORPHANS

Pentazocine is the oldest mixed agonist-antagonist available and may be used orally or parenterally. As with all of the agonist-antagonists, care should be taken not to administer them to patients receiving pure agonist drugs because of the unpredictability of both drugs' effects.

• • •

ANTITUSSIVES

As noted above, the narcotic analgesics are among the most effective drugs available for the suppression of cough. This effect is often achieved at doses below those necessary to produce analgesia. Furthermore, the antitussive effect is also produced by the stereoisomers of opiate molecules, which are devoid of analgesic effects and addiction liability.

The physiologic mechanism of cough is a complex one, and little is known about the specific mechanism of action of the narcotic antitussive drugs. It is likely that both central and peripheral effects come into play.

The opiate derivatives most commonly used as antitussives are dextromethorphan, codeine, levopropoxyphene, and noscapine. While these agents (other than codeine) are largely free of the side-effects associated with the opiates, none of them should be used in patients taking MAO inhibitors (see Table 28–5).

Dextromethorphan is the dextrorotatory stereoisomer of a methylated derivative of levorphanol. It is essentially free of analgesic and addictive properties and produces less constipation than codeine. The usual antitussive dose is 15–30 mg 3–4 times daily. It is available in many over-the-counter products.

Codeine, as noted above, has a useful antitussive action at doses lower than those required for analgesia. Thus, 15 mg is usually sufficient to relieve cough.

Levopropoxyphene is the stereoisomer of the weak opiate agonist dextropropoxyphene. It is devoid of opiate effects, although sedation has been described as a side-effect. The usual antitussive dose is 50–100 mg every 4 hours.

Noscapine is, like papaverine, a nonnarcotic benzylisoquinoline opium alkaloid. It is used only as an antitussive and is claimed to be as effective in this application as codeine. The usual dose is 15–30 mg every 6 hours.

• • •

THE OPIATE ANTAGONISTS

The pure opiate antagonist drugs **naloxone** and **naltrexone** are morphine derivatives with larger substituents at the N position. These agents have a very high affinity for opiate binding sites of the μ receptor type. Their affinity for κ opiate receptors is about one-twentieth of that for μ receptors and even less than for σ receptors.

Pharmacokinetics

Naloxone has poor efficacy when given by the oral route and a short duration of action (1–4 hours) when given by injection. Metabolic disposition is by glucuronide conjugation, like that of the agonist opiates. Naltrexone is well absorbed after oral administration but may undergo rapid first-pass metabolism. It has a half-life of 10 hours, and a single oral dose of 100 mg will block the effects of injected heroin for up to 48 hours.

Pharmacodynamics

When given in the absence of an agonist drug, these antagonists are almost inert. Very large doses of naloxone may cause slight sedation.

In contrast, when given to a morphine-treated subject, the antagonist will completely reverse the opiate effects within 1–2 minutes. This constitutes one of the most dramatic examples of pharmacologic antagonism in medicine. In individuals who are acutely depressed by an overdose of an opiate, the antagonist will effectively normalize respiration, level of consciousness, pupil size, bowel activity, etc. In dependent subjects who appear normal (except for miosis) while taking opiates, naloxone or naltrexone will almost instantaneously precipitate an abstinence syndrome, as described previously.

There is no tolerance to the antagonistic action of these agents, nor does withdrawal after chronic administration precipitate an abstinence syndrome.

Clinical Use

Naloxone is the only pure opiate antagonist available at present. Because it is a pure antagonist, it is preferred over earlier weak agonist-antagonist agents that had been used primarily as antagonists, eg, nalorphine and levallorphan.

The major application of naloxone is in the treatment of acute opiate overdose, as described above; it is the specific antidote for this condition (see also Chapter 58). It is very important that the relatively short duration of action of naloxone be borne in mind when using it for this purpose, since a severely depressed patient may recover after a single dose of naloxone and appear normal, only to relapse into coma after 1–2 hours. The usual dose of naloxone is 0.1–0.4 mg intravenously.

Because of its long duration of action, naltrexone has been proposed as a "maintenance" drug for addicts in treatment programs. A single dose given on alternate days could presumably block all of the effects of a dose of heroin. It might be predicted that this approach to rehabilitation would not be popular with a large percentage of drug users unless they are motivated to become drug-free.

Recent experimental studies suggest that naloxone may be of value in the treatment of shock. Experimental animals with hemorrhagic, endotoxin-induced, and spinal transection shock respond to naloxone with an increase in blood pressure and improved survival rates. The mechanism for this effect is not known, but elevated concentrations of endorphins can be detected in the blood of animals in shock.

• • •

References

Beaver WT: A clinical comparison of the analgesic effects of intramuscular nalbuphine and morphine in patients with postoperative pain. *J Pharmacol Exp Ther* 1978;**204:**487.

Belleville JW et al: Influence of age on pain relief from analgesics. *JAMA* 1971;**217:**1835.

Braude MC et al (editors): *Narcotic Antagonists*. Raven Press, 1974.

Houde RW: Analgesic effectiveness of the narcotic agonist-antagonists. *Br J Clin Pharmacol* 1979;**7(Suppl 3):**297S.

Houde RW, Wallenstein SL, Beaver WT: Clinical measurement of pain. Pages 75–122 in: *Analgetics*. de Stevens G (editor). Academic Press, 1965.

Iwamoto ET, Martin W: Multiple opiate receptors. *Med Res Rev* 1981;**1:**411.

Smith AP, Loh HH: The opiate receptor. In: *Hormonal Proteins and Peptides: β-Endorphin*. Vol 10. Li CH (editor). Academic Press, 1981.

Way EL: Review and overview of four decades of opiate research. Chapter 1 in: *Neurochemical Mechanisms of Opiates and Endorphins*. Loh HH, Ross DH (editors). Vol 20 of: *Advances in Biochemical Psychopharmacology*. Raven Press, 1979.

Way EL, Adler TK: The pharmacologic implications of the fate of morphine and its surrogates. *Pharmacol Rev* 1968;**12:**383.

Drugs of Abuse | 29

Leo Hollister, MD

The term "drug abuse" is an unfortunate one since it connotes social disapproval and may have different meanings to different people. One must also distinguish drug abuse from drug "misuse." Abuse of a drug might be construed as any use of a drug for nonmedical purposes, almost always for altering consciousness. To misuse a drug might be to take it for the wrong indication, in the wrong dosage, or for too long a period, to mention only a few obvious examples. In the context of drug abuse, the drug itself is of less importance than the pattern of use. For example, taking 50 mg of diazepam to heighten the effect of a daily dose of methadone is an abuse of diazepam. On the other hand, taking the same excessive daily dose of the drug but only for its sedative effect is misusing diazepam.

Dependence is a biologic phenomenon. **Psychic dependence** is manifested by compulsive drug-seeking behavior in which the individual uses the drug repetitively for personal satisfaction. Heavy cigarette smoking is an example. **Physical dependence** is present when withdrawal of the drug produces symptoms that are frequently the opposite of those sought by the addict. It has been suggested that the body adjusts to a new level of homeostasis during the period of drug use and reacts in opposite fashion when the new equilibrium is disturbed. Alcohol withdrawal syndrome is perhaps the best-known example, but milder degrees of withdrawal may be observed in people who drink a lot of coffee every day. Psychic dependence almost always precedes physical dependence but does not inevitably lead to it. Cocaine users may be psychically dependent on the drug but show no apparent withdrawal effects when it is stopped. **Addiction** is usually taken to mean a state of physical and psychic dependence, but the word is too imprecise to be useful.

Tolerance signifies a decreased response to the effects of the drug, necessitating ever larger doses to achieve the same effect. Tolerance is closely associated with the phenomenon of physical dependence. It is largely due to compensatory responses that mitigate the drug's pharmacodynamic action. **Metabolic tolerance** due to increased disposition of the drug after chronic use is occasionally reported. **Behavioral tolerance,** an ability to compensate for the drug's effects, is another possible mechanism of tolerance.

Experimental study of drug abuse is difficult for both legal and scientific reasons. The lack of simple animal models is a great disadvantage. The most useful model developed thus far is the self-administration technique in monkeys. Animals are equipped with an intravenous catheter through which a metered dose of the drug under study is administered each time the animal presses a lever. Most agents with significant potential for psychic or physical dependence can readily be detected by this technique. However, this model is both expensive and complex.

Cultural Considerations

Each society accepts certain drugs as licit and condemns others as illicit. In the USA and most of Western Europe, the "national drugs" are caffeine, nicotine, and alcohol. In the Middle East, cannabis may be added to the list of licit drugs, while alcohol is forbidden. Among certain American Indian tribes, peyote, a hallucinogen, may be used licitly for religious purposes. In the Andes of South America, cocaine is used to allay hunger and enhance the ability to perform arduous work at high altitude. Thus, which drugs are licit or illicit or—to use other terminology—"used" or "abused" depends on a social judgment. A major social cost of relegating any substance to the illicit category is the criminal activity that often results, since purveyors of the substance are lured into illegal traffic by the opportunity to make enormous profits while dependent users may resort to robbery, prostitution, and other types of antisocial behavior to support their habits.

Current USA attitudes to drugs of this type are reflected in the Schedule of Controlled Substances (Table 29–1). This schedule is quite similar to those published by international control bodies. They affect principally ethical and law-abiding manufacturers of the drugs and have had little deterrent effect on underground manufacturers or suppliers.

Any use of mind-altering drugs is based on a complicated interplay between 3 factors: the user, the setting in which the drug is taken, and the drug. Thus, the personality of the user and the setting may have a strong influence on what the user experiences. Nonetheless, it is usually possible to identify a pharmacologic "core" of drug effects that will be experienced by almost anyone under almost any circumstances if dosage is adequate.

Table 29–1. Illustrations from Schedule of Controlled Substances, United States Drug Enforcement Agency. Note that the criteria given by the agency do not always reflect the actual pharmacologic properties of the drugs (see text).

Schedule	Criteria	Examples*
I	No medical use; high addiction potential.	Hallucinogens Marihuana Heroin
II	Medical use; high addiction potential.	Morphine, most other narcotic analgesics Cocaine Amphetamines Sedatives such as pentobarbital sodium or methaqualone
III	Medical use; moderate potential for dependence.	Codeine in combination Paregoric Glutethimide, sodium butabarbital
IV	Medical use; low abuse potential.	Phenobarbital Chloral hydrate Benzodiazepines Other sedatives

*List not complete.

SPECIFIC TYPES OF DRUGS OF ABUSE

OPIATES & OPIOIDS

History

The nepenthe (Greek, "free from sorrow") mentioned in the *Odyssey* probably contained opium. Opium smoking was widely practiced in China and the Near East until recently. Isolation of active opium alkaloids as well as the introduction of the hypodermic needle, allowing parenteral use of morphine, increased opiate use in the West. The first of several "epidemics" of opiate use in the USA followed the Civil War. Relief of pain with liberal doses of opiates was one of the few forms of treatment army physicians could offer the gravely wounded, and those lucky enough to survive often found themselves physically dependent. About 4% of adults in the USA used opiates regularly during the postbellum period. By the 1900s, the number had dropped to about one in 400 people in the USA, but the problem was still considered serious enough to justify passage of the Harrison Narcotic Act just before World War I. A new epidemic of opiate use started around 1964 and has remained unabated ever since. Present estimates are that between 400,000 and 600,000 people in the USA are opiate-dependent.

Chemistry & Pharmacology

The most commonly abused opiates are heroin, morphine, oxycodone, and (among health professionals) meperidine. The chemistry and general pharmacology of these agents are presented in Chapter 28.

Tolerance to the mental effects of opiates develops with chronic use. The need for ever-increasing amounts of drug to sustain the desired euphoriant effects—as well as avoid the discomfort of withdrawal—have the expected consequence of strongly reinforcing dependence once it has started. The role of endorphins in opiate dependence is uncertain.

Clinical Aspects

Curiosity and social pressure are the strongest factors in initiating opiate use. Intravenous administration is routine not only because it is the most efficient route but also because it produces a bolus of high concentration of drug that reaches the brain to produce a "rush," followed by euphoria, a feeling of tranquility, and sleepiness ("the nod"). Most doses of heroin available on the street are less than 25 mg and produce effects that last 3–5 hours. Thus, several doses a day are required to forestall manifestations of withdrawal in dependent persons. The trouble and expense of meeting these dose requirements put the dependent person always "on the hustle," either to get money to buy the drug or to find a "connection" with something to sell. Since supplies of heroin are of widely varying potency, the risk of overdosage is always present. And sooner or later in the lives of most heroin abusers, the money runs out or the supplies run out, and the withdrawal syndrome then begins.

Symptoms of opiate withdrawal begin 8–10 hours after the last dose. Many of these symptoms resemble those of increased activity of the sympathetic nervous system. Lacrimation, rhinorrhea, yawning, and sweating appear first. Restless sleep followed by weakness, chills, gooseflesh ("cold turkey"), nausea and vomiting, muscle aches, and involuntary movements ("kicking the habit"), hyperpnea, hyperthermia, and hypertension occur in later stages of the withdrawal syndrome. The acute course of withdrawal may last 7–10 days. A secondary phase of protracted abstinence lasts for 26–30 weeks and is characterized by hypotension, bradycardia, hypothermia, mydriasis, and decreased responsiveness of the respiratory center to carbon dioxide.

Besides the ever-present risk of fatal overdose, a number of other serious complications are associated with opiate dependence. Hepatitis B viral infections are a common complication of sharing contaminated hypodermic syringes. Bacterial infections lead to septic complications such as meningitis, osteomyelitis, and abscesses in various organs. Homicide, suicide, and accidents are more prevalent among heroin abusers than in the general population.

Treatment

Treatment of acute overdoses of opiates may be lifesaving and is described in Chapter 28.

Pharmacologic or psychosocial approaches may be used, either separately or together in long-term treatment of opiate-dependent persons. Unfortunately, widely different opinions are vigorously expounded about which is the preferred type of treatment. Because each treatment method has a self-selected patient population, it is difficult to compare results. Chronic users tend to prefer pharmacologic approaches; those with shorter histories of drug abuse are more amenable to psychosocial interventions.

Pharmacologic treatment is most often used for detoxification. The principles of detoxification are the same for all drugs: to substitute a longer-acting, orally active, pharmacologically equivalent drug for the abused drug, stabilize the patient on that drug, and then gradually withdraw the substituted drug. **Methadone** is admirably suited for such use in opiate-dependent persons. More recently, clonidine, a central α_2-adrenergic receptor agonist, has been used for detoxification. By reducing the outflow of norepinephrine, clonidine might be expected to mitigate many of the signs of sympathetic overactivity. A presumed advantage of clonidine is that it has no narcotic action and is not addicting.

While it is easy to detoxify patients, the recidivism rate (return to abuse of the agent) is extraordinarily high. Methadone maintenance therapy, which substitutes a long-acting orally active opioid for heroin, has been effective. A single dose can be given each day, with the possibility of even less frequent than once-a-day doses for long-term patients. Methadone saturates the opiate receptors and prevents the desired sudden onset of central nervous system effects normally produced by intravenous administration. An even longer-acting methadone homolog, methadyl acetate, may offer additional technical advantages if it proves to be safe.

Use of a narcotic antagonist is rational therapy because blocking the action of self-administered opiates should eventually extinguish the habit. **Naltrexone,** a long-acting orally active pure narcotic antagonist, has been extensively studied. It can be given 3 times a week once dosage reaches levels of 100–150 mg/d. The greatest drawback is that few addicts will accept naltrexone as permanent treatment.

Psychosocial approaches include a variety of techniques. Drug-free communities are based on the assumption that drug use is a symptom of some emotional disturbance or inability to cope with life's stresses. The most common technique employs peer group pressures, emphasizing confrontation. Other techniques include variations on group or individual psychotherapy, didactic approaches, alternative life styles through work or communal living, and a variety of types of medication. Treatment may have to be continued for months or years, with costs depending on the degree to which professional staff is used. Many addicts eventually tire of their habit or "burn out," even without therapy.

BARBITURATES & OTHER SEDATIVES*

History

Bromides were first used as sedatives and anticonvulsants in 1857. They are now obsolete because they cause excessive drowsiness, must be given in doses close to toxic levels, have a slow onset of action, and have the unwanted effect of replacing chloride ion with bromide ion, leading to toxic delirium. Misuse of bromides was common when the drugs were available, but abuse was not.

Chloral hydrate was introduced in 1869 as a hypnotic. Its action is mediated by an active metabolite, trichloroethanol. Although it has the disadvantages of causing gastric irritation and an unpleasant breath odor, it is still used. Possibly because of these drawbacks, chloral hydrate was not widely abused.

Barbiturates were introduced in 1903. Short-acting members of this group have been—and still are—widely abused. Meprobamate was introduced in 1954 as a nonbarbiturate sedative presumably lacking the disadvantages of the older drugs. It turned out to have more similarities to barbiturates than differences. In fact, some of the nonbarbiturate sedative-hypnotics—examples are glutethimide and methaqualone—were worse than barbiturates in many respects, including abuse potential. The current era of **benzodiazepines** began in 1960. In the opinion of many authorities, these drugs are now the sedative-hypnotics of choice. Abuse and physical dependence have been reported but are probably less frequent than with barbiturates.

Chemistry & Pharmacology

The chemical relationships among this class of drugs are reviewed in Chapter 19.

Depending on the dose, these drugs produce sedation, hypnosis, anesthesia, coma, and death. The exact mechanism by which they produce psychic and physical dependence is unclear.

Both barbiturates and benzodiazepines can be classified pharmacokinetically into short- and long-acting compounds. Experience with barbiturates was that most nonmedical use involved short-acting drugs, eg, secobarbital or pentobarbital sodium, and not long-acting ones, eg, phenobarbital. Whether this pattern will be repeated with the benzodiazepines remains to be seen. What has become evident is that the abruptness of onset of withdrawal syndromes as well as their severity is a function of the half-life of the drug. Drugs with half-lives in the range of 8–24 hours produce a rapidly evolving, severe withdrawal syndrome, while those with longer half-lives, such as 48–96 hours, produce a withdrawal syndrome that is slower in onset and less severe but longer in duration. Drugs with half-lives longer than 96 hours usually have a built-in tapering-off action that reduces the possibility of with-

*Alcohol, the oldest and most widely abused drug of any kind, is discussed in Chapter 20.

drawal reactions. Drugs with very short half-lives (less than 4 hours) generally cannot be taken frequently enough to sustain high concentrations of the drug and are rarely associated with withdrawal reactions.

Clinical Aspects

No one knows how many persons are dependent on sedatives. Much of the presumed dependence is psychologic, possibly based on the need for these drugs as a form of "replacement therapy." Physical dependence on benzodiazepines has been documented in little more than 100 instances over the 20 years or so of their use. When one considers that these agents have been among the most widely used drugs in western countries, the problem appears to be almost negligible.

Several patterns of sedative abuse have emerged. People with severe emotional disorders may use these drugs to seek escape into oblivion. Most abusers of sedatives use them to produce an altered mental state with disinhibition in the same way other people—or they themselves—use alcohol. One sometimes sees a pattern of alternating use of sedatives and stimulants, one type of drug being used to counter the effects of the other. A growing trend has been to use sedatives in a pattern of polydrug abuse, which includes most drugs of abuse.

The effects sought by the user are similar to those produced by alcohol—an initial disinhibition followed by drowsiness. Speech may be slurred and incoordination evident. As the goal seems to be to repeat such intoxications frequently, drugs that are eliminated rapidly are preferred.

As these drugs are usually taken orally and the pills or capsules are consistent in drug content, inadvertent fatal overdoses of single agents are rare. Tolerance may develop to the sedative effect but not to the respiratory depressant effect. Thus, if these drugs are used with large amounts of alcohol, another respiratory depressant, fatalities can occur.

The withdrawal syndrome from sedatives is so much like that from alcohol that the 2 types of dependence are classified together (alcohol-barbiturate type). Symptoms and signs of chronic intoxication from short-acting drugs may improve during the first 8 hours after withdrawal but are followed by increasing anxiety, tremors, twitches, and nausea and vomiting for the next 16 hours. Convulsions may occur 16–48 hours after withdrawal. Severe cases are associated with delirium, hallucinations, and other psychosislike manifestations.

In the case of long-acting drugs, the withdrawal syndrome is attenuated. No symptoms may appear for 2–3 days, and initial symptoms may suggest a recrudescence of those originally treated. Only by the fourth or fifth day can one be sure that a withdrawal reaction is under way. Convulsions are a late manifestation when they do occur—often not until the eighth or ninth day. Following this, the syndrome subsides. This slow evolution may allow some patients to recognize what is happening and to abort the syndrome by resuming their drug. As withdrawal is generally mild, other patients may go through the syndrome, knowing that something is wrong but not being entirely sure what is happening.

Treatment

The time-honored principles of treating abstinence syndromes hold for sedative withdrawal as well. If short-acting drugs have been abused, phenobarbital is substituted as the pharmacologically equivalent agent. If long-acting drugs have been used, the same drug may be restarted. The patient is stabilized on whatever dose is required to cause signs and symptoms to abate, and the drug is then gradually withdrawn. The rate of decrement may be 15–25% of the daily dose early in treatment, with later decrements of 5–10%. Complete detoxification can usually be achieved in less than 2 weeks.

No specific treatment programs have been developed for sedative abusers. The problem is so often complicated by abuse of other drugs that it may be more expeditious to put the patient in a program designed for alcoholics or opiate-dependent persons. Patients with psychiatric disorders that can be defined, especially those with depression, may be treated with specific drug treatment for the underlying disorder.

STIMULANTS

History

Caffeine is probably the most widely used social drug worldwide. Most people do not consider it to be a drug, although many, especially as they age, experience disturbing effects on sleep and heart rhythm from too much coffee. A withdrawal syndrome characterized by lethargy, irritability, and headache has been recognized in users of more than 600 mg/d (roughly 6 cups of coffee).

Cocaine has been used for at least 1200 years in the custom of chewing coca leaves by natives of the South American Andes. Coca was first imported to Europe from the western hemisphere in 1580. Cocaine was isolated as the active material in 1860. Its anesthetic properties, especially its topical anesthetic action, were discovered in the 1870s and 1880s. Sigmund Freud was intrigued by the drug and thought it might even be a panacea, but his enthusiasm was dampened by its disastrous effects on a friend who became addicted. A colleague of Freud's, Karl Koller, is credited with first using the drug as a topical anesthetic for eye surgery, a use that still prevails.

Amphetamine was synthesized in the late 1920s and was introduced into medical practice in 1936. Dextroamphetamine is the major member of the class, although many other amphetamines and amphetamine surrogates, such as methamphetamine (Methedrine, "speed"), phenmetrazine (Preludin), and methylphenidate (Ritalin), were subsequently introduced.

Chemistry & Pharmacology

The chemical relationships of the various stimu-

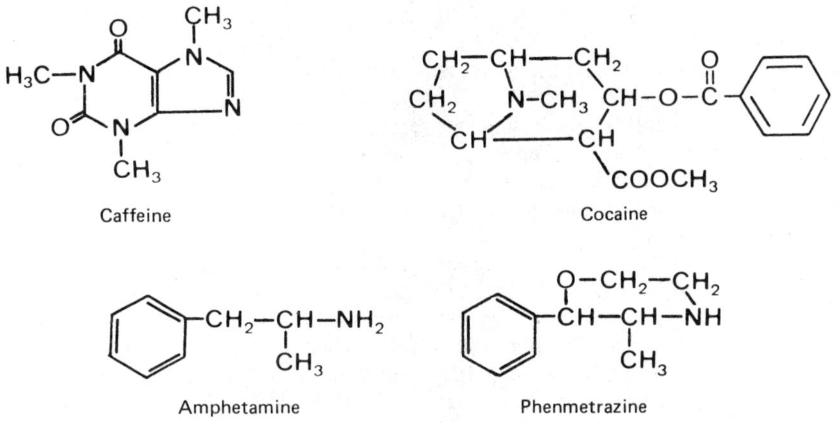

Figure 29–1. Chemical structures of some popular stimulants.

lants are shown in Fig 29–1. Despite their remarkably similar actions, caffeine, cocaine, and amphetamine have very different structures.

Caffeine is thought to increase cAMP concentration by blocking the catabolic enzyme phosphodiesterase, thus increasing the effects of catecholamine neurotransmitters. Another possible mode of action is interaction with receptors for adenosine, a purinergic neurotransmitter structurally similar to caffeine. Cocaine appears to facilitate dopamine neurotransmission by increasing its release and reducing reuptake, and a similar mode of action has been proposed for amphetamines. In addition, amphetamines are weak inhibitors of monoamine oxidase, an action that would increase dopaminergic activity, as well as perhaps being direct dopamine agonists owing to their structural similarity.

Although psychic dependence is strong (cocaine is one of the most strongly reinforcing drugs in self-administration paradigms in animals), it was thought for some time that physical dependence occurred only rarely. However, recent patterns of abuse of these drugs, especially of amphetaminelike agents, have revealed a typical pattern of withdrawal manifested by signs and symptoms opposite to those produced by the drug. Users become sleepy, have a ravenous appetite, are exhausted, and may suffer mental depression. This syndrome may last for several days after the drug is withdrawn. Tolerance develops quickly, so that abusers may take monumental doses compared with those used medically, eg, as anorexiants.

Clinical Aspects

Amphetamine abuse began in the 1940s. The substance was present in substantial amounts in inhalers promoted as nasal decongestants. During World War II, amphetamines were frequently used by military personnel. A huge supply of amphetamines became available to young people in Japan in the postwar period, resulting in an epidemic of abuse that was ultimately curbed by draconian punishments. Meanwhile, in the USA the drug continued to be used in relatively small oral doses, often alternating with barbiturates. In the 1960s, the pattern changed. Methamphetamine became the preferred drug (largely because it was more easily synthesized illicitly), and the preferred route of administration became intravenous injection.

One pattern of amphetamine abuse is called a "run." Repeated intravenous injections are self-administered (as with opiates) to obtain a "rush"—an orgasmlike reaction—followed by a feeling of mental alertness and marked euphoria. Total daily doses as high as 4000 mg have been reported. After several days of such spree use, subjects become paranoid, with a psychosislike state resembling paranoid schizophrenia. Typically, they develop delusions that bugs are crawling under their skin, which leads to characteristic discrete excoriations. Finally, the spree is terminated by exhaustion from lack of sleep and lack of food, followed by the withdrawal syndrome mentioned above.

As is so often the case with social drugs, a pattern of stimulant use has developed in which the drug is thought to enhance sexual pleasure. Although reports are anecdotal and largely unsubstantiated, a better case is made for stimulants in this application than for other agents. Sexual intercourse may be markedly prolonged and orgasm enhanced. Phenmetrazine prescribed as an anorexiant is the current favorite for this use. With chronic use, sexual urges seem to disappear completely.

It is a curious paradox that efforts to regulate the use of drugs by law often lead to the introduction of more dangerous drugs. With the virtual outlawing of amphetamines from legitimate medical practice (based on adverse effects experienced by using doses 2 or 3 orders of magnitude larger than therapeutic doses), cocaine became the substitute. Cocaine may be construed as a highly potent amphetamine ("super-speed") with all of the effects of the latter drug magnified. It is far more likely to lead to dependence than amphetamines, and overdoses leading to death are possible. Cocaine has become the preferred drug of abuse in well-to-do, sophisticated circles. Its great expense limits its use.

Two types of administration of cocaine are current. One may ''snuff'' the drug by sniffing a ''line'' (a measured amount of drug in a folded piece of paper applied to the nose), or one may smoke ''free base.'' Cocaine is supplied as a hydrochloride salt, and free base is made by alkalinizing the salt and extracting with nonpolar solvents. When free base is smoked, entry through the lungs is almost as fast as by intravenous injection, so that effects are even more accentuated. Intravenous injection is rarely used, as the possibility of overdose is considerable. The purity and potency of cocaine available to users varies widely.

The plasma half-life of cocaine is short, so that effects following a single dose persist only for an hour or two. Consequently, the euphoric experience may be repeated many times during the course of a day or night. In this case, as in others, short-acting drugs seem to have greater potential for abuse.

Cocaine may be used sporadically, as at a party, or regularly by those with a self-imposed high level of output, such as rock musicians. It may also be part of the repertoire of the polydrug abuser. A ''speedball'' is a combination of cocaine and heroin taken intravenously, presumably doubling the ''rush'' but extinguishing other effects. Patients in methadone maintenance programs who can no longer get much kick from heroin may turn to cocaine, whose euphoriant effects are not altered by methadone.

Besides the paranoid psychosis associated with chronic use of amphetamines, intravenous injection using contaminated syringes leads to the same infectious complications as with heroin. A specific lesion associated with chronic amphetamine use is necrotizing arteritis, which may involve many small and medium-sized arteries and lead to fatal brain hemorrhage or renal failure. Overdoses of amphetamines are rarely fatal; they can be managed by sedating the patient with haloperidol. Overdoses of cocaine are usually rapidly fatal, victims dying within minutes from respiratory depression and seizures. Those who survive for 3 hours usually recover fully. Intravenous administration of diazepam and propranolol may be the best treatment.

Long-Term Treatment

Subjects with residual emotional disorders, either schizophreniform psychosis or mental depression, may require treatment with antipsychotic or antidepressant drugs. Withdrawal from cocaine could be facilitated by switching to amphetamines followed by gradual withdrawal. No specific treatment programs have been devised for stimulant users. Those who administer these drugs intravenously have more in common with heroin users than any other group and may be suitable for some of the rehabilitative programs devised for opiate-dependent persons.

HALLUCINOGENS

History

Almost every society, however primitive, has found some bark, skin, leaf, vine, berry, or weed that contains ''hallucinogenic'' materials. Although the fortuitous discovery of the properties of lysergic acid diethylamide (LSD) occurred in a chemical laboratory 4 decades ago, this was a case in which scientific art was merely imitating nature. Similar compounds have been found in morning glory seeds, and drugs such as mescaline and psilocybin had long been used by North and Central American Indians in the form of cactus buttons or magical mushrooms. Deliriants, such as the alkaloids in *Atropa belladonna* and *Datura stramonium,* were also known in ancient cultures.

Terminology

Although the term ''hallucinogen'' will be used here, it is not entirely accurate, since hallucinations may be uncommon effects or only part of the overall effects of these drugs. The term ''psychotomimetic'' is often used to connote the possible action of these drugs in mimicking naturally occurring psychoses. However, the state induced by these agents does not closely resemble that of schizophrenia. The term ''psychedelic'' was coined to denote a supposed ''mind-revealing'' aspect of such drug use, but the revelation and insights achieved are not much different than have been claimed with many other disinhibiting drugs, most commonly alcohol.

The drugs we here call hallucinogens are taken for many reasons. The one most widely given by users is that the drugs provide new ways of looking at the world and new insights into personal problems. The former claim implies varying degrees of perceptual distortion, while the latter implies changes in mood and increased introspection. LSD has become the prototypical hallucinogenic drug because of the extent of its use; because it represents a family of drugs that are similar; and because it has been most extensively studied.

Chemistry & Pharmacology

The LSD group of drugs includes **LSD** and related compounds, **mescaline** and related compounds, and **psilocybin** and related compounds. Although these substances differ chemically, they share some chemical features and even more pharmacologic ones (Fig 29–2). LSD is a semisynthetic chemical not known to occur in nature. The monoethyl—rather than the diethyl—amide is found in hallucinogenic morning glory seeds. Mescaline, a phenethylamine derivative, and psilocybin, an indolethylamine derivative, are found in nature. These drugs also have close chemical resemblances to 3 major neurotransmitters: norepinephrine, dopamine, and serotonin.

The mode of action of hallucinogens of the LSD type is uncertain despite much experimental study. Measured electrographically, their effects are to produce a state of hyperarousal of the central nervous system. Neurochemically, LSD seems to work mainly

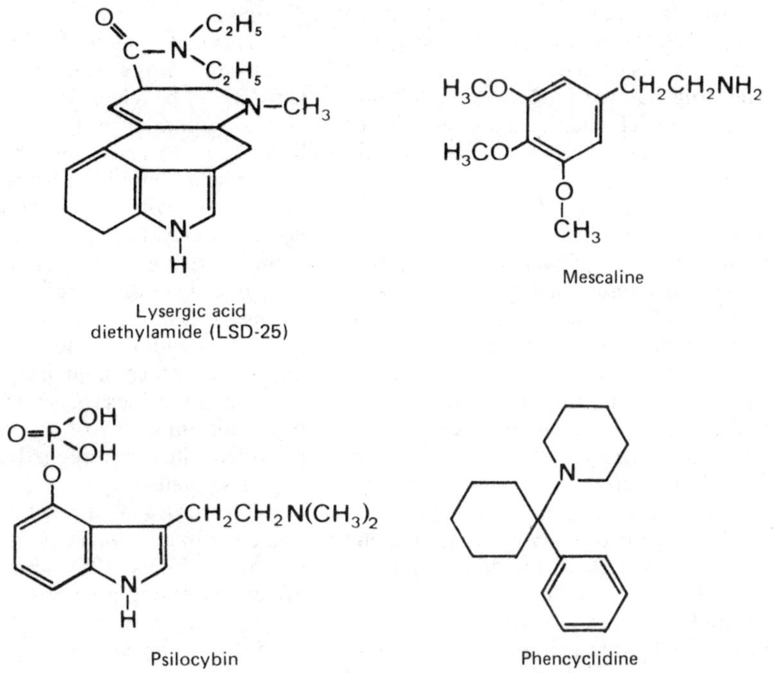

Figure 29–2. Chemical structures of lysergic acid diethylamide (LSD), mescaline, psilocybin, and phencyclidine.

through serotoninergic systems, decreasing activity of this neurotransmitter. It was once thought the drug did this by acting as a false transmitter postsynaptically, replacing the true transmitter. Current opinion is that LSD may act on a presynaptic serotonin receptor, inhibiting the release of serotonin. Decreased turnover of serotonin is manifested by increased brain concentration of serotonin and decreased concentration of its major metabolite, 5-hydroxyindoleacetic acid.

Several amphetamine-mescaline homologs are also hallucinogenic and can be included in the LSD group. They are generally more potent and more dangerous than mescaline, but they resemble the latter drug closely in chemical structure. Their mode of action is presumed to be similar to that of LSD.

The deliriant hallucinogens, exemplified by scopolamine (Chapter 6) and some synthetic centrally acting anticholinergic agents, are different chemically as well as pharmacologically from the LSD group. Their effects seem to be entirely explainable by blockade of central muscarinic receptors. Similar mental effects may be seen during therapeutic or deliberate overdoses of commonly used medications with anticholinergic action, such as antiparkinsonism drugs, tricyclic antidepressants, and antispasmodics. Occasional instances of abuse of these therapeutic agents have occurred.

Phencyclidine (PCP, "angel dust," many other names) is a synthetic phenylcyclohexylamine derivative. There is some question about how it should be classified, since it differs in many ways from other hallucinogens, but its primary use is to obtain hallucinogenic effects. The drug was originally introduced as a "dissociative anesthetic" in 1957. Such anesthetics were presumed to work by making patients insensitive to pain by "separating their bodily functions from their minds" without causing loss of consciousness. Hallucinogenic effects were noted in patients emerging from anesthesia. The drug was withdrawn from use in humans but retained in veterinary practice under the name Sernylan. (The veterinary use has given the drug one of its street names—"hog.") **Ketamine,** a homolog, replaced phencyclidine as an anesthetic for use in humans (see Chapter 22). It too produces some emergent hallucinogenic effects. The first street use of PCP was in 1967, when it quickly gained a reputation as a bad drug. Over the next several years, it was mislabeled, being sold as LSD, THC, and other hallucinogens. Since the 1970s, PCP has become widely accepted and is now the most used hallucinogenic agent. Phencyclidine may be smoked (by mixing the powder with tobacco), "snorted," taken orally, or injected intravenously. Fortunately, a recent trend toward less frequent use of the drug has been noted.

Some of the early investigators of PCP maintained that it provided a much better model of schizophrenia than LSD, mainly through its action in producing a form of sensory isolation. More recent work, however, indicates that the mode of action of PCP is mainly through dopaminergic mechanisms. Dopaminergic transmission is enhanced as a result of reduced uptake of dopamine. Thus, the schizophreniform psychosis may be mediated in a way postulated for true schizophrenia. The drug is unique among hallucinogens in that animals will self-administer it.

Various harmala alkaloids, especially **harmaline,** have been classified as hallucinogens, but very little recent work has been done with these drugs in humans. The drug has the property of inhibiting monoamine oxidase, which could increase activity of dopamine as well as several other biogenic amine neurotransmitters.

Clinical Effects

LSD produces a series of somatic, perceptual, and psychic effects that overlap each other. Dizziness, weakness, tremors, nausea, and paresthesias are prominent somatic symptoms. Blurring of vision, distortions of perspective, organized visual illusions or "hallucinations," less discriminant hearing, and a change in sense of time are common perceptual abnormalities. Impaired memory, difficulty in thinking, poor judgment, and altered mood are prominent psychic effects. Physiologically, LSD produces signs of overactivity of the sympathetic nervous system and central stimulation, manifested by dilated pupils, increased heart rate, mild elevation of blood pressure, tremor, and alertness. Virtually identical effects are produced by mescaline and psilocybin when they are given in equivalent doses. The onset of effects is fairly rapid, but the duration varies with the dose and is usually measured in hours. Phenomena may vary considerably from one user to another owing to such factors as the personality and expectations of the user and the circumstances under which the drug is taken, but the above effects occur in almost everyone. Waxing and waning of effects is typical.

Usual doses of LSD in humans are approximately 1–2 μg/kg, making it one of the most potent pharmacologic agents known. The drug is equally effective parenterally or orally and consequently is almost always taken by mouth. Psilocybin is usually taken in doses of 250 μg/kg and mescaline in doses of 5–6 mg/kg. Despite these differences in potency, the effects are virtually indistinguishable.

Scopolamine and the "JB" series of anticholinergic drugs produce a delirium with fluctuating levels of awareness, disorientation, marked difficulty in thinking, marked loss of memory, and bizarre delusions. If doses are large, these impairments may last for more than a day, with some subjects claiming that several days may elapse before they once again feel confident about their memory. Most subjects, at least under experimental conditions, find these drugs to be unpleasant and have little desire to repeat the experience. Some become frightened during the period of drug effect. Others deliberately seek out and use such drugs repeatedly.

PCP produces detachment, disorientation, distortions of body image, and loss of proprioception. Somatic symptoms and signs include numbness, nystagmus, sweating, rapid heart rate, and hypertension. Effects are dose-dependent. Overdosage has been fatal, as contrasted with the absence of known fatalities directly caused by drugs of the LSD group.

Toxicity

Adverse psychologic consequences of hallucinogenic drugs are common. Panic reactions ("bad trips") may be related to excessive doses; they seem to be less common as the doses of street drugs have become more accurate. They are best managed by simple sedation with a barbiturate or benzodiazepine rather than with a phenothiazine. Simple "talking down" may suffice but is labor-intensive. Acute psychotic or depressive reactions have been precipitated by use of these drugs but usually only in persons with strong predispositions. Acute psychotic reactions are associated with PCP much more commonly than with any of the other hallucinogens. Errors of judgment may lead to reckless acts that threaten life; any person under the influence of one of these drugs should be provided with a nondrugged companion until the effect has dissipated.

Overdoses of the antimuscarinic agents can be treated with infusion of physostigmine. In mild cases, one may simply allow the patient to sleep off the effects by giving a large dose of a hypnotic drug.

Overdoses of PCP are dangerous but can be managed if recognized promptly. PCP is secreted into the stomach, so that removal may be hastened by continual nasogastric suction. Excretion of this basic drug may be hastened by acidification of the urine to pH 5.5. Diazepam can be given to protect against seizures or to curb excitation; antipsychotics aggravate matters at this point. If a prolonged schizophrenialike illness follows acute intoxication, one may consider antipsychotics on a sustained basis.

Treatment

No systematic program of treatment has been devised for abuse of this class of drugs. Users of hallucinogens are likely to stick to this class of drugs rather than proceed to a pattern of polydrug abuse. Separation of the user from the drug culture is probably the best treatment, but it must be voluntarily accepted.

Therapeutic Uses

No therapeutic indication has yet been accepted for any hallucinogen. LSD has been promoted as a cure for alcoholism, but objective evidence of benefit is totally lacking. Facilitation of psychotherapy is another proposed use, again with no substantiation or comparison with other drugs. Although it has been tried in both schizophrenics and depressed individuals, LSD is more likely to precipitate or aggravate these disorders than to alleviate them. Use of the drug in chronic cancer patients was said to diminish the need for opiates, but this work has not been confirmed.

MARIHUANA

History

Use of cannabis has been recorded for thousands of years, especially in eastern countries such as China and India. It was certainly known to the Greeks at the height of their civilization as well as to Arabic nations somewhat later. It is estimated that about 200–300 million people use cannabis in some form. Thus, it is not only one of the oldest but also one of the most widely used of mind-altering drugs. Since the 1960s, the rise in marihuana use in the USA has been remarkable. Although the drug was known in this country prior to that time, there were only a small number of users, mainly from minority groups. It is estimated now that 30–40 million persons in the USA have used the drug and that a substantial number are regular users. Recent reports suggest that the number of youngsters initiated into use of this drug has declined after a steep rise and an increasingly lower age of first use.

Several species of cannabis (hemp) have been named, but botanists are not agreed that more than one species of plant exists; many morphologic variants occur. Some plants are excellent for fiber, being a source of hemp, and rather poor producers of drug; and the converse also is true. These properties are due to genetic differences. The flowers and small leaves of *Cannabis sativa* supply most of the drug. **Marihuana** is a mixture of ground-up plant materials that resembles grass clippings—thus the street name "grass." Extraction of the resin from the plant provides a more potent product: **hashish.**

Chemistry & Pharmacokinetics of Cannabinoids

Three major cannabinoids have been found in cannabis; cannabidiol (CBD), Δ^9-tetrahydrocannabinol (THC), and cannabinol (CBN). The biosynthetic pathway begins with CBD, proceeds to THC, and ends with CBN (Fig 29–3). Thus, one can deduce from the proportions of these cannabinoids in plant material the age of the plant. Many other variants of these structures have been found in cannabis, but with the exception of THC and its homologs no other cannabinoids have definite psychoactivity. The content of THC varies considerably among plants, so that special genetic lines may produce as much as 4–6% THC content in very selected ("manicured") materials. Most plants have a THC content ranging from trace amounts to 1–2%.

The preferred route of administration in western countries is by smoking. The high lipid solubility of THC causes it to be readily trapped on the surfactant lining the lungs. Pharmacokinetic studies indicate that smoking is almost equivalent to intravenous administration except that lower peak plasma concentrations of THC are attained. In some eastern countries, cannabis is taken orally in the form of various confections. The rate of absorption from this route is slow and highly variable, although the duration of action is longer.

THC is extensively metabolized, and new metabolites are still being discovered. One metabolite, 11-hydroxy-THC, is actually more active than the parent compound. However, it is not nearly as abundant, and one must assume that the major part of the activity of cannabis derives from THC itself. The high lipid solubility of the drug leads to extensive sequestration in the lipid compartments of the body, and metabolites may be excreted for as long as a week after a single dose. Whether accumulation of unchanged THC can occur is questionable.

Pharmacodynamics of Cannabinoids

The mechanism of action of THC is not well defined. It has a variety of pharmacologic effects that suggest actions like those of amphetamines, LSD, alcohol, sedatives, atropine, or morphine. Thus, the drug does not fit traditional pharmacologic classifications and must be considered as a separate class.

Small doses of THC may be associated with a

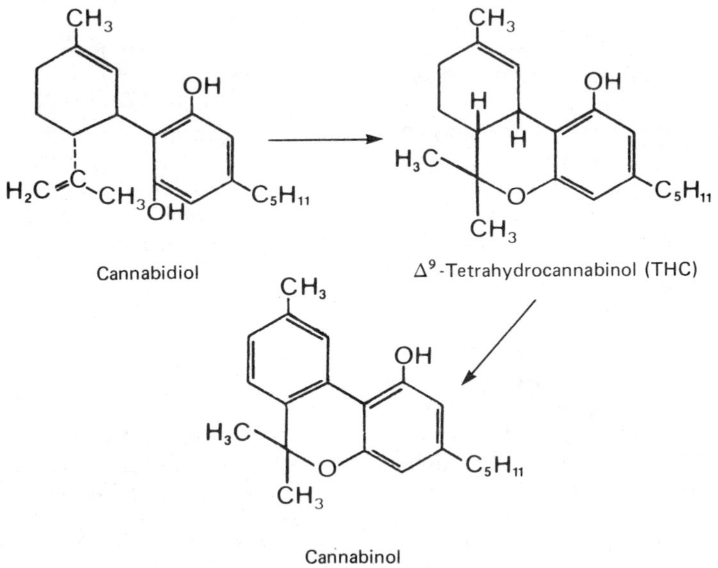

Figure 29–3. Structures of the 3 main cannabinoids in marihuana. Only THC has psychoactivity. C_5H_{11} is *n*-pentyl.

rather definite placebo effect, but large doses are unequivocal in producing the expected range of effects. The expert smoker of marihuana is usually aware of a drug effect after 2 or 3 inhalations. As smoking continues, the effects increase, reaching a maximum about 20 minutes after the smoke has been finished. Most effects of the drug usually have vanished after 3 hours, by which time plasma concentrations are low. Peak effects after oral administration may be delayed until 3–4 hours after drug ingestion but may last for 6–8 hours.

The early stage is one of being "high" and is characterized by euphoria, uncontrollable laughter, alteration of time sense, depersonalization, and sharpened vision. Later, the user becomes relaxed and experiences introspective and dreamlike states if not actual sleep. Thinking or concentrating become difficult, although by force of will the subject can attend.

Two characteristic signs of cannabis intoxication are increased pulse rate and reddening of the conjunctiva. The latter correlates well with the presence of detectable plasma concentrations. Pupil size is not changed. The blood pressure may fall, especially in the upright position. An antiemetic effect may be present. Muscle weakness, tremors, unsteadiness, and increased deep tendon reflexes may also be noted.

Virtually any psychologic test shows impairment if the doses are large enough and the test difficult enough. No distinctive biochemical changes have been found in humans.

Tolerance has been demonstrated in virtually every animal species that has been tested. It is apparent in humans only among heavy long-term users of the drug. Different degrees of tolerance develop for different effects of the drug, with tolerance for the tachycardiac effect developing fairly rapidly. A mild withdrawal syndrome has been noted following very high doses.

Health Hazards

Marihuana has raised concern about possible adverse effects on the health of users, probably because so many are very young. The hazards of use are still controversial and ambiguous, and there are many problems with the studies themselves. First, it is difficult to prove or disprove an adverse reaction for humans in an animal model. Second, users thus far have been mostly young people in excellent general health. Third, cannabis is often used in combination with alcohol or tobacco. And fourth, many investigators have biases for or against the drug.

Three epidemiologic studies in developing countries have failed to find definite evidence of impairment among heavy users of cannabis, but field studies may lack sensitivity. Experimental studies in which subjects have smoked heavily for varying periods have shown a lowered serum testosterone level in men and airway narrowing. Effects on immune mechanisms, chromosomes, and cell metabolism are often contradictory. Effects on the fetus are still uncertain.

Heavy smokers of marihuana may be subject to some of the same problems of chronic bronchitis, airway obstruction, and squamous cell metaplasia as smokers of tobacco cigarettes. Angina pectoris may be aggravated by the speeding of the heart rate, orthostatic hypotension, and increased carboxyhemoglobin. Driving ability is likely to be impaired but is not easily demonstrated with usual testing. "Amotivational syndrome," in which promising young people with obvious social advantages lose interest in school and career and enter the drug culture, is a real phenomenon, but one cannot be sure whether drug use is the cause of the problem or simply a matter of personal choice by a disturbed young man or woman. Acute panic reactions, toxic delirium, paranoid states, and frank psychoses are rare. Brain damage has not been confirmed in humans, although some suggestion of ultrastructural damage has been found in animals.

Therapeutic Uses

Cannabis used to be listed in drug formularies but has not been used medically for some time. Recently, interest in cannabis for therapeutic purposes has revived. A finding of lowered intraocular pressure following oral THC administration has been repeatedly confirmed; it remains to be seen whether preparations of cannabis have any advantages over other forms of treatment for glaucoma. Amelioration of nausea and vomiting associated with cancer chemotherapy appears to be a most promising use, but it is uncertain whether the drug would have any advantage over existing antiemetics. Many homologs of THC have been developed in the search for one that may lack the most offensive side-effect, that of mind alteration, while retaining the desired effects. Not only are these homologs possibly useful for the indications mentioned; they may also be applicable as analgesics, as agents for the relief of muscle spasm, and as anticonvulsants.

Treatment

Few users seek treatment, although many who have stopped using the drug have been pleasantly surprised at the increased clarity of their thinking. Although marihuana has been alleged to be a substitute for alcohol, it is more commonly used along with alcohol; alcoholism complicating marihuana use is rare. Marihuana may be used in a pattern of multiple drug use, in which case treatment may be required for the more dangerous drugs being taken.

INHALANTS

History

The modern discovery of the intoxicant effects of inhalants began with Sir Humphry Davy in 1799, who administered nitrous oxide to himself and others. As other anesthetic gases were introduced, such as chloroform and ether, they were also used socially. Such use persists, with occasional instances of halothane inhalation being added to the anesthetic

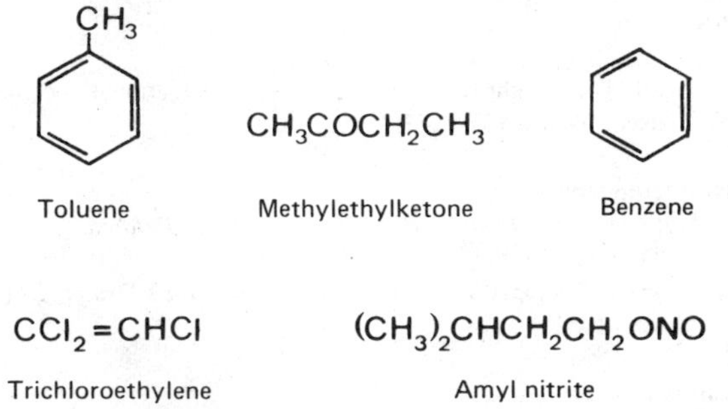

Figure 29–4. Structures of some commonly used inhalants.

gases previously mentioned. In addition to these agents, 3 other patterns of inhalant use are now prevalent: (1) industrial solvents, including a variety of hydrocarbons, such as toluene; (2) aerosol propellants, such as various fluorocarbons; and (3) organic nitrites, such as amyl or butyl nitrite.

Chemistry & Pharmacology

The structures of some inhalants are shown in Fig 29–4. The mode of action of the inhalant anesthetics has been discussed in Chapter 22.

Clinical Aspects

Nitrous oxide is not widely available. When self-administered, it produces difficulty in concentrating, dreaminess, euphoria, numbness and tingling, unsteadiness, and visual and auditory disturbances. It is usually taken as 35% N_2O mixed with oxygen; administration of 100% nitrous oxide may cause asphyxia and death.

Ether and **chloroform** are readily available through chemical supply houses. Cloths soaked with the material are used for inhalation of the fumes. After an initial period of exhilaration, the person often loses consciousness. Ether is highly flammable. Halothane is usually available only to medical or health care personnel.

A variety of **industrial solvents** used as inhalants are on the market and virtually impossible to control. They include gasoline, paint thinner, glue, rubber cement, acrylic paint sprays, shoe polish, and degreasers. The toxic ingredients may be toluene, heptane, hexane, benzene, trichloroethylene, methylethylketone, and others. Because of their ready availability, this group of inhalants is widely used. Aerosol propellants have also been widely available, though manufacturers of products using propellants have recently changed from fluorocarbons to less hazardous materials.

Motives for use of inhalants include peer influence, low cost, ready availability, convenient packaging, quick intoxication of short duration, and mood enhancement. Boys in their early teen years from lower socioeconomic classes are the principal users. They generally also have worse than average problems at school and at home. Psychologic dependence perpetuates the use of inhalants.

The clinical effects of industrial solvent inhalation are short, lasting only 5–15 minutes. Rags or "toques" are soaked in the solvent and the fumes inhaled. Aerosol propellants are usually inhaled from a plastic bag. Euphoria and a relaxed "drunk" feeling are followed by disorientation, slow passage of time, and possibly hallucinations.

Organic nitrites have developed a reputation as a sexual enhancer, a sure way to popularity. Amyl nitrite is used medically in the form of fragile glass ampules covered with cloth. When these are broken, they make a popping sound—hence the nickname "poppers." Street forms of bottled isobutyl nitrite (Locker Room, Rush) are readily available in some areas. Inhalation causes dizziness, giddiness, rapid heart rate, lowered blood pressure, "speeding," and flushing of the skin. The effects last only a few minutes and can readily be repeated.

Toxicity

Chloroform has been implicated in liver and kidney damage. Industrial solvents have produced a variety of adverse effects: liver and kidney damage, peripheral nerve damage and possibly brain damage in animals, bone marrow suppression, and pulmonary disease. Fluorocarbon inhalation has resulted in sudden deaths, either due to ventricular arrhythmias or asphyxiation. Nitrites have been rather safe but might pose hazards for persons with preexisting cardiovascular problems.

• • •

References

General

Pradhan SN, Dutra SN: *Drug Abuse: Clinical and Basic Aspects*. Mosby, 1977.

Ray OA: *Drugs, Society and Human Behavior*. Mosby, 1978.

Opiates

Collier HOJ: Cellular site of opiate dependence. *Nature* 1980;**283:**625.

Goldstein A: Heroin addiction: Sequential treatment employing pharmacologic supports. *Arch Gen Psychiatry* 1976;**33:**353.

Sedatives

Hollister LE (editor): Valium: A discussion of current issues. *Psychosomatics* 1977;**18:**1.

Smith DE, Wesson DR: A new method for treatment of barbiturate dependence. *JAMA* 1970;**213:**294.

Stimulants

Smith DE et al (editors): *Amphetamine Use, Misuse and Abuse*. G.K. Hall, 1979.

Wetli CV, Wright RK: Death caused by recreational cocaine usee. *JAMA* 1979;**241:**2519.

Hallucinogens

Hollister LE: *Chemical Psychoses: LSD and Related Drugs*. Thomas, 1968.

Lewin L: *Phantastics, Narcotic and Stimulating Drugs*. Dutton, 1931.

Cannabis

Milne GM et al (editors): Therapeutic progress in cannabinoid research. *J Clin Pharmacol* 1981;**21(Suppl):**1S.

Nahas GG, Paton WDM (editors): *Marihuana: Biological Effects*. Pergamon, 1979.

Petersen RC: *Marijuana Research Findings: 1980*. NIDA Research Monograph 31, US Government Printing Office, June 1980.

Inhalants

Sharp CW, Carroll LT: *Voluntary Inhalation of Industrial Solvents*. DHEW Publication No. (ADM) 79–779, US Government Printing Office, 1979.

Agents Used in Anemias: Iron, Vitamin B_{12}, & Folic Acid | 30

Curt A. Ries, MD, & Daniel V. Santi, MD, PhD

Iron, vitamin B_{12}, and folic acid are chemically unrelated essential nutrients that are required for normal erythropoiesis. Deficiency of any of these substances results in severe anemia. Iron is required for hemoglobin production; in the absence of adequate iron, small red cells with insufficient hemoglobin are formed, giving rise to microcytic hypochromic anemia. Vitamin B_{12} and folic acid are required for normal DNA synthesis, and deficiency of either of these vitamins results in impaired production and abnormal maturation of erythroid precursor cells, giving rise to the characteristic blood and bone marrow picture known as megaloblastic anemia.

IRON

Basic Pharmacology

Iron forms the nucleus of the iron-porphyrin ring heme, which when combined with appropriate globin chains forms the protein hemoglobin. The structure of hemoglobin allows for reversible binding of oxygen, providing the critical mechanism for oxygen transport from the lungs to other tissues that is essential for humans and other vertebrates. Although iron is also present in small amounts in other important proteins (myoglobin, cytochromes, etc), the vast majority is normally present in hemoglobin; therefore, anemia is the most prominent clinical feature of iron deficiency.

Pharmacokinetics

Iron is normally available in the diet from a wide variety of foods; dietary iron is usually in the form of heme or iron complexed to various organic compounds. Therapeutic iron, on the other hand, is usually given in the form of iron salts or iron complexed to inorganic substances. These different forms of iron differ widely in the amount of iron available for absorption, as discussed below.

Over 90% of the non-storage iron in humans is in hemoglobin. About 6% is in myoglobin, a similar heme-containing protein found in muscle; and the remainder is distributed in trace amounts in cytochromes and other iron-containing enzymes in the tissues and as transport iron in transferrin. In addition to tissue iron, the element is also normally present as storage iron (as ferritin and hemosiderin) in non-iron-deficient individuals. An average healthy 70-kg man has approximately 3500 mg of iron in his body: about 2300 mg in hemoglobin, 200 mg in other tissue iron, and 1000 mg in storage iron. A healthy nonanemic 60-kg woman has proportionately less hemoglobin and other tissue iron, and during her reproductive years she has substantially less storage iron because of iron losses from menstruation and pregnancies.

Iron is normally absorbed in the duodenum and proximal jejunum, although more distal small bowel sites can absorb iron if necessary. The average American diet contains 10–15 mg of elemental iron daily. A normal non-iron-deficient individual absorbs 5–10% of this iron, or about 0.5–1 mg daily. Iron absorption is increased in response to low iron stores or increased iron requirements. Total iron absorption increases to 1–2 mg/d in normal menstruating women and may be as high as 3–4 mg/d in pregnant women. Infants and adolescents also have increased iron requirements during rapid growth periods.

Iron is available in a wide variety of foods but is especially abundant in meat protein. The iron in meat protein is also more available for absorption and can be more efficiently absorbed, since heme iron in meat hemoglobin and myoglobin can be absorbed intact as hemin (the ferric form of heme) without first having to be broken down into free iron. Iron in other foods is often tightly bound to phytates or other complexing agents and may be much less available for absorption. Nonheme iron in foods and iron in inorganic iron salts and complexes must be converted to ferrous ion before it can be absorbed by the intestinal mucosal cells. Such absorption is decreased by the presence of chelators or complexing agents in the intestinal lumen and is increased in the presence of hydrochloric acid and vitamin C. Gastric resection decreases iron absorption by decreasing or eliminating hydrochloric acid production and perhaps even more importantly by removing the site where food is held and digested to make dietary iron more available for absorption by the iron-absorbing areas in the duodenum and proximal jejunum.

Iron is transported across the intestinal mucosal cell by active transport. Absorbed ferrous ion is converted to ferric ion within the mucosal cell, and—together with ferric iron split from hemin—the newly absorbed iron can be made available for immediate transport from the mucosal cell to the plasma via transferrin or can be converted to ferritin and stored in the mucosal cell. In general, when total body iron stores are high and iron requirements by the body are low, newly absorbed iron is diverted into ferritin in the intestinal mucosal cells rather than being transported to other sites. When iron stores are low or iron requirements are high, however, newly absorbed iron is immediately transported from the mucosal cells to the bone marrow for the production of hemoglobin.

Iron is transported in the plasma bound to transferrin, a β-globulin that specifically binds ferric iron. Iron can thus be transported from intestinal mucosal cells or from storage sites in liver or spleen to the developing erythroid cells in bone marrow. Recently, specific receptors for the transferrin-ferric ion complex have been demonstrated on the membranes of maturing erythroid cells (normoblasts) from human bone marrow.

Iron can be stored in 2 forms: ferritin and hemosiderin. Ferritin, the most readily available form of storage iron, is a water-soluble complex consisting of a core crystal of ferric hydroxide covered by a protein shell of apoferritin. Hemosiderin is a particulate substance consisting of aggregates of ferric core crystals partially or completely stripped of apoferritin. Both ferritin and hemosiderin are stored in macrophages in the liver, spleen, and bone marrow; ferritin is also present in intestinal mucosal cells and in plasma. Since the ferritin present in plasma is in equilibrium with storage ferritin in reticuloendothelial tissues, the plasma (or serum) ferritin level can be used to estimate total body iron stores.

There is no mechanism for excretion of iron. Small amounts of iron are lost by exfoliation of intestinal mucosal cells into the stool, and trace amounts are excreted in bile, urine, and sweat. These losses, however, can account for no more than 1 mg of iron per day. Because the body's ability to increase excretion of iron is so limited, regulation of iron balance must be achieved by changing intestinal absorption of iron, depending on the body's needs.

Iron absorption is regulated by the amount of storage iron present, especially the amount of ferritin present in the intestinal mucosal cells, and by the rate of erythropoiesis. Recent studies have shown that increased erythropoiesis is associated with an increase in the number of transferrin receptor sites on developing erythroid cells and that the availability of these receptor sites in some way directly increases the rate of iron absorption. Transferrin and ferritin are both present in intestinal mucosal cells and both appear to regulate iron absorption. Transferrin is increased and ferritin decreased in iron deficiency, promoting increased iron absorption, while transferrin is decreased and ferritin increased in iron overload states, inhibiting further iron absorption.

Clinical Pharmacology of Iron

The only clinical indication for the use of iron preparations is the treatment or prevention of iron deficiency anemia. Iron deficiency is commonly seen in infants, especially premature infants, in children during rapid growth periods, and in pregnant and lactating women. These situations are all associated with increased iron requirements, and individuals in these settings are often routinely supplemented with oral iron to meet the increased need. Iron deficiency also occurs frequently in postgastrectomy states and in patients with severe small bowel disease that results in generalized malabsorption. Iron deficiency in these situations is due to inadequate iron absorption.

The most common cause of iron deficiency in adults, however, is blood loss. Menstruating women lose about 30 mg of iron with each menstrual period; women with heavy or abnormal menstrual bleeding may lose much more. The most common site of unrecognized or occult blood loss is in the gastrointestinal tract. Patients with unexplained iron deficiency anemia must therefore always be evaluated for occult gastrointestinal bleeding, especially to exclude early gastrointestinal cancer, which may present with occult bleeding at a time when the cancer is still surgically curable. Simple nutritional iron deficiency due to inadequate diet is rare in adults and should never be accepted as an explanation of iron deficiency in a patient until a careful search has ruled out occult blood loss and other causes of iron deficiency.

Individuals suspected of being iron-deficient should generally have the diagnosis confirmed before being treated with iron preparations. As iron deficiency develops, storage iron decreases and then disappears; next, serum ferritin decreases; and then serum iron decreases and iron-binding capacity (transferrin) increases, resulting in a decrease in iron-binding (transferrin) saturation. Thereafter, anemia begins to develop. Red cell indices (mean corpuscular volume [MCV]: normal = 80–100 fL; mean corpuscular hemoglobin concentration [MCHC]: normal = 32–36 g/dL) are usually low normal when iron deficiency anemia is mild, but cells become progressively more microcytic and hypochromic as anemia becomes more severe. By the time iron deficiency is diagnosed, serum iron is usually less than 40 μg/dL; total iron-binding capacity (TIBC) is greater than 400 μg/dL; iron-binding saturation is less than 10%; and serum ferritin is less than 12 μg/L. One of the most sensitive ways to detect early iron deficiency is to examine bone marrow stained to detect the presence or absence of storage iron.

The treatment of iron deficiency anemia consists of administration of oral or parenteral iron preparations. Oral iron corrects the deficiency just as rapidly and completely as parenteral iron in most cases if iron absorption from the gastrointestinal tract is normal.

A. Oral Iron Therapy: A wide variety of oral iron preparations are available. Since ferrous iron is most efficiently absorbed, only ferrous salts should be used. Ferrous sulfate, ferrous gluconate, and ferrous fumarate are all effective and inexpensive and are recommended for the treatment of most patients. Supplementation with vitamin C and other nutrients is

Table 30–1. Oral iron preparations.

Preparation	Tablet Size	Elemental Iron Per Tablet	Usual Adult Dose (Tablets Per Day)
Ferrous sulfate, hydrated	320 mg	64 mg	3–6
Ferrous sulfate, desiccated	200 mg	58 mg	3–6
Ferrous gluconate	320 mg	39 mg	5–10
Ferrous fumarate	200 mg	66 mg	3–6
Ferrous fumarate	320 mg	105 mg	2–4

generally not necessary. Sustained-release and enteric-coated iron preparations should not be used, since iron is best absorbed in the duodenum and proximal jejunum.

Different iron salts provide different amounts of elemental iron, as shown in Table 30–1. In an iron-deficient individual, about 50–100 mg of iron can be incorporated into hemoglobin daily, and about 25% of oral iron given as ferrous salt can be absorbed. Therefore, 200–400 mg of elemental iron should be given daily to correct iron deficiency most rapidly. Patients unable to tolerate such large doses of iron can be given lower daily doses of iron, which results in slower—but still complete—correction of iron deficiency.

Treatment with oral iron should be continued for 3–6 months. This will not only correct the anemia but will replenish iron stores. The first measurable response to successful iron therapy can be seen in less than a week, when brisk reticulocytosis occurs, as newly formed hemoglobin-filled red cells from bone marrow enter the bloodstream. The hemoglobin level should increase significantly in 2–4 weeks and should reach normal levels (men = 14–18 g/dL; women = 12–16 g/dL) in 1–3 months. Failure to respond to oral iron therapy may be due to incorrect diagnosis (anemia due to causes other than iron deficiency), continued iron loss (usually secondary to continued blood loss), concurrent chronic inflammation or other illness that suppresses marrow function, or failure of the patient to take or absorb the oral iron.

Common side-effects of oral iron therapy include nausea, epigastric discomfort, abdominal cramps, constipation, and diarrhea. These effects are usually dose-related and can often be overcome by lowering the daily dose of iron or by taking the tablets immediately after or with meals. Some patients have less severe gastrointestinal side-effects with one iron salt than another and benefit from changing preparations. Patients taking oral iron develop black stools; this itself has no clinical significance but may obscure the diagnosis of continued gastrointestinal blood loss.

B. Parenteral Iron Therapy: Parenteral therapy should be reserved for patients with documented iron deficiency unable to tolerate or absorb oral iron and patients with extensive chronic blood loss who cannot be maintained with oral iron alone. This includes patients with various postgastrectomy states and previous small bowel resections, inflammatory bowel disease involving the proximal small bowel, malabsorption syndromes, and chronic heavy bleeding from non-resectable lesions as may occur in hereditary hemorrhagic telangiectasia.

Iron dextran (many trade names) is a stable complex of ferric hydroxide and low-molecular-weight dextran containing 50 mg of elemental iron per milliliter of solution. It can be given either by deep intramuscular injection (using the "Z track" injection technique to avoid local tissue staining) or by intravenous infusion. Adverse effects of parenteral iron therapy include local pain and tissue staining (brown discoloration of the tissues overlying the injection site), headache, light-headedness, fever, arthralgias, nausea and vomiting, back pain, flushing, urticaria, bronchospasm, and, rarely, anaphylaxis and death.

The total amount of parenteral iron required to correct iron deficiency anemia and to replenish iron stores in a 70-kg adult can be calculated as follows: (normal hemoglobin − patient's hemoglobin) × 0.25 = grams of iron required. Most adults with iron deficiency anemia thus require 1–2 g of replacement iron, or 20–40 mL of iron dextran. Although this amount of parenteral iron can be given as 10–20 daily intramuscular injections, most physicians now prefer to give the entire calculated dose in a single intravenous infusion in several hundred milliliters of normal saline over 1–2 hours. Intravenous administration eliminates the local pain and tissue staining that often occur with the intramuscular route and allows delivery of the entire dose of iron necessary to correct the iron deficiency at one time. There is no clear evidence that any of the adverse effects, including anaphylaxis, are more likely to occur with intravenous than with intramuscular administration.

A small test dose of iron dextran should always be given before full intramuscular or intravenous doses are given. A 0.25–0.5-mL dose can be given by deep intramuscular injection or slow intravenous infusion of very dilute solution 30–60 minutes before proceeding with full therapy. If signs or symptoms of an immediate hypersensitivity reaction occur, additional parenteral iron should not be given, and alternative therapy must be considered. Patients with a strong history of allergy and patients who have previously received parenteral iron are more likely to have hypersensitivity reactions following treatment with parenteral iron dextran than those who have not.

Clinical Toxicity

A. Acute Toxicity: Acute iron toxicity is seen almost exclusively in young children who have ingested iron tablets. Although adults appear to be able to tolerate large doses of oral iron without serious consequences, as few as 10 tablets of any of the commonly available oral iron preparations can be lethal in young children. Oral iron preparations should therefore always be stored in "childproof" containers and kept out of the reach of children.

Large amounts of oral iron cause necrotizing gastroenteritis, with vomiting, abdominal pain, and bloody diarrhea followed by shock, lethargy, and dyspnea. Subsequently, improvement is often noted, but this may be followed by severe metabolic acidosis, coma, and death. Urgent treatment of acute iron toxicity is necessary, especially in young children. Gastric aspiration should be performed, followed by lavage with phosphate or carbonate solutions to form insoluble iron salts. Deferoxamine (Desferal), a potent iron chelating compound, should then be instilled into the stomach to bind any remaining free iron in the gut. Deferoxamine should also be given systemically by intermittent intramuscular injection or by continuous intravenous infusion to bind iron that has already been absorbed and to promote its excretion in urine and feces. Appropriate supportive therapy for gastrointestinal bleeding, metabolic acidosis, and shock must also be provided.

B. Chronic Toxicity: Chronic iron toxicity (iron overload), also known as hemochromatosis and hemosiderosis, results when excess iron is deposited in the heart, liver, pancreas, and other organs, leading to organ failure and death. It most commonly occurs in patients with hemochromatosis, an inherited disorder characterized by excessive iron absorption, and in patients who receive many red cell transfusions (each containing 250 mg of iron) over a long period of time. It is doubtful that clinically significant iron overload can occur in normal individuals who chronically ingest excess iron, because of the protective mechanisms that normally regulate iron absorption and because of the very large amounts of total body iron needed before clinical iron overload becomes apparent. However, continued ingestion of excess iron probably contributes to the development of iron overload in patients who have a higher than normal baseline iron absorption, whether due to inherited factors (subclinical hemochromatosis, etc) or to the presence of non-iron deficiency anemias (anemia of chronic disease, hemolytic anemias, etc).

Chronic iron overload in the absence of anemia is most efficiently treated by intermittent phlebotomy. One unit of blood (containing 250 mg of iron) can be removed every week or so until all of the excess iron is removed. Iron chelation therapy using parenteral deferoxamine is much less efficient as well as more complicated, expensive, and hazardous, but it can be useful for severe iron overload that cannot be managed by phlebotomy.

VITAMIN B_{12} & FOLIC ACID

Basic Pharmacology

Vitamin B_{12} and folic acid are chemically unrelated vitamins essential for normal DNA synthesis. Deficiencies lead to impaired DNA synthesis, inhibition of normal mitosis, and abnormal maturation and function of the cells produced. These changes are most apparent in tissues where cells undergo rapid cell division, such as in bone marrow and the gastrointestinal epithelium, but all dividing cells are affected to some degree. Severe anemia is the chief finding in patients with vitamin B_{12} or folic acid deficiency, but pancytopenia (diminished production of red blood cells, white blood cells, and platelets) may occur, and gastrointestinal symptoms are common. Neurologic abnormalities may also occur in vitamin B_{12} deficiency but not in folic acid deficiency.

Anemias caused by vitamin B_{12} and folic acid deficiency have a characteristic appearance of peripheral blood and bone marrow called megaloblastic anemia. Since the underlying defect in megaloblastic anemias is impaired DNA synthesis, there is diminished cell division in the face of continued RNA and protein synthesis. This leads to production of large (macrocytic) red blood cells that have a high RNA: DNA ratio and are defective in the sense that they are highly susceptible to destruction. Morphologically, the bone marrow is hypercellular, with a marked increase in the number of large abnormal early red cell precursors (megaloblasts) but with very few cells maturing beyond this stage to become circulating red cells. The red cells that do form in the bone marrow characteristically show normal cytoplasmic maturation, including normal hemoglobin formation; it is nuclear maturation and cell division that is impaired in the megaloblastic anemias.

Although megaloblastic anemia can theoretically result from any event that impairs DNA synthesis, in practice almost all cases are due to deficiencies of vitamin B_{12} or folic acid. The biochemical and physiologic bases of these deficiencies are now well understood, and it is possible to describe the mechanisms causing these anemias at the molecular level.

Chemistry

A. Vitamin B_{12}: Vitamin B_{12} is made up of a porphyrinlike ring with a central cobalt atom attached to a nucleotide (Fig 30–1). Various ligands may be covalently bound to the cobalt atom, forming various different cobalamins. Deoxyadenosylcobalamin and methylcobalamin are the active forms of the vitamin in humans. Cyanocobalamin and hydroxocobalamin (both available for therapeutic use) and other cobalamins found in food sources must be converted to the above active forms. The ultimate source of vitamin B_{12} is from microbial synthesis; it is not synthesized by animals or plants. The chief dietary source of vitamin B_{12} is microbially derived vitamin B_{12} in meat (especially liver), eggs, and dairy products. Vitamin B_{12} is sometimes called **extrinsic factor** to differentiate it from intrinsic factor, a substance normally secreted by the stomach.

B. Folic Acid: Folic acid (pteroylglutamic acid) is a compound composed of a pteridine heterocycle, *p*-aminobenzoic acid, and glutamic acid (Fig 30–2). Various numbers of glutamic acid moieties may be attached to the pteroyl portion of the molecule, resulting in monoglutamates, triglutamates, or polyglutamates. The fully oxidized pteridine ring of folic acid can undergo reduction, catalyzed by the enzyme dihy-

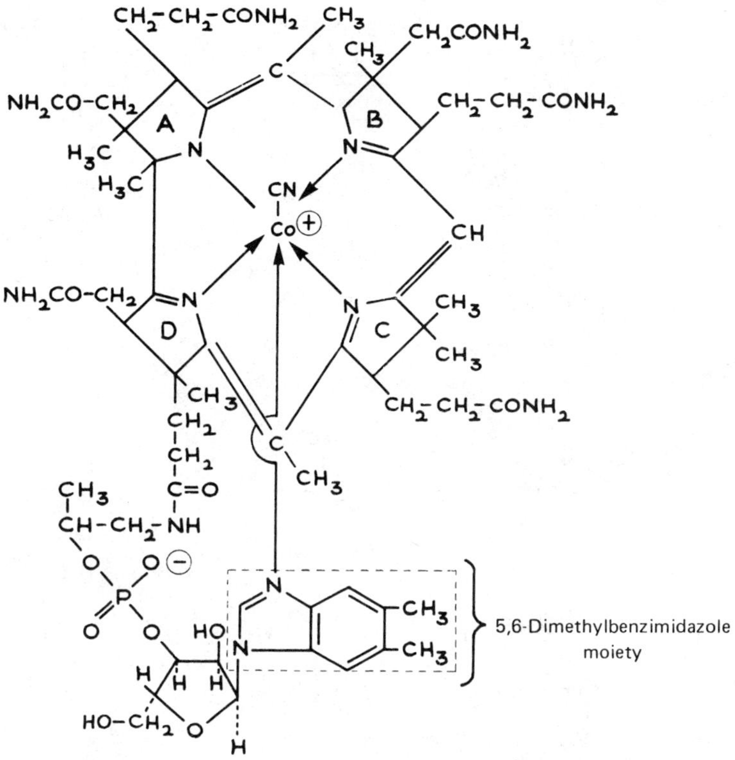

Figure 30–1. Cyanocobalamin; vitamin B_{12} ($C_{63}H_{88}O_{14}N_{14}PCo$). (Reproduced, with permission, from Martin DW, Mayes PA, Rodwell VW: *Harper's Review of Biochemistry,* 18th ed. Lange, 1981.)

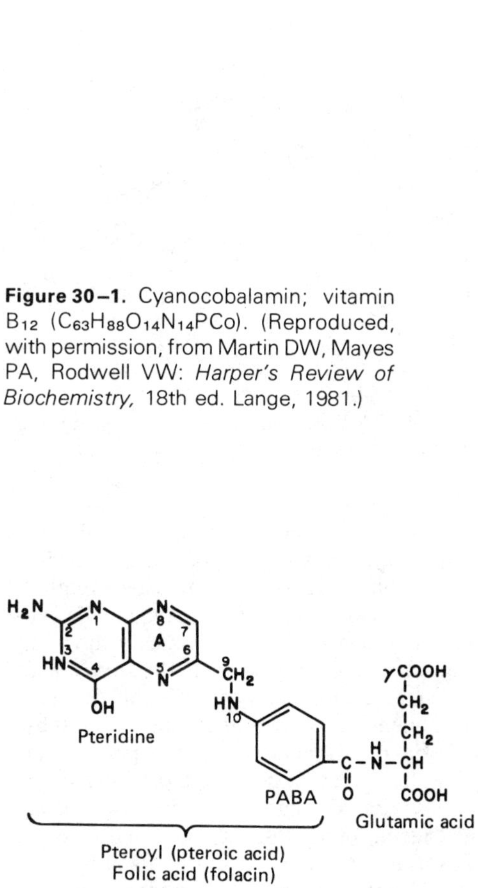

Figure 30–2. The structure and numbering of atoms of folic acid. (Reproduced, with permission, from Martin DW, Mayes PA, Rodwell VW: *Harper's Review of Biochemistry,* 18th ed. Lange, 1981.)

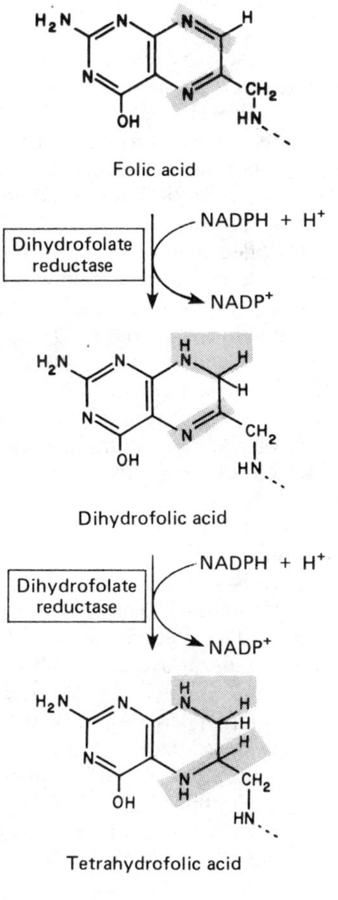

Figure 30–3 (at right). The reduction of folic acid to dihydrofolic acid and dihydrofolic acid to tetrahydrofolic acid by the enzyme dihydrofolate reductase. (Reproduced, with permission, from Martin DW, Mayes PA, Rodwell VW: *Harper's Review of Biochemistry,* 18th ed. Lange, 1981.)

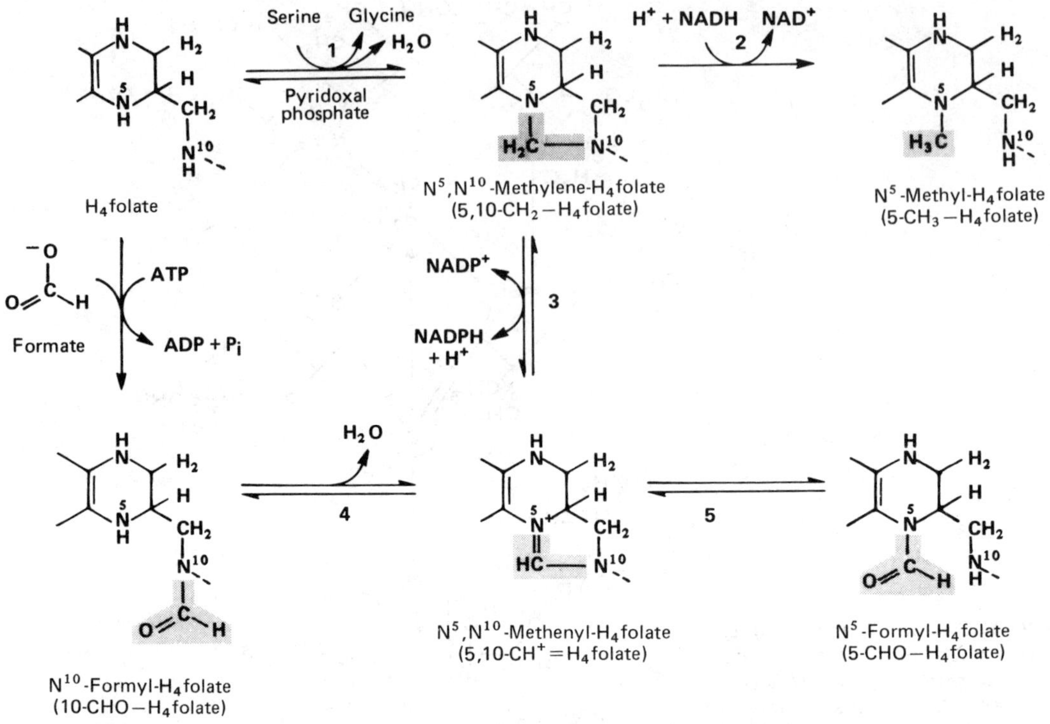

Figure 30–4. The interconversions of 1-carbon moieties attached to tetrahydrofolate. (Reproduced, with permission, from Martin DW, Mayes PA, Rodwell VW: *Harper's Review of Biochemistry,* 18th ed. Lange, 1981.)

drofolate reductase, to give 7,8-dihydrofolic acid (H_2folate) and then to the fully reduced 5,6,7,8-tetrahydrofolic acid (H_4folate) (Fig 30–3). H_4folate can subsequently be transformed to folate cofactors possessing 1-carbon units attached to the 5-nitrogen (5-CH_3–H_4folate and 5-CHO–H_4folate), the 10-nitrogen (10-CHO–H_4folate), or both positions (5,10-CH_2–H_4folate and 5,10-CH^+=H_4folate) (Fig 30–4). The folate cofactors are interconvertible by various enzymic reactions and serve the important biochemical function of donating 1-carbon units at various levels of oxidation. In most instances, H_4folate is regenerated in these reactions and is available for reutilization. Various forms of folic acid are present in a wide variety of plant and animal tissues, the richest sources of which are yeast, liver, kidney, and green vegetables.

Pharmacokinetics

A. Vitamin B_{12}: The average American diet contains 5–30 μg of vitamin B_{12} daily, 1–5 μg of which is usually absorbed. The vitamin is avidly stored, primarily in the liver, with an average adult having a total vitamin B_{12} storage pool of 3000–5000 μg. Only trace amounts of vitamin B_{12} are normally lost in urine and stool. Since the normal daily requirements of vitamin B_{12} are only about 2 μg, it would take about 5 years for all of the stored vitamin B_{12} to be exhausted and for megaloblastic anemia to develop if B_{12} absorption suddenly or gradually stopped.

Vitamin B_{12} in physiologic amounts is absorbed only after it complexes with intrinsic factor. Intrinsic factor is a glycoprotein with a molecular weight of about 50,000 that is secreted by the parietal cells of the gastric mucosa. Intrinsic factor combines with vitamin B_{12} liberated from dietary sources in the stomach and duodenum, and the intrinsic factor-vitamin B_{12} complex is subsequently absorbed in the distal ileum by a highly specific receptor-mediated transport system. Vitamin B_{12} deficiency in humans most often results from malabsorption of vitamin B_{12}, due either to lack of intrinsic factor or to loss or malfunction of the specific absorptive mechanism in the distal ileum.

Once absorbed, vitamin B_{12} is transported to the various cells of the body bound to a plasma glycoprotein, transcobalamin II. Excess vitamin B_{12} is transported to the liver for storage. Significant amounts of vitamin B_{12} are excreted in the urine only when very large amounts are given parenterally, overcoming the binding capacities of the transcobalamins.

B. Folic Acid: The average American diet contains 500–700 μg of folates daily, 50–200 μg of which is usually absorbed, depending on metabolic requirements (pregnant women may absorb as much as 300–400 μg of folic acid daily). Normally, 5–20 mg of folates is stored in the liver and other tissues. Folates are excreted in the urine and stool and are also destroyed by catabolism, so serum levels fall within a few days when intake is diminished. Since body stores of folates are relatively low and daily requirements high, folic acid deficiency and megaloblastic anemia can develop within 1–6 months after the intake of folic acid stops, depending on the patient's nutritional status and the rate of folate utilization.

Unaltered folic acid is readily and completely absorbed in the proximal jejunum. Dietary folates, however, consist primarily of polyglutamate forms of 5-CH_3–H_4folate, with very little unmodified folate present. Before absorption, all but one of the glutamyl residues of the polyglutamates must be hydrolyzed by the enzyme α-L-glutamyl transferase ("conjugase") within the brush border of the intestinal mucosa. The monoglutamate 5-CH_3–H_4folate is subsequently transported into the bloodstream, both by active and passive transport, and then widely distributed throughout the tissues of the body.

Pharmacodynamics

A. Vitamin B_{12}: There are 2 essential enzymic reactions in humans that require vitamin B_{12} (Fig 30–5). In one reaction, deoxyadenosylcobalamin is a required cofactor in the conversion of methylmalonyl-CoA to succinyl-CoA by the enzyme methylmalonyl-CoA mutase. In the face of vitamin B_{12} deficiency, this conversion cannot take place, and the substrate, methylmalonyl-CoA, accumulates. As a result, aberrant fatty acids are synthesized and incorporated into cell membranes. It is believed that incorporation of such nonphysiologic fatty acids into cell membranes of the central nervous system is responsible for the neurologic manifestations of vitamin B_{12} deficiency.

The other enzymic reaction that requires vitamin B_{12} is conversion of 5-CH_3–H_4folate and homocysteine to H_4folate and methionine by the enzyme 5-CH_3–H_4folate-homocysteine methyltransferase (Fig 30–5B). In this reaction, cobalamin and methylcobalamin are interconverted, and the vitamin may be considered a true catalyst. When vitamin B_{12} deficiency occurs, conversion of the major dietary and storage folate, 5-CH_3–H_4folate, to the precursor of folate cofactors, H_4folate, cannot occur. As a result, 5-CH_3–H_4folate accumulates, and a deficiency of folate cofactors necessary for DNA synthesis develops. This accumulation of the body's folate as 5-CH_3–H_4folate and the associated inability to form folate cofactors in vitamin B_{12} deficiency have been referred to as the "methylfolate trap." This is the biochemical step whereby vitamin B_{12} and folic acid metabolism are linked and explains why the megaloblastic anemia of vitamin B_{12} deficiency (but not the neurologic abnormalities) can be partially corrected by folic acid.

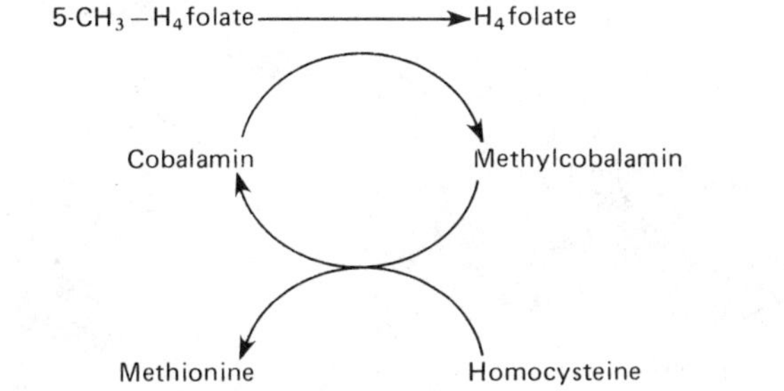

Figure 30–5. Enzymic reactions that use vitamin B_{12}.

B. Folic Acid: As noted above, the ultimate role of the folates is the formation of folate cofactors essential for 1-carbon transfer reactions necessary for DNA synthesis. The de novo synthesis of the purine heterocycle involves 2 enzymic reactions that use folate cofactors. In these, 10-CHO–H_4folate and 5,10-CH^+=H_4folate (Fig 30–4) donate their 1-carbon units to ultimately form carbons 2 and 8 of the purine heterocycle. In both of these reactions, H_4folate is regenerated and can again accept a 1-carbon unit and reenter the H_4folate cofactor pool.

Another essential reaction in which a folate cofactor is necessary is the synthesis of thymidylic acid (2′-deoxythymidylate monophosphate, dTMP), an essential precursor of DNA. In this reaction, the enzyme thymidylate synthetase catalyzes the transfer of the 1-carbon unit of 5,10-CH_2–H_4folate to the 5-position of 2′-deoxyuridylate monophosphate (dUMP) to form dTMP (Fig 30–6). Unlike all of the other enzymic reactions that utilize folate cofactors, in this reaction the cofactor is oxidized to H_2folate, and for each mole of dTMP produced, 1 mol of H_4folate is consumed. In rapidly proliferating tissues, considerable amounts of H_4folate can be consumed in this reaction, and continued DNA synthesis requires continued regeneration of H_4folate by reduction of H_2folate, catalyzed by the enzyme dihydrofolate reductase. The H_4folate thus produced can then reform the cofactor CH_2–H_4folate by the action of serine transhydroxymethylase and thus allow for the continued synthesis of dTMP. The combined catalytic activities of dTMP synthetase, dihydrofolate reductase, and serine transhydroxymethylase are often referred to as the **dTMP synthesis cycle** (Fig 30–7).

Clinical Pharmacology of Vitamin B_{12} & Folic Acid

Vitamin B_{12} and folic acid should be used specifically to treat or prevent deficiencies of these vitamins. There is no evidence that vitamin B_{12} injections have any benefit in persons who do not have vitamin B_{12} deficiency. Supplemental folic acid, however, may be useful in preventing folic acid deficiency in certain high-risk patients with high folate requirements.

The most characteristic clinical manifestation of vitamin B_{12} and folic acid deficiency is megaloblastic

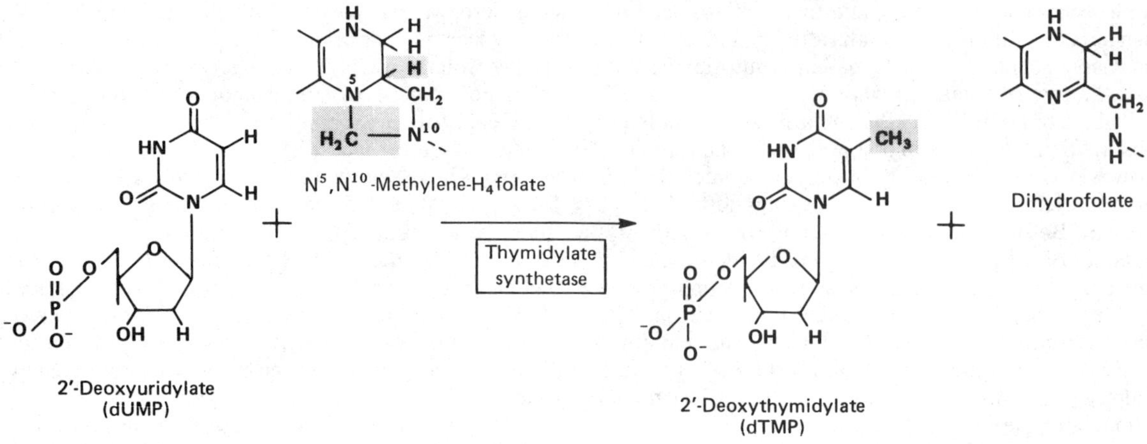

Figure 30–6. The transfer of a methyl moiety from N^5,N^{10}-methylene-H_4folate to deoxyuridylate to generate deoxythymidylate and dihydrofolate (H_2folate). (Reproduced, with permission, from Martin DW, Mayes PA, Rodwell VW: *Harper's Review of Biochemistry,* 18th ed. Lange, 1981.)

anemia. Any patient with macrocytosis, with or without anemia, should be evaluated for possible vitamin B_{12} or folic acid deficiency. Although most patients with neurologic abnormalities caused by vitamin B_{12} deficiency have full-blown megaloblastic anemia when first seen, occasional patients have few if any hematologic abnormalities, and the diagnosis of vitamin B_{12} deficiency may at first be obscure. It is particularly important to differentiate vitamin B_{12} deficiency from other forms of megaloblastic anemia, since treatment with vitamin B_{12} must be continued for life in most cases and the hematologic abnormalities in vitamin B_{12} deficiency may be partially corrected by treatment with large doses of folic acid while the neurologic damage progresses and may become irreversible.

The typical clinical findings in megaloblastic anemia are macrocytic anemia (MCV usually $>$ 120 fL), often with associated mild or moderate leukopenia or thrombocytopenia (or both), and a characteristic hypercellular bone marrow with megaloblastic maturation of erythroid and other precursor cells. Once a diagnosis of megaloblastic anemia is made, it must be determined whether vitamin B_{12} or folic acid deficiency is the cause. (Other causes of megaloblastic anemia are very rare.) This can usually be accomplished by measuring serum levels of the vitamins, although these measurements occasionally give false-positive or false-negative results. Red blood cell folic acid levels are often of greater diagnostic value than serum levels, since serum folic acid levels tend to be quite labile and do not necessarily reflect tissue levels. The Schilling test, which measures absorption and urinary excretion of radioactively labeled vitamin B_{12}, can be used to further define the mechanism of vitamin B_{12} malabsorption when this is found to be the cause of the megaloblastic anemia.

A. Vitamin B_{12}: Vitamin B_{12} deficiency is al-

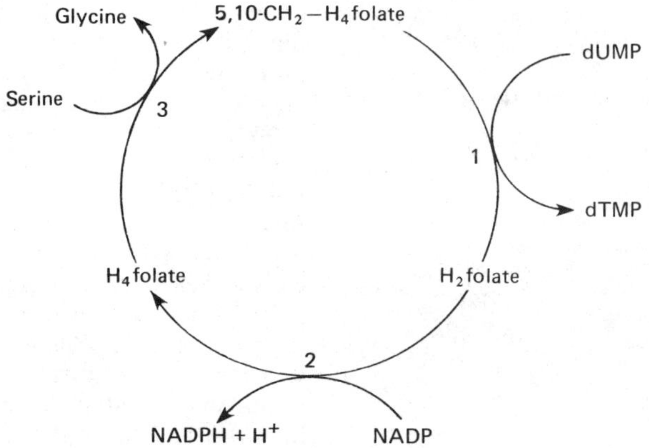

Figure 30–7. dTMP synthesis cycle. (1) dTMP synthetase; (2) H_2folate reductase; (3) serine transhydroxymethylase.

most always caused by malabsorption of vitamin B_{12}, due either to deficiency of intrinsic factor or to defects in the absorption of the vitamin B_{12}-intrinsic factor complex in the distal ileum. The most common causes of vitamin B_{12} deficiency are pernicious anemia, partial or total gastrectomy, and diseases that affect the distal ileum, such as malabsorption syndromes, inflammatory bowel disease, or small bowel resection. Nutritional deficiency of vitamin B_{12} is rare but may be seen in strict vegetarians after many years without meat, eggs, or dairy products.

Pernicious anemia results from defective secretion of **intrinsic factor** by the gastric mucosal cells. It is most common in older individuals of Northern European extraction, but it may occur at any age and in all races. Patients with pernicious anemia have gastric atrophy and fail to secrete hydrochloric acid (as well as intrinsic factor). The Schilling test shows diminished absorption of radioactively labeled vitamin B_{12}, which is corrected when hog intrinsic factor is administered with radioactive B_{12}, since the vitamin can then be normally absorbed. Pernicious anemia is a lifelong disease, and treatment with vitamin B_{12} injections must be continued indefinitely.

Total or partial gastrectomy removes the parietal cell-containing portion of the stomach that secretes intrinsic factor, resulting in vitamin B_{12} malabsorption similar to that seen in pernicious anemia. Since vitamin B_{12} stores may not be exhausted until as long as 5 years after gastrectomy, megaloblastic anemia will not develop until that time; however, many clinicians routinely start patients on vitamin B_{12} injections after gastrectomy to avoid any chance that vitamin B_{12} deficiency will develop later.

Vitamin B_{12} deficiency also occurs when the region of the distal ileum that absorbs the vitamin B_{12}-intrinsic factor complex is damaged, as when the ileum is involved with inflammatory bowel disease or sprue or when the ileum is surgically resected. In these situations, radioactively labeled vitamin B_{12} is not absorbed in the Schilling test, even when intrinsic factor is added. Other rare causes of vitamin B_{12} deficiency include bacterial overgrowth of the small bowel, blind loop syndrome, fish tapeworm, chronic pancreatitis, and thyroid disease. Rare cases of vitamin B_{12} deficiency in children have been found to be secondary to congenital deficiency of intrinsic factor and congenital selective vitamin B_{12} malabsorption due to defects of the receptor sites in the distal ileum.

Since almost all cases of vitamin B_{12} deficiency are caused by malabsorption of the vitamin, parenteral injections of vitamin B_{12} are required for therapy. For patients with potentially reversible diseases (fish tapeworm, sprue, blind loops), the underlying disease should be treated after initial treatment with parenteral vitamin B_{12}. Most patients, however, do not have curable deficiency syndromes and require lifelong treatment with vitamin B_{12} injections.

Vitamin B_{12} for parenteral injection is available as cyanocobalamin or hydroxocobalamin. Hydroxocobalamin is preferred because it is more highly protein-bound and therefore remains longer in the circulation. Initial therapy should consist of 100–1000 μg of vitamin B_{12} intramuscularly daily or every other day for 1–2 weeks to replenish body stores. Maintenance therapy consists of 100–1000 μg intramuscularly once a month for life. If neurologic abnormalities are present, vitamin B_{12} injections should be given every 1–2 weeks for 6 months before switching to monthly injections. Oral vitamin B_{12}-intrinsic factor mixtures and liver extracts should not be used to treat vitamin B_{12} deficiency; however, oral doses of 1000 μg of vitamin B_{12} daily are usually sufficient to treat patients with pernicious anemia who refuse or cannot tolerate the injections.

The hematologic response to treatment with vitamin B_{12} is rapid. The bone marrow usually returns to normal within 48 hours. Reticulocytosis begins on the second or third day and is usually maximal by the fifth to tenth day. Hemoglobin begins to increase in the first week and returns to normal by 1–2 months. Incomplete correction of the anemia may be due to persistence of other deficiencies (ie, combined vitamin B_{12} and iron deficiency) or the presence of inflammatory disease or other disorders that inhibit erythropoiesis.

B. Folic Acid: Folic acid deficiency, unlike vitamin B_{12} deficiency, is often caused by inadequate dietary intake of folates. Elderly patients, poor patients, and food faddists whose diets lack vegetables, eggs, and meat often develop folic acid deficiency. Prolonged cooking of vegetables destroys folates and can lead to folic acid deficiency if this is the only dietary source of this vitamin. Alcoholics and patients with liver disease develop folic acid deficiency because of poor diet and diminished hepatic storage of folates. There is also evidence that alcohol and liver disease interfere with absorption and metabolism of folates. Pregnant women and patients with hemolytic anemia have increased folate requirements and may become folic acid-deficient, especially if their diets are marginal. Patients with sprue and other malabsorption syndromes also frequently develop folic acid deficiency, perhaps because of a lack of intestinal conjugase. Folic acid deficiency is occasionally associated with cancer, leukemia, myeloproliferative disorders, certain chronic skin disorders, and other chronic debilitating diseases. Patients who require renal dialysis also develop folic acid deficiency, because folates are removed from the plasma each time the patient is dialyzed.

Folic acid deficiency can also be caused by drugs that interfere with folate absorption or metabolism. Phenytoin, some other anticonvulsants, oral contraceptives, and isoniazid can cause folic acid deficiency by interfering with folic acid absorption, possibly by inhibiting intestinal folate conjugases. Other drugs such as methotrexate and, to a lesser extent, trimethoprim and pyrimethamine, inhibit dihydrofolate reductase and may result in a deficiency of folate cofactors and ultimately in megaloblastic anemia.

Folic acid is available as tablets containing 0.1, 0.4, 0.8, and 1 mg of pteroylglutamic acid and as a parenteral solution containing 5 mg per milliliter. Parenteral administration is rarely necessary, since oral folic acid is well absorbed even in patients with malabsorption syndromes. A dose of 1 mg of folic acid orally daily is sufficient to reverse megaloblastic anemia, restore normal serum folate levels, and replenish body stores of folates in almost all patients. Therapy should be continued until the underlying cause of the deficiency is removed or corrected. Therapy may be required indefinitely for patients with malabsorption or dietary inadequacy. Folic acid supplementation to prevent folic acid deficiency should be considered in high-risk patients, including pregnant women, alcoholics, and patients with hemolytic anemia, liver disease, certain skin diseases, and patients on renal dialysis.

The response of patients with folate deficiency to treatment with oral folic acid is rapid and complete and similar to the response of the vitamin B_{12}-deficient patient given parenteral vitamin B_{12}. The hemoglobin level should begin to rise within the first week, and the anemia should be completely corrected in 1–2 months.

Clinical Toxicology

Vitamin B_{12} and folic acid have no known toxic effects even when administered in very large amounts. Large doses of both vitamins are promptly excreted in urine and to a lesser extent in stool, so that prolonged tissue exposure to very high levels does not occur. There is no evidence that cyanocobalamin, even in huge doses, causes cyanide poisoning.

• • •

References

Beck WS: Megaloblastic anemias. Chap 103, pp 853–860, in: *Cecil Textbook of Medicine,* 17th ed. Wyngaarden JB, Smith LH (editors). Saunders, 1982.

Brown EB: Iron deficiency anemia. Chap 102.1, pp 844–851, in: *Cecil Textbook of Medicine,* 17th ed. Wyngaarden JB, Smith LH (editors). Saunders, 1982.

Chanarin I: Investigation and management of megaloblastic anemia. *Clin Haematol* 1976;**5:**747.

Chanarin I et al: How vitamin B_{12} acts. *Br J Haematol* 1981; **47:**487.

Dallman PR: Iron deficiency: Diagnosis and treatment. *West J Med* 1981;**134:**496.

Finch CA (editor): Clinical aspects of iron deficiency and excess. *Semin Hematol* 1982;**29(1):**1. [Entire issue.]

Reich PR: Hypochromic anemias. Chap 2, pp 33–64, and Megaloblastic anemias. Chap 3, pp 65–101, in: *Hematology: Pathophysiologic Basis for Clinical Practice.* Little, Brown, 1978.

Drugs Used in Disorders of Coagulation | 31

Robert T. Wall, MD

Over 2500 years ago, a Chinese physician noted of the blood that "when it coagulates within the pulse, the blood ceases to circulate beneficially; when the blood coagulates within the foot, it causes pain and chills." Thus, blood may coagulate too readily. Diseases in which blood cannot coagulate normally, thereby resulting in hemorrhage, have also been recognized for centuries. The pharmacology and clinical applications of drugs used to inhibit coagulation or to correct bleeding disorders are the subjects of this chapter.

PRINCIPLES OF BLOOD COAGULATION

Plasma Coagulation Factors

The modern explanation for blood clotting began with the observation in the 18th century that blood plasma is the source of **fibrinogen,** the major structural component of clotted blood. This 340,000-MW protein circulates in plasma at a concentration of 200–600 mg/dL. Fibrinogen and the other clotting proteins, with the possible exception of factor V and factor VIII, are synthesized in the liver.

Fibrinogen is induced to polymerize when acted upon by thrombin, a protease derived from its plasma precursor prothrombin by the action of other serine proteases found in trace amounts in plasma.

The production of thrombin is normally initiated by contact between plasma and subendothelial structures exposed by injury of the blood vessel wall. Amplification of this initial event to the production of a macroscopic fibrin clot has been called the "waterfall sequence"—a useful metaphor of in vitro coagulation that helps explain the action of drugs on blood coagulation. Two features of this mechanism provide opportunities for inhibition of coagulation by anticoagulant drugs: (1) the serine-active sites common to many of the plasma coagulation factors and (2) the requirement for vitamin K in synthesis of biologically active factors X, VII, and IX and of prothrombin. **Heparin** is a short-acting anticoagulant that exerts its effect at the serine-active site of the coagulation enzymes; it must be administered parenterally. **Warfarin,** a long-acting drug that can be given orally, is the prototype of drugs that act at the vitamin K step in enzyme synthesis. The pharmacology and clinical uses of these drugs are discussed below.

Two major pathways can be identified in the ("cascade") waterfall sequence (Fig 31–1). The more rapidly responding extrinsic pathway is shown at right in the figure. This pathway is initiated by the contact of a cell-derived glycoprotein ("tissue factor"), calcium, and factor VII.

The intrinsic coagulation system is triggered by the contact activation of factor XII (Hageman factor) by a negatively charged surface but does not require the presence of a tissue factor, ie, it is intrinsic to the blood. The **hemophilias** are deficiencies of specific coagulation pathway factors: Lack of factor VIII is responsible for the most common form (hemophilia A); hemophilia B is the result of factor IX deficiency; and deficiency of factor XI is more common in Jewish populations.

There are interactions between the 2 pathways. The initial complex formed in the extrinsic system is able to activate factor IX of the intrinsic system. Thrombin can activate factor VIII, factor V, and factor XIII (fibrin-stabilizing factor). Activated factors XII and IX can each convert factor VII to a form having increased affinity for tissue factor and an enhancing effect on the activation of factor X. Factor Xa can enhance the action of factor VII. It is likely that these points of interaction are biologically important, since a defect in either leads to a bleeding disorder.

Coagulation in vivo has profounder depths of complexity. Specific receptors for certain coagulation factors are present on the blood platelet and the vascular endothelial cell. These are sites for activated factor X, thrombin, and fibrinogen. The platelet binding sites may accelerate the rate of coagulation and protect the clotting proteins from degradation. Platelets also contain factors V, VIII, and fibrinogen in releasable intracellular granules.

Regulation of Coagulation & Fibrinolysis

It is of obvious importance that thrombus formation be confined to the smallest area necessary to achieve hemostasis. The same is true of coagulation occurring in response to bleeding due, for example, to trauma or surgery. Two major systems regulate the process of thrombus formation.

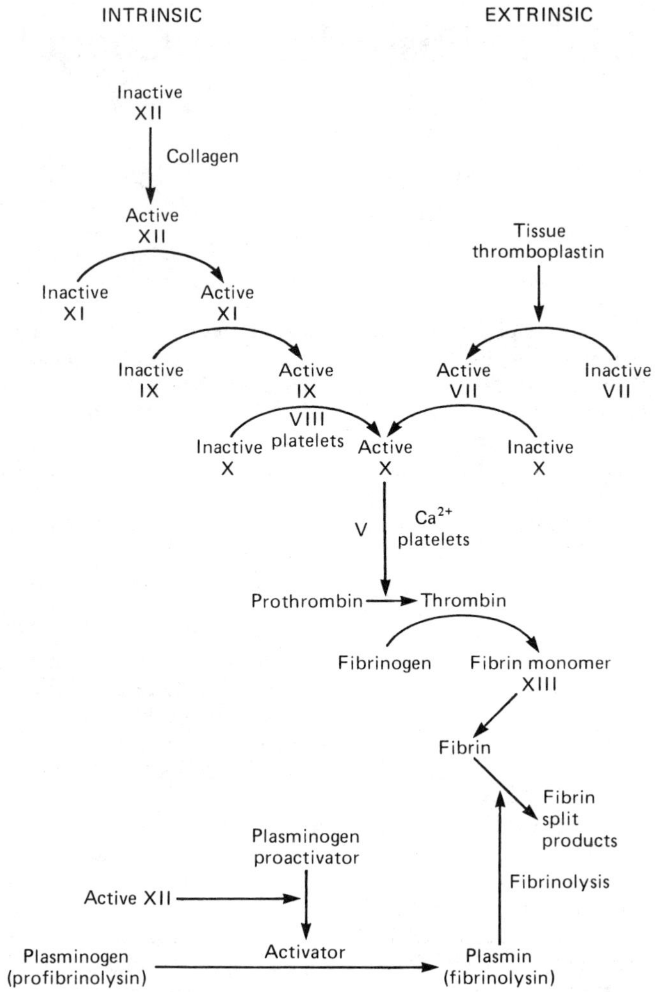

Figure 31–1. Blood coagulation (enzyme cascade scheme). Nearly all the coagulation factors apparently exist as inactive proenzymes that when activated serve to activate the next proenzyme in the sequence. **Synonyms:** Factor I = fibrinogen; II = prothrombin; III = tissue thromboplastin; V = labile factor (proaccelerin); VII = stable factor (proconvertin); VIII = antihemophilic factor (AHG, AHF); IX = plasma thromboplastin component (PTC; Christmas factor); X = Stuart-Prower factor; XI = plasma thromboplastin antecedent (PTA); XII = Hageman factor; XIII = fibrin-stabilizing factor. (Modified from Ganong WF: *Review of Medical Physiology,* 10th ed. Lange, 1981.)

A. Factors That Prevent Fibrin Formation: Plasma contains sufficient protease inhibitors to rapidly inactivate the coagulation proteins if they spill from the site of vessel injury. The major proteins in this system are antithrombin III, α_1-antitrypsin, α_2-macroglobulin, C1 inactivator, and α_2-antiplasmin. If this system is overwhelmed, generalized intravascular clotting might occur—eg, in what has come to be called **disseminated intravascular coagulation** following massive tissue injury, cell lysis, or bacteremia.

B. Factors That Promote Fibrin Destruction: The fibrinolytic system is activated at the onset of blood coagulation by the production of activated factor XII. Injured cells can release activators of the fibrinolytic mechanism as well. The central event in fibrinolysis is cleavage of plasminogen to plasmin, itself a proteolytic enzyme. The major physiologic role of plasmin is proteolysis of fibrin to digest and remodel the thrombus. It may also function to limit extension of thrombosis.

Regulation of the fibrinolytic system could be useful in treating certain coagulation disorders. For example, increasing plasmin generation might be effective therapy for diseases caused by thrombi. Conversely, it seems likely that pharmacologic depression of the fibrinolytic response, by protecting clots from lysis, could decrease bleeding in disorders characterized by failure of hemostasis. The important activators of the fibrinolytic system are **urokinase** and **streptokinase.** The clinically important inhibitor of fibrinolysis is **aminocaproic acid (Amicar).** Heparin does not inhibit plasmin formation.

Platelets & Endothelial Cells

The blood platelets and endothelial cells at the interface of blood and perfused tissue have important primary regulatory effects on blood coagulation. Platelets adhere to damaged vascular structures, become aggregated, and thereby occlude defects in the vessel wall. Platelets also increase the rate of fibrin generation, probably by providing specific binding sites for activated factor X and for thrombin and fibrinogen.

Platelets have a pivotal role in formation of **arterial thrombi,** and inhibition of platelet function is often used to prevent or treat arterial thrombosis. A key observation is that platelets utilize arachidonic acid derivatives (eg, thromboxane A_2) for normal function. Aspirin is the prototype of drugs that interfere with this pathway, and it is now widely used in treatment of thrombosis. The pharmacology and clinical use of aspirin and similar agents will be discussed in the section on arterial thrombosis.

The endothelial cell of the vessel wall provides a major mechanism for preventing blood coagulation, thereby keeping blood in a fluid state under normal conditions. The thromboresistant properties of the endothelial cell are based on unique surface structures as well as on the production of several prostaglandins that inhibit platelet function. The most noteworthy of these is PGI_2, which the endothelial cell produces from arachidonic acid via the cyclooxygenase pathway. PGI_2 (as prostacyclin) has potential as a pharmacologic agent and has been used to prevent thrombosis in hemodialysis and cardiopulmonary bypass machines, but its very short half-life may limit its clinical application.

Laboratory Testing of Coagulation

Clinical analysis of the coagulation mechanism is useful in many clinical conditions and critical in monitoring the use of antithrombotic drugs.

Anticoagulated patient plasma is used to investigate the plasma protein interactions in coagulation. The prothrombin test and the activated partial thromboplastin time (APT) test are particularly useful in drug monitoring. The extrinsic coagulation pathway is studied by the prothrombin test. In this test, patient blood is anticoagulated with 3.8% sodium citrate. The plasma fraction is tested for its capacity to form a fibrin clot by the addition of tissue factor and calcium, and the clot formation time is then compared to a control plasma. Lengthening of the coagulation time ("prothrombin time") can be used to determine the adequacy of anticoagulant therapy. This test is commonly used to monitor patients taking warfarin. The test requires proper controls and is subject to variation from one laboratory to another, because the reagents used may differ. Other tests are the Thrombotest and the P and P (proaccelerin and proconvertin) test, in which factor V is added to decrease the number of potential variables.

The intrinsic coagulation pathway is most commonly investigated clinically by the activated partial thromboplastin (APT) test. In this test, the clotting time of patient plasma is compared to that of control plasma after the addition of a contact activating agent such as kaolin, a phospholipid usually derived from platelets, and calcium. This test is used for the clinical management of patients receiving heparin. The fibrinogen concentration of blood and the coagulation time of plasma exposed to limiting amounts of thrombin (thrombin time) are additional tests for investigating the coagulation system and, in the context of drug therapy, monitoring fibrinolytic treatment.

The euglobulin lysis time is recommended for documenting a state of fibrinolysis during fibrinolytic therapy. It has no other useful clinical application. In this test, the time to lysis of a resuspended and clotted acetic acid-induced precipitate of plasma, the euglobulin fraction, is taken as a measure of systemic fibrinolysis.

The standard template bleeding time is an in vivo test of platelet function. Venous pressure in the arms is raised to 40 mm Hg with a blood pressure cuff on the upper arm. An incision is then made on the forearm with a template to standardize the length and depth of the cut, and the time to cessation of bleeding is recorded.

I. BASIC PHARMACOLOGY OF DRUGS USED TO TREAT THROMBOSIS

HEPARIN

Chemistry & Pharmacokinetics

Heparin is a potent inhibitor of blood coagulation both in vivo and in vitro. It is a naturally occurring glycosaminoglycan obtained from cow lung and pig intestinal mucosa for commercial production. The heparin molecule consists of a repeating disaccharide unit composed of glucosamine and either L-iduronic acid or D-glucuronic acid (Fig 31–2) in chains of variable length but generally in the range of MW 5000–15,000. Heparin is sulfated and highly acidic.

Heparin is generally used as sodium heparin, but calcium heparin is available and equally effective. It is stable in 5% dextrose in saline for 12–24 hours. Unfor-

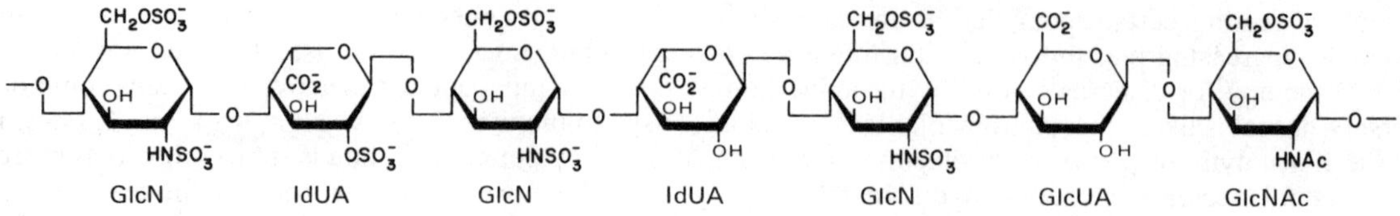

Figure 31–2. Structure of heparin. The polymer section illustrates structural features typical of heparin; however, the sequence of variously substituted repeating disaccharide units has been arbitrarily selected. In addition, non-*O*-sulfated or 3-*O*-sulfated glucosamine residues may also occur. (Modified, redrawn, and reproduced, with permission, from Lindahl U et al: Structure and biosynthesis of heparin-like polysaccharides. *Fed Proc* 1977;**36**:19.)

tunately, good correlation does not exist between the concentration of a given heparin preparation and its effect on coagulation. Heparin is therefore standardized by a bioassay system based on the ability of a preparation to prevent coagulation of sheep plasma under standard conditions. Heparin is administered as so many units based on this biologic assay.

The pharmacokinetics of heparin are complex. Its clearance is best described as a combination of both first-order and zero-order kinetics. Heparin clearance is a function of dosage and varies between individuals (Fig 31–3). Liver disease paradoxically increases heparin elimination; renal failure does not affect it.

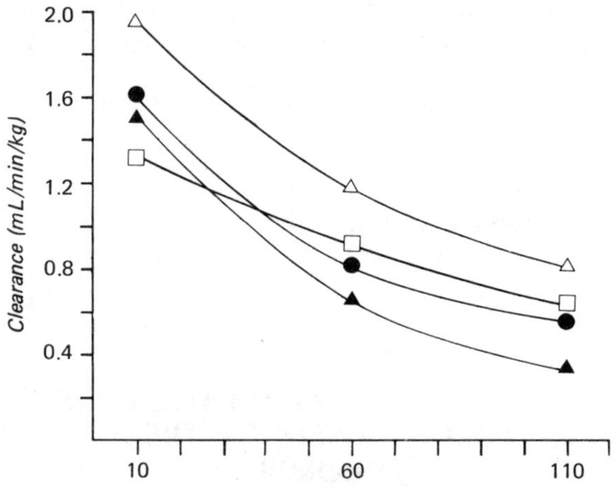

Figure 31–3. Decrease in heparin clearance values for each of 4 normal subjects as a function of dose. Note individual variations. (Modified and reproduced, with permission, from Simon TL et al: *Br J Haematol* 1922;**39**:111.)

Mechanisms of Action

The anticoagulant effect of heparin requires the presence of antithrombin III. This protein, a naturally occurring protease inhibitor, forms a 1:1 complex with thrombin. The rate of complex formation is increased 1000-fold by heparin, and neutralization of thrombin is nearly instantaneous. The heparin-antithrombin III complex can also inhibit activated factors XI, X, IX, and VII.

Administration & Dosage

The plasma concentration of heparin considered to be effective in preventing pulmonary embolism in established venous thrombosis is 0.2 units/mL. This is generally associated with prolongation of the activated partial thromboplastin time to 2–2½ times that of the control. This level of anticoagulant action should be maintained throughout the course of continuous intravenous heparin therapy; when intermittent heparin administration is used, the activated partial thromboplastin time should be measured 3–3½ hours after a dose and the heparin dose modified to achieve prolongation of the test to 2–2½ times the laboratory control. This approach is effective in preventing recurrent thromboembolic events.

Heparin is usually administered by continuous intravenous infusion via an infusion pump. Prolongation of the activated partial thromboplastin time to 2–2½ times the laboratory control usually requires continuous infusion of 10–15 units/kg/h following an initial bolus injection of 5000–10,000 units. The bolus is used to achieve therapeutic steady-state plasma levels more rapidly. Patients with pulmonary embolism may require larger doses, often approaching 25 units/kg/h, because of the increased heparin clearance in this condition. However, the dose required to prolong in vitro clotting time to the therapeutic level may decrease after 3–4 days of heparin therapy.

Heparin may also be administered by intermittent bolus intravenous infusion. The usual dose by this route is 75–100 units/kg every 4 hours. Effective antithrombotic therapy can also be achieved by the subcutaneous injection of 150 units/kg of heparin every 8–12 hours.

Heparin is given in low doses by the subcutaneous route to prevent thrombosis in patients at high risk for developing venous thrombosis such as middle-aged individuals undergoing elective abdominal surgery. For this indication, heparin is administered at a standard dose of 5000 units into the subcutaneous adipose tissue 1–2 hours before surgery and repeated every 12 hours for 7 days.

Other Heparin Effects

The major adverse effect of heparin is bleeding, which occurs in approximately 20% of treatment courses. Serious bleeding occurs less frequently, in perhaps 10% of courses. The risk can be decreased by excluding from heparin therapy patients who have active bleeding sites such as gastric and duodenal ulcers or recent intracerebral bleeding. Regular examination for bleeding, thrice-weekly measurement of the hemoglobin concentration, laboratory control of anticoagulation with dose adjustment to keep the prolongation of the activated partial thromboplastin time less than 2½ times the control, and the use of continuous infusion of heparin rather than high-dose intermittent injection are important additional safety measures.

In 5–10% of patients, heparin may cause a drop in the platelet count, occasionally to dangerously low levels. The mechanism is not known. Discontinuing the heparin is indicated if the platelet count drops below 75,000/μL. Platelet transfusion may be necessary. Heparin from a different animal source can sometimes be substituted without a recurrence of thrombocytopenia. Because of this potential complication, the platelet count should be measured at least twice a week during treatment.

Long-term heparin treatment may result in osteoporosis and hair loss. Heparin does not cross the placenta and thus should not cause bleeding in the fetus or newborn. Excess fetal wastage is observed when mothers receive heparin, but this may reflect the underlying condition rather than heparin itself.

Intravenous injection of heparin accelerates the clearing of postprandial lipemia. This action is due to the release into blood of a lipase from vascular endothelial cells and the liver.

Reversal of Heparin Action

Excess heparin-induced anticoagulation without bleeding can be treated by stopping drug infusion. More vigorous action is required if bleeding occurs. Heparin's action can be neutralized by administration of protamine sulfate, a basic peptide that combines with the acid heparin molecule on a milligram for milligram basis and inhibits its anticoagulant effect. The usual protamine dose is 50 mg given over 10 minutes by the intravenous route. Reversal of anticoagulant effect will be demonstrated in vivo by cessation of bleeding and in vitro by correction of the activated partial thromboplastin test to the normal range.

WARFARIN & THE COUMARIN ANTICOAGULANTS

Chemistry & Pharmacokinetics

The coumarin derivatives are an important class of antithrombotic drugs. Their clinical use can be traced to the discovery of an anticoagulant substance in spoiled sweet clover that produced a profound deficiency of prothrombin and a consequent hemorrhagic disease of cattle. The toxic agent was found to be bishydroxycoumarin (dicumarol). This agent and its congeners, most notably warfarin, have found wide use as rodent poisons as well as in antithrombotic therapy in humans. The group is often referred to as the "oral anticoagulants" because they are well absorbed from the gut.

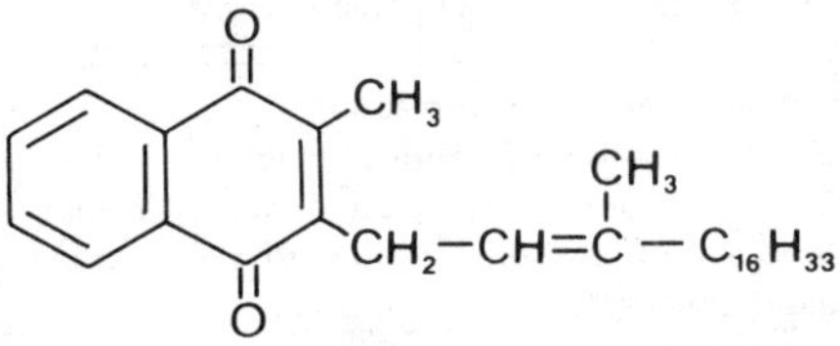

Phytonadione (vitamin K_1)

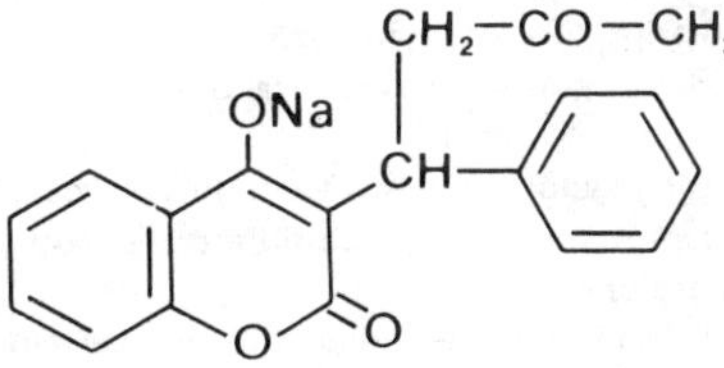

Warfarin

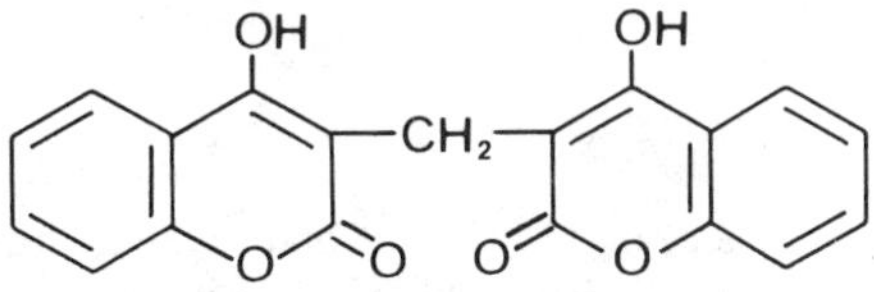

Dicumarol

Figure 31–4. Structural formulas of vitamin K_1 (phytonadione), warfarin sodium, and dicumarol (bishydroxycoumarin).

The structure of the coumarin anticoagulants is similar to that of vitamin K (Fig 31–4). In warfarin, the carbon at position 3 is asymmetric, thereby yielding levorotatory and dextrorotatory optical isomers. The levorotatory (S) isomer of warfarin is 3–5 times more potent than the dextrorotatory (R) isomer. This observation has been useful in understanding the consequences of drug interactions involving warfarin.

Mechanism of Action

The action of coumarin anticoagulants is to block vitamin K-dependent γ-carboxylation of glutamate residues. This action results in production of modified factors VII, IX, X, and prothrombin molecules, which are inactive in promoting coagulation. The cellular basis of vitamin K antagonism is not yet fully understood. It is not a true competitive interaction, although excess vitamin K will overcome a coumarin effect. The reverse also occurs.

Warfarin is the prototype of coumarin anticoagulants. It is rapidly absorbed from the gastrointestinal tract and is generally given orally; an intravenous preparation is available but seldom needed. Peak plasma levels are achieved within 1 hour following ingestion. Food in the stomach decreases the rate of absorption. Racemic warfarin is 99% bound to plasma albumin, and its volume of distribution is that of the

Table 31–1. Common drug interactions with anticoagulants.

Drugs that antagonize coumarin action
Increased catabolism by enzyme induction: Barbiturates, carbamazepine, griseofulvin, glutethimide, rifampin
Reduced absorption from intestine: Cholestyramine
Increased clotting factor synthesis: Vitamin K
Drugs that potentiate coumarin action
Decreased catabolism by enzyme inhibition: Allopurinol, chloramphenicol, cimetidine, disulfiram, ethanol, metronidazole, nortriptyline, phenylbutazone
Reduced availability of vitamin K: Oral broad-spectrum antibiotics
Reduced clotting factor synthesis: Quinidine, salicylates
Increased receptor site affinity: Clofibrate, dextrothyroxine, norethrandrolone
Displacement from protein-binding sites (uncertain significance as a causal mechanism): Chloral hydrate, diazoxide, ethacrynic acid, indomethacin, mefenamic acid, nalidixic acid, phenylbutazone, sulfonamides

albumin space, or 11–12% of body weight. Racemic warfarin has a half-life of 37 ± 15 hours, and the half-life of the R isomer is longer than that of the S form. The R isomer of warfarin is metabolized by oxidation of the ring primarily to 7-hydroxywarfarin. These products are inactive and excreted through both the gastrointestinal tract and the kidney.

Warfarin has important interactions with other drugs that can enhance or antagonize its anticoagulant action. The more commonly encountered interactions are listed in Table 31–1.

Administration & Dosage

Warfarin is generally given as warfarin sodium; the potassium salt has limited bioavailability. Treatment with warfarin is initiated at a dose of 10 mg orally daily as a single dose. An anticoagulant effect is usually observed in 3–4 days. A clinically useful anticoagulant effect can be maintained by chronic administration in the range of 2–15 mg/d. Previously synthesized factors VII, IX, X, and prothrombin must be partially cleared from plasma before the anticoagulant effect of warfarin can become clinically significant. Since the plasma half-lives of these factors are 6, 24, 40, and 60 hours, respectively, several days are required to achieve a steady-state effect.

The anticoagulant effect of warfarin must be closely monitored using tests of the extrinsic pathway. The most commonly used test is the prothrombin time, which should be maintained at 1½–4 times that of the control depending on the source of tissue factor. The therapeutic prothrombin time should be available from the clinical laboratory. Other tests for monitoring warfarin anticoagulation are the Thrombotest and the P and P test, as discussed above. The desired degree of anticoagulation as measured with the Thrombotest is 6–9% of normal activity; the P and P should be maintained at 16–21% of normal levels.

Other Effects

Warfarin can cross the placenta and cause a hemorrhagic disorder in the fetus. Furthermore, proteins with γ-carboxyglutamate residues are found in bone and blood and may be affected by warfarin. The vitamin K antagonist drugs should not be given to a woman in the first trimester of pregnancy, since a serious birth defect characterized by abnormal bone development (chondroplasia punctata) can occur.

Reversal of Action

The anticoagulant action of warfarin can be reversed by discontinuing the drug, administering coagulation factors, and giving large doses of vitamin K. The action taken will depend on the clinical urgency. Modest excesses of anticoagulant therapy may simply require stopping the drug. Recovery of normal coagulation status will depend on the synthetic capacity of the liver, the availability of vitamin K in the gastrointestinal tract, and the rate of clearance of the newly synthesized active coagulation factors. Serious bleeding should be treated by stopping the drug and administering large volumes of fresh-frozen plasma or factor concentrates (see p 355) containing the necessary coagulation proteins.

Analogs & Variants

Other vitamin K antagonists are seldom used to treat thrombotic disorders because they have less favorable pharmacologic properties or greater toxicity. **Dicumarol** (bishydroxycoumarin) (Fig 31–4) is a coumarin derivative with mechanism of action and toxic effects similar to those of warfarin. Dicumarol, however, is slowly and incompletely absorbed after oral administration and frequently causes abdominal pain and cramps. **Phenprocoumon,** an occasionally used coumarin drug, has a half-life of 6 days.

The indandione derivatives are another class of vitamin K antagonists. This group includes **phenindione, diphenadione,** and **anisindione.** These drugs have potentially serious side-effects on kidney and liver and are of little clinical use.

FIBRINOLYTIC DRUGS

Two drugs are available that can rapidly lyse thrombi after coagulation has occurred. This class of drugs is clearly distinct from heparin and the coumarin derivatives, which act to inhibit clot *formation.* It is important to remember that the fibrinolytic drugs create a general lytic state and break down clots formed in defense of bleeding as well as the target thromboemboli.

Basic Pharmacology

Urokinase and **streptokinase** are the prototypes of this class of drug. Streptokinase is an enzyme synthesized by streptococci. Urokinase is found in human urine but is produced commercially from cultured human fetal kidney cells and is readily cleaved to an active protease. The proteolytic activity of urokinase appears to be mediated by an active site containing serine.

These 2 drugs generate plasmin from plasminogen by different mechanisms. Streptokinase forms an activator complex with plasminogen, which in turn converts other plasminogen molecules to plasmin. There is no naturally occurring inhibitor of the activator complex. Urokinase directly converts plasminogen to an active form by enzymatic cleavage of the single-chain plasminogen to the proteolytically active 2-chain plasmin molecule, which in turn can also enzymatically cleave plasminogen to plasmin.

Indications & Dosage

Fibrinolytic agents are used chiefly for the treatment of massive pulmonary embolism. They have also been recommended as initial therapy for venous thrombosis. There is current interest in the use of low doses of streptokinase given by direct infusion into an artery obstructed by a thrombus.

Streptokinase and urokinase for the treatment of venous thromboembolic disease are both administered by intravenous infusion on a fixed-dose schedule. The drugs are provided in lyophilized form. Loading doses of streptokinase (250,000 units) or urokinase (900 units/kg) are given over 30 minutes and 10 minutes, respectively. Urokinase maintenance is given at a dose of 90 units/kg per hour for 24 hours. The streptokinase maintenance dose is 100,000 units per hour for 24 hours. Some clinicians recommend a 72-hour infusion when treating venous thrombosis.

Infused streptokinase combines rapidly with naturally occurring antistreptococcal antibodies as well as with plasminogen and plasmin. Free streptokinase is quickly cleared from the circulation. The streptokinase loading dose is employed to overcome potential antibody neutralization. Increased antibody production to streptokinase will limit the effectiveness of subsequent streptokinase therapy. Allergic reactions occur in 5–10% of patients receiving streptokinase. In 1982, a standard course of streptokinase costs about US $275.00, while urokinase costs 10 times that much.

Since not all patients achieve a lytic state with standard therapy, it is important to monitor the effect of treatment. Shortening of the euglobulin lysis time to less than 30 minutes is thought to be sufficient to define a lytic state. However, neither the extent of shortening of this test nor the degree of prolongation of the standard coagulation tests correlates with the extent of clot lysis.

Fibrinolytic therapy should be followed with anticoagulant therapy—initially with heparin, then followed with warfarin. To minimize the risk of hemorrhage, a delay of 1–2 hours between stopping the fibrinolytic drug and starting heparin is recommended to allow for elimination of the drug.

Treatment of Bleeding During Fibrinolysis

Hemorrhage is the major complication of fibrinolytic therapy. If bleeding occurs, stop the drug and give fibrinogen in the form of fresh-frozen plasma or fibrinogen concentrates (see p 355). Other maneuvers are infusions of aminocaproic acid or tranexamic acid (see p 356), which inhibit plasminogen activation; or of aprotinin (Trasylol), a kallikrein inactivator with antiplasmin activity. Minor skin bleeding may require only local pressure.

DEXTRAN

Dextran is a branched polysaccharide with antithrombotic properties. Although more commonly used as a plasma volume expander in shock or blood loss, it has a limited role in the prevention of venous thrombosis. Available forms of dextran have average molecular weights of 40,000, 70,000, and 75,000. The high-molecular-weight forms, **dextran 70** and **dextran 75,** have been used as antithrombotic agents.

Dextran interferes with normal platelet function and polymerization of fibrin monomers by unknown mechanisms. Adverse effects observed during dextran infusion are blood volume overload, hemorrhage, and allergic reactions.

Drugs That Inhibit Platelet Function

Two potential targets for platelet inhibitory drugs have been identified: arachidonic acid metabolism and platelet cAMP content. Thromboxane A_2 is an arachidonate product that causes platelets to change shape, release their granules, and aggregate. Drugs that antagonize this pathway interfere with aggregation of platelets in vitro and generally prolong the standard template bleeding time. Aspirin is the prototype of this class of drugs. Other nonsteroidal anti-inflammatory drugs affect thromboxane A_2 production and perhaps platelet function but are not often used for this purpose (see Chapter 33). Drugs that appear to act by modulating intraplatelet cAMP concentration generally do not affect template bleeding time.

ASPIRIN

Aspirin is thought to inhibit thromboxane A_2 synthesis by irreversible acetylation of cyclooxygenase. Other salicylates do not have this property. The inhibitory effect on platelet aggregation can be overcome by high concentrations of collagen and moderate doses of thrombin.

The usual antithrombotic dose of aspirin is 325 mg 3–4 times daily. However, there is some concern that this amount of drug may compromise a beneficial clinical effect by inhibiting PGI_2 production from the vascular endothelium (see above). Consequently, lower doses of aspirin are now recommended by many investigators. This approach is based on a theoretical model in which endothelial cell PGI_2 production in vivo is perceived to recover more quickly from a single low aspirin dose than does platelet thromboxane A_2 production, thereby favoring an antithrombotic effect. In a recent study, a long-term 92% decrease in platelet thromboxane production was achieved by a regimen of a single 200-mg dose followed by daily doses of 20–25 mg.

SULFINPYRAZONE

Sulfinpyrazone is a uricosuric drug related to phenylbutazone (see Chapter 33). Since 1965, it has had wide use as an antithrombotic drug. The mechanism of this action of sulfinpyrazone is not known. It decreases the accelerated platelet turnover observed in animal models of arterial thrombosis, but the bleeding time is not prolonged. At high concentrations, sulfinpyrazone can reversibly inhibit cyclooxygenase in vitro. Some studies suggest a protective effect on endothelial cell viability. Dosage is the same as in the treatment of gout (see p 384).

IMIDAZOLE

Imidazole inhibits thromboxane synthetase. This is an attractive target, since the effect is to inhibit thromboxane A_2 production without blocking PGI_2 synthesis. However, it must be anticipated that such a drug might have variable clinical effects, since many cells produce thromboxanes. A number of imidazole derivatives are being tested. No important acute toxic effects have been observed thus far.

Drugs With Other Mechanisms of Action

PROSTAGLANDINS

PGI_2 (prostacyclin) has potent platelet inhibitory effects. The difficulties limiting its application are the short duration of biologic activity of infused PGI_2 (only a few minutes) and the vasodepressor action, which limits the amount that can be given. PGI_2 is able to pass unchanged through the pulmonary circulation.

Prostacyclin has been tested in clinical studies most extensively as an antithrombotic agent for use with hemodialysis and cardiopulmonary bypass machines. The initial dose is generally 4 ng/kg/min. The drug does not affect in vitro coagulation tests. The bleeding time may be prolonged by PGI_2 infusion, but bleeding is not a recognized complication.

THIENPYRIDINES

These are newer compounds with cell actions that distinguish them from the older platelet-inhibiting drugs. The prototype thienpyridine is **ticlopidine.** This drug is a weak inhibitor of aggregation in vitro but a potent inhibitor of platelet function in vivo and prolongs the in vivo bleeding time.

DIPYRIDAMOLE

Dipyridamole (Persantine) is a pyrimidopyrimidine compound that inhibits some platelet functions. Its mechanism of action is not known. High concentrations added in vitro inhibit platelet aggregation, but this effect cannot be demonstrated when the drug is given to experimental subjects. Dipyridamole does not prolong bleeding time. It inhibits phosphodiesterase activity, thereby increasing cAMP levels in the platelet, and this action may be related to its inhibitory effect on platelet function. Unlike aspirin, dipyridamole decreases platelet adhesion to thrombogenic surfaces and can normalize platelet survival in experimental models of arterial thrombosis. The usual dose is 400 mg/d.

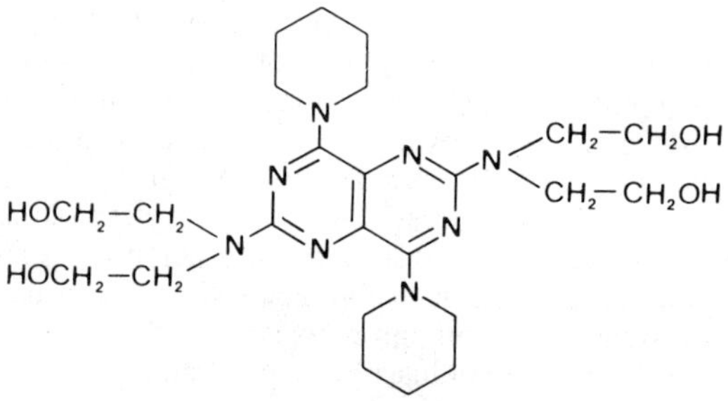

Dipyridamole

II. CLINICAL PHARMACOLOGY OF DRUGS USED TO TREAT THROMBOSIS

VENOUS THROMBOSIS

Antithrombotic Management

A. Prevention: Heparin and dextran are the agents most commonly used to prevent venous thrombosis. The more extensive experience has been with heparin. Dextran is used mainly by orthopedic surgeons doing hip surgery.

The rationale for anticoagulation with these agents is that local thrombin formation is the major event in venous thrombosis. Kinetic analysis of hemostasis in venous thrombosis shows a balanced consumption of platelets and fibrinogen. While platelets may have some pathologic role in venous disease, inhibition of platelet function is not consistently effective in preventing venous thrombosis. Heparin, on the other hand, given as a low-dose intermittent subcutaneous infusion as described above, provides effective prophylaxis under many clinical conditions. Hip and genitourinary surgery and operations on patients with metastatic cancer may be exceptions. Oral anticoagulant prophylaxis is effective for these indications but is not widely used because of the need for close laboratory control and the risk of bleeding. In contrast, full oral anticoagulant therapy is valuable for preventing reinfarction in men over 60 and in patients with prosthetic valves.

B. Treatment of Established Disease: Established venous thrombosis is treated with full anticoagulant doses of heparin and warfarin to prolong in vitro clotting times. Pulmonary embolism is treated in the same manner. A common practice is to treat only those venous clots that occur in or extend into large proximal veins.

Heparin is used as initial therapy and given for 7–10 days—or longer if clinical signs of thrombosis do not subside. The basis for this recommendation is that it takes about 7 days for an experimental thrombus to become adherent to the vein wall, and the risk of early extension of the clot and embolization in patients is lower when heparin is given during the first week compared to oral anticoagulation with warfarin. When heparin is followed by warfarin therapy, the 2 drugs should be overlapped for 2–3 days until therapeutic anticoagulation is obtained with warfarin as defined by tests of the extrinsic clotting system (Thrombotest, P and P, prothrombin time).

There is good evidence that oral anticoagulant therapy with warfarin for several weeks after stopping heparin will decrease the recurrence of venous thromboembolism (Fig 31–5). Current practice is to continue oral anticoagulant therapy with warfarin for 6 weeks to 3 months after hospital discharge. Close laboratory control of anticoagulant therapy is essential.

It must be emphasized that anticoagulant therapy has the potential for causing disability and death. These drugs should be given only for rigorously diagnosed thrombosis or as prophylactic therapy in accepted clinical conditions. Diagnosis of both initial and recurrent events should be based on laboratory investigation, since clinical diagnosis is often in error.

Fibrinolytic Therapy

Many investigators believe that early treatment of life-threatening pulmonary embolism with streptokinase or urokinase will improve survival and perhaps preserve long-term pulmonary function. This approach is now used for some patients with massive embolization who might otherwise be treated with surgical removal of the embolus.

Fibrinolytic therapy is given by a fixed-dose regimen as outlined earlier in this chapter. It is necessary to establish a lytic state, defined as a shortening of the euglobulin lysis time to less than 30 minutes. Streptokinase failures may respond to urokinase. The standard course of fibrinolytic therapy should be followed by anticoagulant therapy with heparin and warfarin. Patients receiving fibrinolytic therapy should not have concomitant invasive procedures. Patients with a history of recent surgery, stroke, metastatic cancer, or underlying hemorrhagic disorders should not be given these drugs.

Streptokinase is often used as initial treatment for major venous thrombosis. The goal of therapy is to preserve vein structure with rapid clot lysis so as to prevent the development of chronic venous insufficiency and the postphlebitic syndrome. Streptokinase is generally given as a 72-hour infusion for this indication. This form of therapy, however, is controversial.

Pregnancy

Warfarin crosses the placenta and can cause de-

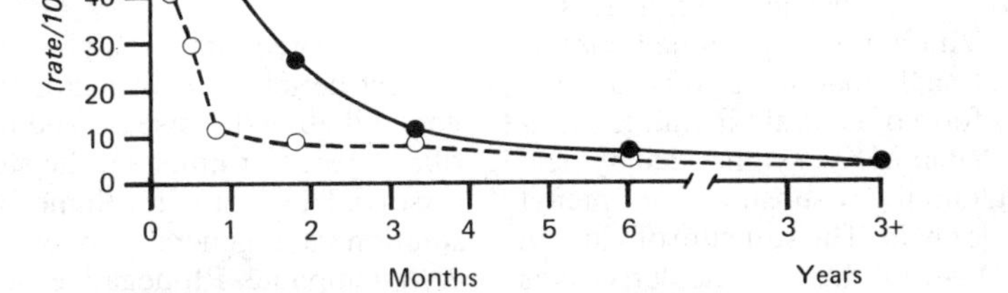

Figure 31–5. Recurrence of venous thromboembolism after discharge from hospital, showing effect of outpatient anticoagulant treatment for 6–12 weeks in reducing recurrence rate. (Modified and reproduced, with permission, from Gallus AS, Hirsch J: *Semin Thromb Hemostas* 1976;2:291.)

velopmental defects when given in the first trimester of pregnancy. It may also cause hemorrhage in the fetus or neonate. For these reasons, venous thromboembolic disease in pregnancy is usually treated with heparin throughout pregnancy, stopping for delivery and reinstituting the drug for a further 2–3 weeks of treatment after delivery. Heparin may be given by intermittent intravenous injection or by subcutaneous injection as described above. Laboratory monitoring of the anticoagulant effect is mandatory.

ARTERIAL THROMBOSIS

Patients with arterial thrombosis have excess consumption of platelets, presumably due to platelet interactions with damaged arterial walls—in contrast to the balanced consumption of both platelets and fibrinogen in venous thrombosis and massive tissue injury. Drug treatment with platelet-inhibiting drugs (aspirin, sulfinpyrazone, dipyridamole) is based on these experimental observations.

• • •

DRUGS USED IN BLEEDING DISORDERS

VITAMIN K

The synthesis of biologically active forms of prothrombin and of factors VII, IX, and X requires vitamin K. Since most of the coagulation factors are synthesized by the liver, severe liver failure with loss of synthetic function will result in a bleeding disorder that cannot be corrected by the administration of vitamin K.

Chemistry & Pharmacology

Vitamin K is a fat-soluble molecule found in liver, egg yolk, and a variety of vegetable oils. Cod liver oil, yellow corn, unpolished rice, and sunflower seeds are poor sources of vitamin K. However, the dietary requirement is low, because the vitamin is also synthesized by bacteria that normally colonize the human intestine.

Vitamin K activity is associated with at least 2 distinct substances. Vitamin K_1 (phytonadione) is 2-methyl-3-phytyl-1,4-naphthoquinone. It is found in plants and is the only form of natural vitamin K available for clinical use. Vitamin K_2, synthesized by bacteria, differs from vitamin K_1 by substitution of prenyl units for the phytyl side chain. The structure of vitamin K_1 is shown in Fig 31–4. Of the quinone derivatives that possess vitamin K activity, the most important is menadione, or vitamin K_3. This compound is not often used in practice.

Vitamins K_1 and K_2 are absorbed from the intestine only if bile salts are present. Vitamin K_3 and its water-soluble derivatives do not require bile salts. All preparations are readily absorbed after intramuscular administration. Removal is by excretion of metabolites in both bile and urine.

The usual oral, subcutaneous, intramuscular, or intravenous dose of vitamin K is 5–20 mg. The duration of therapy depends on the clinical condition being treated. The depressed level of active vitamin K-dependent coagulation factors begins to recover by 6–7 hours after treatment in uncomplicated vitamin K deficiency; factor VII returns to normal first, followed by factors IX and X and prothrombin.

Care must be exercised when administering vitamin K_1 intravenously, since too rapid delivery can produce dyspnea, chest pain, flushing, and death due either to the drug or to the dispersing agents in the preparation.

Vitamin K_1 is now given to all newborns to prevent hemorrhage from vitamin K deficiency in the perinatal period. A single dose of 0.5–1 mg is given by intramuscular administration.

Plasma Fractions

Deficiencies in plasma coagulation factors other than factor XII, high-molecular-weight kininogen, and prekallikrein can lead to bleeding. Spontaneous bleeding may occur when factor concentrations are less than 5% of normal. However, there is variation in the concentration of the various coagulation factors needed for hemostasis (Table 31–2).

Concentrated plasma fractions are available for fibrinogen, factor VII, and factor IX (also containing factors X, prothrombin, and variable factor VII). Factor VIII deficiency (hemophilia A) and factor IX deficiency (hemophilia B) account for about 95% of the heritable coagulation defects. The best use of these therapeutic materials requires specific identification of the deficient factor and quantitation of its plasma level.

Although uncommon, there are a variety of inherited and acquired disorders of platelet function.

FACTOR VIII

There are 2 preparations of concentrated human factor VIII: cryoprecipitate and a lyophilized concentrate.

Cryoprecipitate is a plasma protein fraction used to treat deficiencies of factor VIII in hemophilia and von Willebrand's disease and on occasion to provide fibrinogen. For infusion, the stored cryoprecipitate is dissolved in a small volume of sterile citrate-saline solution and generally pooled with other units of cryoprecipitate. Rh-negative women with potential for childbearing should be treated only with cryoprecipitate from Rh-negative donors because of possible contamination of the product with Rh-positive blood cells. Lyophilized factor VIII concentrates prepared from pooled plasma are also available. These commercially

Table 31–2. Therapeutic materials for the treatment of coagulation disorders.*

Factor No.	Deficiency State	Concentration (Percent), Relative to Normal Plasma, Required for Hemostasis†	Half-Life of Infused Factor	Approximate Recovery in Vivo as Percentage of Infused Dose	Therapeutic Material
I	Afibrinogenemia, defibrination syndrome.	10–25	4–6 days	50	Plasma fibrinogen.
II	Prothrombin deficiency.	40	3–4 days	50–100	Concentrate (factor IX-prothrombin complex).
V	Factor V deficiency.	10–25	24 hours	?50	Plasma.
VII	Factor VII deficiency.	?	4–6 hours	?	Concentrate (some preparations of factor IX).
VIII	Hemophilia A (classic).	10–40	12 hours	50–80	Plasma, cryoprecipitate, and other factor VIII concentrates.‡
	von Willebrand's disease.	20–40	?	?	
IX	Hemophilia B (Christmas disease).	10–40	18–24 hours	25–50	Plasma, cryosupernatant, factor IX-prothrombin complex.
X	Stuart-Prower defect.	10–40	60–70 hours	50–100	Plasma, concentrate (some preparations of factor IX).
XI	PTA deficiency.	?	60–70 hours	Nearly 100	Plasma.
XII	Hageman defect.	...	...	...	Treatment not needed.
XIII	Fibrin-stabilizing factor deficiency.	1–2	6 days	50–100	Plasma.

*Modified and reproduced, with permission, from Biggs R (editor): *Human Blood Coagulation, Haemostasis, and Thrombosis,* 2nd ed. Blackwell, 1976.

†Note that in order to allow for fall-off, the immediate postinfusion level may need to be much higher, varying according to the degree of trauma.

‡Highly purified preparations of factor VIII should not be used in the treatment of von Willebrand's disease without specific evidence of their efficacy.

freeze-dried concentrates may not suffice to treat patients with von Willebrand's disease, since the polymeric structure of the factor VIII in von Willebrand protein that supports platelet adhesion may be lost in the manufacturing process.

An uncomplicated hemorrhage into a joint should be treated with sufficient factor VIII to maintain a level of 4–5% of the normal concentration for 18–24 hours. Soft tissue hematomas require a minimum of 10–15% activity for 4–7 days. Hematuria usually requires 5–10% activity for 2–4 days. Surgery and major trauma will require 30% activity for 7–10 days. Therapy is usually initiated with sufficient factor VIII to achieve a nearly normal concentration in plasma.

Arginine vasopressin (desmopressin acetate; DDAVP) has been used experimentally in patients with mild hemophilia A or von Willebrand's disease to permit performance of minor surgery such as tooth extraction without the requirement for coagulation factor infusion. The drug is given intravenously, 1.5 μg/kg, and repeated doses may be necessary.

FACTOR IX

Freeze-dried concentrates containing prothrombin, factors IX and X, and variable factor VII are marketed by several companies and are available for treating deficiencies of these factors (freeze-dried factor IX-prothrombin complex concentrate). Heparin, usually less than 30 units per bottle, is often added by the manufacturer to inhibit coagulation factors that may have been activated by the manufacturing process.

One unit of factor IX per kilogram will increase the normal plasma level by 1%. Factor VIII concentrates and cryoprecipitate cannot be used to treat deficiencies of vitamin K-dependent factors.

The observation that some preparations of factor IX concentrate contained activated coagulation factors led to the use of these products to treat patients with antibodies to factor VIII or factor IX. In addition to the usual preparations, 2 newer products are available expressly for this purpose. These are Autoplex and FEIBA (Factor Eight Inhibitor Bypassing Activity). The mechanism by which these materials bypass the inhibitor is not established, and they are not uniformly successful in arresting hemorrhage. Inhibitor titers often rise after treatment with these products.

FIBRINOGEN

Fibrinogen can be given in the form of plasma or in a concentrated form as cryoprecipitate, a single unit of which contains 200–400 mg of fibrinogen. Lyophilized concentrates of factor VIII contain a high proportion of fibrinogen and may be used for this purpose.

Fibrinolysis Inhibitors

AMINOCAPROIC ACID

Aminocaproic acid (Amicar)—$H_2NCH_2(CH_2)_3$-CH_2COOH— is a synthetic inhibitor of fibrinolysis. It differs from lysine in the lack of an α-amino group. This drug is a competitive inhibitor of plasminogen activation at a concentration of 10^{-4} M. It is rapidly absorbed from the intestine, with peak plasma levels in 2 hours after an oral dose. It is cleared primarily by the kidney. A plasma level of 10^{-3} M can be obtained by a dose of 24 g daily. A loading dose of 4–6 g is usually given when the drug is to be given intravenously. It should be infused over 30 minutes to avoid hypotension. The usual oral dose is 6 g 4 times daily.

The major clinical indication for aminocaproic acid is as an adjunct in the treatment of hemophilia. It has also been used to treat bleeding due to fibrinolytic therapy and to delay rebleeding from intracranial aneurysms at a dose of 24 g daily. Since aminocaproic acid can prevent plasmin-dependent complement activation, it has been used to treat angioneurotic edema due to deficiency of C1 esterase inhibitor.

When used as an adjunct to tooth extraction in a patient with mild to moderate hemophilia, factor concentrates are given to raise the plasma level to 50% of normal, followed by the administration of aminocaproic acid, 0.1 g/kg. Topical thrombin is often applied to the defect after extraction. Oral therapy in a dose of 24 g daily is continued for 7 days. Factor concentrates are given for bleeding. This regimen may not be sufficient for the safe performance of multiple or difficult extractions.

The most important potential adverse effect of the drug is intravascular thrombosis from inhibition of plasminogen activator activity, but this complication is unusual. Other adverse effects are hypotension, abdominal discomfort, diarrhea, and nasal stuffiness.

TRANEXAMIC ACID

Tranexamic acid (Amstat) is an alicyclic amino acid analog of aminocaproic acid that is an inhibitor of plasminogen activation. It has increased potency and perhaps decreased side-effects compared to those of aminocaproic acid. The loading dose for tranexamic acid is 15 mg/kg, and the maintenance dose is 30 mg/kg every 6 hours. The actions of and indications for tranexamic acid are the same as those of aminocaproic acid.

• • •

References

Albrechtson U et al: Streptokinase treatment of deep venous thrombosis and the post-thrombotic syndrome: Follow-up evaluation of venous function. *Arch Surg* 1981;**116**:33.

Coon WW, Willis PW III: Recurrence of venous thromboembolism. *Surgery* 1973;**73**:823.

Crandon AJ et al: Prophylaxis of postooperative deep vein thrombosis: Selective use of low-dose heparin in high-risk patients. *Br Med J* 1980;**281**:345.

Gallop PM, Lian JB, Hauschka PV: Carboxylated calcium-binding proteins and vitamin K. *N Engl J Med* 1980;**302**:1460.

International Multicentre Trial: Prevention of fatal postoperative pulmonary embolism by low dose heparin. *Lancet* 1975;**2**:45.

Lusker JM et al: Efficacy of prothrombin complex concentrates in hemophiliacs with antibodies to factor VIII: A multicenter therapeutic trial. *N Engl J Med* 1980;**303**:421.

Marder VJ: The use of thrombolytic agents: Choice of patient, drug administration, laboratory monitoring. *Ann Intern Med* 1979;**90**:802.

O'Reilly RA et al: Stereoselective interaction of phenylbutazone with $^{12}C/^{13}C$ warfarin pseudoracemates in man. *J Clin Invest* 1980;**65**:746.

Packham MA, Mustard JE: Clinical pharmacology of platelets. *Blood* 1977;**50**:555.

Rosenberg RD, Armand G, Lam I: Structure-function relationships of heparin species. *Proc Natl Acad Sci USA* 1978;**75**:3065.

Simon TL et al: Heparin pharmacokinetics: Increased requirements in pulmonary embolism. *Br J Haematol* 1978;**39**:111.

Smith JB: The prostanoids in hemostasis and thrombosis: A review. *Am J Pathol* 1980;**99**:743.

Stenflo J et al: Vitamin K dependent modification of glutamic acid residues in prothrombin. *Proc Natl Acad Sci USA* 1974;**71**:2730.

Vermylin J et al: Thromboxane synthetase inhibition as antithrombotic strategy. *Lancet* 1981;**1**:1073.

Wilson JE, Bynum LJ, Parkey RW: Heparin therapy in venous thromboemblism. *Am J Med* 1981;**70**:808.

Agents Used In Hyperlipidemia | 32

Mary J. Malloy, MD, & John P. Kane, MD, PhD

Virtually all of the lipids of human plasma are transported as complexes with protein. With the exception of fatty acids, which are bound chiefly to albumin, the lipids are carried in special macromolecular complexes termed **lipoproteins.** A number of metabolic disorders that involve elevations in plasma lipoprotein concentrations are thus termed **hyperlipoproteinemias.** The term **hyperlipemia** is restricted to those conditions in which levels of triglycerides in plasma are increased.

The 2 major clinical sequelae of the hyperlipoproteinemias are acute pancreatitis and atherosclerosis. Acute pancreatitis occurs in patients with marked hyperlipemia. In such persons, control of triglyceride levels can prevent recurrent attacks of this life-threatening disease.

Atherosclerosis is the leading cause of death in the USA and other western countries. There is a considerable body of evidence linking high levels of certain plasma lipoproteins to accelerated atherogenesis. The lipoproteins that contain apolipoprotein (apoprotein, apo) B-100 have been identified as the vehicles in which cholesterol is transported into the artery wall. The atherogenic lipoproteins are the low-density (LDL), intermediate-density (IDL), and very low density (VLDL) species. Apo B-100 interacts with chondroitin sulfate B, a mucopolysaccharide of the artery wall. This interaction is probably important in the in situ degradation of the lipoproteins. Cholesteryl esters, which are found in the atheroma in cells of smooth muscle origin and in macrophages, also appear in the extracellular matrix and induce collagen production by fibroblasts. Certain other factors also contribute to formation of the atheroma. These include hypertension, which is associated with greater flux of lipoprotein into the subintimal region; low levels of high-density lipoproteins (HDL), which appear to be involved in removal of cholesterol from the atheroma; and smoking.

Atherosclerotic disease of both coronary and peripheral arteries appears to be a dynamic process. Evidence from studies both in animals and in humans suggests that progression of atheroma formation can be slowed or even reversed if elevated serum concentrations of the atherogenic lipoproteins can be reduced to normal. Although definitive studies have not been reported in humans, treatment methods that reduce levels of atherogenic lipoproteins in plasma are justified by the reasonable assumption that limiting exposure to these etiologic agents will retard the progress of the disease.

Many of the hyperlipidemic states are associated with the development of xanthomas. These lesions are produced by deposition of lipid in tendons or skin, may be painful or cosmetically unacceptable to the patient, and are another reason for treating the associated hyperlipidemia.

An understanding of the biology of the lipoproteins and the pathophysiology of the various hyperlipidemic states is essential to the rational choice of treatment regimen.

PATHOPHYSIOLOGY OF HYPERLIPOPROTEINEMIA

NORMAL LIPOPROTEIN METABOLISM

Structure

The major lipoproteins of plasma are spherical particles with hydrophobic core regions containing cholesteryl esters and triglycerides. A monolayer of amphiphilic lipids, chiefly unesterified cholesterol and phospholipids, surrounds the core. Specific proteins (apolipoproteins) that bind noncovalently to the lipids are located on the surface. Certain lipoproteins contain very high molecular weight B apoproteins that do not migrate from one particle to another, as do smaller apolipoproteins. These species (B apoproteins) vary in relative apparent molecular weight and are designated by numbers. Apo B-48, found in chylomicrons and their remnants, is formed in the intestine; apo B-100, found in VLDL, VLDL remnants, and LDL (which are formed from VLDL), arises in the liver.

Smaller apoproteins equilibrate among the lipoproteins. Apo A-I is a cofactor for lecithin:cholesterol acyltransferase (LCAT). Apo C-II is a required cofactor for lipoprotein lipase. Apo D catalyzes the transfer of cholesteryl ester from the HDL subspecies containing LCAT to other lipoproteins. Several isoforms of apo E, based on single amino acid substitutions, are recognized. A normal pattern of these isoforms is

Table 32–1. Major lipoproteins of human serum.

	Electrophoretic Mobility in Agarose Gel	Density Interval (g/cm³)	Core Lipids	Diameter (nm)	Apolipoproteins in Order of Quantitative Importance
High-density (HDL)	Alpha	1.21–1.063	Cholesteryl esters	7.5–10.5	A-I, A-II, C, E, D
Low-density (LDL)	Beta	1.063–1.019	Cholesteryl esters	~ 21.5	B-100
Intermediate-density (IDL)	Beta	1.019–1.066	Cholesteryl esters, triglycerides	25–30	B-100, E, C
Very low density (VLDL)	Prebeta, some "slow prebeta"	< 1.006	Triglycerides, some cholesteryl esters	30–100	C species, B-100, E
Chylomicrons	Remain at origin	< 1.006	Triglycerides, some cholesteryl esters	80–500	B-48, C, E, A-I, A-II

required for uptake of lipoprotein remnants by the liver.

The apoprotein contents of various lipoprotein complexes are set forth in Table 32–1.

Synthesis & Catabolism

A. Chylomicrons: Chylomicrons, the largest of the lipoproteins, are formed in the intestine (Fig 32–1). Partial glycerides and fatty acids resulting from the action of pancreatic lipase on dietary triglyceride in the intestinal lumen form micelles that are absorbed by epithelial cells. There, reesterification to triglycerides occurs. Some cholesterol absorbed with micelles is esterified by the acyl-CoA:cholesterol acyltransferase (ACAT) system and, with the triglyceride, forms the chylomicron core. Phospholipids and free cholesterol, together with newly synthesized apo B-48, A-I, and A-II, form the surface monolayer. The nascent chylomicron enters the extracellular lymph space and travels via the intestinal lymphatics and thoracic duct to the bloodstream.

Triglycerides are removed in extrahepatic tissues chiefly through a common pathway with VLDL that involves hydrolysis by the lipoprotein lipase (LPL) system. Heparin and apo C-II are cofactors for this reaction. More than three-fourths of the free fatty acids (FFA) thus derived enter tissue directly. The remainder enter the plasma FFA pool. A progressive decrease in particle diameter occurs as triglycerides in the core are depleted. Surface lipids, apo A-I, apo A-II, and apo C are returned to HDL. The resultant chylomicron "remnants" are taken up by receptor-mediated endocytosis into hepatic parenchymal cells. The cholesteryl esters are hydrolyzed in lysosomes, and cholesterol is then excreted in bile, oxidized and excreted as bile acids, or secreted into plasma in lipoproteins.

B. Very Low Density Lipoproteins (VLDL): VLDL are secreted by liver and are the principal car-

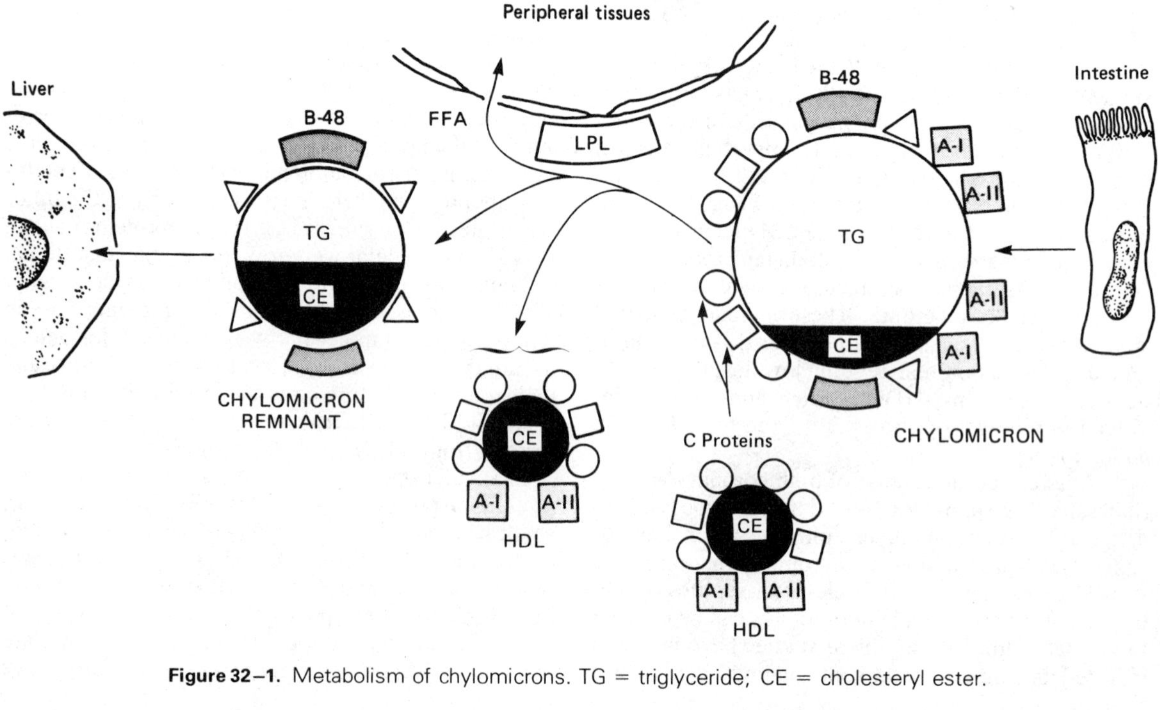

Figure 32–1. Metabolism of chylomicrons. TG = triglyceride; CE = cholesteryl ester.

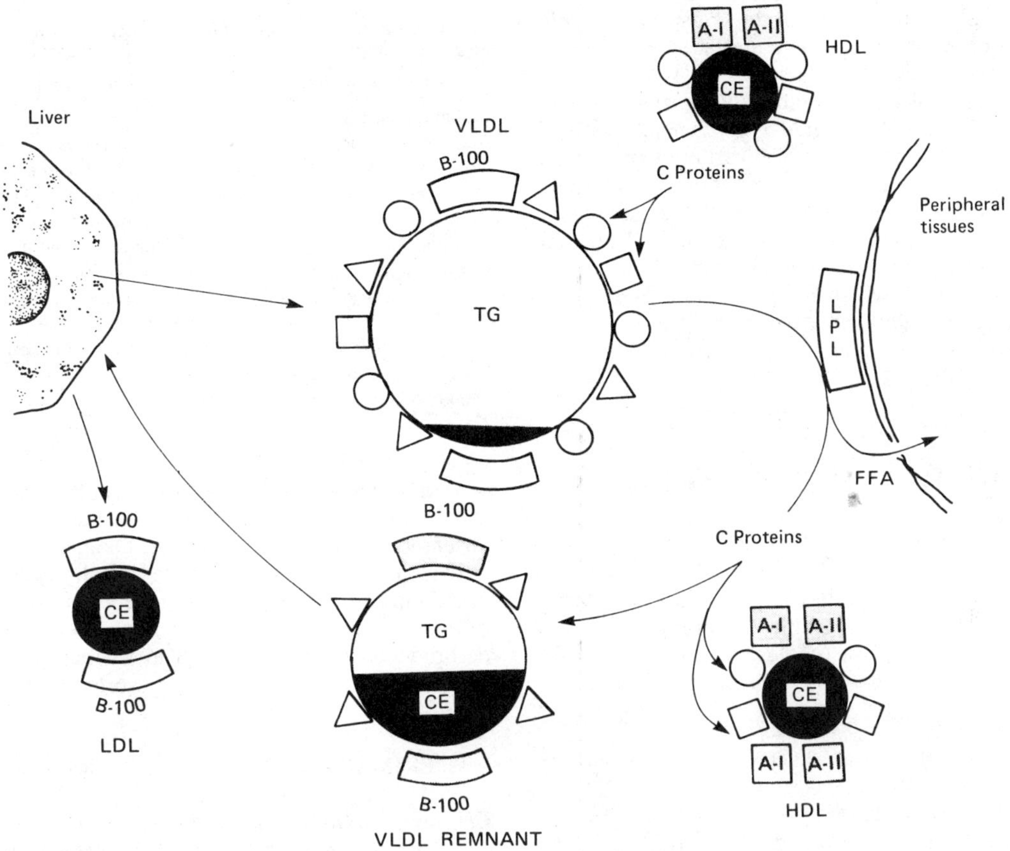

Figure 32–2. Metabolism of very low density lipoproteins. TG = triglyceride; CE = cholesteryl ester.

riers of triglycerides synthesized in liver. VLDL contain apo B-100 but none of the major apoproteins of HDL (Fig 32–2). Some apo C is secreted with the VLDL, and more is acquired from HDL in plasma. Hydrolysis by lipoprotein lipase yields remnant particles that are smaller (25–30 nm in diameter) than those of the chylomicrons (80 nm). Catabolism of VLDL remnants in the liver results in the formation of LDL, which contain mostly cholesteryl esters in the core regions, essentially all of the original complement of apo B-100 from VLDL, and only traces of other apoproteins. The formation of LDL from VLDL explains the clinical phenomenon of the "beta shift," the increase of LDL (β-lipoprotein) in serum as a hypertriglyceridemic state subsides, as in resolving lipemia of diabetes or during treatment with clofibrate. Increased levels of LDL in plasma can thus result from increased secretion of its precursor VLDL as well as from decreased LDL catabolism. In homozygous familial hypercholesterolemia, the liver also appears to secrete an LDL-like lipoprotein directly.

C. Low-Density Lipoproteins (LDL): LDL are apparently catabolized in several ways, including a process of high-affinity receptor-mediated adsorptive endocytosis. The receptors, found in almost all types of cells, are located in "coated pits" of the cell membrane. The apo B binds to the receptor, and an endocytotic vesicle is formed as the coated region invaginates. The vesicles fuse with a lysosome, and apo B is degraded. Cholesteryl esters from the LDL core are hydrolyzed, and the free cholesterol, some of which is used in synthesis of cell membrane, suppresses the de novo formation of cholesterol and leads to down regulation of the LDL receptors. Excess cholesterol is stored, chiefly as cholesteryl oleate.

D. High-Density Lipoproteins (HDL): HDL are secreted from liver in a nascent bilayer disk form. Apolipoproteins E, A-I, and possibly A-II are present in this particle, together with phospholipid and unesterified cholesterol. Through the action of LCAT, the disk form becomes a spherical particle as cholesteryl ester enters the core region between the bilayers. HDL are also formed during catabolism of chylomicrons as surface lipids, and apo A-I and apo A-II dissociate from the chylomicron. Phospholipids and cholesterol released from VLDL hydrolysis also contribute to the formation of HDL. Two major subclasses of HDL, based on flotation properties, have been described: HDL_3 and HDL_2. The HDL_2 content is probably the major reason for the inverse correlation between HDL levels and coronary risk that has been observed in epidemiologic studies. In addition to serving as carriers for the various small apoproteins and delivering cholesterol to the adrenal in support of steroidogenesis, HDL play a major role in the transport of surplus cholesterol away from peripheral tissues. Free cholesterol is transferred to a subspecies of HDL with relatively small molecular weight. "Reverse cholesterol transport" is further mediated by another subspecies of HDL, the esterification-transfer particle that contains LCAT. LCAT catalyzes the formation of cholesteryl esters, which are then transferred with the aid of apo D to LDL and triglyceride-rich lipoproteins. Remnants of the latter normally serve to carry the cholesterol to liver. The ways in which HDL are catabolized are not known, but it appears that peripheral tissues are significantly involved, along with the liver.

Table 32–3. Secondary causes of hyperlipoproteinemia.

Hypertriglyceridemia	Hypercholesterolemia
Diabetes mellitus	Hypothyroidism
Alcohol ingestion	Early nephrosis
Severe nephrosis	Resolving lipemia
Estrogens	Immunoglobulin-lipoprotein complex disorders
Uremia	Hepatic porphyria
Corticosteroid excess	Anorexia nervosa
Hypothyroidism	Cholestasis
Glycogen storage disease	Hypopituitarism
Hypopituitarism	Corticosteroid excess
Acromegaly	
Immunoglobulin-lipoprotein complex disorders	

THE HYPERLIPOPROTEINEMIC STATES

Diagnosis of hyperlipidemia involves a determination that the content of lipids in serum is increased after an overnight fast (cholesterol and triglyceride levels exceeding age- and sex-specific 95th percentile of normal values); differentiation requires identification of the species of lipoproteins that account for the observed increases (Table 32–2). Diagnosis of a specific primary lipoprotein disorder usually necessitates gathering further clinical and genetic data as well as ruling out disorders that can cause secondary hyperlipidemia (Table 32–3). The various patterns of abnormal lipoprotein distribution are described below.

Table 32–2. Drug treatment of hyperlipoproteinemia.

	Single Drug*	Drug Combination
Familial hypertriglyceridemia		
Severe	Nicotinic acid.	
Mild	Clofibrate, nicotinic acid.	
Familial lipoprotein lipase or cofactor deficiency	(Dietary management.)	
Familial dysbetalipoproteinemia	Clofibrate, nicotinic acid.	
Sporadic or unclassified hypertriglyceridemia	Clofibrate, nicotinic acid.	
Familial multiple type hyperlipoproteinemia		
VLDL increased	Nicotinic acid, clofibrate.	
LDL increased	Resin, nicotinic acid.	Resin plus nicotinic acid.
VLDL and LDL increased	Resin, nicotinic acid.	Resin plus nicotinic acid.
Familial hypercholesterolemia		
Heterozygous	Resin.	Resin plus nicotinic acid. Resin plus neomycin.
Homozygous		Resin plus nicotinic acid.
Dietary hypercholesterolemia	Sitosterols.	
Polygenic or unclassified hypercholesterolemia	Resin, nicotinic acid, clofibrate.	

*Where 2 drugs are listed, the first is the preferred drug. Single drug therapy should be evaluated before drug combinations are used, except in the case of homozygous familial hypercholesterolemia, where single drug therapy is known to be ineffective.

PRIMARY HYPERTRIGLYCERIDEMIA

Primary Chylomicronemia

Chylomicrons are not normally present in serum of fasted individuals and generally do not contribute significantly to high levels of triglycerides in serum unless these levels exceed 1000 mg/dL. The autosomal recessive traits of lipoprotein lipase deficiency and lipoprotein lipase cofactor deficiency are usually associated with severe lipemia (2000–25,000 mg/dL triglycerides), which may, however, go undiagnosed until an attack of acute pancreatitis occurs. Patients may have eruptive xanthomas, hepatosplenomegaly, hypersplenism, and lipid-laden foam cells in bone marrow, liver, and spleen. The lipemia is aggravated by estrogens, since they stimulate VLDL production in the liver, and pregnancy may cause marked increases in triglyceride levels in spite of strict dietary control. Although these patients have a predominant chylomicronemia, they may also have moderately elevated VLDL, presenting with a pattern of mixed lipemia. Lipoprotein lipase deficiency is diagnosed by in vitro assay of lipolytic activity in plasma after intravenous injection of heparin; cofactor deficiency is diagnosed by isoelectric focusing or electrophoresis of the VLDL proteins. A presumptive diagnosis of these disorders is justified by demonstrating a precipitous drop in the plasma triglyceride level a few days after sharp restriction of oral fat intake. Marked restriction of the total fat content in the diet provides effective treatment.

Mixed Lipemia

A pattern of mixed lipemia (fasting chylomicronemia and elevated VLDL) usually results from impaired removal of triglyceride-rich lipoproteins, although factors that increase VLDL production aggravate the lipemia because VLDL and chylomicrons are competing substrates for lipoprotein lipase. The primary mixed lipemias probably represent a variety of modes of inheritance. Most patients have the hypertrophic form of obesity with impaired effectiveness of insulin. In addition to obesity, other factors that lead to increased rate of secretion of VLDL also aggravate the lipemia. Eruptive xanthomas, lipemia retinalis, epigastric pain, and overt pancreatitis are variably present, depending on the severity of the lipemia. Treatment is primarily dietary, with restriction of total fat, avoidance of alcohol, and weight reduction to ideal levels. An occasional patient may require treatment with clofibrate or nicotinic acid.

Endogenous Lipemia

Primary increases of VLDL levels probably reflect a number of genetic determinants and are worsened by factors that increase the rate of VLDL secretion from liver, ie, hypertrophic obesity, alcohol ingestion, diabetes, and exogenous estrogens. A major indication for treatment of these patients is the apparent atherogenicity of VLDL. Treatment includes weight reduction to ideal levels, restriction of all types of dietary fat, and avoidance of alcohol. Clofibrate or nicotinic acid usually produces further reduction in triglyceride levels if dietary measures do not reduce them below 600–700 mg/dL.

Multiple Type Hyperlipoproteinemia (Combined Hyperlipidemia)

In kindreds with this disorder, individuals may have elevated levels of VLDL, LDL, or both, and the patterns may change with time. The basic defect is increased production of apo B in VLDL, and factors that increase levels of triglyceride in serum in other disorders do so in this syndrome as well. Elevations of serum cholesterol and triglycerides are usually mild, and xanthomas do not occur. However, drug treatment is warranted because the risk of coronary atherosclerosis is increased, and diet alone usually does not normalize lipid levels. Patients with elevated VLDL respond to nicotinic acid or clofibrate; those with elevated LDL respond to bile acid resins but often have secondary elevations in VLDL, requiring the addition of nicotinic acid.

Disorders in Which Remnant Particles Accumulate

In familial dysbetalipoproteinemia, normal VLDL of prebeta electrophoretic mobility are present. There are also VLDL with beta mobility and remnant particles of intermediate density (IDL). Levels of LDL are usually decreased, probably a reflection of interrupted transformation of VLDL to LDL. There is an apparent defect in the removal of VLDL and chylomicron remnants from plasma. Because these remnants are rich in cholesteryl esters, the level of serum cholesterol may be as high as that of triglycerides. Diagnosis is confirmed by the virtual absence of the E_3 and E_4 isoforms of apo E detected on isoelectric focusing of the apolipoproteins of VLDL. Individuals heterozygous for this disorder may have intensification of lipemia from other causes. Patients often develop tuberous or tuberoeruptive xanthomas or a characteristic planar xanthoma of the palmar creases. Xanthelasma may also occur. The patients are often obese, and some have impaired glucose tolerance. These factors, together with hypothyroidism, aggravate the lipemia. Coronary and peripheral vascular atherosclerotic disease occurs with increased frequency. A weight reduction diet, together with decreased cholesterol and alcohol ingestion, often is sufficient treatment. Occasionally, low doses of clofibrate or nicotinic acid are needed.

PRIMARY HYPERCHOLESTEROLEMIA

Familial Hypercholesterolemia

This disorder is transmitted as an autosomal dominant trait and, although levels of LDL tend to increase throughout childhood, the diagnosis can often be made at birth on the basis of elevated umbilical cord blood cholesterol and a family history of affected first-degree relatives. In heterozygous adults, serum cholesterol levels range from about 325 to 500 mg/dL. Triglycerides are usually normal, tendinous xanthomatosis is often present, and arcus corneae and xanthelasma may occur in the third decade. Coronary atherosclerosis occurs prematurely in these patients, particularly those who also have HDL deficiencies. Homozygous familial hypercholesterolemia, which is often fatal in the second decade, is characterized by very high levels of cholesterol in serum (often exceeding 1000 mg/dL) and early tuberous and tendinous xanthomatosis. These patients may also develop elevated plaquelike xanthomas of the digital webs, buttocks, and extremities.

At least 3 types of defects involving the high-affinity receptor sites for LDL on cell membranes have been recognized in patients with familial hypercholesterolemia. These include receptors with no binding capacity, receptors with impaired capacity, and inability of cells to internalize bound LDL. Homozygotes have no normal receptors; heterozygotes have about half the usual number; and some individuals apparently have combined heterozygosity.

Treatment of the homozygote is very difficult. Repeated plasmapheresis in conjunction with combined drug therapy is currently the most effective method of management. Levels of LDL in compliant heterozygotes can be normalized with a combination of a bile acid-binding resin and nicotinic acid.

Multiple Type Hyperlipoproteinemia

As described above, some persons in kindreds with this disorder have only an elevation in LDL. Xanthomas are absent, and levels of serum cholesterol usually are less than 350 mg/dL. Premature onset of coronary disease is common. Dietary and drug treatment, usually with a bile acid-binding resin, is indicated. It may be necessary to add nicotinic acid to normalize LDL levels or to lower triglycerides should they rise during treatment with the resin.

Other Types of Hypercholesterolemias

Individuals in some kindreds who have elevated LDL concentrations have strikingly favorable responses to dietary management. A polygenic form of hypercholesterolemia occurs, as well as recessive types. Some of the latter individuals may have LDL that contain plant sterols.

Some persons have very high levels of Lp(a) lipoprotein, normally only a minor fraction of circulating lipoproteins, which distributes about the ultracentrifugal density that discriminates HDL from LDL. It contains apo B-100 and appears to be atherogenic. The regimen combining resin and nicotinic acid appears to be effective.

DEFICIENCY OF HDL

Certain rare genetic disorders are associated with extremely low levels of HDL in serum. More commonly, moderate decreases of HDL levels occur in familial distribution. These patients tend to have premature coronary atherosclerosis, and the low HDL levels may be the only identified risk factor. Treatment currently consists only of special attention to avoidance of other risk factors for coronary disease. Nicotinic acid increases HDL cholesterol levels, at least in hyperlipidemic subjects, and may prove to be useful in management of familial hypoalphalipoproteinemia. However, at present, attempting to increase HDL levels with drugs cannot be recommended because the basis for the association between coronary risk in normotriglyceridemic subjects and low levels of HDL is still unclear.

SECONDARY HYPERLIPOPROTEINEMIA

Before the diagnosis of primary hyperlipoproteinemia can be made, secondary causes of the specific phenotype must be considered. The more common conditions that may be associated with hyperlipoproteinemia are summarized in Table 32–3. The lipoprotein abnormality usually resolves with treatment of the underlying disorder.

Certain persons, often with a preexisting mild lipemia, develop severe hypertriglyceridemia when given even small doses of estrogens, such as those in contraceptives. This effect is smaller when the estrogen is used in very low dosage relative to the progestational agent.

Treatment of the hyperlipidemia associated with chronic nephrotic syndrome is probably indicated, since coronary vascular disease is prevalent in these patients. Diet has little effect. Clofibrate is contraindicated, because it may precipitate myopathy. Currently, the drugs of choice are bile acid-binding resins combined with nicotinic acid. Tryptophan supplementation ameliorates hypertriglyceridemia in some nephrotic patients who may be deficient in this amino acid.

The hyperlipidemia associated with cholestasis involves abnormal lipoproteins, including LP-X, vesicular particles rich in unesterified cholesterol and phospholipid; LP-Y, which contains large amounts of triglycerides and carries apo B; and LDL containing unusually large amounts of triglycerides. Neuropathy, caused by xanthomatous involvement of nerves, is an indication for treatment of this hyperlipidemia. Although plasmapheresis is most effective, bile acid-binding resins may be of some value. Clofibrate is contraindicated, since it causes an increase in serum cholesterol in these patients.

DIETARY MANAGEMENT OF HYPERLIPOPROTEINEMIA

When the decision is made to treat hyperlipoproteinemia, dietary measures are always initiated first and may obviate the need for drugs. Cholesterol and saturated fats are the principal dietary factors that influence lipoprotein levels in plasma. Dietary cholesterol primarily contributes to an increase in levels of LDL, but this response varies considerably among individuals. Saturated fats increase the concentration of LDL and, when substituted for polyunsaturated fats, may also produce some increase in VLDL levels.

Lipoprotein levels are also affected, but to a lesser extent, by other dietary factors. Transient increases in VLDL occur when carbohydrate intake is acutely increased. Sucrose and other simple sugars may raise VLDL levels in an occasional hypertriglyceridemic patient. Pectin is probably the only form of dietary fiber that reduces LDL levels appreciably. Alcohol can cause significant hypertriglyceridemia by increasing hepatic secretion of VLDL. HDL levels may be increased by alcohol ingestion. Synthesis and secretion of VLDL are increased by excess caloric intake. Caloric restriction, especially in obese subjects, reduces VLDL triglycerides and also reduces levels of LDL, particularly in persons with combined hyperlipidemia.

Most patients with hyperlipidemia can be managed appropriately with a diet that is restricted in cholesterol and saturated fat but provides calories to achieve and maintain ideal body weight. Total fat calories should be 20–25%, with saturated fats less than 10% of total calories and cholesterol less than 200 mg/d. Reductions in serum cholesterol range from 20 to 30% on this regimen, except in heterozygous familial hypercholesterolemia, where the response is smaller. Increases in complex carbohydrates and fiber are recommended, but large increases in polyunsaturated fats should be avoided. Weight reduction and caloric restriction are especially important for patients with elevated VLDL and IDL. Patients with hypertriglyceridemia should avoid alcohol.

Patients with primary chylomicronemia must consume a diet severely restricted in total fat: 10–15 g/d, of which 5 g should be vegetable oils rich in essential fatty acids. Supplementation of fat-soluble vitamins should be given.

SPECIFIC DRUGS USED IN TREATMENT

Decisions to use drug therapy for hyperlipidemia must be based on the specific physiologic defect and its potential for causing atherosclerosis or pancreatitis. Suggested drug treatments for the principal lipoprotein disorders are presented in Table 32–2. Diet is a necessary adjunct to drug therapy and should be continued for achievement of the full potential of the drug regimen. Drug treatment of hyperlipidemia should be avoided in women who are likely to become pregnant or who are lactating. Children with heterozygous familial hypercholesterolemia may be treated with a bile acid-binding resin, usually after age 7 or 8, when myelination of the central nervous system is essentially complete. Any drug therapy in children is, however, still experimental, and the decision to treat an individual child should be based on the level of plasma LDL, the family history, and the child's age.

NICOTINIC ACID

Nicotinic acid (but not nicotinamide) decreases VLDL and LDL levels in the plasma of patients with a variety of hyperlipidemias.

Chemistry & Pharmacokinetics

Nicotinic acid (niacin) is a water-soluble vitamin with the chemical structure shown below. It is converted in the body to the amide, which is incorporated into nicotinamide adenine dinucleotide (NAD). It is excreted unmodified in the urine and as nicotinamide, N-methyl-2-pyridone-3-carboxamide, N-methyl-2-pyridone-5-carboxamide, and other less abundant metabolites.

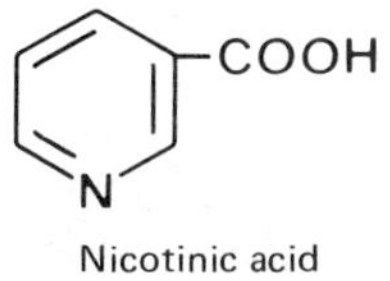

Nicotinic acid

Mechanism of Action

The primary mechanism of action of nicotinic acid probably involves inhibition of VLDL secretion, in turn decreasing production of LDL. Decreased incorporation of amino acids into apo VLDL has been demonstrated. Increased clearance of VLDL via the lipoprotein lipase pathway contributes to the triglyceride-lowering effect of nicotinic acid. The drug has no effect on bile acid production. Excretion of neutral sterols in the stool is increased acutely as cholesterol is mobilized from tissue pools. A new steady state is then reached during chronic administration of the drug. Cholesterogenesis is inhibited, an effect that persists when bile acid-binding resins are given. This synergism provides evidence that the effect of nicotinic acid on cholesterol synthesis is a primary one. Decreased synthesis of cholesterol in liver can increase hepatic uptake of LDL in support of increased bile acid synthesis induced by the resin. The catabolic rate for HDL is decreased, with an associated increase in the HDL_2 subfraction and high levels of HDL cholesterol and apo A-1 in plasma. The processes of atherogenesis or thrombosis may be influenced by the substantial reduction of circulating fibrinogen levels produced by nicotinic acid. This agent is also a potent inhibitor of the intracellular lipase system of adipose tissue, possibly reducing VLDL production by decreasing the flux of free fatty acids to liver. Sustained inhibition of lipolysis has not been established, however.

Therapeutic Uses

In combination with a bile acid-binding resin, nicotinic acid has been found to normalize levels of LDL in patients with heterozygous familial hypercholesterolemia. This drug combination is also indicated in some cases of nephrosis. In severe mixed lipemia, which is incompletely responsive to dietary measures, nicotinic acid often produces marked reduction of triglyceride levels in plasma. It is also useful in lipemic patients with multiple type hyperlipoproteinemia and in those with familial dysbetalipoproteinemia.

Dosage

For combined drug treatment of heterozygous familial hypercholesterolemia, most patients require 6–7.5 g daily orally; more than this should not be given. For other types of hypercholesterolemia and for hypertriglyceridemia, 1.5–3.5 g daily orally is usually sufficient. The drug should be given in divided doses with meals, starting with 100 mg 3 times daily and increasing gradually.

Toxicity

Most persons experience a harmless cutaneous vasodilatation and an uncomfortable sensation of warmth after each dose when the drug is first started or the dose is increased. Taking 0.3 g of aspirin about half an hour beforehand blunts this prostaglandin-mediated effect: Tachyphylaxis to this side-effect usually occurs within a few days at any dose level. The physician should warn the patient to expect this annoying side-effect and should explain why it occurs. Pruritus, rashes, dry skin, and acanthosis nigricans have been reported. Some patients experience nausea and abdominal discomfort. This drug should be avoided in patients with severe peptic disease. Moderate elevations in levels of transaminases or alkaline phosphatase may occur, usually not associated with serious liver toxicity. However, liver function should be monitored regularly. This effect is reversible and is minimized if the daily dose is increased by no more than 2.5 g in a month. Carbohydrate tolerance may be moderately impaired, but this is also reversible. In some patients with latent diabetes, however, this effect may be more evident and incompletely reversible, and nicotinic acid should be used with caution in such persons. Hyperuricemia occurs in about one-fifth of patients receiving nicotinic acid, but it probably becomes symptomatic only in those with preexisting gout. Rarely described conditions associated with the use of nicotinic acid include arrhythmias, mostly atrial, and toxic amblyopia.

CLOFIBRATE

Clofibrate (Atromid-S) decreases levels of VLDL in plasma. Levels of LDL are also decreased in some patients. LDL and HDL levels often increase in hypertriglyceridemic patients during treatment with clofibrate. In some patients with hypertriglyceridemia, there may be marked increases of LDL in plasma as levels of VLDL are reduced, thus increasing the levels of another atherogenic lipoprotein. Bile acid-binding resins may be added to control this effect, or nicotinic acid may be substituted for clofibrate.

Chemistry & Pharmacokinetics

Clofibrate is the ethyl ester of chlorphenoxyisobutyric acid. Upon absorption, the ester group is hydrolyzed, by tissue and plasma esterases, and the anion is transported, mostly bound to albumin, in plasma. Although mainly distributed to the extracellular space, some anion is found in tissues (eg, liver). The drug is excreted in urine as the glucuronide. In humans, its plasma half-life is about 12 hours.

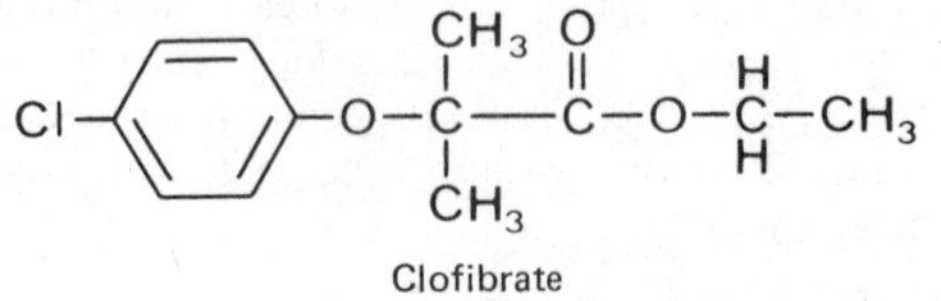

Clofibrate

Mechanism of Action

The principal effect of clofibrate is to increase the clearance of triglyceride-rich lipoproteins via an increase in the activity of lipoprotein lipase. Secretion of VLDL from liver is unaffected in hypertriglyceridemic patients and actually appears to be increased in normotriglyceridemic subjects treated with clofibrate. This flux of LDL precursor could explain the lack of significant synergism in most patients with heterozygous familial hypercholesterolemia treated with a combination of bile acid-binding resin and clofibrate. This combination, however, may have some use in persons with uncharacterized mild elevations of LDL. In hypercholesterolemic patients, body cholesterol pools are decreased as fecal and biliary cholesterol excretions are increased. Fecal excretion of bile acids is reduced. Absorption of cholesterol is unaffected. Cholesterol biosynthesis in liver is inhibited, perhaps as a result of changes in VLDL secretion and catabolism. Fatty acid oxidation by liver may be increased. The content of triglycerides in HDL is reduced by clofibrate, whereas total HDL concentration is often increased. These effects appear to be related to the fall in VLDL concentration.

Therapeutic Uses

Clofibrate usually produces marked reduction in serum triglycerides and triglyceride-rich lipoproteins in patients with familial dysbetalipoproteinemia. VLDL levels are also reduced in individuals with moderately severe endogenous hypertriglyceridemia. Because its primary effect appears to be stimulation of the lipoprotein lipase mechanism, clofibrate has no effect on the lipemia of patients with primary chylomicronemia due to congenital deficiency of lipoprotein lipase. It has variable effect on severe mixed lipemia and is of no value in treating familial hypercholesterolemia. If LDL levels are only moderately elevated, they may be decreased by the use of clofibrate.

Dosage

The usual dose of clofibrate (Atromid-S) is 2 g daily orally in 2 doses; 0.5 g daily may be sufficient in patients with familial dysbetalipoproteinemia.

Toxicity

Nausea and abdominal discomfort are the most common adverse side-effects. Myalgia associated with increased plasma levels of creatine phosphokinase and occasionally involving the myocardium has been reported. This tends to occur more frequently in patients with low serum albumin levels, and clofibrate should therefore be avoided in nephrotic subjects. It should also be given in reduced dosage (if at all) to patients with azotemia. A weak association with gastrointestinal tract carcinoma has been reported, as has a modest increase in the incidence of cholelithiasis. The hypoglycemic effect of sulfonylureas may be enhanced by clofibrate, and it may also potentiate activities of indandione and coumarin anticoagulants by decreasing platelet reactivity. At least at the onset of clofibrate therapy, dosage of these anticoagulants should be reduced by 30–50%. Dermatitis, hepatic dysfunction, and bone marrow depression are rare toxic effects.

Some men taking clofibrate report decreased libido and breast tenderness. Brittle hair and alopecia have also been reported.

GEMFIBROZIL

Gemfibrozil (Lopid) is a newly developed congener of clofibrate that resembles the parent drug pharmacologically.

Chemistry & Pharmacokinetics

The gemfibrozil molecule differs from clofibrate in its aliphatic chain and in the presence of 2 methyl groups rather than a chlorine atom on the phenoxy group. It is supplied as the free carboxylic acid. Gemfibrozil is absorbed quantitatively from the intestine and is tightly bound to plasma proteins. It undergoes enterohepatic circulation and readily passes the placenta. Its plasma half-life is 1½ hours. Seventy percent is eliminated through the kidneys, mostly unmodified. However, the liver modifies a portion of the methyl functions to hydroxymethyl or carboxyl derivatives and some of the compound to a quinol.

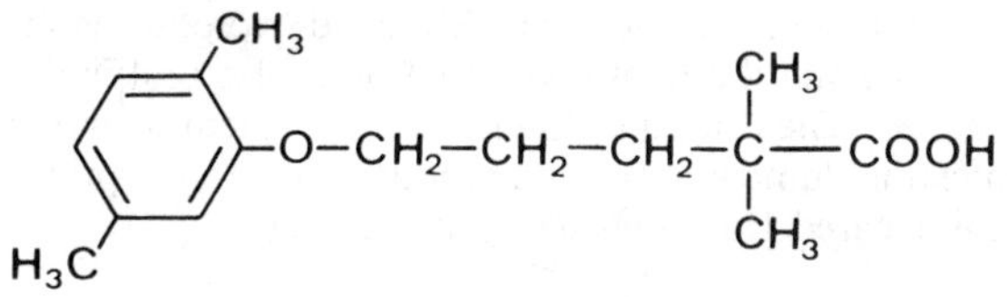

Gemfibrozil

Mechanism of Action

This agent decreases lipolysis in adipose tissue. There is a decrease in levels of VLDL in plasma, attributed in part to a decreased flux of free fatty acids to liver from adipose tissue. Only modest reductions of LDL levels occur, and HDL cholesterol levels increase moderately. Whether the latter effect is greater than with clofibrate is not established. Part of the apparent increase of HDL cholesterol levels is a direct consequence of decreasing the content of triglycerides in plasma with reduction in exchange of triglycerides into HDL in place of cholesterol. Some increase in the protein moiety of HDL has been reported with gemfibrozil.

Therapeutic Uses

The indications for this drug in hypertriglyceridemia are the same as for clofibrate. However, gemfibrozil may be somewhat more effective in reducing triglyceride levels. There is as yet no established indication for attempting to increase HDL levels with drugs, since the effect of doing so on atherosclerotic disease is unknown.

The usual dose of gemfibrozil (Lopid) is 600 mg orally twice daily.

Toxicity

Many of the toxic effects associated with clofibrate appear with this congener also. Skin rashes and gastrointestinal and muscular symptoms have been described. High levels of transaminases or alkaline phosphatase in blood have been reported. A few patients show decreases in white blood count or hematocrit. Gemfibrozil potentiates the action of coumarin or indandione anticoagulants. Doses of these agents must be reduced during therapy with gemfibrozil.

BILE ACID–BINDING RESINS

Colestipol (Colestid) and cholestyramine (Questran) are useful only in hyperlipoproteinemias involving LDL elevations. Patients who have hypertriglyceridemia in addition to elevated LDL may have increased levels of VLDL during treatment with the resins.

Chemistry & Pharmacokinetics

Colestipol and cholestyramine are very large polymeric cationic exchange resins that are insoluble in water. They bind bile acids in the intestinal lumen and prevent their reabsorption. Chloride is released from cationic quaternary ammonium binding sites in exchange for bile acids, but the resin itself is not absorbed.

Mechanism of Action

The bile acids, metabolites of cholesterol, are normally reabsorbed in the jejunum with about 95% efficiency. Their excretion is increased up to 10-fold when the resins are given. This results in lower levels of LDL in plasma because, although cholesterol synthesis by both liver and intestine is increased, the fractional catabolic rate of LDL also increases. The increased catabolism of cholesterol reflects its enhanced conversion to bile acids in liver via 7α-hydroxylation, normally controlled by negative feedback by bile acids. The content of cholesteryl esters in LDL decreases somewhat, and body cholesterol pools are decreased during treatment. It appears that increased uptake of LDL from plasma in patients treated with the resins results from increased numbers of high-affinity LDL receptors on cell membranes, particularly in liver. Hence, the resins are without effect in patients with homozygous familial hypercholesterolemia who have no functioning receptors, but they may be useful in patients with receptor-defective combined heterozygosity.

Therapeutic Uses

The resins are used in treatment of patients with heterozygous familial hypercholesterolemia, producing approximately 20% reduction in LDL cholesterol when used in maximal dosage. Larger reductions at lower dosages may be expected in patients with less severe forms of hypercholesterolemia. If the resins are used to treat LDL elevations in persons with combined hyperlipidemia, they may cause an increase in levels of VLDL that would require the addition of a second agent. The resins are also used in combination with other drugs to achieve a further hypocholesterolemic effect (see below). In addition to their use in hyperlipidemia, they may be helpful in relieving itching in patients who have cholestasis and bile salt accumulation. Since they bind digitalis glycosides, the resins may be used to increase the rate of removal of digitalis from the body in severe digitalis toxicity.

Colestipol (Colestid) and cholestyramine (Questran) are granular preparations available in packets of 5 g and 4 g, respectively, or in bulk. The usual starting dose is 20 g orally daily. Total doses of 30–32 g daily may be needed for maximum effect. The usual dose for a child is 15–20 g daily. The resins are mixed with juice or water and allowed to hydrate for 1 minute. They should be taken in 3 doses, preferably with meals.

Toxicity

The most common complaints are constipation and a bloating sensation, easily relieved by eating bran. Heartburn and diarrhea are occasionally reported. In patients who have preexisting bowel disease or cholestasis, steatorrhea may occur. Bowel obstruction and deficiencies of fat-soluble vitamins have also been reported. Malabsorption of vitamin K may lead to hypoprothrombinemia, and prothrombin time should be measured frequently in patients who are taking resins and anticoagulants. Malabsorption of folic acid has been reported rarely. Increased formation of gallstones, particularly in obese persons, was an anticipated side-effect but has rarely occurred in practice. Another occasional problem is dry flaking skin, which is relieved by application of lanolin. Absorption of certain drugs, including those with neutral or cationic charge as well as anions, may be impaired by the resins. These include digitalis glycosides, chlorothiazide, hydrochlorothiazide, warfarin, tetracycline, vancomycin, thyroxine, iron salts, folic acid, and phenylbutazone. Any medication the patient is taking should be given 1 hour before the resin to ensure adequate absorption.

SITOSTEROLS

Pharmacokinetics & Mechanism of Action

β-Sitosterol is the principal component of a suspension of mixed phytosterols (Cytellin). It is poorly absorbed from the intestine and appears to inhibit both absorption of dietary cholesterol and reabsorption of endogenous cholesterol. The structure of sitosterols is similar to that of cholesterol, differing only in having an ethyl group at carbon 24 of the side chain. Although there is an associated increase in cholesterogenesis when this agent is given, it does produce a decrease in serum levels of cholesterol in some patients. There is recent evidence, however, that it may appreciably reduce HDL cholesterol levels as well.

Therapeutic Uses

Although the effect of this drug on serum cholesterol levels is variable, ranging from no response to moderate reduction, it may be useful in treating patients with mild hypercholesterolemia, particularly those in whom dietary cholesterol plays an important role. It has little or no value when used as a single agent for the treatment of heterozygous familial hypercholesterolemia, but it may potentiate the effect of agents that increase biliary excretion of cholesterol.

The drug is available as sitosterols (Cytellin) in liquid suspension containing 3 g per 15 mL. It is usually given in divided doses with meals. The total daily dose is 3–6 g.

Toxicity

The only reported side-effect has been constipation, which is uncommon. The drug is contraindicated in patients with β-sitosterolemia, who absorb abnormally large amounts of plant sterols.

NEOMYCIN

Pharmacokinetics & Mechanism of Action

This poorly absorbed antibiotic inhibits cholesterol absorption, producing moderate reductions in levels of serum cholesterol. Bile acid excretion is increased, and the total body pool of cholesterol is decreased. The drug may alter micellar structures in the intestinal lumen, accounting for their poor absorption. It is cleared from plasma by the kidney.

Therapeutic Uses

Neomycin is perhaps of greatest value when used in combination with a resin to treat patients with heterozygous familial hypercholesterolemia who cannot tolerate nicotinic acid. In such patients, this combination reduces LDL levels in plasma by approximately 35%.

Dosage

The total daily dose is 0.5–2 g, usually in 2 divided doses with meals.

Toxicity

The dosage of neomycin is limited by severe side-effects. Even at low doses, nausea, abdominal cramps, diarrhea, and malabsorption have been reported. Overgrowth of resistant microorganisms may lead to enterocolitis. In patients with bowel disease, absorption of the drug may be enhanced, so that otic, hepatic, and hematopoietic toxicity will occur with greater frequency. In patients with normal bowel function, these effects are unusual at doses under 2 g daily. Neomycin also impairs absorption of digitalis glycosides. It should not be given to patients with renal disease.

HMG-CoA REDUCTASE INHIBITORS

Several potent competitive inhibitors of cholesterol biosynthesis have been isolated from fungi. Substantial reduction of levels of LDL in plasma has been achieved in human trials with one of them, compactin. The usefulness of these agents will be determined by the outcome of toxicity tests now in progress.

Other Drugs

DEXTROTHYROXINE

Dextrothyroxine (Choloxin) is a synthetic analog of thyroxine that was developed in an attempt to utilize the capacity of levothyroxine to regulate plasma LDL levels while eliminating its hypercalorigenic and related adrenergic effects. It has been shown that thyroxine stimulates the α-hydroxylase reaction, the rate-limiting step in the conversion of cholesterol to bile acids. It also appears to increase the number of high-affinity receptors for LDL on cell membranes and tends to increase fecal excretion of neutral sterol. However, dextrothyroxine apparently retains some calorigenic effects, since its use may be associated with arrhythmias and increased angina pectoris. Decreases of only about 20% in levels of cholesterol in serum of hypercholesterolemic patients have been reported even at higher dosage (6–8 mg daily). The use of dextrothyroxine is indicated only in rare instances in patients with no demonstrable heart disease who cannot tolerate the resins or nicotinic acid.

PROBUCOL

Probucol (Lorelco), introduced fairly recently, does not resemble in chemical structure any of the other agents used to lower lipoprotein levels. Its mechanisms of action are unclear, but it may inhibit cholesterogenesis. It is lipophilic, distributes into adipose tissue, and thus persists in tissues for a long time. An average of 20% of peak blood levels persist 6 months following cessation of treatment. Serious toxicity has been demonstrated in animals (arrhythmias, prolonged Q–T interval). Its utility is further severely limited by its effect on HDL-protein synthesis, substantially reducing HDL cholesterol and apo A-I levels in plasma. It produces only a modest reduction in LDL cholesterol levels.

Treatment With Drug Combinations

Combined drug therapy is useful in the following instances: (1) when VLDL levels are significantly increased during treatment of hypercholesterolemia with a bile acid-binding resin; (2) when LDL and VLDL levels are both elevated initially; and (3) when LDL levels are not normalized with a bile acid sequestrant alone.

CLOFIBRATE/BILE ACID–BINDING RESIN

In familial hypercholesterolemia, this combination produces some decrease in VLDL levels in plasma but offers no advantage over the resins alone in lowering LDL levels in familial hypercholesterolemia. Although clofibrate is said to inhibit cholesterol biosynthesis, it apparently cannot overcome the massively increased cholesterogenesis induced by the resin. There is a theoretic risk of further increasing lithogenicity of bile with this drug combination.

NEOMYCIN/BILE ACID–BINDING RESIN

Serum cholesterol levels in patients with heterozygous familial hypercholesterolemia are reduced by about 35% with this combination, which may be of use in patients who cannot tolerate nicotinic acid (see below).

SITOSTEROLS/BILE ACID–BINDING RESIN

The LDL cholesterol levels of some patients with familial hypercholesterolemia are lowered somewhat more with this combination than with a resin alone.

HMG-CoA REDUCTASE INHIBITORS/ BILE ACID–BINDING RESIN

Highly synergistic effects in lowering LDL cholesterol levels in animals have been reported with this combination. Although the inhibitors are not yet available in the USA, they may hold great promise for the future.

NICOTINIC ACID/BILE ACID–BINDING RESIN

This combination is effective both in controlling VLDL levels (during treatment with resins or in treating disorders in which VLDL and LDL levels are both increased) and in normalizing levels of LDL in patients with familial hypercholesterolemia.

Nicotinic acid, when used alone, has a marked effect on levels of VLDL and chylomicrons and usually normalizes triglyceride levels if they increase when the patient is given a bile acid-binding resin. When VLDL and LDL levels are both increased initially, the doses of nicotinic acid required for treatment in combination with a resin may be as low as 1.5–3 g daily.

The nicotinic acid-colestipol combination is the most effective regimen to date for treating heterozygous familial hypercholesterolemia. This probably reflects (1) the summation of increased catabolism of LDL due to the resin, (2) decreased synthesis of its precursor VLDL attributable to nicotinic acid, and perhaps also (3) the ability of nicotinic acid to inhibit cholesterol biosynthesis in the liver. The nicotinic acid also produces significant elevation in levels of HDL cholesterol, presumably an added beneficial effect of treatment.

Diameters of tendinous xanthomas in patients

with heterozygous familial hypercholesterolemia are significantly reduced during treatment with this regimen, indicating that it is capable of mobilizing cholesterol from tissue sites. Effects on lipoprotein levels are sustained (some patients have now been treated as long as 8 years), and no additional toxicity or side-effect beyond those encountered when the drugs are used singly has developed. In fact, because the resin has acid-neutralizing properties, the gastric irritation produced by the nicotinic acid in some persons is relieved when they take the drugs in combination. The drugs may be taken together, because it has been shown that although nicotinic acid is an anion, it does not bind to the resins, so that its absorption from the intestine is not impeded. Complete normalization of levels of LDL in heterozygous familial hypercholesterolemia is usually attained with daily doses of 6.5 g of nicotinic acid in conjunction with 24–30 g of resin.

Some patients with homozygous familial hypercholesterolemia have a modest decrease in LDL levels when taking this drug combination, but most have had no change.

• • •

References

Differentiation of Hyperlipidemias

Brunzell JD, Bierman EL: Chylomicronemia syndrome: Interaction of genetic and acquired hypertriglyceridemia. *Med Clin North Am* 1982;**66:**455.

Fredrickson DS, Goldstein JL, Brown MS: The familial hyperlipoproteinemias. Pages 604–655 in: *The Metabolic Basis of Inherited Disease,* 4th ed. Stanbury JB, Wyngaarden JB, Fredrickson DS (editors). McGraw-Hill, 1978.

Havel RJ: Classification of the hyperlipidemias. *Annu Rev Med* 1977;**28:**195.

Havel RJ: Familial dysbetalipoproteinemia: New aspects of pathogenesis and diagnosis. *Med Clin North Am* 1982;**66:**441.

Havel RJ (editor): Approach to the patient with hyperlipidemia. *Med Clin North Am* 1982;**66:**319.

Havel RJ, Goldstein JL, Brown MS: Lipoproteins and lipid transport. Pages 393–494 in: *Metabolic Control and Disease,* 8th ed. Bondy PK, Rosenberg LE (editors). Saunders, 1980.

Dietary Treatment

Connor WE, Connor SL: The dietary treatment of hyperlipidemia. *Med Clin North Am* 1982;**66:**485.

Drug Treatment

Grundy SM: Hypertriglyceridemia: Mechanisms, clinical significance, and treatment. *Med Clin North Am* 1982;**66:**519.

Havel RJ, Kane JP: Drugs and lipid metabolism. *Annu Rev Pharmacol Toxicol* 1973;**13:**287.

Havel RJ, Kane JP: Therapy of hyperlipidemic states. *Annu Rev Med* 1982;**33:**417.

Kane JP, Malloy MJ: Treatment of hypercholesterolemia. *Med Clin North Am* 1982;**66:**537.

Kane JP et al: Normalization of low-density lipoprotein levels in heterozygous familial hypercholesterolemia with a combined drug regimen. *N Engl J Med* 1981;**304:**251.

Nonsteroidal Anti-inflammatory Agents; Nonopiate Analgesics; Drugs Used in Gout | 33

Martin A. Shearn, MD

I. NONSTEROIDAL ANTI-INFLAMMATORY AGENTS

Salicylates and other agents used to treat rheumatic disease share the capacity to suppress the signs and symptoms of inflammation. Some of the drugs also exert antipyretic and analgesic effects, but it is their anti-inflammatory properties that make them useful in management of disorders in which pain is related to the intensity of the inflammatory process. Drugs employed for their anti-inflammatory properties are heterogeneous in chemical structure and diverse in mechanism of action.

ASPIRIN

Aspirin and the newer nonsteroidal anti-inflammatory drugs (NSAIDs) (ibuprofen, naproxen, etc) are related chemically in that they are weak organic acids; in addition, they share the important property of inhibiting prostaglandin biosynthesis. They may also decrease the production of free radicals and of superoxide and may interact with adenylate cyclase to alter the cellular concentration of cAMP. Although these drugs effectively inhibit inflammation, there is no evidence that—in contrast to drugs such as gold and penicillamine—they alter the course of an arthritic disorder. Aspirin's long history of use and availability without prescription diminish its glamour compared to that of the newer NSAIDs. However, because of its long history of safety and tolerance, aspirin remains the drug of initial choice for treating the majority of articular and musculoskeletal disorders. Aspirin is also the standard against which all anti-inflammatory agents are measured, and it should not be abandoned unless specific contraindication exists or another NSAID offers a clearly demonstrable advantage.

History

Quinine from cinchona bark is one of the oldest remedies for relief of mild pain and fever. Willow bark was used in folk medicine for years for similar indications. In 1763, Reverend Edmund Stone, in a letter to the president of the Royal Society, described his success in treating fever with a powdered form of the bark of the willow. He had noted that the bitterness of willow bark was reminiscent of the taste of cinchona bark, the source of quinine. The active ingredient of willow bark, salicin, which on hydrolysis yields salicylic acid, was later found in other natural sources. Acetylsalicylic acid was synthesized in 1853, but the drug was not used until 1899, when it was found to be effective in arthritis and well tolerated. The name aspirin was coined from the German word for the compound, *a*cetyl*spir*säure (*Spirea,* the genus of plants from which it was obtained, and *Säure,* the German word for acid). Because of its greater efficacy and lower cost, aspirin rapidly replaced the natural products then in use and has remained one of the most widely employed remedies for over 80 years.

Chemistry & Pharmacokinetics

Salicylic acid is a simple organic acid with a pK_a of 3. Aspirin (acetylsalicylic acid) has a pK_a of 3.5 (Table 1–1). It is about 50% more potent than sodium

Table 33–1. Comparison of aspirin and newer nonsteroidal anti-inflammatory drugs.

	Total Daily Dose for Rheumatoid Arthritis (mg)	Recommended Number of Divided Daily Doses	Plasma Half-Life (hours)	Cost to Patient for 100-Day Supply
Aspirin, generic	4000	3	12	$ 6.00
Benoxaprofen (Oraflex)	400–800	1	28	120.00
Fenoprofen (Nalfon)	2600	4	2	115.00
Ibuprofen (Motrin)	2400	4	2	113.00
Meclofenamate (Meclomen)	400	4	2	95.00
Naproxen (Naprosyn)	750	2	13	83.00
Piroxicam (Feldene)	20	1	45	118.00
Sulindac (Clinoril)	400	2	18	83.00
Tolmetin (Tolectin)	1600	4	1	124.00

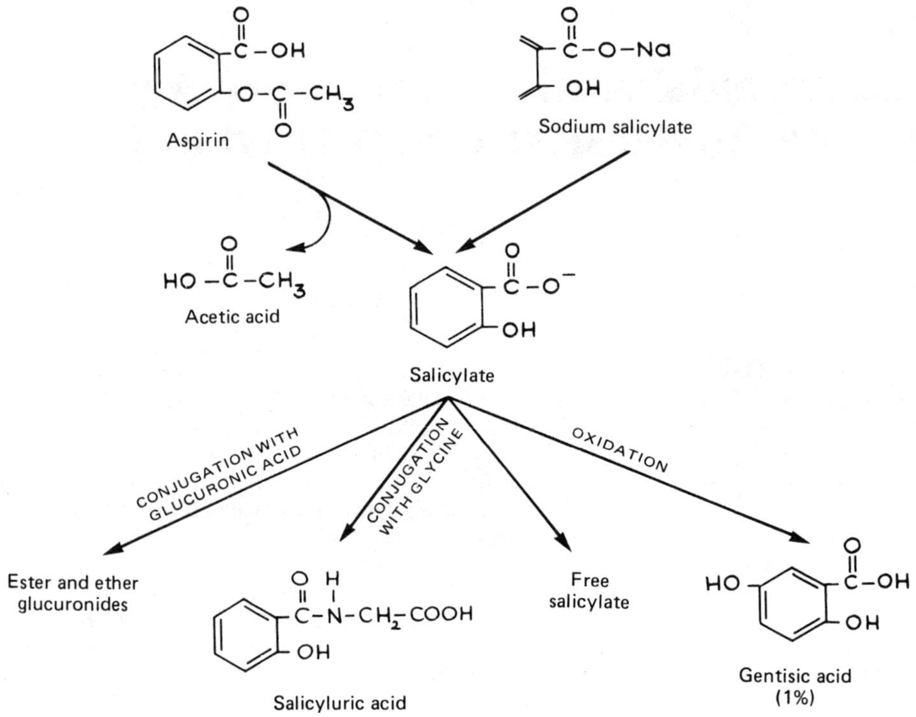

Figure 33–1. Structure and metabolism of the salicylates. (Modified and reproduced, with permission, from Meyers FH, Jawetz E, Goldfien A: *Review of Medical Pharmacology,* 7th ed. Lange, 1980.)

salicylate, although the latter compound causes less gastric irritation.

The salicylates (Fig 33–1) are rapidly absorbed from the stomach and upper small intestine, yielding a peak plasma salicylate level within 1–2 hours. The acid medium in the stomach keeps a large fraction of the salicylate in the nonionized form, promoting absorption. However, when high concentrations of salicylate enter the mucosal cell, the drug may damage the mucosal barrier. If the gastric pH is raised by a suitable buffer to 3.5 or higher, gastric irritation is minimized.

Aspirin is absorbed as such and is hydrolyzed to acetic acid and salicylate by esterases in tissue and blood. Salicylate is bound to albumin, but, as the serum concentration of salicylate increases, a greater fraction remains unbound and available to tissues. Ingested salicylate and that generated by the hydrolysis of aspirin may be excreted unchanged, but most is converted to water-soluble conjugates that are rapidly cleared by the kidney (Fig 33–1). When this pathway becomes saturated, a small increase in aspirin dose results in a large increase in plasma levels. Alkalinization of the urine increases the rate of excretion of free salicylate. When aspirin is used in low doses (600 mg), elimination is in accordance with first-order kinetics and the serum half-life is 3–5 hours. With higher dosage, zero-order kinetics prevail; at anti-inflammatory dosage ($\geq$ 4 g/d), the half-life increases to 15 hours or more. This effect occurs in about a week and is related to saturation of hepatic enzymes that catalyze the formation of salicylate conversion compounds, salicylphenylglucuronide and salicyluric acid.

Pharmacodynamics

A. Anti-Inflammatory Effects: The effectiveness of aspirin is largely due to its capacity to inhibit prostaglandin biosynthesis (see Chapter 16). It does this by irreversibly blocking the enzyme cyclooxygenase (prostaglandin synthetase), which catalyzes the reaction of arachidonic acid to endoperoxide compounds; in high doses, the drug decreases the formation of both the prostaglandins and thromboxane A_2 (Fig 33–2). Aspirin also interferes with the chemical mediators of the kallikrein system (Chapter 15). Aspirin inhibits granulocyte adherence to damaged vasculature, stabilizes lysosomes, and inhibits the migration of polymorphonuclear leukocytes and macrophages into the site of inflammation.

B. Analgesic Effect: Aspirin is most effective in reducing pain of mild to moderate intensity. It alleviates pain of varying causes, such as that of muscular, vascular, and dental origin, postpartum states, arthritis, and bursitis. Aspirin acts peripherally through its effects on inflammation but probably also depresses pain stimuli at a subcortical site.

C. Antipyresis: Aspirin reduces elevated temperature, whereas normal body temperature is only slightly affected. The fall in temperature is related to increased dissipation of heat caused by dilatation of superficial blood vessels. The antipyresis may be accompanied by profuse sweating.

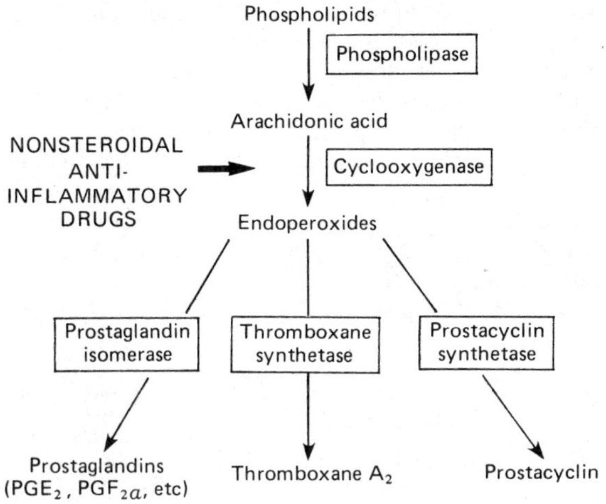

Figure 33–2. Scheme for prostaglandin biosynthesis. (Modified and reproduced, with permission, from Simon LS, Mills JA: Drug therapy: Nonsteroidal anti-inflammatory drugs. *N Engl J Med* 1980;**302**:1179.)

The fever associated with infection is thought to result from the production of prostaglandins in the central nervous system in response to bacterial pyrogens. Aspirin, by blocking this effect, may reset the "temperature control" in the hypothalamus and thereby facilitate heat dissipation by vasodilatation.

D. Central Nervous System Stimulation: Large doses of salicylates cause hyperpnea through a direct effect on the medulla. At high plasma salicylate levels, respiratory alkalosis may occur as a result of the increased ventilation. Later, acidosis supervenes from accumulation of salicylic acid derivatives and depression of the respiratory center.

E. Gastrointestinal Effects: The gastritis that occurs with aspirin may be due to irritation of the gastric mucosa by the undissolved tablet, to absorption in the stomach of nonionized salicylate, or to inhibition of protective prostaglandins. In animals, administration of prostaglandins has prevented gastric erosions, suggesting that the absence of a prostaglandin may make the gastric mucosa more vulnerable.

Vomiting may occur as a result of central nervous system stimulation after absorption of large doses. Upper gastrointestinal bleeding is usually related to erosive gastritis. A small increase in fecal blood loss is routinely associated with aspirin administration; about 1 mL of blood normally lost in the stool daily increases to about 4 mL daily in persons using ordinary aspirin doses and more for higher doses.

Aspirin has never been shown to cause peptic ulcers in humans, and with appropriate therapy, ulcers have been shown to heal while aspirin was taken concomitantly. Nevertheless, because of its irritant properties, aspirin should be taken with effective buffers by individuals with peptic disease.

F. Platelet Effects: Aspirin affects hemostasis. Single doses of aspirin produce a slightly prolonged bleeding time, which doubles if administration is continued for a week. The change is explained by the inhibition of platelet aggregation secondary to inhibition of thromboxane synthesis (Chapter 31). Because thromboxane accelerates platelet aggregation, aspirin inhibits platelet aggregation for up to 8 days—ie, until new platelets are formed.

Aspirin has a longer duration of effect than the many other compounds that inhibit platelet aggregation—clofibrate, phenylbutazone, dipyridamole, tranquilizers, antidepressants, etc. There is no relation between the platelet dysfunction and gastrointestinal bleeding, nor is the hazard of surgery increased in a patient taking aspirin.

G. Other Effects: Aspirin in a daily dose of 2 g or less usually increases serum uric acid levels, whereas doses exceeding 4 g daily decrease urate levels below 2.5 mg/dL. (See Drugs Used in Gout, below.)

Aspirin may cause mild, usually asymptomatic hepatitis, especially in patients with underlying disorders such as systemic lupus erythematosus and juvenile and adult rheumatoid arthritis.

Salicylates may cause reversible decrease of glomerular filtration rate in patients with underlying renal disease, but this may also occur (though rarely) in normal persons.

Aspirin in usual doses has a negligible effect on glucose tolerance. Toxic amounts affect the cardiovascular system directly and may depress cardiac function and dilate peripheral blood vessels. Large doses directly affect smooth muscles.

Therapeutic Uses

A. Analgesia and Anti-Inflammatory Effects: Aspirin is one of the most frequently employed drugs for reducing mild to moderate pain of varied origin. Aspirin is often combined with other mild analgesics, and over 200 such products may be purchased without prescription. These more costly combinations have never been shown to be more effective or less toxic than aspirin alone, and treating poisoning due to overdoses of such combinations is more difficult. Furthermore, the phenacetin contained in many such compounds may cause interstitial nephritis with serious renal impairment. Aspirin is not effective in the treatment of visceral pain such as that associated with acute abdomen, renal colic, pericarditis, or myocardial infarction.

The anti-inflammatory properties of salicylates in high doses are responsible for their recommendation as initial therapy for rheumatoid arthritis, rheumatic fever, and other inflammatory joint conditions. In mild arthritis, many patients can be managed using salicylates as their sole medication.

B. Other Indications:

1. Antipyresis–Except for a few diseases (eg, neurosyphilis, chronic brucellosis), there is no evidence that elevation of body temperature is a useful defense mechanism. Aspirin is the best available drug for reducing fever when doing so is desirable.

2. Inhibition of platelet aggregation–Aspirin has been shown to decrease the incidence of transient ischemic attacks in men and has been used as a prophylactic agent for this purpose. Its efficacy in reducing the incidence of coronary thrombosis has not been proved.

3. Cataract–Preliminary studies suggest that aspirin may reduce cataract formation.

Dosage

The optimal analgesic or antipyretic dose of aspirin is less than the 0.6-g oral dose commonly used. Larger doses may prolong but will not increase the effect. The usual dose may be repeated every 4 hours and smaller doses (0.3 g) every 3 hours. The dose for children is 50–75 mg/kg/d in divided doses.

The average anti-inflammatory dose of 4 g daily can be tolerated by most adults. For children, 50–75 mg/kg/d usually produces adequate blood levels. Blood levels of 15–30 mg/dL are associated with anti-inflammatory effects. A simple reliable method for determining salicylate blood levels is available, and

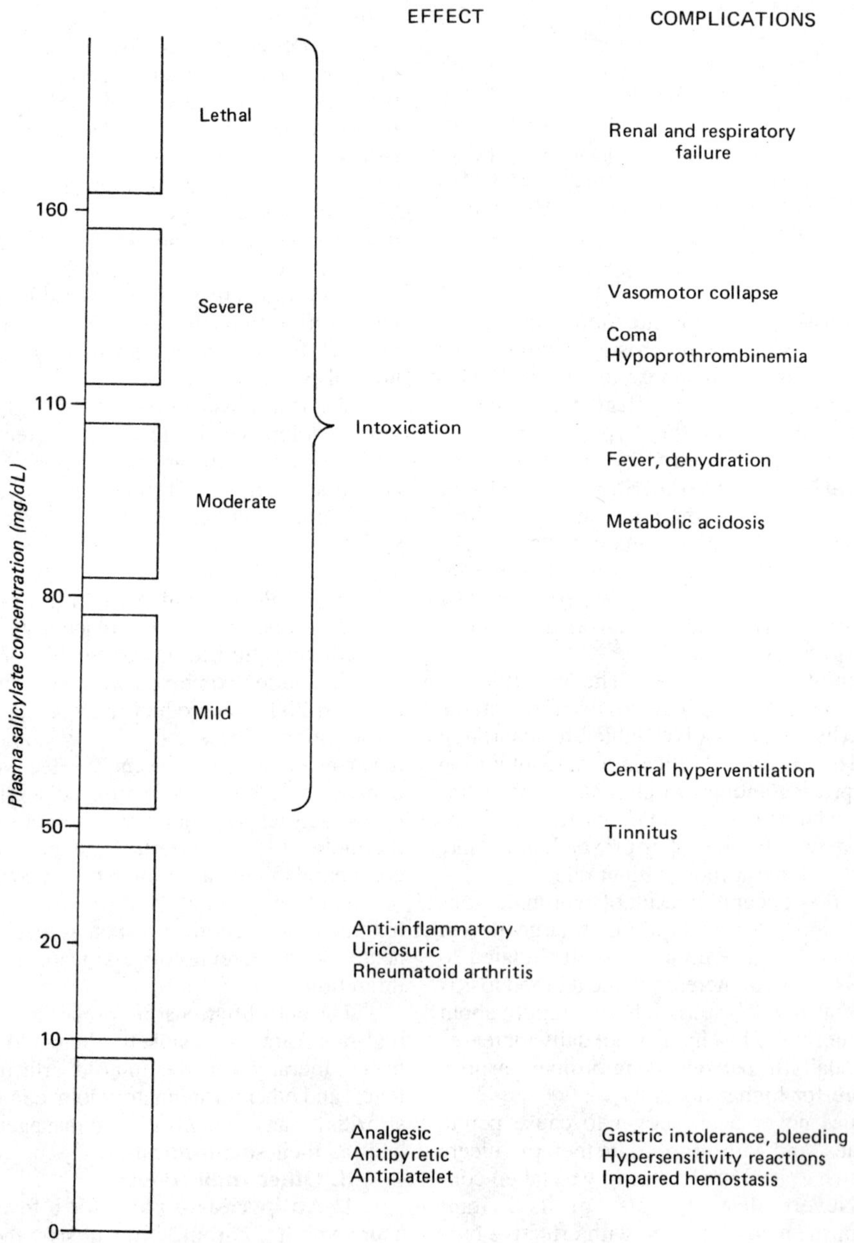

Figure 33–3. Approximate relationships of plasma salicylate levels to pharmacodynamics and complications. (Modified and reproduced, with permission, from Hollander J, McCarty D Jr: *Arthritis and Allied Conditions.* Lea & Febiger, 1972.)

the drug can thus be titrated to the proper level. Because of the long half-lives (about 12 hours) of aspirin and its metabolites, frequent dosing is not necessary when daily doses of 4 g or more are required. A convenient method is to give the total amount divided into 3 doses taken after meals.

The relationship of salicylate blood levels to therapeutic effect and toxicity is illustrated in Fig 33–3.

Preparations Available

Aspirin is available from many different manufacturers, and although it may vary in texture and appearance, the content of aspirin is constant. A disintegration test is part of the official standard, and there is little evidence that differences among tablets have clinical significance. The most popular buffered aspirin does not contain sufficient alkali to modify gastric irritation, and there is no evidence that these more expensive preparations are associated with higher blood levels, greater clinical effectiveness, or a lower incidence of side-effects. Enteric-coated aspirin (Ecotrin, etc) may be suitable for patients in whom buffering fails to control gastritis, since the coating prevents the tablet from dissolving in the stomach and the drug is absorbed in the alkaline medium of the small intestine. Therapeutic blood levels with this preparation may be similar to those achieved with the same doses of regular aspirin. Enteric coating increases the cost of aspirin, but these products are still less costly than the newer NSAIDs. The use of cimetidine to counteract gastric acidity increases the cost considerably and adds another drug with potential side-effects.

Adverse Effects

At the usual dosage, the main adverse effect is gastric intolerance. This effect can be minimized with suitable buffering (taking aspirin with meals followed by a glass of water or antacids). With higher doses, patients may experience "salicylism"—tinnitus, decreased hearing, and vertigo—reversible by reducing the dosage.

The effect of aspirin on renal function and on the liver has been mentioned earlier. Hypersensitivity reactions may occur in patients with asthma and nasal polyps and may be associated with bronchoconstriction and shock. Aspirin is contraindicated in patients with hemophilia. Aspirin is not recommended for pregnant women. Although a relationship to peptic ulcer disease has not been proved, aspirin is best avoided in patients with active peptic ulcer.

Overdosage Toxicity

Aspirin is such a common household drug that it is a frequent cause of poisoning in young children. Serious intoxication results when the amount ingested exceeds 150–175 mg/kg of body weight.

Most aspirin is sold and used without prescription. The drug must be kept out of reach of children and in the child-resistant container in which it is dispensed. Colorful, flavored, and liquid preparations should be kept in locked cabinets.

When overdosing occurs, either accidentally or with suicidal intent, gastric lavage is advised (Chapter 58). Hyperthermia may be treated with alcohol sponges or ice packs. It is important to maintain a high urine volume and to treat acid-base abnormalities. In severe toxic reactions, ventilatory assistance may be required. Sodium bicarbonate infusions may be employed to alkalinize the urine, which will increase the amount of salicylate excreted.

Drug Interactions

Drugs that enhance salicylate intoxication include acetazolamide and ammonium chloride. Alcohol increases gastrointestinal bleeding produced by salicylates. Aspirin displaces a number of drugs from protein-binding sites in the blood. These include tolbutamide, chlorpropamide, nonsteroidal anti-inflammatory agents, methotrexate, phenytoin, and probenecid. Corticosteroids may decrease salicylate concentration. Aspirin reduces the pharmacologic activity of spironolactone, antagonizes the effect of heparin, competes with penicillin G for renal tubular secretion, and inhibits the uricosuric effect of sulfinpyrazone and probenecid.

NEWER NONSTEROIDAL ANTI-INFLAMMATORY DRUGS

The side-effects of aspirin—especially the gastric irritation that occurs when large doses are employed—have led to the search for alternative compounds. Starting with ibuprofen in 1974, several drugs with aspirinlike properties (designated nonsteroidal anti-inflammatory drugs, NSAIDs) have been approved for use in the USA for the treatment of rheumatoid arthritis or osteoarthritis (Table 33–1). Over 50 drug applications for NSAIDs are on file with the FDA. Although aspirin is an NSAID, this term has come into use to designate the newer aspirin substitutes.

Chemistry

The NSAIDs (Fig 33–4) are grouped in 6 major classes: (1) propionic acid derivatives, (2) indole derivatives, (3) fenamates, (4) pyrrolealkanoic acids, (5) pyrazolone derivatives, and (6) oxicams. This chemical diversity yields such a broad range of pharmacokinetic characteristics that these properties are best discussed in connection with the individual agents.

Pharmacodynamics

The anti-inflammatory activity of the NSAIDs is similar in mechanism to that of aspirin and is mediated chiefly through inhibition of biosynthesis of prostaglandins. Inflammation is reduced by decreasing the

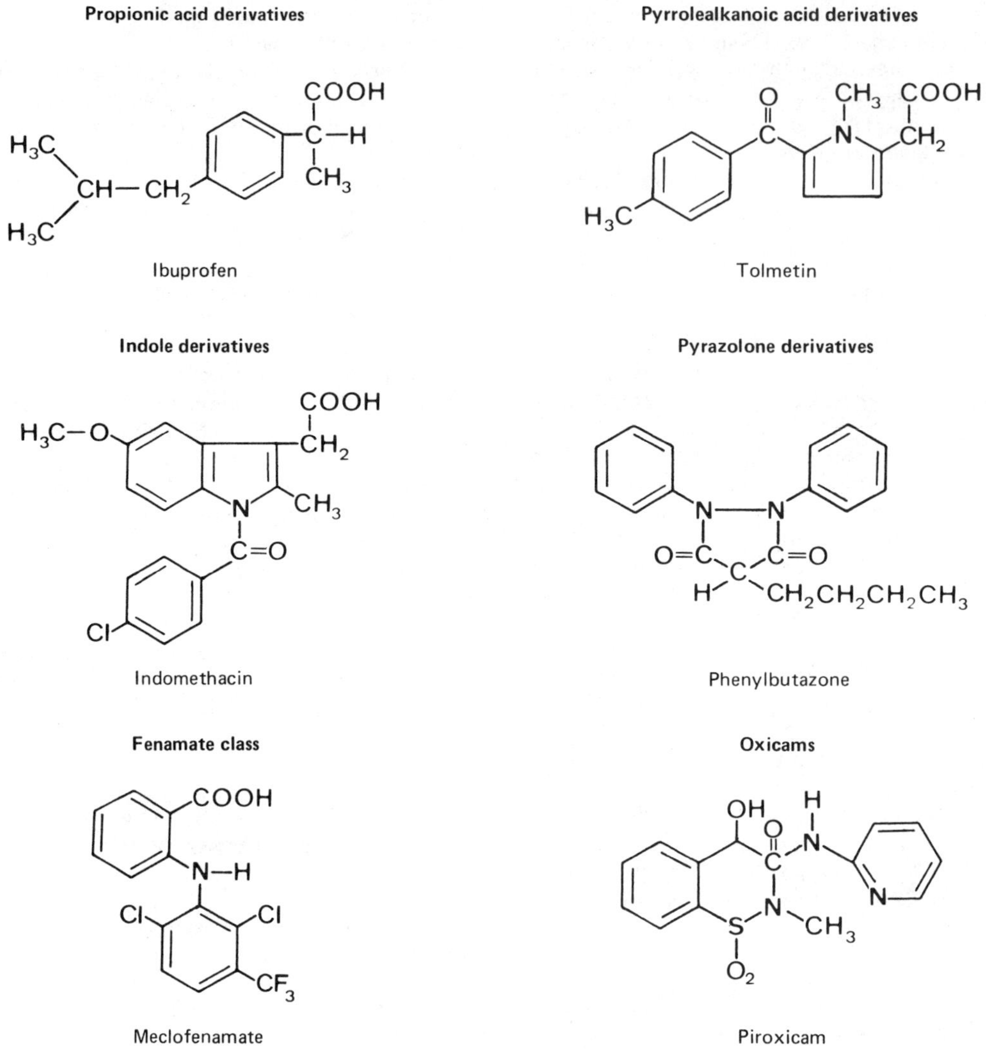

Figure 33–4. Chemical structures of some NSAIDs.

release of mediators from granulocytes, basophils, and mast cells. The NSAIDs decrease the sensitivity of vessels to bradykinin and histamine, affect lymphokine production from T lymphocytes, and cause vascular constriction. To varying degrees, all are inhibitors of prothrombin synthesis; all are analgesic, anti-inflammatory, and antipyretic; and all inhibit platelet aggregation. They are all gastric irritants as well. Nephrotoxicity has increasingly been observed for all of the drugs for which extensive experience has been reported.

Phenylpropionic Acid Derivatives

IBUPROFEN

Ibuprofen (Motrin, Rufen) is a simple derivative of phenylpropionic acid. In doses of about 2400 mg daily, ibuprofen is equivalent to 4 g of aspirin in anti-inflammatory effect. The drug is usually prescribed in lower doses, at which it is analgesic but inferior as an anti-inflammatory agent. The half-life is 3½ hours. Ibuprofen is metabolized in the liver, and less than 10% is excreted unchanged. Gastrointestinal irritation and bleeding occur, although less frequently than with aspirin. The use of ibuprofen concomitantly with aspirin may decrease the total anti-inflammatory effect. The drug is contraindicated in individuals with nasal polyps, angioedema, and bronchospastic reactivity to aspirin. In addition to the gastrointestinal symptoms (which can be modified by ingestion with meals), rash, pruritus, tinnitus, dizziness, headache, anxiety, aseptic meningitis, and fluid retention have been reported. Interaction with anticoagulants is uncommon. Serious hematologic effects include agranulocytosis and aplastic anemia; effects on the kidney include acute renal failure, interstitial nephritis, and nephrotic syndrome.

NAPROXEN, FENOPROFEN, BENOXAPROFEN

Naproxen (Anaprox, Naprosyn) is a naphthylpropionic acid that binds to plasma protein and has a long half-life (13 hours). Antacids delay its absorption. Naproxen is excreted in the urine as an inactive glucuronide metabolite. Like ibuprofen, naproxen competes with aspirin for plasma protein-binding sites. It also prolongs prothrombin time.

Fenoprofen (Nalfon) has a short half-life (2 hours) so that multiple dosing is required. The dose for inflammatory arthritis is 600–800 mg 4 times daily.

Side-effects and drug interactions of naproxen and fenoprofen are similar to those of ibuprofen, ie, nephrotoxicity, jaundice, nausea, dyspepsia, peripheral edema, rash, pruritus, central nervous system and cardiovascular effects, and tinnitus.

Benoxaprofen (Oraflex) differs from the preceding propionic acid derivatives in having a much longer half-life (25–32 hours) and hepatic toxicity that has, at the time of this writing, caused its withdrawal from the market. Because of its long half-life, the drug accumulates in the body when given on a daily basis. The drug is highly bound to plasma proteins and excreted primarily by the kidneys as the glucuronide conjugate. In addition to causing gastrointestinal side-effects like the other NSAIDs, benoxaprofen is associated with a higher-than-average incidence of severe hepatic damage and significant phototoxic responses to sunlight: burning and itching of exposed skin and onycholysis (separation of the terminal portions of the fingernails and toenails from the nail beds).

Indole Derivatives

INDOMETHACIN

Indomethacin (Indocin), introduced in 1963, is more toxic but in certain circumstances more effective than aspirin or any of the other NSAIDs (Fig 33–4). In the laboratory, it is the most potent of the inhibitors of prostaglandin synthesis. Indomethacin is well absorbed after oral administration and highly bound to plasma proteins. Metabolism occurs in the liver, and unchanged drug and inactive metabolites are excreted in bile and urine. The serum half-life is 2 hours.

Clinical Uses

Indomethacin is not suggested for general use as an analgesic. Except for the treatment of patent ductus arteriosus (discussed below), it should not be used in children. It is useful in special situations, including acute gouty arthritis, ankylosing spondylitis, and osteoarthritis of the hip and has also been effective in extra-articular inflammatory conditions such as pericarditis and pleurisy and in Bartter's syndrome. In acute gout, indomethacin has virtually replaced colchicine as the initial medication (see section on gout).

A special investigational application of indomethacin is in the management of patent ductus arteriosus in premature infants.

Adverse Reactions

Indomethacin produces a high incidence of dose-related toxic effects. At higher dosage levels, at least a third of patients have reactions requiring discontinuance of the medication. The gastrointestinal effects may include abdominal pain, diarrhea, gastrointestinal hemorrhage, and pancreatitis. Severe headache is experienced by 20–25% of patients and may be associated with dizziness, confusion, and depression. Rarely, psychosis with hallucinations has been reported. Hepatic abnormalities are rare. Serious hematologic reactions have been noted, including thrombocytopenia and aplastic anemia. Coronary vasoconstriction has been demonstrated. Hyperkalemia has been reported and is related to inhibition of the effect of prostaglandins on the kidney. A number of interactions with other drugs have been reported (see Appendix I). Use of indomethacin should be avoided in patients with nasal polyps or angioedema, in whom asthma may be precipitated. The drug is contraindicated in pregnancy and should be used with caution in persons with psychiatric disorders or peptic disease.

SULINDAC

Sulindac (Clinoril), a sulfoxide, is a prodrug, closely related to indomethacin. The drug is effective only after it is converted by liver enzymes to a sulfide, which is excreted in bile and then reabsorbed from the intestine. The enterohepatic cycling prolongs the duration of action to about 16 hours.

The indications and adverse reactions are similar to those of other NSAIDs. Stevens-Johnson epidermal necrolysis syndrome, thrombocytopenia, agranulocytosis, and nephrotic syndrome have all been observed. The average dose for inflammatory arthritis is 200 mg twice daily.

Fenamate Agents

MECLOFENAMATE

Meclofenamate (Meclomen), a recently released NSAID, reaches a peak plasma level in 30–60 minutes, with a half-life of 2 hours. It is excreted in the urine, largely as the glucuronide conjugates. Although long-term experience is lacking, meclofenamate appears to have adverse effects similar to those of related agents and to have no advantage over them. This drug enhances the effect of oral anticoagulants.

Meclofenamate is contraindicated in pregnancy; its efficacy and safety have not been established for young children.

In inflammatory arthritis, the recommended dosage is 200–400 mg daily divided into 4 equal doses.

MEFENAMIC ACID

Mefenamic acid (Ponstel) possesses analgesic properties but is probably less effective than aspirin as an anti-inflammatory agent and is clearly more toxic. It should not be used for longer than 1 week and never in children.

Pyrrolealkanoic Acids

TOLMETIN

Tolmetin (Tolectin) is similar to aspirin in effectiveness in juvenile and adult rheumatoid arthritis and osteoarthritis. The drug has a short half-life (60 minutes), which means that it must be given repeatedly. It is one of the most expensive NSAIDs.

Pyrazolone Derivatives

PHENYLBUTAZONE

Phenylbutazone (Butazolidin) rapidly gained favor after its introduction in 1949 for the treatment of rheumatoid arthritis, ankylosing spondylitis, acute gouty arthritis, and various musculoskeletal disorders. It has potent anti-inflammatory properties and is thus still commonly prescribed, even though aspirin and newer NSAIDs are superior in most applications.

The package insert lists a panoply of adverse effects. The most serious are agranulocytosis and aplastic anemia, which have led to a number of deaths. Phenylbutazone has also caused hemolytic anemia, nephrotic syndrome, optic neuritis, deafness, serious allergic reactions, exfoliative dermatitis, and hepatic and renal tubular necrosis. The main indications for phenylbutazone are for the short-term therapy of such painful conditions as acute gouty arthritis and superficial thrombophlebitis.

Oxicams

PIROXICAM

Piroxicam (Feldene) is a new NSAID of novel structure (Fig 34–4). It has a half-life of 45 hours, permitting once-daily dosing, which should favor compliance. It is rapidly absorbed in the stomach and reaches 80% of its peak plasma concentration in 1 hour. It is excreted as the glucuronide conjugate and to a small extent unchanged.

The efficacy and adverse effects of piroxicam appear similar to those of other NSAIDs used in the treatment of rheumatoid arthritis and ankylosing spondylitis. The drug is new, and evaluation of its risks and value compared with other agents now in use will require more time and experience.

• • •

CLINICAL PHARMACOLOGY OF THE NSAIDs

Most patients with inflammatory joint disorders benefit from aspirin when administered in sufficient doses (4 g or more) and when special attention is given to lessening gastric irritation by proper buffering. About 15% of patients develop troublesome side-effects from aspirin; it is primarily for these patients that NSAIDs are indicated. As a group, these newer agents tend to cause less gastric irritation, and the dosing schedule of some is simpler (one tablet once or twice daily). In choosing an agent, it is worth remembering that the cost to the patient is $74–124 for a 100-day supply of the newer agents compared to about $6 for generic over-the-counter aspirin (Table 33–1). In addition, a reliable method for determining salicylate blood levels is available to establish therapeutic range, which is not true for the newer drugs. These advantages must be weighed against easier dosage schedules, better compliance, and lower incidence of gastric irritation with some of the newer agents. Surveys show that most patients with inflammatory arthritis receive NSAIDs without an adequate trial of salicylates, yet none of these newer drugs have proved more effective than aspirin in controlled studies. Moreover, although less gastrointestinal irritation has been shown for most of them, some are proving more toxic in other ways.

The NSAIDs have been responsible for many instances of acute renal failure and nephrotic syndrome, which develops insidiously and is neither dose-dependent nor related to duration of drug use. Patients rarely have symptoms suggestive of a hypersensitivity reaction, so the condition may go undetected until advanced.

If the decision is made to use an NSAID, it is important to consider adverse effects, cost, and dosing schedules. It is not possible to know which patient will respond in a specific way to which NSAID, for some patients derive benefit from one and not from another. How much of this variability of response is related to the agent per se, to individual differences in metabolism of the drug, or to a placebo effect is difficult to evaluate. When compliance is a problem, drugs such as piroxicam, sulindac, and naproxen are useful because only one or 2 doses are required daily. If a patient is taking a hypoglycemic agent or warfarin, ibuprofen or tolmetin might be considered, since, unlike sulindac, they do not potentiate the effect of the hypoglycemic drugs or warfarin. Hypersensitivity to one of the phenylalkanoic acids, however, should preclude use of the others in that group. Dosing schedules listed for the drugs are those recommended by the manufacturer, but it is becoming clear that some patients require and may tolerate higher doses. Until blood level assays become available, it is probably safest to use the dosages as listed.

SLOW-ACTING ANTI-INFLAMMATORY AGENTS

ANTIMALARIAL DRUGS (Chloroquine, Hydroxychloroquine)

The pharmacology of the 4-aminoquinoline derivatives is fully discussed in Chapter 54. Chloroquine (Aralen) and hydroxychloroquine (Plaquenil) have been used in the treatment of rheumatoid arthritis and systemic lupus erythematosus since the 1950s, and their efficacy in inducing remission has been confirmed in carefully controlled studies. Rheumatoid factor declines after prolonged chloroquine use; however, there is no evidence that chloroquine decreases the progression of erosive bone lesions as is observed with gold.

The mechanism of anti-inflammatory action of chloroquine and hydroxychloroquine in rheumatic disorders is unclear. They suppress the responsiveness of T lymphocytes to mitogens, interfere with the replication of viruses, decrease leukocyte chemotaxis, stabilize lysosomal membranes, inhibit DNA and RNA synthesis, and trap free radicals. The action of chloroquine is not apparent until after a latent period of 4–12 weeks. The drug is often useful as an adjunct to treatment with NSAIDs and has no adverse interaction with other antirheumatic agents.

Adverse Effects

These are described in Chapter 54.

Indications

Antimalarials are often administered to patients with rheumatoid arthritis who have not responded optimally to salicylates and NSAIDs. In addition to their use in rheumatoid arthritis, antimalarials have been used successfully for their anti-inflammatory effect in juvenile rheumatoid arthritis, Sjögren's syndrome, and systemic lupus erythematosus (in which they have a beneficial effect on both joint and skin findings). The antimalarial drugs should not be used in psoriatic arthritis because of the possible development of exfoliative dermatitis.

Dosage

Hydroxychloroquine, available in tablets of 200 mg (155 mg of base), is the preferred drug. Initial dosage is 2 tablets orally daily. Once clinical improvement is established, the dose can often be decreased to one tablet daily.

GOLD

Gold compounds were introduced for treatment of rheumatoid arthritis in the 1920s, but it was not until 1960, following a report of a large double-blind trial, that the efficacy of gold salts in the management of rheumatoid arthritis was clearly established. Subsequent controlled studies have confirmed the value of the drug and have demonstrated that these agents *retard the progression of bone and articular destruction* determined roentgenographically. In this regard, gold salts have special value in treating rheumatoid arthritis. Further impetus to the popularity of gold salts has been the demonstration that the drug may be continued for years, allaying earlier fears of toxicity from accumulation.

Chemistry

The 2 most commonly administered gold preparations are gold sodium thiomalate (Myochrysine) and aurothioglucose (Solganal). Both are administered intramuscularly as water-soluble gold salts containing 50% elemental gold. An oral gold preparation (auranofin) that appears to be as effective as intramuscular gold and better tolerated is presently being tested.

Pharmacokinetics

Gold salts are approximately 95% bound to plasma protein during transport by the blood. Although they tend to concentrate in synovial membranes, gold salts are also concentrated in the liver, kidney, spleen, adrenal glands, lymph nodes, and bone marrow. Following intramuscular injection, peak levels are reached in 2–6 hours; 40% is excreted within a week, about two-thirds in the urine and one-third in the feces. One month after intramuscular injection of 50 mg, 75–80% of the drug has been eliminated. Certain tissue compartments such as the epithelial cells of the renal tubules, which have a particular affinity for gold, show its presence many years after therapy has ceased. Most studies have failed to show a correlation between serum gold concentration and either therapeutic effect or toxicity.

Pharmacodynamics

The precise manner in which gold salts produce

their beneficial effects in patients with rheumatoid arthritis and allied disorders is unknown. Gold alters the morphologic and functional capabilities of human macrophages; this may be its major mode of action. Other effects ascribed to gold include inhibition of lysosomal enzyme activity, reduction of histamine release from mast cells, inactivation of the first component of complement, suppression of phagocytic activity of the polymorphonuclear leukocytes, and inhibition of the Shwartzman phenomenon.

Indications

Gold therapy is indicated for active rheumatoid arthritis in patients who have been given an adequate trial of therapy with NSAIDs for a period of 3–4 months and continue to show active synovitis. Patients who later in the course of their disease show active inflammation and erosive changes are also candidates for gold. Patients with rheumatoid arthritis in the presence of Sjögren's syndrome and those with juvenile rheumatoid arthritis may also be considered, whereas the usefulness of gold in the treatment of psoriatic arthritis is less clear.

The major contraindications to gold are a confirmed history of previous toxicity from the drug, pregnancy, serious impairment of liver or renal function, and blood dyscrasias. Gold is not given in conjunction with penicillamine, because this chelator will remove much of the administered gold.

Adverse Effects

Approximately one-third of patients receiving gold salts experience some form of toxicity. Dermatitis, which is usually pruritic, is the most common side-effect, occurring in 15–20% of patients. Eosinophilia may precede or be associated with cutaneous lesions. Hematologic abnormalities, including thrombocytopenia, leukopenia, and pancytopenia, occur in 1–10% of patients. Aplastic anemia, although rare, may be fatal. About 8–10% of patients develop proteinuria that may progress to nephrotic syndrome in a few cases. Other side-effects include stomatitis, a metallic taste in the mouth, skin pigmentation, enterocolitis, cholestatic jaundice, peripheral neuropathy, pulmonary infiltrates, and corneal deposition of gold. Nitritoid reactions (sweating, faintness, flushing, and headaches) may occur, especially with gold thiomalate, and are presumably due to the vehicle rather than the gold salts themselves. Transient aggravation of arthritic symptoms may occur after injections of gold.

Method of Administration

The usual practice is to give 50 mg intramuscularly weekly until a total of 1000 mg has been injected (unless there is no response by the time 600–700 mg has been given, in which case the drug can be stopped). If 1 g is given without serious adverse effects and a favorable response is observed, the drug can be continued indefinitely in lengthening intervals of 2, 3, then 4 weeks. Clinical response usually requires a few months to become evident and may be delayed for as long as 4 months. Urinalysis and blood and platelet counts should be performed every other week and liver function tests less frequently. Patients should avoid strong light and be warned to promptly report any skin or mucous membrane lesions. Gold should be stopped if dermatitis occurs but may be reintroduced cautiously if dermatitis then clears. Nephrosis, thrombocytopenia, leukopenia, and exfoliative dermatitis require cessation of gold therapy, and reintroduction of the drug is contraindicated. Penicillamine and dimercaprol have been used to treat toxicity with varying success. Improvement may be expected in 60–70% of patients who tolerate the drug.

PENICILLAMINE

Penicillamine, a metabolite of penicillin, is an analog of the amino acid cysteine. The drug is available as the D or L isomer; it is the D form that is used clinically.

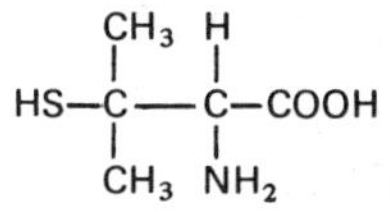

Penicillamine

Pharmacokinetics

Radiolabeling studies indicate that about half of orally administered penicillamine is absorbed. Peak serum concentrations occur in 1–2 hours; 80% of the plasma penicillamine is protein-bound. Absorption is enhanced if the drug is administered 1½ hours after meals. Free penicillamine and its metabolites may be found in urine and feces. About 60% of the drug is excreted in 24 hours. No satisfactory method is available for determining blood levels.

Pharmacodynamics

Penicillamine suppresses arthropathy in experimental animal models and has been shown to dissociate lymphocyte membrane receptors. It may interfere with the synthesis of DNA, collagen, and mucopolysaccharides. Rheumatoid factor titer falls following administration of the drug, probably reflecting disruption of disulfide bonds of macroglobulins but perhaps also reflecting a basic action of the drug on the immune system. The mechanism of penicillamine's action in rheumatoid arthritis is unclear.

Indications

Penicillamine is similar to gold in its latency period (3–4 months) and in its anti-inflammatory properties and like gold, may retard the progression of bone and articular destruction. About 70% of patients who tolerate the drug are improved, and complete remissions have been observed. Penicillamine is reserved for patients with active, progressive erosive rheumatoid disease not controlled by conservative therapy. Penicillamine is usually prescribed for patients who have not responded to gold therapy. Penicillamine is not useful in seronegative arthropathies. Caution is required when administering other drugs simultaneously, because penicillamine impedes absorption of many drugs and prevents them from reaching therapeutic levels.

Adverse Reactions

The side-effects of penicillamine limit its usefulness. Animal studies have shown inhibition of wound healing and evidence of muscle and blood vessel damage. In humans, side-effects are reduced by giving lower doses and by slow progression to maintenance dosages. Proteinuria is encountered in 20% of patients. Immune complex nephritis has been seen in 4% of patients; it is often reversible when the drug is withdrawn. Leukopenia and thrombocytopenia may occur at any time and may herald aplastic anemia. Most deaths related to penicillamine are due to aplastic anemia. Skin and mucous membrane reactions, the most common side-effects, may occur at any time during therapy and may respond to lowering the dose. Drug fever, which may be seen as an early response to penicillamine, is often associated with cutaneous eruptions.

Loss of taste perception or a metallic taste may develop. The blunting of taste perception relates to zinc chelation. Anorexia, nausea, and vomiting occur.

A variety of autoimmune diseases, including myasthenia gravis, Goodpasture's syndrome, lupus erythematosus, hemolytic anemia, and thyroiditis may be seen. The drug must be discontinued permanently when any of these conditions is encountered.

Mammary hyperplasia, alopecia, and psychologic changes have also been observed.

Penicillamine is contraindicated in pregnancy and in the presence of renal insufficiency and should not be given in combination with gold, cytotoxic drugs, or phenylbutazone.

Side-effects necessitating cessation of the drug occur in about 40% of patients. Blood counts (including platelet count) and urinalysis are performed twice a month for 4–6 months, then monthly. The drug should be stopped if the platelet count falls below 100,000/μL or the white count below 3000/μL. A history of penicillin allergy is not a contraindication to penicillamine. Patients who develop renal involvement, drug fever, autoimmune syndromes, and hematologic problems should not be rechallenged with the drug.

Dosage

Penicillamine (Cuprimine, Depen) is taken orally 1½ hours after meals. If clinical benefits are to occur, they should be apparent by 6 months. Treatment begins with 125 mg or 250 mg daily for 1–3 months; if no side-effects are seen and improvement does not occur, the dose is doubled. If therapeutic effects are absent after 3–4 months, the dose is increased at monthly intervals up to 750 mg daily (250 mg 3 times daily), which it is rarely necessary to exceed. When therapy is discontinued after improvement, most patients relapse within 6 months.

EXPERIMENTAL ANTIRHEUMATIC AGENTS

LEVAMISOLE

Levamisole (Ketrax), a drug employed for the treatment of helminthic infections (especially *Ascaris lumbricoides*), was found to have immunostimulant properties that led to its trial in rheumatic diseases, in which immune *enhancement* was considered (paradoxically) to be of potential benefit. Levamisole restored impaired cellular immune responses in arthritis induced by adjuvant injection in rats. The drug increases chemotaxis and phagocytosis of macrophages and polymorphonuclear leukocytes and appears to enhance T lymphocyte function, especially in situations where delayed hypersensitivity is impaired.

Pharmacokinetics

Levamisole is administered orally and is rapidly absorbed, reaching peak blood levels at 2 hours. The plasma half-life is about 4 hours; the drug is metabolized by the liver and excreted mainly in urine and to a lesser degree in feces.

Indications

Levamisole has proved in randomized double-blind studies to be effective in rheumatoid arthritis. It decreases inflammatory changes while simultaneously lowering the erythrocyte sedimentation rate and the titer of rheumatoid factor.

Adverse Reactions

Reactions occur in up to 20% of patients. Rash is the most common side-effect, but more toxic reactions include leukopenia, agranulocytosis, and thrombocytopenia. Influenzalike illnesses, mouth ulcers, and nausea and vomiting also occur. Reversible immune complex glomerulonephritis has been reported.

Dosage

The usual dosage schedule for levamisole is 40–50 mg orally daily for the first week, increased to 80–100 mg daily for the second week and 120–150 mg daily thereafter. Administering 150 mg on 3 consecutive days and none the rest of the week has proved as effective as daily dosing. Like gold and penicillamine, there is a latent period of 3–4 months before clinical improvement is observed. The FDA has not yet approved levamisole for treatment of rheumatic diseases in the USA.

IMMUNOSUPPRESSIVE DRUGS

The immunosuppressive agents (see Chapter 57) have been employed for over 4 decades in the therapy of rheumatic diseases. The drugs are considered experimental, and their current use is largely restricted to certain life-threatening disorders or seriously crippling diseases with reversible lesions after conventional therapy has failed. Because of their toxic potential, they should be employed only by physicians completely familiar with their actions. Reliable methods of selecting one drug instead of another are not available, and acceptable controlled studies demonstrating efficacy in humans are lacking for most of the drugs.

Drugs for which there is adequate experience include the alkylators mechlorethamine, cyclophosphamide, and chlorambucil; the purine antagonist azathioprine; and the folate antagonist methotrexate.

Immunosuppressive agents have been shown to be effective in some patients, especially those with vasculitis syndromes, such as Wegener's granulomatosis and panarteritis. They are useful in lupus nephritis, in seropositive progressive rheumatoid arthritis, and occasionally in patients with other rheumatic diseases. Because of the severity of side-effects—especially the oncogenic effects and bone marrow depression—immunosuppressive drugs should be given only after safer agents have been tried.

GLUCOCORTICOID AGENTS

The pharmacology of corticosteroids and their effect on inflammation are discussed in Chapter 37. The indications for management of rheumatic disease are briefly discussed here.

Rheumatoid Arthritis

The effect of prednisone on rheumatoid arthritis is prompt and dramatic. However, the prolonged use of the drug leads to serious, disabling side-effects. Corticosteroids do not alter the course of the disease, and bone and cartilage destruction continues while inflammation is decreased. Corticosteroids may be administered for certain serious extra-articular manifestations such as pericarditis or eye involvement or during periods of exacerbation. When prednisone is required for long-term therapy, the dosage should not exceed 10 mg daily, and gradual reduction of the dose should be encouraged. Alternate-day corticosteroid therapy is unsuccessful in arthritis: patients become symptomatic on the day they do not take the drug.

Intra-articular corticosteroids are often helpful to alleviate painful symptoms and, when successful, are preferable to increasing the dosage of systemic medication.

Cranial Arteritis & Polymyalgia Rheumatica

Patients with headache, jaw claudication, and other symptoms of cranial arteritis should be started on prednisone, 60 mg daily. The dose is maintained for several months, then decreased to the lowest level compatible with normal erythrocyte sedimentation rate. In polymyalgia rheumatica without cranial artery symptoms and negative temporal artery biopsy, 15 mg daily often suffices.

Necrotizing Vasculitis

Prednisone, 60 mg daily, is indicated, although cyclophosphamide appears to be of equal or possibly greater effectiveness.

Systemic Lupus Erythematosus

Prednisone is used for complications such as hemolytic anemia, thrombocytopenic purpura, and involvement of lung, brain, heart, and kidney. Articular symptoms may respond to more conservative therapy.

Polymyositis-Dermatomyositis

Corticosteroids are usually effective in doses of 60 mg daily, which are tapered in accordance with improvement and reduction of muscle enzymes.

Mixed Connective Tissue Disease

Lower doses are usually required than in lupus erythematosus and depend on the site and degree of involvement.

Scleroderma

Corticosteroids are usually of little benefit.

Wegener's Granulomatosis

Although corticosteroids may be used, cyclophosphamide is the preferred agent.

II. NONOPIATE ANALGESIC AGENTS

For the treatment of mild to moderate pain when an anti-inflammatory effect is not necessary, the drugs discussed below have been used.

Para-Aminophenol Derivatives

PHENACETIN

Phenacetin can no longer be prescribed in the USA and has been removed from many over-the-counter analgesic combinations such as Anacin and Empirin Compound. However, it is still present in a number of proprietary analgesics in this country and is in common use in many other parts of the world. The association between the excessive use of analgesic combinations—especially those that contain phenacetin—and the development of renal failure has been recognized for almost 30 years. Estimates of the percentage of patients with end-stage renal disease resulting from this kind of analgesic abuse range from 5 to 15%. After prohibition of the use of phenacetin in proprietary analgesics in Finland, Scotland, and Canada, the number of new cases of analgesic nephropathies in those countries decreased significantly.

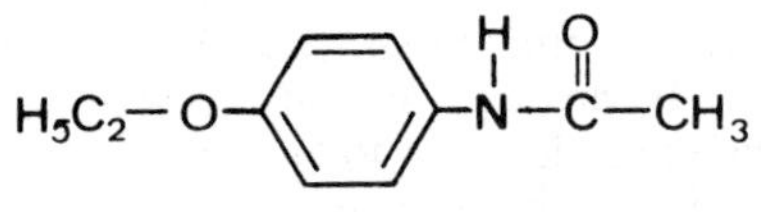

Phenacetin
(acetophenetidin)

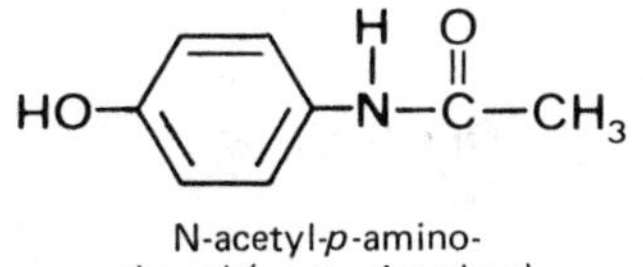

N-acetyl-*p*-amino-
phenol (acetaminophen)

ACETAMINOPHEN

Acetaminophen (Tempra, Tylenol, etc) is the active metabolite of phenacetin responsible for its analgesic effect. It is a weak prostaglandin inhibitor and possesses no significant anti-inflammatory effects.

Pharmacokinetics

Acetaminophen is administered orally. Absorption is related to the rate of gastric emptying, and peak blood concentrations are usually reached in 30–60 minutes. Acetaminophen is slightly bound to plasma proteins and is partially metabolized by hepatic microsomal enzymes and converted to acetaminophen sulfate and glucuronide, which are pharmacologically inactive (Fig 3–10). Less than 5% is excreted unchanged. A minor but highly active metabolite (N-acetyl-*p*-benzoquinone) is important in large doses because of its toxicity to both liver and kidney. The half-life of acetaminophen is 2–3 hours and is relatively unaffected by renal function. With toxic quantities or liver disease, the half-life may be increased 2-fold or more.

Pharmacologic Effects

Although equivalent to aspirin as an effective analgesic and antipyretic agent, acetaminophen differs by its lack of anti-inflammatory properties. It does not affect uric acid levels and lacks platelet-inhibiting properties. The drug is useful in mild to moderate pain such as headache, myalgia, postpartum pain, and other circumstances in which aspirin is an effective analgesic. Acetaminophen alone is inadequate therapy for inflammatory conditions such as rheumatoid arthritis, although it may be used as an analgesic adjunct to anti-inflammatory therapy. For mild analgesia, acetaminophen is the preferred drug in patients allergic to aspirin or when salicylates are poorly tolerated. It is preferable to aspirin in patients with hemophilia or a history of peptic ulcer and in those in whom bronchospasm is precipitated by aspirin. Unlike aspirin, acetaminophen does not antagonize the effects of uricosuric agents; it may be used concomitantly with probenecid in the treatment of gout. Concomitant use with aspirin may increase blood levels of the latter drug.

Dosage

Acute pain and fever may be managed by 325–500 mg 4 times daily and proportionately less for children. Steady-state conditions are attained within a day.

Adverse Effects

In therapeutic doses, a mild increase in hepatic enzymes may occasionally occur in the absence of jaundice: this is reversible when the drug is withdrawn. With larger doses, dizziness, excitement, and disorientation are seen. Ingestion of 15 g of acetaminophen may be fatal, death being caused by severe hepatotoxicity with central lobular necrosis, sometimes associated with acute renal tubular necrosis (Chapter 58). Early symptoms of hepatic damage include nausea, vomiting, diarrhea, and abdominal pain. Therapy is much less satisfactory than for aspirin overdose. In addition to supportive therapy, measures that have proved encouraging are the provision of sulfhydryl groups to neutralize the toxic metabolites. Acetylcysteine (Mucomyst) has been used for this purpose.

Hemolytic anemia and methemoglobinemia, reported with the use of phenacetin, have rarely been noted with acetaminophen. Interstitial nephritis and papillary necrosis, serious complications of phenacetin, although anticipated with widespread chronic use of acetaminophen, have not occurred despite the fact that about 80% of phenacetin is rapidly metabolized to acetaminophen. Gastrointestinal bleeding does not occur. Caution should be exercised in patients with liver disease.

Zomepirac

Zomepirac (Zomax) is a nonsteroidal anti-inflammatory agent recently released for treatment of mild to moderately severe pain. It is a close analog of tolmetin and thus possesses antipyretic and anti-inflammatory properties. However, its value lies in its capacity to relieve relatively severe pain without being addictive.

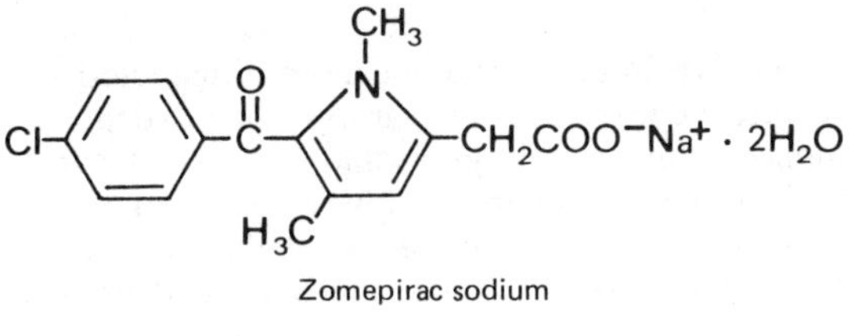

Zomepirac sodium

Pharmacokinetics

Zomepirac is administered orally. Food and antacids inhibit absorption. Peak plasma levels occur within 1 hour, and the half-life is approximately 4 hours. The onset of analgesia occurs in about 30 minutes and reaches a maximum in 1–2 hours, with a duration of 4–6 hours. The agent is highly bound (more than 98%) to plasma proteins, and elimination is primarily through the kidneys.

Mechanism of Action

Zomepirac is an NSAID and, like the other agents in this class, inhibits prostaglandin synthetase (cyclooxygenase). Its analgesic properties may derive in part from an effect on pain receptors. However, this does not explain why zomepirac possesses stronger analgesic properties than other NSAIDs. Whether an additional central effect exists is not known. The drug does not bind to opiate receptors and is not antagonized by naloxone.

Indications

Zomepirac is indicated in patients with mild to moderate pain who fail to respond to aspirin or acetaminophen. It is also indicated for patients with pain of greater severity, such as pain following oral surgery, postpartum pain, and dysmenorrhea, and has been shown to be more effective than 60 mg of codeine with or without aspirin. The analgesic effect does not increase with doses greater than 100 mg.

Dosage

The recommended dosage of zomepirac is 100 mg every 4–6 hours. Neither tolerance nor addiction has been reported.

Adverse Effects

The most common adverse effects are abdominal pain, nausea, and dyspepsia. Gastrointestinal bleeding is rare. Headache, tinnitus, hearing loss, and insomnia may occur, as well as other side-effects seen with the NSAIDs, including depression of renal function, increased blood pressure, fluid accumulation, rash, and prolonged bleeding time. Zomepirac causes asthma in predisposed patients. The drug should be used with caution in patients with renal or cardiac failure, hypertension, and hypersensitivity to aspirin. It is not recommended during pregnancy or for children or nursing mothers.

III. DRUGS USED IN GOUT

Gout is a familial metabolic disease characterized by recurrent episodes of acute arthritis due to deposits of monosodium urate in joints and cartilage. Formation of uric acid calculi in the kidneys may also occur. Gout is associated with high serum levels of uric acid, a poorly soluble substance that is the major end product of purine metabolism. In most mammals, uricase converts uric acid to the more soluble allantoin; this enzyme is absent in humans.

The treatment of gout is aimed at relieving the acute gouty attack and preventing recurrent gouty episodes and urate lithiasis. Before therapy for gout is started, patients in whom hyperuricemia is associated with gout and urate lithiasis must be clearly distinguished from those that have only hyperuricemia. In an asymptomatic person with hyperuricemia, the efficacy of long-term drug treatment is unproved. Uric acid levels may be elevated up to 2 standard deviations above the mean for a lifetime without adverse consequences in some individuals.

COLCHICINE

Colchicine is an alkaloid isolated from the autumn crocus, *Colchicum autumnale*. Its structure is shown in Fig 33–5.

Pharmacokinetics

Colchicine is absorbed readily after oral administration and reaches peak plasma levels within 2 hours. Metabolites of the drug are excreted in the intestinal tract and urine.

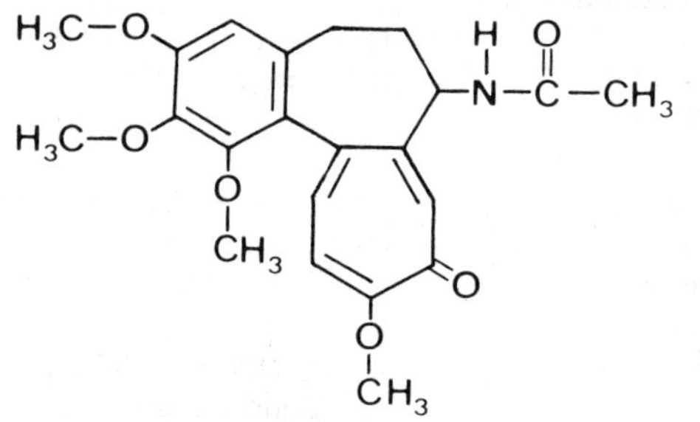

Colchicine

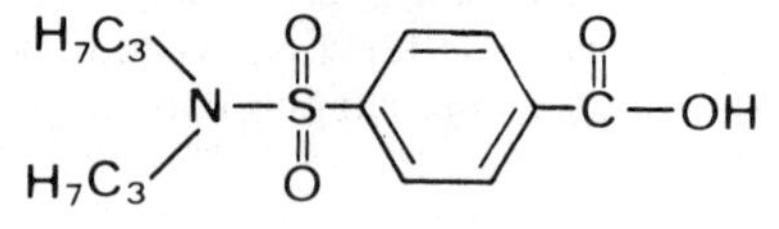

Probenecid

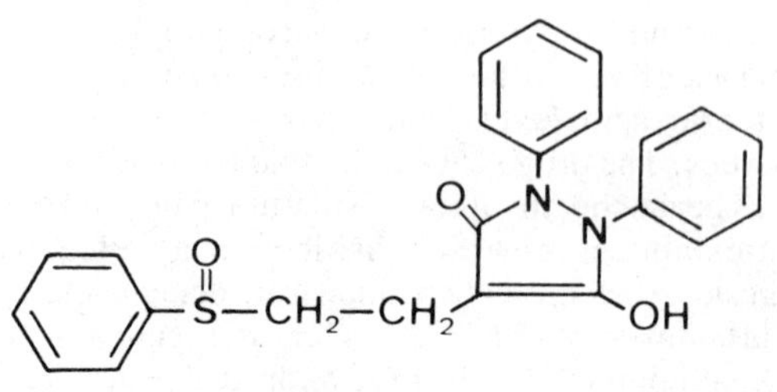

Sulfinpyrazone

Figure 33–5. Colchicine and uricosuric drugs.

Pharmacodynamics

Colchicine dramatically relieves the pain and inflammation of gouty arthritis in 12–24 hours without altering the metabolism or excretion of urates and without other analgesic effects. Colchicine is effective in this disorder by means of its anti-inflammatory properties. Gouty arthritis is produced by the deposition of urate crystals in synovial tissue. An inflammatory process results through activation of the kallikrein-kinin system, plasminogen, and complement. Phagocytosis of crystals by polymorphonuclear leukocytes and discharge of proteolytic enzymes results in decreased pH, which further increases urate deposition and intensifies inflammation. Colchicine apparently exerts its anti-inflammatory effects through binding to the microtubular protein tubulin, preventing its polymerization and leading to inhibition of leukocyte migration and phagocytosis.

Clinical Use

Colchicine has been the traditional drug used for alleviating the inflammation of acute gouty arthritis. Although colchicine is more specific in gout than the NSAIDs, other agents (eg, indomethacin) are often employed because of the troublesome diarrhea associated with colchicine therapy. Colchicine is preferred for the prophylaxis of recurrent episodes of gouty arthritis, is effective in preventing attacks of acute Mediterranean fever, and may have a mild beneficial effect in sarcoid arthritis.

Dosage

For terminating an attack of gout, the initial dose of colchicine is usually 0.5 or 1 mg, followed by 0.5 mg every 2 hours until pain is relieved or nausea and diarrhea appear. The total dose can be given intravenously, if necessary, but it should be remembered that as little as 8 mg in 24 hours may be fatal.

The prophylactic dose of colchicine is 0.5 mg 1–3 times daily.

Adverse Effects

Colchicine may occasionally cause nausea, vomiting, and abdominal pain. Colchicine may rarely cause hair loss and bone marrow depression as well as peripheral neuritis and myopathy.

Acute intoxication after ingestion of large (nontherapeutic) doses of the alkaloid is characterized by burning throat pain, bloody diarrhea, shock, hematuria, and oliguria. Fatal ascending central nervous system depression has been reported. Treatment is supportive.

NSAIDs IN GOUT

Indomethacin may be used as initial treatment of gout or as an alternative drug when colchicine is unsuccessful or causes too much discomfort. Indomethacin is the agent most often used today to treat acute gout. Three to 4 doses of 50 mg every 6 hours are given; when a response occurs, the dosage is reduced to 25 mg 3 or 4 times daily for about 5 days.

Phenylbutazone also is effective in the treatment of acute attacks of gout. Because the drug is used for a few days only, the serious side-effects of phenylbutazone are rarely a problem in this application. The usual initial dose is 400 mg followed by 200 mg every 6 hours until the attack subsides. Phenylbutazone should not be continued after 3 days.

The newer NSAIDs are also being used with success in the acute episode. Ibuprofen in doses of 2400 mg daily has alleviated attacks. However, there is no evidence that these agents will prove to be as effective or as safe as the older drugs.

URICOSURIC AGENTS

Probenecid (Benemid) and sulfinpyrazone (Anturane) are uricosuric drugs employed to decrease the body pool of urate in patients with tophaceous gout or in those with increasingly frequent gouty attacks. In a patient who excretes large amounts of uric acid, the uricosuric agents should be avoided so as not to precipitate the formation of uric acid calculi.

Chemistry

Uricosuric drugs are organic acids (Fig 34–5) and, as such, act at the anionic transport sites of the renal tubule (Chapter 13). Sulfinpyrazone is a metabolite of an analog of phenylbutazone.

Pharmacokinetics

Probenecid is completely reabsorbed by the renal tubules and is metabolized very slowly. Sulfinpyrazone or its active hydroxylated derivative is rapidly excreted by the kidneys. Even so, the duration of its effect after oral administration is almost as long as that of probenecid.

Pharmacodynamics

Uric acid is freely filtered at the glomerulus (Fig 33–6). Like many other weak acids, uric acid is then completely reabsorbed in the proximal convoluted tubule and finally secreted by another system for the transport of organic acids in the proximal tubule. Drugs with a greater affinity for the carriers involved in these tubular transport mechanisms might therefore saturate the anion transport capacity at either the reabsorbing or the secreting sites. An additional secretory site is located more distally in the tubule.

Small doses of uricosuric agents may preferentially reduce proximal secretion and have a uric acid–retaining effect, but therapeutic doses block reabsorption in the proximal tubules and greatly increase the urinary output of uric acid. They also inhibit reabsorption of secreted uric acid at the postsecretory site. (The salicylates are unsatisfactory because large doses are required to reach a uricosuric effect; smaller doses cause a net retention of uric acid. They should not be used even as analgesics in patients with gout.) The

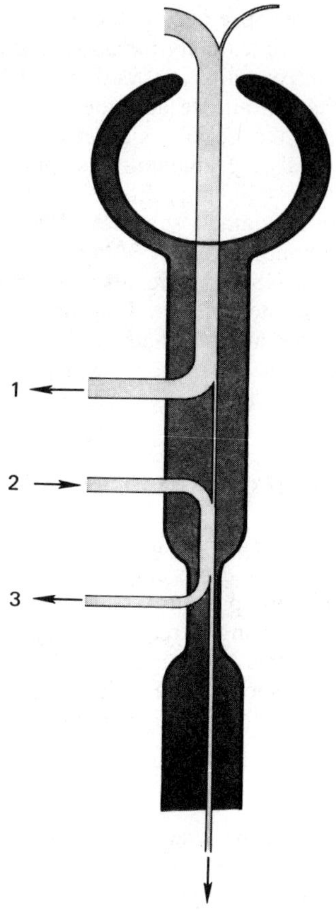

Figure 33–6. Renal handling of uric acid and sites of action of drugs. (Reproduced, with permission, from Meyers FH, Jawetz E, Goldfien A: *Review of Medical Pharmacology,* 7th ed. Lange, 1980.)

secretion of other organic acids—eg, penicillin—is reduced by uricosuric agents. Probenecid was originally developed as an agent to prolong penicillin blood levels.

As the urinary excretion of uric acid increases, the plasma level may not be greatly reduced, but the size of the urate pool decreases. In patients who respond favorably, tophaceous deposits of urate will be reabsorbed, with relief of arthritis and remineralization of bone. With the ensuing increase in uric acid excretion, a predisposition to the formation of renal stones is augmented rather than decreased; therefore, the urine volume should be maintained at a high level and—at least early in treatment—the urine pH kept above 6.0 by the administration of alkali.

Clinical Use

Uricosuric therapy should be initiated if several acute attacks of gouty arthritis have occurred, when evidence of tophi appears, or when plasma levels of uric acid in patients with gout are so high that tissue damage is almost inevitable. Therapy should not be started until 2–3 weeks after an acute attack.

Sulfinpyrazone has also been suggested for preventing sudden death after myocardial infarction, but questions have been raised about the methodology of the study.

Dosage

Probenecid is usually started at a dosage of 0.5 g orally daily in divided doses, progressing to 1 g daily after 1 week. Sulfinpyrazone is started at a dosage of 200 mg orally daily, progressing to 400–800 mg daily. It should be given in divided doses with food to reduce gastrointestinal side-effects.

Adverse Reactions

Side-effects do not provide a basis for preferring one or the other of the uricosuric agents. Both of these organic acids cause gastrointestinal irritation, but sulfinpyrazone is more active in this regard. Probenecid is more likely to cause allergic dermatitis, but a rash may appear after the use of either compound. Nephrotic syndrome has resulted from the use of probenecid. Both sulfinpyrazone and probenecid may (though rarely) cause aplastic anemia.

Contraindications & Cautions

It is essential to maintain a large urine volume to minimize the possibility of stone formation.

ALLOPURINOL

An alternative to increasing uric acid excretion in the treatment of gout is to reduce its synthesis by inhibiting xanthine oxidase with allopurinol (Zyloprim).

Chemistry

The structure of allopurinol, an isomer of hypoxanthine, is shown in Fig 33–7.

Pharmacokinetics

Allopurinol is approximately 80% absorbed after oral administration. Like uric acid, allopurinol is itself metabolized by xanthine oxidase. The resulting compound, alloxanthine, retains the capacity to inhibit xanthine oxidase and has a long enough duration of action so that allopurinol need be given once a day only.

Pharmacodynamics

Dietary purines are not an important source of uric acid. The quantitatively important amounts of purines are formed from amino acids, formate, and carbon dioxide in the body. Those purine ribonucleotides not incorporated into nucleic acids and those derived from the degradation of nucleic acids are converted to xanthine or hypoxanthine and oxidized to uric acid. When this last step is inhibited by allopurinol (Fig 33–7), there is a fall in the plasma urate level and a decrease in the size of the urate pool with a concurrent rise in the more soluble xanthine and hypoxanthine.

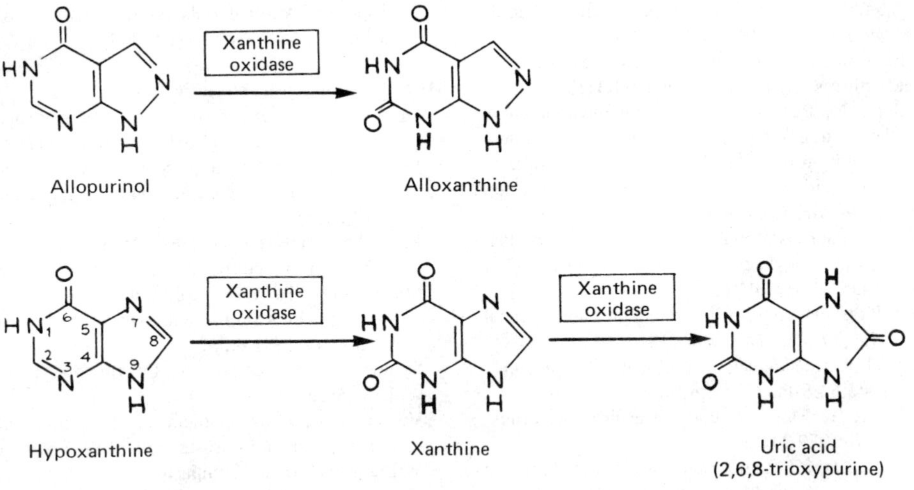

Figure 33–7. Inhibition of uric acid synthesis by allopurinol. (Modified and reproduced, with permission, from Meyers FH, Jawetz E, Goldfien A: *Review of Medical Pharmacology,* 7th ed. Lange, 1980.)

Therapeutic Use

Treatment of gout with allopurinol, as with uricosuric agents, is begun with the expectation that it will be continued for years if not for life. Allopurinol for the treatment of gout is indicated in the following circumstances: (1) in chronic tophaceous gout, in which reabsorption of tophi is more rapid than with uricosuric agents; (2) in patients with gout whose 24-hour urinary uric acid on purine-free diet exceeds 1.1 g; (3) when probenecid or sulfinpyrazone cannot be used because of side-effects or allergic reactions, or when they are providing less than optimal therapeutic effect; (4) for recurrent renal stones; (5) in patients with renal functional impairment; or (6) when serum urate levels are grossly elevated. Aside from gout, allopurinol is indicated to prevent the massive uricosuria following therapy of blood dyscrasias that could otherwise lead to renal calculi.

Adverse Effects

Acute attacks of gouty arthritis occur early in treatment with allopurinol when urate crystals are being withdrawn from the tissues and plasma levels are below normal. To prevent acute attacks, colchicine should be given during the initial period of therapy with allopurinol unless allopurinol is being used in combination with probenecid or sulfinpyrazone. Gastrointestinal intolerance, including nausea and vomiting and diarrhea, may occur. Peripheral neuritis and necrotizing vasculitis, depression of bone marrow elements, and, rarely, aplastic anemia may also occur. Hepatic toxicity and interstitial nephritis have been reported. An allergic skin reaction characterized by pruritic maculopapular lesions develops in 3% of patients. Isolated cases of exfoliative dermatitis have been reported.

Interactions & Contraindications

When chemotherapeutic mercaptopurines are being given concomitantly, their dose must be reduced by about 25%. Allopurinol may also increase the effect of cyclophosphamide. Allopurinol inhibits the metabolism of probenecid and oral anticoagulants and may increase hepatic iron concentration. Safety in children and during pregnancy has not been established.

Dosage

The initial dose of allopurinol is 100 mg daily. A daily dose of 300 mg is reached in 3 weeks and is adequate for most patients.

Colchicine, 0.5 mg twice daily, should be given during the first weeks of allopurinol therapy to control the gouty arthritis episodes that sometimes occur.

• • •

References

General

Roe RL: Drug therapy in rheumatic diseases. *Med Clin North Am* 1977;**61:**405.

Simon LS, Mills JA: Drug therapy: Nonsteroidal anti-inflammatory drugs. (2 parts.) *N Engl J Med* 1980; **302:**1179, 1237.

Salicylates

Abrishami MA, Thomas J: Aspirin intolerance: A review. *Ann Allergy* 1977;**39:**28.

Aspirin Myocardial Infarction Study Research Group: A randomized, controlled trial of aspirin in persons recovered from myocardial infarction. *JAMA* 1980;**243:**661.

Cohen LS: Clinical pharmacology of acetylsalicylic acid. *Semin Thromb Hemostas* 1976;**2:**146.

Cotlier E, Sharma YR: Aspirin and senile cataracts in rheumatoid arthritis. (Letter.) *Lancet* 1981;**1:**338.

Furst DE, Gupta N, Paulus HE: Salicylate metabolism in twins: Evidence suggesting a genetic influence and induction of salicylurate formation. *J Clin Invest* 1977;**60:**32.

Gabow PA et al: Acid-base disturbances in the salicylate-intoxicated adult. *Arch Intern Med* 1978;**138:**1343.

Graham GG et al: Patterns of plasma concentrations and urinary excretion of salicylate in rheumatoid arthritis. *Clin Pharmacol Ther* 1977;**22:**410.

Kimberly RP, Plotz PH: Aspirin-induced depression of renal function. *N Engl J Med* 1977;**296:**418.

Levy G: Clinical pharmacokinetics of aspirin. (Symposium.) *Pediatrics* 1978;**62(5-Part 2 Suppl):**867.

Moncada S, Vane JR: Mode of action of aspirin-like drugs. *Adv Intern Med* 1979;**24:**1.

Orozco-Alcala JJ, Baum J: Regular and enteric coated aspirin: A reevaluation. *Arthritis Rheum* 1979;**22:**1034.

Silvoso GR et al: Incidence of gastric lesions in patients with rheumatic disease on chronic aspirin therapy. *Ann Intern Med* 1979;**91:**517.

Trang LE: Prostaglandins and inflammation. *Semin Arthritis Rheum* 1980;**9:**153.

Other Nonsteroidal Drugs (NSAIDs)

Benoxaprofen. (Editorial.) *Br Med J* 1982;**285:**459.

Bowers DE: Naproxen in rheumatoid arthritis: A controlled trial. *Ann Intern Med* 1975;**83:**470.

Bunch TW, O'Duffy JD: Disease-modifying drugs for progressive rheumatoid arthritis. *Mayo Clin Proc* 1980;**55:**161.

Donnelly P, Lloyd K, Campbell H: Indomethacin in rheumatoid arthritis: An evaluation of its anti-inflammatory and side effects. *Br Med J* 1967;**1:**69.

Famaey JP: Recent developments about non-steroidal anti-inflammatory drugs and their mode of action. *Gen Pharmacol* 1978;**9:**155.

Findling JW: Indomethacin-induced hyperkalemia in three patients with gouty arthritis. *JAMA* 1980;**244:**1127.

Indomethacin for patent ductus arteriosus. *Med Lett Drugs Ther* (Oct 30) 1981;**23:**95.

Kantor TG: Ibuprofen. *Ann Intern Med* 1979;**91:**877.

Pharmacology, efficacy and safety of a new class of anti-inflammatory agents: A review of piroxicam. *Am J Med* 1982;**72;**1. [Entire issue.]

Slow-Acting Anti-Inflammatory Drugs (Remission-Inducing Drugs)

Bluhm GB: The treatment of rheumatoid arthritis with gold. *Semin Arthritis Rheum* 1975;**5:**147.

International Workshop and Symposium on Gold Salts in the Rheumatic Diseases, Montreal, Feb 5, 1979. *J Rheumatol* 1979;**6(Suppl 5):**1.

Kean WF, Anastassiades TP: Long term chrysotherapy: Incidence of toxicity and efficacy during sequential time periods. *Arthritis Rheum* 1979;**22:**495.

Lyle WH: Penicillamine. *Clin Rheum Dis* 1979;**5:**569.

Mackenzie AH: An appraisal of chloroquine. *Arthritis Rheum* 1970;**13:**280.

Proceedings: International Symposium on Penicillamine, Miami, May 8–9, 1980. *J Rheumatol* 1981;**8(Suppl 7):**1.

Stein HB et al: Adverse effects of D-penicillamine in rheumatoid arthritis. *Ann Intern Med* 1980;**92:**24.

Zvaifler NJ: Antimalarials in the treatment of rheumatoid arthritis. *Mod Treat* 1971;**8:**769.

Miscellaneous Antirheumatic Drugs

Drew SI et al: Levamisole-associated neutropenia and autoimmune granulocytotoxins. *Ann Rheum Dis* 1980;**39:**59.

Dwosh IL et al: Azathioprine in early rheumatoid arthritis: Comparison with gold and chloroquine. *Arthritis Rheum* 1977;**20:**685.

Fauci AS et al: Cyclophosphamide therapy of severe systemic necrotizing vasculitis. *N Engl J Med* 1979;**301:**235.

Shearn MA, Tu WH: Proliferative glomerulonephritis associated with levamisole therapy of rheumatoid arthritis. *J Rheumatol* 1981;**8:**55.

Symoens J, Schuermans Y: Levamisole. *Clin Rheum Dis* 1979;**5:**603.

Veys EM et al: Levamisole as basic treatment of rheumatoid arthritis: Longterm evaluation. *J Rheumatol* 1981;**8:**45.

Williams HJ et al: Comparison of high and low dose cyclophosphamide therapy in rheumatoid arthritis. *Arthritis Rheum* 1980;**23:**527.

Wolff SM et al: Wegener's granulomatosis. *Ann Intern Med* 1974;**81:**513.

Nonopiate Analgesic Drugs

Baird WM, Turek D: Comparison of zomepirac, APC with codeine, codeine and placebo in the treatment of moderate and severe postoperative pain. *J Clin Pharmacol* 1980;**20:**243.

Gonwa TA, Hamilton RW, Buckalew VM Jr: Chronic renal failure and end-stage renal disease in Northwest North Carolina. *Arch Intern Med* 1981;**141:**462.

Koch-Weser J: Drug therapy: Acetaminophen. *N Engl J Med* 1979;**295:**1297.

Lewis JR: Zomepirac sodium: A new nonaddicting analgesic. *JAMA* 1981;**246:**377.

Pruss TP et al: Evaluation of the analgesic properties of zomepirac. *J Clin Pharmacol* 1980;**20:**216.

Slattery JT, Levy G: Acetaminophen kinetics in acutely poisoned patients. *Clin Pharmacol Ther* 1979;**25:**184.

Drugs Used in Gout

Boss GR, Seegmiller JE: Hyperuricemia and gout: Classification, complications and management. *N Engl J Med* 1979;**300:**1459.

Chawla SK et al: Allopurinol hepatotoxicity: Case report and literature review. *Arthritis Rheum* 1977;**20:**1546.

Landgrebe AR, Nyham WL, Coleman M: Urinary-tract stones resulting from the excretion of oxypurinol. *N Engl J Med* 1975;**292:**626.

Levinson DJ, Sorensen LB: Renal handling of uric acid in normal and gouty subjects: Evidence for a 4-component system. *Ann Rheum Dis* 1980;**39:**173.

Liang MH, Fries JF: Asymptomatic hyperuricemia: The case for conservative management. *Ann Intern Med* 1978;**88:**666.

Rodnan GP et al: Allopurinol and gouty hyperuricemia: Efficacy of a single daily dose. *JAMA* 1975;**231:**1143.

Schweitz MC, Nashel DJ, Alepa P: Ibuprofen in the treatment of acute gouty arthritis. *JAMA* 1978;**239:**34.

Seegmiller JE: Human aberrations of purine metabolism and their significance for rheumatology. *Ann Rheum Dis* 1980;**39:**103.

Wright DG et al: Efficacy of intermittent colchicine therapy in familial Mediterranean fever. *Ann Intern Med* 1977;**86:**165.

Introduction to Endocrine Pharmacology | 34

Henry R. Bourne, MD

When a drug is made by the patient's body, rather than by a pharmaceutical chemist, we call it a hormone. Endocrine drugs, like many other drugs, act by mimicking or interfering with chemical signals that mediate normal biologic regulation. Because hormones are synthesized in discrete anatomic sites and circulate in the blood, these chemical signals are particularly amenable to experimental manipulation and chemical analysis. Consequently, as will be explained in subsequent chapters, the physiologic and even molecular mechanisms of many endocrine drugs have been specifically identified. This chapter will describe the cellular mechanisms involved in endocrine regulation in an idealized system and is intended to serve as a basis for understanding the actions and uses of drugs described in later chapters.

THERAPEUTIC USES & SITES OF ACTION OF ENDOCRINE DRUGS

The clinical uses of endocrine drugs can be summarized as follows:

(1) To repair a deficiency of a specific hormone (or of its normal effect): The first triumphs of clinical endocrinology came from observations that extracts of certain glands—eg, adrenal, thyroid, and pancreatic islet cells—could restore normal physiologic function in animals from which the glands had been surgically removed. Administration of hormones to treat specific deficiencies still constitutes one of the most gratifying and effective modes of drug therapy in modern clinical medicine.

(2) To compensate for excess or inappropriate effect of a specific hormone: When surgical removal of a hyperfunctioning gland is not possible or must be delayed, drugs can often be used to decrease the secretion or effects of the excess hormone.

(3) To alter (or test) the functional integration of an endocrine system: Many endocrine responses are controlled by feedback loops (see below). By stimulation or pharmacologic blockade of one component in the loop, it is often possible to alter the hormonal response of a second component. Oral contraceptives employ this principle in preventing ovulation. Diagnostically, the same principle may be used to identify the site of a pathologic lesion, eg, in determining whether excess endogenous cortisol is due to a tumor in the pituitary or adrenal gland.

(4) Treatment of nonendocrine disease by stimulation or blockade of normally functioning endocrine responses: With the exception of diabetes mellitus, most classic endocrine diseases are relatively rare. Accordingly, endocrine drugs are most commonly used in treatment of nonendocrine disorders—as in therapy of asthma with glucocorticoids, breast cancer with sex steroids, or hypertension with mineralocorticoid antagonists. Subsequent chapters describe many additional examples of each of these uses of endocrine drugs.

In order to understand how endocrine drugs work, it is useful first to review the basic mechanism of endocrine regulation and the 3 general sites of drug action in an idealized endocrine system: the hormone-producing cell, the circulating hormone itself, and the target cell or tissue on which the hormone acts (Fig 34–1).

HORMONE-PRODUCING CELL

These specialized cells may be localized in a discrete gland or dispersed (like pancreatic islet cells) throughout a larger organ. Such cells may synthesize a peptide hormone, eg, insulin or parathyroid hormone, from larger precursor polypeptides and store the hormone in intracellular granules for release on demand. Alternatively, they may respond to stimulation by increasing synthesis of a hormone that is immediately secreted, as in the case of steroid hormones. Hormone secretion may be regulated by another hormone (eg, corticotropin and cortisol); by neural influences (cholinergic stimulation of catecholamine release from the adrenal medulla); by the concentration of a circulating ion or metabolite (ionized calcium and parathyroid hormone, glucose and glucagon); or by all 3 kinds of regulation (as is the case with the insulin-secreting beta cells of pancreatic islets).

In most cases, synthesis or secretion of a hormone is negatively regulated by one or more mechanisms that sense an effect of the hormone produced. Such negative feedback loops may be relatively simple (ele-

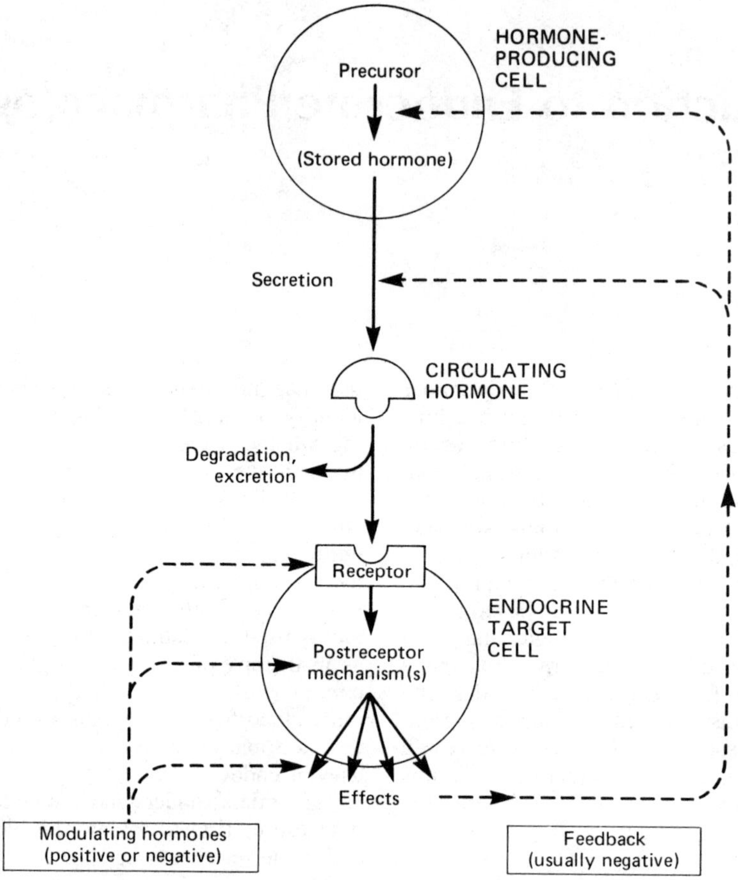

Figure 34–1. An idealized endocrine system, showing potential sites of action of endocrine drugs.

vated blood glucose → increased insulin secretion → reduction of blood glucose → decreased insulin secretion) or may involve multiple interacting pathways in different organs (as exemplified by relations between renin, angiotensin, aldosterone, and blood volume and concentration of Na^+ and K^+).

CIRCULATING HORMONE

As is the case with all drugs, the chemical structure of a hormone determines its distribution among tissues, its susceptibility to enzymatic degradation, and its excretion from the body. In addition, certain hormones (eg, cortisol, sex steroids) are transported in blood by specific carrier proteins. Any of these processes may alter the concentration of a hormone in blood and its accessibility to the target cell and thereby alter its effects.

ENDOCRINE TARGET CELL

Each target cell possesses its own complement of specific hormone receptors capable of discriminating between the appropriate hormone and other circulating molecules. Binding of the hormone to cell receptors initiates a sequence of postreceptor events that results in the characteristic hormonal response of that cell—lipolysis, thermogenesis, production of a second hormone, etc. In addition, the cell's responsiveness to one hormone in many cases can be modified by additional hormones, which may act by altering the receptors for the first hormone or the enzymes involved in postreceptor mediation of the hormonal effect. Thus, for example, glucocorticoids can regulate responsiveness of many tissues to insulin, and thyroid hormones can alter responsiveness of the cardiovascular system to catecholamines.

The 3 components of this idealized endocrine system present a multitude of potential sites of drug action. The remainder of this chapter surveys these sites in order to introduce concepts that underlie the actions of currently useful endocrine drugs and to suggest opportunities for development of new drugs.

DRUG ACTIONS ON HORMONE-PRODUCING CELLS

Table 34–1 lists drugs that are clinically useful because of their primary actions on hormone-producing cells. These drugs are divided into 2 groups depending on whether they act via hormone receptors or not.

The drugs listed in group A in Table 34–1 are used as *hormones* to produce effects normally produced by endogenous hormones. Thus, corticotropin and thyrotropin are used to test the ability of their target glands to produce cortisol and thyroid hormones, respectively. Conversely, triiodothyronine (T_3) or dexamethasone (a potent synthetic analog of cortisol) is used to determine whether the pituitary's stimulation of thyroid or adrenocortical hormone production can be appropriately suppressed by the hormonal product of the target gland. These negative feedback loops are described in more detail in Chapters 36 and 37. (***Note:*** In addition to their use in endocrine tests, T_3 and dexamethasone are used clinically for their direct effects on tissues.)

The other 3 drugs in group A are used in therapy rather than in tests of endocrine function. Estrogens and progestins act as contraceptives by suppressing pituitary production of gonadotropins, which are necessary for induction of ovulation. These effects of oral contraceptives take advantage of the negative feedback regulation normally exerted by sex steroids on the pituitary. The efficacy of these contraceptives results from altering the timing and extent of normal pituitary suppression (see Chapter 38). Growth hormone promotes growth, in part, by stimulating hepatic production of somatomedins (Chapter 35) and is used in replacement therapy for pituitary dwarfism. Bromocriptine acts as a dopaminergic agonist to prevent pituitary release of prolactin. Although this drug is used to prevent pathologic galactorrhea (eg, caused by autonomously prolactin-secreting pituitary cells), it acts by augmenting a normal regulatory pathway that is mediated by dopamine.

Table 34–1. Drugs used for their primary action on hormone-producing cells.

Drug	Action	Clinical Use
Group A: Drugs that act via hormone receptors.		
Growth hormone	Increases somatomedin release.	Pituitary dwarfism.
Corticotropin	Increases cortisol release.	Test adrenal responsiveness.
Thyrotropin	Increases production of T_4 and T_3.	Test thyroid responsiveness.
Oral contraceptives	Decrease gonadotropin production.	Prevent ovulation.
T_3	Decreases thyrotropin production.	Test integrity of pituitary-thyroid axis.
Dexamethasone	Decreases corticotropin production.	Test integrity of pituitary-thyroid axis.
Bromocriptine	Decreases prolactin secretion.	Galactorrhea.
Group B: Drugs that do not act via hormone receptors.		
Iodide, thionamides	Decrease production of T_4 and T_3.	Thyrotoxicosis.
Sulfonylureas	Increase insulin production.	Diabetes mellitus.
Metyrapone	Decreases cortisol production.	Test integrity of pituitary-adrenal axis.
Aminoglutethimide	Decreases cortisol production.	Cushing's syndrome.
Mitotane (*o,p'*-DDD)	Destroys adrenocortical cells.	Adrenal carcinoma.
Streptozocin	Destroys pancreatic islet cells.	Pancreatic islet cell carcinoma.

Thus, all the drugs in group A act via hormone receptors that are essential control points in normal regulatory pathways. These drugs were discovered by the classic methods of endocrinology: surgical extirpation of a gland and demonstration that an extract of the gland can restore a normal endocrine function, followed eventually by isolation of the pure hormone and, in some cases, by synthesis of a congener of the hormone.

In contrast, none of the drugs in group B act via normal hormone receptors, and most of them were discovered serendipitously, as a result of investigations not directed toward understanding endocrine regulation. For example, the sulfonylureas—now widely used in treating maturity-onset diabetes (Chapter 39)—were developed because of the clinical observation that a sulfonamide caused hypoglycemia in the course of treatment of typhoid fever. Similarly, goiters in rabbits fed a diet composed largely of cabbage led to discovery of the thionamides. Prototypes of this class of drug—now extremely useful in suppressing thyrotoxicosis—were isolated from cabbage seeds (Chapter 36).

Such fortuitous advances suggest that hormone-producing cells contain many potential sites at which synthesis or secretion of hormones can be specifically altered by drugs. Even when the specific drug is already available, it is not always easy to determine exactly where these sites are. Thus, despite considerable research, it is still not clear, at a molecular level, how sulfonylureas stimulate insulin release or precisely how the thionamides block incorporation of iodine into thyroid hormones (see Chapters 36 and 39). Similarly, although mitotane and streptozocin are cytotoxic to many cell types, they show considerable specificity in killing tumors derived from adrenal cortex and pancreatic islets, respectively. This specificity must indicate quite specific molecular targets in the 2 cell types, although the molecules involved are unknown.

The molecular sites of action of aminoglutethimide and metyrapone are well established. These drugs inhibit specific enzymatic steps in the biosynthesis of cortisol (Chapter 37). Pharmacologic inhibition of cortisol production provides additional probes for testing the integrity of the pituitary-adrenal axis and may also be useful in preventing or decreasing the deleterious effects of excess cortisol in some patients (eg, when Cushing's syndrome is caused by ectopic corticotropin in an inoperable lung carcinoma).

None of the agents in group B specifically affect the endocrine function of cells that produce peptide hormones such as parathyroid hormone, growth hormone, calcitonin, or the pituitary trophic hormones. Such drugs will eventually be developed as a result of continuing advances in understanding the molecular mechanisms involved in synthesis, storage, and release of these hormones.

We have contrasted drugs that alter hormone production by acting on hormone receptors (group A) with those that act on nonreceptor components of the hormone-producing cell (group B). Development of agents in the first group directly followed characterization of normal hormones, which provided chemical structures to be copied or modified. Consequently, these drugs possess the advantage of biologic specificity, selected by evolution.

Drugs in the second group have exactly the opposite potential advantage: Because they do *not* act through hormone receptors, their potential actions are not confined to those of endogenous hormones. Thus, in spite of the fact that no known hormone directly inhibits production of thyroid hormones, it was possible to develop drugs like the thionamide propylthiouracil that have precisely this effect.

A survey of endocrine diseases reveals obvious clinical needs for new agents that might be added to the list in group B. For example, a new drug (analogous to mitotane) that selectively kills parathyroid cells or a drug (analogous to aminoglutethimide) that specifically inhibits synthesis of parathyroid hormone would rapidly find a place in the therapy of parathyroid tumors or primary or secondary hyperparathyroidism, respectively. Similarly, a drug that specifically inhibits synthesis of gonadotropins without producing the potentially undesirable effects of sex steroids would be an obvious candidate for use as an oral contraceptive in both men and women.

PHARMACOLOGIC IMPORTANCE OF THE METABOLISM, DISTRIBUTION, & EXCRETION OF HORMONES

In principle, the effect of a natural hormone could be regulated by varying its rate of production, its rate of degradation, or the sensitivity of its target cell. With few exceptions, nature appears to have concentrated on the first and last of these mechanisms. In most endocrine systems, investigation has failed to uncover physiologically meaningful regulation of the rate of clearance of a hormone from the compartment in which it acts.* Nonetheless, the rate of clearance of a hormone or hormone congener from the bloodstream can be of crucial clinical importance, because it helps to determine the rate of onset and the duration of action of exogenously administered hormones.

Thyroid hormones exemplify this principle. Thus, the maximal effect of a given daily dose of T_3 (plasma half-life less than 2 days) occurs much sooner than does the maximal effect of thyroxine (plasma half-life more than 7 days). Correspondingly, the effects of thyroid hormone dissipate much more rapidly upon withdrawal of T_3 than when thyroxine administration is stopped. The clinical implications of these differences are examined in Chapter 36.

The very much shorter plasma half-lives of most peptide hormones create a different set of therapeutic problems. Thus, hormone replacement therapy with insulin (plasma half-life 9 minutes) would be impossible if insulin could not be injected in forms that release active hormone into the bloodstream over several hours. The therapeutic challenge posed by varying metabolic requirements for insulin over the course of a day—depending upon ingestion of carbohydrate, exercise, etc—has stimulated development of short-, intermediate-, and long-acting insulin preparations. The specific characteristics of these preparations must be thoroughly understood by both the physician and the diabetic patient (see Chapter 39).

As a therapeutic strategy, deliberate manipulation of the metabolism and distribution of endogenous hormones and endocrine drugs is just beginning to be explored. The pharmacology of catecholamines, refined over more than 4 decades, provides many examples of such a strategy (see Chapters 7–9). These include the following: (1) specific enzyme inhibitors that increase the concentration of endogenous neurohormone (monoamine oxidase inhibitors); (2) structural modification of catecholamine congeners to bypass metabolizing enzymes (eg, terbutaline, which is not a substrate for catechol-O-methyltransferase); (3) structural modifications that enhance gastrointestinal absorption or distribution to specific sites such as the brain (eg, amphetamine); (4) administration of a precursor of specific neurohormone or congener (methyldopa, levodopa); and (5) coadministration of an enzyme inhibitor (carbidopa) with a catecholamine precursor (levodopa) to reduce accumulation of the active drug (dopamine) at receptors where an effect is not desired.

This general strategy can be more easily pursued with chemically simple hormones—biogenic amines, steroids, etc—than with the peptide hormones, for obvious reasons. Thus, development of peptide hormone congeners that can be administered orally presents a difficult challenge. Similarly, it will be difficult to design congeners of insulin, parathyroid hormone, or gonadotropins that are simultaneously resistant to biodegradation, nonantigenic, and effective at appro-

*Norepinephrine, the sympathetic neurotransmitter, is a possible exception in that presynaptic reuptake of the transmitter is regulated by norepinephrine itself. This reuptake process is a determinant of the extent and duration of stimulation of postsynaptic receptors, as described in Chapter 4.

priate receptor sites. The development of captopril, a specific inhibitor of the protease that generates angiotensin II and degrades bradykinin (see Chapters 9 and 15), suggests that it should be possible to develop specific inhibitors of the proteolytic synthesis or degradation of other peptide hormones.

DRUGS THAT ACT ON THE ENDOCRINE TARGET CELL

Most endocrine drugs act directly on endocrine target cells by binding to receptors for endogenous hormones. The mechanisms of action and therapeutic uses of these drugs vary greatly in complexity. In the simplest case, the drug substitutes for a deficient hormone and may indeed be chemically identical to the hormone. The therapeutic strategies followed in administering most endocrine drugs are more complex. These include administration of supraphysiologic doses of hormones, use of hormone congeners with enhanced receptor specificity (greater than observed with the normal hormone), and use of hormone antagonists. In addition, hormones and hormone antagonists that bind to one class of receptor can be used to modulate the effects of hormones that act through a different class of receptor. After a review of the postreceptor mechanisms by which different classes of receptors produce their effects, the pharmacologic and therapeutic principles that underlie all these strategies will be considered, proceeding from the simplest case to the most complex.

POSTRECEPTOR MECHANISMS OF HORMONE ACTION

The mechanisms of action of hormones fall into 2 general groups: **Gene-active hormones** promote synthesis of specific messenger RNA (mRNA) and thus increase synthesis of key proteins whose activities produce the effects seen in the target cell. **Membrane-active hormones** employ several mechanisms to change the activities of enzymes and proteins that have already been synthesized.

Gene-Active Hormones

The steroid hormones (glucocorticoids, mineralocorticoids, sex steroids, and vitamin D metabolites) all act by a common general mechanism, as depicted in Fig 34–2. The hormone enters the cytoplasm, where it binds to a specific receptor. The steroid-receptor complex then undergoes an activation process that enables it to enter the nucleus, where it binds to sites on chromatin and regulates transcription of specific gene sequences into RNA. The RNA molecules are processed to form mRNAs, which leave the nucleus and bind to ribosomes where their nucleotide sequences are translated into the corresponding amino acid sequences of specific enzymes and pro-

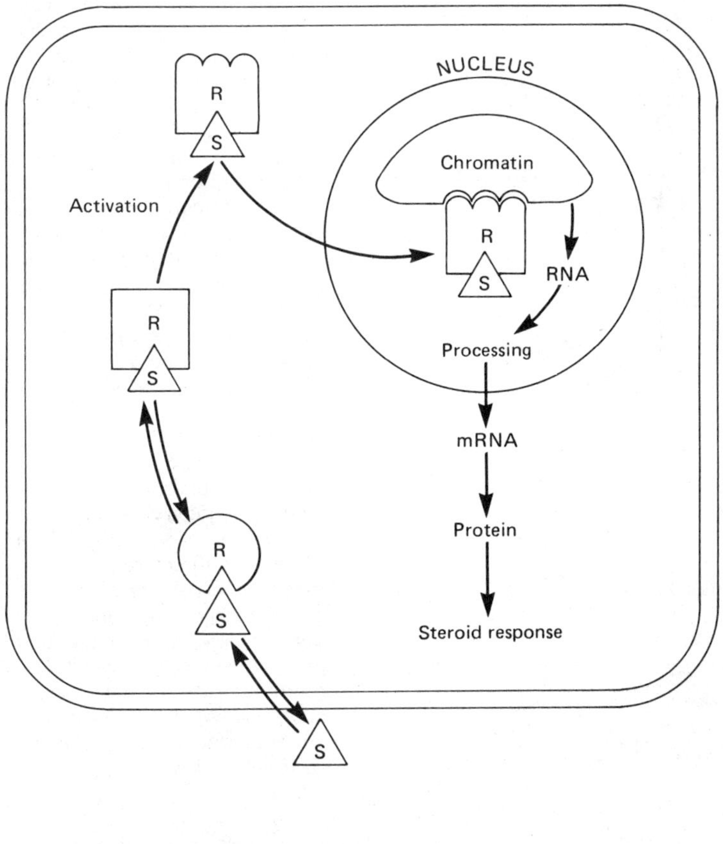

Figure 34–2. Mechanism of action of steroid hormones in mammalian cells. The steroid hormone (S) binds reversibly to a cytoplasmic receptor (R), and the steroid-receptor complex undergoes an irreversible activation step that allows it to enter the nucleus, where it activates transcription of specific genes into RNA. After processing in the nucleus, the corresponding mRNAs code for ribosomal synthesis of the specific proteins that mediate the steroid response.

teins. Note that the specificity of action of a steroid hormone thus depends upon the type of steroid receptor involved. Once it has formed a complex with hormone, each type of steroid receptor is able to activate the transcription of a limited number of specific genes. Thus, although a cell may possess both glucocorticoid and sex steroid receptors, the 2 different classes of hormone will induce synthesis of different sets of mRNAs and proteins.

Thyroid hormones act by a similar mechanism. The sequence of events differs from that shown for steroid hormones in that the thyroid hormones bind to receptors that are already present in the nucleus, so that the cytoplasmic binding and receptor activation steps are omitted. Thyroid hormones also bind with some specificity to sites in the plasma membrane, cytoplasm, and mitochondria. Because some experimentally observed effects of these hormones do not require de novo protein synthesis, these effects may be mediated by extranuclear receptors via mechanisms that do not alter gene expression.

Two important therapeutic implications follow from the mechanisms of action of the gene-active hormones: (1) As a class, all of these hormones produce their effects after a characteristic lag period of 30 minutes to several hours—a period that is required for synthesis of new proteins. An increase in blood concentration of these hormones will produce an increased effect after a similar lag period. This means that the gene-active hormones cannot be expected to alter a pathologic state within minutes—eg, glucocorticoids will not immediately relieve the symptoms of acute bronchial asthma. (2) When tissues are exposed for a brief period to increased concentrations of these hormones in plasma, the effects characteristically persist for hours or days. This may be due in part to high affinity of hormone for receptor (which means that the agonist dissociates slowly from the receptor once it has been bound). The persistence of effect is also due to the relatively slow turnover of most enzymes and proteins, which can remain active in cells for hours or even days after they have been synthesized. In this way, a cell or tissue can "remember" that it came in contact with a gene-active hormone at an earlier time. Therapeutically, this means that the beneficial (or toxic) effects of a gene-active hormone will usually decrease slowly when the administration of the hormone is discontinued and that there will not be a simple temporal correlation between plasma concentration of the hormone and its effects.

Membrane-Active Hormones

Many hormones—including most peptide hormones, the biogenic amines, and the prostaglandins—combine with receptors in the plasma membrane. These hormones produce their effects on target cells by a diverse set of mechanisms. The best-established mechanism involves synthesis of an intracellular "second messenger," cyclic 3′,5′-adenosine monophosphate (cyclic AMP, cAMP) (Fig 34–3). The hormone-receptor complex interacts with a guanine nucleotide-binding membrane protein, which in turn

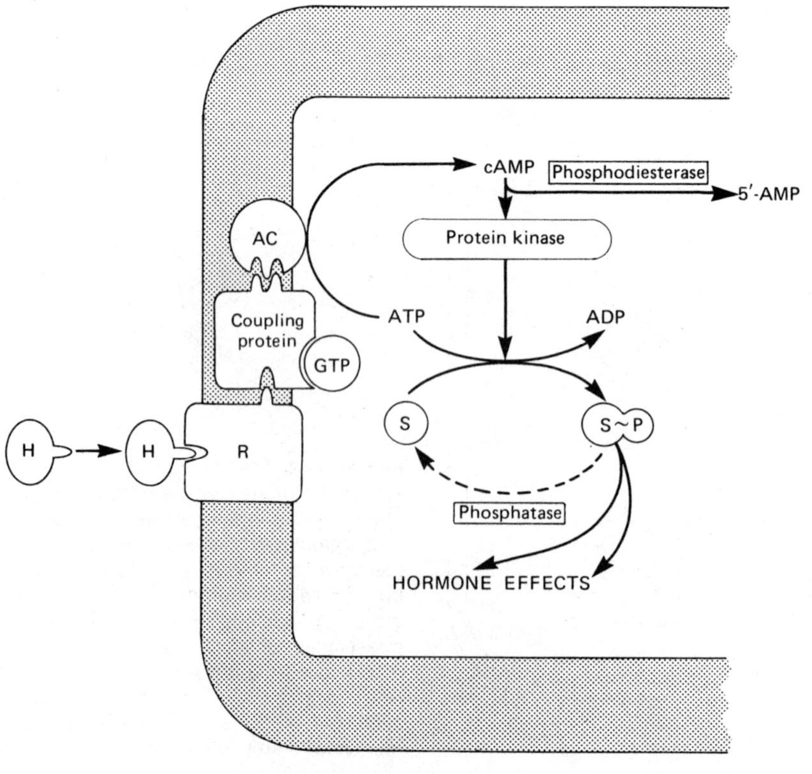

Figure 34–3. Cyclic AMP (cAMP) as an intracellular second messenger for hormones. The diagram depicts an idealized cell containing the enzymes involved in mediating the actions of hormones that work via cAMP. Hormone (H) binds to its membrane receptor (R), triggering the guanosine triphosphate (GTP)-dependent activation of adenylate cyclase (AC) by a membrane-bound coupling protein. cAMP synthesized by adenylate cyclase diffuses through the cytoplasm and activates cAMP-dependent protein kinase, which in turn catalyzes the phosphorylation of specific substrate proteins (S), usually enzymes. Altered activity of the phosphorylated substrates, denoted S~P, produces the characteristic effects of cAMP (and therefore of the hormone) in a particular cell. The stimulatory action of hormones is opposed by cyclic nucleotide phosphodiesterase, which degrades cAMP, and by phosphatases, which dephosphorylate substrates of cAMP-dependent protein kinase.

stimulates conversion of intracellular ATP to cAMP by a third membrane-bound protein, the enzyme adenylate cyclase. Within the cell, cAMP relays the hormonal message by combining with its own receptor, cAMP-dependent protein kinase. Activated by cAMP, the protein kinase catalyzes phosphorylation of specific enzymes, thus stimulating or inhibiting their activities. Either directly or through a series of subsequent metabolic steps, altered activities of these enzymes produce the characteristic effect of a hormone on its target cell.

The cAMP-dependent phosphorylation mechanism produces very rapid responses to hormone (ie, within seconds), because it only requires activation of enzymes already present in the cell. Similarly, disappearance of the hormone is rapidly followed by disappearance of its effect, owing to degradation of intracellular cAMP by cyclic nucleotide phosphodiesterases and dephosphorylation of kinase substrates by phosphatases. This quick-on, quick-off mechanism is well suited for moment-to-moment regulation of physiologic responses to rapid changes in the environment—as in the "fight-or-flight" sympathetic response, which involves several cAMP-mediated processes (cardioacceleration, glycogenolysis, lipolysis, etc).

Table 34–2 lists the membrane-active hormones that are thought to act by stimulating cAMP synthesis and an additional group of hormones that are not. (Note that some hormones, such as the catecholamines, appear in both groups, because some of their actions are clearly mediated by cAMP, while others are not.) In general, the actions of hormones that do not work via cAMP are not well understood. For example, it is not known whether insulin stimulates glucose uptake via a second messenger analogous to cAMP or whether the insulin receptor directly interacts with a glucose transport protein in the membrane. Some hormones in this second group appear to act by increasing intracellular concentrations of chemical signals such as calcium ion or cyclic 3′,5′-guanosine monophosphate (cGMP). Certain of these hormones also *decrease* cAMP synthesis in some tissues (eg, insulin and prostaglandin E_1 in adipose tissue, α-adrenergic amines in platelets).

Table 34–2. Postreceptor mechanisms of action of membrane-active hormones.*

cAMP as "Second Messenger"	Mechanism Not Established
Adrenocorticotropic hormone (ACTH)	Angiotensin
Calcitonin	Catecholamines (α-adrenergic)
Catecholamines (β-adrenergic)	Chorionic somatomammotropin (placental lactogen, PL)
Chorionic gonadotropin (hCG)	Epidermal growth factor (EGF)
Follicle-stimulating hormone (FSH)	Fibroblast growth factor (FGF)
Glucagon	Growth hormone
Histamine (H_2)	Histamine (H_1)
Luteinizing hormone (LH)	Insulin
Luteinizing hormone-releasing hormone (LHRH)	Nerve growth factor (NGF)
Lipotropin (LPH)	Oxytocin
Melanocyte-stimulating hormone (MSH)	Prolactin
Nerve growth factor (NGF)	Prostaglandin $F_{2\alpha}$
Prostacyclin, prostaglandin E_1	Somatomedin
Thyrotropin-releasing hormone (TRH)	Somatostatin
Thyroid-stimulating hormone (TSH)	Vasopressin (ADH)
Vasopressin (ADH)	

*Modified and reproduced, with permission, from Baxter JD, McLeod KM: Molecular basis for hormone action. In: *Duncan's Diseases of Metabolism.* Bondy PK, Rosenberg LE (editors). Saunders, 1980.

Although the biochemical mechanisms of hormone action are the subject of intensive investigation, relatively few drugs act to block or enhance the actions of hormones at sites distal to the hormone receptor. The methylxanthines caffeine and theophylline inhibit cyclic nucleotide phosphodiesterases and may produce some of their effects, such as bronchodilation, by blocking intracellular degradation of cAMP.

Despite the lack of drugs that act specifically on postreceptor mechanisms, the multiplicity of these mechanisms has important therapeutic implications. Many important homeostatic functions are regulated by more than one hormone and often by both gene-active and membrane-active hormones. When excess or deficiency of one of these hormones is difficult to treat directly, indirect therapy based on the actions of a second hormone can often be effective. The therapeutic uses of such hormone-hormone interactions are discussed in a later section of this chapter.

THERAPY BASED ON RECEPTOR SPECIFICITY OF THE TARGET CELL

Whatever their ultimate mechanism of action on the target cell, hormones and hormone analogs derive their therapeutic usefulness from specific interactions with hormone receptors. Receptor specificity allows direct replacement of a missing hormone, use of hormone analogs with greater potency or specificity than the natural hormone, and use of hormone antagonists.

Hormone Replacement Therapy

Conceptually, treatment of endocrine deficiency disorders appears quite straightforward, now that the chemical structures of most hormones are well established and they are available in pure form. Clinically, however, effective therapy is not always simple.

In order to design an effective replacement regimen, the physician must first understand the hormone's role in normal regulation. What is the hormone's normal plasma concentration? What is the normal rate of its secretion? What are the environmental and physiologic stresses that require increased secretion of the hormone in a normal person? What additional problems in a sick patient may modify either end organ responsiveness to the hormone or its metabolism and thus alter the effectiveness or toxicity of the exogenously administered agent?

Right or wrong answers to these questions may dramatically affect the outcome of insulin replacement therapy in diabetes—determining the frequency of life-threatening ketoacidosis or hypoglycemic coma and perhaps influencing the incidence and severity of vascular complications of this disease (Chapter 39). In a more subtle fashion, knowing that the normal adrenal produces 10–20 times more cortisol under conditions of severe stress may avert disaster when a patient with adrenal insufficiency is subjected to major surgery or develops pneumonia (Chapter 37). Many similar examples are presented in subsequent chapters.

Enhanced Specificity of Hormonal Agonists

Some endocrine drugs are used in an "extraphysiologic" fashion to produce an effect not usually observed in a normally regulated endocrine system rather than to replace a missing hormone. In this more complex situation, the physician often seeks to induce an intense pharmacologic effect in certain tissues and risks producing toxic effects in other target tissues. A cardinal example is the use of glucocorticoids for their anti-inflammatory, immunosuppressive, or lympholytic actions. The glucocorticoids may be life-saving, but they also can produce a host of dangerous toxicities that include acute psychosis, increased catabolism of protein, arrested growth (in children), hyperglycemia, cataracts, retention of salt and water, etc (see Chapter 37).

To avoid or minimize such toxic effects, 2 therapeutic strategies may be used. The first of these—simple to describe, often difficult to use in practice—is to administer the hormonal agonist (eg, the glucocorticoid) in the lowest dose and for the shortest period possible. In every case, the drug dosage should be reduced or discontinued as soon as the disorder—bronchial asthma, Crohn's disease, thrombocytopenic purpura, whatever—is amenable to less dangerous treatment.

The second strategy takes advantage of the fact that a single hormone or hormone analog may interact with more than one kind of receptor. If one of these receptors mediates the desired therapeutic effect while a second receptor is responsible for a toxic effect, the chemist may be able to design a synthetic agonist that selectively binds to the first receptor. Thus, in comparison to the natural hormone cortisol, synthetic steroids such as prednisone and dexamethasone have much greater affinity for glucocorticoid receptors and much lower affinity for mineralocorticoid receptors. This "improvement on nature" can reduce or eliminate one of the toxic effects of adrenal steroids—retention of salt and water.

Exploitation of this kind of receptor selectivity has been most successful with chemically simple hormones such as the adrenal steroids and catecholamines. The diversity of receptors for many other hormones—including histamine, dopamine, endogenous opioids, vasopressin, and even insulin—is just beginning to be explored.

Hormone Antagonists

Disorders of hormone excess present obvious potential opportunities for use of specific hormone antagonists. Here again, the chemically simple hormones have been exploited most successfully, as with the use of α- and β-adrenergic antagonists in treatment of pheochromocytoma. In treating more common diseases, hormone antagonists are used to block regulatory pathways that may be physiologically normal but are nonetheless deleterious to the patient suffering from a nonendocrine disorder—eg, propranolol for hypertension, cimetidine for peptic ulcer, tamoxifen to block estrogen actions that may support growth of breast cancer, or spironolactone to block the sodium-retaining effects of aldosterone in congestive heart failure.

Useful antagonists to most of the peptide hormones have proved more difficult to synthesize, probably owing to their chemical complexity. Saralasin, an angiotensin II antagonist, is finding restricted use in the diagnosis of some kinds of hypertension (Chapter 9). Antagonists (or partial agonists) to corticotropin, luteinizing hormone-releasing hormone, glucagon, oxytocin, and parathyroid hormone have been used experimentally in animals or isolated cells but not yet in humans. Obstacles to development of such antagonist drugs include chemical complexity, the fact that they often turn out to be partial agonists (like tamoxifen and saralasin), and—especially with peptides—the difficulty of finding a drug that is effective when administered orally.

Hormone-Hormone Interactions

Virtually every important homeostatic function is regulated by more than one control system. In most cases, as with regulation of arterial blood pressure or the concentration of plasma glucose, it is possible to delineate a finely tuned network of multiple synergistic and antagonistic controls, mediated by autonomic nerves and hormones. In pathologic states where the therapeutic strategies discussed above prove inadequate, it is often possible to take advantage of these redundant regulatory mechanisms by administering hormones or hormone antagonists.

The cardiovascular and metabolic effects of excess thyroid hormone, for example, can produce a medical emergency that is difficult to treat. No specific receptor antagonist to thyroid hormone is available; drugs that suppress synthesis and release of thyroid hormone act too slowly to provide the immediate relief that may be necessary; and thyroid surgery in the thyrotoxic state is extremely dangerous. In such a situation, propranolol, a β-adrenergic antagonist, can swiftly reduce many of the signs and symptoms caused by excess thyroid hormone and allow time for other therapy to take effect. The physiologic basis of this therapy is fairly well understood: Thyroid hormones and β-adrenergic catecholamines normally regulate many functions, such as heart rate, in the same direction; in addition, thyroid hormones increase the sensitivity of the heart to β-adrenergic stimuli (see Chapters 8 and 36).

In the other direction, synergistic actions of hormones can sometimes be used to treat a hormone deficiency when direct replacement of the hormone is difficult or impossible. Examples include the use of mineralocorticoids to maintain blood pressure in patients with autonomic insufficiency and the use of vitamin D metabolites to elevate serum calcium in hypoparathyroidism.

Note that each of these examples involves a physiologic synergism between a gene-active and a membrane-active hormonal signal (thyroid hormone and catecholamines, mineralocorticoids and catecholamines, vitamin D and parathyroid hormone). The existence of multiple hormonal controls, acting through distinct postreceptor mechanisms, allows the physician to treat disorders that are not yet amenable to more "specific" therapy.

• • •

References

Baxter JD, McLeod KM: Molecular basis for hormone action. Chap 4, pp 104–160, in: *Duncan's Diseases of Metabolism*. Bondy PK, Rosenberg LE (editors). Saunders, 1980.

Bernal J, Refetoff S: The action of thyroid hormone. *Clin Endocrinol (Oxf)* 1977;**6**:227.

Chan L, O'Malley BW: Steroid hormone action: Recent advances. *Ann Intern Med* 1978;**89**:694.

Roth J, Grunfeld C: Endocrine systems: Mechanisms of disease, target cells, and receptors. Chap 2, pp 15–72, in: *Textbook of Endocrinology*. Williams RL (editor). Saunders, 1981.

Sutherland EW: Studies on the mechanism of hormone action. *Science* 1972;**177**:401.

Williams RL: *Textbook of Endocrinology*. Saunders, 1981.

35 | Hypothalamic & Pituitary Hormones

David C. Klonoff, MD, & John H. Karam, MD

Neuroendocrine control of metabolism, growth, and certain aspects of reproduction is mediated by a combination of neural and endocrine systems located in the hypothalamus and pituitary gland. The pituitary gland weighs an average of about 0.6 g and rests in the bony sella turcica under a layer of dura mater. It is connected to overlying brain by a stalk from the hypothalamus containing neurosecretory fibers surrounded by a complex of blood vessels, including a portal venous system that drains the hypothalamus and perfuses the anterior pituitary.

The pituitary gland consists of an anterior lobe (adenohypophysis), intermediate lobe, and posterior lobe (neurohypophysis), which under hypothalamic influence release a number of hormones that either control the secretion of other endocrine glands or affect metabolic actions of target tissues directly (Table 35–1).

The secretion of anterior lobe hormones is regulated by factors formed in the median eminence of the hypothalamus and carried to the adenohypophysis by the hypothalamic-hypophyseal portal venous system (Fig 35–1). These factors are small peptides that function as releasing or inhibiting hormones. The structures of several of these peptides have been determined, thus permitting the synthesis of the natural hormones as well as of experimentally modified forms.

The posterior lobe hormones are synthesized in the hypothalamus and transported via the neurosecretory fibers in the stalk of the pituitary to the posterior lobe, from which they are released into the circulation.

The hormones of the intermediate lobe (Table 35–1) have melanocyte-stimulating properties that are important in animals that utilize skin color changes as adaptive mechanisms. They have not been identified as discrete hormones in humans and therefore have no role at present in clinical pharmacology.

Therapeutic preparations of pituitary and hypothalamic peptide hormones are usually synthetic; a few are purified from human sources. Their applications lie in 3 areas: (1) as replacement therapy for hormone deficiency states; (2) as drug therapy for a variety of disorders using pharmacologic doses to elicit a hormonal effect that is not present at physiologic blood levels; and (3) as diagnostic tools for performing stimulation tests to diagnose hypo- or hyperfunctional endocrine states.

Table 35–1. Pituitary hormones.*

Name and Source	Principal Actions
Anterior lobe	
Growth hormone (GH, somatotropin, STH)	Accelerates body growth.
Adrenocorticotropic hormone (ACTH, corticotropin)	Stimulates adrenocortical secretion and growth.
Thyroid-stimulating hormone (TSH, thyrotropin)	Stimulates thyroid secretion and growth.
Follicle-stimulating hormone (FSH)	Stimulates ovarian follicle growth in female and spermatogenesis in male.
Luteinizing hormone (LH, interstitial cell–stimulating hormone, ICSH)	Stimulates ovulation and luteinization of ovarian follicles in female and testosterone secretion in male.
Prolactin (luteotropic hormone, LTH, luteotropin, lactogenic hormone, mammotropin)	Stimulates secretion of milk and maternal behavior. Maintains corpus luteum in female rodents but apparently not in other species.
β-Lipotropin (β-LPH)	?
Intermediate lobe	
α- and β- Melanocyte-stimulating hormones (α- and β-MSH; referred to collectively as melanotropin or intermedin)	Expand melanophores.
Posterior lobe	
Vasopressin (antidiuretic hormone, ADH)	Promotes water retention.
Oxytocin	Causes milk ejection.

*Reproduced, with permission, from Ganong WF: *Review of Medical Physiology,* 10th ed. Lange, 1981.

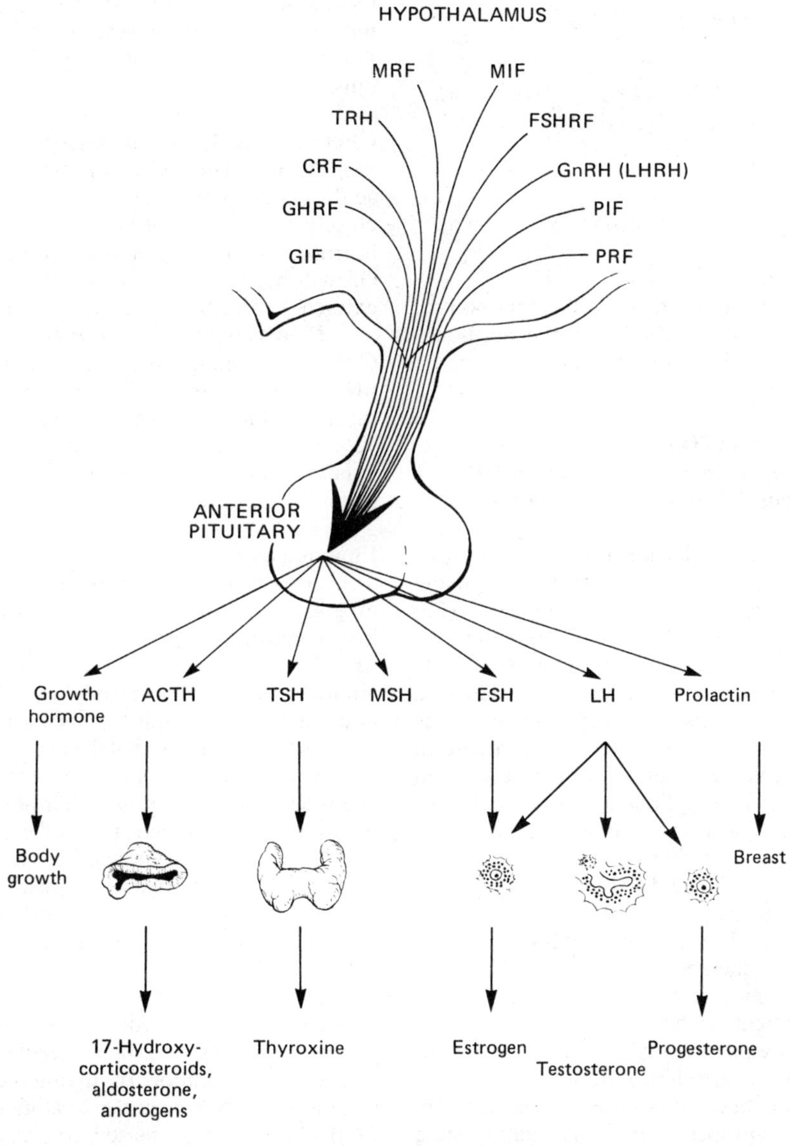

Figure 35–1. Hypothalamic releasing factors and actions of anterior pituitary hormones. GHRF, growth hormone–releasing factor; GIF (somatostatin); CRF, corticotropin-releasing factor; TRH, thyrotropin-releasing hormone; MRF, melanocyte-releasing factor; MIF, melanocyte-inhibiting factor; FSHRF, follicle-stimulating hormone–releasing factor; GnRH (LHRH), gonadotropin-releasing hormone, luteinizing hormone–releasing hormone; PIF, prolactin-inhibiting factor; and PRF, prolactin-releasing factor.

HYPOTHALAMIC & ANTERIOR PITUITARY HORMONES

Hypothalamic regulatory hormones that have been identified and (in most cases) synthesized include a growth hormone-inhibiting factor (somatostatin), thyrotropin-releasing hormone, corticotropin-releasing factor, gonadotropin-releasing hormone (GnRH, LHRH), and prolactin-inhibiting factor (PIF, now known to be dopamine).

Six anterior pituitary hormones are recognized: growth hormone, thyrotropin, adrenocorticotropin, follicle-stimulating hormone, luteinizing hormone, and prolactin.

It also appears that certain hormones from the thyroid, adrenal cortex, and gonads inhibit hypophyseal-pituitary release of their respective tropic hormones, while neurotransmitters such as serotonin, norepinephrine, and dopamine directly influence the secretion of the hypothalamic hormones by the peptidergic neurons of the median eminence.

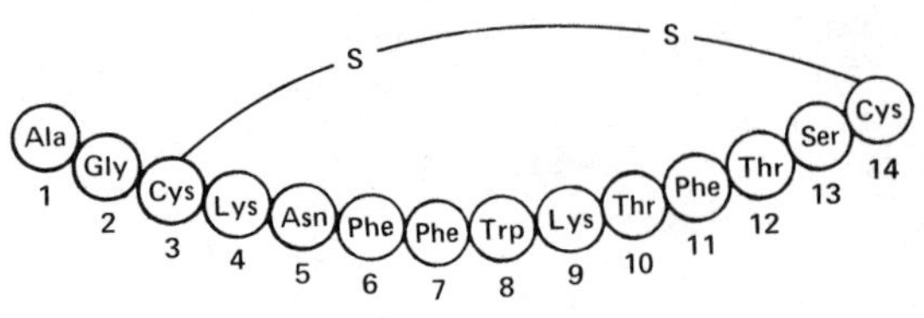

Figure 35–2. Amino acid sequence of somatostatin.

In the discussion below, the hypothalamic control peptides are paired with their pituitary target hormones in the order in which they are listed above.

SOMATOSTATIN (Growth Hormone–Inhibiting Hormone, GIF, Somatotropin Release–Inhibiting Factor)

Somatostatin, a tetradecapeptide, has been isolated from the hypothalamus and other parts of the central nervous system. It has been sequenced (Fig 35–2) and synthesized. This substance has been shown to inhibit growth hormone release in response to a wide variety of stimuli in normal individuals. It produces a decrease in circulating insulin levels and interferes with the ability of thyrotropin-releasing hormone to cause thyrotropin release. Somatostatin has also been identified in the pancreas and other sites in the gastrointestinal tract. It has been shown to inhibit the release of glucagon, insulin, and gastrin.

Exogenously administered somatostatin is rapidly cleared from the circulation, with an initial half-life of 1–3 minutes. The kidney appears to play an important role in its metabolism and excretion.

Somatostatin can effectively inhibit growth hormone release in patients with acromegaly. However, it is of no use in the treatment of this disorder because of its lack of specificity and short duration of action.

Peptides have been synthesized that partially separate the various properties of somatostatin, and a 7-aminoheptanoic acid derivative containing only 4 of the 14 amino acids of somatostatin has been found to block the effect of somatostatin.

A 28-amino-acid peptide called prosomatostatin isolated from intestine and hypothalamus is believed to be the precursor of somatostatin. It is 10 times more potent than somatostatin in inhibiting insulin secretion in rats, but its effect on glucagon secretion is only twice that of somatostatin. Its greater potency and prolonged action make prosomatostatin more useful than somatostatin in testing hormonal control mechanisms.

GROWTH HORMONE (Somatotropin, GH)

Growth hormone is a peptide hormone produced by the anterior pituitary. Growth hormone has direct metabolic effects on lipolysis in adipose tissue and on insulin action and indirect anabolic effects mediated through another class of factors known as somatomedins.

Chemistry & Pharmacokinetics

A. Structure: Growth hormone is a 191-amino-acid peptide with 2 sulfhydryl bridges. Its structure closely resembles those of prolactin and the placental hormone human chorionic somatomammotropin. Growth hormone for pharmacologic use is presently extracted from human cadaver pituitaries.

B. Absorption, Metabolism, and Excretion: Circulating endogenous growth hormone has a half-life of 20–25 minutes and is predominantly cleared by the liver. Human growth hormone can be dissolved in a 15% w/v gelatin solution and administered intramuscularly, with peak levels occurring in 2–4 hours and active blood levels persisting for 36 hours.

Pharmacodynamics

Growth hormone has both metabolic and anabolic effects. The metabolic consequence of a pharmacologic dose of growth hormone is an initial insulin-like effect with increased tissue uptake of glucose and amino acids and decreased lipolysis. Within a few hours there is a peripheral insulin-antagonistic effect with impaired glucose uptake and increased lipolysis.

The major anabolic consequence of a pharmacologic dose of growth hormone is longitudinal growth. The anabolic effects of growth hormone are mediated indirectly via another class of peptide hormones, the somatomedins, or insulinlike growth factors. Growth hormone stimulates synthesis of somatomedins (predominantly in the liver); somatomedins promote uptake of sulfate into cartilage and are probably the actual mediators of the cellular processes associated with bone growth. This growth can be traced back to the molecular level, where increased incorporation of thymidine into DNA and uridine into RNA occur (indicating cellular proliferation) along with increased conversion of proline to hydroxyproline (indicating cartilage synthesis).

It has long been recognized that growth hormone deficiency leads to inadequate somatomedin production and dwarfism. There are also states of dwarfism in which elevated plasma growth hormone levels fail to induce adequate production of somatomedins.

Clinical Pharmacology

Timely growth hormone replacement therapy will permit achievement of full predicted adult height in children with growth hormone deficiency. Criteria for diagnosis of growth hormone deficiency usually include (1) stature more than 2 SD below the mean for age and sex, (2) growth velocity (measured over 1 year) below the 25th percentile for age, and (3) impaired growth hormone secretion during an insulin tolerance test. The prevalence of congenital growth hormone deficiency is approximately one in 4000. Congenital growth hormone deficiency can result from lesions affecting the hypophyseal-pituitary region such as craniopharyngiomas but is most often due to lack of hypothalamic growth hormone-releasing factors, resulting in pituitary dwarfism. In the newborn, hypoglycemia and even seizures can occur in the absence of growth hormone.

In addition to isolated growth hormone deficiency, congenital deficiencies of multiple pituitary hormones occur with approximately equal frequency. Affected children will respond with normal growth to administration of growth hormone plus appropriate other pituitary replacement preparations. Acquired growth hormone deficiency, which is often accompanied by multiple hormone deficiencies, may also respond well to growth hormone plus other hormone replacements as needed provided the underlying disease process can be controlled.

Preparations & Dosage

Animal preparations of growth hormone are ineffective in humans. Treatment of children with human growth hormone has been limited by the scarcity of the hormone as well as its expense.

Commercially available growth hormone (somatropin) freeze-extracted from human pituitaries comes in vials containing 4 IU (Crescormon) or 10 IU (Asellacrin). Specific activity of these preparations is approximately 21 IU per milligram of protein.

Initial recommended therapy is 0.05–0.1 unit/kg intramuscularly 3 times weekly. Maximal growth is achieved with the largest dose, but current supplies of the preparation are not adequate to support such use.

Stimulated by the great medical need for a larger supply of growth hormone, a massive research effort has recently been successful in producing a biosynthetic human growth hormone through recombinant DNA technology. The expressed product contains the same amino acid sequence as human growth hormone, except for the addition of a methionyl residue at the N-terminal end. By all of the indices measured in short-term studies, synthetic methionyl human growth hormone is equipotent with pituitary human growth hormone and justifies current optimism that adequate supplies of growth hormone will soon be available to meet clinical needs.

Toxicity & Contraindications

Growth hormone prepared in national pituitary centers may cause antibody formation in up to 2% of patients, with subsequent resistance and lack of augmented growth. Somatropin powder for injection prepared from frozen pituitaries has a lower incidence of antibody formation. A patient whose initial response to growth hormone begins to fail should be tested for antibodies and changed from acetone- to freeze-extracted hormone therapy if titers are present. There is a theoretic possibility of transmitting hepatitis through the freezing technique, although this has not actually been reported.

Growth hormone is contraindicated in patients with actively growing pituitary tumors. Patients receiving growth hormone should be screened regularly for diabetes. If growth slows, in the absence of a rising titer of antibodies, they should be tested for deficiencies of other pituitary hormones. Untreated hypothyroidism or excessive glucocorticoid replacement therapy can impair growth.

THYROTROPIN-RELEASING HORMONE (TRH)

Thyrotropin-releasing hormone, or protirelin, is a tripeptide hormone found in the hypothalamus as well as in other parts of the brain. TRH is secreted into the portal venous system and stimulates the pituitary to produce thyrotropin, which in turn stimulates the thyroid to produce thyroxine (T_4). TRH stimulation of thyrotropin is blocked by thyroxine and stimulated by lack of thyroxine such that the extent of thyrotropin response to TRH stimulation forms the basis for using TRH as a diagnostic agent in the evaluation of hyperthyroid and hypothyroid states.

Chemistry & Pharmacokinetics

A. Structure: TRH is (pyro)Glu-His-Pro-NH_2.

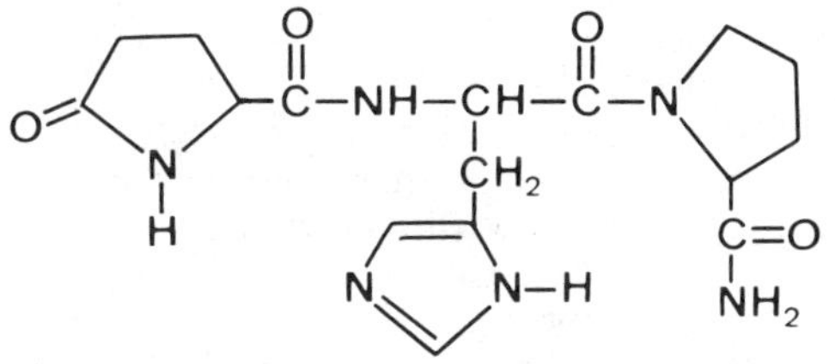

Thyrotropin-releasing hormone (protirelin)

B. Absorption, Metabolism, and Excretion: TRH is usually administered intravenously. Rapid plasma inactivation occurs, with a half-life of 4–5 minutes.

Pharmacodynamics

TRH stimulates pituitary production of thyrotropin, possibly through stimulation of adenylate cyclase. TRH stimulation of thyrotropin may be blocked by pretreatment with thyroxine, corticosteroids, and somatostatin. TRH stimulation of prolactin production is not blocked.

Peak serum thyrotropin levels occur 20–30 minutes after an intravenous TRH injection in healthy individuals. In hyperthyroidism, high serum thyroxine levels blunt the thyrotropin response to TRH. In primary hypothyroidism, thyrotropin levels start high, and the pituitary response to TRH may be quite large, with a particularly brisk outpouring of additional thyrotropin. In secondary (pituitary) hypothyroidism, serum thyrotropin levels start low and fail to rise after TRH administration. In tertiary (hypothalamic) hypothyroidism, the baseline serum thyrotropin level may be low or normal, and the thyrotropin response to TRH may be delayed.

TRH infusion leads to stimulation of prolactin release by the pituitary in healthy individuals but has no effect on cells producing growth hormone or ACTH. In certain types of pituitary tumors, however, the neoplastic cells may respond abnormally to TRH by releasing growth hormone (in acromegaly), by releasing ACTH (in Cushing's disease), or by failing to release prolactin (in prolactinoma).

Clinical Pharmacology

TRH is used only for diagnostic purposes. A TRH infusion test is the most sensitive method for diagnosing mild hyperthyroidism and mild hypothyroidism in the minimally symptomatic patient with equivocal serum thyroxine or thyrotropin levels. In spite of overlap in the responses between various hyper- and hypothyroid states and normals, the test is quite valuable in some patients.

A blunted thyrotropin response to TRH occurs in approximately half of euthyroid patients with Graves' exophthalmopathy, whereas orbital mass lesions are associated with a normal thyrotropin response.

TRH infusion has also been suggested as a test for differentiating unipolar and bipolar depressions. However, a blunted thyrotropin response can occur in many psychiatric disorders, making such a test useless.

Preparations & Dosage

TRH is available as protirelin (Relefact TRH, Thypinone) in ampules for intravenous injection. The dosage is 500 μg for adults and 7 $\mu g/kg$ for children age 6 or older but not to exceed the adult dose. A baseline thyrotropin level should be obtained, followed by 3 further determinations at 15, 30, and 60 minutes postinfusion.

Toxicity

Up to 50% of patients tested may note side-effects lasting for a few minutes: nausea, an urge to urinate, light-headedness, a metallic taste, or abdominal discomfort. Transient hypertension may occur.

THYROID-STIMULATING HORMONE (Thyrotropin, TSH)

Thyrotropin is an anterior pituitary hormone that regulates thyroid function by stimulating production of thyroxine. Diagnostic use of thyrotropin in various states of borderline thyroid function has been largely supplanted by measurement of the baseline thyrotropin concentration and its response to TRH as well as by sensitive radionuclide scanning methods. Therapeutic use of thyrotropin in conjunction with ^{131}I ablation is established in selected cases of thyroid carcinoma to enhance thyroid radioiodine uptake.

Chemistry & Pharmacokinetics

A. Structure: Thyrotropin consists of 2 peptides (α and β), each containing branched carbohydrate side chains. Therapeutic thyrotropin is prepared from bovine anterior pituitaries. There is 70% homology between human and bovine TSH-α subunits and 90% homology between human and bovine TSH-β subunits. The TSH-α subunit sequence in humans is virtually identical to that of the α subunit of FSH, LH, and hCG.

B. Absorption, Metabolism, and Excretion: Thyrotropin is administered intramuscularly or subcutaneously. Its half-life is approximately 1 hour, with degradation occurring in the kidneys. However, unlike gonadotropins, little thyrotropin appears in the urine.

Pharmacodynamics

Thyrotropin stimulates thyroid cell adenylate cyclase activity. Increased cAMP production causes increased iodine uptake and, ultimately, increased production of thyroid hormones. Increased thyroid size and vascularity follow thyrotropin administration.

Clinical Pharmacology

A. Diagnostic Uses: Radioiodine uptake following thyrotropin uptake has been used to distinguish primary and secondary hypothyroidism from the euthyroid state. This method has been largely replaced by TRH stimulation of thyrotropin production, which is quicker, less expensive, and easier to interpret.

B. Therapeutic Uses: Thyrotropin has a role in the therapy of metastatic thyroid carcinoma. Following a tumoricidal dose of ^{131}I, the patient is maintained on triiodothyronine for 10 weeks and then taken off hormone replacement for 3 weeks. Finally, the patient is given thyrotropin, 5–10 units subcutaneously daily for 3–7 days, in an attempt to elicit iodine uptake by remaining metastatic tissue. Additional ^{131}I is then administered if needed.

Preparations & Dosage

Thyrotropin (Thytropar) is derived from beef pituitaries and is intended for intramuscular or subcutaneous administration. A dose of 5 units per day for 3 days is used for diagnostic purposes; 5–10 units per day for 3–7 days is used in conjunction with ^{131}I ablation of thyroid carcinoma.

Toxicity

Local soreness at the injection site is common. Nausea, vomiting, thyroid tenderness, allergic symptoms, and symptoms of hyperthyroidism may occur. This drug should be used cautiously in the presence of heart disease or adrenocortical insufficiency.

CORTICOTROPIN-RELEASING FACTOR (CRF)

This hypothalamic peptide contains 41 amino acids. It has been chemically synthesized and proved to have corticotropin-releasing action on cultured pituitary cells. This effect is associated with cAMP generation. The hormone-releasing action of CRF is specific for corticotrophs (cells that synthesize corticotropin), since only ACTH and β-endorphin release occurs, with no observed effect on growth hormone or thyrotropin secretion. Glucocorticoids prevent the release of ACTH by cultured pituitary corticotrophs in response to CRF. A pharmacologic use has not yet been established for this peptide, but it may provide a means of differentiating hypothalamic versus pituitary causes of ACTH deficiency or excess. Furthermore, its availability will permit the development of radioimmunoassays to elucidate its physiologic role and its contribution to the pathogenesis of Cushing's disease.

ADRENOCORTICOTROPIN
(Corticotropin, ACTH)

Adrenocorticotropin is a peptide hormone produced in the anterior pituitary. Its primary endocrine function is to stimulate synthesis and release of adrenocortical hormones. Pharmacologic administration of corticotropin results in increased production not only of cortisol but of adrenal androgens and mineralocorticoids as well. Corticotropin can be used therapeutically, but its primary usefulness is in the assessment of adrenocortical responsiveness. A substandard adrenocortical response to exogenous corticotropin administration indicates adrenocortical insufficiency.

Chemistry & Pharmacokinetics

A. Structure: Human ACTH is a single polypeptide chain of 39 amino acids (Fig 35–3). The N-terminal portion containing amino acids 1–24 is necessary for full biologic activity. The remaining amino acids (25–39) confer species specificity. Therapeutic ACTH preparations are derived from porcine pituitaries and differ in structure from human ACTH only in the nonessential 25–39 region. Synthetic human $ACTH_{1-24}$ is known as cosyntropin (Cortrosyn). The N-terminal amino acids 1–13 are identical to melanocyte-stimulating hormone (α-MSH), which has been found in animals but not humans. In states of excessive pituitary ACTH secretion, hyperpigmentation, due to the α-MSH activity intrinsic to ACTH, may be noted.

ACTH from animal sources is assayed biologically by measuring the depletion of adrenocortical ascorbic acid that follows subcutaneous administration of the ACTH. Synthetic ACTH can be assayed by weight. The steroidogenic activity of 1 unit of porcine ACTH is approximately equal to that of 10 μg of cosyntropin.

B. Absorption, Metabolism, and Excretion: Both porcine and synthetic corticotropin are well absorbed by the intramuscular route. Corticotropin cannot be administered orally because of gastrointestinal proteolysis.

The biologic half-lives of $ACTH_{1-39}$ and $ACTH_{1-24}$ are under 20 minutes. Tissue uptake occurs in the liver and kidneys. $ACTH_{1-39}$ is transformed into a biologically inactive substance with a structure similar to that of $ACTH_{1-39}$, probably by modification of a side chain. ACTH is not excreted in the urine in significant amounts.

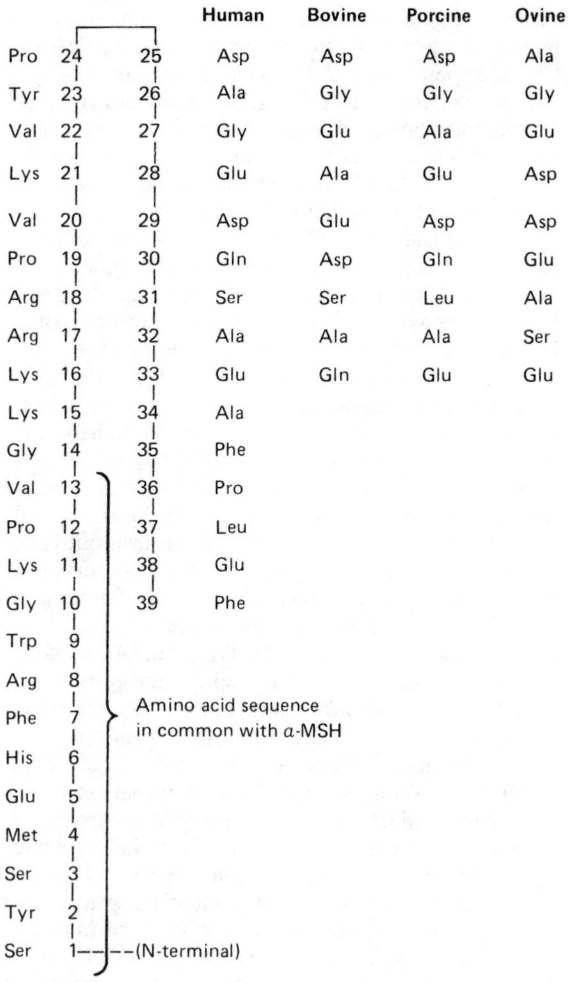

Figure 35–3. Amino acid sequences of human, bovine, porcine, and ovine adrenocorticotropin.

The effects of a long-acting repository form of porcine corticotropin persist for up to 18 hours with an ACTH-gelatin complex, and up to several days with an ACTH-zinc hydroxide complex.

Pharmacodynamics

ACTH stimulates the adrenal cortex to produce glucocorticoids, mineralocorticoids, and androgens. ACTH increases the activity of cholesterol esterase, the enzyme that catalyzes the rate-limiting step of steroid hormone production: cholesterol → pregnenolone. ACTH also stimulates adrenal hypertrophy and hyperplasia. In pharmacologic doses, corticotropin may cause adipose tissue lipolysis and increased skin pigmentation.

Clinical Pharmacology

A. Therapeutic Uses: Corticotropin may be prescribed for patients with normal adrenal function when increased glucocorticoid concentrations are desired. Chronic use of ACTH has been proved successful in allergic disorders, asthma, rheumatoid arthritis, inflammatory bowel disease, infantile spasms (hypsarhythmia), and multiple sclerosis. In choosing between ACTH and glucocorticoids, side-effects should be considered, since their effectiveness is similar.

Advantages of ACTH over glucocorticoids include less suppression of the hypothalamic-pituitary axis and less growth suppression in children. Disadvantages of ACTH compared to glucocorticoids, in addition to the necessity for parenteral administration, include a higher incidence of side-effects attributable to increased adrenal mineralocorticoid and androgen production (hypertension, hirsutism, and acne); the requirement for a state of adrenal responsiveness; and the hyperpigmentation that may occur with prolonged administration of high doses. On balance, the disadvantages of ACTH appear to outweigh its advantages, making glucocorticoids the drugs of choice in chronic conditions where anti-inflammatory or immunosuppressive therapy is warranted.

B. Diagnostic Uses: ACTH stimulation of the adrenals will fail to elicit an appropriate response in states of adrenal insufficiency. A rapid test for ruling out adrenal insufficiency employs cosyntropin (see below). Plasma cortisol levels are measured before and either 30 or 60 minutes following an intramuscular or intravenous injection of 0.25 mg of cosyntropin. A normal plasma cortisol response is a stimulated increment exceeding 7 μg/dL and a peak level exceeding 18 μg/dL. A subnormal response indicates primary or secondary adrenocortical insufficiency that can be differentiated using plasma ACTH levels (which are increased in primary adrenal insufficiency and decreased in the secondary form).

A normal response to ACTH testing excludes the necessity for daily glucocorticoid maintenance therapy but does not necessarily predict a normal pituitary response to stress. If elective surgery is contemplated in a patient with possible hypothalamic-pituitary-adrenal axis suppression, further testing with insulin-induced hypoglycemia or metyrapone is warranted; alternatively, the patient should be empirically treated with glucocorticoids.

The plasma 17-hydroxyprogesterone level rises in response to rapid ACTH infusion in patients with congenital adrenal hyperplasia due to 21-hydroxylase deficiency. Detection of the carrier state for this gene may be possible using this method, since heterozygotes also show enhanced production of 17-hydroxyprogesterone with ACTH infusion.

Preparations & Dosage

Porcine corticotropin is available in vials containing 25, 40, and 80 units per milliliter for parenteral use. Repository preparations containing gelatin for intramuscular or subcutaneous use or zinc hydroxide for intramuscular use only are available in vials containing 40 or 80 units/mL. Cosyntropin (Cortrosyn) (synthetic human $ACTH_{1-24}$) is available in vials of 0.25 mg for intravenous or intramuscular use. ACTH may be used therapeutically in doses of 10–20 units 4 times daily. Repository ACTH, 40–80 units, may be administered every 24–72 hours. Cosyntropin, 0.25 mg (= 25 units), is used for diagnostic studies.

Toxicity & Contraindications

The toxicity of ACTH resembles that of the glucocorticoids. The occasional development of antibodies to animal ACTH or to depot cosyntropin (a preparation not currently available in the USA) has produced anaphylactic reactions or refractoriness to ACTH therapy in a few individuals. Painful swelling occurs at the injection site more often with the zinc hydroxide depot preparation than with the gelatin preparation.

Contraindications are similar to those of glucocorticoids. Use of ACTH during pregnancy should be minimized. When immediate effects are desired, glucocorticoids are preferable.

GONADOTROPIN-RELEASING HORMONE (GnRH; Luteinizing Hormone–Releasing Hormone [LHRH])

Gonadotropin-releasing hormone is a decapeptide structure—(pyro)Glu-His-Trp-Ser-Tyr-Gly-Leu-Arg-Pro-Gly-NH_2—produced in the hypothalamus that controls the release of the gonadotropins FSH and LH.

Infusion of GnRH effects a rise in LH levels within 30 minutes plus a less rapid and less pronounced rise in FSH levels. cAMP is generated in cultured pituitary cells exposed to GnRH and is thought to contribute to the mechanism by which GnRH releases gonadotropins (Chapter 34).

Clinical Pharmacology

GnRH has been used successfully to induce ovulation in women with hypothalamic or so-called idiopathic amenorrhea as well as polycystic ovary syndrome. In males, this hormone has been used to stimulate spermatogenesis. Gonadotropin secretion is maximal when the GnRH infusion is intermittent rather than continuous. GnRH administered continuously has been used to inhibit gonadotropin production in precocious puberty.

GnRH infusion has been used as a diagnostic test to measure pituitary responsiveness. Serum FSH and LH levels usually rise markedly in response to GnRH infusion in hypothalamic hypogonadism. However, lack of a pituitary response may be seen in either pituitary or hypothalamic hypogonadal states. Therefore, GnRH stimulation is probably inadequate to distinguish pituitary from hypothalamic hypogonadism.

Toxicity

Ovarian hyperstimulation and multiple births appear to be much less common with GnRH than with gonadotropin therapy. Potential problems may appear with more widespread use.

FOLLICLE-STIMULATING HORMONE (FSH)

Follicle-stimulating hormone is a glycoprotein hormone produced in the anterior pituitary. It is composed of 2 peptide chains that, along with LH, regulate gonadal function. The principal function of FSH is to stimulate gametogenesis and follicular development in women and spermatogenesis in men.

A naturally modified form of FSH is available for therapeutic use. The urine of postmenopausal women contains a substance with FSH-like properties but with 4% of the potency and a different dose-response curve. There is also an LH-like substance in such urine. The use of these excreted menotropins (postmenopausal gonadotropins) is discussed below.

FSH acts on the immature follicular cells of the ovary and induces development of the mature follicle and oocyte. In the testes, FSH acts on the Sertoli cells and stimulates their production of androgen-binding protein.

LUTEINIZING HORMONE (LH)

Luteinizing hormone is a glycoprotein hormone consisting of 2 chains and, like FSH, is produced by the anterior pituitary. LH is primarily responsible for regulation of gonadal steroid hormone production. No LH preparation is presently available for clinical use. Human chorionic gonadotropin—with an almost identical structure—is available and can be used as a luteinizing hormone substitute in many gonadotropin-deficient states.

LH acts on the testicular Leydig cell to stimulate testosterone production. In the ovary, LH acts in concert with FSH to stimulate follicular development. LH acts on the mature follicle to induce ovulation, and it stimulates the corpus luteum in the luteal phase of the menstrual cycle to produce progesterone and androgens.

HUMAN MENOPAUSAL GONADOTROPINS (hMG)

Human menopausal gonadotropins are a mixture of partially catabolized human FSH and LH extracted from the urine of postmenopausal women. The commercial preparation of hMG, or menotropins (Pergonal), is biologically standardized for FSH and LH content. It is used in states of infertility to stimulate ovarian follicle development in women and spermatogenesis in men. In both sexes, it must be used in conjunction with a luteinizing hormone, ie, human chorionic gonadotropin (hCG), to permit ovulation and implantation in women and testosterone production and full masculinization in men.

Pharmacokinetics

Over a 14-day course of daily hMG administration intended to mimic the follicular phase of the ovarian cycle in women with hypothalamic amenorrhea, FSH levels gradually rise to twice their baseline level, and LH levels increase to 1½ times the baseline.

Pharmacodynamics

Ovarian follicular growth and maturation will occur during hMG treatment of gonadotropin-deficient women. Ovulation requires administration of chorionic gonadotropin when adequate follicular maturation has occurred.

In men with gonadotropin deficiencies, pretreatment with chorionic gonadotropin produces external sexual maturation; addition of a course of hMG will stimulate spermatogenesis and lead to fertility.

Clinical Pharmacology

hMG is indicated for pituitary or hypothalamic hypogonadism with infertility. Anovulatory women with the following conditions may benefit from hMG: primary amenorrhea, secondary amenorrhea, polycystic ovary syndrome, and anovulatory cycles.

Over 50% of men with hypogonadotropic hypogonadism become fertile after hMG administration.

Preparations & Dosage

An ampule of menotropins (Pergonal) contains 75 IU of FSH and 75 IU of LH. By bioassay, 1 IU of LH is approximately equivalent to 0.5 IU of hCG. hMG is administered intramuscularly.

A. Women: One ampule is administered daily for 9–12 days until evidence of adequate follicular maturation is present. Serum estradiol levels and a cervical examination should be performed daily. When appropriate follicular maturation has occurred, hMG is discontinued; the following day, hCG, 10,000 IU, is administered intramuscularly to induce ovulation.

B. Men: Following pretreatment with 4000–5000 IU of hCG 3 times weekly for up to 6 months in order to achieve masculinization, menotropins is administered as one ampule weekly in combination with hCG, 2000 IU twice weekly. At least 4 months of combined treatment are usually necessary before spermatozoa appear in the ejaculate.

Toxicity & Contraindications

Overstimulation of the ovary can lead to uncomplicated ovarian enlargement in approximately 20% of patients. This usually resolves spontaneously. The "hyperstimulation syndrome" occurs in 0.5–4% of patients. It is characterized by hMG-induced ovarian enlargement, ascites, hydrothorax, and hypovolemia, sometimes to the point of shock. Hemoperitoneum (from a ruptured ovarian cyst), fever, or arterial thromboembolism can occur. The frequency of multiple births is approximately 20%. A reported 25% incidence of spontaneous abortions may be due to earlier diagnosis of pregnancy in treated than in untreated patients, with recognition of very early abortion. There may, however, be abnormal development and premature degeneration of corpus luteum in some treated patients. Gynecomastia occasionally occurs in men.

hMG should be administered only by a physician experienced in treating infertility. Before treatment of women, a thorough gynecologic evaluation must be performed to rule out uterine, tubal, or ovarian disease as well as pregnancy. In cases of irregular bleeding, uterine cancer should be ruled out.

HUMAN CHORIONIC GONADOTROPIN (hCG)

Human chorionic gonadotropin is a hormone produced by the human placenta and excreted into the urine, whence it is extracted and purified. The function of hCG is to stimulate the ovarian corpus luteum to produce progesterone and maintain the placenta. hCG is very similar to LH in structure and is used to treat both men and women with LH deficiency.

Chemistry & Pharmacokinetics

A. Structure: hCG is a glycoprotein consisting of an alpha chain virtually identical to that of FSH, LH, and TSH and a beta chain of 147 amino acids that resembles that of LH except for the presence of a carboxy terminal sequence of 30 amino acids not present in LH.

Pharmacokinetics

hCG is well absorbed after intramuscular administration and has a biologic half-life of 8 hours, compared to 30 minutes for LH. The difference may lie in the high sialic acid content of hCG compared to LH. hCG is apparently modified in the serum prior to urinary excretion, because the half-life measured by immunoassay far exceeds that measured by bioassay.

Pharmacodynamics

hCG stimulates production of gonadal steroid hormones. The interstitial and corpus luteal cells of the female produce progesterone, and the Leydig cells of the male produce testosterone. hCG can be used to mimic a midcycle LH surge and trigger ovulation in a hypogonadotropic woman.

hCG has no established effect on fat mobilization, fat distribution, or appetite. It has been advocated without justification as an adjunct to dietary management in obese patients.

Clinical Pharmacology

A. Diagnostic Uses: In prepubertal boys with undescended gonads, a truly retained (cryptorchid) testis can be distinguished from a retracted (pseudocryptorchid) one using hCG. Testicular descent during a course of hCG administration usually foretells permanent testicular descent at puberty, when circulating LH levels rise. Lack of descent usually means that orchiopexy will be necessary at puberty to preserve spermatogenesis.

B. Therapeutic Uses: As described above, hCG can be used in combination with human menotropins to induce ovulation in women with secondary hypogonadism or to induce spermatogenesis in men with secondary hypogonadism.

Preparations & Dosage

Lyophilized powder preparations are available. The dosages for female and male infertility are described under hMG dosage. For prepubertal cryptorchidism, a dosage of 500–4000 units 3 times weekly for up to 6 weeks has been advocated.

Toxicity & Contraindications

Reported side-effects include headache, depression, edema, precocious puberty, gynecomastia, or (rarely) production of antibodies to hCG.

hCG should be administered for infertility only by a physician with experience in this field. Androgen-dependent neoplasia and precocious puberty are contraindications to its use.

PROLACTIN

Prolactin is a glycoprotein hormone produced in the anterior pituitary whose structure resembles that of growth hormone. Prolactin is the principal hormone responsible for lactation. Milk production is stimulated by prolactin when appropriate circulating levels of estrogens, progestins, corticosteroids, and insulin are present. Deficiency of prolactin—which can occur in states of pituitary deficiency—is manifested only by failure to lactate. In hypothalamic destruction, prolactin levels may be elevated as a result of impaired transport of prolactin-inhibiting factor (dopamine) to the pituitary. Hyperprolactinemia can produce galactorrhea and hypogonadism and may be associated with symptoms of a pituitary mass. No preparation is available for use in prolactin-deficient patients. For patients with symptomatic hyperprolactinemia, inhibition of prolactin secretion can be achieved with bromocriptine, a dopamine agonist (see below).

BROMOCRIPTINE

Although bromocriptine is not a hormone, it has important inhibitory effects on the pituitary that warrant its discussion here.

Bromocriptine is an ergot derivative with dopamine agonist properties that lowers circulating prolactin levels. Its chemical structure and pharmacokinetic features are presented in Chapter 14.

Bromocriptine decreases pituitary prolactin secretion through dopaminergic action on the pituitary at 2 central nervous system loci: (1) It decreases dopamine turnover in the tuberoinfundibular neurons of the arcuate nucleus, generating increased hypothalamic dopamine; and (2) it acts directly on pituitary dopamine receptors to inhibit spontaneous prolactin release and that evoked by thyrotropin-releasing hormone. Bromocriptine stimulates pituitary growth hormone release in normal subjects and—paradoxically, and for unknown reasons—suppresses growth hormone release in acromegalics.

Clinical Pharmacology

A. Amenorrhea/Galactorrhea: Bromocriptine is approved in the USA for short-term treatment of amenorrhea/galactorrhea associated with various hyperprolactinemic states other than pituitary tumors. Idiopathic hyperprolactinemia responds well to bromocriptine. Upon cessation of therapy, hyperprolactinemia and galactorrhea generally recur.

B. Physiologic Lactation: Bromocriptine suppresses the prolactin secretion that occurs after parturition or abortion and is used to prevent breast engorgement when breast feeding is not desired.

C. Prolactin-Secreting Adenomas: Although not yet approved in the USA for this purpose, bromocriptine is gaining wide acceptance as initial treatment for prolactinomas. Significant reduction in both tumor size and serum prolactin levels can be demonstrated with bromocriptine treatment. For definitive therapy of such tumors, eventual surgical excision with or without radiation therapy remains necessary, because the effects of long-term bromocriptine therapy are not known, and expansion of these tumors may occur if bromocriptine is discontinued.

D. Acromegaly: Although not approved for this indication in the USA, bromocriptine has also been used for acromegaly. Acromegalic patients demonstrate improvement of symptoms less frequently than those with prolactinomas and rarely achieve clinical remissions. There may also be dissociation between clinical improvement and plasma growth hormone levels, which may fall but rarely to normal. The role of bromocriptine in acromegaly remains to be determined.

E. Parkinson's Disease: The use of bromocriptine in Parkinson's disease is discussed in Chapter 25.

Preparations & Dosage

Bromocriptine (Parlodel) is supplied as 2.5-mg tablets. For amenorrhea/galactorrhea or prevention of physiologic lactation, 2.5–10 mg in divided doses taken with meals is used, and this dose is generally adequate to treat prolactin microadenomas. For larger prolactinomas, daily doses up to 20 mg may be needed, and even higher doses are required in acromegaly. Doses should be increased by no more than 2.5–5 mg/d.

Toxicity & Contraindications

Doses up to 10 mg daily may cause nausea, light-headedness, orthostatic hypotension, or constipation. Doses above 10 mg daily may cause cold-induced peripheral digital vasospasm, neuropsychiatric symptoms, or, rarely, peptic ulcer.

Animal experiments demonstrating teratogenicity of bromocriptine have not been confirmed by human studies, but bromocriptine should not be used during pregnancy. Women with infertility due to idiopathic hyperprolactinemia who have continued to take bromocriptine after conception have not been shown to deliver a higher rate of malformed offspring than do controls. Contraceptive measures may be needed when bromocriptine-induced restoration of fertility is likely to occur, as in treatment of amenorrhea/galactorrhea.

POSTERIOR PITUITARY HORMONES

Two posterior pituitary hormones are known: vasopressin and oxytocin. Their structures are very similar (Fig 35–4), and they probably have a common phylogenetic precursor. Secretion of posterior pituitary hormones is not regulated by hypothalamic releasing factors, as is the case with anterior pituitary hormones. Posterior pituitary hormones are synthesized in the hypothalamus and then transported intracellularly to the posterior pituitary, from which they are released into the circulation.

OXYTOCIN

Oxytocin is a peptide secreted by the posterior pituitary that elicits milk ejection in lactating women. In therapeutic doses, oxytocin can be used to induce uterine contractions and maintain labor; however, at physiologic blood levels, the contribution of this hormone to parturition is probably small.

Chemistry & Pharmacokinetics

A. Structure: Oxytocin is a 9-amino-acid pep-

S——S (bridge between positions 1 and 6)
Cys-Tyr-Phe-Gln-Asn-Cys-Pro-Arg-Gly-NH_2
1 2 3 4 5 6 7 8 9

Arginine vasopressin

S——S (bridge between positions 1 and 6)
Cys-Tyr-Ile-Gln-Asn-Cys-Pro-Leu-Gly-NH_2
1 2 3 4 5 6 7 8 9

Oxytocin

Figure 35–4. Arginine vasopressin and oxytocin. In some species, lysine is substituted for arginine in position 8 of the vasopressin molecule. (Reproduced, with permission, from Ganong WF: *Review of Medical Physiology,* 10th ed. Lange, 1981.)

tide composed of a 6-membered disulfide ring and a 3-membered tail containing the carboxy terminus. Oxytocin and vasopressin differ by only one amino acid residue each from vasotocin, which is the only posterior pituitary hormone found in nonmammalian vertebrates.

B. Absorption, Metabolism, and Excretion: Oxytocin is usually administered intravenously for stimulation of labor, although buccal absorption is possible. Oxytocin is inactive if swallowed, because it is destroyed in the stomach and intestine. Oxytocin is not bound to plasma proteins and is catabolized by the kidneys and liver, with a circulating half-life of 5 minutes.

Pharmacodynamics

Oxytocin alters transmembrane ionic currents in myometrial smooth muscle cells to produce sustained uterine contraction. The sensitivity of the uterus to oxytocin increases during pregnancy. Oxytocin-induced myometrial contractility can be inhibited by β-adrenergic agonists, magnesium sulfate, or inhalation anesthetics. Oxytocin also causes contraction of myoepithelial cells surrounding mammary alveoli, which leads to milk ejection. Without oxytocin-induced contraction, normal lactation cannot occur. Oxytocin is a weak antidiuretic acting at the same renal tubular location as vasopressin.

Clinical Pharmacology

A. Therapeutic Uses: Oxytocin is used for induction and reinforcement of labor in women with mild preeclampsia near term, uterine inertia, and incomplete abortion. The drug should not be used for elective induction of labor in the absence of these indications. Oxytocin can also be used for control of postpartum uterine hemorrhage. Impaired milk ejection may respond to oxytocin.

B. Diagnostic Uses: Oxytocin infusion near term will produce uterine contractions that decrease the fetal blood supply. The fetal heart rate response to a standardized oxytocin challenge test provides information about placental circulatory reserve. An abnormal response suggests intrauterine growth retardation and may warrant immediate cesarean delivery.

Preparations & Dosage

Oxytocin is available in vials (Pitocin, Syntocinon), for parenteral use, as buccal tablets (Pitocin), and as oxytocin nasal spray (Syntocinon). Intravenous oxytocin should be administered via an infusion pump with appropriate fetal monitoring. For induction of labor, an initial infusion rate of 1 mU/min is gradually increased up to 5–20 mU/min until a physiologic contraction pattern is established. For postpartum uterine bleeding, 10–40 units is added to 1 L of 5% dextrose, and the infusion rate is titrated to control uterine atony. Alternatively, 10 units can be given intramuscularly after delivery of the placenta. To induce lactation, one puff is sprayed into each nostril in the sitting position 2–3 minutes before nursing.

Toxicity & Contraindications

Among the reported adverse reactions are maternal deaths due to hypertensive episodes, uterine rupture, and water intoxication and fetal deaths. Afibrinogenemia has been reported.

Contraindications include fetal distress, prematurity, abnormal fetal presentation, cephalopelvic disproportion, and other predispositions for uterine rupture.

VASOPRESSIN
(Antidiuretic Hormone, ADH)

Vasopressin is a peptide hormone released by the posterior pituitary in response to rising plasma tonicity or falling blood pressure. Vasopressin possesses antidiuretic and vasopressor properties. A deficiency of this hormone results in diabetes insipidus (Chapters 13 and 15).

Chemistry & Pharmacokinetics

A. Structure: Vasopressin is a nonapeptide with a 6-amino-acid ring and a 3-amino-acid side chain. The residue at position 8 is arginine in humans and most other mammals except pigs and related species, whose vasopressin contains lysine at position 8 (Fig 35–4).

B. Absorption, Metabolism, and Excretion: Vasopressin must be administered parenterally. Intravenous, intramuscular, or inhalational routes of administration may be selected. The half-life of circulating ADH is approximately 20 minutes, with renal and hepatic catabolism via reduction of the disulfide bond and peptide cleavage. A small amount of vasopressin is excreted as such in the urine, but urinary clearance is less than 5% of that of creatinine and does not reflect plasma levels.

Pharmacodynamics

The antidiuretic effect of vasopressin is mediated through activation of cAMP in renal collecting duct cells, leading to an increase in permeability and increased resorption of water from the filtrate. Vasopressin is a vasoconstrictor of splanchnic vessels, which makes it useful in certain types of gastrointestinal bleeding. Unfortunately, vasopressin may also cause coronary artery vasoconstriction and can result in myocardial depression.

Clinical Pharmacology

Vasopressin is the treatment of choice for pituitary diabetes insipidus (Chapter 13). Vasopressin infusion is also effective in some cases of esophageal variceal bleeding and of colonic diverticular bleeding. It is much less effective in bleeding caused by gastric or small intestine mucosal damage.

Preparations & Dosage

Four preparations are in common use.

A. Aqueous Vasopressin: Aqueous vasopressin

(Pitressin Synthetic) is a short-acting preparation for intramuscular, subcutaneous, or intravenous administration. The dose is 5–10 units subcutaneously or intramuscularly every 3–6 hours for transient diabetes insipidus; 0.1–0.5 units/min intravenously for gastrointestinal bleeding.

B. Vasopressin Tannate in Oil: Vasopressin (Pitressin) tannate in oil is a long-acting form for intramuscular injection. The dosage is 2.5–5 units every 24–72 hours.

C. Lysine Vasopressin: Lypressin (Diapid) is a short-acting nasal spray. The dosage is 10–20 units sprayed deeply into one or both nostrils every 4–6 hours.

D. Desmopressin Acetate: Desmopressin acetate (DDAVP)—1-desamino-8-D-arginine vasopressin—is a long-acting synthetic analog of vasopressin for nasal administration. It is usually the preferred form for chronic therapy, although it is the most expensive. The dosage is 10–40 μg/d (0.1–0.4 mL) in 2 or 3 divided doses, usually as 0.1 mL (10 μg) inhaled deeply through a flexible graduated plastic nasal tube into a single nostril once at bedtime and once during the day. Ten micrograms of desmopressin is equivalent to 40 IU of vasopressin.

Toxicity & Contraindications

Headache, nausea, abdominal cramps, and allergic reactions have been reported. Overdosage can result in hyponatremia.

Vasopressin should be used cautiously in patients with coronary artery disease. Drugs known to potentiate the effects of vasopressin include chlorpropamide, clofibrate, and carbamazepine. Inhalation of vasopressin may be ineffective when nasal congestion is present.

• • •

References

Anoussakis C, Skopelitis P: HCG stimulation test in prepubertal boys with cryptorchidism. *J Pediatr* 1978;**93:**630.

Axelrod L: Glucocorticoid therapy. *Medicine* 1976;**55:**39.

Chechval MC, Mehan DJ: Chorionic gonadotropins in the treatment of the subfertile male. *Fertil Steril* 1979;**31:**666.

Cobb WE et al: Neurogenic diabetes insipidus: Management with DDAVP. *Ann Intern Med* 1978;**88:**183.

Crowley WF et al: The biologic activity of a potent analogue of gonadotropin-releasing hormone in normal and hypogonadotropic men. *N Engl J Med* 1980;**302:**1052.

Donald RA: ACTH and related peptides. *Clin Endocrinol (Oxf)* 1980;**12:**491.

Fogel MR et al: Continuous intravenous vasopressin in active upper gastrointestinal bleeding. *Ann Intern Med* 1982;**96:**565.

Frasier SD et al: A dose-response curve for human growth hormone. *J Clin Endocrinol Metab* 1981;**53:**1213.

Hammond CB et al: Ovulation induction with luteinizing hormone-releasing hormone in amenorrheic, infertile women. *Am J Obstet Gynecol* 1979;**135:**924.

Harman SM et al: Evaluation of pituitary gonadotropic function in men: Value of luteinizing hormone-releasing hormone response versus basal luteinizing hormone level for discrimination of diagnosis. *J Clin Endocrinol Metab* 1982;**54:**196.

Hintz RL et al: Biosynthetic methionyl human growth hormone is biologically active in adult man. *Lancet* 1982;**1:**1276.

Hyek A, Peake GT: Growth and somatomedin-C responses to growth hormone in dwarfed children. *J Pediatr* 1981;**99:**868.

Jackson IMD: Thyrotropin-releasing hormone. *N Engl J Med* 1982;**306:**145.

Larsen PR: Thyroid-pituitary interaction. *N Engl J Med* 1982;**306:**23.

Lin C-C et al: Oxytocin challenge test and intrauterine growth retardation. *Am J Obstet Gynecol* 1981;**140:**282.

Lindsay AN et al: Growth hormone deficiency in twins: Three cases with normal co-twins. *Pediatrics* 1982;**69:**486.

Malone DNS, Strong JA: The present status of corticotrophin therapy. *Practitioner* 1972;**208:**329.

Mauseth RS et al: Detection of heterozygotes for congenital adrenal hyperplasia: 21-Hydroxylase deficiency. A comparison of HLA typing and 17-OH progesterone response to ACTH infusion. *J Pediatr* 1980:**97:**749.

McCann SM: Luteinizing-hormone-releasing hormone. *N Engl J Med* 1977;**296:**797.

Milner RDG et al: Experience with human growth hormone in Great Britain: The report of the MRC working party. *Clin Endocrinol* 1979;**11:**15.

Nicholson WE et al: Adrenocorticotropic hormone biotransformation, clearance and catabolism. *Endocrinology* 1978; **103:**1344.

Parkes D: Drug therapy: Bromocriptine. *N Engl J Med* 1979; **301:**873.

Rodriguez-Arnao MD et al: Effects of prosomatostatin on growth hormone and prolactin response to arginine in man. *Lancet* 1981;**1:**353.

Rudman D et al: Children with normal-variant short stature: Treatment with human growth hormone for six months. *N Engl J Med* 1981;**305:**123.

Sairan MR, Li CH: Human pituitary thyrotropin: The primary structure of the α and β subunits. *Can J Biochem* 1977; **55:**755.

Schwartz M et al: The use of human menopausal and chorionic gonadotropins for induction of ovulation. *Am J Obstet Gynecol* 1980;**138:**801.

Singer WD et al: The effect of ACTH therapy upon infantile spasms. *J Pediatr* 1980;**96:**485.

Taliadouros GS et al: Biological and immunological characterization of crude commercial human choriogonadotropin. *J Clin Endocrinol Metab* 1982;**54:**1002.

Wang CF, Gemzell C: The use of human gonadotropins for the induction of ovulation in women with polycystic ovarian disease. *Fertil Steril* 1980;**33:**479.

36 | Thyroid & Antithyroid Drugs

Francis S. Greenspan, MD, & Betty J. Dong, PharmD

Because of its anatomic prominence, the thyroid was one of the first of the endocrine glands to be correctly associated with the clinical conditions caused by its malfunction. However, the fact that this gland releases 2 very different types of hormones was not appreciated until recently. This chapter discusses the pharmacology of the thyroid hormones essential for growth and development and for regulation of energy metabolism: thyroxine and triiodothyronine. The second type of thyroid hormone, calcitonin, is important in the regulation of calcium metabolism and is discussed in Chapter 40.

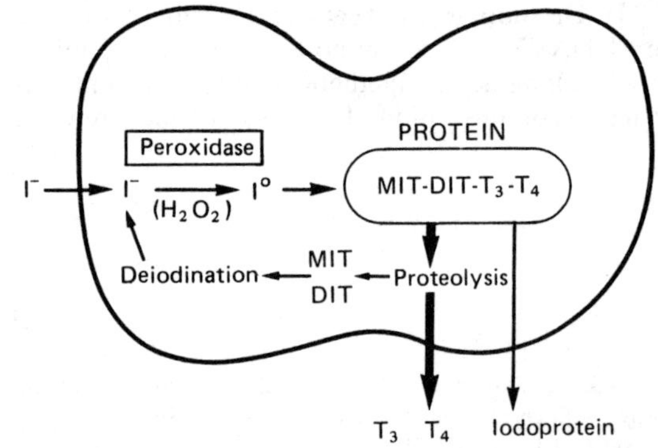

Figure 36–1. Hormone synthesis in the thyroid gland. I^-, iodide ion; I°, oxidized iodine; MIT, monoiodotyrosine; DIT, diiodotyrosine; T_3, triiodothyronine; and T_4, thyroxine. (Modified and reproduced, with permission, from Greenspan FS. In: *Gynecologic Endocrinology,* 3rd ed. Gold JJ, Josimovich JB [editors]. Harper & Row, 1980.)

THYROID PHYSIOLOGY

The normal thyroid gland secretes sufficient amounts of the thyroid hormones—triiodothyronine (T_3) and tetraiodothyronine (T_4, thyroxine)—to maintain normal growth and development, normal body temperature, and normal energy levels. These hormones contain 59% and 65% (respectively) of iodine as an essential part of the molecule.

Iodide Metabolism

Nearly all of the iodide (I^-)* intake is via the gastrointestinal tract in the form of food, water, or medication. The recommended daily adult intake is 150 μg. This ingested iodide is rapidly absorbed and enters an extracellular fluid pool. The thyroid gland removes about 75 μg a day from this pool for hormone secretion, and the balance is excreted in the urine. If iodide intake is increased, the fractional iodine uptake by the thyroid is diminished.

Biosynthesis of Thyroid Hormones

Once taken up by the thyroid gland, iodide undergoes a series of enzymatic reactions that convert it into active thyroid hormone (Fig 36–1). The first step is the transport of iodide into the thyroid gland, called **iodide trapping.** This can be inhibited by such anions as SCN^-, BF_4^-, NO_3^-, and ClO_4^-. Iodide is then oxidized to iodine, in which form it rapidly iodinates tyrosine residues within the thyroglobulin molecule to form monoiodotyrosine (MIT) and diiodotyrosine (DIT). This process is called **iodide organification.** Two molecules of DIT combine within the thyroglobulin molecule to form L-thyroxine (T_4). One molecule of MIT and one molecule of DIT will combine to form T_3. In addition to thyroglobulin, other proteins within the gland may be iodinated, but these iodoproteins do not have hormonal activity. Thyroid hormones are released from thyroglobulin by pinocytosis and proteolysis of thyroglobulin at the apical colloid border. The colloid droplets of thyroglobulin merge with lysosomes containing proteolytic enzymes, which hydrolyze thyroglobulin and release T_4, T_3, MIT, and DIT. The MIT and DIT are deiodinated, and the iodine is reutilized. The ratio of T_4 to T_3 within thyroglobulin is approximately 5:1, so that most of the hormone released is thyroxine. Most of the T_3 circulating in the blood is derived from peripheral metabolism of thyroxine (see below).

Transport of Thyroid Hormones

T_4 and T_3 in plasma are reversibly bound to protein, primarily thyroxine-binding globulin (TBG); T_3 is bound primarily to TBG and to albumin. About 0.04% of total T_4 and 0.4% of T_3 exist in the free form.

*In this chapter, "iodine" is used to refer to all forms of the element. Iodide refers only to the ionic form, I^-.

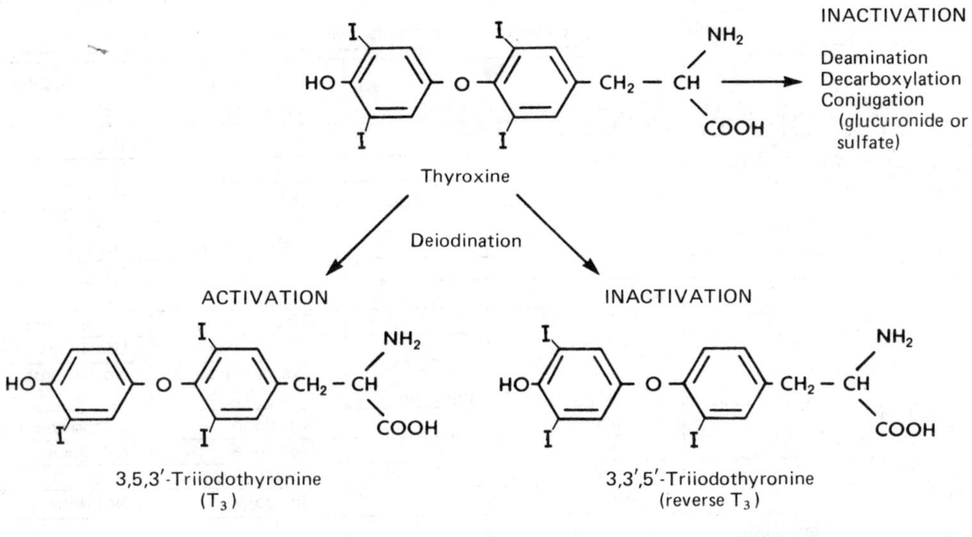

Figure 36–2. Peripheral metabolism of thyroxine. (Modified and reproduced, with permission, from Greenspan FS. In: *Gynecologic Endocrinology,* 3rd ed. Gold JJ, Josimovich JB [editors]. Harper & Row, 1980.)

Many physiologic and pathologic states and drugs affect T_4, T_3, and thyroid transport. However, the actual levels of free hormone generally remain normal, reflecting feedback control.

Peripheral Metabolism of Thyroid Hormones

A small amount of thyroxine is biologically inactivated by deamination, decarboxylation, or conjugation and excretion as a glucuronide or sulfate. The primary pathway for the peripheral metabolism of thyroxine, however, is deiodination. Deiodination of T_4 may occur by monodeiodination of the outer ring, producing 3,5,3'-triiodothyronine (T_3), which is 3–4 times more potent than T_4. Alternatively, deiodination may occur in the inner ring, producing 3,3',5'-triiodothyronine (reverse T_3, or rT_3), which is metabolically inactive (Fig 36–2).

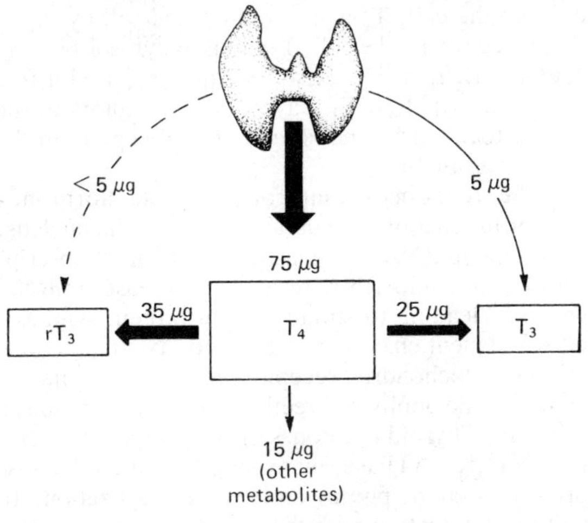

Figure 36–3. Quantitative aspects (per day) of thyroid hormone production and metabolism in normal adults.

Fig 36–3 shows the amounts of thyroid hormone produced and metabolized per day in normal adults. Normal levels of thyroid hormone in the serum are listed in Table 36–1. The low serum levels of T_3 (Table 36–1) and rT_3 in normal individuals are due to the high metabolic clearances of these 2 compounds.

Control of Thyroid Function

The tests used to evaluate thyroid function are listed in Table 36–2.

A. Thyroid-Pituitary Relationships: Control of thyroid function via the thyroid-pituitary feedback is discussed in Chapter 35. Briefly, hypothalamic cells secrete thyrotropin-releasing hormone (TRH). TRH is secreted into capillaries of the pituitary portal venous system, and in the pituitary gland TRH stimulates the synthesis and release of thyroid-stimulating hormone (TSH). TSH in turn stimulates an adenylate cyclase mechanism in the thyroid cell to increase the synthesis and release of T_4 and T_3. These thyroid hormones, in a negative feedback fashion, act in the pituitary to block the action of TRH and in the hypothalamus to inhibit

Table 36–1. Summary of thyroid hormone kinetics.

Kinetic Variable	T_4	T_3
Volume of distribution	10 L	40 L
Extrathyroidal pool	800 μg	54 μg
Daily production	80 μg	30 μg
Fractional turnover per day	10%	60%
Metabolic clearance per day	1.1 L	24 L
Half-life (biologic)	7 days	1½ days
Serum levels	5–12 μg/dL	80–180 ng/dL
Amount bound	99.96%	99.6%
Amount free	0.04%	0.4%
Biologic potency	1	4
Oral absorption	65%	95%

Table 36–2. Normal values for thyroid function tests.

Name	Normal Value	Results in Hypothyroidism	Results in Hyperthyroidism
Total thyroxine by RIA (T_4 [RIA])	5–12 μg/dL	Low	High
Total triiodothyronine by RIA (T_3 [RIA])	80–180 ng/dL	Normal or low	High
Resin T_3 uptake (RT_3U)	25–35%	Low	High
Free thyroxine index (FT_4I)	1.3–4.2	Low	High
Free T_3 index (FT_3I)	20–63	Normal or low	High
Thyrotropic hormone (TSH)	0–10 μU/mL	High	Low
^{123}I Uptake at 24 hours	5–35%	Low	High
Antithyroglobulin antibodies (Atg-ab)	Not detectable	Often present	Usually present
Antimicrosomal antibodies (Am-ab)	Titer less than 1:100	Often present	Usually present
Thyrotropin-releasing hormone test (TRH)	Three- to 5-fold rise in serum TSH 15–30 minutes after injection	Exaggerated rise	No response
Isotope scan with ^{123}I or $^{99m}TcO_4$	Normal pattern	Not done	Diffusely enlarged gland
Thin needle aspiration biopsy (TNA)	Normal pattern	Not done	Not done
Serum thyroglobulin	< 50 ng/mL*	Low	High
Serum calcitonin	< 200 pg/mL*	Not done	Not done

*Results may vary with different laboratories.

the synthesis and secretion of TRH. Other hormones or drugs may also affect the release of TRH or TSH.

B. Autoregulation of the Thyroid Gland: The thyroid gland also regulates its uptake of iodide and thyroid hormone synthesis by intrathyroidal mechanisms that are independent of TSH. These mechanisms are primarily related to the level of iodine in the blood. Large doses of iodine inhibit iodide organification. In certain disease states, this can result in inhibition of thyroglobulin iodination and thyroid hormone synthesis.

C. Abnormal Thyroid Stimulators: In Graves' disease (see below), lymphocytes secrete a thyroid-stimulating immunoglobulin (TSI). This immunoglobulin is probably bound to the TSH receptor site and turns on the gland in exactly the same fashion as TSH itself. The duration of the effect, however, is much longer than that of TSH.

I. BASIC PHARMACOLOGY OF THYROID & ANTITHYROID DRUGS

THYROID HORMONES

Chemistry

The structural formulas of thyroxine (T_4) and triiodothyronine (T_3) as well as reverse triiodothyronine (rT_3) are shown in Fig 36–2. All of these naturally occurring molecules are levo (L) isomers. The synthetic dextro (D) isomer of thyroxine, dextrothyroxine, has approximately 4% of the biologic activity of the L isomer as evidenced by its ability to suppress TSH secretion and correct hypothyroidism.

Mechanism of Action

The precise mechanism of action of thyroid hormone is still controversial. The detection of high-affinity binding sites for T_3 and T_4 in the nucleus, mitochondria, and plasma membranes suggests multiple sites of action rather than a single site.

Large numbers of receptors are found in the most hormone-responsive tissues (pituitary, liver, kidney, heart, skeletal muscle, lung, and intestine), while few receptor sites occur in hormone-unresponsive tissues (spleen, testes). The brain, which lacks an anabolic response to T_3, contains an intermediate number of receptors. In agreement with their biologic potencies, the affinity of the receptor site for T_4 is about 10 times lower than that for T_3. The number of nuclear receptors may be altered to preserve body homeostasis. For example, starvation lowers both circulating T_3 and T_3 receptors.

A model for the 3 sites of thyroid hormone action is depicted in Fig 36–4. In this model, thyroid hormone T_3 binds to a receptor protein in the cell membrane and increases the uptake of glucose and amino acid into the cell. T_3 can also enter the cell by diffusion. Once within the cell, T_3 binds to cytosol-binding protein (CBP), which exists in equilibrium with free T_3. In the cell, free T_3 may bind to receptors in the inner mitochondrial membrane or to receptors in the nuclear chromatin.

The responses that follow these hormone-receptor interactions are quite diverse. In the nucleus, an increase in RNA polymerase activity and transcription of DNA into RNA results in increased mRNA synthesis, leading to stimulation of protein synthesis and subsequent enzyme and cell activity. Interactions with the mitochondrial receptor may affect regulation of energy metabolism directly and protein synthesis indirectly. Thyroid hormones directly stimulate membrane Na^+,K^+-ATPase, increasing Na^+ and K^+ transport (the sodium pump) and oxygen utilization. In addition, interaction with the cell membrane receptor results in increased uptake of amino acids and glucose independent of protein synthesis.

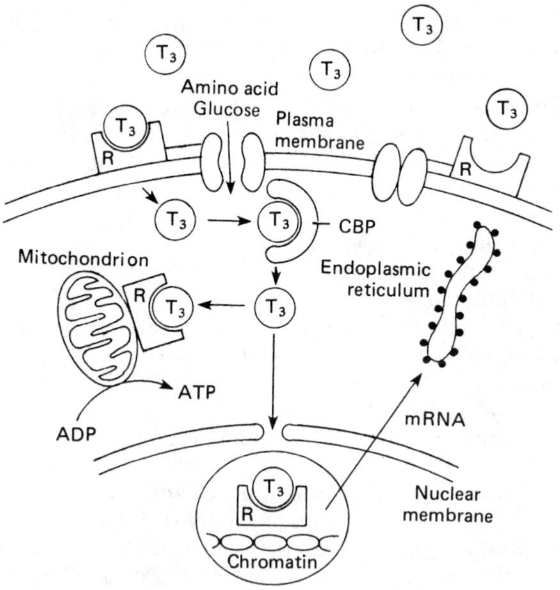

Figure 36–4. Proposed mechanism of thyroid hormone action. Thyroid hormone (in this case triiodothyronine or T_3) binds to receptor proteins (R) on the cell surface and increases the uptake of glucose and amino acids. T_3 also enters the cell where it reacts with cytoplasmic binding proteins (CBP) and receptors on chromatin and mitochondria. In the nucleus, the T_3-receptor complex leads to the synthesis of new protein. (Courtesy of JA Williams.)

Most of the effects of thyroid on metabolic processes appear to be mediated by activation of nuclear receptors that lead to increased formation of RNA and subsequent protein synthesis. For example, increased formation of the protein Na^+,K^+-ATPase and the consequent increase in ATP turnover and oxygen consumption are responsible for some of the calorigenic effects of thyroid hormones. This is consistent with the observation that the action of thyroid is manifested in vivo after a time lag of hours or days after its administration.

Effects of Thyroid Hormones

The thyroid hormones are responsible for optimal growth, development, function, and maintenance of all body tissues (Table 36–3). Since T_3 and T_4 are qualitatively similar, they may be considered as one hormone in the discussion that follows.

Thyroid hormone is critical for nervous, skeletal, and reproductive tissues. Its effects depend upon protein synthesis as well as potentiation of the secretion and action of growth hormone. Thyroid deprivation in early life results in irreversible mental retardation and dwarfism—symptoms typical of congenital cretinism.

Effects on growth and calorigenesis are accompanied by a pervasive influence on metabolism of drugs as well as carbohydrates, fats, proteins, and vitamins. Many of these changes are dependent upon or modified by activity of other hormones. Con-

Table 36–3. Summary of thyroid hormone effects.

System	Thyrotoxicosis	Hypothyroidism
Skin and appendages	Warm moist skin; sweating, heat intolerance; fine, thin hair; Plummer's nail.	Pale, cool, puffy skin; dry and brittle hair; brittle nails.
Eyes, facial	Retraction of upper lid with wide stare.	Drooping of eyelids, periorbital edema, loss of temporal aspects of eyebrows; puffy nonpitting facies; large tongue.
Cardiovascular	Increased peripheral vascular resistance, heart rate, stroke volume, cardiac output, pulse pressure; increased inotropic/chronotropic effects, arrhythmias, high-output congestive heart failure, angina.	Decreased peripheral vascular resistance, heart rate, stroke volume, cardiac output, pulse pressure; low-output congestive heart failure; ECG: bradycardia, prolonged P–R interval, flat T wave, low voltage; pericardial effusion.
Respiratory	Dyspnea, decreased vital capacity.	Pleural effusions; hyperventilation and CO_2 retention.
Gastrointestinal	Increased appetite; increased frequency of bowel movements; hypoproteinemia.	Decreased appetite; decreased bowel movements, ascites.
Central nervous system	Nervousness, hyperkinesia; emotional lability.	Lethargy, general slowing of mental processes; neuropathies.
Musculoskeletal	Weakness; fatigue; increased deep tendon reflexes; osteoporosis; hypercalcemia.	Stiffness and muscle fatigue; decreased deep tendon reflexes; increased alkaline phosphatase, LDH, SGOT.
Renal	Mild polyuria; increased renal blood flow, glomerular filtration rate.	Decreased renal blood flow, glomerular filtration rate; impaired water excretion.
Hematopoietic	Increased erythropoiesis, anemia.	Decreased production of erythropoietin; anemia.
Reproductive	Menstrual irregularities; decreased fertility; increased gonadal steroid metabolism.	Hypermenorrhea; infertility; decreased libido, impotence, and oligospermia; decreased steroid metabolism.
Metabolic	Increased basal metabolic rate, negative nitrogen balance; hyperglycemia; increased free fatty acids; decreased cholesterol and triglycerides; increased hormone degradation; increased requirements for fat- and water-soluble vitamins; increased drug detoxification.	Decreased basal metabolic rate, slightly positive nitrogen balance; delayed degradation of insulin with increased sensitivity; increased cholesterol and triglycerides; decreased hormone degradation; decreased requirements for fat- and water-soluble vitamins; decreased drug detoxification.

versely, the secretion and degradation rates of virtually all other hormones, including catecholamines, cortisol, estrogens, testosterone, and insulin, are affected by thyroid status.

Many of the manifestations of thyroid hyperactivity resemble sympathetic nervous system overactivity, although catecholamine levels are not increased. Possible explanations have included an increased number of beta-adrenergic receptor sites or enhanced amplification of the beta-adrenergic signal without an increase in the number of receptor sites. Changes in catecholamine-stimulated adenylate cyclase activity as measured by cAMP are found with changes in thyroid activity. The most dramatic effects of this catecholamine hyperactivity are seen in the cardiovascular system. Other clinical symptoms reminiscent of excessive epinephrine activity and partially alleviated by adrenergic antagonists include lid lag and retraction, tremor, excessive sweating, anxiety, nervousness, and muscle weakness. The opposite constellation of symptoms is seen in hypothyroidism.

Pharmacokinetics

Data on oral absorption of thyroid hormones are derived from administration of exogenous hormones. T_4 is absorbed best in the ileum and colon and is modified by intraluminal contents such as plasma proteins, food, and intestinal flora. Oral absorption in humans ranges from 35 to 80% (average, 65%; see Table 36–1). In contrast, T_3 is almost completely absorbed (95%) and minimally interfered with by intraluminal binding proteins. T_4 and T_3 absorption appears not to be affected by mild hypothyroidism but may be impaired in severe myxedema with ileus. These factors are important in switching from oral to parenteral therapy. For parenteral use, the intravenous route is preferred for both hormones (even though no commercial intravenous preparation of T_3 is available).

In patients with hyperthyroidism, the metabolic clearance rates of T_4 and T_3 are increased and the half-life decreased; the opposite is true in patients with hypothyroidism. Drugs such as phenobarbital that induce hepatic microsomal enzymes increase the metabolism of both T_4 and T_3. However, despite this change, the normal hormone concentration is maintained in euthyroid patients as a result of compensatory hyperfunction of the thyroid. A similar compensation occurs if binding sites are altered. If TBG sites are increased by pregnancy, estrogens, or oral contraceptives, there is an initial shift of hormone from the free to the bound state and a decrease in its metabolic clearance until the normal hormone concentration is reached. Thus, the concentration of total and bound hormone will increase, but the concentration of free hormone and the steady-state clearance will remain normal. The reverse occurs when thyroid binding sites are decreased.

Thyroid Preparations

Available preparations can be classified as either synthetic (levothyroxine, liothyronine, liotrix) or of animal origin (desiccated thyroid, thyroglobulin).

Thyroid USP is derived primarily from pork thyroid glands, although beef and sheep are also used. Because the USP requires only that desiccated thyroid contain between 0.17% and 0.23% organic iodine by weight and says nothing about the appropriate T_4:T_3 ratio, potency may vary from one lot to the next. The disadvantages of thyroid USP outweigh the advantage of low cost and include protein antigenicity, product instability, and difficulty in laboratory monitoring. Thyroglobulin (Proloid) is a purified extract of hog gland, standardized biologically to give a T_4:T_3 ratio of 2.5:1. It offers no advantages over desiccated thyroid and is more expensive. Sixty-five milligrams (1 gr) of thyroglobulin is equivalent to 65 mg of desiccated thyroid.

Levothyroxine sodium (Levothroid, Synthroid, etc) is the drug of choice for replacement and suppression therapy. Advantages include stability, uniform potency, low cost, lack of allergenic foreign protein, easy interpretation of laboratory values, and a half-life of 7 days, so that once-daily administration is feasible. Absorption is variable (approximately 65%) and is increased by fasting. Generic preparations should probably not be used until problems of erratic bioavailability are corrected. T_4 for intravenous use is available when indicated. Sixty-five milligrams (1 gr) of desiccated thyroid is equivalent to 100 μg of levothyroxine.

Liothyronine (Cytomel, Cytomine) is often used as a diagnostic agent in the T_3 suppression test and when short-term suppression of TSH is necessary. Although it is 3–4 times more active than T_4, it is not recommended for routine replacement because of its shorter half-life (1½ days) and higher cost and the difficulty of using conventional laboratory tests to monitor adequacy of replacement. Serum TSH is the only laboratory index that can be used to monitor T_3 replacement. T_3 should not be used for replacement therapy in patients with cardiac disease, since therapy is so difficult to monitor and the potential for cardiotoxicity so great. T_3 for intravenous use is not commercially available but can be prepared by dissolving crystalline liothyronine in a few drops of 0.1 N sodium hydroxide. The solution is then diluted with about 5 mL of sterile 1% human serum albumin in 0.85% saline, mixed by swirling, and then sterilized by passage through a Millipore filter.

Liotrix (Euthroid, Thyrolar) is a combination of synthetic T_4 and T_3 in a standard ratio of 4:1. It is an expensive form of thyroid medication but is stable, has predictable potency, lacks antigenicity, and is easily monitored. Furthermore, since a significant amount of T_4 is peripherally converted to T_3, the rationale that it is better because it mimics normal secretion is not valid. It is also important to note that Euthroid is 20% more potent than Thyrolar when corresponding milligram equivalents are compared.

The shelf life of the synthetic hormone preparations is excellent, particularly if they are stored in a dark bottle to minimize spontaneous deiodination. If desiccated thyroid is kept dry and free from moisture, potency is better preserved.

ANTITHYROID AGENTS

Reduction of thyroid activity and hormone effects can be accomplished by agents that interfere with the production of thyroid hormones; by agents that modify the tissue response to thyroid hormones; or by glandular destruction with radiation or surgery. "Goitrogens" are agents that suppress secretion of T_3 and T_4 to subnormal levels and thereby increase TSH to produce goiter. The antithyroid compounds used clinically include the thionamides, iodides, and radioactive iodine, which will be discussed later.

THIONAMIDES

The thionamides—propylthiouracil and methimazole (Tapazole)—are major drugs for treatment of thyrotoxicosis. In the United Kingdom, carbimazole, which is converted to methimazole in vivo, is widely used. Methimazole is about 10 times more active than propylthiouracil.

The chemical structures of these compounds are shown in Fig 36–5. The thiocarbamide group (see below) is essential for antithyroid activity.

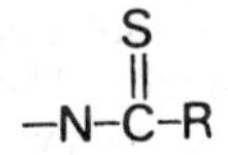

Pharmacokinetics

Propylthiouracil is rapidly absorbed, reaching peak serum levels after 1 hour. The bioavailability of 50–80% may be due to incomplete absorption or a large first-pass effect in the liver. The volume of distribution approximates total body water with accumulation in the thyroid gland. Most of an ingested dose of propylthiouracil is excreted by the kidney as the inactive glucuronide within 24 hours.

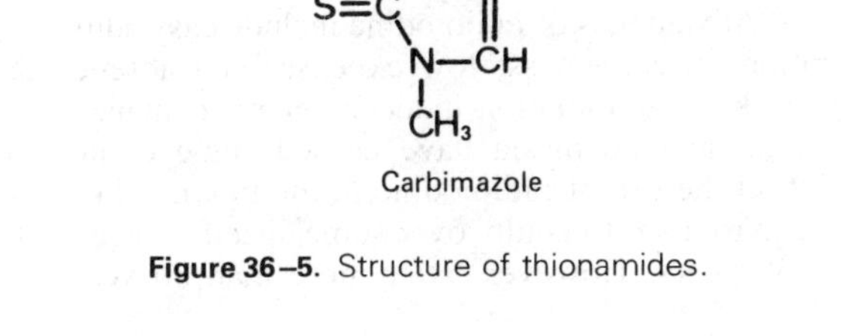

Figure 36–5. Structure of thionamides.

In contrast, methimazole is completely absorbed but at variable rates. It is readily accumulated by the thyroid gland and has a volume of distribution similar to that of propylthiouracil. Excretion is slower than with propylthiouracil, 65–70% of a dose is recovered in the urine in 48 hours.

The short plasma half-life of these agents (1½ hours for propylthiouracil and 6 hours for methimazole) has little bearing on the duration of the antithyroid action or the dosing interval, since both agents are accumulated by the thyroid gland. For propylthiouracil, giving the drug every 6 hours is reasonable since a single 100-mg dose can inhibit 60% of iodine organification for 7 hours. Likewise, for methimazole, giving the drug every 8 hours is reasonable since a single 10-mg dose of methimazole inhibits over 90% of iodine organification for 8 hours. Since a single 30-mg dose of methimazole exerts an antithyroid effect for longer than 24 hours, a single daily dose may be effective in the management of mild to moderate hyperthyroidism.

Both thionamides cross the placental barrier and are concentrated by the fetal thyroid, so that caution must be employed while using these drugs in pregnancy. Methimazole appears to cross the placenta more readily than propylthiouracil. Recent data suggest that propylthiouracil is not secreted in breast milk and so can be used when breast feeding is elected.

Pharmacodynamics

The thionamides act by multiple mechanisms. The major action is to prevent hormone synthesis by inhibiting the thyroid peroxidase-catalyzed reactions to block iodine organification. In addition, they block coupling of the iodotyrosines—primarily the formation of DIT. They do not block uptake of iodide by the gland. Propylthiouracil and (to a much lesser extent) methimazole inhibit the peripheral deiodination of T_4 and T_3. An immunosuppressive action has also been suggested. Since the synthesis rather than the release of hormones is affected, the onset of these agents is slow, often requiring 3–4 weeks before stores of T_4 are depleted.

Preparations

Propylthiouracil is available in 50-mg tablets and methimazole (Tapazole) in 5- and 10-mg tablets for oral administration. Since methimazole is water-soluble, both oral liquid and intravenous preparations can be prepared. In contrast, propylthiouracil is very insoluble and not suitable for intravenous use. A suspension of propylthiouracil can be compounded by dissolving tablets in carboxymethylcellulose flavored with cherry syrup.

Toxicity

Adverse reactions to the thionamides occur in about 3–12% of treated patients. Most reactions occur early. The most common side-effect is a maculopapular pruritic rash, at times accompanied by systemic signs such as fever. Rare adverse effects include an urticarial rash, vasculitis, arthralgia, a lupuslike reaction, cholestatic jaundice, lymphadenopathy, hypoprothrombinemia, and polyserositis. Leukopenia, which is dose-dependent, should be differentiated from that occurring in Graves' disease. The most dangerous complication is agranulocytosis, which may require antibiotic therapy but usually subsides when the drug is discontinued. The incidence is about 0.4% for propylthiouracil and 0.1% for methimazole. The cross-sensitivity between propylthiouracil and methimazole is not clear.

ANION INHIBITORS

Monovalent anions such as perchlorate (ClO_4), pertechnetate (TcO_4), and thiocyanate (SCN^-) can block uptake of iodide by the gland through competitive inhibition of the iodide transport mechanism. Since these effects can be overcome by large doses of iodides, their effectiveness is somewhat unpredictable.

Most of these agents, because of their toxicity, are used clinically only for diagnostic purposes. Potassium perchlorate was used clinically in the treatment of thyrotoxicosis until it was shown to cause aplastic anemia.

IODIDES

Iodides have been known since the 1920s to have multiple effects on the thyroid gland. Prior to the introduction of the thionamides in the 1940s, iodides were the major antithyroid agents; today they are rarely used as sole therapy.

Pharmacodynamics

Iodides have several actions on the thyroid. They inhibit organification (see physiology section), inhibit hormone release, and decrease the size and vascularity of the hyperplastic gland. In susceptible individuals, iodides can induce hyperthyroidism (jodbasedow) or precipitate hypothyroidism.

In pharmacologic doses (> 6 mg daily), the major action of iodides is to inhibit hormone release, possibly through thyroglobulin proteolysis. Rapid improvement in symptoms occurs within 2–7 days—hence the value of iodide therapy in thyroid storm. In addition, iodides decrease the vascularity, size, and fragility of a hyperplastic gland, making the drugs valuable as preoperative preparation for surgery.

Preparations

Stable iodine is available either as Lugol's solution (5% iodine and 10% potassium iodide) containing 8 mg of iodide per drop or as the more palatable saturated solution of potassium iodide (SSKI), containing 50 mg of iodide per drop. Parenteral preparations of sodium iodide, 1 and 2 g/10 mL, are also available. Disadvantages of iodide therapy include an increase in intraglandular stores of iodine, which may delay onset of thionamide therapy or prevent use of radioactive iodine therapy for several weeks. Thus, iodides should be initiated after onset of thionamide therapy and avoided if treatment with radioactive iodine seems likely. Iodide should not be used alone, since its withdrawal may produce severe exacerbation of thyrotoxicosis in an iodine-enriched gland. Chronic use of iodides in pregnancy should be avoided, since they cross the placenta and can cause fetal goiter.

Toxicity

Adverse reactions to iodine (iodism) are uncommon and in most cases reversible upon discontinuation. They include acneiform rash (similar to that of bromism), swollen salivary glands, mucous membrane ulcerations, conjunctivitis, rhinorrhea, drug fever, metallic taste, bleeding disorders, and, rarely, anaphylactoid reactions.

IPODATE

A most promising agent (now investigational) in the clinical treatment of hyperthyroidism is ipodate sodium (Oragrafin), an iodinated contrast medium that contains 61.4% iodine and can inhibit conversion of T_4 to T_3 in the liver, kidney, pituitary, and brain. When administered in a dose of 3 g orally every third day to thyrotoxic patients, improvement occurs in both subjective and objective symptoms, ie, decreased pulse rate and increased weight. The prolonged effect of suppressing T_4 as well as T_3 levels suggests that inhibition of hormone release due to the iodine released from ipodate may be an additional mechanism of action. Since ipodate is relatively nontoxic, it may prove to be useful in the treatment of thyrotoxicosis.

RADIOACTIVE IODINE

^{131}I is the only isotope used for treatment of thyrotoxicosis. Administered orally in solution as sodium ^{131}I, it is rapidly absorbed, concentrated by the thyroid, and incorporated into storage follicles. Its therapeutic effect depends on emission of beta rays with an effective half-life of 5 days and a penetration range of 400–2000 μm. Within a few weeks after treatment, destruction of the thyroid parenchyma occurs as evidenced by epithelial swelling and necrosis, follicular disruption, edema, and leukocyte infiltration. Advantages of radioiodine include easy administration, effectiveness, low expense, and absence of pain. Fears of radiation-induced genetic damage, leukemia, and neoplasia have caused some clinics to restrict the use of radioiodine in the treatment of hyperthyroidism to adults over some specified age such as 35 years. However, after more than 30 years of clinical experience with radioiodine, these fears have not been realized. Radioactive iodine should not be administered to pregnant women or nursing mothers, since it crosses the placenta and is excreted in breast milk.

ADRENERGIC BLOCKING AGENTS

Since many of the symptoms of thyrotoxicosis mimic those associated with adrenergic stimulation, agents that deplete adrenergic catecholamines such as guanethidine—or agents such as beta-blockers that impair the tissue response at the receptor site—are useful therapeutic adjuncts. Beta-adrenergic blocking drugs are the agents of choice because they are effective in patients refractory to guanethidine and reserpine. Propranolol has been the drug in this group most widely used and studied in the therapy of thyrotoxicosis. For a more complete discussion of this important class of drugs, see Chapter 8.

DIET-INDUCED THYROID DISEASE

Naturally occurring goitrogens of the Brassicaceae family include cabbage, turnips, rutabagas, and mustards. Thiocyanate is present in cabbage, and the others contain progoitrins that become goitrogenic when acted upon by enzymes present in the plant or in intestinal bacteria. These agents rarely produce goiter or hypothyroidism unless consumed raw in large quantities by susceptible individuals.

II. CLINICAL PHARMACOLOGY OF THYROID & ANTITHYROID DRUGS

HYPOTHYROIDISM

Hypothyroidism is a syndrome resulting from deficiency of thyroid hormones manifested by a general slowing of almost all body functions. In infants and children, there is striking retardation of growth and development, with resulting dwarfism and irreversible mental retardation. In adults, hypothyroidism is manifested largely by reversible slowing down of all body functions (Table 36–3).

The etiology and pathogenesis of hypothyroidism are outlined in Table 36–4. Hypothyroidism can occur with or without thyroid enlargement (goiter). The most common cause of hypothyroidism in the USA at this time is probably Hashimoto's thyroiditis, an immunologic disorder in genetically predisposed individuals. There is evidence of humoral immunity in the presence of antithyroid antibodies (see above) and lymphocyte sensitization to thyroid antigens. The laboratory diagnosis of hypothyroidism in the adult is easily made by the combination of a low T_4, low RT_3U, low free thyroxine index, and elevated serum TSH (Table 36–2). Antithyroid antibodies are often positive, indicating underlying thyroiditis.

Table 36–4. Etiology and pathogenesis of hypothyroidism.

Cause	Pathogenesis	Goiter	Degree of Hypothyroidism
Hashimoto's thyroiditis	Autoimmune destruction of thyroid.	Present early, absent later	Mild to severe
Drug-induced*	Block hormone formation.	Present	Mild to moderate
Dyshormonogenesis	Impaired synthesis of T_4 due to enzyme deficiency.	Present	Mild to severe
Radiation ^{131}I, x-ray	Destruction of gland.	Absent	Severe
Congenital (cretinism)	Athyreosis, or ectopic thyroid.	Absent	Severe
Secondary (TSH deficit)	Pituitary or hypothalamic disease.	Absent	Mild

*Iodides, lithium, fluoride, thionamides, aminosalicylic acid, phenylbutazone, etc.

Management of Hypothyroidism

Except for hypothyroidism caused by drugs (Table 36–4), which can be treated by simply removing the depressant agent, the general strategy of replacement therapy is appropriate. The most satisfactory preparation is levothyroxine (Levothroid, Synthroid, etc). Infants and children require somewhat more T_4 per kilogram of body weight than adults. The average dose for an infant 1–6 months of age is about 10 μg/kg, whereas the average dose for an adult is about 2.25 μg/kg. There is some variability in the absorption of thyroxine, so this dosage may vary from patient to patient. Because of the long half-life of thyroxine, the dose need be given only once daily. Children should be monitored for normal growth and development. Serum TSH and free thyroxine levels should be measured at regular intervals and maintained within a normal range. It takes about 6–8 weeks after starting a given dose of thyroxine to reach steady-state levels in the bloodstream. Thus, dosage changes should be made slowly.

In long-standing hypothyroidism, in older patients, and in patients with underlying cardiac disease, it is imperative to start treatment with reduced dosage. In such adult patients, levothyroxine is given in a dose of 0.0125–0.025 mg/d for 2 weeks, increasing by 0.025 mg every 2 weeks until euthyroidism or drug toxicity is observed. In older patients, the heart is very sensitive to the level of circulating thyroxine, and if angina pectoris or cardiac arrhythmia develops, it is essential to reduce the dose of thyroxine immediately. In younger patients or those with very mild disease, full replacement therapy may be started immediately.

The toxicity of thyroxine is directly related to the hormone level. In children, restlessness, insomnia, and accelerated bone maturation and growth may be signs of thyroxine toxicity. In adults, increased nervousness, heat intolerance, episodes of palpitation and tachycardia, or unexplained weight loss may be the presenting symptoms of thyroid toxicity. If these symptoms are present, it is important to monitor the free thyroxine index (Table 36–2), which will determine whether the symptoms are due to excess thyroxinemia.

Special Problems in Management of Hypothyroidism

A. Myxedema and Coronary Artery Disease: Since myxedema frequently occurs in older persons, it is often associated with underlying coronary artery disease. In this situation, the low levels of circulating thyroid hormone actually protect the heart against increasing demands that could result in angina pectoris or myocardial infarction. Correction of myxedema must be done cautiously to avoid provoking arrhythmia, angina, or acute myocardial infarction.

B. Myxedema Coma: Myxedema coma is an end state of untreated hypothyroidism. It is associated with progressive weakness, stupor, hypothermia, hypoventilation, hypoglycemia, hyponatremia, water intoxication, shock, and death. Symptoms usually develop quite slowly, with a gradual onset of lethargy, progressing to stupor or coma.

The pathophysiology of myxedema coma involves 3 major aspects: (1) CO_2 retention and hypoxia associated with decreased sensitivity of the respiratory center; (2) fluid and electrolyte imbalance with hyponatremia; and (3) marked hypothermia, with body temperatures as low as 24 °C (75 °F). Serum tests are consistent with severe hypothyroidism (see above).

Management of myxedema coma is an acute medical emergency. The patient should be treated in the intensive care unit, since intubation and mechanical ventilation may be required. Associated illnesses such as infection or heart failure must be treated by appropriate therapy. Patients with myxedema coma absorb drugs poorly. It is therefore important to give all preparations intravenously. Intravenous fluids should be administered with caution to avoid excessive water intake. These patients have large pools of free T_3 and T_4 binding sites in their sera that must be filled before there is adequate free thyroxine to affect tissue metabolism. Accordingly, the treatment of choice in myxedema coma is to give a loading dose of levothyroxine intravenously—usually 300–400 μg initially, followed by 50 μg daily. Intravenous hydrocortisone is indicated if the patient has associated adrenal or pituitary insufficiency but is probably not necessary in most patients with primary myxedema. Narcotics and sedatives must be used with extreme caution.

Clinically, improvement is evidenced by an increase in body temperature and arousal from the comatose state. Once the patient is able to breathe normally, assisted mechanical ventilation can be removed, and steady improvement will ensue.

C. Hypothyroidism and Pregnancy: Hypothyroid females frequently have anovulatory cycles and are therefore relatively infertile until restoration of the euthyroid state. This has led to the widespread use of thyroid hormone for infertility, although there is no evidence for its usefulness in this situation unless the patient is clearly hypothyroid. In a pregnant hypothyroid patient receiving thyroxine, it is extremely important that the daily dose of thyroxine be maintained. In most cases, the dose in the nonpregnant state is the same as that in the pregnant state, and no change in dose is required. Because of the elevated maternal TBG, the free thyroxine index (FT_4I) (Table 36–2) must be used to monitor maternal thyroxine dosages.

HYPERTHYROIDISM

Hyperthyroidism, or thyrotoxicosis, is the clinical syndrome that results when tissues are exposed to high levels of thyroid hormone.

GRAVES' DISEASE

The most common form of hyperthyroidism is Graves' disease, or diffuse toxic goiter. The presenting signs and symptoms of Graves' disease are set forth in Table 36–3.

Pathophysiology

Graves' disease is considered to be an autoimmune disorder in which there is a genetic defect in suppressor T lymphocytes, and helper T lymphocytes stimulate B lymphocytes to synthesize antibodies to thyroidal antigens. One such antibody (thyroid-stimulating immunoglobulin, or TSI) is directed against the TSH receptor site in the thyroid cell membrane and has the capacity to stimulate the thyroid cell.

Laboratory Diagnosis

In most patients, T_3, T_4, RT_3U, and FT_4I will all be elevated (Table 36–2). Radioiodine uptake is usually markedly elevated as well. Antithyroglobulin antibodies, antimicrosomal antibodies, and TSI are also present.

Management of Graves' Disease

The 3 primary methods for controlling hyperthyroidism are antithyroid drug therapy, surgical thyroidectomy, and destruction of the gland with radioactive iodine.

A. Antithyroid Drug Therapy: Drug therapy is most useful in young patients with small glands and mild disease. Either propylthiouracil or methimazole is administered until the disease undergoes spontaneous remission, which may take from 1 year to 15 years.

This is the only therapy that leaves an intact thyroid gland, but it does require a long period of treatment and observation, and there is a 60–70% incidence of relapse.

Antithyroid drug therapy is usually begun with large divided doses, shifting to single-dose maintenance therapy when the patient becomes clinically euthyroid. Therapy is frequently started with propylthiouracil, 100–150 mg every 6 hours, and then, after 4–8 weeks, reduction of the dose to 100 or 200 mg once daily. Propylthiouracil inhibits the conversion of T_4 to T_3, so it brings the level of activated thyroid hormone down more quickly than does methimazole. However, methimazole has a longer duration of action and is more useful if one is striving to achieve a single daily dose regimen. The best clinical guide to remission is reduction in the size of the goiter. Laboratory tests most useful in monitoring the course of therapy are serum T_3 by RIA and FT_4I (Table 36–2).

Reactions to antithyroid drugs have been described above. A minor rash can often be controlled by antihistamine therapy. The more severe reaction of agranulocytosis is heralded by a sore throat or high fever. Thus, all patients receiving antithyroid drugs are instructed that if they develop sore throat or fever they must immediately discontinue the drug and seek a physician, who should obtain a throat culture and white and differential counts and then institute appropriate antibiotic therapy. Cholestatic jaundice, hepatocellular toxicity, exfoliative dermatitis, and acute arthralgia are rare adverse reactions to antithyroid drugs also requiring cessation of drug therapy.

B. Thyroidectomy: Subtotal thyroidectomy is the treatment of choice for patients with very large glands or multinodular goiters. Patients are treated with antithyroid drugs until euthyroid (about 6 weeks). In addition, for 2 weeks prior to surgery, they receive saturated solution of potassium iodide, 5 drops twice daily, to diminish vascularity of the gland and simplify surgery. About 50–60% of patients will require thyroid supplementation following subtotal thyroidectomy.

C. Radioactive Iodine: Radioiodine therapy utilizing ^{131}I is the preferred treatment for most patients over 21 years of age. In patients without heart disease, the therapeutic dose may be given immediately in a range of 80–100 $\mu Ci/g$ of estimated thyroid weight corrected for uptake. In patients with underlying heart disease or relatively large glands, it is desirable to treat with antithyroid drugs until euthyroid before giving ^{131}I. The medication is then stopped for 7–10 days; radioiodine uptake is determined; and a dose of 120–150 $\mu Ci/g$ of estimated thyroid weight is administered. Iodides should be avoided to assure maximal ^{131}I uptake. Six to 12 weeks following the administration of radioiodine, the gland will shrink in size and the patient will usually become euthyroid. A second dose may be required in some patients. The major complication of radioiodine therapy is hypothyroidism, which occurs in about 80% of patients. Serum FT_4I and TSH levels should be monitored. When hypothyroidism develops, prompt replacement with levothyroxine, 0.15–0.2 mg orally daily, is instituted.

D. Adjuncts to Antithyroid Therapy: During the acute phase of thyrotoxicosis, beta-adrenergic blocking agents are extremely helpful. Propranolol, 10–40 mg orally every 6 hours, will control tachycardia, hypertension, and atrial fibrillation. Propranolol is gradually withdrawn as serum thyroxine levels return to normal. Adequate nutrition and vitamin supplements are essential. Barbiturates accelerate T_4 breakdown (by hepatic enzyme induction) and may be helpful both as a sedative and to lower T_4 levels.

TOXIC UNINODULAR GOITER & TOXIC MULTINODULAR GOITER

These forms of hyperthyroidism occur often in older women with nodular goiters. T_4 and resin T_3 uptake are often normal, but T_3 by RIA is strikingly elevated. Single toxic adenomas can be managed with either surgical excision of the adenoma or with radioiodine therapy. Toxic multinodular goiter is usually associated with a large goiter and best treated by preparation with propylthiouracil followed by subtotal thyroidectomy.

SUBACUTE THYROIDITIS

During the acute phase of viral infection of the thyroid gland, thyroid hormones are produced that result in transient thyrotoxicosis. This syndrome has been called "spontaneously resolving hyperthyroidism." Supportive therapy is usually all that is necessary, such as propranolol for tachycardia and aspirin to control local pain and fever.

THYROTOXICOSIS FACTITIA

This is due to excessive ingestion of thyroid hormones, either accidentally or purposely. Treatment consists of supportive therapy and discontinuing excessive medication.

SPECIAL PROBLEMS

Thyroid Storm

Thyroid storm, or thyrotoxic crisis, is sudden acute exacerbation of all of the symptoms of thyrotoxicosis, presenting as a life-threatening syndrome. The clinical manifestations are variable in intensity but reflect hypermetabolism and excessive adrenergic response. Fever is present, often associated with flushing and sweating. Tachycardia is common, often with atrial fibrillation, high pulse pressure, and occasionally heart failure. Central nervous system symptoms include marked agitation, restlessness, delirium, and coma. Gastrointestinal symptoms include nausea, vomiting, diarrhea, and jaundice. Death may occur from heart failure and shock.

Vigorous management is mandatory. Propranolol, 1–2 mg slowly intravenously or 40–80 mg orally every 6 hours, is helpful to control the severe cardiovascular manifestations. If propranolol is contraindicated by the presence of severe heart failure or asthma, reserpine, 1 mg orally, intramuscularly, or intravenously every 6–12 hours, or guanethidine, 1–2 mg/kg orally in divided doses, may help control hypertension and tachycardia. Release of thyroid hormones from the gland is retarded by the administration of sodium iodide, 1 g intravenously over a 24-hour period, or saturated solution of potassium iodide, 10 drops orally daily. Hormone synthesis is blocked by the administration of propylthiouracil, 250 mg orally every 6 hours. If the patient is unable to take propylthiouracil by mouth, methimazole may be prepared for intravenous administration in a dose of 25 mg every 6 hours. Hydrocortisone, 50 mg intravenously every 6 hours, will protect the patient against shock and will block the conversion of T_4 to T_3, bringing down the level of thyroactive material in the blood quickly.

Supportive therapy is essential to control fever, heart failure, and any underlying disease process that may have precipitated the acute storm. In rare situations, where the above methods are not adequate to control the problem, plasmapheresis or peritoneal dialysis has been used to lower the levels of circulating thyroxine.

Ophthalmopathy

Although severe ophthalmopathy is rare, it is difficult to treat. Management requires effective treatment of the thyroid disease, usually by total surgical excision or ^{131}I ablation of the gland. In addition, local therapy may be necessary, eg, elevation of the head to diminish periorbital edema and artificial tears to relieve corneal drying. For the severe, acute inflammatory reaction, a short course of prednisone, 100 mg orally daily for about a week and then 100 mg every other day, tapering the dose over a period of 6–12 weeks, may be effective.

Dermopathy

Dermopathy or pretibial myxedema will often respond to topical corticosteroids applied to the involved area and covered with an occlusive dressing.

Thyrotoxicosis During Pregnancy

Radioiodine is contraindicated during pregnancy because it crosses the placenta and injures the fetal thyroid. In the first trimester, the patient can be prepared with propylthiouracil and a subtotal thyroidectomy performed safely during the middle trimester. It is essential to give the patient a thyroid supplement during the balance of the pregnancy. Alternatively, the patient can be treated with antithyroid drugs during the pregnancy, and the decision regarding long-term management can be made after delivery. The dosage of antithyroid drugs must be kept to the minimum necessary for control of the disease, because these drugs cross the placenta and may affect the function of the fetal thyroid gland.

Neonatal Graves' Disease

Graves' disease may occur in the newborn infant, either due to passage of TSI through the placenta, stimulating the thyroid gland of the neonate, or to genetic transmission of the trait to the fetus. Laboratory studies reveal an elevated free thyroxine index, a markedly elevated T_3, and a *low* TSH, in contrast to the normal infant, in whom TSH is *elevated* at birth. TSI is usually found in the serum of both the child and the mother.

If caused by maternal TSI, the disease is usually self-limited and subsides over a period of 4–12 weeks, coinciding with the fall in the infant's TSI level. However, treatment is necessary because of the severe metabolic stress the infant is subjected to. Therapy includes propylthiouracil in a dose of 5–10 mg/kg/d in divided doses at 8-hour intervals; Lugol's solution (8 mg of iodide per drop), 1 drop every 8 hours; and propranolol, 2 mg/kg/d in divided doses. Careful supportive therapy is essential. If the infant is very ill, prednisone, 2 mg/kg/d orally in divided doses, will help block conversion of T_4 to T_3. These medications are gradually reduced as the clinical picture improves and can be discontinued by 6–12 weeks.

NONTOXIC GOITER

Nontoxic goiter is a syndrome of thyroid enlargement without excessive thyroid hormone production. Enlargement of the thyroid gland is usually due to TSH stimulation from inadequate thyroid hormone synthesis. The most common cause of nontoxic goiter worldwide is iodide deficiency, but in the USA it is Hashimoto's thyroiditis. Less common causes include dietary goitrogens, dyshormonogenesis, and neoplasms (see below).

Goiter due to iodide deficiency is best managed by prophylactic administration of iodide. The optimal daily iodide intake is 150–300 μg. Iodized salt and iodate used as preservatives in flour and bread are excellent sources of iodine in the diet. In areas where it is difficult to introduce iodized salt or iodate preservatives, a solution of iodized poppyseed oil has been administered intramuscularly to provide a long-term source of inorganic iodine.

Goiter due to ingestion of goitrogens in the diet is managed by elimination of the goitrogen or by adding sufficient thyroxine to shut off TSH stimulation. Similarly, in Hashimoto's thyroiditis and dyshormonogenesis, adequate thyroxine therapy—0.15–0.2 mg/d orally—will suppress pituitary TSH and result in slow regression of the goiter as well as correction of hypothyroidism.

THYROID NEOPLASMS

Neoplasms of the thyroid gland may be benign (adenomas) or malignant. Thin needle aspiration biopsy has proved effective for differentiation of benign from malignant disease. Some adenomas will regress following thyroxine therapy; those that do not should be rebiopsied or surgically removed. Management of thyroid carcinoma requires a near-total thyroidectomy, postoperative radioiodine therapy in selected instances, and lifetime replacement with levothyroxine.

• • •

References

Physiology & Pharmacology

Brennan MD: Series on pharmacology in practice. 5. Thyroid hormones. *Mayo Clin Proc* 1980;**55:**33.

Hershman JM, Bray GA (editors): *The Thyroid: Physiology and Treatment of Disease*. Pergamon, 1979.

Marchant B, Lees JFH, Alexander WD: Antithyroid drugs. *Pharmacol Ther* [*B*] 1978;**3:**305.

Miller LJ, Gorman CA, Go VLW: Gut-thyroid interrelationships. *Gastroenterology* 1978;**75:**901.

Shenfield GM: Influence of thyroid dysfunction on drug pharmacokinetics. *Clin Pharmacokinet* 1981;**6:**275.

Sterling K: Thyroid hormone action at the cell level. (2 parts.) *N Engl J Med* 1979;**300:**117, 173.

Hypothyroidism

Evered D, Hall R (editors): *Hypothyroidism and Goitre*. Vol 8 of: *Clinics in Endocrinology and Metabolism*. Saunders, 1979.

Fisher DA et al: Results of screening one million North American infants. *J Pediatr* 1979;**94:**700.

Maeda M et al: Changes in serum triiodothyronine, thyroxine and thyrotropin during treatment with thyroxine in severe primary hypothyroidism. *J Clin Endocrinol Metab* 1976;**43:**10.

Odell WD, Fisher DA: Treatment of hypothyroidism. Pages 92–110 in: *Diagnosis and Treatment of Common Thyroid Diseases*. Selenkow HA, Hoffman F (editors). Excerpta Medica International Congress Series No. 227, 1971.

Rees-Jones RW, Rolla AR, Larsen PR: Hormonal content of thyroid replacement preparations. *JAMA* 1980;**243:**549.

Urbanic RC, Mazzaferri EL: Thyrotoxic crisis and myxedema coma. *Heart Lung* 1978;**7:**435.

Hyperthyroidism

Bierwaltes WH: The treatment of hyperthyroidism with iodine-131. *Semin Nucl Med* 1978;**8:**95.

Braverman LE: Thyrotoxicosis: Therapeutic considerations. *Clin Endocrinol Metab* 1978;**7:**221.

Burrow GN: Hyperthyroidism during pregnancy. *N Engl J Med* 1978;**298:**150.

Dobyns BM: Prevention and management of hyperthyroid storm. *World J Surg* 1978;**2:**293.

Gorman CA: The presentation and management of endocrine ophthalmopathy. *Clin Endocrinol Metab* 1978;**7:**67.

Vanderlaan WP: Antithyroid drugs in practice. *Mayo Clin Proc* 1972;**41:**962.

Volpe R: The pathogenesis of Graves' disease: An overview. *Clin Endocrinol Metab* 1978;**7:**3.

Nontoxic Goiter, Nodules, & Cancer

Clark OH: Thyroid nodules and thyroid cancer: Surgical aspects. *West J Med* 1980;**133:**1.

Miller JM, Hamburger JI, Kim S: Diagnosis of thyroid nodules: Use of fine needle aspiration and needle biopsy. *JAMA* 1979;**241:**481.

Papapetrou PD et al: Long-term treatment of Hashimoto's thyroiditis with thyroxine. *Lancet* 1972;**2:**1045.

Stanbury JB: Familial goiter. Page 206 in: *The Metabolic Basis of Inherited Disease,* 4th ed. Stanbury JB, Wyngaarden JB, Frederickson DS (editors). McGraw-Hill, 1978.

37 | Adrenocorticosteroids & Adrenocortical Antagonists

Alan Goldfien, MD

The natural adrenocortical hormones are steroid molecules produced and released by the adrenal cortex. Both natural and synthetic corticosteroids are used for both diagnosis and treatment of disorders of adrenal function. They are also used—in much larger quantities—for treatment of a variety of inflammatory and immunologic disorders.

Secretion of adrenocortical steroids is controlled by the pituitary release of corticotropin (ACTH). Secretion of the salt-retaining hormone aldosterone is also under the influence of angiotensin. Corticotropin has some actions that do not depend upon its effect on adrenocortical secretion. However, its pharmacologic value as an anti-inflammatory agent and its use in testing adrenal function depend on its trophic action. Therefore, its pharmacology will be discussed with the adrenocortical hormones.

Antagonists of the synthesis or action of ACTH and the adrenocortical steroids are important in the treatment of several tumors. These agents are described at the end of this chapter.

I. ADRENOCORTICOSTEROIDS

The adrenal cortex releases a large number of steroids into the circulation. Some have minimal biologic activity and function primarily as precursors, and there are some for which no function has been established. The hormonal steroids may be classified as those having important effects on intermediary metabolism (glucocorticoids), those having principally salt-retaining activity (mineralocorticoids), and those having androgenic or estrogenic activity (see Chapter 38). In humans, the major glucocorticoid is cortisol and the most important mineralocorticoid is aldosterone. Quantitatively, dehydroepiandrosterone (DHEA) is the major androgen, since about 20 mg is secreted daily, partly as the sulfate. However, both DHEA and androstenedione are very weak androgens. A small amount of testosterone is secreted by the adrenal and may be of greater importance as an androgen. Little is known about the estrogens secreted by the adrenal. However, it has been shown that the adrenal androgens such as testosterone and androstenedione can be converted to estrone in small amounts by nonendocrine tissues and that they constitute the major endogenous source of estrogen in women after menopause and in those in whom ovarian function is abnormal.

THE NATURALLY OCCURRING GLUCOCORTICOIDS; CORTISOL (Hydrocortisone)

Pharmacokinetics

The major glucocorticoid in humans is cortisol. It is synthesized from cholesterol (as shown in Fig 37–1) by the cells of the zona fasciculata and zona reticularis and released into the circulation under the influence of ACTH. The mechanisms controlling its secretion are discussed in Chapter 35.

In the normal adult in the absence of stress, about 20 mg of cortisol is secreted daily. The rate of secretion changes in a circadian rhythm (Fig 37–2). In plasma, cortisol is bound to plasma proteins. Corticosteroid-binding globulin (CBG), an α_2-globulin synthesized by the liver, binds 95% of the circulating hormone under normal circumstances. The remainder is free or loosely bound to albumin and is available to exert its effect on target cells. When plasma cortisol levels exceed 20–30 μg/dL, CBG is saturated and most of the excess is loosely bound to albumin.

The half-life of cortisol in the circulation is normally about 90–110 minutes; it may be increased when large amounts are present or in hypothyroidism. Cortisol is removed from the circulation in the liver, where it is reduced and conjugated to form water-soluble compounds that are excreted into the urine (Fig 37–3). The side chain (C20 and C21) is removed from about 5–10% of the cortisol, and the resulting compounds are further metabolized and excreted into the urine as 11-oxy 17-ketosteroids.

In some species (eg, the rat), corticosterone is the major glucocorticoid. It is less firmly bound to protein and therefore metabolized more rapidly. The pathways of its degradation are similar to those of cortisol.

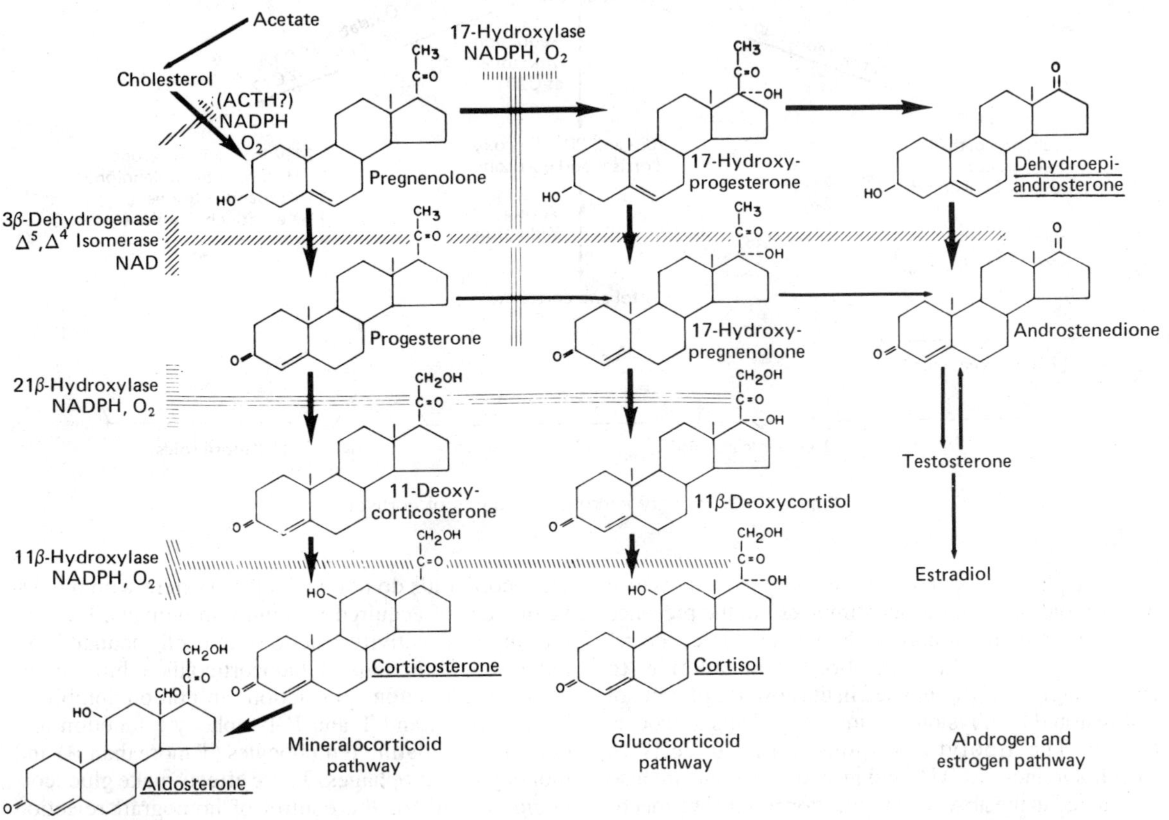

Figure 37–1. Outline of major pathways in adrenocortical hormone biosynthesis. The major secretory products are underlined. Pregnenolone is the major precursor of corticosterone and aldosterone, and 17-hydroxypregnenolone is the major precursor of cortisol. The enzymes and cofactors for the reactions progressing down each column are shown on the left and from the first to the second column at the top of the figure. When a particular enzyme is deficient, hormone production is blocked at the points indicated by the shaded bars. (Modified after Welikey, Mulrow, et al; reproduced, with permission, from Ganong WF: *Review of Medical Physiology,* 10th ed. Lange, 1981.)

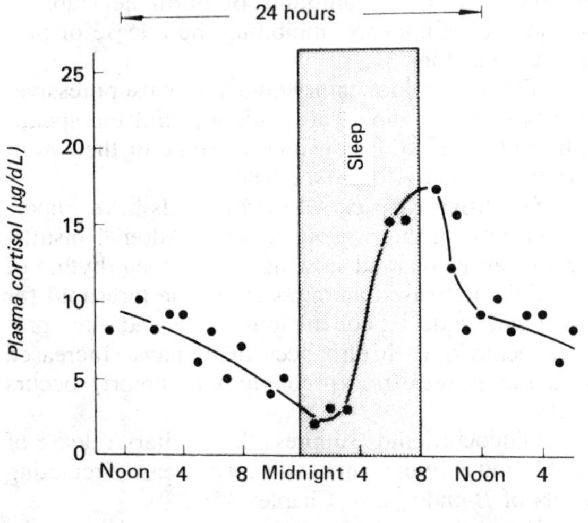

Figure 37–2. Circadian rhythm of plasma cortisol (free and protein-bound). (After Liddle, 1966.)

Pharmacodynamics

A. Mechanism of Action: Natural and synthetic glucocorticoids and anti-inflammatory steroids bind to specific intracellular receptors upon entering target tissues. The macromolecular complex thus formed is transported into the nucleus, where it interacts with chromosomal constituents to alter gene expression. These hormones alter the regulation of many cellular processes, including enzyme synthesis and activity, membrane permeability, transport processes, and structure (see Chapter 34).

B. Physiologic Effects: The glucocorticoids have widespread effects because they influence the function of most cells in the body. The major metabolic consequences of glucocorticoid secretion or administration are due to direct actions of these hormones in the cell. However, some important effects are the result of homeostatic responses by insulin and glucagon. Although many of the effects are dose-related and become magnified when large amounts are administered for therapeutic purposes, there are also "permissive" effects. In other words, many normal reactions

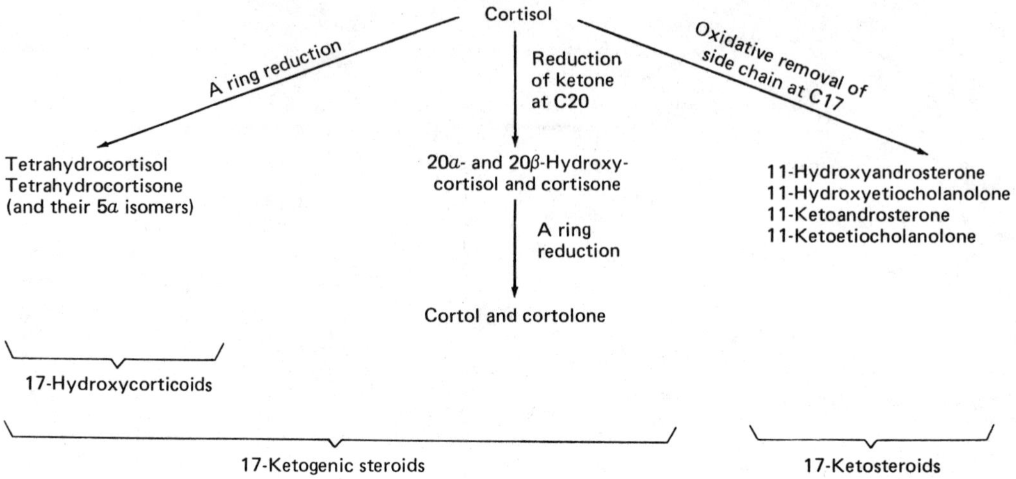

Figure 37–3. Primary excretion products of cortisol.

that take place at a significant rate only in the presence of corticoids are not further stimulated in the presence of larger amounts of corticoids. For example, the response of vascular and bronchial muscle to catecholamines is diminished in the absence of cortisol and restored by physiologic amounts of this glucocorticoid. The lipolytic responses of fat cells to catecholamines, ACTH, and growth hormone are also attenuated in the absence of glucocorticoid. The mechanism of these effects has not been determined.

C. Metabolic Effects: The glucocorticoids have important dose-related effects on carbohydrate, protein, and fat metabolism. The same effects are responsible for some of the serious adverse effects associated with their use in therapeutic doses. Glucocorticoids stimulate—and are required for—gluconeogenesis in the fasted state and in diabetes. Glucocorticoids also increase amino acid uptake by the liver and kidney and increase the activity of enzymes required for gluconeogenesis.

Glucocorticoids increase liver glycogen deposition by stimulating glycogen synthetase activity and increasing glucose production from protein. The increase in glucose levels also stimulates insulin release.

Glucocorticoids inhibit the uptake of glucose by fat cells, leading to increased lipolysis. However, the increased insulin secretion described above stimulates lipogenesis, leading to a net increase in fat deposition.

D. Catabolic Effects: Although glucocorticoids stimulate protein and RNA synthesis in the liver, they have catabolic effects in lymphoid and connective tissue, muscle, fat, and skin. Supraphysiologic amounts of glucocorticoids lead to decreased muscle mass and weakness. Catabolic effects on bone are the cause of osteoporosis in Cushing's syndrome and constitute a major limitation in the long-term therapeutic use of glucocorticoids. In children, the catabolic effects of excessive amounts of glucocorticoid reduce growth. This effect is not prevented by growth hormone.

E. Immunosuppressive Effects: Although glucocorticoids do not generally interfere with the development of acquired immunity in humans, they inhibit hypersensitivity reactions and cell-mediated immunologic functions. Glucocorticoids inhibit complement activation and action, migration inhibition factor (MIF), and T and B lymphocyte function and decrease circulating lymphocytes (T more than B) and monocyte macrophages. These effects make glucocorticoids useful for the control of homograft rejection reactions in organ transplant patients. They also reduce the amount of antigen released by the grafted tissue, delay revascularization, and interfere with sensitization of antibody-forming cells.

F. Anti-Inflammatory Effects: Corticosteroids have the capacity to dramatically reduce the manifestations of inflammation. As noted above, there is a reduction in circulating immunocompetent cells and macrophages. Bactericidal activity and interferon production are inhibited, and fever and pyrogen reactions are reduced. Large amounts of hormone stabilize lysosomal membranes, inhibiting the release of proteolytic enzymes.

The anti-inflammatory (and immunosuppressive) effects of these agents are widely useful therapeutically but are also responsible for some of their most serious adverse effects (see below).

G. Other Effects: Glucocorticoids have important effects on the nervous system. Adrenal insufficiency causes marked slowing of the alpha rhythm of the EEG. Increased amounts lower the threshold for electrically induced convulsions in rats and often produce behavioral disturbances in humans. Increased intracranial pressure (pseudotumor cerebri) occurs rarely.

Glucocorticoids suppress the pituitary release of ACTH and β-lipotropin but do not decrease circulating levels of β-endorphin (Chapter 35).

Large doses of glucocorticoids stimulate excessive production of acid and pepsin in the stomach and may cause peptic ulcer. They facilitate fat absorption and appear to antagonize the effect of vitamin D on calcium absorption. The glucocorticoids also have important effects on the hematopoietic system, decreasing the number of lymphocytes, eosinophils, and basophils while increasing the number of neutrophils, platelets, and red blood cells.

In the absence of physiologic amounts of cortisol, renal function (particularly glomerular filtration) is impaired and there is an inability to excrete a water load.

SYNTHETIC ADRENOCORTICOSTEROIDS

ACTH and steroids having glucocorticoid activity have become important agents for use in the treatment of many inflammatory and allergic disorders. This has stimulated the search for and development of many steroids with anti-inflammatory activity.

Pharmacokinetics

A. Source: Although the natural corticosteroids can be obtained from animal adrenals, they are usually synthesized from cholic acid (obtained from cattle) or steroid sapogenins, diosgenin in particular, found in plants of the Liliaceae and Dioscoreaceae families. Further modifications of these steroids have led to the marketing of a large group of synthetic steroids with special characteristics that are pharmacologically and therapeutically important (Table 37–1).

B. Metabolism: The metabolism of the naturally occurring adrenal steroids has been discussed above. The synthetic corticosteroids for oral use (Table 37–1) are in most cases rapidly and completely absorbed when given by mouth. Although they are transported and metabolized in a fashion similar to the endogenous steroids, important differences exist.

Alterations in the molecule influence the degree of protein binding, side chain stability, rate of reduction, and end products. Halogenation at the 9 position, unsaturation of the Δ1-2 bond of the A ring, and methylation at the 2 or 16 position will prolong the half-life by more than 50%. The 11-hydroxyl group also appears to inhibit destruction, since the half-life of 11-deoxycortisol is half that of cortisol. The Δ1 compounds are excreted in the free form.

Pharmacodynamics

The actions of the synthetic steroids are similar to those of cortisol (see above). They bind to the specific intracellular receptor protein and produce the same effects with different ratios of glucocorticoid to mineralocorticoid potency (Table 37–1).

Clinical Pharmacology

A. Diagnosis and Treatment of Disturbed Adrenal Function:

1. Adrenocortical insufficiency (Addison's disease)–Chronic adrenocortical insufficiency (addisonism) is characterized by hyperpigmentation, weak-

Table 37–1. Some commonly used natural and synthetic corticosteroids for general use.

Agent	Activity: Anti-inflammatory	Activity: Topical	Activity: Salt-Retaining	Equivalent Oral Dose (mg)	Forms Available
Short-acting glucocorticoids					
Hydrocortisone (cortisol) (11β,17,21-trihydroxy-4-pregnene-3,20-dione)	1	1	1	20	Oral, injectable, topical.
Cortisone (17,21-dihydroxy-4-pregnene-3,11,20-trione)	0.8	0	0.8	25	Oral, injectable, topical.
Prednisone (17,21-dihydroxy-1,4-pregnadiene-3,11,20-trione)	4	0	0.3	5	Oral.
Prednisolone (11β,17,21-trihydroxy-1,4-pregnadiene-3,20-dione)	5	4	0.3	5	Oral, injectable, topical.
Fluocortolone (6α-fluoro-11β,21-dihydroxy-16α-methyl-1,4-pregnadiene-3,20-dione)*				5	Oral, topical.
Methylprednisolone (6α-methylprednisolone)	5	5	0	4	Oral, injectable, topical.
Meprednisone (16β-methylprednisone)	5		0	4	Oral, injectable.*
Intermediate-acting glucocorticoids					
Triamcinolone (acetonide) (9α-fluoro-16α-hydroxyprednisolone) (16,17-acetonide)	5	5†	0	4	Oral, injectable, topical.
Paramethasone (6α-fluoro-16α-methylprednisolone)	10		0	2	Oral, injectable.*
Fluprednisolone (6α-fluoroprednisolone)	15	7	0	1.5	Oral.
Long-acting glucocorticoids					
Betamethasone (9α-fluoro-16β-methylprednisolone)	25–40	10	0	0.6	Oral, injectable, topical.
Dexamethasone (9α-fluoro-16α-methylprednisolone)	30	10	0	0.75	Oral, injectable, topical.
Mineralocorticoids					
Fludrocortisone (9α-fluorohydrocortisone)	10	10	250	2	Oral, injectable, topical.
Desoxycorticosterone (11-deoxycorticosterone)	0	0	20	0	Oral, injectable.

*Outside USA.
†Acetonide: Up to 100.

ness, fatigue, weight loss, hypotension, and inability to maintain the blood glucose level with fasting. In such individuals, minor noxious, traumatic, or infectious stimuli may produce acute adrenal insufficiency with shock and finally death.

In adrenal insufficiency, whether primary or following adrenalectomy, about 20–30 mg of cortisol must be given daily, with increased amounts during periods of stress. This must be supplemented by an appropriate amount of salt-retaining hormone such as desoxycorticosterone (DOC) or fludrocortisone. It is for this reason that glucocorticoids devoid of salt-retaining activity are not indicated for these patients.

Aldosterone is not used for replacement therapy, since the supply is too small. However, desoxycorticosterone pivalate (trimethylacetate) given in monthly injections and fludrocortisone given orally are excellent preparations for this purpose.

When a rapidly acting intravenous preparation is needed for the management of acute adrenal insufficiency (or to prevent adrenal insufficiency during major stress such as surgery), the water-soluble hemisuccinate of cortisol is ideal. Intramuscular administration of cortisol or cortisone or their acetates is not satisfactory because the rate of absorption is unpredictable and the onset of effect is too slow for emergency use.

2. Adrenocortical hyperfunction–

a. Congenital adrenal hyperplasia–This group of disorders is characterized by specific defects in the synthesis of cortisol. The most common is a decrease in or lack of 21-hydroxylase activity. As can be seen in Fig 37–1, this would lead to a reduction in cortisol synthesis and produce a compensatory increase in ACTH release. If sufficient enzyme activity is present, a normal amount of cortisol will be produced in response to the increased level of ACTH, but the gland will become hyperplastic and produce abnormally large amounts of precursors such as 17-hydroxyprogesterone that can be diverted to the androgen pathway, leading to virilization. Metabolism of this compound in the liver leads to pregnanetriol, which is characteristically excreted into the urine in large amounts in this disorder.

If the defect is in 11-hydroxylation, hypertension is prominent. When 17-hydroxylation is defective in the adrenals and gonads, hypogonadism will be present. However, increased amounts of 11-deoxycorticosterone (DOC) (see below) are formed and the signs and symptoms associated with mineralocorticoid excess—such as hypertension and hypokalemia—are found.

Cortisol and cortisone have been used in the treatment of congenital adrenal hyperplasia. Since ACTH suppression is an important objective of therapy, slowly absorbed parenteral preparations can be given in smaller amounts than the oral preparations, which are rapidly absorbed and metabolized and must be given in divided doses. When treating these patients, larger doses of cortisone (25–100 mg daily intramuscularly, depending upon age) can be given for 5–10 days to achieve adequate suppression of adrenal secretion. The dose is then reduced to 4–6 mg/d and adjusted to maintain a low urinary ketosteroid excretion. Treatment with orally administered hydrocortisone in a dose of 25 mg/d/m^2 of body surface or less can be used as the basis of therapy. Undesirable effects are minimized by giving the larger part of the dose in the morning. The dose must also be adjusted over the long course of therapy to permit normal growth, since excessive amounts of glucocorticoids inhibit linear growth in children. In some infants, salt-retaining hormone therapy is also required.

b. Cushing's syndrome–Cushing's syndrome is usually the result of bilateral adrenal hyperplasia secondary to a pituitary adenoma but occasionally is due to tumors of the adrenal gland or ectopic production of ACTH by other tumors. The manifestations are those associated with the presence of excessive glucocorticoids. When changes are marked, a rounded, plethoric face and trunk obesity are striking in appearance. In general, the manifestations of protein loss are severe and include muscle wasting, thinning of the skin, striae, easy bruisability, poor wound healing, and osteoporosis. Other serious disturbances include mental disorders, hypertension, and diabetes. This disorder is treated by surgical removal of the tumor producing the hormone, irradiation or removal of a pituitary microadenoma producing ACTH, or resection of hyperplastic adrenals. These patients must receive large doses of cortisol during and following the surgical procedure. Doses of 300 mg of soluble hydrocortisone are given as a continuous intravenous infusion on the day of surgery. The dose must be reduced slowly to normal replacement levels, since rapid reduction in dose may produce symptoms including fever and joint pain. If adrenalectomy has been performed, long-term maintenance is similar to that outlined above for adrenal insufficiency.

c. Hyperaldosteronism–Primary hyperaldosteronism usually results from the excessive production of aldosterone by an adrenal adenoma. It may result from abnormal secretion of hyperplastic glands or from a malignant tumor. The clinical findings of hypertension, polyuria, polydipsia, weakness, and tetany are related to the continued renal loss of potassium, which leads to hypokalemia, alkalosis, and hypernatremia.

In contrast to patients with secondary hyperaldosteronism (see below), these patients have low (suppressed) levels of plasma renin activity and angiotensin II. When treated with desoxycorticosterone acetate (20 mg intramuscularly daily for 3 days), they fail to retain sodium and their secretion of aldosterone is not significantly reduced. They are generally improved when treated with spironolactone, and their response to this agent is of diagnostic value.

3. Use of glucocorticoids for diagnostic purposes–It is sometimes necessary to suppress the production of ACTH in order to identify the source of a particular hormone or to establish whether or not its production is influenced by the secretion of ACTH. In these circumstances, it is advantageous to employ a very potent substance such as dexamethasone or betamethasone. Although these preparations are no more effective, the use of small quantities reduces the possibility of confusion in the interpretation of hormone assays in blood or urine. For example, if complete suppression is achieved by the use of 50 mg of cortisol, the urinary 17-hydroxycorticoids will be 15–18 mg/24 h, since one-third of the dose is recovered in urine as 17-hydroxycorticoid. If 1.5 mg of dexamethasone is employed, the excretion will be only 0.5 mg/24 h.

Suppression of the adrenal with glucocorticoids and of the ovary with estrogens can be useful in locating the source of androgen production in a hirsute woman if the effect on testosterone levels in blood can be measured before and during hormone administration.

B. Adrenocorticosteroids and Stimulation of Lung Maturation in the Fetus: Lung maturation in the fetus is regulated by the fetal secretion of cortisol. Treatment of the mother with large doses of glucocorticoid reduces the incidence of respiratory distress syndrome in infants delivered prematurely. When delivery is anticipated before 34 weeks of gestation, betamethasone, 12 mg, followed by an additional dose of 12 mg 18–24 hours later, is commonly used. Protein binding of this corticosteroid is less than that of cortisol, allowing increased transfer across the placenta to the fetus. Corticosteroid levels achieved in the fetus are equivalent to those observed when the fetus is stressed. The safety of this treatment in patients with severe preeclampsia or hypertension—or diabetes with renal complications—has not been established.

C. Adrenocorticosteroids and Nonadrenal Disorders: Cortisol and its synthetic analogs have been found to be useful in the treatment of a diverse group of diseases unrelated to any known disturbance of adrenal function. The usefulness of corticosteroids in these disorders is a function of their ability to suppress inflammatory and immune responses as described above. In disorders in which host response is the cause of the major manifestations of the disease, these agents are useful. In instances where the inflammatory or immune response is important in controlling the pathologic process, therapy with corticosteroids may be dangerous but justified, if used in conjunction with specific therapy for the disease process, to prevent irreparable damage from an inflammatory response.

Since the corticosteroids are not usually curative, the pathologic process may progress while clinical manifestations are suppressed. Therefore, systemic therapy with these drugs should be undertaken with great care and only when the seriousness of the disorder warrants their use and less hazardous measures have been exhausted.

In general, attempts should be made to bring the disease process under control using short-acting agents as well as all ancillary measures possible to keep the dose low. Where possible, alternate-day therapy should be utilized (see p 427). Therapy should not be decreased or stopped abruptly. When prolonged therapy is anticipated, it is helpful to obtain chest films and a tuberculin test. The presence of diabetes, peptic ulcer, osteoporosis, and psychologic disturbances should be excluded, and cardiovascular function should be assessed.

The following supplemental measures should be considered: The diet should be rich in potassium and low in sodium to prevent electrolyte disturbances. Caloric management to prevent obesity should be instituted. High protein intake is required to compensate for the loss due to the increased breakdown of protein from gluconeogenesis. Antacids should be used 3–4 times daily in patients prone to epigastric distress. Where osteoporosis is of concern, the use of physical therapy, fluorides, androgens, and vitamin D (with careful monitoring of serum calcium levels) has been recommended.

1. Some therapeutic indications for glucocorticoids in nonadrenal disorders–

- Allergic disorders (angioneurotic edema, asthma, bee stings, contact dermatitis, drug reactions, allergic rhinitis, hay fever, serum sickness, urticaria)
- Arthritis, bursitis, and tenosynovitis
- Collagen vascular disorders (giant cell arteritis, lupus erythematosus, mixed connective tissue syndromes, polymyositis, polymyalgia rheumatica, rheumatoid arthritis, temporal arteritis)
- Hematologic disorders (acquired hemolytic anemia, acute allergic purpura, leukemia, autoimmune hemolytic anemia, idiopathic thrombocytopenic purpura, lymphoblastic leukemia, multiple myeloma)
- Eye diseases (acute uveitis, allergic conjunctivitis, choroiditis, optic neuritis)
- Gastrointestinal diseases (inflammatory bowel disease, nontropical sprue, regional enteritis, subacute hepatic necrosis, ulcerative colitis)
- Hypercalcemia (immunosuppression [transplants], carcinoma, sarcoidosis)
- Malignant exophthalmos and subacute thyroiditis
- Neurologic diseases
- Pulmonary diseases (aspiration pneumonia, bronchial asthma, prevention of infant respiratory distress syndrome, sarcoidosis)
- Renal diseases (certain nephrotic syndromes)
- Infection (gram-negative septicemia, shock; occasionally helpful to suppress excessive inflammation)
- Skin disorders (atopic dermatitis, dermatoses [see above], lichen simplex chronicus [localized neurodermatitis], mycosis fungoides, pemphigus, seborrheic dermatitis, xerosis)

Toxicity

The benefits obtained from the use of the compounds vary considerably. They must be carefully weighed in each patient against the widespread effects on every part of the organism. The major undesirable effects of the glucocorticoids are not toxic effects but exaggerations of their hormonal actions (see above) and lead to the clinical picture of iatrogenic Cushing's syndrome.

When the glucocorticoids are used for short periods (less than 1 week), it is unusual to see serious side-effects even with moderately large doses. However, behavioral changes and acute peptic ulcers are occasionally observed.

A. Adrenal Suppression: When corticosteroids are administered for a period of months or years, adrenal suppression occurs and the patient should be given supplementary therapy at times of severe stress such as accidental trauma or surgery. The degree of adrenal unresponsiveness is a function of the dose and the length of time the patient has been treated. The dose is a less important variable when the threshold for suppression has been exceeded. With very rare exceptions, recovery occurs when the drug is withdrawn; however, after prolonged suppression, a state of relative insufficiency may persist for 6–9 months or longer.

Treatment with ACTH does not significantly reduce the suppression of pituitary-adrenal function. The problem can be approached by treating the patient with an amount of steroid that is slightly less than the replacement dose. This will not prevent the return of adrenal function but will provide support for the patient in the interim. The dose can be augmented during periods of acute stress.

B. Metabolic Effects: Most patients who are given daily doses of 100 mg of cortisol or more (or the equivalent amount of synthetic steroid) for longer than 2 weeks undergo a series of changes that have been termed iatrogenic Cushing's syndrome. The rate of development is a function of the dose. The appearance of the face is altered by rounding, puffiness, and plethora. Fat tends to be redistributed from the extremities to the trunk and face. There is an increased growth of fine hair over the thighs and trunk and sometimes the face. Acne may increase or appear, and insomnia and increased appetite are noted. In the treatment of dangerous or disabling disorders, these changes may not require cessation of therapy. However, the underlying metabolic changes accompanying them can be very serious by the time they become obvious. The continuing breakdown of protein and diversion of amino acids to glucose production increase the need for insulin and over a period of time result in **weight gain;** fat deposition; muscle wasting; thinning of the skin, with striae and bruising; hyperglycemia; and eventually the development of **osteoporosis** and **diabetes.** When diabetes occurs, it is treated by diet and insulin. These patients are often resistant to insulin but rarely develop ketoacidosis. In general, patients treated with corticosteroids should be on high-protein diets, and increased potassium and anabolic steroids should be used when required.

C. Other Complications: Other serious complications include the development of **peptic ulcers** and their complications. The clinical findings associated with other disorders, particularly bacterial and mycotic infections, may be masked by the corticosteroids, and patients must be carefully watched to avoid serious mishap when large doses are used. Some patients develop a myopathy the nature of which is unknown. The frequency of myopathy is greater in patients treated with triamcinolone. The administration of this drug as well as of methylprednisolone has been associated with nausea, dizziness, and weight loss in some patients. It is treated by changing drugs, reducing dosage, and increasing the potassium and protein intake.

Psychosis may occur, particularly in patients receiving large doses of corticosteroids. Long-term therapy is associated with the development of posterior subcapsular **cataracts.** Increased intraocular pressure is common, and **glaucoma** may be induced. **Benign intracranial hypertension** also occurs. In doses of 45 $mg/m^2/d$ or more, **growth retardation** occurs in children.

When given in greater than physiologic amounts, steroids such as cortisone and hydrocortisone, which have mineralocorticoid effects in addition to glucocorticoid effects, cause some sodium and fluid retention and loss of potassium. In patients with normal cardiovascular and renal function, this leads to a **hypokalemic, hypochloremic alkalosis** and eventually a rise in blood pressure. In patients with hypoproteinemia, renal disease, or liver disease, edema may also occur. In patients with heart disease, even small degrees of sodium retention may lead to congestive heart failure. These effects can be minimized by sodium restriction and judicious use of potassium supplements. Many of the synthetic steroids have so little mineralocorticoid effect that these problems can be avoided. However, for the same reason, such compounds are not indicated for replacement therapy in adrenal insufficiency.

Children with asthma treated for prolonged periods with these steroids have been reported to develop cataracts with increased frequency. Periodic slit lamp examination is indicated in such patients.

Contraindications & Cautions

A. Special Precautions: Patients receiving these drugs must be observed carefully for the development of hyperglycemia, glycosuria, sodium retention with edema or hypertension, hypokalemia, peptic ulcer, osteoporosis, and hidden infections. In order to minimize undesirable effects, periodic clinical examination with determination of plasma glucose and serum potassium is useful. A high-protein diet and adequate calcium intake are necessary. In patients with limited cardiac reserve, sodium restriction may be required. When more than physiologic amounts of steroids have been used, sudden cessation of therapy should be avoided in order to prevent an acute exacerbation of the disease process or symptoms of adrenal insufficiency.

The dosage should be kept as low as possible and intermittent dosage (eg, alternate-day) employed when satisfactory therapeutic results can be obtained on this schedule. In patients being maintained on relatively low doses of corticosteroids, supplementary therapy may be required at times of stress such as when surgical procedures are performed or accidents occur.

B. Contraindications: These agents must be used with the greatest of caution in patients with the following disorders:

1. Peptic ulcer–In the presence of active peptic ulcer disease, these steroids may cause hemorrhage or perforation. In patients with previous ulceration, activation is likely. Careful dietary control and antacids should be used when corticosteroids must be given to these patients. Cimetidine may be useful.

2. Heart disease or hypertension with congestive heart failure–Measures to avoid the accumulation of extracellular fluid should be utilized. The concomitant use of potassium-wasting diuretics may create serious problems in patients receiving digitalis.

3. Infections–Since natural indicators of and defenses against infection are attenuated, great care is required even when antibiotics are used. Antituberculosis therapy may be required even in patients with inactive tuberculosis. Ophthalmic herpes simplex (see below) is particularly dangerous in the presence of corticosteroids.

4. Psychoses–Serious behavioral disturbances may occur in patients on steroid therapy, and prior disturbances are thought to predispose patients to acute psychoses.

5. Diabetes–Since these agents increase glucose production, more insulin may be required. However, the corticosteroids rarely cause acidosis or coma unless complications (such as an infection) occur.

6. Osteoporosis.

7. Glaucoma may be made worse by corticosteroid therapy.

8. Herpes simplex involving the cornea is particularly destructive in patients receiving corticosteroid therapy.

Selection of Drug & Dosage Schedule

Since these preparations differ with respect to relative anti-inflammatory and mineralocorticoid effect (Table 37–1), duration of action, cost, and dosage forms available, these factors should be taken into account in selecting the drug to be used.

A. ACTH Versus Adrenocortical Steroids: In patients with normal adrenals, ACTH has been used to induce the endogenous production of cortisol to obtain similar effects. However, when exogenous ACTH is given, the total amount of cortisol released by the adrenal can only be measured in retrospect. Furthermore, following ACTH administration the adrenal also increases its output of other hormones, including the androgens, which may not be desirable. Therefore, except when the increase in androgens is desirable, the use of ACTH as a therapeutic agent is probably unjustified. Instances in which ACTH has been claimed to be more effective than glucocorticoids are probably due to the administration of smaller amounts of corticoids than were produced by the dosage of ACTH.

B. Dosage: In determining the dose to be used, the physician must consider the seriousness of the disease, the amount of drug likely to be required to obtain the desired effect, and the duration of therapy. In some diseases, the amount required for maintenance of the desired therapeutic effect is less than the dose needed to obtain the initial effect, and the lowest possible dose for the needed effect should be determined by gradually lowering the dose until an increase in signs or symptoms is noted.

Many types of dosage schedules have been used in administering glucocorticoids. When it is necessary to maintain continuously elevated plasma corticosteroid levels in order to suppress ACTH, a slowly absorbed parenteral preparation or small doses at frequent intervals are required. The opposite situation exists with respect to the use of corticosteroids in the treatment of inflammatory and allergic disorders. The same total quantity given in a few doses may be more effective than when given in many smaller doses or in a slowly absorbed parenteral form. In addition, the other less desirable effects of the hormone may be less marked because there is a recovery period between each dose. The intermittent use of large doses of shorter-acting corticosteroids has been very helpful in the chronic treatment of disorders such as asthma and the nephrotic syndrome. When used in this manner, very large amounts (eg, 100 mg prednisone daily) can sometimes be administered with only minimal side-effects. The transition to an alternate-day schedule can be made after the disease process is under control. It should be done gradually and with additional supportive measures between doses. A typical schedule for a patient maintained on 50 mg of prednisone daily would be as follows:

Day	1: 50 mg	7: 75 mg
	2: 40 mg	8: 5 mg
	3: 60 mg	9: 70 mg
	4: 30 mg	10: 5 mg
	5: 70 mg	11: 65 mg
	6: 10 mg	12: 5 mg
		etc

When selecting a drug for use in large doses, a shorter-acting synthetic steroid with little mineralocorticoid effect is advisable. If possible, it should be given as a single morning dose.

Methylprednisolone in doses of 1 g given intravenously over 30–60 minutes at monthly intervals has been reported to be useful in treatment of rheumatoid arthritis in a few cases. The indications for this mode of therapy are not established.

C. Special Dosage Forms: The use of local therapy such as topical preparations for skin disease, ophthalmic forms for eye disease, intra-articular injections for joint disease, and hydrocortisone enemas for ulcerative colitis provides a means of delivering large amounts of steroid to the diseased tissue without serious systemic effects.

Beclomethasone dipropionate administered as an aerosol containing a microcrystalline suspension in doses of 400 μg daily has been found to be effective in the treatment of asthma. In this dose, endogenous adrenal function is not significantly depressed, and systemic effects are minimal. This agent and its metabolites are excreted mainly in feces. The switch from therapy with systemic glucocorticoids to aerosol therapy with beclomethasone must be undertaken with caution, since adrenal insufficiency will occur if adrenal function is suppressed. In such patients, a slow, graded reduction of systemic therapy should accompany the institution of aerosol administration. During an acute attack, the aerosol is not a dependable route of administration. The possibility of local atrophic changes with long-term use has not been excluded. Mycotic infections occur in 5–10% of patients, and most patients have positive oral cultures for *Candida albicans*.

Beclomethasone dipropionate and flunisolide are available as nasal sprays for the treatment of allergic rhinitis. They are effective at doses that in most patients result in plasma levels too low to influence adrenal function. Beclomethasone is administered as a powder delivered as an aerosol; flunisolide is provided as 0.025% solution sprayed by a hand-activated pump. The dose of beclomethasone is 400 μg daily; of flunisolide, 200 μg daily. Both are given in divided doses 2–4 times daily.

MINERALOCORTICOIDS (Aldosterone, Desoxycorticosterone, Fludrocortisone)

The most important mineralocorticoid in humans is aldosterone. However, small amounts of desoxycorticosterone (DOC) are also formed and released. Although the amounts are normally insignificant, DOC is of some importance therapeutically. Its actions, effects, and metabolism are similar to those described below for aldosterone. Fludrocortisone, a synthetic corticosteroid, is the most commonly used salt-retaining hormone.

ALDOSTERONE

Aldosterone is synthesized mainly in the zona glomerulosa of the adrenal cortex. Its structure and synthesis are illustrated in Fig 37–1.

The rate of aldosterone secretion is subject to several influences. ACTH produces a moderate stimulation of its release, but this effect is not sustained for more than a few days in the normal individual. Although aldosterone is no less than one-third as effective as cortisol in suppressing ACTH, the minute quantities of aldosterone produced by the adrenal cortex prevent it from participating in any feedback relationship in the control of ACTH secretion.

After hypophysectomy, aldosterone secretion gradually falls to about half the normal rate, which means that other factors are able to maintain and perhaps regulate its secretion. Independent variations between cortisol and aldosterone secretion can also be demonstrated by means of lesions in the nervous system such as decerebration, which decreases the secretion of hydrocortisone while increasing the secretion of aldosterone.

One of the important stimuli of aldosterone secretion is a reduction in blood volume, whether due to hemorrhage, dietary sodium restriction, or sodium loss following administration of diuretics (Fig 37–4). These stimuli lead to a decrease in mean renal arterial pressure that is associated with an increase in the release of renin by the cells of the juxtaglomerular apparatus. The enzyme renin then acts upon a circulating α_2-globulin (renin substrate), releasing angioten-

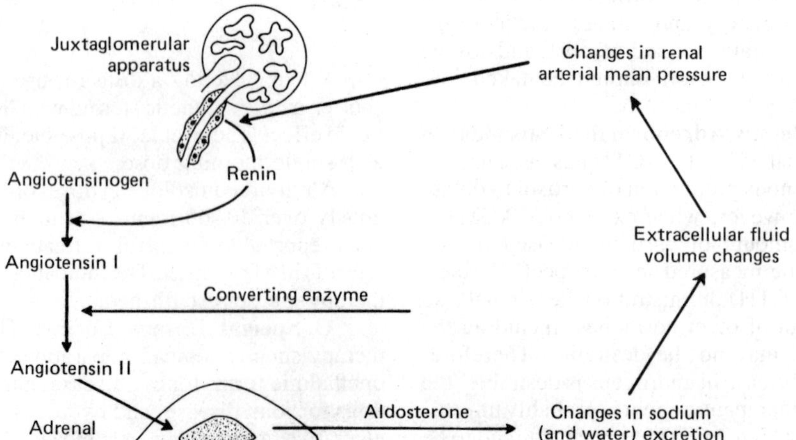

Figure 37–4. A postulated feedback mechanism regulating aldosterone secretion. (Reproduced, with permission, from Ganong WF: *Review of Medical Physiology,* 10th ed. Lange, 1981.)

sin I, which is then converted to angiotensin II. Angiotensin is a powerful stimulant of aldosterone production, only a few micrograms being required to show an effect in humans (Chapter 15). A metabolite of angiotensin II, the heptapeptide formed by the removal of asparagine from the N-terminus, is also a potent stimulator of aldosterone production.

Physiologic & Pharmacologic Effects

Aldosterone and other steroids with mineralocorticoid properties induce the reabsorption of sodium from urine by the distal renal tubules in exchange for potassium and hydrogen ion. Sodium reabsorption in the sweat and salivary glands, gastrointestinal mucosa, and across cell membranes in general is also increased. Excessive levels of aldosterone produced by tumors or overdosage with other mineralocorticoids lead to hypernatremia, hypokalemia, metabolic alkalosis, increased plasma volume, and hypertension.

Aldosterone has a delayed action on sodium transport. Recent experiments indicate that its action is dependent upon the synthesis of an enzyme required by the transport mechanism. The hormone appears to stimulate the formation of nuclear RNA, which in turn serves the induction of enzyme synthesis.

Metabolism

Aldosterone is secreted at the rate of 100–200 μg/d in normal individuals with a moderate dietary salt intake. The plasma level in males (resting supine) is about 0.007 μg/dL. The half-life of aldosterone injected in tracer quantities is 15–20 minutes, and it does not appear to be firmly bound to serum proteins.

The metabolism of aldosterone is similar to that of cortisol, about 50 μg/24 h appearing in the urine as conjugated tetrahydroaldosterone. Approximately 5–15 μg/24 h is excreted free or as the 3-oxo glucuronide.

DESOXYCORTICOSTERONE (DOC)

DOC, which also serves as a precursor of aldosterone (Fig 37–1), is normally secreted in amounts of about 200 μg/d. Its half-life when injected into the human circulation is about 70 minutes. Preliminary estimates of its concentration in plasma are approximately 0.03 μg/dL. The control of its secretion differs from that of aldosterone in that the secretion of DOC is primarily under the control of ACTH. Although the response to ACTH is enhanced by dietary sodium restriction, a low-salt diet does not increase DOC secretion.

FLUDROCORTISONE (Florinef)

This compound, a potent glucocorticoid and mineralocorticoid, has become the most widely used mineralocorticoid. Doses of 0.1 mg 2–7 times weekly have potent salt-retaining activity and are used in the treatment of adrenocortical insufficiency but are too small to have important anti-inflammatory effects.

The clinical uses of fludrocortisone are discussed in the section on adrenocortical insufficiency. The available preparations are listed in Table 37–1.

• • •

ALDOSTERONE ANTAGONISTS

In addition to agents that interfere with aldosterone synthesis such as amphenone B (see below), there are steroids that compete with aldosterone for binding sites and decrease its effect peripherally. Progesterone is mildly active in this respect. However, it has been found that substitution of a 17-spironolactone group for the C20-C21 side chain of desoxycorticosterone results in a compound capable of blocking the sodium-retaining effect of aldosterone.

Spironolactone (Aldactone) is a 7α-acetylthiospironolactone. Little is known about its metabolism. The onset of activity is slow, and the effects last for 2–3 days after the drug is discontinued. It is used in the treatment of primary hyperaldosteronism in doses of 50–100 mg/d in divided doses. This agent will reverse many of the findings of hyperaldosteronism. It has been useful in establishing the diagnosis in some patients and in ameliorating the signs and symptoms when surgical removal of an adenoma is delayed. When used diagnostically for the detection of hyperaldosteronism in hypokalemic patients with hypertension, doses of 400–500 mg/d for 4–8 days—with an adequate intake of sodium and potassium—will restore potassium levels to or toward normal. This agent is also useful in preparing these patients for surgery. Doses of 300–400 mg/d for 2 weeks are used for this purpose and may reduce the incidence of cardiac arrhythmias.

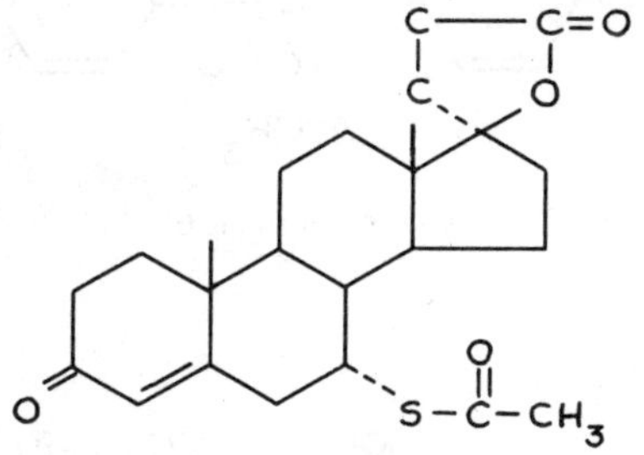

Spironolactone
(3-[3-oxo-7α-acetylthio-17β-hydroxy-4-androsten-17α-yl] propionic acid γ-lactone)

Spironolactone is also used in treatment of hirsutism in women. Doses of 200 mg/d cause a reduction in the density, diameter, and rate of growth of facial hair in patients with idiopathic hirsutism or hirsutism secondary to androgen excess. The effect can usually be seen in 2 months and becomes maximal in about 6 months. It may be due to inhibition of androgen production and action at the hair follicle.

Spironolactone has limited usefulness as a diuretic (Chapter 13).

Side-effects reported for spironolactone include hyperkalemia, menstrual abnormalities, gynecomastia, sedation, headache, gastrointestinal disturbances, and skin rashes.

II. ANTAGONISTS OF ADRENOCORTICAL AGENTS

MITOTANE

Suppression of adrenal steroidogenesis with DDT derivatives is a rational research objective but the results so far have not been as expected. Mitotane (*o,p'*-DDD, Lysodren; 2,2-bis[*o*-chlorophenyl-*p*-chlorophenyl]-1,1-dichloroethane) produces adrenal atrophy in dogs and will interfere with biosynthetic pathways (Fig 37–5). Doses of up to 10 g daily have been administered to patients with carcinoma of the adrenal. The production of corticosteroids was reduced, and in a few patients some reduction in tumor size was noted. However, severe toxic effects, including central nervous system depression, tremors, and skin and gastrointestinal disturbances, limit the effective use of this experimental compound.

AMPHENONE B

Amphenone B is a more potent inhibitor of synthesis than mitotane, blocking hydroxylation at the 11, 17, and 21 positions (Fig 37–5). It does not have a destructive effect on the tissue, and the synthetic block leads to increased production of ACTH and hyperplasia of the gland. It is considered too toxic for use in humans. Amphenone causes central nervous system depression and gastrointestinal tract and skin disorders, and impairs liver and thyroid function.

METYRAPONE

Metyrapone (Metopirone) (Fig 37–5) has a more selective effect at low doses than either mitotane or amphenone B. It inhibits 11-hydroxylation, interfering with cortisol and corticosterone synthesis and leading to secretion of 11-deoxycortisol. In the presence of a normal pituitary gland, there is a compensatory increase in 11-deoxycortisol production. This response is a measure of the capacity of the anterior pituitary to produce ACTH and has been adapted for clinical use. Although the toxicity of metyrapone is much lower than that of the above agents, it does produce transient dizziness and gastrointestinal disturbances. This agent has not been widely used for the treatment of Cushing's syndrome. However, in doses of 0.25 g twice daily to 1 g 4 times daily, metyrapone can reduce cortisol production to normal levels in some patients with adrenal tumors, ectopic ACTH syndromes, and hyperplasia. It may be useful in the management of severe manifestations of cortisol excess while the cause is being determined or in conjunction with radiation or surgical treatment. The major side-effects observed are salt and water retention and hirsutism resulting from diversion of precursor to DOC and androgen synthesis.

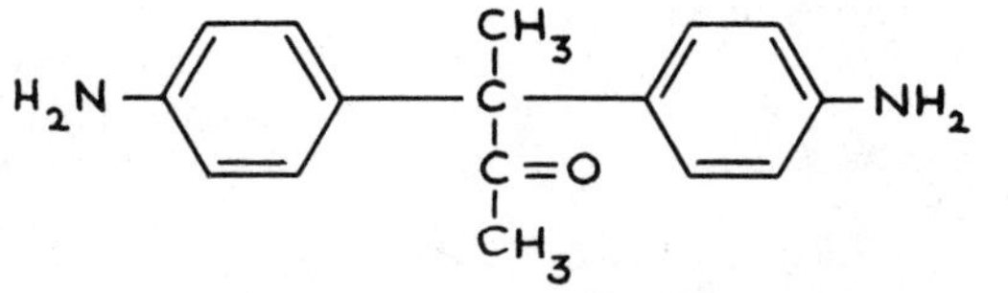

Amphenone B

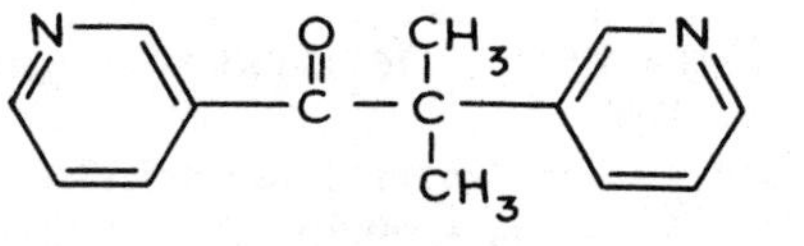

Metyrapone (Su 4885)

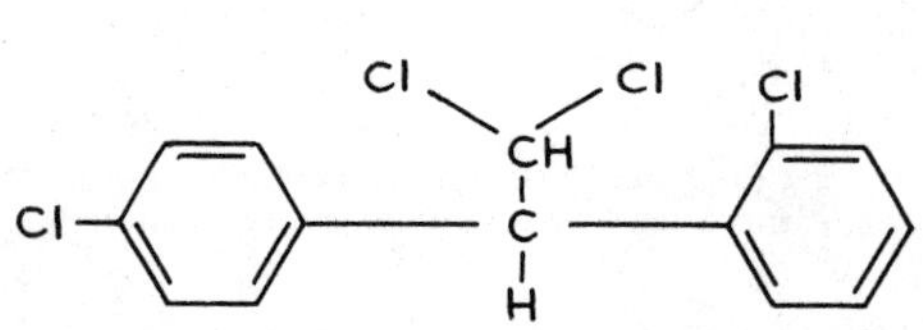

Mitotane (*o,p'*-DDD; dichlorodiphenyldichloroethane)

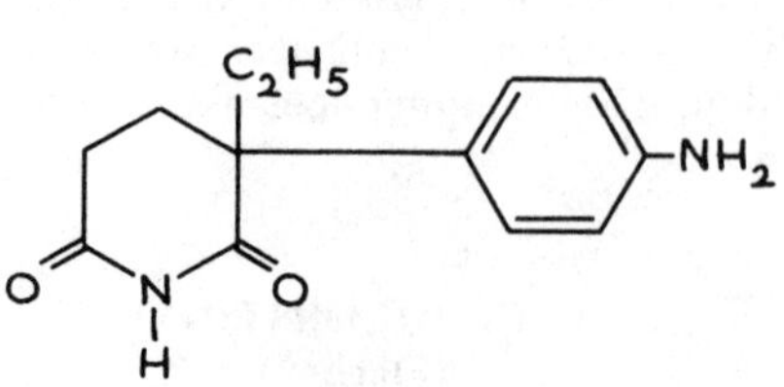

Aminoglutethimide

Figure 37–5. Adrenocortical antagonists.

Metyrapone is most commonly used in tests of adrenal function. The blood levels of 11-deoxycortisol and the urinary excretion of 17-hydroxycorticoids are measured before and after administration of the compound. Normally, there is a 2-fold or greater increase in the urinary 17-hydroxycorticoid excretion. A dosage of 300–500 mg every 4 hours for 6 doses is commonly used, and urine collections are made on the day before and the day after treatment. In patients with Cushing's syndrome, a normal response to metyrapone indicates that the cortisol excess is not the result of adrenal carcinoma or autonomous adenoma, since secretion by such tumors produces suppression of ACTH and atrophy of normal adrenal cortex.

Adrenal function may also be tested by administering metyrapone, 2–3 g orally at midnight, and measuring the level of ACTH or 11-deoxycortisol in blood drawn at 8:00 AM, or by comparing the excretion of 17-hydroxycorticosteroids in the urine during the 24-hour periods preceding and following administration of the drug.

In patients with suspected or known lesions of the pituitary, this procedure is a means of estimating the ability of the gland to produce ACTH.

AMINOGLUTETHIMIDE

Aminoglutethimide (Cytadren) (Fig 37–5) blocks the conversion of cholesterol to pregnenolone and causes a reduction in the synthesis of all hormonally active steroids (Fig 37–1). It has been used in conjunction with dexamethasone to reduce or eliminate estrogen and androgen production in patients with carcinoma of the breast. In doses of 1 g daily it was well tolerated; however, with higher doses, lethargy was a common effect. This drug may prove to be useful in reducing steroid secretion in patients with adrenocortical malignancy. It has been shown to enhance the metabolism of dexamethasone. During treatment, the half-life of ^{3}H-dexamethasone was reduced from 264 to 120 minutes.

• • •

References

Axelrod L: Glucocorticoid therapy. *Medicine* 1976;**55:**39.

Bartter FC (editor): *The Clinical Use of Aldosterone Antagonists*. Thomas, 1960.

Baxter JD, Rousseau GG (editors): *Glucocorticoid Action*. Monographs on Endocrinology. Vol 12. Springer-Verlag, 1979.

Bethune JE: *The Adrenal Cortex*. A Scope Monograph. Upjohn, 1974.

Bongiovanni AM, Root AW: The adrenogenital syndrome. (3 parts.) *N Engl J Med* 1963;**268:**1283, 1342, 1391.

Brook CGD et al: Experience with long-term therapy in congenital adrenal hyperplasia. *J Pediatr* 1974;**85:**12.

Burdick KH, Poulsen B, Place VA: Extemporaneous formulation of corticosteroids for topical usage. *JAMA* 1970;**211:**462.

Byyny RL: Withdrawal from glucocorticoid therapy. *N Engl J Med* 1976;**295:**30.

Cope CL: *Adrenal Steroids and Disease*. Lippincott, 1972.

Cumming DC et al: Treatment of hirsutism with spironolactone. *JAMA* 1982;**247:**1295.

Davis JO, Freeman RH: Mechanisms regulating renin release. *Physiol Rev* 1976;**56:**1.

Edelman IS, Fimognari GM: On the biochemical mechanism of action of aldosterone. *Recent Prog Horm Res* 1968;**24:**1.

Fauci AS, Dale DC, Balow JE: Glucocorticosteroid therapy: Mechanisms of action and clinical considerations. *Ann Intern Med* 1976;**84:**304.

Graber AL et al: Natural history of pituitary-adrenal recovery following long-term suppression with corticosteroids. *J Clin Endocrinol Metab* 1965;**25:**11.

Hahn TJ: Corticosteroid-induced osteopenia. *Arch Intern Med* 1978;**138:**882.

Hutter AM Jr, Kayhoe DE: Adrenal cortical carcinoma: Results of treatment with o,p'DDD in 138 patients. *Am J Med* 1966;**41:**581.

Jeffcoate WJ et al: Metyrapone in long-term management of Cushing's disease. *Br Med J* 1977;**2:**215.

Jubiz W et al: Plasma metyrapone, adrenocorticotropic hormone, cortisol, and deoxycortisol levels: Sequential changes during oral and intravenous metyrapone administration. *Arch Intern Med* 1970;**125:**468.

Kaplan NM: Assessment of pituitary ACTH secretory capacity with Metopirone [metyrapone]. *J Clin Endocrinol Metab* 1963; **23:**945.

Morimoto Y, Yagura T, Yamamura Y: The effect of prolonged administration of beclomethasone dipropionate inhaler on adrenocortical functions in bronchial asthma. *J Med* 1977; **8:**1.

Myles AB, Daly JR: *Corticosteroid and ACTH Treatment*. Williams & Wilkins, 1974.

Reid IA, Ganong WF: Control of aldosterone secretion. Pages 265–292 in: *Hypertension*. Genest J, Koiw E, Kuchel O (editors). McGraw-Hill, 1976.

Santen RJ, Lipton A, Kendall J: Successful medical adrenalectomy with amino-glutethimide. *JAMA* 1974;**230:**1661.

Scoggins RB, Kliman B: Percutaneous absorption of corticosteroids: Systemic effects. *N Engl J Med* 1965;**273:**831.

Slaunwhite W Jr, Sandberg A: Transcortin: A corticosteroid-binding protein of plasma. *J Clin Invest* 1959;**38:**384.

Thorn GW: Clinical considerations in the use of corticosteroids. *N Engl J Med* 1966;**274:**775.

Thorn GW, Lauler DP: Clinical therapeutics of adrenal disorders. *Am J Med* 1972;**53:**673.

Zachmann M et al: Effect of aminoglutethimide on urinary cortisol and cortisol metabolites in adolescents with Cushing's syndrome. *Clin Endocrinol* 1977;**7:**63.

38 | The Gonadal Hormones & Inhibitors

Alan Goldfien, MD

I. THE OVARY (Estrogens, Progestins, Other Ovarian Hormones, Oral Contraceptives, Other Uses of Estrogens & Progestins, & Ovulation-Inducing Agents)

The ovary has important gametogenic functions that are integrated with its complex hormonal activity. Our present understanding of these functions, their interrelationships, and the differences from one species to another is incomplete. In the human female, the gonad is relatively quiescent during the period of rapid growth and maturation. At puberty, the ovary begins a 30- to 40-year period of cyclic function called the menstrual cycle because of the regular episodes of bleeding that are its most obvious manifestation. It then fails to respond to gonadotropins secreted by the anterior pituitary gland, and the cessation of cyclic bleeding that occurs is called the menopause.

The nature of the mechanism responsible for the onset of ovarian function at the time of puberty is thought to be neural in origin, because the immature gonad can be stimulated by gonadotropins already

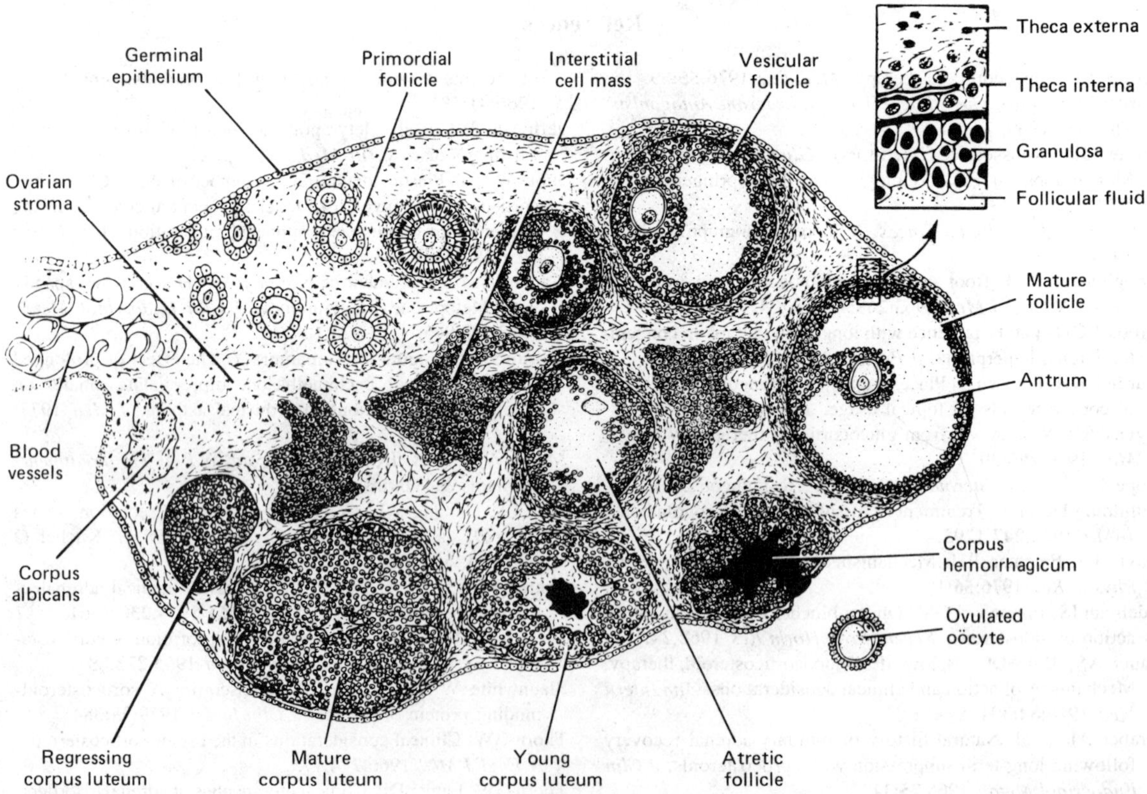

Figure 38–1. Diagram of a mammalian ovary, showing the sequential development of a follicle, formation of a corpus luteum, and, in the center, follicular atresia. A section of the wall of a mature follicle is enlarged at the upper right. The interstitial cell mass is not prominent in primates. (After Patten and Eakin. Reproduced, with permission, from Gorbman A, Bern AL: *Textbook of Comparative Endocrinology.* Wiley, 1962.)

present in the hypothalamus and because the pituitary is responsive to hypothalamic gonadotropin-releasing hormones. The maturation of centers such as the amygdala in the brain may release an inhibition of the cells in the median eminence of the hypothalamus, allowing them to produce gonadotropin-releasing hormone (GnRH, LHRH), which stimulates the release of follicle-stimulating hormone (FSH) and luteinizing hormone (LH) (see Chapter 35). At first, small amounts of these latter 2 hormones are released, and the limited quantities of estrogens secreted in response to FSH cause breast development, alterations in fat distribution, and a growth spurt associated with epiphyseal closure in the long bones. The small amounts of androgens produced by the ovary and adrenal contribute to the appearance of axillary and pubic hair at this time.

After a year or two, sufficient estrogen is produced to induce endometrial changes and periodic bleeding. After the first few cycles, which may be anovulatory, normal cyclic function is established.

At the beginning of each cycle, a variable number of follicles, each containing an ovum, begin to enlarge in response to FSH. After 5 or 6 days, one of the follicles begins to develop more rapidly. The granulosa cells of this follicle multiply and, under the influence of LH, synthesize estrogens and release them at an increasing rate. The estrogens appear to inhibit FSH release, which may lead to regression of the smaller, less mature follicles and produces local stimulation of the maturing follicle. The ovum undergoes meiotic reduction division at this time. This structure is called the ovarian follicle and consists of an ovum surrounded by a fluid-filled antrum lined by granulosa and theca cells (Fig 38–1). The estrogen secretion reaches a peak just before midcycle and stimulates the brief surge in LH and FSH release that precedes (and causes) ovulation. At the time of ovulation, the granulosa cells are beginning to secrete progesterone. When the follicle ruptures, the ovum is released into the abdominal cavity near the uterine tube.

Following the above events, the cavity of the ruptured follicle fills with blood, and the luteinized theca and granulosa cells proliferate and replace the blood to form the corpus luteum. The cells of this structure produce estrogens and progesterone for the remainder of the cycle, or longer if pregnancy occurs. The maintenance of a functioning corpus luteum requires the elaboration of prolactin in the rodent. However, in the human female the structure is supported by the presence of LH. Its life can be prolonged by chorionic gonadotropin, and, when the ovum is fertilized and implants in the endometrium, it produces sufficient amounts of chorionic gonadotropin to maintain the corpus luteum for a prolonged period of time.

If pregnancy does not occur, the corpus luteum begins to degenerate and ceases hormone production. The cause of luteolysis is unknown. Most other hormonal events occurring during the normal ovarian cycle can be explained on the basis of feedback regulation. The endometrium, which proliferated during the follicular phase and developed its glandular structure during the luteal phase, is shed in the process of menstruation. These events are summarized in Fig 38–2.

The ovary normally ceases its gametogenic and endocrine function with time. This change is accompanied by a cessation in uterine bleeding (menopause) and occurs at a mean age of 52 years in the USA. Although the ovary ceases to secrete estrogen, many women maintain significant levels of estrogen by converting adrenal steroids such as androstenedione to estrone and estradiol in nonendocrine tissues.

Disturbances in Ovarian Function

The control of ovarian function is complex. It involves several parts of the brain, including the hypothalamus and the limbic system. Under normal circumstances, the hypothalamic neurons producing GnRH secrete this substance in pulses at regular intervals, leading to pulsatile secretion of LH and FSH by the pituitary; these hormones in turn control follicular development, ovulation, and hormone production in the ovary. Disturbances of cyclic function are common even during the peak years of reproduction. A minority of these result from inflammatory or neoplastic processes that destroy the uterus, ovaries, or pituitary, but the causes of most menstrual problems are poorly understood. Many of the minor disturbances leading to periods of amenorrhea or anovulatory cycles are functional in nature and self-limited. They are often associated with emotional or environmental changes and are thought to represent temporary disorders in the centers in the brain that control the secretion of the hypothalamic releasing factors. Amenorrhea is at times associated with inappropriate lactation, indicating a loss of the inhibitory influence of the hypothalamus on the pituitary secretion of prolactin. This disturbance occurs commonly in women who have used hormonal contraceptives. Pituitary adenomas are not uncommon in patients with galactorrhea. In some patients, the biosynthesis of estrogens is deranged in a fashion that allows increased amounts of androgens, including testosterone, to be secreted by the ovary. This produces hirsutism in association with menstrual disturbances. Normal ovarian function can be modified by androgens produced by the adrenal cortex or tumors arising from it. The ovary also gives rise to androgen-producing neoplasms such as arrhenoblastomas and Leydig cell tumors and estrogen-producing granulosa cell tumors.

THE ESTROGENS

Estrogenic activity is shared by a large number of chemical substances. In addition to the variety of steroidal estrogens derived from animal sources, nonsteroidal estrogens have been synthesized. Many phenols are estrogenic, and estrogenic activity has

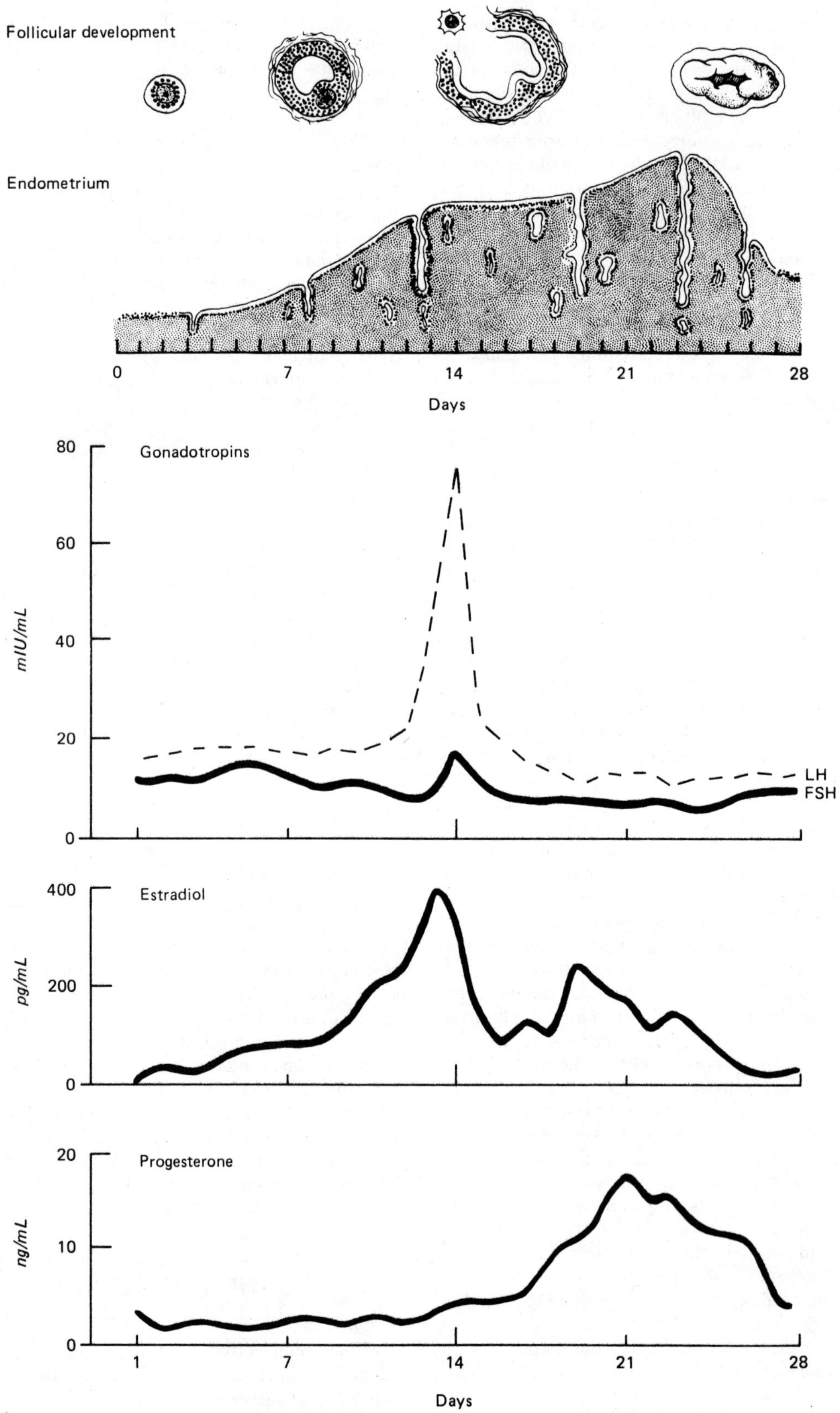

Figure 38–2. The menstrual cycle, showing pituitary and ovarian hormones and histologic changes.

been identified in such diverse forms of life as those found in the sediments of the seas and certain species of clover.

The Natural Estrogens

The major estrogens produced by women are estradiol, estrone, and estriol (Fig 38–3). Estradiol appears to be the major secretory product of the ovary. Although some estrone is produced in the ovary, most of it (and estriol) is formed in the liver from estradiol or formed in peripheral tissues from androstenedione and other androgens. As noted above, during the first part of the menstrual cycle estrogens are produced in the ovarian follicle by the theca cells. After ovulation, the estrogens as well as progesterone are synthesized by the granulosa cells of the corpus luteum, and the pathways of biosynthesis are slightly different. The biosynthetic pathways during both of these phases are illustrated in Fig 38–3.

During pregnancy, a large amount of estrogen is synthesized by the fetoplacental unit. Neither the placenta nor the fetal adrenal contains all the enzymes necessary for this synthesis, and there is a remarkable coordination of activity leading to the production of this hormone. The pathways involved and the locations of the enzymes are shown in Fig 38–4. The estriol synthesized by the fetoplacental unit is released into the maternal circulation and excreted into the urine. Repeated assay of maternal urinary estriol excretion has been useful in the assessment of fetal well-being.

One of the most prolific natural sources of estrogenic substances is the stallion, which liberates more of this hormone than the pregnant mare or pregnant human woman. The equine estrogens—equilenin and equilin—and their congeners are unsaturated in the B as well as the A ring and are excreted in large quantities in urine, from which they can be recovered and used for medicinal purposes.

In normal women, estradiol is produced at a rate that varies during the cycle. Plasma levels of estradiol vary during the menstrual cycle (Fig 38–2) from a low of 50 pg/mL to as high as 350–850 pg/mL at the time of the preovulatory peak. When released into the circulation, estradiol binds strongly ($K_d = 5 \times 10^{-9}$) to an α_2-globulin (sex hormone-binding globulin [SHBG]) and to albumin with less affinity. Estradiol is converted by the liver and other tissues to estrone and estriol and their 2-hydroxylated derivatives and other metabolites (Fig 38–3). The catechol estrogens compete for catechol-O-methyltransferase and in high concentration inhibit the inactivation of catecholamines by the enzyme. Estrogens are also excreted in the breast milk of nursing mothers.

Synthetic Estrogens

A variety of chemical alterations have been produced in the natural estrogens. The most important

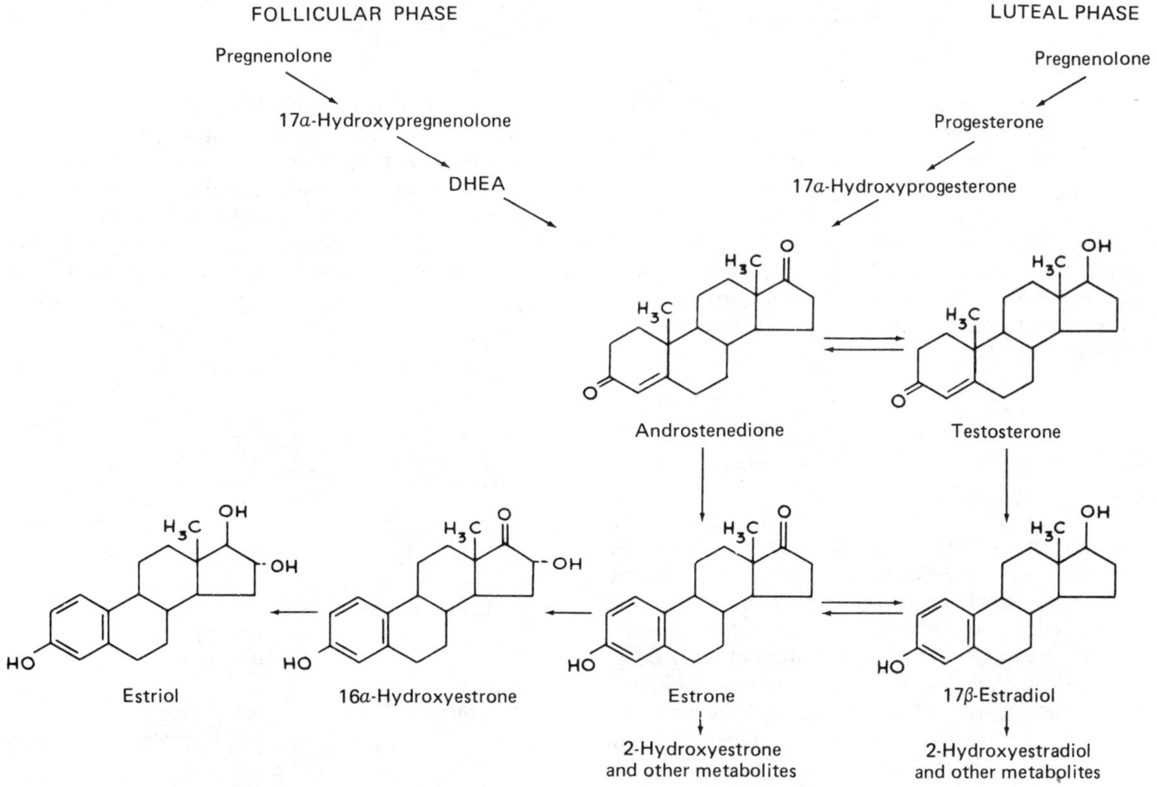

Figure 38–3. Biosynthesis and metabolism of estrogens.

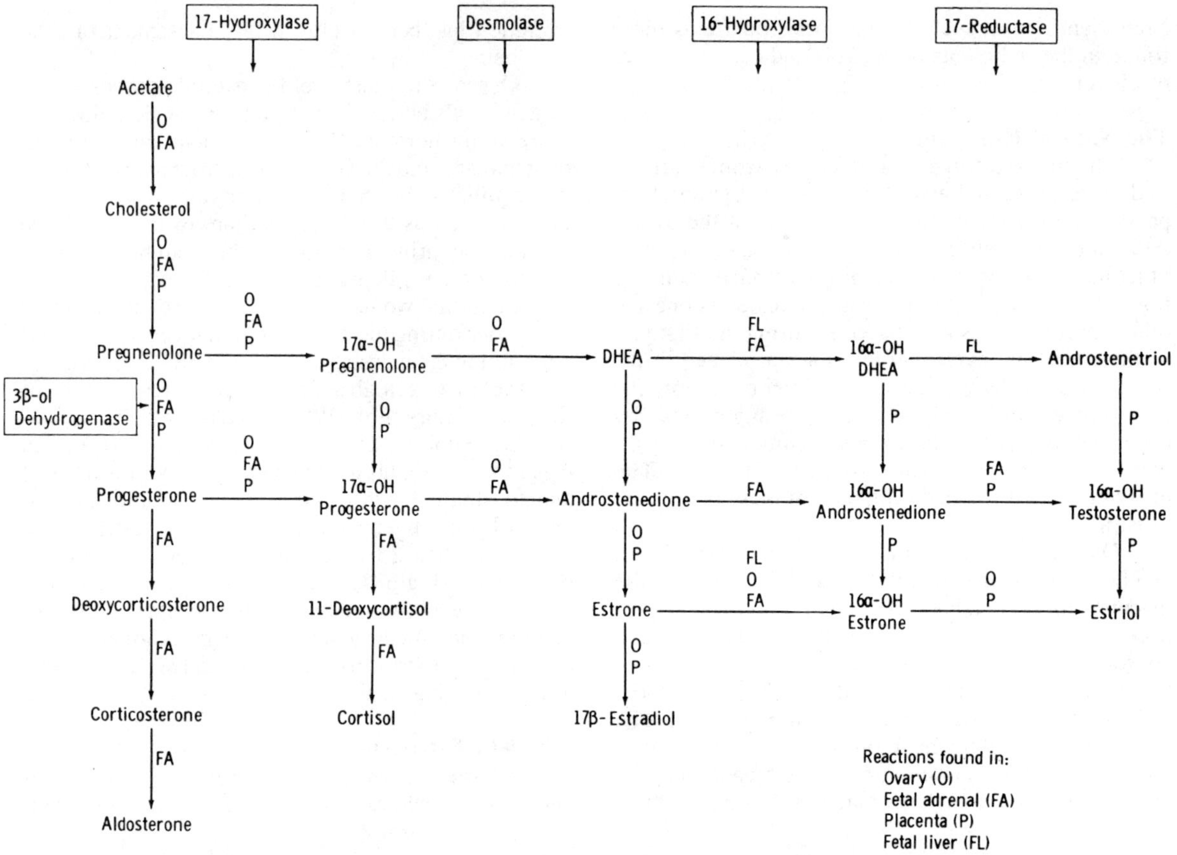

Figure 38–4. Steroid biosynthesis in the fetus and placenta.

effect of these alterations has been to increase the effectiveness of the estrogens when administered orally. Some structures are shown in Fig 38–5. Those with therapeutic uses are listed in Table 38–1.

In addition to the steroidal estrogens, a variety of nonsteroidal compounds with estrogenic activity have been synthesized and used clinically. These include dienestrol, benzestrol, hexestrol, methestrol, methallenestril, and chlorotrianisene. Some structures are shown in Fig 38–5.

Physiologic Effects

The estrogens are required for the normal maturation of the female. They stimulate the development of the vagina, uterus, and uterine tubes as well as the secondary sex characteristics. They stimulate stromal development and ductal growth in the breast and are responsible for the accelerated growth phase and the closing of the epiphyses of the long bones that occurs at puberty. They contribute to the growth of the axillary and pubic hair and alter the distribution of body fat so as to produce typical female body contours, including some accumulation of body fat around the hips and breasts. Larger quantities also stimulate development of pigmentation in the skin, most prominent in the region of the nipples and areola and in the genital region.

In addition to its growth effects on the uterine muscle, estrogen also plays an important role in the development of the endometrial lining. Continuous exposure to estrogens for prolonged periods leads to an abnormal hyperplasia of the endometrium that is usually associated with abnormal bleeding patterns. When the estrogen production is properly coordinated with the production of progesterone during the normal

Table 38–1. Commonly used estrogens.

	Average Replacement Dose
Ethinyl estradiol	0.01–0.05 mg/d
Micronized estradiol	1–2 mg/d
Estradiol	0.2–0.5 mg/d
Estradiol cypionate	2–5 mg every 3–4 weeks
Estradiol valerate	2–20 mg every other week
Piperazine estrone sulfate	1.25–5 mg/d
Conjugated, esterified, or mixed estrogenic substances:	
Oral	0.3–2.5 mg/d
Injectable	0.2–20 mg/d
Topical	. . .
Diethylstilbestrol	0.1–0.5 mg/d
Quinestrol	0.1–0.2 mg/week
Dienestrol	. . .
Chlorotrianisene	12–25 mg/d
Methallenestril	3–9 mg/d

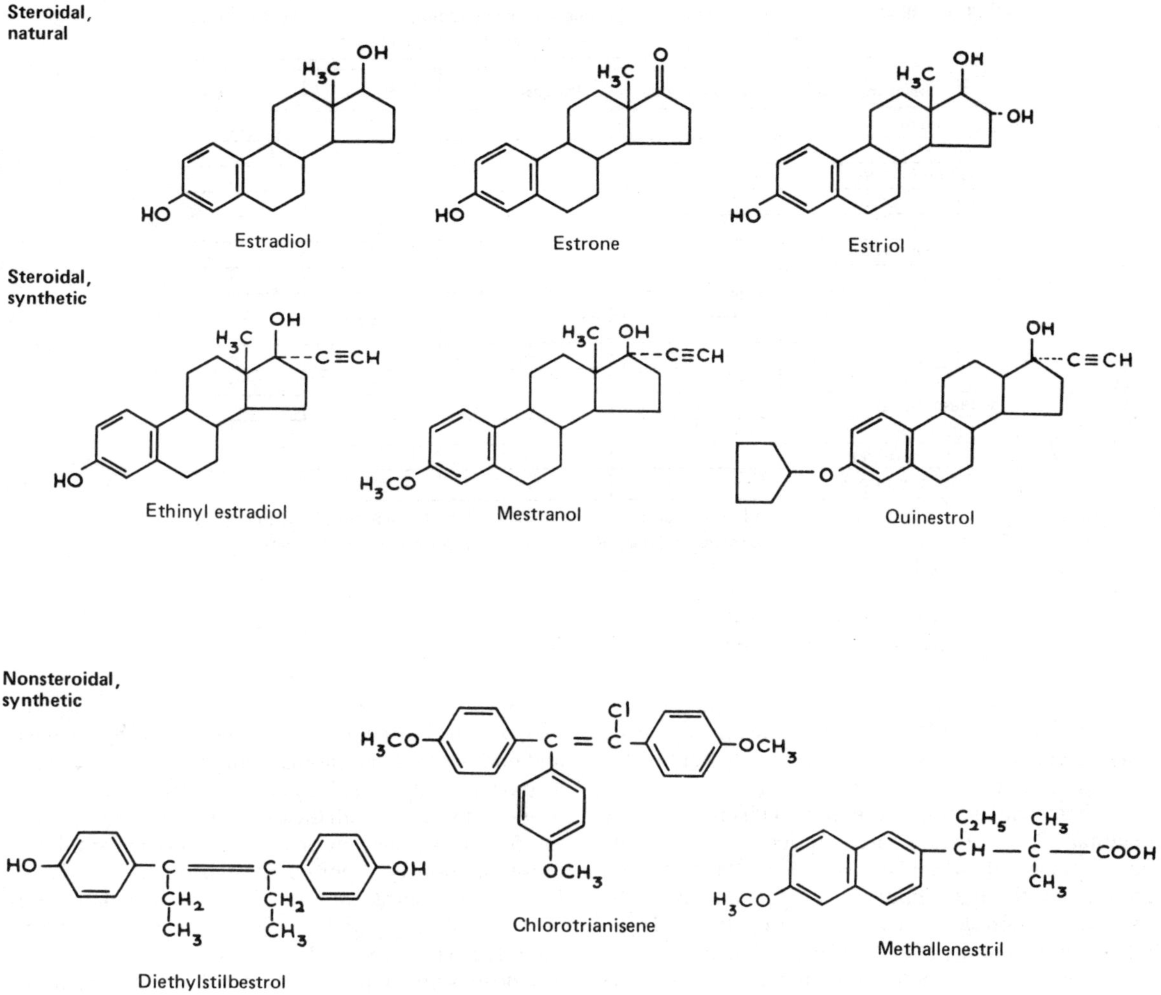

Figure 38–5. Compounds with estrogenic activity.

human menstrual cycle, regular periodic bleeding and shedding of the endometrial lining occur.

Estrogens have a number of important metabolic effects. They seem to be partially responsible for the maintenance of the normal structure of the skin and blood vessels in women. Estrogens decrease the rate of resorption of bone by antagonizing the effect of parathyroid hormone on bone but do not stimulate bone formation. Estrogens may have important effects on intestinal absorption because they reduce the motility of the bowel. In addition to stimulating the synthesis of enzymes leading to uterine growth, they alter the production and activity of many other enzymes in the body. In the liver, metabolism of α_2-globulin is altered, so that there is a higher circulating level of this group of proteins (Table 38–2). This results in an increase in thyroxine, estrogen, testosterone, iron, copper, and other transport proteins.

Estrogens enhance the coagulability of blood. Many changes in factors influencing coagulation have been reported, including increased circulating levels of factors II, VII, IX, and X. Increased plasminogen levels and decreased platelet adhesiveness have been found.

Alterations in the composition of the plasma lipids caused by estrogens are characterized by an increase in the alpha lipoproteins, a slight reduction in the beta lipoproteins, and a reduction in plasma cholesterol levels. Plasma triglyceride levels are increased (Table 38–3).

Estrogens have many other effects. They are responsible for estrous behavior in animals and influence libido in humans. They facilitate the loss of intravascular fluid into the extracellular space, producing edema. The resulting decrease in plasma volume causes a compensatory retention of sodium and water by the kidney. Estrogens also modulate sympathetic nervous system control of smooth muscle function.

Clinical Uses

A. Primary Hypogonadism: Estrogens have been used extensively for replacement therapy in

Table 38–2. The effects of testosterone, progesterone, estradiol, and pregnancy on plasma proteins.* (↑ = increased, ↓ = decreased, — = unchanged.)

Measurement	Testosterone	Progesterone	Estradiol	Pregnancy
Serum proteins	—	—	↓	↓
TBPA†	↑	—	↓	↓
Albumin	—	—	↓	↓
Orosomucoid	. . .	—	↓	↓
TBG‡	↓	—	↑	↑
Trypsin inhibitor	—	—	↑	↑
CBG§	↓	—	↑	↑
Transferrin	↓	—	—	↑
Ceruloplasmin	—	—	↑	↑
Haptoglobin	—	—	↓	—
Immunoglobulins	—	—	—	—
Plasminogen	—	—	↑	↑
Fibrinogen	↓	—	↑	↑
Renin substrate	. . .	—	↑	↑
Plasma amino acids	↑	↓	↑	. . .

*Modified and reproduced, with permission, from Salhanick HA, Kipnis DM, Vande Wiele RL (editors): *Metabolic Effects of Gonadal Hormones and Contraceptive Steroids.* Plenum Press, 1969.

†Thyroxine-binding prealbumin.

‡Thyroxine-binding globulin.

§Corticosteroid-binding globulin.

estrogen-deficient patients. The estrogen deficiency may be due to primary failure of development of the ovaries, castration, or menopause.

Treatment of primary hypogonadism is usually begun at 11–13 years of age in order to stimulate the development of secondary sex characteristics and menses, to stimulate optimal growth, and to avoid the psychologic consequences of delayed puberty. Treatment consists mainly of the administration of estrogens and progestins, but androgens and anabolic agents have also been used in these patients to stimulate growth. However, with the latter hormones, the final height achieved was not greater than when estrogens alone were used. Furthermore, acne, hirsutism, clitorimegaly, and premature closure of the epiphyses have occurred as unwanted effects of androgens and anabolic agents. Progestins are advisable in conjunction with estrogens, because long-term replacement therapy with estrogen alone, even when used cyclically in modest doses, has been associated with an increase in the incidence of endometrial hyperplasia and endometrial carcinoma. Oral contraceptives have also been used for replacement therapy. Experience is limited; however, with the use of preparations containing 50 μg of estrogen or less, side-effects similar to those previously reported have been observed (see Hormonal Contraception). Estrogen in small doses (0.3 mg of conjugated estrogens; 5 μg of ethinyl estradiol) can be given on the first 21 days of each month. The dose is gradually increased to 2–4 times the initial dose over the next 2 years. The smallest dose required to maintain a normal rate of maturation is used. After 6 months of therapy—or sooner if breakthrough bleeding occurs—5 mg of medroxyprogesterone should be given on the last 10 days of estrogen treatment cycles (days 12–21).

B. Hormonal Therapy in Postmenopausal Women: Estrogens are widely used after the menopause. The need for and response to estrogen are quite variable, and many symptoms and disorders in

Table 38–3. Some effects of oral contraceptives on plasma lipids (Dec 1968).*

	Estrogen	Progestin	Cholesterol	Phospholipid	Triglyceride
	All	. . .	↓	↑	↑
	. . .	All	—	—	—
Provest	Ethinyl estradiol	Medroxyprogesterone	—	↑	↑
Volidan	Ethinyl estradiol	Megestrol	—	↑	↑
Anovlar	Ethinyl estradiol	Norethisterone	↓	sl ↓	?↑
Enovid	Mestranol	Norethynodrel	—	. . .	↑
Ovulen	Mestranol	Ethynodiol	—	↑	↑

*Modified and reproduced, with permission, from Salhanick HA, Kipnis DM, Vande Wiele RL (editors): *Metabolic Effects of Gonadal Hormones and Contraceptive Steroids.* Plenum Press, 1969.

menopausal women are probably unrelated to its deficiency. Hot flushes, sweating, and atrophic vaginitis are generally relieved by estrogens, and many patients experience some increased sense of well-being, but depression and other psychopathologic states are seldom improved.

The role of estrogens in the prevention and treatment of osteoporosis has been carefully studied. The amount of bone present is maximal in the young active adult and begins to decline in middle age in men and women. The development of osteoporosis depends on the amount of bone present at the start of this process as well as activity. Since estrogen opposes the resorption caused by parathyroid hormone, bone loss is accelerated at the time of the menopause (artificial or natural). Estrogen therapy has been shown to reduce this loss. However, estrogens do not increase bone formation and cannot repair the process by increasing bone formation. Factors other than change in estrogen secretion are important in the development of osteoporosis.

The major indications for hormonal therapy in menopausal women are the treatment of hot flushes, atrophic vaginitis, and a high risk of osteoporosis. The risk of osteoporosis is highest in smokers who are thin, Caucasian, and inactive and have a low calcium intake and a strong family history of osteoporosis. Estrogens should be used in the smallest dose consistent with relief of symptoms. In women who have not undergone hysterectomy, treatment should be given for a period of 3 weeks, with a week of rest in between, and a progestational agent for the last 10–13 days of estrogen administration. Studies indicate that 10 mg/d of medroxyprogesterone for 10–14 days markedly reduces the risk of endometrial carcinoma in these patients. The recommended dosages of estrogen are 0.3–1.2 mg/d of conjugated estrogen or 0.01–0.02 mg/d of ethinyl estradiol. Doses in the middle of this range have been shown to be maximally effective in preventing the decrease in bone density occurring at menopause. From this point of view, it is important to begin therapy as soon as possible after the menopause for maximum effect.

Patients at low risk of developing osteoporosis who manifest only mild atrophic vaginitis can be treated with topical preparations. This route of application is also useful in the treatment of urinary tract symptoms in these patients. It is important to realize, however, that locally administered estrogens are almost completely absorbed into the circulation.

In patients in whom estrogen replacement therapy is contraindicated, such as those with estrogen-sensitive tumors, relief of vasomotor symptoms can be obtained by the use of progestational agents. In these patients, calcium supplements are useful in bringing the total daily calcium intake up to 1500 mg. Fluoride in adequate amounts can increase bone density, but the effects on bone strength have not been assessed. Vitamin D therapy can be useful when calcium intake is less than optimal.

C. Other Uses: Estrogens combined with progestins can be used to suppress ovulation in patients with intractable dysmenorrhea or when suppression of ovarian function is used in the treatment of hirsutism and amenorrhea due to excessive secretion of androgens by the ovary. Under these circumstances, marked suppression is needed, and oral contraceptives containing 80–100 μg of estrogen are usually recommended (Table 38–5).

Estrogens have been used to stop excessive uterine bleeding due to endometrial hyperplasia. Repeated doses of 20 μg of ethinyl estradiol every few hours or the administration of 20 mg of conjugated estrogens intravenously have been useful in arresting blood loss temporarily.

Adverse Effects

A large number of adverse effects of variable severity have been reported with the therapeutic use of estrogens. Many other effects reported in conjunction with hormonal contraceptives may be related to their estrogen content. These are discussed on pp 447–449.

Estrogen therapy has now become the major cause of postmenopausal bleeding. Unfortunately, vaginal bleeding at this time of life may be due to carcinoma of the endometrium, and a large number of women have been and will be subjected to dilatation and curettage of the uterus unnecessarily. In order to avoid this complication, patients should be treated with the smallest amount of estrogen possible. It should be given cyclically so that bleeding, when it occurs, will be more likely to occur during the withdrawal period. Endometrial hyperplasia that leads to this bleeding can be prevented by administration of a progestational agent for several days with the last doses of estrogen in each cycle. For example, the patient may take 0.3–0.6 mg of conjugated estrogens for the first 20 days of each month, and 10 mg of medroxyprogesterone can be added on days 18, 19, and 20. This will usually produce regular and predictable withdrawal bleeding. Endometrial hyperplasia and consequent bleeding can also be minimized by combining the estrogen with an androgen such as methyltestosterone in doses of 5 mg daily. The long-term metabolic effects of androgens in postmenopausal women have not been adequately assessed.

Nausea and breast tenderness are common and can be minimized by using the smallest effective dose of estrogen. They may be more marked at the beginning of therapy. The presence of cystic mastitis or fibroids that increase in size during treatment may also interfere with the use of estrogen. Hyperpigmentation also occurs. Estrogen therapy is associated with an increase in frequency of migraine headaches as well as cholestasis, hypertension, and gallbladder disease.

The relationship of estrogen therapy to cancer continues to be the subject of intensive investigation. Although it has not been possible to establish that there is an increased risk in the incidence of breast cancer, it is not clear that it is safe to use these agents in patients considered to be at high risk for this tumor. Many studies have been published showing an increased risk of endometrial carcinoma in patients taking estrogens. The risk seems to vary with the dose and duration of treatment: 15 times as great in patients taking large doses of estrogen for 5 or more years, in contrast with 2–4 times greater in patients receiving lower doses for short periods. Several recent studies indicate that the concomitant use of a progestin not only prevents this increased risk but actually reduces the incidence of endometrial cancer below that in the general population.

A number of papers have appeared reporting the occurrence of adenocarcinoma of the vagina in young women whose mothers were treated with large doses of diethylstilbestrol early in pregnancy. There is no good indication for its use at that time, and it should be avoided. It is not known whether other estrogens have a similar effect or whether this is peculiar to diethylstilbestrol. This agent should be limited to use in the treatment of cancer (eg, prostate) or to use as a "morning after" contraceptive (see p 449).

Cautions

Since the risks of estrogen therapy cannot be accurately assessed at present, these agents should be used with caution in postmenopausal women with symptoms. Both physician and patient should be alert to the manifestations of thrombophlebitis and cerebral and retinal thrombosis. If these occur or are suspected, estrogens should be discontinued. They should be used with caution in patients with epilepsy, migraine, asthma, recurrent depression, and cardiac and renal failure. Estrogens can cause exacerbation of symptoms in patients with porphyria. They may activate endometriosis.

Estrogens may influence tests of endocrine and liver function (see Hormonal Contraception).

The vaginal route of administration should not be considered to have only local effects, since the hormone is well absorbed by this route.

Contraindications

Estrogens should not be used in patients with estrogen-dependent neoplasms such as carcinoma of the endometrium or in patients with known or suspected carcinoma of the breast. They should be avoided in patients with undiagnosed genital bleeding, liver disease, or a history of thromboembolic disorder.

Preparations & Dosages

The commonly used natural and synthetic preparations and equivalent dosages are given in Table 38–1.

THE PROGESTINS

PROGESTERONE

Progesterone is the most important progestin in humans. In addition to having important hormonal effects, it serves as a precursor to the estrogens, androgens, and adrenocortical steroids. It is synthesized in the ovary, testis, and adrenal from acetate, cholesterol, and pregnenolone, as shown in Fig 38–6. Large amounts are also synthesized and released by the placenta during pregnancy (Fig 38–4).

In the ovary, progesterone is produced primarily by the corpus luteum and secreted in amounts of 20–30 mg/d during the luteal phase. Normal males appear to secrete 1–5 mg of progesterone daily, resulting in plasma levels of about 0.03 μg/dL. The level is only slightly higher in the female during the follicular phase of the cycle, when only a few milligrams per day of progesterone are secreted. During the luteal phase, 20–30 mg/d are released into the circulation and the plasma levels range from 0.5 to more than 2 μg/dL (Fig 38–2).

Progesterone is rapidly absorbed following administration by any route. Its half-life in the plasma is approximately 5 minutes, and small amounts are stored temporarily in body fat. It is almost completely metabolized in one passage through the liver, and for that reason it is quite ineffective when administered orally.

In the liver, progesterone is metabolized to pregnanediol and conjugated with glucuronic acid. It is excreted into the urine as pregnanediol glucuronide (Fig 38–6). The amount of pregnanediol in the urine has been used as an index of progesterone secretion. It has been very useful in spite of the fact that the proportion of secreted progesterone converted to this compound varies from day to day and from individual to individual. Although a variety of biologic assays have been used for the measurement of progesterone in the past, several excellent methods including double-isotope derivative techniques, gas chromatographic techniques, and ligand-binding assays are now available.

In addition to progesterone, 20α- and 20β-hydroxyprogesterone (20α- or 20β-hydroxy-4-pregnene-3-one) are also found. These compounds have about one-fifth the progestational activity of progesterone in humans and other species. Little is known of the role of these compounds, but 20α-hydroxyprogesterone is produced in large amounts in some species and may be of some importance biologically.

The effects of progesterone on lipid and protein metabolism are summarized in Tables 38–2 and 38–3. Progesterone has important effects on carbohydrate metabolism. A dose of 50 mg intramuscularly daily can reproduce the increased insulin levels and decreased response of blood glucose levels to insulin observed in normal pregnancy.

Progesterone can compete with aldosterone at the

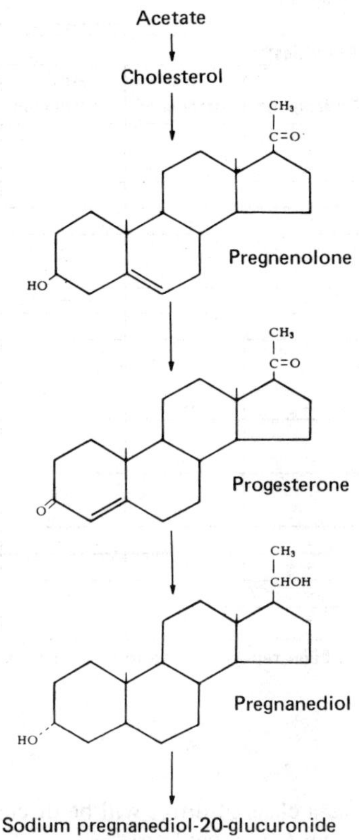

Figure 38–6. Biosynthesis of progesterone and major pathway for its metabolism. Other metabolites are also formed. (Reproduced, with permission, from Ganong WF: *Review of Medical Physiology,* 10th ed. Lange, 1981.)

renal tubule, causing a decrease in Na^+ reabsorption. This leads to an increased secretion of aldosterone by the adrenal cortex (eg, in pregnancy). Progesterone increases the body temperature in humans. The mechanism of this effect is not known, but an alteration of the temperature-regulating centers in the hypothalamus has been suggested. Progesterone also alters the function of the respiratory centers. The ventilatory response to CO_2 is increased (synthetic progestins with an ethinyl group do not have respiratory effects). This leads to a measurable reduction in arterial and alveolar P_{CO_2} during pregnancy and in the luteal phase of the menstrual cycle. Progesterone and related steroids also have hypnotic effects on the brain.

Progesterone is responsible for the alveolobular development of the secretory apparatus in the breast. It also causes the maturation and secretory changes in the endometrium that are seen following ovulation (Fig 38–2).

Progesterone decreases the plasma levels of many amino acids and leads to increased urinary nitrogen excretion. It has been found to induce changes in the smooth endoplasmic reticulum and its functions in experimental animals.

Other effects are noted in the section on oral contraceptives, below.

SYNTHETIC PROGESTATIONAL AGENTS

A variety of progestational compounds have now been synthesized. Some of these are active when given by mouth. They are not a uniform group of compounds, and all of them differ from progesterone in one or more respects. Table 38–4 lists many of these compounds.

In general, the compounds related to progesterone can produce a secretory endometrium and maintain pregnancy in animals. They antagonize aldosterone-induced sodium retention (see above) and have no androgenic or estrogenic effects. The remaining compounds produce a decidual change in the endometrial stroma, do not support pregnancy in test animals, are more effective gonadotropin inhibitors, and may have minimal estrogenic and androgenic or anabolic activity.

Therapeutic Uses

The major use of progestational hormones is for hormonal contraception (see below). However, they are useful in producing long-term ovarian suppression for other purposes. When used alone in large doses parenterally (eg, medroxyprogesterone acetate, 150 mg intramuscularly every 90 days), prolonged anovulation and amenorrhea are produced. This procedure has been employed in the treatment of dysmenorrhea, endometriosis, hirsutism, and bleeding disorders when estrogens are contraindicated. The major problem with this regimen is the prolonged time required for ovulatory function to return after cessation of therapy in some patients. It should not be used for patients planning a pregnancy in the near future.

Progestins do not appear to have any place in the therapy of threatened or habitual abortion. Early reports of the usefulness of these agents resulted from the unwarranted assumption that after several abortions the likelihood of repeated abortions was over 90%. When progestational agents were administered to patients with previous abortions, a salvage rate of 80% was obtained. It is now recognized that similar patients abort only 20% of the time even when untreated.

In some patients with "threatened" abortion, it has been noted that progesterone production is decreased. It is likely that the decrease in progesterone reflects damage to the placenta or fetus and is another result of the events leading to abortion rather than the cause of the abortion. Administration of progesterone in these circumstances does not appear to be useful and may result in delaying recognition of an abortion that has occurred. Progesterone and progestational agents administered early in pregnancy have been incriminated in the masculinization of the external genitalia in the female fetus and induction of congenital anomalies. Prolonged postpartum bleeding has been reported in some patients treated with repository medroxyprogesterone or hydroxyprogesterone caproate and, when used in women with "threatened" abortion, may cause a delay in the expulsion of a dead fetus.

Table 38–4. Activities of progestational agents.

	Activities*					
	Duration of Action	Estrogenic	Androgenic	Anti-estrogenic	Anti-androgenic	Anabolic
Progesterone and derivatives						
Progesterone	1 d	–	–	+	–	–
Dydrogesterone	1–3 d	–	–	+	–	–
Hydroxyprogesterone caproate	8–14 d	sl	sl	–	–	–
Medroxyprogesterone acetate	Tablets: 1–3 d Injectable: 4–12 weeks	–	+	+	–	–
Chlormadinone acetate	...	–	–	+	+	–
Megestrol acetate	1–3 d	–	–	+	+	–
17α-Ethinyl testosterone derivatives						
Testosterone derivatives						
Dimethisterone	1–3 d	–	–	sl	–	–
19-Nortestosterone derivatives						
Norethynodrel†	1–3 d	+	–	–	–	–
Lynestrenol (Not available in USA)	1–3 d	+	+	–	–	+
Norethindrone†	1–3 d	sl	+	+	–	+
Norethindrone acetate†	1–3 d	sl	+	+	–	+
Ethynodiol diacetate†	1–3 d	sl	+	+	–	–
dl-Norgestrel†	1–3 d	–	+	+	–	+

*Interpretation: + = active; – = inactive; sl = slight activity. Activities have been reported in various species using various end points and may not apply to humans.
†See Table 38–5.

Progesterone and medroxyprogesterone have been used in the treatment of women who have difficulty in conceiving and who demonstrate a slow rise in basal body temperature. Some investigators believe that these patients suffer from a relative luteal insufficiency, and progesterone or related compounds are given to replace the deficiency. There is no convincing evidence that this treatment is effective. The successes reported are impossible to distinguish from placebo effects in the absence of satisfactory controls.

Diagnostic Uses

Progesterone can also be used as a test of estrogen secretion. The administration of progesterone, 150 mg/d, or medroxyprogesterone, 10 mg/d for 5–7 days, is followed by withdrawal bleeding in amenorrheic patients only when the endometrium has been stimulated by estrogens. A combination of estrogen and progestin can be given to test the responsiveness of the endometrium in patients with amenorrhea.

Contraindications, Cautions, & Adverse Effects

See Hormonal Contraception, below.

COMBINATIONS OF ESTROGENS & PROGESTINS

Since estrogens and progestins are often used in combination with one another, a variety of combined preparations are available. Most of them have been designed for use as oral contraceptives, and their properties as a class of drugs will be discussed below (see Hormonal Contraception).

DANAZOL

Danazol (Danocrine), an isoxazole derivative of ethisterone (17α-ethinyl testosterone) with weak progestational and androgenic activities, is used to suppress ovarian function. Danazol inhibits the midcycle surge of LH and FSH and can prevent the compensatory increase in LH and FSH following castration in animals, but it does not significantly lower or suppress basal LH or FSH levels in normal women. Danazol binds to androgen, progesterone, and glucocorticoid receptors and can translocate into the nucleus the androgen receptor to initiate androgen-specific RNA synthesis. It does not bind to intracellular estrogen receptors, but it does bind to sex hormone-binding globulin (SHBG) and corticosteroid-binding globulins (CBG). It inhibits the cholesterol-cleaving enzyme, 3-α-hydroxysteroid dehydrogenase, 17-α-hydroxysteroid dehydrogenase, 17,21-lyase, 17α-hydroxylase, 11β-hydroxylase, and 21-hydroxylase, but it does not inhibit aromatase. It increases the mean clearance rate of progesterone, probably by displacing the hormone from binding proteins, and may have similar effects on other active steroid hormones. Ethisterone, a major metabolite, has both progestational and mild androgenic effects.

Danazol is slowly metabolized in humans, having a half-life of over 15 hours. This results in stable circulating levels when the drug is administered twice daily. It has been found to be highly concentrated in the liver, adrenals, and kidneys and is excreted in both feces and urine.

Danazol has been employed as an inhibitor of gonadal function and has found its major use in the treatment of endometriosis. For this purpose, it is usually administered at a starting dose of 400 mg/d, and in those patients who do not respond it can be increased to 600 or 800 mg. In patients requiring larger doses, the dose can usually be reduced after several months without a return of symptoms.

Danazol has also been used for the treatment of fibrocystic disease of the breast. It has been effective in some patients for the relief of severe cyclic breast pain and tenderness but should be reserved for use in patients in whom analgesics and other drugs have failed.

The major side-effects are weight gain, edema, decreased breast size, acne and oily skin, increasing growth of hair, deepening of the voice, headache, hot flushes, changes in libido, and muscle cramps. Although mild side-effects are very common, it is seldom necessary to discontinue the drug because of them.

Danazol should be used with great caution in patients with hepatic dysfunction, since it has been reported to produce mild to moderate hepatocellular damage in some patients, as evidenced by enzyme changes. It is also contraindicated during pregnancy and breast feeding, as it may produce urogenital abnormalities in the offspring.

OTHER OVARIAN HORMONES

The normal ovary produces small amounts of androgens, including testosterone, androstenedione, and dehydroepiandrosterone. Only testosterone has a significant amount of biologic activity, although androstenedione can be converted to estrone in peripheral tissues. The normal woman produces a total of less than 200 μg of testosterone in 24 hours, and about one-third of this is probably formed in the ovary directly. The physiologic significance of these small amounts of androgens is not established, but they may be partly responsible for normal hair growth at puberty and may have other important metabolic effects. The androgen production by the ovary may be markedly increased in some abnormal states, usually in association with amenorrhea as noted above.

The ovary also produces one or more substances similar to the inhibin produced by the testis that decreases the pituitary release of FSH.

RELAXIN

Relaxin is a polypeptide that has been extracted from the ovary. In certain animal species, it appears to play an important role at the time of parturition. It causes relaxation of the pelvic ligaments and softening of the uterine cervix.

In women, relaxin has been measured by immunoassay. Levels were highest immediately after the LH surge and during menstruation. A physiologic role for this hormone has not been established.

Clinical trials with relaxin have been carried out in patients with dysmenorrhea. Relaxin has also been administered to patients in premature labor and during prolonged labor. The therapeutic value of this hormone has not been established.

HORMONAL CONTRACEPTION (Oral Contraceptives)

A large number of oral contraceptives containing estrogens or progestins (or both) are now available for clinical use. These preparations vary chemically and, as might be expected, have many properties in common, but they exhibit definite differences. Experience with some of the drugs has been much greater than with others, and more differences may emerge as further experience accumulates.

Three types of preparations have been used for oral contraception: (1) combinations of estrogens and progestins; (2) the sequential use of estrogens followed by progestins; and (3) continuous progestin therapy without concomitant administration of estrogens. Only combination products and progestin-only products are currently marketed.

The preparations for oral use are all well absorbed, and the metabolism of the drugs is not known to be profoundly altered by simultaneous administration. Little information is available concerning the turnover time and excretion of some of these compounds.

Pharmacologic Effects

A. Mechanism of Contraceptive Action: The combinations of estrogens and progestins and the sequential agents appear to exert their effect largely through inhibition of ovulation. The combination agents containing estrogens and progestins also produce a change in the cervical mucus, in the uterine endometrium, and in the motility and secretion in the uterine tubes, all of which decrease the likelihood of conception and implantation. The continuous use of progestins alone does not inhibit ovulation. The other factors mentioned, therefore, play a major role in the prevention of pregnancy when these agents are used.

B. Effects on the Ovary: Chronic use of combination or sequential agents appears to depress ovarian function. The gross appearance of the ovary is that of relative inactivity; there is a minimum of follicular development; and corpora lutea, larger follicles, stromal edema, and other morphologic features normally seen in ovulating women are absent. In general, the amounts of the endogenous estrogens excreted in the urine are less than those observed in normal menstruating women, and pregnanediol excretion is

Table 38–5. Oral contraceptive agents in use. The estrogen-containing compounds are arranged in order of increasing content of estrogen (ethinyl estradiol and mestranol have similar potencies). The relative progestational potencies are shown in the last column.

	Estrogen (mg)	Progestin (mg)	PP*
Combination tablets			
Loestrin 1/20 Zorane 1/20	Ethinyl estradiol 0.02	Norethindrone acetate 1.0	4
Loestrin 1.5/30 Zorane 1.5/30	Ethinyl estradiol 0.03	Norethindrone acetate 1.5	6
Ovcon 35	Ethinyl estradiol 0.035	Norethindrone 0.4	0.8
Brevicon Modicon	Ethinyl estradiol 0.035	Norethindrone 0.5	1
Lo/Ovral	Ethinyl estradiol 0.03	dl-Norgestrel 0.3	18
Ovral	Ethinyl estradiol 0.05	dl-Norgestrel 0.5	30
Norlestrin 1/50 Zorane 1/50	Ethinyl estradiol 0.05	Norethindrone acetate 1.0	4
Norlestrin 2.5/50	Ethinyl estradiol 0.05	Norethindrone acetate 2.5	10
Demulen	Ethinyl estradiol 0.05	Ethynodiol diacetate 1.0	30
Ovcon 50	Ethinyl estradiol 0.05	Norethindrone 1.0	2
Norinyl 1/50 Ortho-Novum 1/50	Mestranol 0.05	Norethindrone 1.0	2
Norinyl 1/80 Ortho-Novum 1/80	Mestranol 0.8	Norethindrone 1.0	2
Norinyl-2 Ortho-Novum-2	Mestranol 0.1	Norethindrone 2.0	4
Ovulen	Mestranol 0.1	Ethynodiol diacetate 1.0	30
Enovid 5	Mestranol 0.075	Norethynodrel 5.0	11
Enovid E	Mestranol 0.1	Norethynodrel 2.5	6
Daily progestin tablets			
Micronor Nor-QD	...	Norethindrone 0.35	0.7
Ovrette	...	dl-Norgestrel 0.075	3

*Progestational potency.

not usually increased in the latter phase of the cycle. It is not known whether the few instances in which pregnanediol excretion is elevated are due to escape ovulation in these patients or whether corpora lutea have been formed without ovulation. Although cystic follicles have been described in patients being treated with oral contraceptives, the ovaries usually become smaller even when enlarged before therapy.

The great majority of patients return to normal menstrual patterns when therapy is terminated. About 75% will ovulate in the first posttreatment cycle, and 97% by the third posttreatment cycle. Patients with a history of irregular cycles seem more liable to the development of amenorrhea following cessation of therapy.

About 2% of patients remain amenorrheic for periods of up to several years after therapy has been concluded, and the prevalence of amenorrhea, often with galactorrhea, is higher in women who have used this form of contraception.

These preparations have important effects on the genital tract. The cytologic findings on vaginal smears vary depending on the preparation used. For example, with the use of sequential regimens a high maturation index—ie, cornified epithelium—is noted until the progestational drug is added during the last 5 days. With almost all of the combined drugs, a low maturation index is found because of the presence of progestational agents.

C. Effects on the Uterus: These agents have important effects on the uterus. After prolonged use, the cervix may show some hypertrophy and polyp formation. There are also important effects on the cervical mucus. Normally, through the menstrual cycle, there is an increasing amount of clear liquefied mucus that is altered by the secretion of progesterone following ovulation. At that time it becomes thick and less copious and contains much cellular debris. This sequence is not much altered by the sequential preparations; however, the combined products as well as continuous progesterone therapy produce the expected changes in the mucus.

Initially there is some stimulation of the uterine muscle, resulting in some softening and increase in size. This effect is neither common nor marked and is due to the estrogens. The endometrial changes vary markedly with the preparation. With sequential agents the sequence of changes does not vary greatly from normal. During the last 5 days, progressive progestational effects on the glandular tissues are observed. In contrast to this, agents containing both estrogens and progestins produce a stromal deciduation toward the end of the cycle. The agents containing the 19-nor compounds—particularly those with the smaller amounts of estrogen—tend to produce more glandular atrophy and usually less bleeding, whereas combination agents containing progestins that produce more physiologic changes in the endometrium (eg, medroxyprogesterone) are associated with spotting between periods and more bleeding at the time of menses. The flow during menses tends to be slightly heavier than or similar to that prior to therapy when sequential regimens are used.

Although studies in rodents suggest that the development of the blastocyst and the endometrium must be very precisely matched for implantation to occur, pregnancies occur in some patients who omit a few tablets or when the medication was begun too late in a given cycle to prevent ovulation.

Although studies in humans are not available, animal experiments indicate that alterations in the transport of the gamete through the uterine tube are produced by estrogens and progestins. The effect on germ cell transport is thought by some to be an important mechanism for the impairment of fertility, particularly with the use of low-dosage continuous progestin therapy as noted above.

D. Effects on the Breast: Stimulation of the breasts occurs in most patients receiving estrogen-containing agents. Some enlargement is generally noted. The administration of estrogens and combinations of estrogens and progestins tends to suppress lactation. When the doses are small, the effects on breast feeding are not appreciable. However, when postpartum mothers are examined, milk is found in the breasts of fewer patients taking oral contraceptives than in untreated mothers. Preliminary studies of the transport of the oral contraceptives into the breast milk suggest that only small amounts of these compounds are found, and they have not been considered to be of importance.

E. Other Effects of the Oral Contraceptives: The state of knowledge about these effects is incomplete at present, even though they reflect effects of either estrogens or progestins that have been used for many years. The possible consequences of these compounds have been brought to our attention more forcefully because of the large and growing number of normal individuals using them. In some cases the effects are known to be secondary to the estrogens and in other cases to the progestins. However, in many instances the agent responsible for the effects is not known. Various effects may be more pronounced with one of the preparations than with others.

1. Central nervous system effects–The central nervous system effects of the oral contraceptives have not been well studied in humans. A variety of effects of estrogen and progesterone have been noted in animals. Estrogens tend to lower the threshold of excitability in the brain, whereas progesterone tends to increase it. The thermogenic action of progesterone and some of the synthetic progestins is also thought to be in the central nervous system. The suppression of ovarian function that results from inhibition of gonadotropin secretion is also thought to be due to an influence on the hypothalamus or other parts of the nervous system.

It is very difficult to evaluate any behavioral or emotional effects of these compounds. Although the incidence of pronounced changes in mood, affect, and behavior reported in most studies is low, milder changes are common. These changes are variable and therefore difficult to evaluate in relation to the pharmacologic effects of the drug. They may be psychologically induced by the act of using contraception or the circumstances surrounding it. However, it is possible that the changes in neuronal activity and thresholds produced by these drugs may lead to changes conditioned by other factors.

2. Effects on endocrine function–The effects on the endocrine system are not well understood at present. The inhibition of pituitary gonadotropin secretion has been mentioned. Estrogens are known to alter adrenal structure and function. In humans, a few changes are of note. Estrogens increase the plasma concentration of the α_2-globulin that binds hydrocortisone (cortisol-binding globulin). This does not appear to lead to any chronic alteration in the rate of secretion of cortisol, but plasma concentrations may be more than double the levels found in untreated individuals. It has also been observed that the ACTH response to the administration of metyrapone (see Chapter 35) is attenuated by estrogens and the oral contraceptives.

These preparations cause alterations in the angiotensin-aldosterone system. Plasma renin activity has been found to increase, and there is an increase in aldosterone secretion. The relationship between these alterations and the hypertension that occurs in some patients taking oral contraceptives is not clear.

Thyroxine-binding globulin is increased. As a result, the plasma protein-bound iodine (PBI) and butanol-extractable iodine (BEI) levels are increased to those commonly seen during pregnancy. Since more of the thyroxine is bound, red cell T_3 uptake of radioactive iodine is not altered. The free thyroxine level in these patients is also normal.

3. Hematologic effects–Serious thromboembolic phenomena occurring in women taking oral contraceptives have stimulated a great many studies of the effects of these compounds on blood coagulation. A clear picture of such effects has not yet emerged. The oral contraceptives do not consistently alter bleeding or clotting time. Preliminary indications are that the changes observed are similar to those reported in pregnancy. There is an increase in factors VII, VIII, IX, and X. Increased amounts of coumarin derivatives are required to produce a reduction in prothrombin time in patients taking oral contraceptives. Vitamin K-dependent clotting activity is increased in vitro only after the storage of blood for 16 hours in plastic tubes.

In addition to the changes in clotting factors, there are important changes in serum proteins. There is an increase in the α_2-globulins that affects the concentrations of hormones and other serum constituents that are protein-bound (Table 38–2). There is an increase in serum iron and total iron-binding capacity similar to that reported in patients with hepatitis.

Significant alterations in the cellular components of blood have not been reported with any consistency. However, the platelet aggregation response to catecholamines is increased. A number of patients have been reported to develop folic acid deficiency anemias. Preliminary studies indicate that the oral contraceptives inhibit the conversion of polyglutamic folate (found in food) to the monoglutamic folate that can be absorbed in the gastrointestinal tract. This can be reversed by supplementary folic acid or cessation of oral contraceptives.

4. Hepatic effects–The liver plays an important role in the inactivation and conversion to water-soluble conjugates of the estrogens and progestins used in oral contraceptives. These hormones have profound effects on the function of the liver in other respects. Some of these effects are deleterious and will be considered below under Adverse Reactions.

The effects on serum proteins noted above result from the effects of the estrogens on the synthesis of the various α_2-globulins and fibrinogen. Serum haptoglobins that also arise from the liver are depressed rather than increased by estrogen.

Some of the effects on carbohydrate and lipid

metabolism are probably influenced by changes in liver metabolism. However, detailed studies of these changes have not been reported.

Important alterations in drug excretion and metabolism are also found in the liver. Estrogens in the amounts seen during pregnancy or used in oral contraceptive agents delay the clearance of sulfobromophthalein and reduce bile flow. These alterations result from impairment of the transfer of cholephilic substances from hepatic cells into the bile. Some of these effects of estrogens and progestins may be indirectly induced or due to metabolites of the hormones rather than the hormones themselves. These changes may cause the observed increase in cholelithiasis associated with use of these agents.

These agents increase the saturation of cholesterol in bile. The proportion of cholic acid in bile acids is increased while the proportion of chenodeoxycholic acid is decreased.

5. Effects on lipid metabolism–(Table 38–3.) The effects on lipid metabolism are potentially important in evaluating the long-term use of these compounds. There are conflicting reports about the effects of the oral contraceptive drugs containing mixtures of estrogens and progestins.

The available studies indicate that estrogens increase serum triglycerides and free and esterified cholesterol. Phospholipids are also increased, as are high-density lipoproteins. Low-density lipoproteins usually decrease. Although the effects are marked with doses of 100 mg of mestranol or ethinyl estradiol, doses of 50 mg or less have minimal effects. The progestins (particularly the 19-nortestosterone derivatives) tend to antagonize the effects of estrogen. Preparations containing small amounts of estrogen and a progestin may slightly decrease triglycerides and high-density lipoproteins.

6. Effects on carbohydrate metabolism–The administration of oral contraceptives produces alterations in carbohydrate metabolism similar to those observed in pregnancy. There is a reduction in the rate of absorption of carbohydrates from the gastrointestinal tract. Many individuals exhibit decreases in glucose tolerance; others, although their glucose tolerance has not been altered, have been shown to secrete increased amounts of insulin following the ingestion or injection of glucose. In general, these changes have been more marked in patients with a family history of diabetes. Since estrogens are known to enhance the secretion of growth hormone by the pituitary, it has been suggested that this may be responsible for some of the observed effects. Studies in experimental animals indicate that estrogens stimulate islet cell function and increase the ability of the pancreas to secrete insulin. Progesterone, on the other hand, clearly interferes with insulin action. Preliminary observations indicate that both effects occur in women. Although the changes in glucose tolerance are reversible on discontinuing medication, the implications of long-term treatment in patients who inherit the trait for diabetes is not known.

7. Cardiovascular effects–These agents cause small increases in cardiac output associated with higher systolic and diastolic blood pressure and heart rate. Pathologic increases in blood pressure have been reported in a small number of patients. This may be related to the enhancement of plasma renin activity as a result of oral contraceptive drugs. The pressure returns to normal when treatment is terminated. Although the magnitude of the change is small in many patients, it is marked in others. It is important that blood pressure be followed in each patient. An increase in blood pressure has been reported to occur in few postmenopausal women treated with estrogens alone.

Although not found consistently, venous engorgement has been reported in some patients. Changes in the connective tissue in the arteries of rodents have been reported, but the significance of these changes is not known. Plasma from women taking oral contraceptives stimulates arterial smooth muscle in tissue culture. It is postulated that this effect enhances the atherosclerotic process.

8. Effects on the skin–The oral contraceptives have been noted to increase pigmentation of the skin of patients (chloasma). This effect seems to be enhanced in women who have dark complexions and by exposure to ultraviolet light. Some of the androgenlike progestins may increase the production of sebum. The sequential oral contraceptive preparations as well as estrogens often decrease sebum production. This may be due to suppression of the ovarian production of androgens. Estrogens also decrease pore size and lead to acne in some patients.

Clinical Uses

The most important use of the estrogens and progestins is for oral contraception. A large number of preparations are available for this specific purpose. They are specially packaged to provide for ease of administration. In general, they are very effective; when these agents are taken according to directions, the risk of conception is extremely small. The pregnancy rate is estimated to be about 0.5–1 per 100 woman years at risk with combination agents; the pregnancy rate is slightly higher for the sequential preparations. When these agents are not taken as directed and one or more doses are missed, there appears to be a significantly higher pregnancy rate in patients taking the formerly available sequential agents than when the combinations are employed. Contraceptive failure has been observed in some patients taking phenytoin or antibiotics.

Progestins and estrogens are also useful in the treatment of endometriosis. When severe dysmenorrhea is the major symptom, the suppression of ovulation with estrogen may be followed by painless periods. However, in most patients this approach to therapy is inadequate. The long-term administration of large doses of progestins or combinations of progestins and estrogens prevents the periodic breakdown of the endometrial tissue and in some cases will lead to endometrial fibrosis and prevent the reactivation of implants for prolonged periods.

As is true with most hormonal preparations, many of the side-effects are physiologic or pharmacologic effects of the drugs that are objectionable only because they are not pertinent to the situation for which they are being used. Therefore, the product containing the smallest amounts of hormones should be selected for use.

Adverse Reactions

The incidence of serious known side-effects associated with the use of these drugs is low. There are a number of reversible changes in intermediary metabolism. However, the long-term effects of such changes as an increase in plasma triglycerides or decrease in glucose tolerance cannot be assessed as yet. Minor side-effects are frequent, but most are mild and many are transient. Although it is not often necessary to discontinue medication for these, as many as one-third of all patients started on oral contraception with combined or sequential agents discontinue therapy for reasons other than a desire to become pregnant.

Common minor problems may respond to simple changes in pill formulation. A brief summary of some symptoms and suggested changes is as follows:

(1) Nausea, breast tenderness, edema, chloasma: Decrease estrogen content.

(2) Early and midcycle spotting, decreased flow or amenorrhea: Increase estrogen content or decrease progestin content (or both).

(3) Weight gain, hair growth, depression, tiredness: Decrease progestin content.

(4) Excessive bleeding, late cycle spotting: Increase progestin content or decrease estrogen content (or both).

A. Mild Side-Effects:

1. Nausea, mastalgia, breakthrough bleeding, and edema are related to the amount of estrogen in the preparation. They were more common with the sequential preparations because of the larger amounts of estrogen present and can often be alleviated by a shift to a combination agent or to a preparation containing smaller amounts of estrogen or to agents containing progestational compounds with androgenlike effects.

2. Changes in serum proteins and other effects on endocrine function (see above) must be taken into account when thyroid, adrenal, or pituitary function is being evaluated. Increases in sedimentation rate are thought to be due to increased levels of fibrinogen.

3. Psychologic changes are often transient and are not predictable with any of the preparations. In general, most patients "feel better" because they are relieved of anxiety about becoming pregnant. Some patients experience premenstrual-like symptoms of irritability and depression throughout the cycle.

4. Headache is mild and often transient. Migraine is often made worse and has been reported to be associated with an increased frequency of cerebrovascular accidents. When this occurs, or when migraine has its onset during therapy with these agents, treatment should be discontinued.

5. Libido is increased or decreased in a few patients and unchanged in the majority. Similar changes have been observed with placebo therapy.

6. Withdrawal bleeding sometimes fails to occur—most often with combination preparations—and may cause confusion with regard to pregnancy. If this is disturbing to the patient, a different preparation may be tried or other methods of contraception used.

B. More Annoying Side-Effects: Any of the following may require discontinuation of oral contraceptives:

1. Breakthrough bleeding is the most common problem in using progestational agents alone for contraception. It occurs in as many as 25% of patients. It is more frequently encountered in patients taking low-dose preparations than in those taking combination pills with higher levels of progestin and estrogen.

2. Weight gain is more common with the combination agents containing androgenlike progestins. It can usually be controlled by shifting preparations with less progestin effect or by dieting.

3. Increased skin pigmentation may be distressing in dark-skinned women. It tends to increase with time, the incidence being about 5% at the end of the first year and about 40% after 8 years. It is thought to be exacerbated by vitamin B deficiency. It is often reversible upon discontinuance of medication, but in occasional cases the pigmentation disappears very slowly.

4. Acne may be exacerbated by agents containing androgenlike progestins, whereas agents containing large amounts of estrogen frequently cause marked improvement in acne.

5. Hirsutism may also be aggravated by the 19-nortestosterone derivatives, and the combination containing nonandrogenic progestins is preferred.

6. Ureteral dilatation similar to that observed in pregnancy has been reported, and bacteriuria is more frequent.

7. Vaginal infections are more common and more difficult to treat in patients who are receiving oral contraceptives.

8. Amenorrhea after discontinuation–Following cessation of administration of oral contraceptives, 95% of patients with normal menstrual histories resume normal periods and all but a few resume normal cycles during the next few months. However, some patients remain amenorrheic for several years. Many of these patients also have galactorrhea. Patients who have had menstrual irregularities before taking oral contraceptives are particularly susceptible to prolonged amenorrhea when the agents are discontinued.

C. Severe Side-Effects:

1. Vascular disorders–Thromboembolism was one of the earliest of the serious unanticipated effects to be reported and has been the most thoroughly studied.

a. Venous thromboembolic disease–Epidemiologic studies indicate that about one patient per thousand woman years not using oral contraceptives will develop superficial or deep thromboembolic disease. The overall incidence of these disorders in patients taking oral contraceptives is about 3 per thousand woman years. The risk for this disorder is increased during the first month of contraceptive use and remains constant for several years or more. The risk returns to normal within a month when use is discontinued. The risk of venous thrombosis or pulmonary embolism among women with predisposing conditions may be higher than that in normal women.

The incidence of this complication is related to the estrogen content of oral contraceptives. Lowering the estrogen content from a dosage of 100–150 μg to a dosage of 50–80 μg reduced the incidence of pulmonary embolism by 50% or more. The most recent studies of contraceptives containing 30 μg of estrogen indicate that the risk of death from pulmonary embolism is even lower with these low-dose preparations. There is no clear relationship between progestin content and the incidence of this complication. The risk of superficial or deep thromboembolic disease in patients treated with oral contraceptives is not related to age, parity, mild obesity, or cigarette smoking. However, some studies indicate a genetic susceptibility to this disorder and suggest that oral contraceptives multiply the effect. Decreased venous blood flow, endothelial proliferation in veins and arteries, and increased coagulability of blood resulting from changes in platelet coagulation and fibrinolytic systems contribute to the increased incidence of thrombosis. The major plasma inhibitor of thrombin, antithrombin 3, is substantially decreased during oral contraceptive use. This change occurs in the first month of treatment and lasts as long as treatment persists, reversing within a month thereafter.

b. Myocardial infarction–Early studies indicated that myocardial infarction occurs more frequently in oral contraceptive users without relation to the duration of use. However, more recent studies suggest that risk of infarction is not increased in past users who used these agents for less than 5 years. The risk is related to the dose of estrogen and is significantly lower in women using low-dose estrogen compounds.

The use of oral contraceptives is associated with a higher risk of myocardial infarction in women who smoke more than 15 cigarettes per day, who have a history of preeclampsia or hypertension, or who have hyperlipoproteinemia or diabetes. Since 40% of women 20–50 years of age smoke 15 or more cigarettes a day, this becomes clinically very important. The risk attributable to oral contraceptives in women 30–39 years of age who do not smoke is about 4 cases per 100,000 users per year, as compared to 185 cases per 100,000 among women 40–44 who smoke heavily. The association with myocardial infarction is thought to involve acceleration of atherogenesis, decreased glucose tolerance, decreased levels of high-density lipoproteins and increased levels of low-density lipoproteins, and increased platelet aggregation. However, facilitation of coronary arterial spasm may also play a role in some of these patients. The progestational component of oral contraceptives decreases high-density lipoprotein cholesterol, although the estrogenic component has also been found to increase it. The net difference, therefore, will depend entirely on the specific composition of the pill used and the patient's susceptibility to the particular effects. Preparations containing norgestrel 0.5 mg and norethindrone acetate 2.5 mg have been reported to have strong antiestrogenic effects and decrease high-density lipoprotein cholesterol, while some of the others have no effect.

c. Cerebrovascular disease–The risk of strokes is concentrated in women over 35. It is increased in current users but not in past users. However, subarachnoid hemorrhages have been found to be increased among both current and past users and may increase with time. The risk of thrombotic or hemorrhagic stroke attributable to oral contraceptives is about 37 cases per 100,000 users per year. Ten percent of these strokes were fatal, and most of the fatal ones were due to subarachnoid hemorrhage. Insufficient data are available on which to base an assessment of the effects of smoking and other risk factors. However, it is thought that the pattern of risk is similar to that seen for myocardial infarction.

Elevations in blood pressure may also increase the risk, since there is a 3- to 6-fold increase in the incidence of overt hypertension in women taking oral contraceptives.

In summary, available data indicate that oral contraceptives increase the risk of various cardiovascular disorders at all ages and among both smokers and nonsmokers. However, this risk appears to be concentrated in women 35 years of age or older who are heavy smokers. It is clear that the presence of these risk factors must be considered in each individual patient for whom oral contraceptives are considered.

2. Gastrointestinal disorders–Many cases of cholestatic jaundice have been reported in patients taking progestin-containing drugs. The differences in incidence of these disorders from one population to another suggest that genetic factors may be involved.

The jaundice caused by these agents is similar to that produced by other 17-alkyl-substituted steroids. It is most often observed in the first 3 cycles and is particularly common in women with a history of cholestatic jaundice during pregnancy. Liver biopsies taken from such women show bile thrombi in the canaliculi and occasional focal necrosis. Serum alkaline phosphatase and SGPT are increased. Sulfobromophthalein retention and serum enzyme changes observed in some patients may indicate liver damage.

Jaundice and pruritus disappear 1–8 weeks after the drug is discontinued.

These agents have also been found to increase the incidence of symptomatic gallbladder disease, including cholecystitis and cholangitis. This is probably the result of the alterations in bile described above.

It also appears that the incidence of hepatic adenomas is increased in women taking oral contraceptives. Ischemic bowel disease secondary to thrombosis of the celiac and superior and inferior mesenteric arteries and veins has also been reported in women using these drugs.

3. Depression–Depression of sufficient degree to require cessation of therapy occurs in about 6% of patients treated with some preparations.

In addition to the above effects, a number of other adverse reactions have been reported for which a causal relationship has not been established. These include alopecia, erythema multiforme, erythema nodosum, and other skin disorders.

Contraindications & Cautions

These drugs are contraindicated in patients with thrombophlebitis, thromboembolic phenomena, and cerebrovascular disorders or a past history of these conditions. They should not be used to treat vaginal bleeding when the cause is unknown. They should be avoided in patients with known or suspected tumor of the breast or other estrogen-dependent neoplasm.

Since these preparations have caused aggravation of preexisting disorders, they should be avoided or used with caution in patients with liver disease, asthma, eczema, migraine, diabetes, hypertension, optic neuritis, retrobulbar neuritis, or convulsive disorders.

These agents—as well as progestational agents alone—increase the incidence of congenital abnormalities when taken early in pregnancy. Therefore, they should not be used as a means of diagnosing pregnancy.

The oral contraceptives may produce edema, and for that reason they should be used with great caution in patients in congestive failure or in whom edema is otherwise undesirable or dangerous.

Estrogens may increase the rate of growth of fibroids. Therefore, for women with these tumors, agents with the smallest amounts of estrogen and the most androgenic progestins should be selected. The use of progestational agents alone for contraception might be especially useful in such patients (see below).

At present, these agents are contraindicated in adolescents in whom epiphyseal closure has not yet been completed.

Since the long-term consequences of the changes in lipid and carbohydrate metabolism are unknown, and since estrogens are such potent carcinogens in some mammals, the precise risks involved in the prolonged use of these doses of estrogenic and progestational agents cannot be accurately assessed. This fact (and the known risks) should be explained to all patients for whom these drugs are prescribed.

Contraception with progestins or estrogens alone. Small doses of progestins administered orally can be used for contraception. They are particularly suited for use in patients for whom estrogen administration is undesirable. They are about as effective as intrauterine devices or combination pills containing 20–30 μg of ethinyl estradiol. There is a high incidence of abnormal bleeding. The use of infrequent injections of long-acting progestins (see above) such as medroxyprogesterone acetate has also found limited usefulness. The use of large doses of oral progestins at the time of intercourse is under study.

Diethylstilbestrol in doses of 25 mg twice a day for 5 days, beginning preferably within 24 hours and not later than 72 hours after exposure, is effective in preventing pregnancy. However, this form of contraception should not be used routinely or frequently, since serious questions about the teratogenic potency of this compound have been raised. Because of the possibility that diethylstilbestrol may cause vaginal cancer in the offspring of mothers treated later in pregnancy, the voluntary termination of pregnancy should be considered when conception occurs in these patients. Side-effects include nausea, vomiting, headache, dizziness, breast tenderness, and abdominal and leg cramps.

Health Benefits of Hormonal Contraceptives

It has become apparent during the last decade that reduction in the dose of the constituents of oral contraceptives has markedly reduced mild and severe adverse effects. Treatment with these agents has reduced the risk of endometrial cancer and iron deficiency anemia by 50%. Furthermore, the incidence of benign breast disease, functional ovarian cysts, premenstrual tension, and dysmenorrhea is significantly reduced.

It is clear, in view of these and other benefits, that hormonal contraception with these agents is a good choice in young women who do not smoke.

ANTIESTROGENS

TAMOXIFEN

Tamoxifen (Nolvadex) is a competitive inhibitor of estradiol at the receptor and is being used in the palliative treatment of advanced breast cancer in postmenopausal women. It is a nonsteroidal agent that is given orally. Peak plasma levels are reached in a few hours. It has an initial half-life of 7–14 hours in the circulation and is predominantly excreted by the liver. It is dispensed as the citrate in the form of tablets containing the equivalent of 10 mg tamoxifen. It is used in doses of 10–20 mg twice daily. Hot flashes and nausea and vomiting occur in 25% of patients, and many other adverse effects are observed.

CLOMIPHENE

Clomiphene citrate (Clomid) is a weak estrogen that also acts as a competitive inhibitor of endogenous estrogens. It has found use as an ovulation-inducing agent (see below).

OVULATION-INDUCING AGENTS

CLOMIPHENE CITRATE

Interest in the discovery of antiestrogenic compounds has been stimulated by the increasing need for antifertility compounds. Several of the synthetic estrogens have been shown to have significant antiestrogen properties. They are able to successfully compete for binding sites, yet have weaker hormonal properties. Clomiphene citrate (Clomid) is one such compound. It is closely related to other pharmacologically active compounds such as the estrogen chlorotrianisene (Fig 38–5) and the cholesterol inhibitor triparanol.

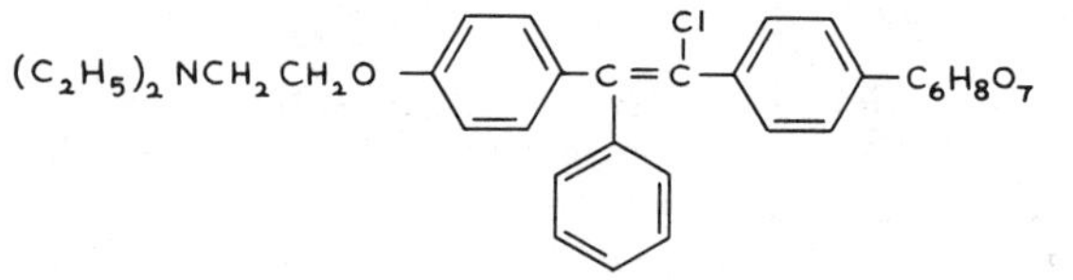

Clomiphene citrate

This compound is active when taken orally, since it is readily absorbed. Very little is known about its metabolism, but available studies indicate that about half of the compound is excreted into the stools within 5 days after administration. Studies of the metabolism of clomiphene have been more extensive in animals. In monkeys the half-life of clomiphene citrate, when given intravenously, is approximately 48 hours. When 90% of the dose has been eliminated from the body, the liver, gallbladder, and bile have the highest concentrations of the remaining compound. It has been suggested that clomiphene is slowly excreted from an enterohepatic pool.

Pharmacologic Effects

A. Mechanisms of Action: Clomiphene citrate is a weak estrogen. The estrogenic effects are best demonstrated in animals with marked gonadal deficiency. Clomiphene has also been shown to effectively inhibit the action of stronger estrogens. In humans it leads to an increase in the secretion of gonadotropins and estrogens.

B. Effects: The pharmacologic importance of this compound rests on its ability to stimulate ovulation in women with amenorrhea and other ovulatory disorders. The mechanism by which ovulation is produced is not known. It has been suggested that it blocks an inhibitory influence of estrogens on the hypothalamus and increases the production of gonadotropins. Clomiphene will not work in the absence of a pituitary gland capable of producing gonadotropins. It has been shown in the rat that crystals of this compound implanted in the pituitary have no effect, whereas those implanted in parts of the median eminence are able to induce ovulation. The observation that this compound can induce ovulation in patients with very low estrogen levels does not support the hypothesis that it works by breaking a feedback inhibition. However, it does stimulate gonadotropin production by the pituitary by an action on the hypothalamus.

Clinical Uses

Clomiphene citrate is used for the treatment of disorders of ovulation in patients wishing to become pregnant. In general, a single ovulation is induced by a single course of therapy, and the patient must be treated repeatedly until pregnancy is achieved, since normal ovulatory function does not usually resume. The compound is of no use in patients with ovarian or pituitary failure.

Standardized procedures for the use of clomiphene as a testing substance have not been established. This substance can serve as a useful test of the ability of the pituitary gland to secrete gonadotropins.

When clomiphene is administered in doses of 100 mg daily for 5 days, a rise in plasma LH and FSH is observed several days after starting. In patients who ovulate, the initial rise is followed by a second rise of gonadotropin levels just prior to ovulation.

Adverse Reactions

The most common side-effects in patients treated with this drug are hot flushes, which resemble those experienced by menopausal patients. They tend to be mild and disappear when the drug is discontinued. There have been occasional reports of eye symptoms due to intensification and prolongation of after-images. These are generally of short duration. Headache, constipation, allergic skin reactions, and reversible hair loss have been reported occasionally.

The effective use of clomiphene is associated with some stimulation of the ovaries and usually with ovarian enlargement. The degree of enlargement tends to be greater and its incidence higher in patients who have enlarged ovaries at the beginning of therapy.

A variety of other symptoms such as nausea and vomiting, increased nervous tension, depression, fatigue, breast soreness, weight gain, urinary frequency, and heavy menses have also been reported. However, these appear to be due to the hormonal changes associated with an ovulatory menstrual cycle rather than a result of the medication. The incidence of multiple pregnancy is approximately 10%.

Clomiphene has not been shown to have an adverse effect in human pregnancy. However, since the only current indication for clomiphene therapy is to achieve pregnancy, existing pregnancy is a contraindication to its use.

Contraindications & Cautions

Special precautions should be observed in patients with enlarged ovaries. These women are thought to be more sensitive to this drug and should receive small doses. Any patient who complains of abdominal symptoms should be carefully examined. The maximum ovarian enlargement occurs after the 5-day course has been completed, and many patients can be shown to have a palpable increase in ovarian size by the seventh to tenth days.

Special precautions must also be taken in patients who have visual symptoms associated with clomiphene therapy, since these symptoms may make activities such as driving more hazardous.

Dosages

The recommended dose of clomiphene citrate (Clomid) at the beginning of therapy is 50 mg/d for 5 days. If ovulation occurs, this same course may be repeated until pregnancy is achieved. If ovulation does not occur, the dose is doubled to 100 mg/d for 5 days. If ovulation and menses occur, the next course can be started on the fifth day of the cycle. Experience to date suggests that patients who do not ovulate after 3 courses of 100 mg/d of clomiphene are not likely to respond to continued therapy. However, such patients occasionally respond to slightly larger doses or more prolonged treatment schedules. The combined use of clomiphene and bromocriptine in normal prolactinemic women has also been successful in the induction of ovulation.

About 80% of patients with anovulatory disorders or amenorrhea can be expected to respond by having ovulatory cycles. Approximately half of these patients will become pregnant. In the patients in whom pregnancy is achieved, the incidence of early abortion seems to be slightly increased. Although a variety of congenital defects have been described in the children resulting from these pregnancies, the incidence does not appear to be greater than occurs spontaneously. Clomiphene has also been used in combination with menotropins to reduce the amount of the latter required to induce ovulation.

BROMOCRIPTINE

In some amenorrheic women, an elevated level of prolactin appears to be the causative factor. These patients may have prolactin-secreting tumors or "empty sella" syndrome, which should be excluded before treatment is begun. The criteria for selecting medical, surgical, and radiation therapy for prolactinomas have not been firmly established.

Bromocriptine (Parlodel), an ergot alkaloid (Chapter 14), acts by binding to dopaminergic receptors in the pituitary and inhibits prolactin secretion. In 90% or more of patients, treatment leads to the onset of menses in 3–5 weeks. The usual dose required is 2.5 mg 2 or 3 times a day. Prolactin levels should be depressed to normal if treatment is adequate.

The long-term use of bromocriptine to induce regression of pituitary tumors is under study. Preliminary results indicate that at least in some patients, tumors can be shown to regress.

HUMAN MENOPAUSAL GONADOTROPIN (hMG, Menotropins)

Because of antibody formation and species differences in response, animal preparations of FSH have not been very useful in humans. Studies are currently in progress utilizing partially purified extracts of human pituitary glands or pooled urine obtained from postmenopausal women that contains both FSH and LH activity. The LH content is estimated by observing changes in the weight of the ventral prostate in hypophysectomized immature rats or depletion of ascorbic acid from the ovaries of immature rats. An ovarian augmentation assay is available for measuring FSH content. The pituitary extracts are available in only a few laboratories, but hMG is now more widely available.

Clinical Uses

hMG—in conjunction with human chorionic gonadotropin (hCG); see p 404—is used to stimulate ovulation in patients who do not ovulate but have potentially functional ovarian tissue. It has been successful in the induction of ovulation in patients with hypopituitarism and other defects in gonadotropin secretion. It has also been used in patients with amenorrhea or anovulatory cycles and in patients in whom ovulatory disturbances are associated with galactorrhea or hirsutism. Ovarian failure should be excluded in patients considered for therapy. Since therapy is difficult and expensive, it is useful to look for the existence of other factors such as obstruction of the uterine tubes or abnormalities in sperm production by the husband. The acceptability of multiple birth by the patient must be considered.

Preparations of human menopausal gonadotropin can stimulate spermatogenesis in males with isolated gonadotropin deficiency. Using hMG in conjunction with HCG (see Chapter 35), endocrine and gametogenic function has been restored in a few of these patients.

Contraindications & Cautions

hMG is a potentially dangerous agent and should be administered only after thorough acquaintance with its use and by physicians experienced in dealing with endocrine disturbances and problems of reproductive function. Careful selection of patients is required.

This preparation should not be used in early pregnancy (which may be difficult to diagnose in patients with irregular cycles), or in patients with ovarian failure except as a diagnostic procedure. In patients with pituitary and other intracranial tumors, the primary disease process should be treated before undertaking therapy with hMG. hMG should not be used in patients with other causes of infertility than lack of ovulation.

Adverse Reactions

The most common problem encountered is excessive ovarian stimulation. Ovarian enlargement is

Table 38–6. Results of treatment with hMG.

Pregnancy Achieved	Multiple Pregnancy		Aborting	Hyper-stimulation Syndrome
	Twins	Triplets, Etc		
25–40%	10–20%	5–10%	20–30%	0.5–1.5%

common. When marked (hyperstimulation syndrome), it may be accompanied by pain, ascites, and pleural effusion. Arterial thromboembolism has been reported in 2 patients. Occasional patients experience swelling and fever along with discomfort at the injection site. Undesirable results of therapy include the high incidence of multiple pregnancy and abortion (Table 38–6). The frequency of birth defects has not been elevated in the offspring of patients who have succeeded in carrying their pregnancies to term.

The typical outcome of therapy in suitably selected patients treated by experienced physicians is shown in Table 38–6.

It is clear that this mode of therapy is complicated, time-consuming, and expensive. It should not be undertaken lightly but can be very helpful to the proper patient after simpler therapeutic methods have failed.

II. THE TESTIS (Androgens & Anabolic Steroids)

The testis, like the ovary, has both gametogenic and endocrine functions. The gametogenic function of the testes is controlled largely by the secretion of FSH by the pituitary. High concentrations of androgens locally are also required for sperm production in the seminiferous tubules. The Sertoli cells in the seminiferous tubules may be the source of the estradiol produced in the testes. The androgens are produced in the interstitial or Leydig cells found in the spaces between the seminiferous tubules.

In humans the most important androgen secreted by the testis is testosterone. The pathways of synthesis of testosterone in the testes are similar to those previously described in the ovary and the adrenal (Fig 38–7).

In the male, approximately 8 mg of testosterone is produced daily. About 95% is produced by the Leydig cells and only 5% by the adrenal. The testis also secretes small amounts of another potent androgen, dihydrotestosterone, as well as androstenedione and dehydroepiandrosterone, which are weak androgens. Pregnenolone and progesterone and their 17-hydroxylated derivatives are also released in small amounts. Plasma levels of testosterone in males are about 0.6 μg/dL after puberty and do not appear to vary significantly with age. Testosterone is also present in the plasma of women in concentrations of approximately 0.03 μg/dL and is derived in approximately equal parts from the ovaries, the adrenals, and by the peripheral conversion of other hormones.

About 65% of circulating testosterone is bound to sex hormone-binding globulin (SHBG), a specific protein produced by the liver. This protein is increased in plasma by estrogen, by thyroid hormone, and in patients with cirrhosis of the liver. It is decreased by androgen and growth hormone and is lower in obese individuals. Most of the remaining testosterone is

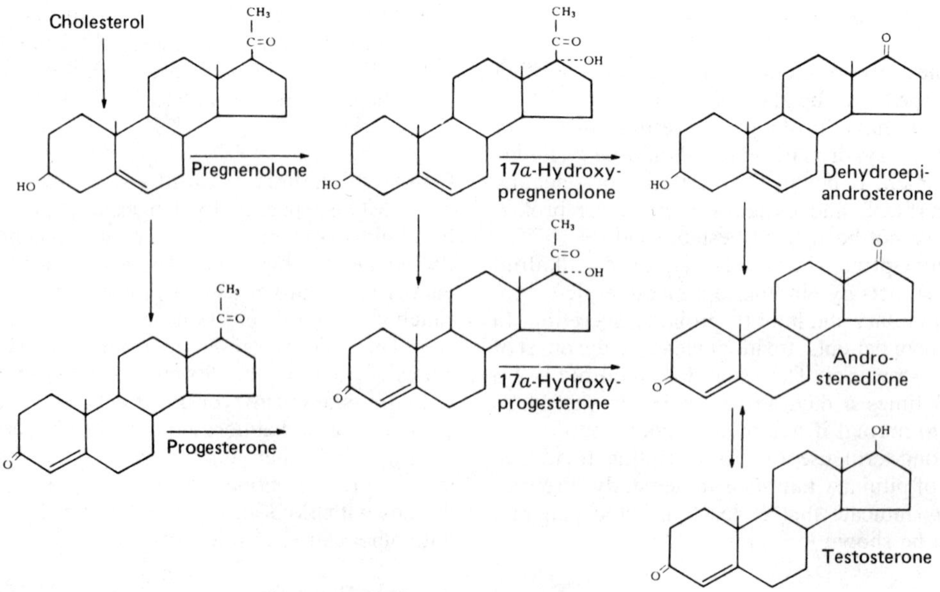

Figure 38–7. Biosynthesis of testosterone. (Reproduced, with permission, from Ganong WF: *Review of Medical Physiology,* 8th ed. Lange, 1977.)

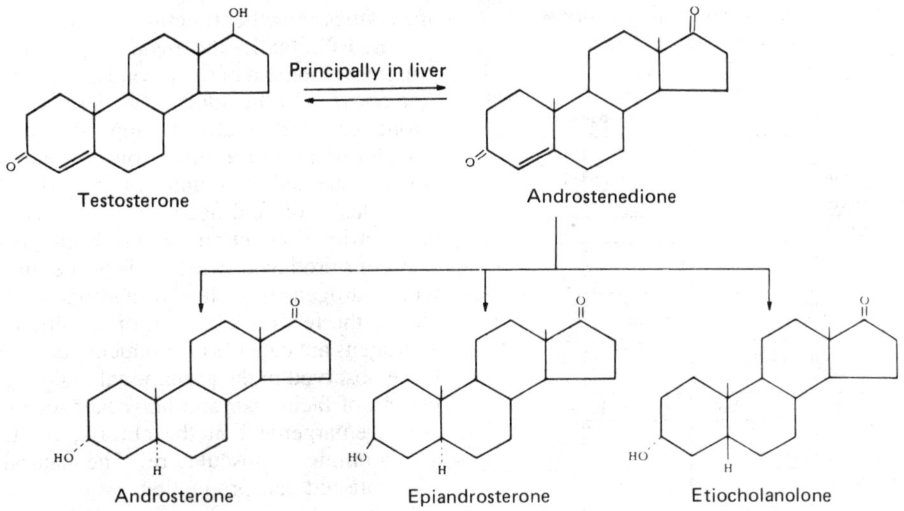

Figure 38–8. Metabolism of testosterone. (Reproduced, with permission, from Ganong WF: *Review of Medical Physiology,* 8th ed. Lange, 1977.)

bound to albumin. However, approximately 2% remains free and available to enter cells and bind to intracellular receptors.

Metabolism

In many target tissues, testosterone is converted to dihydrotestosterone by the enzyme 5α-reductase. In these tissues, dihydrotestosterone is the major androgen. The conversion of testosterone to estradiol also occurs in some tissues, including the hypothalamus, and may be of importance in regulating gonadal function.

The major pathway for the degradation of testosterone in humans is illustrated in Fig 38–8. In the liver, the reduction of the double bond and ketone in the A ring, as is seen in other steroids with a Δ^4-ketone configuration in the A ring, leads to the production of inactive substances such as androsterone and etiocholanolone that are then conjugated and excreted into the urine.

Androstenedione and dehydroepiandrosterone (Fig 38–7) are also produced in significant amounts in humans, although largely in the adrenal rather than in the testes. These compounds do not have significant androgenic activity, but they are to a large extent metabolized in the same fashion as testosterone. Both compounds—but particularly androstenedione—can be converted by peripheral tissues to estrone in very small amounts (1–5%).

Control of Secretion

Gonadotropin-releasing hormone (GnRH, LHRH) binds to membrane receptors activating adenylate cyclase and causes the secretion of LH and smaller amounts of FSH by gonadotropin-producing cells in the pituitary.

LH stimulates the production of steroids by activating membrane receptors of the Leydig cells in the testis. LH release is in turn regulated by androgens, which suppress LH release at the pituitary. Estrogens formed locally from circulating androgens inhibit the hypothalamic release of GnRH. Inhibin, a nonsteroid hormone produced by the Sertoli cells of the testis, inhibits the release of FSH by the pituitary.

Physiologic Effects

In the normal male, testosterone is responsible for the many changes that occur in puberty. In addition to the general growth-promoting properties of androgens on the body tissues, these hormones are responsible for penile and scrotal growth. Changes in the skin include the appearance of pubic hair, axillary hair, and beard hair. The sebaceous glands become more active, and the skin tends to become thicker and oilier. The larynx grows and the vocal cords become thicker, leading to a lower pitched voice. Skeletal growth is stimulated and epiphyseal closure accelerated. Other effects include growth of the prostate and seminal vesicles, darkening of the skin, and increased skin circulation. Psychologic and behavioral changes also occur.

Synthetic Steroids With Androgenic & Anabolic Action

Testosterone, when administered by mouth, is rapidly absorbed. However, it is largely converted to inactive metabolites, and only about one-sixth of the dose administered is available in active form. Testosterone can be administered parenterally, but it has a more prolonged absorption time and greater activity when esterified. Methyltestosterone and fluoxymesterone are active when given by mouth.

Testosterone and its derivatives have been used for their anabolic effects as well as for the replacement of testosterone deficiency. Although testosterone and other known active steroids can be isolated in pure form and measured by weight, biologic assays are still

Table 38–7. Androgens: Preparations available and relative androgen/anabolic activity.

	Androgenic/Anabolic Activity
Testosterone	1:1
Testosterone cypionate	1:1
Testosterone enanthate	1:1
Testosterone propionate	1:1
Methyltestosterone	1:1
Methandriol	1:2
Methandriol dipropionate	1:2
Fluoxymesterone	1:2
Methandrostenolone (metandienone)	1:3
Oxymetholone	1:3
Ethylestrenol	1:4–1:8
Oxandrolone	1:3–1:13
Nandrolone phenpropionate	1:3–1:6
Nandrolone decanoate	1:2.5–1:4
Stanozolol	1:3–1:6
Dromostanolone propionate	1:3–1:4

used in the investigation of new compounds. In some of these studies in animals, the anabolic effects of the compound—as measured by trophic effects on muscles or the reduction of nitrogen excretion—may be dissociated from the other androgenic effects. This has led to the marketing of a substantial group of compounds that are supposed to have marked anabolic activity associated with only weak androgenic effects. This dissociation does not appear to be complete, and in humans it is less marked than in the animals used for testing (Table 38–7). Though they may be less virilizing than equivalent doses of testosterone, doses of these drugs large enough to promote nitrogen retention can also produce unwanted androgenic effects.

Pharmacologic Effects

A. Mechanisms of Action: Testosterone acts intracellularly in target cells. In skin, prostate, seminal vesicles, and epididymis, it is converted to 5α-dihydrotestosterone by the enzyme 5α-reductase. In these tissues, dihydrotestosterone is the dominant androgen. The distribution of this enzyme in the fetus is different and has important developmental implications.

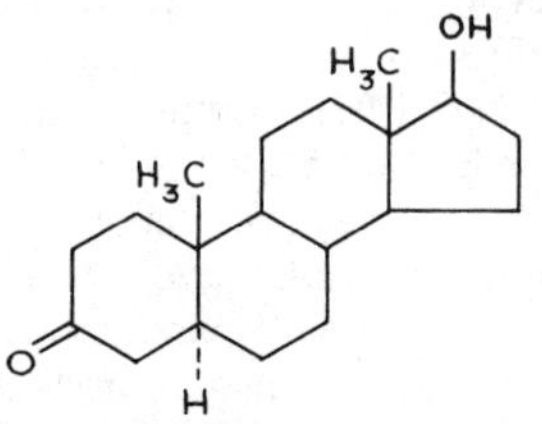

5α-Dihydrotestosterone (androstanolone, stanolone, DHT)

Testosterone and dihydrotestosterone bind to the cytosol androgen receptor, initiating a series of events leading to a variety of intracellular processes, including growth, differentiation, and synthesis of a variety of enzymes and other functional proteins (Chapter 34).

B. Effects: In the male at puberty, androgens cause development of the secondary sex characteristics (see above). In the adult male, large doses of testosterone or its derivatives suppress the secretion of gonadotropins and result in some atrophy of the interstitial tissue and the tubules of the testes. Since fairly large doses of androgens are required to suppress gonadotropic secretion, it has been postulated that estrogens produced in the testis (either in combination with androgens or instead of androgens) are responsible for the feedback control of secretion. In women, androgens are capable of producing changes similar to those observed in the prepubertal male. These include growth of facial hair and body hair, deepening of the voice, enlargement of the clitoris, frontal baldness, and prominent musculature. The natural androgens stimulate red cell production.

The administration of androgens reduces the excretion of nitrogen into the urine, indicating an increase in protein synthesis or decrease in protein breakdown within the body. This effect is much more pronounced in women and children than in normal men.

Clinical Uses

A. Androgen Replacement Therapy in Men: Androgens are used to replace or augment endogenous androgen secretion in hypogonadal men (Table 38–8). Even in the presence of hypogonadotropism, androgens are used rather than gonadotropin except when normal spermatogenesis is to be achieved. When androgen deficiency occurs prior to completion of sexual maturation, large doses of androgens are required, and orally administered androgens are not sufficiently efficacious. In these patients, therapy should begin using testosterone enanthate or cypionate in doses of 200 mg intramuscularly every 1–2 weeks until maturation is complete. The dose can then be reduced to 200 mg at 2- to 3-week intervals. Testosterone propionate, though potent, is not practical for long-term use. The development of polycythemia or hypertension may require some reduction in dose.

Table 38–8. Androgen preparations for replacement therapy.

	Route of Administration	Dose
Methyltestosterone	Oral	25–50 mg/d
	Sublingual (buccal)	5–10 mg/d
Fluoxymesterone	Oral	2–10 mg/d
Testosterone propionate	Sublingual (buccal)	5–20 mg/d
	Intramuscular	10–50 mg 3 times weekly
Testosterone enanthate	Intramuscular	200 mg every 1–2 weeks until maturation is complete, then every 2–3 weeks for maintenance.
Testosterone cypionate	Intramuscular	
Testosterone pellets	Subcutaneous	450 mg every 4–6 months

In patients with hypopituitarism, androgens are not added to the treatment regimen until puberty, at which time they are instituted in gradually increasing doses to achieve the growth spurt and the development of secondary sex characteristics.

B. Gynecologic Disorders: Androgens are used occasionally in the treatment of certain gynecologic disorders, but the undesirable effects in women are such that they must be used with great caution. Androgens have been used to reduce breast engorgement during the postpartum period, usually in conjunction with estrogens. For example, 4 mL of a preparation containing 90 mg/mL of testosterone enanthate and 4 mg/mL of estradiol are useful for this purpose when given at the onset of the second stage of labor.

Androgens are sometimes given in combination with estrogens for replacement therapy in the postmenopausal period in an attempt to eliminate the endometrial bleeding that may occur when only estrogens are used. They are also used for the chemotherapy of breast tumors in premenopausal women.

C. Use as Protein Anabolic Agents: Androgens and anabolic steroids have been used in conjunction with dietary measures and exercises in an attempt to reverse protein loss after trauma, surgery, or prolonged immobilization and in patients with debilitating diseases.

D. Anemia: Large doses of androgens have been employed in the treatment of refractory anemias and have resulted in some increase in reticulocytosis and hemoglobin levels. The large amounts required prevent this from being a useful method of therapy in women.

E. Osteoporosis: Androgens and anabolic agents have been used in the treatment of osteoporosis, either alone or in conjunction with estrogens. The benefits of androgens in these patients have not been substantiated by careful studies.

F. Use as Metabolic Stimulators: These agents have been used to stimulate growth in prepubertal boys. If the drugs are used carefully, these children will probably achieve their expected adult height (and sooner than normal). If treatment is too vigorous, the patient may grow rapidly at first but will not achieve full stature because of the accelerated epiphyseal closure that occurs. It is difficult to control this type of therapy adequately even with frequent x-ray examination of the epiphyses, since the action of the hormones on epiphyseal centers may continue for many months after therapy is discontinued.

Adverse Reactions

The adverse effects of these compounds are due largely to their masculinizing actions and are most noticeable in women and prepubertal children. In women, the administration of more than 200–300 mg of testosterone per month is usually associated with hirsutism, acne, depression of menses, clitoral enlargement, and deepening of the voice. These effects may occur with even smaller doses in some women. Some of the androgenic steroids exert progestational activity leading to endometrial bleeding. These hormones also alter serum lipids and could conceivably increase susceptibility to atherosclerotic disease of the vessels in women. Except under the most unusual circumstances, androgens should not be used in infants. Recent studies in animals suggest that administration of androgens in early life may have profound effects on maturation of central nervous system centers governing sexual development, particularly in the female. Administration of these drugs to pregnant females may lead to masculinization of the external genitalia in the infant. Although the above-mentioned effects may be less marked with the anabolic agents, they do occur.

Sodium retention and edema are not common but must be carefully watched for in patients with heart and kidney disease.

Most of the synthetic androgens and anabolic agents are 17-alkyl-substituted steroids. Administration of drugs with this structure is associated with increase in sulfobromophthalein retention and SGOT levels. Alkaline phosphatase values are also elevated. These changes usually occur early in the course of treatment, and the degree is proportionate to the dose. Bilirubin levels occasionally increase until clinical jaundice is apparent. The cholestatic jaundice is reversible upon cessation of therapy, and permanent changes do not occur. In older males, prostatic hyperplasia may develop, causing urinary obstruction.

Contraindications & Cautions

The use of androgenic steroids is contraindicated in pregnant women or women who may become pregnant during the course of therapy.

Androgens should not be administered to male patients with carcinoma of the prostate or breast.

Until more is known about the effects of these hormones on the central nervous system in developing children, they should be avoided in infants and young children.

Special caution is required in giving these drugs to children to produce a growth spurt.

Care should be exercised in the administration of these drugs to patients with renal or cardiac disease predisposed to edema. If sodium and water retention occurs, it will respond to diuretic therapy.

Methyltestosterone therapy is associated with creatinuria, but the significance of this finding is not known.

Caution: Several cases of hepatocellular carcinoma have been reported in patients with aplastic anemia treated with androgen anabolic therapy.

III. ANTIANDROGENS

The potential usefulness of antiandrogens for the treatment of patients producing excessive amounts of testosterone has led to the search for effective drugs that can be used for this purpose. Two approaches to the problem have met with limited success experimentally.

Several compounds have been developed that inhibit the 17-hydroxylation of progesterone or pregnenolone, thereby preventing the action of the side chain-splitting enzyme and the further transformation of these steroid precursors to active androgens. A few of these compounds have been tested clinically but have been too toxic for prolonged use.

Another approach has been the development of steroids that are chemically similar and act as competitive inhibitors. A few of these have been tried in patients on a limited basis.

Cyproterone and cyproterone acetate are effective antiandrogens that inhibit the action of the androgens at the target organ. The acetate form has a marked progestational effect that suppresses the feedback enhancement of LH and FSH, leading to a more effective antiandrogen effect. These compounds have been used to decrease excessive sexual drive and are being studied in other conditions in which the reduction of androgenic effects would be useful.

IV. HORMONAL CONTRACEPTION IN THE MALE

A large number of studies conducted over the past few decades have been unsuccessful in identifying an effective oral contraceptive for men. Various androgens, including testosterone and testosterone enanthate, in doses of 400 mg per month, will produce azoospermia in less than half of the men treated. Minor adverse reactions, including gynecomastia and acne, were encountered. Testosterone in combination with danazol was well tolerated but no more effective than testosterone alone. Androgens in combination with a progestin such as depomedroxyprogesterone acetate were no more effective. Cyproterone acetate, a very potent progestin, will also produce oligospermia but has not produced reliable contraception. Potent analogs of GnRH are also under study.

GOSSYPOL

Extensive trials of this cottonseed derivative are being conducted in China. This compound destroys elements of the seminiferous epithelium but does not alter the endocrine function of the testis.

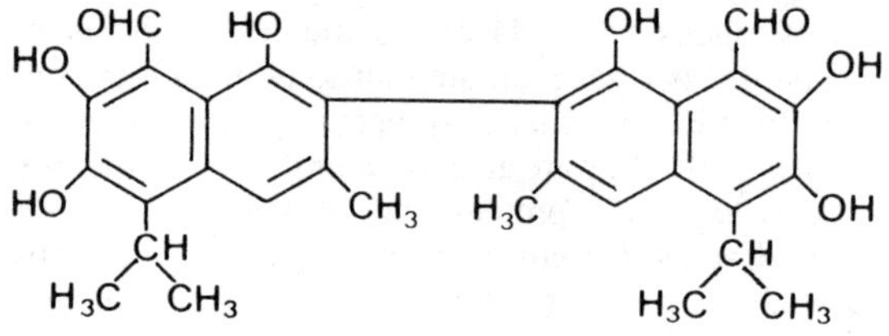

Gossypol

Large numbers of men have been treated with 20 mg/d of gossypol or gossypol acetic acid for 2 months, followed by a maintenance dose of 60 mg a week. On this regimen, 99% of men developed sperm counts below 4 million per milliliter. Preliminary data indicate that recovery (return of normal sperm count) following discontinuation of gossypol administration is more apt to occur in men whose counts do not fall to extremely low levels and when administration is not continued for over 2 years. Hypokalemia is the major side-effect and may lead to transient paralysis.

• • •

References

Androgens II and antiandrogens. Vol 35, part 2, in: *Handbook of Experimental Pharmacology*. (New series.) Springer, 1974.

Antunes CMF et al: Endometrial cancer and estrogen use. *N Engl J Med* 1979;**300:**9.

Barbieri RL, Ryan KJ: Danazol: Endocrine pharmacology and therapeutic applications. *Am J Obstet Gynecol* 1981;**141:**453.

Beck P: Contraceptive steroids: Modifications of carbohydrate and lipid metabolism. *Metabolism* 1973;**22:**841.

Belchetz PE et al: Hypophyseal responses to continuous and intermittent delivery of hypothalamic gonadotropin-releasing hormone. *Science* 1978;**202:**631.

Bibbo M et al: Follow-up study of male and female offspring of DES-exposed mothers. *Obstet Gynecol* 1977;**49:**1.

Bingel AS, Benoit PS: Oral contraceptives: Therapeutics versus adverse reactions, with an outlook for the future. (2 parts.) *J Pharm Sci* 1973;**62:**179, 349.

Bradley BD et al: Serum high-density-lipoprotein cholesterol in women using oral contraceptives, estrogen and progestins. *N Engl J Med* 1978;**299:**17.

Cann CE et al: Spinal mineral loss by quantitative computed tomography in oophorectomized women. *JAMA* 1980; **244:**2056.

Carter DE et al: Effect of oral contraceptives on drug metabolism. *Clin Pharmacol Ther* 1974;**15:**22.

Christiansen C et al: Prevention of early postmenopausal bone loss. *Eur J Clin Invest* 1980;**10:**273.

Conte FA, Grumbach MM: Estrogen use in children and adolescents: A survey. *Pediatrics* 1978;**62(6-Part 2):**1091.

Dmowski WP: Endocrine properties and clinical application of danazol. *Fertil Steril* 1979;**31:**237.

Franchimont P et al: Effects of oral testosterone undecanoate in hypogonadal male patients. *Clin Endocrinol* 1978;**9:**313.

Garattini S, Berendes HW: *Pharmacology of Steroid Contraceptive Drugs*. Raven Press, 1977.

Goldzieher JW, Dozier TS, de la Pena A: Plasma levels and pharmacokinetics of ethynyl estrogens in various populations. 1. Ethynylestradiol. *Contraception* 1980;**21:**1.

Griffin JE, Wilson JD: The syndromes of androgen resistance. *N Engl J Med* 1980;**302:**198.

Gusberg SB: Current concepts in cancer: The changing nature of endometrial cancer. *N Engl J Med* 1980;**302:**729.

Hahn HB Jr, Hayles AB, Albert A: Medroxyprogesterone [Provera] and constitutional precocious puberty. *Mayo Clin Proc* 1964;**39:**182.

Hammond CS et al: Effects of long-term estrogen replacement therapy. *Am J Obstet Gynecol* 1979;**133:**525.

Heaney RP, Recker RR, Saville PD: Menopausal changes in calcium balance performance. *J Lab Clin Med* 1978;**92:**953.

Hertz R: Physiologic effects of androgens and estrogens in man. *Am J Med* 1956;**21:**671.

Huggins GR, Guintoli RL: Oral contraceptives and neoplasia. *Fertil Steril* 1979;**32:**1.

Jeppsson S, Johansson EDB: Medroxyprogesterone acetate, estradiol, FSH and LH in peripheral blood after intramuscular administration of Depo-Provera to women. *Contraception* 1976;**14:**461.

Jewelewicz R: Management of infertility resulting from anovulation. *Am J Obstet Gynecol* 1975;**122:**909.

Jick H, Dinan B, Rothman KJ: Non-contraceptive estrogens and non-fatal myocardial infarction. *JAMA* 1978;**239:**1406.

Jick H, Dinan B, Rothman KJ: Oral contraceptives and non-fatal myocardial infarction. *JAMA* 1979;**239:**1403.

Jick H et al: Myocardial infarction and other vascular diseases in young women: Role of estrogens and other factors. *JAMA* 1978;**240:**2548.

Jick H et al: Replacement estrogens and endometrial cancer. *N Engl J Med* 1979;**300:**218.

Johnson FL et al: Association of androgenic-anabolic steroid therapy with development of hepatocellular carcinoma. *Lancet* 1972;**2:**1273.

Larsson-Cohn U et al: Lipoprotein changes may be minimized by proper composition of a combined oral contraceptive. *Fertil Steril* 1981;**35:**172.

Linde R et al: Reversible inhibition of testicular steroidogenesis and spermatogenesis by a potent gonadotropin-releasing hormone agonist in normal men. *N Engl J Med* 1981;**305:**663.

Mann JI, Inman WHW: Oral contraceptives and death from myocardial infarction. *Br Med J* 1975;**2:**245.

Mann JI et al: Myocardial infarction in young women with special reference to oral contraceptive practice. *Br Med J* 1975;**2:**241.

Meema S, Bunker ML, Meema HE: Preventive effect of estrogen on postmenopausal bone loss. *Arch Intern Med* 1975;**135:**1436.

Mishell DR Jr: Noncontraceptive health benefits of oral contraceptives. *Am J Obstet Gynecol* 1982;**142:**809.

Nachtigall LE et al: Estrogen replacement therapy. 1. A ten year prospective study in the relationship to osteoporosis. *Obstet Gynecol* 1979;**53:**277.

Neumann F: Pharmacology and potential use of cyproterone acetate. *Horm Metab Res* 1977;**9:**1.

Nieschlag E, Wickings EJ, Breuer H: Chemical methods for male fertility control. *Contraception* 1981;**23:**1.

Nora JJ et al: Exogenous progestogen and estrogen implicated in birth defects. *JAMA* 1978;**240:**837.

Progesterone, progestational drugs and antifertility agents. Section 48 in: *International Encyclopedia of Pharmacology and Therapeutics*. Tausk M (editor). Permagon Press, vol 1, 1971; vol 2, 1972.

Rigberg SV, Brodsky I: Potential roles of androgens and the anabolic steroids in the treatment of cancer: A review. *J Med* 1975;**6:**271.

Riggs LB et al: Effect of the fluoride/calcium regimen on vertebral fracture occurrence in postmenopausal osteoporosis. *N Engl J Med* 1982;**306:**446.

Robboy SJ, Bradley R: Changing trends and prognostic features in endometrial cancer associated with exogenous estrogen therapy. *Obstet Gynecol* 1979;**54:**269.

Rosemberg E (editor): *Gonadotropin Therapy in Female Infertility*. International Congress Series No. 266. Excerpta Medica, 1973.

Royal College of General Practitioners: *Oral Contraceptives and Health*. Pitman, 1974.

Salhanick HA, Kipnis DM, Vande Wiele RL (editors): *Metabolic Effects of Gonadal Hormones and Contraceptive Steroids*. Plenum Press, 1969.

Schwartz NB, Channing CP: Evidence for ovarian "inhibin": Suppression of the secondary rise in serum follicle stimulating hormone levels in proestrus rats by injection of porcine follicular fluid. *Proc Natl Acad Sci USA* 1977;**74:**5721.

Shapiro AG, Thomas T, Epstein M: Management of hyperstimulation syndrome. *Fertil Steril* 1977;**28:**237.

Shapiro S et al: Oral-contraceptive use in relation to myocardial infarction. *Lancet* 1979;**1:**743.

Spellacy WN, Buhi WC, Birk SA: Effect of estrogen treatment for one year on carbohydrate and lipid metabolism in women with normal and abnormal glucose tolerance test results. *Am J Obstet Gynecol* 1978;**131:**87.

Stadel BV: Oral contraceptives and cardiovascular disease. (2 parts.) *N Engl J Med* 1981;**305:**612, 672.

Van Keep PA, Lauritzen C (editors): *Ageing and Estrogens*. Frontiers of Hormone Research, vol 2. Karger, 1973.

Weiss G et al: Distribution of relaxin in women during pregnancy. *Obstet Gynecol* 1978;**52:**569.

Weiss NS, Sayvetz TA: Incidence of endometrial cancer in relation to the use of oral contraceptives. *N Engl J Med* 1980;**302:**551.

Wise AJ, Gross MA, Schalch DS: Quantitative relationships of the pituitary-gonadal axis in postmenopausal women. *J Lab Clin Med* 1973;**81:**28.

Wolstenholme GEW, O'Connor M (editors): Endocrinology of the testis. *Ciba Found Colloq Endocrinol* 1967;**16:**1.

Yen SSC et al: Circulating estradiol, estrone and gonadotropin levels following the administration of orally active 17α-estradiol in postmenopausal women. *J Clin Endocrinol Metab* 1975;**40:**518.

Ziel HK, Finkle WD: Increased risk of endometrial carcinoma among users of conjugated estrogens. *N Engl J Med* 1975;**293:**1167.

39 | Pancreatic Hormones & Antidiabetic Drugs

John H. Karam, MD

The endocrine pancreas in the adult human consists of approximately 1 million islets of Langerhans interspersed throughout the pancreatic gland. Within the islets, at least 4 hormone-producing cells have been identified (Table 39–1). Their hormone products include **insulin,** the storage and anabolic hormone of the body; **glucagon,** the hyperglycemic factor that mobilizes glycogen stores; **somatostatin,** a universal inhibitor of secretory cells; and **pancreatic polypeptide,** a small protein that facilitates digestive processes by a mechanism not yet clarified.

Table 39–1. Pancreatic islet cells and their secretory products.

Cell Types	Approximate Percent of Islet Mass	Secretory Products
A cell (alpha)	20	Glucagon, proglucagon.
B cell (beta)	75	Insulin, C-peptide, proinsulin.
D cell (delta)	3–5	Somatostatin.
F cell (PP cell)*	<2	Pancreatic polypeptide (PP).

*Within pancreatic polypeptide-rich lobules of adult islets, located in the posterior portion of the head of the human pancreas, glucagon cells are scarce (less than 0.5%), and F cells make up as much as 80% of the cells.

INSULIN

Chemistry

Insulin is a small protein with a molecular weight of 5734. It contains 51 amino acids arranged in 2 chains (A and B) linked by disulfide bridges; there are species differences in the amino acids of both chains (Fig 39–1). Within the B cell, insulin precursor is produced by DNA/RNA-directed synthesis. Initially, proinsulin, a long single-chain protein molecule, is processed within the Golgi apparatus and packaged into granules, where it is hydrolyzed into insulin and a residual connecting segment called the C-peptide by removal of 4 amino acids (shown in dashed lines in Fig 39–2). Insulin and C-peptide are secreted in equimolar amounts in response to all insulin secretogogues; a small quantity of unprocessed or partially hydrolyzed proinsulin is released as well. Neither proinsulin nor C-peptide is known to have any physiologic function. Granules within the B cell store the insulin in the form of crystals consisting of 2 atoms of zinc and 6 molecules of insulin. The entire human pancreas contains up to 8 mg of insulin, representing approximately 200 biologic "units." Originally, the unit was defined on the basis of the hypoglycemic activity of insulin in rabbits. With improved purification techniques, the unit is presently defined on the basis of weight, and present insulin standards used for assay purposes are 25 units per milligram.

Insulin Degradation

The liver and kidney are the 2 main organs that remove insulin from the circulation, presumably by hydrolysis of the disulfide connections between the A and B chains through the action of glutathione insulin transhydrogenase (insulinase). After this reductive cleavage, further degradation by proteolysis occurs. The liver normally clears the blood of approximately 60% of the insulin released from the pancreas by virtue of its location as the terminal site of portal vein blood flow, with the kidney removing 35–40% of the endogenous hormone. However, in insulin-treated diabetics receiving subcutaneous insulin injections, this ratio is reversed, with as much as 60% of exogenous insulin being cleared by the kidney and the liver removing no more than 30–40%. The half-life of circulating insulin is 3–5 minutes.

Measurement of Circulating Insulin

The radioimmunoassay of insulin, developed in 1960, permits detection of insulin in picogram quantities, which is below the capabilities of ordinary chemical methods of peptide analysis. The assay is based on antibodies developed in guinea pigs against bovine or pork insulin. Because of the similarities between these 2 insulins and human insulin, the assay successfully measures the human hormone.

With this assay, basal insulin values of 5–15 μU/mL are found in normal humans, with a peak rise to 60–90 μU during meals. Similar assays for measuring all of the known peptide hormones of the endocrine pancreas (including C-peptide and proinsulin) have been developed.

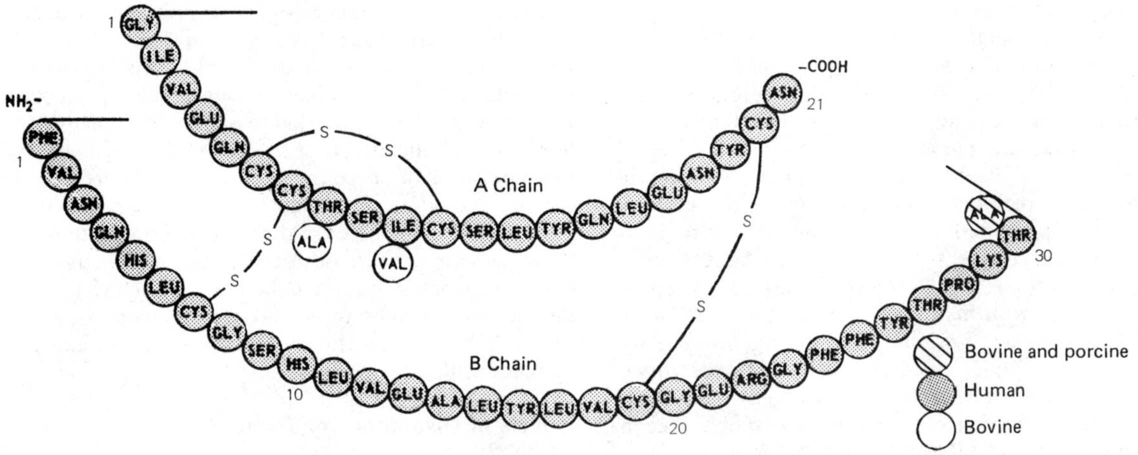

Figure 39–1. Structure of human insulin, with differences in amino acid sequences of porcine and bovine insulin.

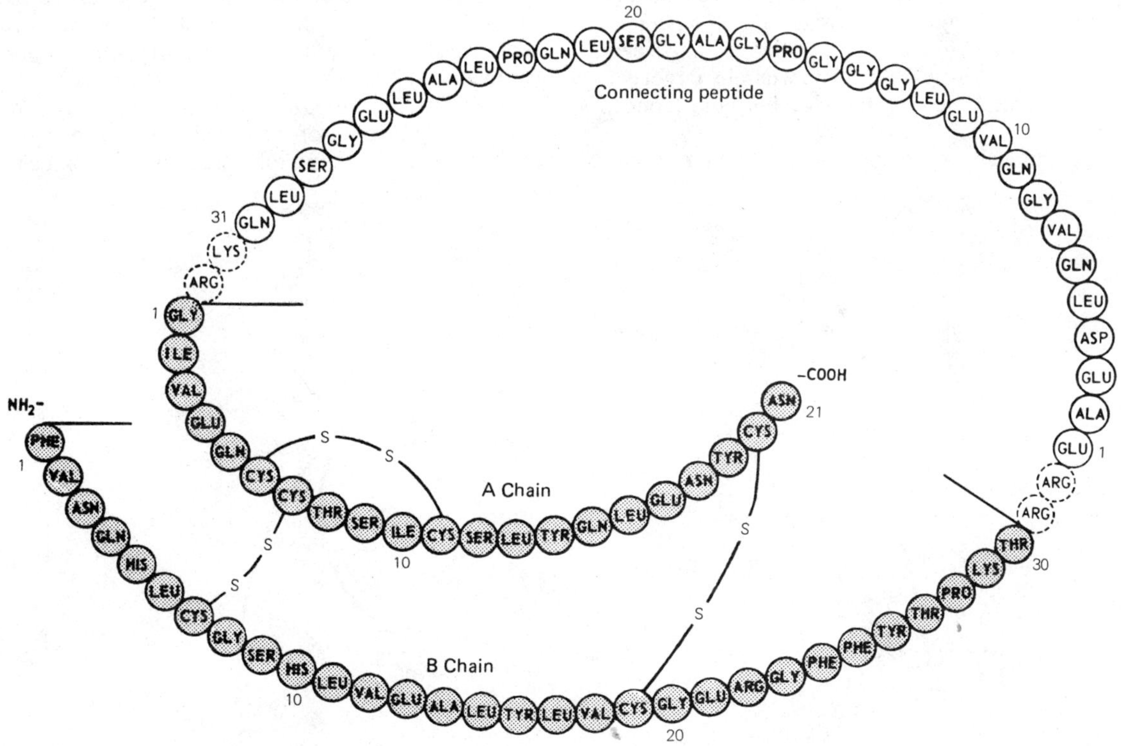

	1	2	3	4	5	6	7	8	9	10	11	12	13	14	15	16
Human:	Glu	Ala	Glu	Asp	Leu	Gln	Val	Gly	Gln	Val	Glu	Leu	Gly	Gly	Gly	Pro
Porcine:	Glu	Ala	Glu	Asn	Pro	Gln	Ala	Gly	Ala	Val	Glu	Leu	Gly	Gly	Gly	Leu
Bovine:	Glu	Val	Glu	Gly	Pro	Gln	Val	Gly	Ala	Leu	Glu	Leu	Ala	Gly	Gly	Pro

	17	18	19	20	21	22	23	24	25	26	27	28	29	30	31
Human:	Gly	Ala	Gly	Ser	Leu	Gln	Pro	Leu	Ala	Leu	Glu	Gly	Ser	Leu	Gln
Porcine:	Gly	—	Gly	—	Leu	Gln	Ala	Leu	Ala	Leu	Glu	Gly	Pro	Pro	Gln
Bovine:	Gly	Ala	Gly	—	—	—	—	—	Gly	Leu	Glu	Gly	Pro	Pro	Gln

Figure 39–2. Structure of human proinsulin. Comparisons of human, porcine, and bovine C-peptides are shown in the accompanying diagram. Identical residues are shown in boxes.

Biologic Effect of Insulin

Insulin promotes the storage of fat as well as glucose (both sources of energy) within specialized target cells (Fig 39–3) and influences cell growth and the metabolic functions of a wide variety of tissues. Once insulin has entered the circulation, it is taken up by specialized receptors that have been found on the membranes of most tissues. However, the biologic responses promoted by these insulin-receptor complexes have been identified in only a few target tissues, eg, liver, muscle, and adipose tissue. The receptors bind insulin with high specificity and affinity in the picomolar range. Various hormonal agents (eg, hydrocortisone) lower the affinity of insulin receptors to insulin; growth hormone in excess increases this affinity slightly. The concentration of these specific receptor molecules as well as their affinity for binding insulin seems to be affected by the concentration of insulin molecules to which they are exposed. In clinical situations associated with elevated blood levels of circulating insulin, such as obesity or insulinoma, the concentration of insulin receptors is reduced. This phenomenon of ''down regulation'' of insulin receptors seems to provide an intrinsic mechanism whereby target cells limit their response to excessive hormone concentrations.

Traditionally, it had been thought that a ''second messenger'' was generated by the combination of insulin with its membrane receptor to initiate both rapid (transport) effects of insulin and more sustained (anabolic) effects. The inability to identify a second messenger for insulin has led to a consideration that at least the anabolic effects of insulin result from cellular internalization of the complex of insulin with its receptor and activation of intracellular processes by some portion of this complex. Although internalization of these complexes has been documented, it remains controversial whether this phenomenon contributes to further action of insulin or is merely a means of limiting further effects of insulin by removing insulin and its receptor within scavenger lysosomes.

Effects of Insulin on Its Target Cells

(Table 39–2)

A. Action of Insulin on Liver: The first major organ endogenous insulin reaches via the portal circulation is the liver, where it acts to increase storage of glucose as glycogen and to reset the liver to the fed state by reversing a number of catabolic mechanisms associated with the postabsorptive state: glycogenolysis, ketogenesis, and gluconeogenesis. These effects are brought about in part through the induction, by insulin, of increased synthesis of pyruvate kinase, phosphofructokinase, and glucokinase,

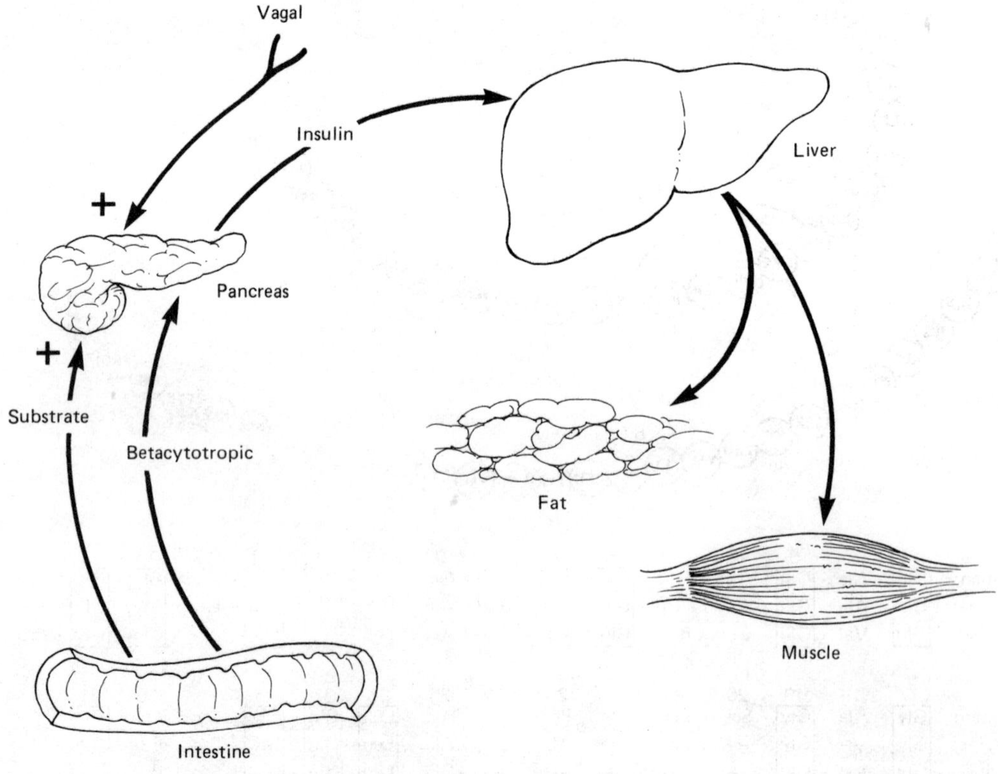

Figure 39–3. Insulin promotes synthesis (from circulating nutrients) and storage of glycogen, triglycerides, and protein in its major target tissues: liver, fat, and muscle. The release of insulin from the pancreas is stimulated by increased blood glucose, vagal nerve stimulation, and other factors (see text).

Table 39–2. Endocrine effects of insulin.

Effect on liver:
Reversal of catabolic features of insulin deficiency
Inhibits glycogenolysis.
Inhibits conversion of fatty acids and amino acids to keto acids.
Inhibits conversion of amino acids to glucose.
Anabolic action
Promotes glucose storage as glycogen (induces glucokinase and glycogen synthetase, inhibits phosphorylase).
Increases triglyceride synthesis and very low density lipoprotein formation.
Effect on muscle:
Increased protein synthesis
Increases amino acid transport.
Increases ribosomal protein synthesis.
Increased glycogen synthesis
Increases glucose transport.
Induces glycogen synthetase and inhibits phosphorylase.
Effect on adipose tissue:
Increased triglyceride storage
Lipoprotein lipase is induced and activated by insulin to hydrolyze triglycerides from lipoproteins.
Glucose transport into cell provides glycerol phosphate to permit esterification of fatty acids supplied by lipoprotein transport.
Intracellular lipase is inhibited by insulin.

and the repression of gluconeogenic enzymes, including pyruvate carboxylase, phosphoenolpyruvate carboxykinase, fructose bisphosphatase, and glucose 6-phosphatase. In addition, insulin decreases urea production, protein catabolism, and cAMP in the liver and increases potassium and phosphate uptake by the organ.

B. Effect of Insulin on Muscle: Insulin promotes protein synthesis by increasing amino acid transport and by stimulating ribosomal activity. It also promotes glycogen synthesis to replace glycogen stores expended by muscle activity. This is accomplished by increasing glucose transport into the muscle cell, inducing glycogen synthetase, and inhibiting phosphorylase. Approximately 500–600 g of glycogen is stored in muscle tissue of a 70-kg male.

C. Effect of Insulin on Adipose Tissue: The most efficient means of storing energy is in the form of triglyceride depots. This provides 9 kcal per gram of stored substrate and, unlike glycogen, does not require water to maintain it within cells. A normal 70-kg man has 12–14 kg of fat in storage, chiefly in adipose tissue.

Insulin acts to reduce circulating free fatty acids and to promote triglyceride storage in adipocytes by 3 primary mechanisms: (1) induction of lipoprotein lipase, which actively hydrolyzes triglycerides from circulating lipoproteins; (2) glucose transport into cells to generate glycerophosphate as a metabolic product, which permits esterification of fatty acids supplied by lipoprotein hydrolysis; and (3) reduction of intracellular lipolysis of stored triglyceride by a direct inhibition of intracellular lipase. These effects appear to involve suppression of cAMP production, and dephosphorylation of the lipases in the fat cell.

Characteristics of Available Insulin Preparations

Commercial insulin preparations differ in a number of ways, including differences in the animal species from which they are obtained; their purity, concentration, and solubility; and the time of onset and duration of their biologic action. In the past few years, a number of additional preparations have been added to the list of available insulins. As a result, in 1982, at least 42 different insulin preparations are available for purchase in the USA. When human insulin becomes available, the number of products may be reduced.

A. Principal Types and Duration of Action of Insulin Preparations: Three principal types of insulins are available: (1) short-acting, with rapid onset of action; (2) intermediate-acting; and (3) long-acting, with slow onset of action (Fig 39–4) (Table 39–3). Short-acting insulin is a crystalline zinc-insulin complex provided in soluble form and dispensed as a clear

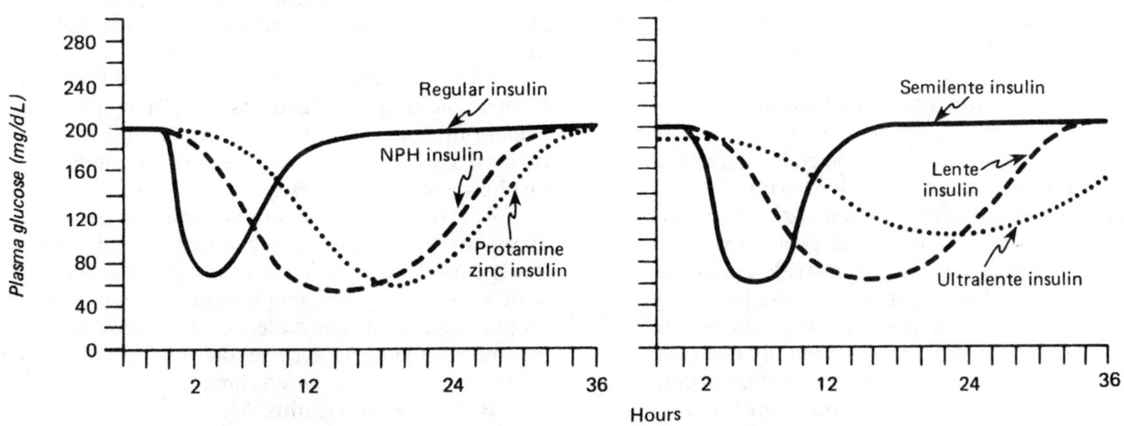

Figure 39–4. Extent and duration of action of various types of insulin (in a fasting diabetic).

Table 39–3. Insulin: Sources and activity.

Type of Preparations	Animal Source	Activity (hours) Peak	Duration*
Rapid-acting			
Insulin injection USP (regular, crystalline zinc)	Beef, pork, or mixture	½–3	5–7
Insulin zinc suspension USP (prompt, semilente)	Beef, pork, or mixture	1–4	12–16
Intermediate-acting			
Isophane insulin suspension USP (NPH insulin)	Beef, pork, or mixture	8–12	18–24
Insulin zinc suspension USP (lente)	Beef, pork, or mixture	8–12	18–24
Long-acting			
Protamine zinc insulin suspension USP (PZI)	Beef, pork, or mixture	8–16	24–36
Insulin zinc suspension extended USP (ultralente)	Beef or mixture	8–16	24–36

*The duration of action is increased with increasing doses.

solution at neutral pH. All other commercial insulins have been modified to provide prolonged action and are dispensed as turbid suspensions at neutral pH with either protamine in phosphate buffer (protamine zinc and NPH insulin) or varying concentrations of zinc in acetate buffer (ultralente, lente, and semilente insulins). Treatment with protamine zinc insulin or semilente preparations is currently decreasing, and almost no clinical indications for their use exist. Conventional subcutaneous insulin therapy presently consists of split-dose injections of mixtures of short-acting and intermediate-acting insulins (NPH or lente) or multiple doses of short-acting insulin preprandially in association with any of 3 insulin suspensions (NPH, lente, or ultralente) whose prolonged duration of action provides overnight basal insulin levels.

1. Short-acting insulin–Regular insulin is a short-acting soluble crystalline zinc insulin whose effect appears within 15 minutes of subcutaneous injection and lasts 5–7 hours. It is the only type of insulin that can be administered intravenously or by infusion pumps. Short-acting soluble insulin is particularly useful for intravenous therapy in the management of diabetic ketoacidosis and when the insulin requirement is changing rapidly, such as after surgery or during acute infections.

2. Lente and ultralente insulin–Lente insulin is a mixture of 30% semilente (an amorphous precipitate of insulin with zinc ions in acetate buffer that has a relatively rapid onset of action) with 70% ultralente insulin (a poorly soluble crystal of zinc and beef insulin that has a delayed onset and prolonged duration of action). These 2 components provide a combination of relatively rapid absorption, with sustained long action making lente insulin a useful therapeutic agent. While both beef and pork insulin can readily form zinc crystals in acetate buffer under the conditions employed, only the beef insulin has the proper hydrophobic alignment within the crystal to provide the delayed, sustained release of insulin characteristic of ultralente. Zinc crystals of pork insulin dissolve more rapidly, and while the appearance of the crystals is virtually identical to that of zinc crystals of beef insulin, the onset of action is earlier and the duration shorter. Accordingly, there is no ultralente insulin made of porcine insulin alone. Until data become available on onset and duration of action of the more recently developed pure pork forms of lentelike insulin (Monotard, from Novo; and Pork Lente Iletin II, from Lilly), one must assume that their time course may be less sustained than that of lente insulin containing beef crystals of ultralente.

Lente insulin is the most widely used of the lente series of insulins, particularly in combination with regular insulin, which has a more rapid onset of action than the semilente component. Ultralente has a very slow onset of action with a prolonged duration, and its administration once or twice daily has been advocated to provide a basal level of insulin comparable to that achieved by basal endogenous insulin secretion or the overnight infusion rate programmed into insulin pumps. There has recently been a resurgence of use of ultralente insulin in combination with multiple injections of regular insulin as a means of attempting optimal control in patients with insulin-dependent diabetes.

3. NPH (neutral protamine Hagedorn, or isophane) insulin–NPH insulin is an intermediate-acting insulin wherein the onset of action is delayed by combining appropriate amounts of insulin and protamine so that neither is present in an uncomplexed form ("isophane"). Protamine isolated from the sperm of rainbow trout is a mixture of 6 major and some minor compounds of similar structure. They appear to be arginine-rich peptides with an average molecular weight of approximately 4400. To form an isophane complex (one in which neither component retains any free binding sites), approximately a 1:10 ratio by weight of protamine to insulin is required—eg, 0.3–0.4 mg of protamine to 4 mg of insulin (100 units). This represents approximately 6 molecules of insulin per molecule of protamine. In the complex, asparagine (the terminal amino acid on insulin's A chain) combines with an arginine-binding site on protamine. After subcutaneous injection, proteolytic enzymes degrade the protamine to permit absorption of insulin.

The onset and duration of action of NPH insulin is comparable to that of lente insulin (Table 39–3); it is usually mixed with regular insulin and given at least twice daily for insulin replacement in patients with insulin-dependent diabetes.

4. Mixtures of insulins–Since intermediate-acting insulins require several hours to reach adequate therapeutic levels, their use in insulin-dependent diabetic patients requires supplements of regular insulin preprandially. For convenience, these may be mixed together in the same syringe and injected subcutaneously in split dosage before breakfast and supper.

B. Species of Insulin: Most commercial insulin in the USA contains beef insulin as its chief component. Beef insulin differs by 3 amino acids from human insulin, whereas only a single amino acid distinguishes pork and human insulins. The beef hormone is slightly more antigenic in humans than is pork insulin. The most commonly prescribed preparations in the USA are standard mixtures containing 70% beef and 30% pork insulin. However, supplies of "monospecies" pork or beef insulin are commercially available and are particularly useful in patients with conditions in which pure monospecies insulin may be indicated, such as insulin allergy or insulin resistance (see below). Recent advances in the mass production of human insulin by recombinant DNA techniques are quite promising, and biosynthetic human insulin has been prepared by inserting a copy of the transcribing portion of the human insulin gene into *E coli*. A semisynthetic human insulin has also been produced by chemical modification of pork insulin, in which the carboxy terminal alanine of the B chain has been replaced by threonine. Both of these human insulin preparations have proved to be safe and effective during short-term trials in nondiabetic human volunteers, and long-term clinical trials are presently in progress to determine their efficacy, safety, and immunogenicity in diabetic patients. At present, semisynthetic human insulin (derived from porcine insulin) is commercially available as Actrapid and Monotard human insulin in the United Kingdom.

C. Purity of Insulin: Recent improvements in purification techniques (using gel columns) have considerably reduced contaminating proteins with molecular weights greater than that of insulin. These include proinsulin and partially cleaved proinsulins that are metabolically inactive yet capable of inducing anti-insulin antibodies. Further purification with chromatography can virtually eliminate these larger proteins and markedly lower the concentration of smaller peptide contaminants. When proinsulin content is less than 10 parts per million, manufacturers are entitled by FDA regulations in the USA to label the insulin as "purified."

In the process of purifying insulin, most of the other islet cell hormones such as glucagon, somatostatin, pancreatic polypeptide, and vasoactive intestinal peptide are removed, so that purified insulin contains much less than 1 ppm of these hormonal contaminants, while standard insulins contain less than 5 ppm. However, some insulin molecules undergo desamidation of asparagine and glutamine residues during purification and storage, so that even purified insulins may contain up to 0.1% desamido insulin. This material apparently has full biologic activity and does not increase the immunogenicity of insulin.

D. Concentration: Currently, most insulins are available in a concentration of 100 units/mL (U100), and all are dispensed in 10-mL vials. To accommodate children and occasional adults who may require small quantities, U40 insulin continues to be produced. For use in rare cases of severe insulin resistance in which large quantities of insulin are required, a limited supply of U500 regular porcine insulin is available.

Insulin Delivery Systems

Automated administration of soluble insulin by "closed loop" systems (blood glucose-controlled insulin infusion systems) has recently been successful in acute situations such as management of diabetic ketoacidosis or maintaining insulin balance of diabetics undergoing surgery. Chronic use of such systems is prevented by the need for uninterrupted aspiration of blood to reach an external glucose sensor and by the size of the computerized insulin pump system used on present models.

Research into smaller "open loop" methods of insulin delivery (insulin reservoir and pump programmed to deliver regular insulin at a calculated rate without a glucose sensor) has resulted in readily portable pumps for subcutaneous, intravenous, or intraperitoneal infusion. As methods for self-monitoring of blood glucose are increasingly accepted by patients, these pump systems are becoming less "open loop" and therefore potentially more useful for managing insulin-dependent diabetics. However, at present, intensive therapy using conventional daily administration of multiple subcutaneous injections of soluble, rapid-acting insulin and a single daily injection of long-acting insulin appears to provide blood glucose control as effective as either type of loop system.

Treatment With Insulin

The current classification of diabetes mellitus identifies a group of patients who have virtually no insulin secretion and whose survival is dependent on administration of exogenous insulin. This "insulin-dependent" group represents only about 10% of the diabetic population. Most diabetics do not require exogenous insulin for survival but may need exogenous supplementation of their endogenous secretion to achieve optimum health.

Complications of Insulin Therapy

A. Hypoglycemia:

1. Mechanisms and diagnosis–Hypoglycemic reactions are the most common complication of insulin therapy. They may result from a delay in taking a meal, unusual physical exertion, or a dose of insulin that is too large for immediate needs. With more patients attempting "tight" control without frequent capillary blood glucose home monitoring, hypoglycemia is likely to become an even more frequent complication.

In older diabetics and those taking longer-acting insulins, autonomic warning signals of hypoglycemia are less frequent, and the manifestations of insulin excess are mainly those of impaired function of the central nervous system, ie, mental confusion, bizarre behavior, and ultimately coma. More rapid development of hypoglycemia from the effects of regular insulin causes signs of autonomic hyperactivity, both adrenergic (tachycardia, palpitations, sweating, tremulousness) and parasympathetic (nausea, hunger), that may progress to convulsions and coma. All of the manifestations of hypoglycemia are rapidly relieved by glucose administration.

An identification bracelet, necklace, or card in the wallet or purse should be carried by every diabetic receiving hypoglycemic drug therapy.

2. Treatment–All of the manifestations of hypoglycemia are rapidly relieved by glucose administration. In a case of mild hypoglycemia in a patient who is conscious and able to swallow, orange juice, glucose, or any sugar-containing beverage or food may be given. If more severe hypoglycemia has produced unconsciousness or stupor, the treatment of choice is to give 20–50 mL of 50% glucose solution by intravenous infusion over a period of 2–3 minutes. If intravenous therapy is not available, 1 mg of glucagon injected intramuscularly will usually restore consciousness within 15 minutes to permit ingestion of sugar. Family members or others in the household should be taught how to give glucagon when the need arises. If the patient is stuporous and glucagon is not available, small amounts of honey or syrup can be inserted within the buccal pouch. In general, however, oral feeding is contraindicated in unconscious patients.

B. Immunopathology of Insulin Therapy: At least 5 molecular classes of insulin antibodies may be produced during the course of insulin therapy in diabetes: IgA, IgD, IgE, IgG, and IgM. There are 2 major types of immune disorders in these patients:

1. Insulin allergy–Insulin allergy, an immediate type hypersensitivity, is a rare condition in which local or systemic urticaria is due to histamine release from tissue mast cells sensitized by anti-insulin IgE antibodies. In severe cases, anaphylaxis results. A subcutaneous nodule appearing several hours later at the site of insulin injection and lasting for up to 24 hours has been attributed to an IgG-mediated complement-binding Arthus reaction. Because sensitivity is often to noninsulin protein contaminants, the new highly purified insulins have markedly reduced the incidence of insulin allergy, especially local reactions. When allergy to beef insulin is present, a species change (eg, to pure pork insulin) may correct the problem. Antihistamines, corticosteroids, and even desensitization may be required, especially for systemic hypersensitivity.

2. Immune insulin resistance–All insulin-treated patients develop a low titer of circulating IgG anti-insulin antibodies that neutralize the action of insulin to a small extent. In some diabetic patients, principally those with some degree of tissue insensitivity to insulin (such as occurs in obese diabetics) and a history of interrupted insulin therapy, a high titer of circulating IgG anti-insulin antibodies develops. This results in extremely high insulin requirements—often more than 200 units daily. This is often a self-limited condition and may clear spontaneously after several months. However, in cases where the circulating antibody is specifically more reactive with beef insulin—a more potent antigen in humans than pork insulin—switching to a less antigenic (pork) insulin may make possible a dramatic reduction in insulin dosage or may at least shorten the duration of immune resistance. Other forms of therapy include sulfated beef insulin (a chemically modified form of beef insulin containing an average of 6 sulfate groups per molecule) and immunosuppression with corticosteroids. In some adults, the foreign insulin can be completely discontinued and the patient maintained on diet alone with oral sulfonylureas. This is possible only when the circulating antibodies do not effectively neutralize the patient's own insulin.

C. Lipodystrophy at Injection Sites: Atrophy or hypertrophy of subcutaneous fatty tissue leading to scarring may occur at the site of injection. This complication has become rare since the development of highly concentrated, pure insulin preparations of neutral pH. Injection of these preparations directly into the atrophic area often results in restoration of normal contours.

ORAL HYPOGLYCEMIC AGENTS

In the USA, the only oral medications available for treating hyperglycemia in non-insulin-dependent diabetics are the class of compounds known as sulfonylureas, which increase the release of endogenous insulin. In other countries, a much wider choice of preparations is available, including a more potent "second-generation" group of sulfonylureas and a second class of compounds, the biguanides, that reduce blood glucose even in the absence of pancreatic B cell function. Biguanides were removed from the market in the USA in 1977, because the use of phenformin was reported to be associated with lactic acidosis.

Sulfonylureas

In 1955, sulfonylurea drugs became widely available for treatment of non-insulin-dependent diabetics. The compounds are arylsulfonylureas with substitutions on the benzene and urea groups. Table 39–4 depicts the chemical structures of the 4 sulfonylureas used in the USA and 2 representative "second-generation" preparations of higher potency that are used in other countries.

Mechanism of Action

At least 3 mechanisms of sulfonylurea action have been proposed: (1) release of insulin from B cells, (2) reduction of serum glucagon levels, and (3) an extrapancreatic effect to increase the number of insulin receptors.

A. Insulin Release From Pancreatic B Cells: When therapy is started, release of preformed insulin is stimulated by sulfonylureas by an unknown mechanism. Insulin synthesis is not stimulated and may even be reduced. Release of insulin in response to the major physiologic stimulus—glucose—is enhanced. There is evidence, however, that after prolonged sulfonylurea therapy, serum insulin levels are no longer increased by the drug and may even be decreased. This

Table 39–4. Sulfonylureas.

Sulfonylurea	**Chemical Structure**	**Daily Dose**	**Duration of Action (hours)**
Tolbutamide (Orinase)	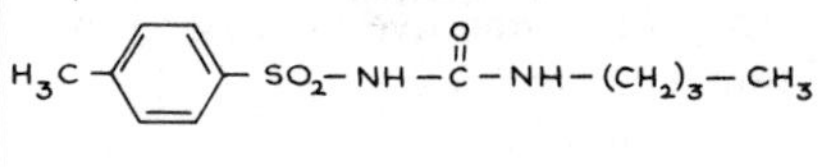	0.5–2 g in divided doses	6–12
Tolazamide (Tolinase)	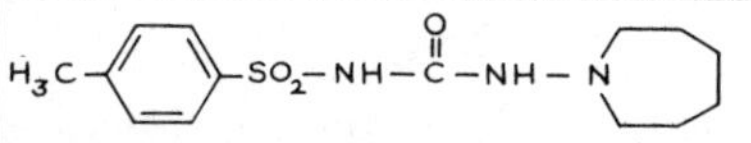	0.1–1 g as single dose or in divided doses	10–14
Acetohexamide (Dymelor)	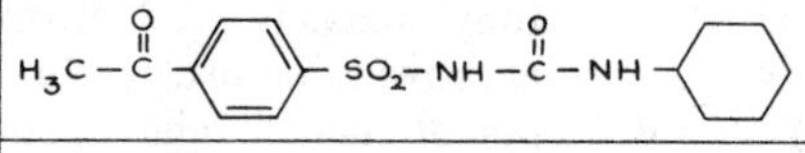	0.25–1.5 g as single dose or in divided doses	12–24
Chlorpropamide (Diabinese)	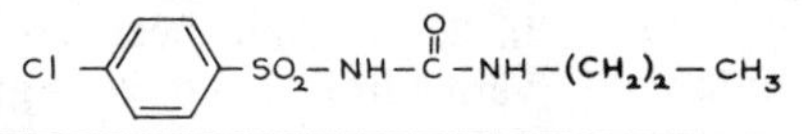	0.1–0.5 g as single dose	Up to 60
Glyburide* [Glibenclamide] * (many products)	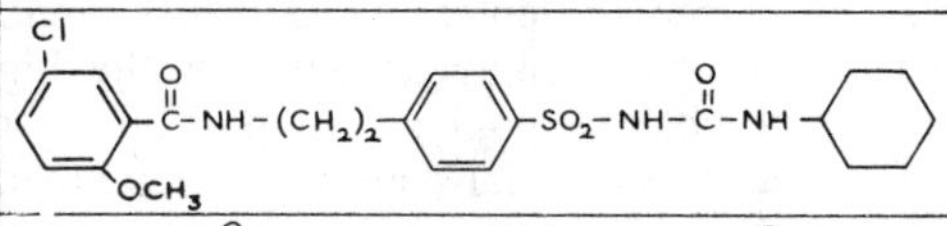	0.0025–0.02 g	10–24
Glipizide* [Glydiazinamide]* (Glibenese, Mindiab, Minodiab)*	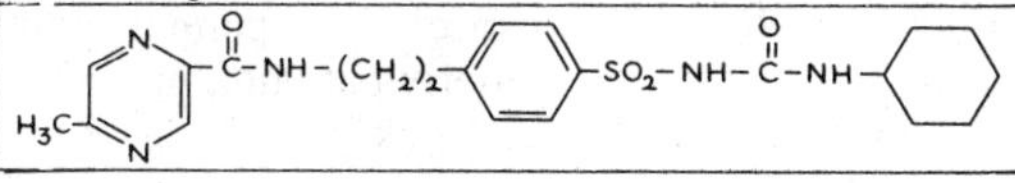	0.0025–0.02 g	3–8

*Outside USA.

observation is complicated by the fact that most such data are obtained from oral glucose tolerance testing—an unphysiologic measure of pancreatic response to a glucose load. After mixed meals containing protein as well as carbohydrate, the beneficial effect of chronic sulfonylurea treatment is generally associated with increased levels of serum insulin.

B. Reduction of Serum Glucagon Concentrations: It is now established that chronic administration of sulfonylureas to non-insulin-dependent diabetics reduces serum glucagon levels. This could contribute to the hypoglycemic effect of the drugs. The mechanism for this suppressive effect of sulfonylureas on glucagon levels is unclear but may involve a direct action on pancreatic A cell secretion or an indirect homeostatic response to enhanced insulin release or insulin effectiveness.

C. Increase in Numbers of Insulin Receptors: There is evidence that increased binding of insulin to tissue receptors occurs during sulfonylurea therapy. As shown in Fig 2–6, an increase in receptor number can increase the effect achieved with a given concentration of agonist; such an action by the sulfonylureas would potentiate the effect of the patient's low levels of insulin as well as that of exogenous insulin. However, in juvenile-onset insulin-dependent diabetics with no endogenous insulin secretion, therapy with sulfonylureas has yet to be shown to improve blood glucose control or enhance sensitivity to administered insulin.

Efficacy & Safety of the Sulfonylureas

In 1970, the University Group Diabetes Program (UGDP) reported that the number of deaths due to cardiovascular disease in diabetic patients treated with tolbutamide was excessive compared to either insulin-treated patients or those receiving placebos. Controversy persists about the validity of the conclusions reached by the UGDP, because of the heterogeneity of the population studied and certain features of the experimental design such as the use of a fixed dose of tolbutamide.

TOLBUTAMIDE

Tolbutamide (Orinase) is supplied in tablets of 250 and 500 mg. It is well absorbed but rapidly oxidized in the liver. Its duration of effect is relatively short (6–10 hours). Tolbutamide is best administered in divided doses (eg, 500 mg before each meal and at bedtime); however, some patients require only 1 or 2 tablets daily. Acute toxic reactions are rare; skin rash occurs infrequently. Prolonged hypoglycemia has been reported rarely, mostly in elderly people or in patients receiving certain drugs (eg, dicumarol, phenylbutazone, or some of the sulfonamides). These drugs apparently compete for oxidative enzymes in the liver, resulting in higher levels of unmetabolized, active tolbutamide in the circulation.

CHLORPROPAMIDE

Chlorpropamide (Diabinese) is supplied in tablets of 100 and 250 mg. This drug, with a half-life of 32 hours, is slowly metabolized; approximately 20–30% is excreted unchanged in the urine. Chlorpropamide also interacts with the drugs mentioned above that depend on hepatic oxidative catabolism, and it is contraindicated in patients with hepatic or renal insufficiency. The average maintenance dose is 250 mg daily, given as a single dose in the morning. Prolonged hypoglycemic reactions are more common than with tolbutamide, particularly in elderly patients, in whom chlorpropamide therapy should be monitored with special care. Doses in excess of 250 mg daily increase the risk of jaundice, which is uncommon at lower doses. Patients with a genetic predisposition who are taking chlorpropamide may experience a hyperemic flush when alcohol is ingested. Dilutional hyponatremia has been recognized as a complication of chlorpropamide therapy in some patients. This appears to result from both a stimulation of vasopressin secretion and a potentiation of its action at the renal tubule by chlorpropamide. The antidiuretic effect of chlorpropamide appears to be independent of the sulfonylurea part of its structure, since 3 other sulfonylureas (acetohexamide, tolazamide, and glyburide) have diuretic effects in man. Hematologic toxicity (transient leukopenia, thrombocytopenia) occurs in less than 1% of patients.

ACETOHEXAMIDE

Acetohexamide (Dymelor) is supplied in tablets of 250 and 500 mg. Its duration of action is 10–16 hours—intermediate between tolbutamide and chlorpropamide. Therapeutic doses consist of 0.25–1.5 g daily in one or 2 doses. Liver metabolism is rapid, but the metabolite produced remains active. Side-effects are similar to those of the other sulfonylurea drugs.

TOLAZAMIDE

Tolazamide (Tolinase) is supplied in tablets of 100, 250, and 500 mg. It is comparable to chlorpropamide in potency but has a shorter duration of action, similar to that of acetohexamide. Tolazamide is more slowly absorbed than the other sulfonylureas, and its effect on blood glucose does not appear for several hours. Its half-life is about 7 hours. Tolazamide is metabolized to several compounds that retain hypoglycemic effects. If more than 500 mg per day is required, the dose should be divided and given twice daily. Doses larger than 1000 mg daily do not further improve the degree of blood glucose control.

GLYBURIDE

Glyburide (Micronase), the newest of the sulfonylureas, is used in other countries but is not yet approved for use in the USA. Although it is more potent than the other agents, no qualitative differences in action have been documented. Effective dosage varies from 2.5 to 20 mg; unfamiliarity with its great potency (100 times greater than that of tolbutamide) may account for the high incidence of severe hypoglycemic reactions, with occasional fatalities. Special caution is recommended when using this drug, especially in patients with cardiovascular disease or in elderly patients, in whom hypoglycemia carries a special risk.

Biguanides

The structure of biguanides is shown in Table 39–5.

Phenformin was discontinued in the USA because of its association with lactic acidosis and because there was no documentation of any long-term benefit from its use. Metformin, buformin, and phenformin continue to be used elsewhere, although in some areas the indications for biguanide therapy are being reevaluated.

Mechanism of Action

An explanation of the mechanism of action of biguanides remains elusive. Its blood glucose-lowering action does not depend on the presence of functioning pancreatic B cells. Glucose is not lowered in normal subjects after an overnight fast, but postprandial blood glucose levels are considerably lower during phenformin administration. Patients with maturity-onset diabetes have considerably less fasting hyperglycemia as well as postprandial hyperglycemia

Table 39–5. Biguanides.

Biguanide	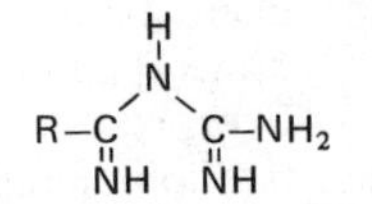	Daily Dose	Duration of Action (hours)
Phenformin (DBI, Meltrol)	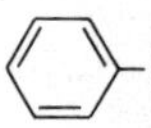 $-(CH_2)_2-NH-$	0.025–0.15 g as single dose or in divided doses	4–6 8–14
Buformin*	$CH_3-(CH_2)_3-NH-$	0.05–0.3 g in divided doses	. . .
Metformin*	$(CH_3)_2-N-$	1–3 g in divided doses	. . .

*In clinical use outside USA.

after biguanides; however, hypoglycemia during biguanide therapy is essentially unknown. These agents might therefore be more appropriately termed "euglycemic" rather than hypoglycemic agents. Currently proposed mechanisms of action include (1) direct stimulation of glycolysis in peripheral tissues, with increased glucose removal from blood; (2) reduced hepatic gluconeogenesis; (3) slowing of glucose absorption from the gastrointestinal tract; and (4) inhibition of plasma glucagon levels.

Metabolism & Excretion

Phenformin is bound to plasma protein, and therapeutic dose levels range from 100 to 250 ng/mL. The half-life is approximately 11 hours. Phenformin is about one-third metabolized by hydroxylation of its benzene ring and thereby rendered biologically inactive; the remainder is excreted in the active unmetabolized form. In patients with renal insufficiency, unmetabolized phenformin accumulates in high concentration and thereby increases the risk of lactic acidosis, which appears to be a dose-related complication.

Clinical Use of Biguanides

Biguanides have been most often prescribed for patients with refractory obesity whose hyperglycemia is due to ineffective insulin action. Another indication for its use is in certain nonobese adult-onset diabetics in whom sulfonylurea therapy alone is less effective than when combined with phenformin.

Phenformin is contraindicated in patients with renal disease, alcoholism, hepatic disease, or conditions predisposing to tissue anoxia, such as chronic cardiopulmonary dysfunction, because of an increased risk of lactic acidosis induced by this drug in the presence of these diseases.

In the UGDP study, phenformin given in a dosage of 100 mg daily showed no favorable effects in comparison with a control group of placebo-treated patients. A slight increase in heart rate and blood pressure was noted in the phenformin-treated diabetics, and an increased risk of cardiovascular mortality was reported.

GLUCAGON

Chemistry & Metabolism

Glucagon is synthesized in the A cells of the pancreatic islets of Langerhans (Table 39–1). Glucagon is a polypeptide—identical in all mammals—consisting of a single chain of 29 amino acids (Fig 39–5), with a molecular weight of 3485. Selective proteolytic cleavage converts a large precursor molecule of approximately MW 18,000 to glucagon. One of the precursor intermediates consists of a 100-amino-acid polypeptide called **glicentin,** which contains the glucagon sequence interposed between peptide extensions.

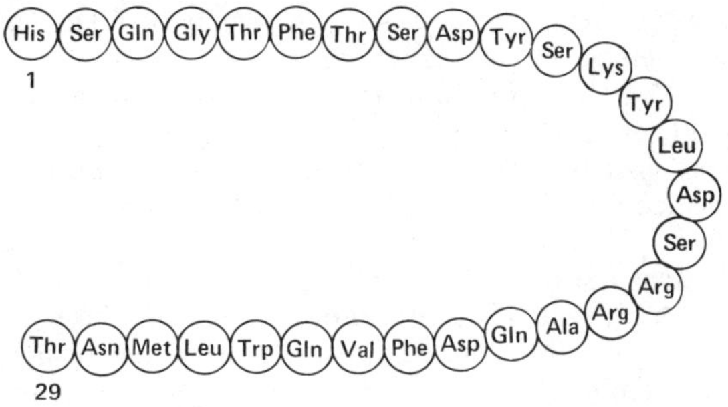

Figure 39–5. Amino acid sequence of glucagon polypeptide.

Glucagon is extensively degraded in the liver and kidney as well as in plasma, and at its tissue receptor sites. Because of its rapid deactivation by plasma, chilling of the collecting tubes and addition of antiproteolytic enzymes such as aprotinin are necessary when samples of blood are collected for immunoassay of circulating glucagon. Its half-life in plasma is between 3 and 6 minutes, which is similar to that of insulin.

"Gut Glucagon"

Glicentin immunoreactivity has been found in cells of the small intestine as well as in pancreatic A cells and in effluents of perfused pancreas. The intestinal cells secrete **enteroglucagon,** a family of glucagonlike polypeptides, of which glicentin is a member. Unlike the pancreatic A cell, these intestinal cells lack the enzymes to convert glucagon precursors to true glucagon by removing the carboxy terminal extension from the molecule. Accordingly, the enteroglucagons do not react with antibody directed against the carboxy terminus of glucagon.

The function of the enteroglucagons has not been clarified, although smaller precursors can bind hepatic glucagon receptors where they exert partial activity.

Pharmacologic Effects of Glucagon

A. Metabolic Effects: The first 6 amino acids at the N-terminus of the glucagon molecule bind to specific receptors on liver cells. This leads to an increase in production of cAMP, which facilitates catabolism of stored glycogen and increases gluconeogenesis and ketogenesis. The immediate pharmacologic result of glucagon infusion is to raise blood glucose at the expense of stored hepatic glycogen. There is no effect on skeletal muscle glycogen, presumably because of the lack of glucagon receptors on skeletal muscle. Pharmacologic amounts of glucagon cause release of insulin from normal pancreatic B cells, catecholamines from pheochromocytoma, and calcitonin from medullary carcinoma cells.

B. Cardiac Effects: Glucagon has been shown to have an inotropic and chronotropic effect on the heart.

However, it has not proved to be clinically useful in the management of cardiac failure.

C. Effects on Smooth Muscle: Glucagon has also been used extensively in radiology as an aid to x-ray visualization of the bowel, because large doses produce a profound relaxation of the intestine.

Clinical Uses

A. Severe Hypoglycemia: The major use of glucagon is for emergency treatment of severe hypoglycemic reactions in insulin-dependent patients when unconsciousness prohibits oral feedings (see p 464).

B. Endocrine Diagnosis: Several diagnostic tests use glucagon to diagnose endocrine pathophysiologic processes. In patients with insulin-dependent diabetes mellitus, a standard test of pancreatic B cell secretory reserve utilizes 1 mg of glucagon administered as an intravenous bolus. Since insulin-treated patients develop circulating anti-insulin antibodies that interfere with radioimmunoassays of insulin, measurements of C-peptide are used to indicate B cell secretion. Normal persons achieve a standard serum concentration of pancreatic C-peptide within 10 minutes of the injection, and in insulin-treated diabetics various degrees of B cell insufficiency can be quantitated. Most long-standing insulin-dependent diabetics show no C-peptide response to glucagon.

In patients with suspected endocrine tumors such as insulinoma, pheochromocytoma, or medullary carcinoma of the thyroid, a bolus of 0.5–1 mg of glucagon intravenously is occasionally effective in discharging hormonal products from a tumor, although negative tests may not rule out the diagnosis.

Adverse Reactions

Transient nausea and occasional vomiting can result from glucagon administration. These are generally mild, and glucagon is relatively free of severe adverse reactions.

• • •

References

Albisser AM et al: An artificial endocrine pancreas. *Diabetes* 1974;**23:**389.

Berger M et al: Absorption kinetics and biologic effects of subcutaneously injected insulin preparations. *Diabetes Care* 1982;**5:**77.

Deckert T: Intermediate-acting insulin preparations: NPH and lente. *Diabetes Care* 1980;**3:**623.

Galloway JA: Insulin treatment for the early 80's: Facts and questions about old and new insulins and their usage. *Diabetes Care* 1980;**3:**615.

Galloway JA et al: Factors influencing the absorption, serum insulin concentration, and blood glucose response, after injections of regular insulin and various insulin mixtures. *Diabetes Care* 1981;**4:**366.

Goldstein DE et al: Clinical application of glycosylated hemoglobin measurements. *Diabetes* 1982;**31(Suppl 3):**70.

Greenfield MS et al: Effect of sulfonylurea treatment on in vivo insulin secretion and action in patients with non-insulin-dependent diabetes mellitus. *Diabetes* 1982;**31:**307.

Grodsky GM et al: Pancreatic action of the sulfonylureas. *Fed Proc* 1977;**36:**2714.

Karam JH, Matin SB, Forsham PH: Antidiabetic drugs after the University Group Diabetes Program. *Annu Rev Pharmacol* 1975;**15:**351.

Marliss EB et al: Present and future expectations regarding insulin infusion systems. *Diabetes Care* 1981;**4:**325.

Peterson CM (editor): Symposium on optimal insulin delivery. *Diabetes Care* 1982;**5(Suppl 1):**1.

Seltzer HS: Efficacy and safety of oral hypoglycemic agents. *Annu Rev Med* 1980;**31:**261.

Skillman TG, Feldman JF: The pharmacology of sulfonylureas. *Am J Med* 1981;**70:**361.

Skyler JS: A plethora of insulins. *Diabetes Care* 1980;**3:**638.

Soeldner JS: Treatment of diabetes mellitus by devices. *Am J Med* 1981;**70:**183.

Tattersal RB, Gale EAM: Patient self-monitoring of blood glucose and refinements of conventional insulin treatment. *Am J Med* 1981;**70:**177.

Unger RH: Meticulous control of diabetes: Benefits, risks, and precautions. *Diabetes* 1982;**31:**479.

Agents That Affect Bone Mineral Homeostasis | 40

Daniel D. Bikle, MD, PhD

I. BASIC PHARMACOLOGY

Calcium and phosphate, the major mineral constituents of bone, are also 2 of the most important minerals for general cellular function. Accordingly, the body has evolved a complex set of mechanisms by which calcium and phosphate homeostasis is carefully maintained. Approximately 98% of the 1–2 kg of calcium and 85% of the 1 kg of phosphorus in the human adult is found in bone, the principal reservoir for these minerals. This function is dynamic, with constant remodeling of bone and ready exchange of bone mineral with that in the extracellular fluid. Bone also serves as the principal structural support for the body and provides the space for hematopoiesis. Thus, abnormalities in bone mineral homeostasis can lead not only to a wide variety of cellular dysfunction (eg, tetany, coma, muscle weakness) but also to disturbances in structural support of the body (eg, osteoporosis with fractures) and loss of hematopoietic capacity (eg, infantile osteopetrosis).

Calcium and phosphate enter the body from the intestine. The average American diet provides 600–1000 mg of calcium per day, of which approximately 100–250 mg is absorbed. This figure represents net absorption, since both absorption (principally in the duodenum and upper jejunum) and secretion (principally in the ileum) occur. The amount of phosphorus in the American diet is about the same as that of calcium. However, the efficiency of absorption (principally in the jejunum) is greater, ranging from 70 to 90% depending on intake. In the steady state, renal excretion of calcium and phosphate balances intestinal absorption. In general, over 95% of filtered calcium and 85% of filtered phosphate is reabsorbed by the kidney. The movement of calcium and phosphate across the intestinal and renal epithelia is closely regulated. Intrinsic disease of intestine (eg, nontropical sprue) or kidney (eg, chronic renal failure) disrupts bone mineral homeostasis.

Two hormones serve as the principal regulators of calcium and phosphate homeostasis: the polypeptide parathyroid hormone (PTH) and the steroid vitamin D. Vitamin D is a prohormone, rather than a true hormone, since it must be further metabolized to gain biologic activity. Other hormones—calcitonin, prolactin, growth hormone, insulin, thyroid hormone, glucocorticoids, and sex steroids—influence calcium and phosphate homeostasis under certain physiologic circumstances and can be considered secondary regulators. Deficiency or excess of these secondary regulators within a physiologic range does not produce the disturbance of calcium and phosphate homeostasis observed in situations of deficiency or excess PTH and vitamin D. However, certain of these secondary regulators—especially calcitonin, glucocorticoids, and estrogens—are useful therapeutically and will be discussed in subsequent sections.

In addition to these regulators, calcium and phosphate themselves, other ions such as sodium and fluoride, and a variety of drugs (diphosphonates, mithramycin, and thiazides) also alter calcium and phosphate homeostasis. This chapter is concerned with the pharmacology of these agents.

PRINCIPAL HORMONAL REGULATORS OF BONE MINERAL HOMEOSTASIS

PARATHYROID HORMONE

Parathyroid hormone (PTH) is a single-chain polypeptide hormone composed of 84 amino acids. It is produced in the parathyroid gland in a precursor form of 115 amino acids, the remaining 31 N-terminal amino acids being cleaved off prior to secretion. Within the gland is a calcium-sensitive protease capable of cleaving the intact hormone into fragments. Biologic activity resides in the N-terminal region such that synthetic 1–34 PTH is fully active. Loss of the first two N-terminal amino acids eliminates activity.

The metabolic clearance rate of intact PTH in dogs has been estimated to be 20 mL/min/kg, with a half-time of disappearance measured in minutes. Most of the clearance occurs in the liver and kidney. The biologically inactive C-terminal fragments produced during metabolism of the intact hormone have a much lower clearance rate, especially in renal failure. This accounts, in part, for the very high PTH values often observed in patients with renal failure when measured by radioimmunoassays directed against the C-terminal region of the molecule. The appearance of N-terminal fragments of PTH in the blood is difficult to demonstrate, consistent with the observations that only small amounts of such fragments are released into the blood and that their clearance is high.

PTH regulates calcium and phosphate flux across cellular membranes in bone and kidney, resulting in increased serum calcium and decreased serum phosphate. In bone, PTH leads to increased activity and number of osteoclasts, the cells responsible for bone resorption. This action increases bone turnover or bone remodeling, a specific sequence of cellular events initiated by osteoclastic bone resorption and followed by osteoblastic bone formation. Although both bone resorption and bone formation are enhanced by PTH, the net effect of excess PTH is to increase bone resorption. Preliminary evidence indicates that PTH in low doses may actually increase bone formation without first stimulating bone resorption. This raises the possibility of direct effects of PTH on both osteoblasts and osteoclasts, which differ depending on the concentration of hormone. Although cAMP is involved in the action of PTH on bone cells, other mediators (including calcium) probably play a role.

In the kidney, PTH increases the ability of the nephron to reabsorb calcium and magnesium but reduces its ability to reabsorb phosphate, amino acids, bicarbonate, sodium, chloride, and sulfate. Although PTH markedly stimulates the renal production and excretion of cAMP and cAMP reproduces a number of the renal actions of PTH, cAMP may not be the sole mediator of PTH action on the kidney. Another important action of PTH on the kidney is its stimulation of 1,25-dihydroxyvitamin D (1,25[OH]$_2$D) production.

Recent evidence has called attention to vasoactive and cardiotropic actions of PTH. These observations may explain the ability of PTH to increase the glomerular filtration rate acutely. Whether such actions are involved in the apparent association of hyperparathyroidism and hypertension remains to be determined.

VITAMIN D

Vitamin D is a secosteroid produced in the skin from 7-dehydrocholesterol under the influence of ultraviolet irradiation. Vitamin D is also found in certain foods and is used to supplement dairy products. Both the natural form (vitamin D$_3$, cholecalciferol) and the plant-derived form (vitamin D$_2$, ergocalciferol) are present in the diet. These forms differ in that ergocalciferol contains a double bond (C22–23) and an additional methyl group in the side chain. This difference in humans apparently is of little physiologic consequence, and the following comments apply equally well to both forms of vitamin D.

Vitamin D is really a prohormone and serves as precursor to a number of biologically active metabolites (Fig 40–1). Vitamin D is first hydroxylated in the

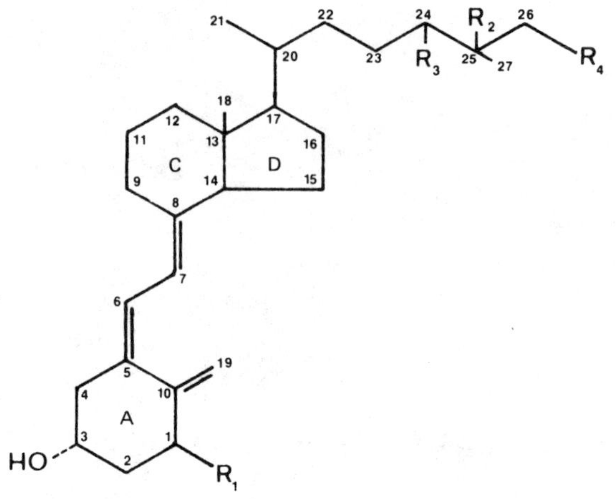

Figure 40–1. The structure of vitamin D$_3$. R$_1$–R$_4$ represent the sites of principal hyroxylation by which vitamin D$_3$ is converted to biologically active metabolites. R$_1$ = 1α(OH); R$_2$ = 25(OH); R$_3$ = 24(OH); R$_4$ = 26(OH). The letters in the rings (A, C, D) and the carbon numbering are derived from the steroid nucleus of 7-dehydrocholesterol.

liver to form 25-hydroxyvitamin D (25[OH]D). This metabolite is further converted in the kidney to a number of other forms the best-studied of which are 1,25-dihydroxyvitamin D (1,25[OH]$_2$D), 24,25-dihydroxyvitamin D (24,25[OH]$_2$D), 25,26-dihydroxyvitamin D (25,26[OH]$_2$D), 1,24,25-trihydroxyvitamin D (1,24,25[OH]$_3$D), 1,25,26-trihydroxyvitamin D (1,25,26[OH]$_3$D), and the 25(OH)D-26,23-lactone. Only vitamin D, 25(OH)D (as calcifediol), and 1,25(OH)$_2$D (as calcitriol), are available for clinical use, although clinical studies with 24,25(OH)$_2$D are under way. The regulation of vitamin D metabolism is complex, involving calcium, phosphate, and a variety of hormones the most important of which is PTH.

Vitamin D and its metabolites circulate in plasma tightly bound to a carrier protein, the vitamin D-binding protein. This α-globulin binds 25(OH)D and 24,25(OH)$_2$D with comparable high affinity and vitamin D and 1,25(OH)$_2$D with lower affinity. In normal subjects, the terminal half-life of injected calcifediol is 23 days, whereas in anephric subjects it is longer (42 days). The half-life of 24,25(OH)$_2$D is probably similar. Tracer studies with vitamin D have shown a rapid clearance from the blood. The liver appears to be the principal organ for clearance. Excess vitamin D is stored in adipose tissue. The metabolic clearance rate of calcitriol in humans indicates a rapid turnover, with a terminal half-life measured in hours.

The mechanism of action of the vitamin D metabolites remains under active investigation. However, calcitriol is well established as the most potent agent with respect to stimulation of intestinal calcium and phosphate transport and bone resorption. Calcitriol appears to act on the intestine both by induction of new protein (calcium-binding protein) and by modulation of calcium flux across the brush border and mitochondrial membranes by a means that does not require new protein synthesis. The molecular action of calcitriol on bone has received less attention, but it does appear to require protein synthesis. The metabolites 25(OH)D and 24,25$(OH)_2$D are far less potent stimulators of intestinal calcium and phosphate transport or bone resorption. However, 25(OH)D appears to be more potent than 1,25$(OH)_2$D in stimulating renal reabsorption of calcium and phosphate and may be the major metabolite regulating calcium flux and contractility in muscle. Recent evidence suggests that the main physiologic action of 24,25$(OH)_2$D is to stimulate bone formation. Specific cytosol receptors for 1,25$(OH)_2$D exist in target tissues that transport this metabolite into the nucleus. However, the role and even the existence of cellular receptors for 25(OH)D and 24,25$(OH)_2$D remain controversial.

INTERACTION OF PTH & VITAMIN D

A summary of the principal actions of PTH and vitamin D on the 3 main target tissues—intestine, kidney, and bone—is presented in Table 40–1. The net effect of PTH is to raise serum calcium and reduce serum phosphate; the net effect of vitamin D is to raise both. As is the case with other endocrine systems also, regulation of calcium and phosphate homeostasis is achieved through a variety of feedback loops. Calcium is the principal regulator of PTH secretion; as serum calcium levels rise, PTH secretion falls. Phosphate regulates PTH secretion indirectly, by forming complexes with calcium in the serum. Since it is the ionized concentration of calcium that is detected by the parathyroid gland, increases in serum phosphate levels reduce the ionized calcium and lead to stimulation of PTH secretion. Such feedback regulation is appropriate to the net effect of PTH to raise serum calcium and reduce serum phosphate levels. Likewise, both calcium and phosphate at high levels reduce the amount of 1,25$(OH)_2$D produced by the kidney and increase the amount of 24,25$(OH)_2$D produced. Since 1,25$(OH)_2$D raises serum calcium and phosphate, whereas 24,25$(OH)_2$D has less effect, such feedback regulation is again appropriate.

A different type of interaction is observed between PTH secretion and vitamin D metabolism. PTH stimulates 1,25$(OH)_2$D production and may reduce 24,25$(OH)_2$D production by the kidney. Conversely, 24,25$(OH)_2$D appears to suppress PTH secretion, whereas 1,25$(OH)_2$D does not if serum calcium is fixed. These interactions suggest a feed-forward or amplification interaction between PTH secretion and 1,25$(OH)_2$D production such that these hormone levels can rise or fall together if required to maintain normal serum calcium levels.

Table 40–1. Actions of PTH and vitamin D on gut, bone, and kidney.

	PTH	Vitamin D
Intestine	Increased calcium and phosphate absorption (by increased 1,25$[OH]_2$D production).	Increased calcium and phosphate absorption (by 1,25$[OH]_2$D).
Kidney	Decreased calcium excretion, increased phosphate excretion.	Calcium and phosphate excretion may be decreased by 25(OH)D and 1,25$(OH)_2$D.
Bone	Calcium and phosphate resorption increased by high doses. Low doses may increase bone formation.	Increased calcium and phosphate resorption by 1,25$(OH)_2$D. Bone formation may be increased by 24,25$(OH)_2$D.
Net effect on serum levels	Serum calcium increased, serum phosphate decreased.	Serum calcium and phosphate both increased.

THE SECONDARY HORMONAL REGULATORS OF BONE MINERAL HOMEOSTASIS

A number of hormones modulate the actions of PTH and vitamin D in regulating bone mineral homeostasis. Compared to PTH and vitamin D, the physiologic impact of such secondary regulation on bone mineral homeostasis is minor. However, in pharmacologic amounts, a number of these hormones have actions on the bone mineral homeostatic mechanisms that can be exploited therapeutically.

CALCITONIN

The calcitonin secreted by the parafollicular cells of the mammalian thyroid (and by piscine ultimobranchial bodies) is a single-chain polypeptide hormone with 32 amino acids and a molecular weight of 3600. A disulfide bond between positions 1 and 7 is essential for biologic activity. Calcitonin is produced in these glands from a precursor with MW 15,000. The circulating forms of calcitonin are multiple, ranging in size from the monomer (MW 3600) to forms with an apparent molecular weight of 60,000. Whether such heterogeneity includes precursor forms or covalently linked oligomers is not known. Because of its heterogeneity, calcitonin is standardized by bioassay in rats. Activity is compared to a standard maintained by the British Medical Research Council (MRC) and expressed as MRC units.

Human calcitonin monomer has a half-life of about 10 minutes with a metabolic clearance rate of 8–9 mL/kg/min. Salmon calcitonin has a longer half-life and a reduced metabolic clearance rate (3 mL/kg/min). Much of the clearance occurs in the kidney, although little intact calcitonin appears in the urine.

The principal effects of calcitonin are to lower serum calcium and phosphate by actions on bone and kidney. Calcitonin inhibits osteoclastic bone resorption. Although bone formation is not impaired at first after calcitonin administration, with time both formation and resorption of bone are reduced. Thus, the early hope that calcitonin would prove useful in restoring bone mass has not been realized. In the kidney, calcitonin reduces both calcium and phosphate reabsorption as well as reabsorption of other ions, including sodium, potassium, and magnesium. Although calcitonin stimulates cAMP formation in both bone and kidney, a requirement for cAMP in mediating these actions is not established. PTH also stimulates cAMP accumulation in these tissues, yet the effects of PTH and calcitonin are generally antagonistic. Other tissues are also affected by calcitonin. Calcitonin in pharmacologic amounts decreases gastrin secretion and reduces gastric acid output while increasing secretion of sodium, potassium, chloride, and water in the gut. Pentagastrin is a potent stimulator of calcitonin secretion (as is hypercalcemia), suggesting a possible physiologic relationship between gastrin and calcitonin. In the adult human, no readily demonstrable problem develops in cases of calcitonin deficiency (thyroidectomy) or excess (medullary carcinoma of the thyroid). However, the ability of calcitonin to acutely block bone resorption and lower serum calcium makes it a useful drug for the treatment of Paget's disease and hypercalcemia.

GLUCOCORTICOIDS

Glucocorticoid hormones alter bone mineral homeostasis by antagonizing vitamin D-stimulated intestinal calcium transport, by blocking bone collagen synthesis, and by increasing PTH-stimulated bone resorption (although this last action is not universally accepted). Although these observations underscore the negative impact of glucocorticoids on bone mineral homeostasis, these hormones have proved useful in 2 situations involving bone mineral homeostasis: in the intermediate term treatment of hypercalcemia and as a diagnostic test of the cause of hypercalcemia.

ESTROGENS

Estrogens can prevent accelerated bone loss during the immediate postmenopausal period. Estrogens do not restore bone in the patient who already has osteoporosis. The prevailing hypothesis to explain these observations is that estrogens reduce the bone-resorbing action of PTH. The renal response to PTH may also be altered by estrogens. Estrogen administration leads to an increased $1,25(OH)_2D$ level in blood, but estrogens have no direct effect on $1,25(OH)_2D$ production in vitro. Conceivably, most—if not all—of the observed increase in $1,25(OH)_2D$ levels with estrogen therapy reflects the increase in vitamin D-binding protein and may not be associated with increased $1,25(OH)_2D$ production or free $1,25(OH)_2D$ levels. The principal therapeutic application for estrogen administration in disorders of bone mineral homeostasis is the treatment or prevention of postmenopausal osteoporosis.

NONHORMONAL AGENTS AFFECTING BONE MINERAL HOMEOSTASIS

DIPHOSPHONATES

The diphosphonates are analogs of pyrophosphate in which the P–O–P bond has been replaced with a nonhydrolyzable P–C–P bond (Fig 40–2). Only ethane-1-hydroxy-1,1-diphosphonate (EHDP, etidronate) is available for clinical use, although other forms are undergoing clinical trials. The diphosphonates owe their clinical usefulness and toxicity to their ability to retard formation and dissolution of hydroxyapatite crystals within and without the skeletal system.

The results from animal studies indicate that 1–10% of an oral dose of etidronate is absorbed. Nearly half of the absorbed drug accumulates in bone; the remainder is excreted unchanged in the urine. That portion bound to bone is retained for weeks, depending on the turnover of bone itself.

Etidronate and the other diphosphonates exert a variety of effects on bone mineral homeostasis. Their physicochemical properties of reducing hy-

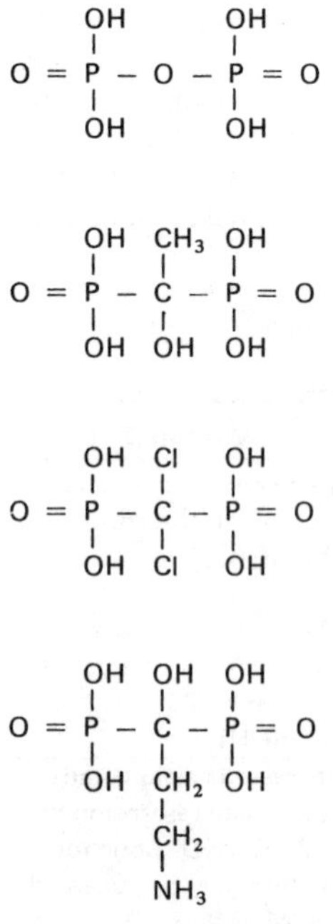

Inorganic pyrophosphoric acid

Ethane-1-hydroxy-1,1-diphosphonic acid (EHDP)

Dichloromethane diphosphonic acid (Cl_2MDP)

3-Amino-1-hydroxy-propane-1,1-diphosphonic acid (AHPDP)

Figure 40–2. The structure of pyrophosphate and the 3 diphosphonates that have been most studied. EHDP (etidronate), Cl_2MDP, and AHPDP.

droxyapatite formation and dissolution make them clinically useful. However, the diphosphonates exert a variety of other cellular effects, including inhibition of $1,25(OH)_2D$ production, inhibition of intestinal calcium transport, metabolic changes in bone cells such as inhibition of glycolysis, inhibition of cell growth, and changes in acid and alkaline phosphatase. These effects vary depending on the diphosphonate being studied and may account for some of the clinical differences observed in the effects of the various diphosphonates on bone mineral homeostasis.

MITHRAMYCIN

Mithramycin is a cytotoxic antibiotic (see Chapter 56) that has been used clinically for 2 disorders of bone mineral metabolism: Paget's disease and hypercalcemia. The cytotoxic properties of the drug appear to involve its binding to DNA and interruption of DNA-directed RNA synthesis. The reasons for its usefulness in the treatment of Paget's disease and hypercalcemia are unclear but may relate to the need for protein synthesis to sustain bone resorption. The doses required to treat Paget's disease and hypercalcemia are about one-tenth the amounts required to achieve cytotoxic effects.

THIAZIDES

The chemistry and pharmacology of this family of drugs are covered in Chapter 13. The principal application of thiazides in the treatment of bone mineral disorders is in reducing renal calcium excretion by some mechanism that is presently unclear. It may be that thiazides increase the effectiveness of parathyroid hormone in stimulating reabsorption of calcium by the renal tubules. They may also act on calcium reabsorption secondarily by increasing sodium reabsorption in the proximal tubule, thus reducing sodium delivery to the distal tubule. Thiazides have proved to be quite useful in reducing the hypercalciuria and incidence of stone formation in subjects with idiopathic hypercalciuria. Part of their efficacy in reducing stone formation may also lie in their ability to decrease urine oxalate excretion and increase urine magnesium and zinc levels (both of which inhibit calcium oxalate stone formation).

FLUORIDE

Fluoride is the only clinically available agent known to increase bone formation in the presence of adequate calcium, phosphate, and vitamin D without stimulating bone resorption. When used in patients with osteoporosis in conjunction with adequate dietary calcium, some increase in bone density has been observed. The mechanism by which fluoride stimulates bone formation is poorly understood. However, its use is accompanied by an increase in alkaline phosphatase activity, suggesting a direct stimulation of osteoblasts (the bone cells containing alkaline phosphatase that are responsible for new bone formation).

II. CLINICAL PHARMACOLOGY

Disorders of bone mineral homeostasis generally present with abnormalities in serum or urine calcium levels (or both), often accompanied by abnormal serum phosphate levels. These abnormal mineral concentrations may themselves cause symptoms requiring immediate treatment (eg, malignant hypercalcemia or tetany). More commonly, they serve as clues to an underlying disorder in hormonal regulators (eg, primary hyperparathyroidism), target tissue response (eg, chronic renal failure), or drug abuse (eg, vitamin D intoxication). In such cases, treatment of the underlying disorder is of prime importance.

Since bone and kidney play central roles in bone mineral homeostasis, conditions that alter bone mineral homeostasis usually affect either or both of these tissues secondarily. Effects on bone can result in osteoporosis (abnormal loss of bone; remaining bone histologically normal), osteomalacia (abnormal bone formation due to inadequate mineralization), or osteitis fibrosa (excessive bone resorption with fibrotic replacement of resorption cavities). Biochemical markers of skeletal involvement include changes in serum levels of the skeletal isoenzyme of alkaline phosphatase (reflecting osteoblastic activity) and urine levels of hydroxyproline (reflecting osteoclastic activity). The kidney becomes involved when the calcium-times-phosphate product in serum exceeds the point at which ectopic calcification occurs (often in renal parenchyma) or when the calcium-times-oxalate (or phosphate) product in urine exceeds saturation, leading to nephrocalcinosis and nephrolithiasis. Subtle early indicators of such renal involvement include polyuria, nocturia, and hyposthenuria. Radiologic evidence of nephrocalcinosis and stones is not available until later. The degree of the ensuing renal failure is best followed by a decline in creatinine clearance.

ABNORMAL SERUM CALCIUM & PHOSPHATE LEVELS

Hypercalcemia

The major causes of hypercalcemia (other than thiazide therapy) are hyperparathyroidism and cancer with or without bone metastases. Less common causes are hypervitaminosis D, sarcoidosis, thyrotoxicosis, milk-alkali syndrome, adrenal insufficiency, and immobilization. With the possible exception of hypervitaminosis D, these latter disorders seldom require emergency lowering of serum calcium. A number of approaches are used to manage the hypercalcemic crisis.

SALINE DIURESIS

In hypercalcemia of sufficient severity to produce symptoms, rapid reduction of serum calcium is required. The first steps include rehydration with saline and diuresis with furosemide. Most patients presenting with severe hypercalcemia have a substantial component of prerenal azotemia owing to dehydration, which prevents the kidney from compensating for the rise in serum calcium by excreting more calcium in the urine. Therefore, the initial infusion of 500–1000 mL/h of saline to reverse the dehydration and restore urine flow can by itself substantially lower serum calcium. The addition of a loop diuretic such as furosemide (Chapter 13) not only enhances urine flow but floods the distal tubule with sodium, which competes with calcium for reabsorption at this site. Monitoring central venous pressure is important to forestall the development of congestive heart failure and pulmonary edema in predisposed subjects. In many subjects, saline diuresis will suffice to reduce serum calcium levels to a point at which more definitive diagnosis and treatment of the underlying condition can be achieved. If this is not the case or if more prolonged medical treatment of hypercalcemia is required, the following agents are available (discussed in order of preference).

CALCITONIN

Calcitonin has proved useful as ancillary treatment in a large number of patients. Calcitonin by itself seldom restores serum calcium to normal, and refractoriness frequently develops. However, its lack of toxicity permits frequent administration at high doses (200 MRC units or more). An effect on serum calcium is observed within 4–6 hours and lasts for 6–10 hours. Calcimar (salmon calcitonin) is available for parenteral administration only.

MITHRAMYCIN

Because of its toxicity, mithramycin is not the drug of first choice for the treatment of hypercalcemia. However, when other forms of therapy fail, a 25–50 μg/kg dose given intravenously usually lowers serum calcium substantially within 24–48 hours. This effect can last for several days. This dose can be repeated as necessary. The most feared toxic effect is sudden thrombocytopenia followed by hemorrhage. Hepatic and renal toxicity can also occur. Hypocalcemia, nausea, and vomiting may limit therapy. Use of this drug must be accompanied by careful monitoring of platelet counts, liver and kidney function, and serum calcium levels.

PHOSPHATE

Giving intravenous phosphate is probably the fastest and surest way to reduce serum calcium, but it is a hazardous procedure if not done properly. Intravenous phosphate should probably be used only after other methods of treatment (calcitonin, saline diuresis with furosemide, and mithramycin) have failed to control symptomatic hypercalcemia. Phosphate must be given slowly (50 mmol or 1.5 g elemental phosphorus over 6–8 hours) and the patient switched to oral phosphate (1–2 g elemental phosphorus daily) as soon as symptoms of hypercalcemia have cleared. The risks of intravenous phosphate therapy include sudden hypocalcemia, ectopic calcification, acute renal failure, and hypotension. Oral phosphate can also lead to ectopic calcification and renal failure if serum calcium and phosphate levels are not carefully monitored, but the risk is less and the time of onset much longer. Phosphate is available in oral and intravenous forms as the sodium or potassium salt. Amounts required to provide 1 g of elemental phosphorus are as follows:

- Intravenous:
  - In-Phos: 40 mL
  - Hyper-Phos-K: 15 mL
- Oral:
  - Fleet's Phospho-Soda: 6.2 mL
  - Neutra-Phos: 300 mL
  - Phos-Tab: 6 tablets

GLUCOCORTICOIDS

Glucocorticoids have no role in the acute treatment of hypercalcemia. However, the chronic hypercalcemia of sarcoidosis, vitamin D intoxication, and certain cancers (particularly multiple myeloma and related lymphoproliferative diseases) may respond within several days to glucocorticoid therapy. Prednisone in doses of 30–60 mg orally daily is generally used, although equivalent doses of other glucocorticoids are effective. The rationale for the use of glucocorticoids in these diseases differs, however. The hypercalcemia of sarcoidosis appears to be secondary to increased production of $1,25(OH)_2D$, possibly by the sarcoid tissue itself. Glucocorticoid therapy directed at the reduction of sarcoid tissue results in restoration of normal serum calcium and $1,25(OH)_2D$ levels. The treatment of hypervitaminosis D with glucocorticoids probably does not alter vitamin D metabolism significantly but is thought to reduce vitamin D-mediated intestinal calcium transport. An action of glucocorticoids to reduce vitamin D-mediated bone resorption has not been excluded, however. The effect of glucocorticoids on the hypercalcemia of cancer is probably 2-fold. The malignancies responding best to glucocorticoids (ie, multiple myeloma and related lymphoproliferative diseases) are sensitive to the lytic action of glucocorticoids, so part of the effect may be related to decreased tumor mass and activity. Glucocorticoids have also been shown to inhibit the effectiveness of osteoclast activating factor, a humoral substance elaborated by multiple myeloma and related cancers that stimulates osteoclastic bone resorption. Other causes of hypercalcemia—particularly primary hyperparathyroidism—do not respond to glucocorticoid therapy. In theory, if glucocorticoids potentiated PTH-stimulated bone resorption, as has been observed in vitro, one would expect to see aggravation (not amelioration) of hypercalcemia with glucocorticoid administration in persons with primary hyperparathyroidism.

This difference in response of the various forms of hypercalcemia to glucocorticoids forms the basis for the glucocorticoid suppression test, in which the response of serum calcium to a 10-day course of prednisone, 60 mg orally daily, helps differentiate the hypercalcemia of primary hyperparathyroidism from other causes such as sarcoidosis, vitamin D intoxication, and certain cancers. This test may be misleading and should not be used as a substitute for more specific tests for primary hyperparathyroidism such as serum immunoreactive PTH determinations.

Hypocalcemia

The main features of hypocalcemia are neuromuscular—tetany, paresthesias, laryngospasm, muscle cramps, and convulsions. The major causes of hypocalcemia in the adult are hypoparathyroidism, vitamin D deficiency, renal failure, and malabsorption. Neonatal hypocalcemia is a common disorder that usually resolves without therapy. The roles of PTH, vitamin D, and calcitonin in the neonatal syndrome are under active investigation. Large infusions of citrated blood can produce hypocalcemia by the formation of citrate-calcium complexes. Calcium and vitamin D (or its metabolites) form the mainstay of treatment of hypocalcemia.

CALCIUM

A number of calcium preparations are available for intravenous, intramuscular, and oral use. Calcium gluceptate (0.9 mEq calcium/mL), calcium gluconate (0.45 mEq calcium/mL), and calcium chloride (0.68–1.36 mEq calcium/mL) are available for intravenous therapy. Calcium gluconate is the preferred form because it is less irritating to veins. Oral preparations include calcium carbonate (40% calcium), calcium lactate (13% calcium), calcium phosphate (25% calcium), and calcium chloride (27% calcium). Calcium carbonate is often the preparation of choice because of its high percentage of calcium, ready availability (eg, Tums), low cost, and antacid properties. Combinations of vitamin D and calcium are available, but treatment must be tailored to the individual patient and individual disease, a flexibility lost by fixed-dosage combinations. Treatment of severe symptomatic hypocalcemia can be accomplished with slow infusion of 5–20 mL of 10% calcium gluconate. Rapid infusion can lead to cardiac arrhythmias. Less severe hypocalcemia is best treated with oral forms sufficient to provide approximately 400–800 mg of elemental calcium (1–2 g calcium carbonate per day). Dosage must be adjusted to avoid hypercalcemia and hypercalciuria.

VITAMIN D

When rapidity of action is required, $1,25(OH)_2D$ (calcitriol), 0.25–1 μg daily, is the vitamin D metabolite of choice, since it is capable of raising serum calcium within 24–48 hours. Calcitriol also raises serum phosphate, although this action is usually not observed early in treatment. The combined effects of calcitriol and all other vitamin D metabolites and analogs on both calcium and phosphate make careful monitoring of these mineral levels especially important to avoid ectopic calcification secondary to an abnormally high serum calcium-times-phosphate product. Since the choice of the appropriate vitamin D metabolite or analog for long-term treatment of hypocalcemia depends on the nature of the underlying disease, further discussion of vitamin D treatment will be found under the headings of the specific diseases.

Hyperphosphatemia

Hyperphosphatemia is a frequent complication of renal failure but is also found in all types of hypoparathyroidism (idiopathic, surgical, and pseudo), vitamin D intoxication, and the rare syndrome of tumoral calcinosis. Emergency treatment of hyperphosphatemia is seldom necessary but can be achieved by dialysis or glucose and insulin infusions. In general, control of hyperphosphatemia involves restriction of dietary phosphate plus the use of phosphate binding fels such as $Al(OH)_3$-containing antacids.

Hypophosphatemia

A variety of conditions are associated with hypophosphatemia, including primary hyperparathyroidism, vitamin D deficiency, idiopathic hypercalcemia, vitamin D-resistant rickets, various other forms of renal phosphate wasting (eg, Fanconi's syndrome), overzealous use of $Al(OH)_3$-containing antacids, and parenteral nutrition with inadequate phosphate content. Theoretically, hypophosphatemia should lead to a reduction in the intracellular levels of high-energy organic phosphates (eg, ATP) and interfere with normal hemoglobin-to-tissue oxygen transfer by decreasing red cell 2,3-diphosphoglycerate levels. However, clinically significant acute effects of hypophosphatemia are not well described, and emergency treatment is not indicated. The long-term effects of hypophosphatemia include proximal muscle weakness and abnormal bone mineralization (osteomalacia). Therefore, hypophosphatemia should be avoided during other forms of therapy and treated in conditions such as vitamin D-resistant rickets of which it is a cardinal feature. Oral forms of phosphate available for use are listed above in the section on hypercalcemia.

SPECIFIC DISORDERS INVOLVING THE BONE MINERAL REGULATING HORMONES

PRIMARY HYPERPARATHYROIDISM

This rather common disease, if associated with symptoms and significant hypercalcemia, is best treated surgically. Oral phosphate has been tried but cannot be recommended.

HYPOPARATHYROIDISM

In the absence of PTH (idiopathic or surgical hypoparathyroidism) or a normal target tissue response to PTH (pseudohypoparathyroidism), serum calcium falls and serum phosphate rises. In such patients, $1,25(OH)_2D$ levels are usually low, presumably reflecting the lack of stimulation by PTH of $1,25(OH)_2D$ production. The skeletons of patients with idiopathic or surgical hypoparathyroidism are normal except for a slow turnover rate. A number of patients with pseudohypoparathyroidism appear to have osteitis fibrosa, suggesting that the normal or high PTH levels found in such patients are capable of acting on bone but not on the kidney. The distinction between pseudohypoparathyroidism and idiopathic hypoparathyroidism is made on the basis of normal or high PTH levels but deficient renal response (ie, diminished excretion of cAMP or phosphate) in patients with pseudohypoparathyroidism.

The principal therapeutic concern is to restore normocalcemia and normophosphatemia. Under most circumstances, vitamin D (25,000–100,000 units 3 times per week) and dietary calcium supplements suffice. More rapid increments in serum calcium can be achieved with calcitriol, although it is not clear that this metabolite offers a substantial advantage over vitamin D itself for long-term therapy. Many patients treated with vitamin D develop episodes of hypercalcemia. This complication is more rapidly reversible with cessation of therapy using calcitriol rather than vitamin D. This would be of importance to the patient in whom such hypercalcemic crises are common. Dihydrotachysterol and 25(OH)D have not received much study as therapy for hypoparathyroidism, although both should be effective. Whether they offer advantages over vitamin D sufficient to justify their added expense remains to be seen.

NUTRITIONAL RICKETS

Vitamin D deficiency, once thought to be rare in this country, is being recognized more often, especially in the pediatric and geriatric populations. Part of this problem seems to be due to avoidance of meat and dairy products by some individuals, who also dress in a way that reduces sunlight exposure. In older adults, a similar combination of poor nutrition and limited sunlight results in vitamin D deficiency. This problem can be avoided by daily intake of 400 units of vitamin D and treated by somewhat higher doses (4000 units per day). No other metabolite is indicated. The diet should also contain adequate amounts of calcium and phosphate.

CHRONIC RENAL FAILURE

The major problems of chronic renal failure that impact on bone mineral homeostasis are the loss of $1,25(OH)_2D$ and $24,25(OH)_2D$ production, the retention of phosphate that reduces ionized calcium levels, and the secondary hyperparathyroidism which results. With the loss of $1,25(OH)_2D$ production, less calcium is absorbed from the intestine and less bone is resorbed under the influence of PTH. As a result, usually, hypocalcemia develops, furthering the development of hyperparathyroidism. The bones show a mixture of osteomalacia and osteitis fibrosa. Some patients may become hypercalcemic from 2 causes other than overzealous treatment with calcium supplements and high dialysate calcium levels. The most common cause of hypercalcemia is the development of severe secondary (sometimes referred to as tertiary) hyperparathyroidism. In such cases, the PTH level in blood is very high. Serum alkaline phosphatase levels also tend to be high. Treatment often requires parathyroidectomy. A less common circumstance leading to hypercalcemia is development of a form of osteomalacia characterized by a profound decrease in bone cell activity and loss of the calcium buffering action of bone. In the absence of kidney function, any calcium absorbed from the intestine accumulates in the blood. Therefore, such patients are very sensitive to the hypercalcemic action of $1,25(OH)_2D$. These individuals generally have a high serum calcium but nearly normal alkaline phosphatase and PTH levels.

The choice of vitamin D preparation to be used in the setting of chronic renal failure in the dialysis patient depends on the type and extent of bone disease and hyperparathyroidism. No consensus has been reached regarding the advisability of using any vitamin D metabolite in the predialysis patient. $1,25(OH)_2D$ (calcitriol) will rapidly correct hypocalcemia and at least partially reverse the secondary hyperparathyroidism and osteitis fibrosa. Many patients with muscle weakness and bone pain gain an improved sense of well-being. Dihydrotachysterol, an analog of $1,25(OH)_2D$, is also available for clinical use. Dihydrotachysterol appears to be as effective as calcitriol, differing principally in its time course of action: calcitriol increases serum calcium in 1–2 days, whereas dihydrotachysterol requires 1–2 weeks. For an equipotent dose (0.2 mg dihydrotachysterol versus 0.5 μg calcitriol), dihydrotachysterol costs about one-fourth as much as calcitriol. A minor disadvantage of dihydrotachysterol is the inability to measure it in serum. Neither dihydrotachysterol nor calcitriol corrects the osteomalacic component of renal osteodystrophy in the majority of patients, and neither should be used in patients with hypercalcemia, especially if the bone disease is primarily osteomalacic. The recently introduced drug calcifediol (25[OH]D) may be used to advantage when osteomalacia is a significant component of the bone disease. This metabolite appears to stimulate bone formation more effectively than calcitriol. Furthermore, calcifediol is less effective than calcitriol in stimulating intestinal calcium transport, so that hypercalcemia is less of a problem with calcifediol. Like dihydrotachysterol, calcifediol requires several weeks to restore normocalcemia in hypocalcemic individuals with chronic renal failure. Presumably because of the inability of the diseased kidney to metabolize calcifediol to more active metabolites, high doses (50–100 μg daily) must be given to achieve the supraphysiologic serum levels required for therapeutic effectiveness.

Vitamin D has been used in treating renal osteodystrophy. However, patients with a substantial degree of renal failure who are thus unable to convert vitamin D to its active metabolites usually are refractory to vitamin D. Its use is decreasing as more effective alternatives become available. Regardless of the drug employed, careful attention to serum calcium and phosphate levels is required. Calcium supplements (dietary and in the dialysate) and phosphate restriction (dietary and with oral ingestion of phosphate binders) should be employed along with the use of vitamin D metabolites. Monitoring serum PTH and alkaline phosphatase levels is useful in determining whether therapy is correcting or preventing secondary hyperparathyroidism. Although not generally available, percutaneous bone biopsies for quantitative histomorphometry are becoming increasingly important in choosing appropriate therapy and following the effectiveness of such therapy. Unlike the rapid changes in serum values, changes in bone morphology require months to years. Monitoring serum levels of the vitamin D metabolites has only recently become possible.

INTESTINAL OSTEODYSTROPHY

A number of gastrointestinal and hepatic diseases result in disordered calcium and phosphate homeostasis that ultimately leads to bone disease. The bones in such patients show a combination of osteoporosis and osteomalacia. Osteitis fibrosa does not occur (as it does in renal osteodystrophy). The common features that appear to be important in this group of diseases are malabsorption of calcium and vitamin D. Liver disease may, in addition, reduce the production of 25(OH)D from vitamin D, although the importance of this in all but patients with terminal liver failure remains in dispute. The malabsorption of vitamin D is probably not limited to exogenous vitamin D. The liver secretes into bile a substantial number of vitamin D metabolites and conjugates that are reabsorbed in (presumably) the distal jejunum and ileum. Interference with this process could deplete the body of endogenous vitamin D metabolites as well as limit absorption of dietary vitamin D.

In mild forms of malabsorption, vitamin D (25,000–50,000 units 3 times per week) should suffice to raise serum levels of 25(OH)D into the normal range. Many patients with severe disease do not respond to vitamin D. Clinical experience with the other metabolites is limited, but both calcitriol and calcifediol have been used successfully in doses similar to those recommended for treatment of renal osteodystrophy. Theoretically, calcifediol should be the drug of choice under these conditions, since no impairment of the renal metabolism of 25(OH)D to $1,25(OH)_2D$ and $24,25(OH)_2D$ exists in these patients. Both calcitriol and calcifediol may be of importance in reversing the bone disease. As in the other diseases discussed, treatment of intestinal osteodystrophy with vitamin D and its metabolites should be accompanied by appropriate dietary calcium supplementation and monitoring of serum calcium and phosphate levels.

OSTEOPOROSIS

Osteoporosis can be defined as an abnormal loss of bone predisposing to fractures. This occurs most commonly during the postmenopausal period in females but can be seen in older males. Osteoporosis can also result from a variety of drugs (glucocorticoids) or endocrinopathies (thyrotoxicosis, hyperparathyroidism) or can occur without obvious cause (idiopathic). The postmenopausal form of osteoporosis is accompanied by lower $1,25(OH)_2D$ levels and reduced intestinal calcium transport. This form of osteoporosis appears to be due to estrogen deficiency and is best treated with cyclic doses of estrogen. It is important to note that the most rapid loss of bone occurs within the first 5 years after menopause and that administration of estrogens after this time will be less effective. Furthermore, if estrogen therapy is discontinued, a period of accelerated bone loss will occur. Thus, treatment with estrogens should be started prior to the onset of osteoporosis (ie, in the perimenopausal period) and continued for life. Since continuous estrogen therapy is associated with increased risk of endometrial carcinoma, the recommendation to treat all postmenopausal women with estrogens has not been universally accepted. Recent evidence indicates that cyclic estrogen therapy in combination with a progestational agent reduces or eliminates this added risk of cancer. Therefore, estrogens should be administered for 21 of 28 days in the lowest effective dose (eg, 0.625 mg of conjugated estrogens or 25–50 μg of ethinyl estradiol), with addition of a progestational agent on days 14–21 (eg, 10 mg of medroxyprogesterone acetate). This may reinitiate menstrual bleeding, so the patient must be advised of this in advance. Other complications of estrogen therapy such as hypertension and thrombophlebitis must also be kept in mind when such treatment is initiated.

To counter the reduced intestinal calcium transport, vitamin D therapy is often employed in addition to dietary calcium supplementation. There is no clear evidence that pharmacologic doses of vitamin D are of much additional benefit beyond cyclic estrogens and calcium supplementation. Studies are under way in which calcitriol and calcifediol are being tried in an effort to restore bone or to prevent further bone loss, but definitive results are not yet available. Fluoride in large doses (50 mg of sodium fluoride in divided doses per day), in addition to cyclic estrogens and calcium, seems to stimulate new bone formation without first increasing bone resorption. It is too early to conclude that the results achieved with high doses of fluoride in the treatment of postmenopausal osteoporosis justify the high incidence of side-effects (nausea and vomiting, arthralgias).

The cause of idiopathic osteoporosis in men is not known. Treatment usually consists of giving vitamin D and dietary calcium supplements, but little information is available about its efficacy. It is important to exclude more treatable forms of osteoporosis such as that accompanying corticosteroid therapy, alcohol abuse, hyperparathyroidism, thyrotoxicosis, or occult nutritional osteomalacia.

VITAMIN D–RESISTANT RICKETS

This X-linked recessive disorder is manifested by the appearance of rickets and hypophosphatemia in children. The disease can present in adulthood, presumably reflecting either less severe disease or a missed diagnosis in childhood. The main defect appears to be an abnormality in renal phosphate reabsorption. Phosphate is critical to normal bone mineralization; when phosphate stores are deficient, a clinical and pathologic picture resembling vitamin D-deficient rickets develops. However, such children fail to respond to the usual doses of vitamin D employed in the treatment of nutritional rickets. A defect in $1,25(OH)_2D$ production by the kidney has also been suggested by some investigators, because the serum $1,25(OH)_2D$ levels tend to be low relative to the degree of hypophosphatemia observed. This combination of low serum phosphate and low or low-normal serum $1,25(OH)_2D$ provides the rationale for treating such patients with oral phosphate (1–3 g daily) and large doses of vitamin D (25,000–100,000 units daily). Recently, some groups have used calcitriol with good effect (0.25–1 μg daily). Reports of such combination therapy are encouraging in this otherwise debilitating disease.

VITAMIN D–DEPENDENT RICKETS

This entity actually represents 2 different diseases (types I and II). Both present as childhood rickets that does not respond to conventional doses of vitamin D. Type I vitamin D-dependent rickets is due to an isolated deficiency of $1,25(OH)_2D$ production. This condition can be treated with vitamin D (4000 units daily) or calcitriol (0.25–0.5 μg daily). Type II vitamin D-dependent rickets is caused by a target tissue defect in response to $1,25(OH)_2D$. The serum levels of $1,25(OH)_2D$ are very high in type II but not in type I. Treatment with large doses of calcitriol has been claimed to be effective in restoring normocalcemia. Such patients are totally refractory to vitamin D. One recent report indicates a reversal of resistance to calcitriol when $24,25(OH)_2D$ was given. These diseases are rare.

NEPHROTIC SYNDROME

Patients with nephrotic syndrome can lose vitamin D metabolites into their urine, presumably by loss of the vitamin D-binding protein. Such patients may have very low 25(OH)D levels. At least some of them develop bone disease. It is not yet clear what value vitamin D therapy has in such patients, since this complication of the nephrotic syndrome has only recently been recognized, and therapeutic trials with vitamin D (or any other vitamin D metabolite) have not yet been carried out. Since the problem is not related to vitamin D metabolism, one would not anticipate any advantage in using the more expensive vitamin D metabolites in place of vitamin D itself.

IDIOPATHIC HYPERCALCIURIA

This syndrome, characterized by hypercalciuria and nephrolithiasis with normal serum calcium and PTH levels, has been identified in 3 subgroups of patients: (1) hyperabsorbers, patients with increased intestinal absorption of calcium, resulting in high-normal serum calcium, low-normal PTH, and a secondary increase in urine calcium; (2) renal calcium leakers, patients with a primary decrease in renal reabsorption of filtered calcium, leading to low-normal serum calcium and high-normal serum PTH; and (3) renal phosphate leakers, patients with a primary decrease in renal reabsorption of phosphate, leading to stimulation of $1,25(OH)_2D$ production, increased intestinal calcium absorption, increased ionized serum calcium, low-normal PTH levels, and a secondary increase in urine calcium. There is some disagreement about this classification, but many such patients present with mild hypophosphatemia, and oral phosphate has been used with some success to reduce stone formation. However, a clear role for phosphate in the treatment of this disorder has not been established. Therapy with hydrochlorothiazide, 50 mg twice daily, is recommended, although equivalent doses of other thiazide diuretics work as well. Loop diuretics such as furosemide and ethacrynic acid should not be used, since they increase urinary calcium excretion. The major toxicity of thiazide diuretics, besides hypokalemia and hyperglycemia, is hypercalcemia. This is seldom more than a biochemical observation unless the patient has a disease such as hyperparathyroidism in which bone turnover is accelerated. Accordingly, one should screen patients for such disorders before starting thiazide therapy and monitor serum and urine calcium when therapy has begun. An alternative to thiazides is allopurinol. Some studies indicate that hyperuricosuria is associated with idiopathic hypercalcemia and that a small nidus of urate crystals could lead to the calcium oxalate stone formation characteristic of idiopathic hypercalciuria. Allopurinol, 300 mg daily, may reduce stone formation by reducing uric acid excretion.

OTHER DISORDERS OF BONE MINERAL HOMEOSTASIS

PAGET'S DISEASE OF BONE

Paget's disease is a localized bone disease characterized by uncontrolled osteoclastic bone resorption with secondary increases in bone formation. This new bone is poorly organized, however. The cause of Paget's disease is obscure, although recent studies suggest that a slow virus may be involved. The disease is fairly common, although symptomatic bone disease is less common. The biochemical parameters of elevated serum alkaline phosphatase and urinary hydroxyproline are useful for diagnosis. Along with the characteristic radiologic and bone scan findings, these biochemical determinations provide good markers by which to follow therapy. The goal of treatment is to reduce bone pain and stabilize or prevent other problems such as progressive deformity, hearing loss, high-output cardiac failure, and immobilization hypercalcemia. Calcitonin can be used as sole treatment or in combination with diphosphonates for this disease. Treatment failures may respond to mithramycin. Calcitonin is administered subcutaneously or intramuscularly in doses of 50–100 MRC units every day or every other day. Higher or more frequent doses have been advocated when this initial regimen is ineffective. Improvement in bone pain and reduction in serum alkaline phosphatase and urine hydroxyproline levels require weeks to months. Often a patient who responds well initially will lose the response to calcitonin. This refractoriness is not correlated with the development of antibodies.

Sodium etidronate is the only diphosphonate currently available for clinical use. The recommended dosage is 5 mg/kg of the sodium salt daily by oral administration. Long-term (months to years) remission may be expected in patients who respond to etidronate. Treatment should not exceed 6 months per course but can be repeated after 3 months if necessary. The principal toxicity of etidronate is the development of osteomalacia and increased incidence of fractures when the dose is raised substantially above 5 mg/kg. Other diphosphonates such as dichloromethane diphosphonate or aminohydroxypropane diphosphonate are less toxic in this regard. Some patients treated with etidronate develop bone pain similar in nature to the bone pain of osteomalacia. This subsides after stopping the drug.

The use of a potentially lethal cytotoxic drug such as mithramycin in a generally benign disorder like Paget's disease is recommended only when other less toxic agents (calcitonin, etidronate) have failed and the symptoms are debilitating. Insufficient clinical data on long-term use of mithramycin are available to determine its usefulness for extended therapy. However, short courses involving 15–25 μg/kg intravenously for 5–10 days followed by 15 μg/kg intravenously each week have been used to control the disease.

ENTERIC OXALURIA

Patients with short bowel syndromes associated with fat malabsorption can present with renal stones composed of calcium and oxalate. Such patients characteristically have normal or low urine calcium levels but elevated urine oxalate levels. The major reasons for the development of oxaluria in such patients are thought to be decreased availability of luminal calcium (which is bound to fat) to bind to oxalate to prevent its absorption and increased production of oxalate by enteric flora acting on the increased supply of nutrients reaching the colon. Although one would ordinarily avoid treating a patient with calcium oxalate stones with calcium supplementation, this is precisely what is done in patients with enteric oxaluria. One to 2 g of calcium carbonate can be given daily in divided doses, with careful monitoring of urinary calcium and oxalate to be certain that urinary oxalate falls without a dangerous increase in urinary calcium.

• • •

References

Austin LA, Heath HH III: Calcitonin: Physiology and pathophysiology. *N Engl J Med* 1981;**304:**269.

Bikle DD: The vitamin D endocrine system. *Adv Intern Med* 1981;**27:**45.

Bikle DD et al: The intestinal response to vitamin D. *Rev Physiol Biochem Pharmacol* 1981;**89:**64.

Coburn JW, Massry SG (editors): Uses and actions of 1,25 dihydroxyvitamin D_3 in uremia. *Contrib Nephrol* 1980;**18:**1.

Dambacher MD, Binswanger U, Fischer JA: Diagnosis and treatment of primary hyperparathyroidism. *Urol Res* 1979;**7:**171.

Forscher BK, Arnaud CD (editors): The third F. Raymond Keating, Jr., memorial symposium: Parathyroid hormone, calcitonin and vitamin D. *Am J Med* 1974;**56:**743 and **57:**1.

Fraser DR: Regulation of the metabolism of vitamin D. *Physiol Rev* 1980;**60:**551.

Lei DBM, Zawada ET, Kleeman CR: The pathophysiology and clinical aspects of hypercalcemic disorders. *West J Med* 1978;**129:**278.

Long RG: Hepatic osteodystrophy: Outlook good but some problems unsolved. *Gastroenterology* 1980;**78:**644.

Pak CYC (editor): Symposium on urolithiasis. *Kidney Int* 1978;**13:**341.

Parfitt AM: The action of parathyroid hormone on bone: Relation to bone remodeling and turnover, calcium homeostasis, and metabolic bone disease. (4 parts.) *Metabolism* 1976;**25:**809, 909, 1033, 1157.

Puschett JB: Renal tubular effects of parathyroid hormone. *Clin Orthop* 1978;**135:**249.

Riggs BL: Postmenopausal and senile osteoporosis: Current concepts of etiology and treatment. *Endocrinol Jpn* 1979;**26(Suppl):**31.

Wallach S (editor): Paget's disease symposium. *Clin Orthop* 1977;**127:**1.

Principles of Antimicrobial Drug Action | 41

Ernest Jawetz, MD, PhD

An ideal antimicrobial drug exhibits **selective toxicity.** This term implies that the drug is harmful to a parasite without being harmful to the host. In many instances, selective toxicity is relative rather than absolute and implies that a drug may damage a parasite in a concentration that can be tolerated by the host.

Selective toxicity may be a function of a specific receptor required for drug attachment, or it may depend on the inhibition of biochemical events that exist in or are essential to the parasite but not the host. For a large majority of antimicrobial drugs, the mechanism of action is not completely understood. However, for purposes of discussion, it is convenient to present antimicrobial mechanisms under 4 distinct headings:

(1) Inhibition of cell wall synthesis.

(2) Alteration in the permeability of cell membrane or active transport across cell membrane.

(3) Inhibition of protein synthesis (ie, inhibition of translation and transcription of genetic material).

(4) Inhibition of nucleic acid synthesis.

ANTIMICROBIAL ACTION THROUGH INHIBITION OF CELL WALL SYNTHESIS (Bacitracin, Cephalosporins, Cycloserine, Penicillins, Ristocetin, Vancomycin)

In contrast to animal cells, bacteria possess a rigid outer layer, the cell wall. It maintains the shape of microorganisms and "corsets" the bacterial cell, which possesses an unusually high internal osmotic pressure.

The internal pressure is 3–5 times greater in gram-positive than in gram-negative bacteria. Injury to the cell wall (eg, by lysozyme) or inhibition of its formation may lead to lysis of the cell. In a hypertonic environment (eg, 20% sucrose), damaged cell wall formation leads to formation of spherical bacterial "protoplasts" from gram-positive organisms or "spheroplasts" from gram-negative organisms, which are limited by the fragile cytoplasmic membrane. If such flexible cells are placed in an environment of ordinary tonicity, they take up fluid rapidly and may explode.

The cell wall contains a chemically distinct complex polymer "mucopeptide" ("murein," "peptidoglycan") consisting of polysaccharides and a highly cross-linked polypeptide. The polysaccharides regularly contain the amino sugars N-acetylglucosamine and acetylmuramic acid. The latter is found only in bacteria. To the amino sugars are attached pentapeptide chains. The final rigidity of the cell wall is imparted by cross-linking of the peptide chains (eg, through pentaglycine bonds) as a result of "transpeptidation" reactions carried out by several enzymes. The peptidoglycan layer is much thicker in the cell wall of gram-positive bacteria than in the cell wall of gram-negative bacteria.

All penicillins and all cephalosporins (β-lactam antibiotics) are selective inhibitors of bacterial cell wall synthesis. While this is only one of many different activities of these drugs, it is perhaps the best understood. The initial step in drug action consists of binding of the drug to cell receptors. These are surface proteins (3–8 or more in number), and some are transpeptidation enzymes. Different receptors may possess different affinity for a drug, and each may mediate a different mode of action. For example, attachment of penicillin to one protein receptor may result chiefly in abnormal elongation of the cell, whereas attachment to another may lead to a cell wall defect at the periphery. After a β-lactam antibiotic has attached to the receptor, the transpeptidation reaction is inhibited and peptidoglycan synthesis is blocked. The next step probably involves the removal or inactivation of an inhibitor of autolytic enzymes in the cell wall. This activates the lytic enzyme in some microorganisms and may result in lysis in an isotonic environment. In a hypertonic environment (eg, 20% sucrose), the microbes may change to protoplasts or spheroplasts covered only by the fragile cell membrane. In such cells, synthesis of proteins and nucleic acids may continue for some time.

Inhibition of the transpeptidation enzymes by the penicillins and cephalosporins may be due to a structural similarity of these drugs to acyl-D-alanyl-D-alanine. The transpeptidation reaction involves the loss of a D-alanine from the pentapeptide.

The remarkable lack of toxicity of β-lactam antibiotics to mammalian cells must be attributed to the absence of a bacterial type cell wall, with its peptidoglycan, in animal cells. The difference in susceptibility of gram-positive and gram-negative bacteria to various penicillins or cephalosporins probably depends on structural differences in their cell walls (eg, amount of peptidoglycan, presence of receptors and lipids, nature of cross-linking, activity of autolytic enzymes) that determine penetration, binding, and activity of the drugs.

Some derivatives of 6-β-amidinopenicillanic acid, eg, mecillinam, are far more active against gram-negative than against gram-positive bacteria. They do not affect final transpeptidation reactions in cell wall synthesis but act by other mechanisms; they may exhibit synergism with several penicillins.

Susceptibility of bacteria to β-lactam antibiotics depends on various structural and functional characteristics. In order to reach receptors, the drugs must permeate the outer layers of the cell envelope. In gram-negative bacteria, there is an outer phospholipid membrane that may hinder passage of these drugs. Hydrophilic molecules (eg, ampicillin, amoxicillin) may pass more readily than penicillin G. In gram-positive bacteria, the phospholipid membrane is lacking and its barrier function is absent.

The number and type of receptor proteins vary in different species. They are under chromosomal control, and mutation may alter their number or their affinity to drugs.

Some bacteria may be inhibited by β-lactam drugs as peptidoglycan formation is inhibited, but they may fail to lyse. This "tolerance" may be due to a lack of activation of autolytic enzymes (hydrolases) in the cell wall. This in turn may be a function of the presence or absence of precursors or of the nature of the enzyme inhibitor.

The most important clinically encountered mechanism of insusceptibility to β-lactam drugs is the production by the bacteria of β-lactamases. These enzymes break the β-lactam ring and nullify the biologic effect of the drug.

There are many types of β-lactamases, most of them under the genetic control of plasmids. Such gene-bearing plasmids are widespread among staphylococci and enteric gram-negative rods. Some β-lactamases can be firmly bound by compounds such as clavulanic acid and by certain penicillins (eg, cloxacillin) and can thus be prevented from attacking hydrolyzable penicillins (eg, ampicillin). Certain β-lactam antibiotics are resistant to β-lactamases because their β-lactam ring is protected by methoxy or other groups (eg, methicillin, cefoxitin). Such antibiotics can attack β-lactamase-producing bacteria, inhibit their transpeptidation, or lyse them. The basis for the resistance of some bacteria to the latter type of drug (eg, methicillin-resistant staphylococci) is not well understood. It may depend on varying affinity of receptors for the drug.

Several other drugs, including bacitracin, vancomycin, and ristocetin, inhibit early steps in the biosynthesis of the peptidoglycan. Since the early stages of synthesis take place inside the cytoplasmic membrane, these drugs must penetrate the membrane to be effective. For these drugs, the inhibition of peptidoglycan synthesis is not the sole mode of antibacterial action.

Cycloserine, an analog of D-alanine, interferes also with peptidoglycan synthesis. This drug blocks the action of alanine racemase, an essential enzyme in the incorporation of D-alanine in the pentapeptide of peptidoglycan. Phosphonopeptides also inhibit enzymes needed for early steps in the synthesis of peptidoglycans.

ANTIMICROBIAL ACTION THROUGH INHIBITION OF CELL MEMBRANE FUNCTION
(Amphotericin B, Colistin, Nystatin, Polymyxins)

The cytoplasm of all living cells is bounded by the cytoplasmic membrane, which serves as a selective permeability barrier, carries out active transport functions, and thus controls the internal composition of the cell. If the functional integrity of the cytoplasmic membrane is disrupted, purine and pyrimidine nucleotides, proteins, and ions escape from the cell, and cell damage or death ensues. The cytoplasmic membrane of certain bacteria and fungi can be more readily disrupted by certain agents than can the membranes of animal cells. Consequently, selective chemotherapeutic activity is possible.

Good examples of this mechanism are the polymyxins acting on gram-negative bacteria (polymyxins selectively act on membranes rich in phosphatidyl ethanolamine and act like cationic detergent) and the polyene antibiotics acting on fungi. However, polymyxins are inactive against fungi, and polyenes are inactive against bacteria. This is because ergosterol is present in the fungal cell membrane and absent in the bacterial cell membrane. Polyenes require ergosterol as a receptor in the fungal cell membrane, prior to exerting their effect. Bacterial cell membranes do not contain that sterol and (presumably for this reason) are resistant to polyene action—a good example of cell individuality and of selective toxicity. Fungi that are resistant to polyenes exhibit a decrease in membrane ergosterol or a modification in its structure, so that it combines less well with the drug. The antifungal imidazoles impair the integrity of fungal cell membranes by inhibiting the biosynthesis of membrane lipids.

ANTIMICROBIAL ACTION THROUGH INHIBITION OF PROTEIN SYNTHESIS
(Chloramphenicol, Erythromycins, Lincomycins, Tetracyclines; Aminoglycosides: Amikacin, Gentamicin, Kanamycin, Neomycin, Streptomycin, Tobramycin, Etc)

It is established that chloramphenicol, tetracyclines, aminoglycosides, erythromycins, and lincomycins can inhibit protein synthesis in bacteria. Puromycin is an inhibitor of protein synthesis in animal and other cells. The concepts of protein synthesis are undergoing rapid change, and the precise mechanism of action is not fully established for these drugs.

Bacteria have 70S ribosomes, whereas mammalian cells have 80S ribosomes. The subunits of each type of ribosome, their chemical composition, and their functional specificities are sufficiently different to explain why antimicrobial drugs can inhibit protein synthesis in bacterial ribosomes without having a major effect on mammalian ribosomes.

In normal microbial protein synthesis, the mRNA message is simultaneously "read" by several ribosomes that are strung out along the mRNA strand. These are called polysomes.

Aminoglycosides

The mode of action of streptomycin has been studied far more than that of other aminoglycosides (kanamycin, neomycin, gentamicin, tobramycin, amikacin, etc), but probably all act similarly. The first step is the attachment of the aminoglycoside to a specific receptor protein (P 12 in the case of streptomycin) on the 30S subunit of the microbial ribosome. Second, the aminoglycoside blocks the normal activity of the "initiation complex" of peptide formation (mRNA + formyl methionine + tRNA). Third, the mRNA message is misread on the "recognition region" of the ribosome, and, as a result, the wrong amino acid is inserted into the peptide, resulting in a nonfunctional protein. Fourth, aminoglycoside attachment results in the breakup of polysomes and their separation into "monosomes" incapable of protein synthesis. These activities occur more or less simultaneously, and the overall effect is usually an irreversible event—killing of the cell.

Chromosomal resistance of microbes to aminoglycosides principally depends on the lack of a specific protein receptor on the 30S subunit of the ribosome. Plasmid-dependent resistance to aminoglycosides depends on the production by the microorganism of adenylylating, phosphorylating, or acetylating enzymes that destroy the drugs. A third type of resistance consists of a "permeability defect," perhaps due to absence of active transport of the aminoglycoside into the cell so that the drug cannot reach the ribosome. This is—at least sometimes—plasmid-mediated.

Tetracyclines

Tetracyclines bind to the 30S subunit of microbial ribosomes. They inhibit protein synthesis by blocking the attachment of charged aminoacyl-tRNA. Thus, they prevent introduction of new amino acids into the nascent peptide chain. The action is usually bacteriostatic and reversible upon withdrawal of the drug. Resistance to tetracyclines results from changes in permeability of the microbial cell envelope. In susceptible cells, the drug is concentrated from the environment by an energy-dependent process of active transport and does not readily leave the cell. In resistant cells, the drug either is not actively transported into the cell or leaves it so rapidly that inhibitory concentrations are not maintained. This is often plasmid-controlled. Mammalian cells do not actively concentrate tetracyclines.

Chloramphenicol

Chloramphenicol attaches to the 50S subunit of the ribosome. It interferes with the binding of new amino acids to the nascent peptide chain, largely because chloramphenicol inhibits peptidyl transferase. Chloramphenicol is mainly bacteriostatic, and growth of microorganisms resumes (ie, drug action is reversible) when the drug is withdrawn. Microorganisms resistant to chloramphenicol produce the enzyme chloramphenicol acetyl transferase, which destroys drug activity. The production of this enzyme is usually under control of a plasmid.

Macrolides (Erythromycins)

These drugs bind to the 50S subunit of the ribosome and can compete with lincomycins for binding sites (a 23S rRNA). Macrolides may interfere with formation of initiation complexes for peptide chain synthesis or may interfere with aminoacyl translocation reactions. Some macrolide-resistant bacteria lack the proper receptor on the ribosome (through methylation of the rRNA); this may be under plasmid or chromosomal control.

Lincomycins (Clindamycin)

Lincomycins bind to the 50S subunit of the microbial ribosome and resemble macrolides in antibacterial activity and mode of action. There may be mutual interference between these drugs, presumably because they share the same receptor. Chromosomal mutants are resistant by virtue of lacking the proper binding site on the 50S subunit.

ANTIMICROBIAL ACTION THROUGH INHIBITION OF NUCLEIC ACID SYNTHESIS
(Nalidixic Acid, Novobiocin, Pyrimethamine, Rifampin, Sulfonamides, Trimethoprim)

Drugs such as the actinomycins are effective inhibitors of DNA synthesis. Actually, they form complexes with DNA by binding to the deoxyguanosine residues. The DNA-actinomycin complex inhibits the DNA-dependent RNA polymerase and blocks mRNA formation. Actinomycin also inhibits DNA virus replication. Mitomycins result in the firm cross-linking of complementary strands of DNA and subsequently block DNA replication. Both actinomycins and mitomycin inhibit bacterial as well as animal cells but are not sufficiently selective to be employed in antibacterial chemotherapy.

Rifampin inhibits bacterial growth by binding strongly to the DNA-dependent RNA polymerase of bacteria. Thus, it inhibits bacterial RNA synthesis.

Nalidixic acid and oxolinic acid, used mainly as urinary antiseptics, are potent inhibitors of DNA synthesis. However, it is not known whether their antibacterial action depends solely on this effect.

For many microorganisms, *p*-aminobenzoic acid (PABA) is an essential metabolite. It is used by them as a precursor in the synthesis of folic acid in the pathway leading to the synthesis of nucleic acids. The specific mode of action of PABA probably involves an adenosine triphosphate (ATP)-dependent condensation of a pteridine with PABA to yield dihydropteroic acid, which is subsequently converted to folic acid. Sulfonamides are structural analogs of PABA and inhibit dihydropteroate synthetase.

Sulfonamides can enter into the reaction in place of PABA and compete for the active center of the enzyme. As a result, nonfunctional analogs of folic acid are formed, preventing further growth of the bacterial cell. The inhibiting action of sulfonamides on bacterial growth can be counteracted by an excess of PABA in the environment (competitive inhibition). Animal cells cannot synthesize folic acid and must depend upon exogenous sources. Some bacteria, like animal cells, are not inhibited by sulfonamides. Many other bacteria, however, synthesize folic acid as mentioned above and consequently are susceptible to inhibition by sulfonamides.

Tubercle bacilli are not inhibited markedly by sulfonamides, but their growth is inhibited by PAS (*p*-aminosalicylic acid). Conversely, most sulfonamide-susceptible bacteria are resistant to PAS. This suggests that the receptor site for PABA differs in different types of organisms.

Trimethoprim (3,4,5-trimethoxybenzyl pyrimidine) inhibits the dihydrofolic acid reductase of bacteria 50,000 times more efficiently than the same enzyme of mammalian cells. This enzyme reduces dihydrofolic to tetrahydrofolic acid, a stage in the sequence leading to the synthesis of purines and ultimately of DNA. Sulfonamides and trimethoprim produce sequential blocking of this pathway, resulting in marked enhancement (synergism) of activity. Such sulfonamide (5 parts) + trimethoprim (1 part) mixtures have been used in a variety of clinical infections.

Pyrimethamine (Daraprim) also inhibits dihydrofolate reductase, but it is more active against the mammalian cell enzyme and therefore more toxic than trimethoprim. Pyrimethamine plus sulfonamides is the current treatment of choice in toxoplasmosis and some other protozoal infections.

Many different chemicals that can interfere with the synthesis of viral nucleic acids have been employed for chemoprophylaxis and chemotherapy of viral infections. These are discussed in some detail in Chapter 48, and their mechanism of action is presented there.

• • •

RESISTANCE TO ANTIMICROBIAL DRUGS

There are many different mechanisms by which microorganisms might exhibit resistance to drugs. The following are fairly well supported by evidence:

(1) Microorganisms produce enzymes that destroy the active drug. ***Examples:*** Staphylococci resistant to penicillin G produce a β-lactamase that destroys the drug. Other β-lactamases are produced by gram-negative rods. Gram-negative bacteria resistant to aminoglycosides (by virtue of a plasmid) produce adenylylating, phosphorylating, or acetylating enzymes that destroy the drug. Gram-negative bacteria may be resistant to chloramphenicol if they produce a chloramphenicol acetyl transferase.

(2) Microorganisms change their permeability to the drug. ***Examples:*** Tetracyclines accumulate in susceptible bacteria through active transport through the cell membrane. Resistant bacteria lack this mechanism. Resistance to polymyxins is probably associated with a change in permeability to the drugs. Streptococci have a natural permeability barrier to aminoglycosides. This can be partly overcome by the simultaneous presence of a cell wall-active drug, eg, a penicillin. Resistance to amikacin and some other aminoglycosides may depend on a lack of permeability to the drugs, apparently due to impaired active transport across cell membranes.

(3) Microorganisms develop an altered structural target for the drug (see also ¶ [5]). ***Examples:*** Chromosomal resistance to aminoglycosides is associated with the loss (or alteration) of a specific protein on the 30S subunit of the bacterial ribosome that serves as a receptor in susceptible organisms. Erythromycin-resistant organisms have an altered receptor site on the 50S subunit of the bacterial ribosome, resulting from methylation of a 23S ribosomal RNA.

(4) Microorganisms develop an altered metabolic pathway that bypasses the reaction inhibited by the drug. ***Example:*** Some sulfonamide-resistant bacteria do not require extracellular PABA but, like mammalian cells, can utilize preformed folic acid.

(5) Microorganisms develop an altered enzyme that can still perform its metabolic function but is much less affected by the drug than the enzyme in the susceptible organism. ***Example:*** In some sulfonamide-susceptible bacteria, dihydropteroate synthetase has a much higher affinity for sulfonamide than for PABA. In sulfonamide-resistant mutants, the opposite is the case.

Origin of Drug Resistance

The origin of drug resistance may be genetic or nongenetic.

A. Nongenetic Origin: Active replication of bacteria is usually required for most antibacterial drug actions. Consequently, microorganisms that are metabolically inactive (nonmultiplying) may be resistant to drugs. However, their offspring are fully susceptible. ***Example:*** Mycobacteria often survive in tissues for many years after infection yet are restrained by the host's defenses and do not multiply. Such "persisting" organisms are resistant to treatment and cannot be eradicated by drugs. However, if they start to multiply (eg, following corticosteroid treatment of the patient), they are fully susceptible to the same drug.

Microorganisms may lose the specific target structure for a drug for several generations and thus be resistant. ***Example:*** Penicillin-susceptible organisms may change to L forms (protoplasts) during penicillin administration. Lacking most cell wall, they are then resistant to cell wall-inhibitor drugs (penicillins, cephalosporins) and may remain so for several generations as "persisters." When these organisms revert to their bacterial parent forms by resuming cell wall production, they are again fully susceptible to penicillin.

B. Genetic Origin: The vast majority of drug-resistant microbes have emerged as a result of genetic changes and subsequent selection processes. Genetic changes may be chromosomal or extrachromosomal.

Bacteria contain chromosomes made of a double-stranded circular molecule of DNA. These chromosomes are supercoiled and folded within the cell to allow for orderly segregation into the daughter cells. Bacterial chromosomes replicate semiconservatively and sequentially. In some bacteria, replication is known to proceed bidirectionally.

1. Chromosomal resistance–This develops as a result of spontaneous mutation in a locus that controls susceptibility to a given antimicrobial. The presence of the drug serves as a selecting mechanism to suppress susceptibles and promote the growth of drug-resistant mutants. Spontaneous mutation occurs with a frequency of 10^{-12} to 10^{-7} and thus is an infrequent cause for the emergence of clinical drug resistance within a given patient. Chromosomal mutants are most commonly resistant by virtue of a change in a structural receptor for a drug. Thus, the P 12 protein on the 30S subunit of the bacterial ribosome serves as a receptor for streptomycin attachment. Mutation in the gene that controls that structural protein results in streptomycin resistance. A narrow region of the bacterial chromosome contains structural genes that code for a number of drug receptors, including those for erythromycin, tetracycline, lincomycin, aminoglycosides, etc. Mutation may also result in a loss of penicillin receptors in some microbial species, making the mutant penicillin-resistant.

2. Extrachromosomal resistance–Bacteria also contain extrachromosomal genetic elements called plasmids (or episomes). Plasmids are circular DNA molecules, have 1–3% of the weight of the bacterial chromosome, may exist free in the bacterial cytoplasm, or may be integrated into the bacterial chromosome. Some carry their own genes for replication and transfer. Others rely on genes in other plasmids.

R factors are a class of plasmids that carry genes for resistance to one—and often several—antimicrobial drugs and heavy metals. Plasmid genes for antimicrobial resistance often control the formation of enzymes capable of destroying antimicrobial drugs. Thus, plasmids determine resistance to penicillins and cephalosporins by carrying genes for the formation of β-lactamases. Plasmids code for enzymes that destroy chloramphenicol (acetyl transferase); enzymes that acetylate, adenylylate, or phosphorylate various aminoglycosides; enzymes that determine the permeability of the cell envelope to tetracyclines; and others.

Genetic material and plasmids can be transferred by the following mechanisms:

a. Transduction–Plasmid DNA is enclosed in a bacterial virus and transferred by the virus to another bacterium of the same species. ***Example:*** The plasmid carrying the gene for β-lactamase production can be transferred from a penicillin-resistant to a susceptible staphylococcus if carried by a suitable bacteriophage. Similar transduction occurs in salmonellae.

b. Transformation–Naked DNA passes from one cell of a species to another cell, thus altering the genotype of the latter. This can occur spontaneously or through laboratory manipulation, such as in recombinant DNA technology.

c. Bacterial conjugation–A unilateral transfer of genetic material between bacteria of the same or different genera occurs during a mating (conjugation) process. This is mediated by a fertility (F) factor that results in the extension of sex pili from the donor (F^+) cell to the recipient. Plasmid or other DNA is transferred through these protein tubules from the donor to the recipient cell. A series of closely linked genes, each determining resistance to one drug, may thus be transferred from a resistant to a susceptible bacterium. Such a resistance transfer factor (RTF) is the commonest method of spread of multidrug resistance among various genera of gram-negative bacteria.

d. Translocation or transposition–An exchange of short DNA sequences (transposons) occurs between one plasmid and another or between a plasmid and a portion of the bacterial chromosome within a bacterial cell.

Cross-Resistance

Microorganisms resistant to a certain drug may also be resistant to other drugs that share a mechanism of action or attachment. Such relationships exist mainly between agents that are closely related chemically (eg, polymyxin B-colistin; erythromycin-oleandomycin; neomycin-kanamycin), but they may also exist between unrelated chemicals (erythromycin-lincomycin). In certain classes of drugs, the active nucleus of the chemical is so similar among many congeners (eg, tetracyclines) that full cross-resistance is to be expected.

• • •

References

Blumberg PM, Strominger JL: Interaction of penicillin with the bacterial cell: Penicillin binding proteins and penicillin-sensitive enzymes. *Bacteriol Rev* 1974;**38:**291.

Buchanan CE, Strominger JL: Altered penicillin-binding components in penicillin-resistant mutants of *Bacillus subtilis. Proc Natl Acad Sci USA* 1976;**73:**1816.

Davies J: General mechanisms of antimicrobial resistance. *Rev Infect Dis* 1979;**1:**23.

Davies J, Courvalin P: Mechanisms of resistance to aminoglycosides. *Am J Med* 1977;**62:**868.

Falkow S: *Infectious Multiple Drug Resistance*. Pion Ltd, 1975.

Finland M: Emergence of antibiotic resistance in hospitals 1935–75. *Rev Infect Dis* 1979;**1:**4.

Jacobs MR et al: Emergence of multiply resistant pneumococci. *N Engl J Med* 1978;**299:**735.

Jawetz E: Antimicrobial drugs: Mechanisms and factors influencing their action. Chap 1, pp 3–10, in: *Antimicrobial Therapy*, 3rd ed. Kagan BM (editor). Saunders, 1980.

Pestka S: Inhibitors of ribosome function. *Annu Rev Microbiol* 1971;**25:**487.

Salton MRJ, Tomasz A: Mode of action of antibiotics on microbial walls and membranes. *Ann NY Acad Sci* 1974;**235:**5. [Entire issue.]

Tipper DJ: Mode of action of beta-lactam antibiotics. *Rev Infect Dis* 1979;**1:**39.

Tomasz A: From penicillin-binding proteins to the lysis and death of bacteria: A 1979 view. *Rev Infect Dis* 1979;**1:**434.

Penicillins & Cephalosporins | 42

Ernest Jawetz, MD, PhD

PENICILLINS

In 1929, Fleming reported his observation that colonies of staphylococci lysed on a plate that had become contaminated with a *Penicillium* mold. His efforts to extract the bacteriolytic substance failed, but in 1940 Chain, Florey, and their associates succeeded in producing significant quantities of the first penicillins from cultures of *Penicillium notatum*. Fermentation methods improved rapidly, so that by 1949 virtually unlimited quantities of penicillin were available for clinical use. Of the several fermentation products, penicillin G proved to be the best.

The 2 principal limitations of penicillin G were its susceptibility to destruction by β-lactamase (penicillinase) and its relative inactivity against most gram-negative bacteria. A research assault on these problems organized by Chain, Rolinson, and Batchelor led, in 1957, to the isolation of 6-aminopenicillanic acid in bulk amounts. Thus began the development of a long series of semisynthetic penicillins. This resulted in the selective design of drugs resistant to β-lactamase, stable to acid pH, and active against both gram-positive and gram-negative bacteria.

Penicillins and cephalosporins are large groups of drugs that share features of chemistry, mechanism of action, pharmacologic and clinical effects, and immunologic characteristics. These drugs are referred to as β-lactam drugs or cell wall inhibitors.

Chemistry

All penicillins share the basic structure shown in Fig 42–1. There is a thiazolidine ring (A) attached to a β-lactam ring (B) that carries a free amino group (C). Acidic radicals (R) can be attached to the amino group and can be separated from the amino group by bacterial and other amidases. The structural integrity of the 6-aminopenicillanic acid nucleus is essential to the biologic activity of the molecules. If the β-lactam ring is enzymatically cleaved by bacterial β-lactamases (penicillinases), the resulting product, penicilloic acid, is devoid of antibacterial activity. However, it carries an antigenic determinant of the penicillins, acts as a sensitizing structure when attached to host proteins, and can be used as skin testing material when attached to peptide chains. Products of alkaline hydrolysis of the penicillins also contribute to sensitization.

The attachment of different radicals (R) to the free amino group of 6-aminopenicillanic acid determines the essential pharmacologic properties of the resulting molecules. Clinically important penicillins available in 1982 fall into several groups: (1) Highest activity against gram-positive organisms but susceptible to hydrolysis by β-lactamases, eg, penicillin G. (2) Relatively resistant to staphylococcal β-lactamases but of lower activity against gram-positive organisms and inactive against gram-negatives, eg, nafcillin, methicillin. (3) Relatively high activity against both gram-negative and gram-positive organisms but destroyed by β-lactamases, eg, carbenicillin, ticarcillin. (4) Relatively stable to gastric acid and suitable for oral administration, eg, penicillin V, ampicillin, cloxacillin.

Some representatives of each group are shown in Fig 42–1, with a few distinguishing characteristics. Newer derivatives of β-amidinopenicillanic acid (eg, mecillinam) are also being investigated. Their antibacterial mechanism is different from that of β-lactam drugs.

Most penicillins are dispensed as the sodium or potassium salt of the free acid. Potassium penicillin G contains about 1.7 mEq of K^+ per million units of penicillin (2.8 mEq/g). Nafcillin contains Na^+, 2.8 mEq/g. Procaine salts (procaine penicillin) and benzathine salts (benzathine penicillin; Bicillin) are employed to provide repository forms for intramuscular injection.

In dry crystalline form, penicillin salts are stable for long periods (eg, for years at 4 °C). Solutions lose their activity rapidly (eg, 24 hours at 20 °C) and must be prepared fresh for administration.

Antimicrobial Activity of Beta-Lactam Drugs

Penicillins and cephalosporins share general mechanisms of antibacterial action that involve damage to the cell wall of bacteria. These complex mechanisms are incompletely understood and may not be the same for all drugs. Only a simplified outline is presented here. (See also Chapter 41.)

The initial step in penicillin action consists of binding of the drug to cell receptors. At least some of these receptor proteins are transpeptidation enzymes. After attachment of the drug, penicillins and cephalosporins inhibit the activity of various transpeptidation enzymes, and transpeptidation reactions are blocked. As a result, the synthesis of cell wall peptidoglycan

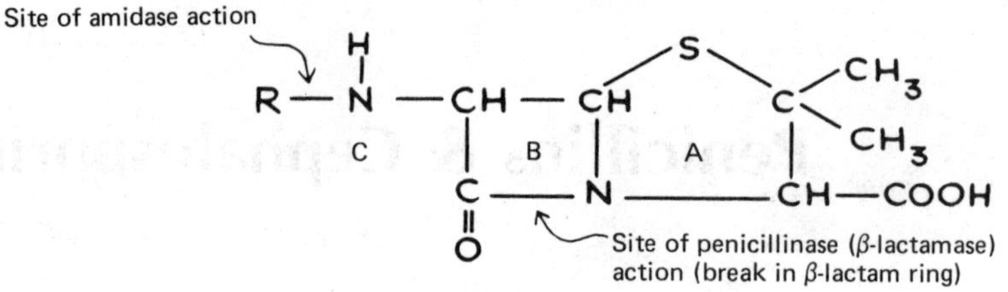

6-Aminopenicillanic acid

The following structures can each be substituted at R to produce a new penicillin.

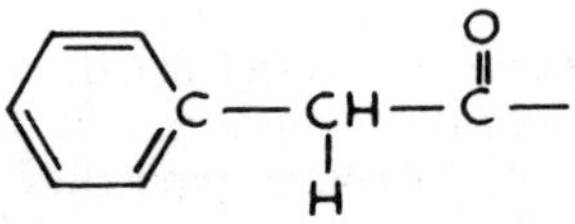

Penicillin G (benzylpenicillin):
High activity against gram-positive bacteria. Low activity against gram-negative bacteria. Acid-labile. Destroyed by β-lactamase. 60% protein-bound.

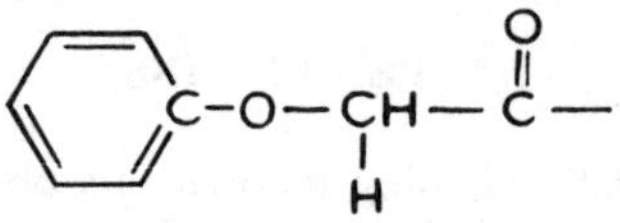

Penicillin V (phenoxymethyl penicillin):
Similar to penicillin G but relatively acid-resistant and can be taken orally.

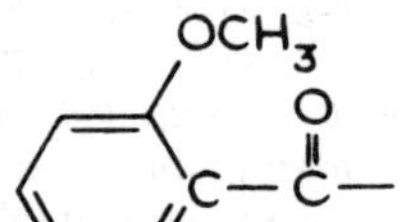

Methicillin (dimethoxyphenylpenicillin):
Lower activity than penicillin G but resistant to β-lactamase. Acid-labile. 40% protein-bound.

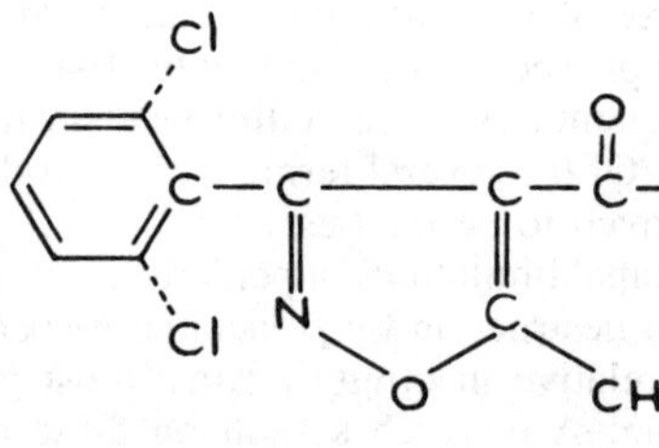

Oxacillin; cloxacillin (one Cl in structure); dicloxacillin (2 Cls in structure); flucloxacillin (one Cl and one F in structure) (isoxazolyl penicillins):
Similar to methicillin in β-lactamase resistance, but acid-stable. Can be taken orally. Highly protein-bound (95–98%).

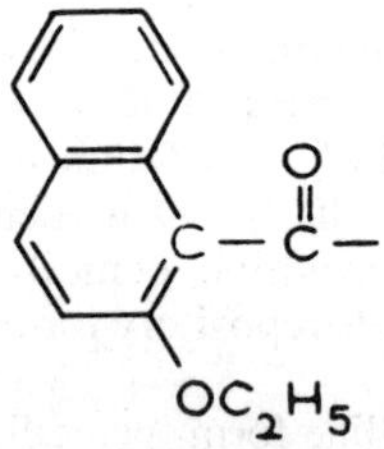

Nafcillin (ethoxynaphthamidopenicillin):
Similar to isoxazolyl penicillins. Less strongly protein-bound (90%). Can be given by mouth or by vein. Resistant to staphylococcal β-lactamase.

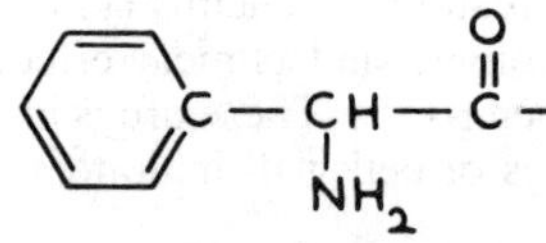

Ampicillin (alpha-aminobenzylpenicillin):
Similar to penicillin G (destroyed by β-lactamase) but acid-stable and more active against gram-negative bacteria. Carbenicillin has –COONa instead of $-NH_2$ group.

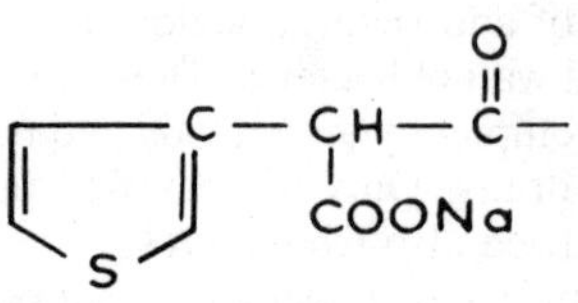

Ticarcillin:
Similar to carbenicillin but gives higher blood levels.

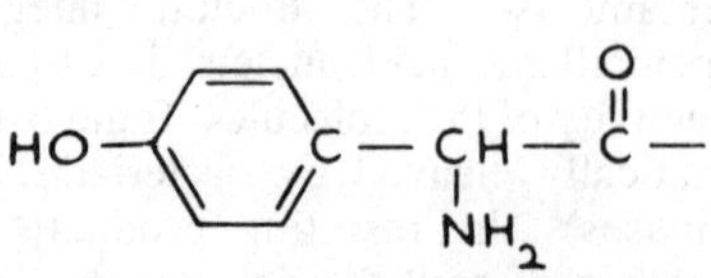

Amoxicillin:
Similar to ampicillin but better absorbed, gives higher blood levels.

Figure 42–1. Structures of some penicillins.

remains incomplete. The next step in the action of these drugs probably involves removal or inactivation of an inhibitor of autolytic enzymes in the cell wall. This activates the lytic enzymes and may result in lysis of the organism if the environment is isotonic. In a markedly hypertonic environment (eg, 20% sucrose), the cells change to protoplasts or spheroplasts, covered only by the fragile cell membrane. In such forms, the synthesis of proteins and nucleic acids may continue for some time.

Penicillins and cephalosporins can be bactericidal only if active peptidoglycan synthesis takes place. Metabolically inactive cells are unaffected.

Different penicillins possess different quantitative activity against certain organisms. Whereas 0.002–0.5 μg/mL of penicillin G is lethal for a majority of susceptible gram-positive bacteria, nafcillin and other β-lactamase-resistant penicillins are 10–100 times less active against the same organisms. While ampicillin, 0.01–0.5 μg/mL, is active against most organisms susceptible to penicillin G, it is also active against gram-negative non-β-lactamase-producing organisms in similar concentrations. The susceptibility of microorganisms is in part generic and in part a characteristic of individual strains. The difference in susceptibility of gram-positive and gram-negative organisms must depend in part on the frequency and avidity of drug receptors; on the relative amount of peptidoglycan present (gram-positive organisms usually possess far more); on the amount of lipids in the cell wall; and on other chemical differences that determine binding, penetration, and resistance to lysis or rupture. The gram-negative neisseriae are as susceptible to penicillin G as many gram-positive organisms.

The activity of penicillin G was originally defined in units. Crystalline sodium penicillin G contains approximately 1600 units/mg (1 unit = 0.6 μg; 1 million units of penicillin = 0.6 g). Most semisynthetic penicillins are prescribed in gram doses only.

Resistance

Resistance to penicillins falls into several distinct categories.

A. Certain bacteria (eg, many *Staphylococcus aureus*, some *Haemophilus influenzae* and gonococci, most gram-negative enteric rods) produce β-lactamases (penicillinases), enzymes that inactivate some penicillins by breaking the β-lactam ring. The genetic control of β-lactamase production—there are about 50 different such enzymes—resides in transmissible plasmids (see Chapter 41). Other penicillins (eg, nafcillin) and cephalosporins are β-lactamase-resistant because the β-lactam ring is protected by parts of the R side chain. Such penicillins are active against β-lactamase-producing organisms.

B. Other bacteria do not produce β-lactamases but are resistant to the action of penicillins either because they lack specific receptors or because of lack of permeability of outer layers, so that the drug cannot reach the receptors.

C. Some bacteria may be insusceptible to the killing action of penicillins because the autolytic enzymes in the cell wall are not activated. Such "tolerant" organisms (staphylococci, *Listeria*) are inhibited but not killed.

D. Organisms that lack cell walls (*Mycoplasma*, L forms) or are metabolically inactive are insusceptible to penicillins and other cell wall inhibitors because they do not synthesize peptidoglycans.

E. Some bacteria (eg, *Staphylococcus* sp) may be resistant to the action of β-lactamase-resistant penicillins, eg, methicillin. The mechanism of this resistance is unclear; it is independent of any β-lactamase production, and its frequency varies greatly with time and place.

Absorption, Metabolism, & Excretion

After parenteral administration, absorption of most penicillins is complete and rapid. Because of the irritation and consequent local pain produced by the intramuscular injection of large doses, administration by the intravenous route (intermittent bolus addition to a continuous drip) is often preferred. After oral administration, absorption differs greatly for different penicillins, depending in part on their acid stability and protein binding. In order to minimize binding to foods, oral penicillins should not be preceded or followed by food for at least 1 hour.

After absorption, penicillins are widely distributed in body fluids and tissues. Penicillins are lipid-insoluble and do not enter living cells well. With parenteral doses of 3–6 g (5–10 million units) of penicillin G, injected in divided doses into a continuous infusion or by intramuscular injections, average serum levels of the drug reach 1–10 units (0.6–6 μg)/mL. A rough relationship of 6 g given parenterally per day yielding serum levels of 1–6 μg/mL also applies to other penicillins. Highly protein-bound penicillins (eg, oxacillin, dicloxacillin) tend to produce lower levels of free drug in serum than less protein-bound penicillins (eg, penicillin G, ampicillin). However, the relevance of protein binding to clinical efficacy of drug is not fully understood.

Special dosage forms of penicillin have been designed for delayed absorption to yield low blood and tissue levels for long periods. The outstanding example is benzathine penicillin G. After a single intramuscular injection of 1.5 g (2.4 million units), serum levels in excess of 0.03 unit/mL are maintained for 10 days and levels in excess of 0.005 unit/mL for 3 weeks. The latter is sufficient to protect against β-hemolytic streptococcal infection; the former to treat an established infection with these organisms. Procaine penicillin also has delayed absorption, yielding levels for 24 hours after intramuscular injection.

In many tissues, penicillin concentrations are equal to those in serum. Lower levels are found in the eye, the prostate, and the central nervous system. However, with active inflammation of the meninges, as in bacterial meningitis, penicillin levels in the cerebrospinal fluid exceed 0.2 μg/mL with a daily parenteral dose of 12 g. Thus, pneumococcal and meningococcal meningitis may be treated with systemic penicillin and there is no need for intrathecal injection. It is probable that high levels of penicillins in the cerebrospinal fluid in meningitis are due to (1) increased permeability of meninges, (2) inhibition of active transport of penicillin from the cerebrospinal fluid, which occurs normally, or (3) some binding of penicillin to cerebrospinal fluid proteins. Absorbed penicillins also reach pleural, pericardial, and joint fluids well, so that local injection is rarely warranted.

Most of the absorbed penicillin is rapidly excreted by the kidneys into the urine; small amounts are excreted by other channels. About 10% of renal excretion is by glomerular filtration and 90% by tubular secretion, to a maximum of about 2 g/h in an adult. The normal half-life of penicillin is ½–1 hour; in renal failure, it may be up to 10 hours. Ampicillin is secreted more slowly than penicillin G. Nafcillin is excreted 80% into the biliary tract and only 20% by tubular secretion; therefore, it is little affected by renal failure. Tubular secretion can be partially blocked by probenecid (Benemid) to achieve higher systemic and cerebrospinal fluid levels. Renal clearance is less efficient in the newborn, so that proportionately smaller doses result in higher systemic levels that are maintained longer than in the adult.

Renal excretion of penicillin results in very high levels in the urine. Thus, systemic daily doses of 6 g of penicillin may yield urine levels of 500–3000 μg/mL—enough to suppress not only gram-positive but also many gram-negative bacteria in the urine (provided they produce little β-lactamase).

Penicillin is also excreted into sputum and milk to levels of 3–15% of those present in the serum. This is the case in both humans and cattle. The presence of penicillin in the milk of cows treated for mastitis presents a problem in allergy.

Clinical Uses

Penicillins are by far the most widely effective and the most extensively used antibiotics. All oral penicillins should be given away from meal times (1 hour before or 1–2 hours after), to reduce binding and acid inactivation. Oxacillin is most strongly bound to food (ie, protein-bound), dicloxacillin somewhat less so. Blood levels of all penicillins can be raised by simultaneous administration of probenecid, 0.5 g every 6 hours orally (10 mg/kg every 6 hours), which impairs tubular secretion.

A. Penicillin G is the drug of choice for infections caused by pneumococci, streptococci, meningococci, non-β-lactamase-producing staphylococci and gonococci, *Treponema pallidum* and many other spirochetes, *Bacillus anthracis* and other gram-positive rods, clostridia, *Actinomyces, Listeria,* and *Bacteroides* (except *Bacteroides fragilis*). Most of these infections respond to daily doses of penicillin G, 0.6–5 million units (0.36–3 g). Intermittent intramuscular injection is the usual method of administration. Much larger amounts (6–50 g daily) can be given by injection during a 20-minute period every 4–6 hours into an intravenous infusion. Such a procedure is useful in serious or complicated infections due to these organisms. Oral administration of **penicillin V** is indicated only in minor infections—eg, of the respiratory tract or its associated structures, especially in children (pharyngitis, otitis, sinusitis)—in a daily dose of 1–4 g. Oral administration is subject to so many variables that it should not be relied upon in seriously ill patients. Many non-β-lactamase-producing gonococci have developed partial resistance to penicillin, requiring 1–3 units/mL for inhibition. Treatment of such gonorrhea now requires procaine penicillin, 4.8 million units once, with probenecid, 1 g orally. In gonococcal prostatitis, arthritis, salpingitis, or other closed lesions, 10 million units must be given daily for 4–14 days, combined with drainage when needed. When β-lactamase-producing gonococci are present, alternative drugs, eg, spectinomycin or tetracycline, must be used.

Penicillin G is inhibitory for enterococci *(Streptococcus faecalis),* but the simultaneous administration of an aminoglycoside is often necessary for bactericidal effects, eg, in enterococcal endocarditis. In urinary tract infections, large doses of penicillin G (eg, 1–10 million units intramuscularly) may provide sufficiently high levels in the urine to inhibit relatively resistant gram-negative coliform bacteria and, in particular, *Proteus mirabilis*. However, such treatment is likely to fail in the presence of large numbers of bacteria producing large amounts of β-lactamase.

B. Benzathine penicillin G is a salt of very low water solubility for intramuscular injection that yields low but prolonged drug levels. A single injection of 1.2 million units intramuscularly is satisfactory for treatment of beta-hemolytic streptococcal pharyngitis. A similar injection given intramuscularly once every 3–4 weeks provides satisfactory prophylaxis against reinfection with beta-hemolytic streptococci. Benzathine penicillin G (2.4 million units intramuscularly once a week for 1–3 weeks) is effective in the treatment of early or latent syphilis. This drug should never be given by mouth.

C. Ampicillin, Amoxicillin, Carbenicillin, Ticarcillin: These drugs differ from penicillin G in having greater activity against gram-negative bacteria, but they are inactivated by β-lactamases.

Ampicillin, 500 mg orally every 6–8 hours, is used to treat common urinary tract infections with gram-negative coliform bacteria or mixed secondary bacterial infections of the respiratory tract (sinusitis, otitis, bronchitis). Ampicillin is also sometimes given for infections in which penicillin G is the drug of choice but oral therapy is preferred (eg, in acute uncomplicated gonorrhea, 3.5 g once, with probenecid). Ampicillin, 300 mg/kg/d intravenously, is a current choice for bacterial meningitis in children, especially if the disease is caused by *H influenzae*. However, in some locations, β-lactamase-producing *H influenzae* are emerging, which means that ampicillin is ineffective and chloramphenicol must be used.

Ampicillin is ineffective against *Enterobacter, Pseudomonas,* and indole-positive *Proteus* infections. In invasive *Salmonella* infections (eg, typhoid), ampicillin, 6–12 g/d intravenously, can suppress signs and symptoms and eliminate organisms from some carriers. In typhoid and paratyphoid fevers, ampicillin is an alternative to chloramphenicol or trimethoprim-sulfamethoxazole. However, it is not beneficial in noninvasive *Salmonella* gastroenteritis and may even prolong carriage and shedding. An exception may be salmonellosis in severely malnourished children. In enterococcal sepsis or endocarditis, ampicillin may be more active than penicillin G when combined with an aminoglycoside.

Amoxicillin is similar to ampicillin but is somewhat better absorbed from the gut. The same applies to the esters pivampicillin and bacampicillin. These 3 drugs are comparable in spectrum, activity, and side-effects to ampicillin but can be given somewhat less frequently (eg, amoxicillin, 500 mg 3 times daily, instead of ampicillin, 500 mg 4 times daily).

Carbenicillin resembles ampicillin but has more activity against *Pseudomonas* and *Proteus* organisms, although *Klebsiella* are usually resistant. In susceptible populations of *Pseudomonas,* resistance to carbenicillin may emerge rapidly. Therefore, in *Pseudomonas* sepsis (eg, burns, immunosuppressed patients), carbenicillin, 12–30 g/d intravenously (300–500 mg/kg/d), is usually combined with an aminoglycoside, eg, gentamicin, 5–7 mg/kg/d intramuscularly, to delay emergence of resistance and perhaps to obtain synergistic effects. Carbenicillin contains Na^+, 4.7 mEq/g. Carbenicillin indanyl sodium is acid-stable and can be given orally in urinary tract infections.

Ticarcillin resembles carbenicillin in single and combined activity, but the dose may be lower, eg, 200–300 mg/kg/d intravenously. Hetacillin is converted to ampicillin and should not be used.

D. Beta-Lactamase-Resistant Penicillins: These are relatively resistant to destruction by staphylococcal β-lactamases. The sole indication for their use is infection by β-lactamase-producing staphylococci.

Oxacillin, cloxacillin, dicloxacillin, or nafcillin, 0.25–0.5 g every 4–6 hours by mouth, is suitable for treatment of mild localized staphylococcal infections (50–100 mg/kg/d for children). All of these drugs are relatively acid-stable and reasonably well absorbed from the gut. They are all highly protein-bound (95–98%). Food interferes with their absorption, and the drugs must be administered 1 hour away from meals.

For serious systemic staphylococcal infections, nafcillin, 8–12 g/d, is administered intravenously, usually by introducing 1–2 g during 20–30 minutes every 2–4 hours into a continuous infusion of 5% dextrose in water. The dose for children is 50–100 mg/kg/d. Methicillin is employed similarly but at present is believed to be more nephrotoxic than nafcillin and therefore employed less often.

Adverse Reactions

The penicillins undoubtedly possess less direct toxicity than any other antibiotics. Most of the serious side-effects are due to hypersensitivity.

A. Allergy: All penicillins are cross-sensitizing and cross-reacting. Any preparation containing penicillin may induce sensitization, including foods or cosmetics. In general, sensitization occurs in direct proportion to the duration and total dose of penicillin received in the past. The responsible antigenic determinants appear to be degradation products of penicillins, particularly penicilloic acid and products of alkaline hydrolysis bound to host protein. Skin tests with penicilloylpolylysine, with alkaline hydrolysis products, and with undegraded penicillin will identify many hypersensitive individuals. Among positive reactors to skin tests, the incidence of subsequent penicillin reactions is high. Although many persons develop IgG antibodies to antigenic determinants of penicillin, the presence of such antibodies does not appear to be correlated with allergic reactivity (except rare hemolytic anemia), and serologic tests have little predictive value. A history of a penicillin reaction in the past is not reliable; about 5–8% of people claim such a history in the USA. However, in such cases, penicillin should be administered with caution or a substitute drug given.

About 10–15% of persons with a past history of a penicillin reaction have an allergic reaction when given penicillin again. Less than 1% of persons who previously received penicillin without incident will have an allergic reaction when given penicillin again. The incidence of allergic reactions in small children is negligible.

Allergic reactions may occur as typical anaphylactic shock (very rare—0.5% of recipients), typical serum sickness type reactions (now rare—urticaria, fever, joint swelling, angioneurotic edema, intense pruritus, and respiratory embarrassment occurring 7–12 days after exposure), and a variety of skin rashes, oral lesions, fever, interstitial nephritis (an autoimmune reaction to a penicillin-protein complex), eosinophilia, hemolytic anemia and other hematologic disturbances, and vasculitis.

At times, individuals known to be hypersensitive to penicillin can tolerate the drug during corticosteroid administration. "Desensitization" with gradually increasing doses of penicillin is rarely indicated. Most patients allergic to penicillins can be treated with alternative drugs. Anaphylactic reactions are less common after oral penicillin administration than after parenteral administration.

B. Toxicity: Since the action of penicillin is directed against a unique bacterial structure, the cell wall, it is virtually without effect on animal cells. The toxic effects of penicillin G are due to the direct irritation caused by intramuscular or intravenous injection of exceedingly high concentrations (eg, 1 g/mL). Such concentrations may cause local pain, induration, thrombophlebitis, or degeneration of an accidentally injected nerve. All penicillins are irritating to the central nervous system and greatly increase the excitability of neurons. For that reason, no more than 20,000 units can be given intrathecally on any one day, but there is little indication for intrathecal administration at present. In rare cases, a patient receiving high doses (eg, more than 20 million units of penicillin G daily) has exhibited signs of cerebrocortical irritation as a result of the passage of unusually large amounts of penicillin into the central nervous system. With doses of this magnitude, direct cation toxicity (Na^+, K^+) can also occur (see Chemistry, above), particularly in patients with renal failure.

Large doses of penicillins given orally may lead to gastrointestinal upset, particularly nausea, vomiting, and diarrhea. This is more pronounced with the broad-spectrum forms (ampicillin, amoxicillin) than with other penicillins. Oral therapy may also be accompanied by luxuriant overgrowth of staphylococci, *Pseudomonas, Proteus,* or yeasts, which may occasionally cause enteritis. Superinfections in other organ systems may occur with penicillins as with any antibiotic therapy. Methicillin, nafcillin, and other penicillins have occasionally caused granulocytopenia, especially in children. Methicillin causes nephritis more commonly than does nafcillin: The tubular basement membrane protein serves to bind penicillin, and antibody to the carrier-hapten antigen forms a complex, with binding of complement. Carbenicillin can cause hypokalemic alkalosis and transaminase elevation in serum. It can also induce hemostatic defects leading to bleeding tendency. Ampicillin frequently causes skin rashes, some of which are not allergic in nature.

Problems Relating to the Use of the Penicillins

The penicillins are by far the most widely used antibiotics. Several thousand tons of these drugs have been administered to humans during the past 40 years. Therefore, penicillins have been responsible for some of the most drastic consequences of antibiotic misuse.

A significant proportion (perhaps 1–5%) of the population of many countries has become hypersensitive. In many cases, there is no doubt that sensitization has occurred when penicillin was administered without proper indication. It would be desirable to have penicillin-hypersensitive individuals definitely identified, but hypersensitivity may be temporary.

The saturation of certain environments (eg, hospitals) with penicillin has produced a selection pressure against penicillin-sensitive microorganisms and resulted in greater numbers of penicillin-resistant organisms. In the 1950s, hospitals were an important site for the proliferation and selection of β-lactamase-producing staphylococci; subsequently, they led to outbreaks of sepsis in newborn nurseries and surgical units. Now β-lactamase-producing staphylococci prevail everywhere; they cause about 80% of community-acquired staphylococcal infections.

The suppression of normal flora creates a partial void that is regularly filled with drug-resistant, prevalent organisms. Penicillins are administered to a high proportion of patients in hospitals. These patients are made selectively susceptible to superinfections with microorganisms derived from the hospital environment (*Proteus, Pseudomonas, Enterobacter, Serratia,* yeasts, staphylococci, etc). Such organisms become established in organ systems where the normal flora has been suppressed (eg, the respiratory tract, gut, skin) and can cause disease processes there.

Plasmids that control β-lactamase production are being distributed with increasing frequency among different genera of microorganisms. *Neisseria gonorrhoeae* has recently acquired such plasmids, probably from *Haemophilus* sp. In West Africa and in the Philippines, outbreaks of β-lactamase-producing gonococci are seen. Local endemic foci have also been found in the USA (eg, Los Angeles), presenting problems for their control.

Although pneumococci have long been considered an example of total and regular susceptibility to penicillins, this is no longer entirely true. In New Guinea and South Africa, outbreaks of relatively penicillin-resistant pneumococci have been observed, causing pneumonia and meningitis. The pneumococci do not appear to produce β-lactamase, but up to 6 μg/mL of penicillin G may be necessary to kill them. Such concentrations of penicillin cannot be obtained in the central nervous system, and the mortality rate has consequently been high. Sporadic cases of similar resistance have been observed in the USA.

CEPHALOSPORINS

Fungi of *Cephalosporium* sp yielded several antibiotics that resembled penicillins but were resistant to β-lactamase and were active against both gram-positive and gram-negative bacteria. Methods were eventually developed for the large-scale production of the common nucleus, 7-aminocephalosporanic acid. This made possible the synthesis of many derivatives, the cephalosporins. A bewildering array of semisynthetic cephalosporins has been developed. In addition to the synthetics derived from cephalosporanic acid, the cephamycins (fermentation products of *Streptomyces*) have very similar properties, as do totally synthetic new drugs such as moxalactam.

Chemistry

The nucleus of the cephalosporins, 7-aminocephalosporanic acid, bears a close resemblance to 6-aminopenicillanic acid and also to the nucleus of the cephamycin antibiotics. The intrinsic antimicrobial activity of natural cephalosporins is low, but the attachment of various R_1 and R_2 groups has yielded drugs of good therapeutic activity and low toxicity.

The cephalosporins have molecular weights of 400–450. They are soluble in water and relatively stable to pH and temperature changes. They vary in resistance to β-lactamases. The sodium salt of cephalothin contains 2.4 mEq Na^+ per gram.

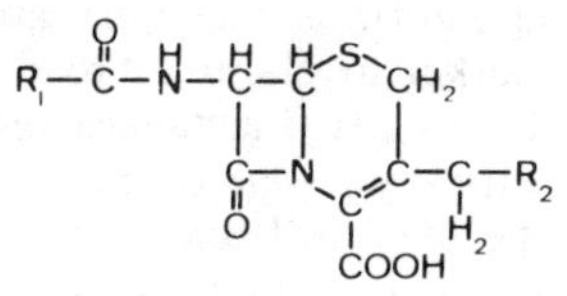

7-Aminocephalosporanic acid

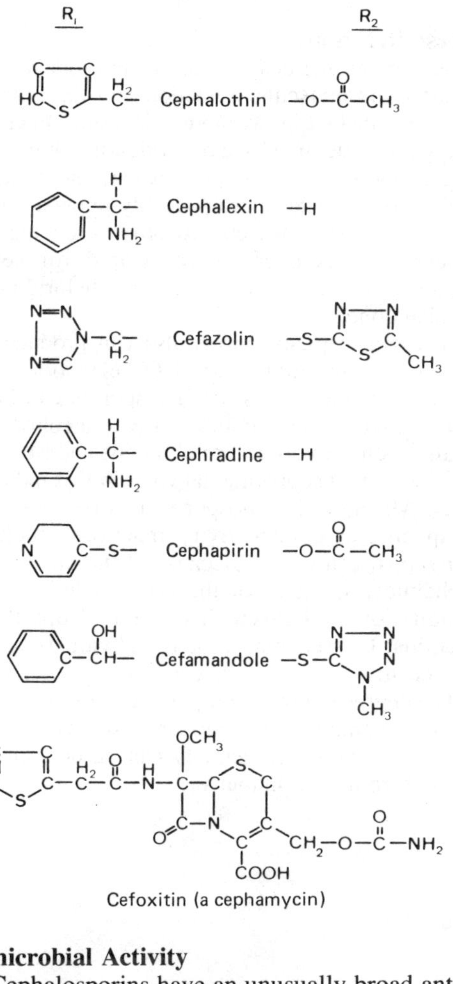

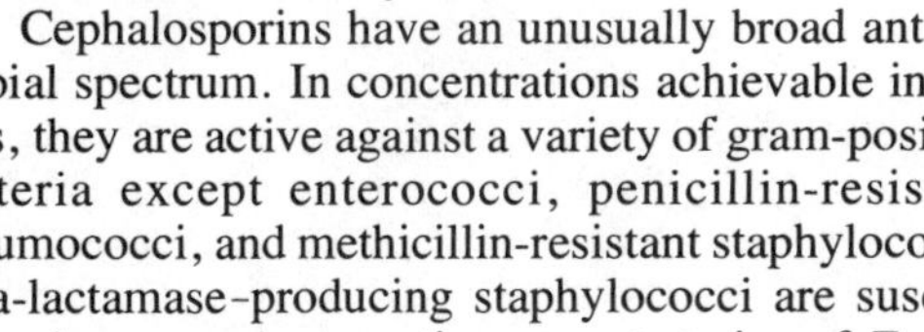

Cefoxitin (a cephamycin)

Antimicrobial Activity

Cephalosporins have an unusually broad antimicrobial spectrum. In concentrations achievable in tissues, they are active against a variety of gram-positive bacteria except enterococci, penicillin-resistant pneumococci, and methicillin-resistant staphylococci. Beta-lactamase-producing staphylococci are susceptible. Among gram-negatives, most strains of *Escherichia coli, Klebsiella* sp, and *Proteus* sp are susceptible, and some strains of *Enterobacter, Serratia,* and *Pseudomonas*. There are substantial differences between different drugs also in their activity against anaerobes, including *B fragilis*. The more recent arrivals, eg, cefamandole, cefoxitin, cefuroxime, and moxalactam have a broader spectrum than the earlier drugs.

The mechanism of action of cephalosporins is analogous to that described for penicillins. The receptors are similar or identical proteins, but different drugs may bind to different receptors. Transpeptidation enzymes are inhibited, resulting in blockage of terminal cross-linking of bacterial cell wall peptidoglycan. Autolytic enzymes in cell wall may be activated. It appears that the mechanism is not identical for every drug and for every bacterial species.

Resistance to cephalosporins is often mediated by bacterial β-lactamases (many different enzymes) or by lack of bacterial permeability to the drug. Absence of the proper receptors may play a role.

Absorption, Distribution, & Excretion

Of the more than 20 cephalosporins available in the USA in 1982, only 4 (cephalexin, cephradine, cefaclor, cefadroxil) are sufficiently well absorbed after oral intake to give systemic levels or urine levels suitable for treatment. The other drugs in this class are usually given intravenously because intramuscular injection is too painful. Commonly, a bolus of 0.5–2 g is added 4–8 times daily to an intravenous drip, resulting in serum levels ranging from 10 to 40 μg/mL. The serum half-life typically ranges from 30 to 90 minutes. There are significant variations between individual drugs.

Cephalosporins are distributed widely into tissues and body fluids, including pleural, pericardial, and synovial fluids. However, there is little or no penetration into the central nervous system or across the placenta. The earlier cephalosporins have been singularly unsuccessful in the treatment of meningitis.

Cephalosporins are excreted mainly by glomerular filtration and tubular secretion into the urine, where levels may reach 200–2000 μg/mL. Tubular blocking agents (eg, probenecid) may increase serum levels substantially. Those cephalosporins containing acetyl groups in the R_2 position (cephalothin, cephapirin) are deacetylated in the liver; the metabolic product is less biologically active. In renal failure, the dose must be reduced, since the excretion of cephalosporins may be markedly impaired, and high fluid and tissue levels may exert toxic effects. Levels of cephalosporins in bile are similar to those in serum.

Clinical Uses

Cephalosporins can be considered for the following major applications:

(1) Suspected bacteremia due to an unknown organism (most likely *Staphylococcus, Klebsiella,* coliform bacteria, *Proteus,* or *Pseudomonas*), especially in debilitated or immunosuppressed patients. A cephalosporin is usually given together with an aminoglycoside.

(2) Selected "surgical prophylaxis." A cephalosporin is given parenterally for 2–6 hours before and 12–24 hours after a surgical procedure that has more than a 5% risk of infection.

(3) Mixed infections, especially those including anaerobes, involving chest, abdomen, or pelvis.

(4) Penicillinase-producing *N gonorrhoeae* and other special infections. An alternative choice in urinary tract infections.

(5) Gram-negative rod bacterial meningitis may be treated with moxalactam or other recent cephalosporins.

A. Oral Administration: Cephalexin and cephradine seem virtually identical in terms of absorption, levels in blood (10 μg/mL after 0.5 g every 6 hours), protein binding (20%), antimicrobial activity, and excretion in urine. Use is limited to infections of the urinary tract (levels in urine may reach 500 μg/mL) or to minor infections of the respiratory tract (otitis, sinusitis, tracheobronchitis) caused by susceptible organisms. Cefadroxil (1 g every 12 hours) has similar indications. Cefaclor is similar to these drugs but is also active against β-lactamase-producing *H influenzae*. It is given 3–4 times daily in a dose of 15–30 mg/kg/d (up to 1 g/d for children).

B. Parenteral Administration:

1. Intramuscular–Cefazolin, cefamandole, cefoxitin, cefotaxime, and others may be given by this route in the same dose as intravenously. However, pain on injection may be a major objection to this route of administration.

2. Intravenous–Typically, a portion of the daily dose (below) is added as a bolus every 4–8 hours to an intravenous infusion. Cefazolin, 4 g/d (50–100 mg/kg/d), has been used for surgical prophylaxis because it gives unusually high and prolonged levels. Cephalothin, 6–12 g/d (50–200 mg/kg/d), yields somewhat lower serum levels, but it is highly resistant to staphylococcal β-lactamase. Cephapirin is similar. Cefamandole, 6–12 g/d (75–200 mg/kg/d), is often active against *Klebsiella, Enterobacter, Proteus,* and anaerobes. Cefoxitin is similar but is claimed to be preferred in *B fragilis* infections and is considered an alternative drug for penicillinase-producing *N gonorrhoeae*. With all of these drugs, individual strains may exhibit resistance.

Laboratory tests for susceptibility of a given isolate may occasionally be helpful. Cefotaxime, 4–12 g/d (50–200 mg/kg/d), is the 1981 arrival on the United States market to claim a broader spectrum, enhanced activity, greater β-lactamase resistance, and greater clinical efficacy. *None* of the earlier cephalosporins should be used in bacterial meningitis. The latest drugs—especially moxalactam, cefotaxime, and cefoperazone—may be suitable for treating meningitis caused by gram-negative enteric bacteria.

Adverse Reactions

A. Toxicity: Local irritation can produce severe pain after intramuscular injection and thrombophlebitis after repeated intravenous injection. Other toxic reactions include anaphylaxis, urticaria, skin rashes, fever, eosinophilia, granulocytopenia, and hemolytic anemia. Some of these are probably hypersensitivity reactions (see below). Renal toxicity producing tubular necrosis has been demonstrated for several cephalosporins. For this reason, cephaloridine has been abandoned.

The oral cephalosporins also can produce diarrhea, nausea, vomiting, and SGOT elevation.

Some of the newest cephalosporins can have a disulfiramlike effect if combined with alcohol. They may also induce hypoprothrombinemia and a bleeding tendency, so that supplemental vitamin K is indicated.

B. Allergy: Cephalosporins can be sensitizing, and specific hypersensitivity reactions, including anaphylaxis, can occur. Because of the difference in the chemical structure of the drug nucleus, the antigenicity of cephalosporins differs from that of penicillins. Consequently, many individuals who are hypersensitive to penicillins can tolerate cephalosporins. The degree of cross-allergenicity between penicillins and cephalosporins remains controversial (6–16%). Some cross-antigenicity can be demonstrated both in vitro and in humans.

• • •

References

Barza M: Antimicrobial spectrum, pharmacology and therapeutic use of penicillins. *Am J Hosp Pharm* 1977;**34:**57.

Border WA et al: Antitubular basement membrane antibodies in methicillin-associated interstitial nephritis. *N Engl J Med* 1974;**291:**381.

Brown CH et al: The hemostatic defect produced by carbenicillin. *N Engl J Med* 1974;**291:**265.

Buchanan CE, Strominger JL: Altered penicillin-binding components in penicillin-resistant mutants of *Bacillus subtilis*. *Proc Natl Acad Sci USA* 1976;**73:**1816.

Finegold SM et al: Comparative trial of bacampicillin and amoxicillin in bacterial infections of the lower respiratory tract. *Rev Infect Dis* 1981;**3:**150.

Grose WE et al: Some pharmacologic features of cefamandole. *Clin Pharmacol Ther* 1976;**20:**579.

Heseltine PN et al: Cefoxitin: Clinical evaluation in thirty-eight patients. *Antimicrob Agents Chemother* 1977;**11:**427.

Kancir LM et al: Adverse reactions to methicillin and nafcillin during treatment of serious *Staphylococcus aureus* infections. *Arch Intern Med* 1978;**138:**909.

Landesman SH et al: Gram-negative bacillary meningitis: New therapy and changing concepts. *Arch Intern Med* 1982; **142:**939.

Love LJ et al: Randomized trial of empiric antibiotic therapy with ticarcillin in combination with gentamicin, amikacin, or netilmicin in febrile patients with granulocytopenia and cancer. *Am J Med* 1979;**66:**603.

Mangi RJ et al: Development of meningitis during cephalothin therapy. *Ann Intern Med* 1973;**78:**347.

Murray BE, Moellering RC Jr: Cephalosporins. *Annu Rev Med* 1981;**32:**559.

Neu HC: Comparative studies of cefoxitin and cephalothin: An overview. *Rev Infect Dis* 1979;**1:**144.

Parker CW: Drug allergy. (3 parts.) *N Engl J Med* 1975;**292:**511, 732, 957.

Parry MF et al: Nafcillin nephritis. *JAMA* 1973;**225:**178.

Petz LD: Immunologic cross reactivity between penicillins and cephalosporins: A review. *J Infect Dis* 1978;**137(Suppl):**S74.

Phillips JA et al: Ampicillin-associated diarrhea. *Pediatrics* 1976;**58:**869.

Reyes MP et al: Granulocytopenia associated with carbenicillin. *Am J Med* 1973;**54:**413.

Rolinson GN: 6-APA and the development of the beta-lactam antibiotics. *J Antimicrob Chemother* 1979;**5:**7.

Rudolph AH, Price EV: Penicillin reactions among patients in venereal disease clinics. *JAMA* 1973;**223:**499.

Scheifele DW et al: Evaluation of rapid β-lactamase test for detecting ampicillin-resistant strains of *Hemophilus influenzae* type b. *Pediatrics* 1976;**58:**382.

Spector R, Lorenzo AV: Inhibition of penicillin transport from the cerebrospinal fluid after intracisternal inoculation of bacteria. *J Clin Invest* 1974;**54:**316.

Tipper DJ: Mode of action of beta-lactam antibiotics. *Rev Infect Dis* 1979;**1:**39.

43 | Chloramphenicol & Tetracyclines

Ernest Jawetz, MD, PhD

CHLORAMPHENICOL

Chloramphenicol was first isolated from cultures of *Streptomyces venezuelae* in 1947 and was synthesized in 1949. It is the only available representative of its chemical type and the only completely synthetic antibiotic of importance to be produced commercially.

Chemistry

Crystalline chloramphenicol is a neutral, stable compound with the following structure:

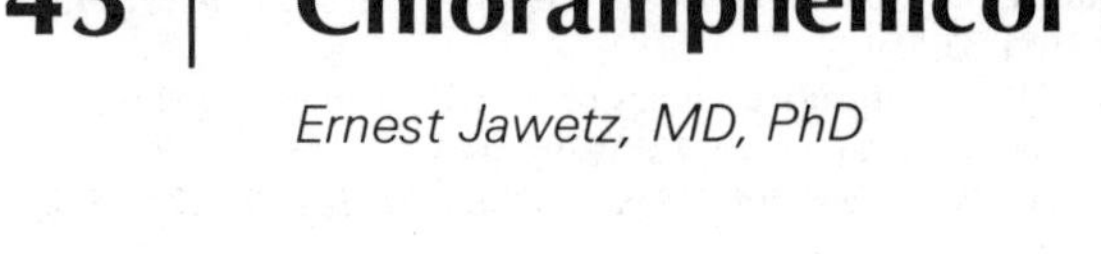

Chloramphenicol

It consists of colorless crystals with an intensely bitter taste. It is highly soluble in alcohol and poorly soluble in water. Saturated aqueous solutions (0.25%) keep their activity for many months at refrigerator or room temperature if protected from light. Chloramphenicol succinate is highly soluble in water and is hydrolyzed in tissues with the liberation of free chloramphenicol; it is used for parenteral injection.

Antimicrobial Activity

Chloramphenicol is a potent inhibitor of microbial protein synthesis and has little effect on other microbial metabolic functions. Chloramphenicol binds reversibly to a receptor site on the 50S subunit of the bacterial ribosome. There it interferes markedly with the incorporation of amino acids into newly formed peptides by blocking the action of peptidyl transferase (see Chapter 41). Chloramphenicol also inhibits mitochondrial protein synthesis of mammalian bone marrow cells but does not greatly affect other intact cells.

Chloramphenicol is bacteriostatic for many bacteria and for rickettsiae but is clinically ineffective against chlamydiae. Its action is reversible by removal of the drug. Most gram-positive bacteria are inhibited by chloramphenicol in concentrations of 1–10 μg/mL, and many gram-negative bacteria are inhibited by concentrations of 0.2–5 μg/mL. *Haemophilus influenzae* and many strains of *Bacteroides* are highly susceptible, and for them chloramphenicol may be bactericidal. Some salmonellae are susceptible, but plasmid-mediated resistance to chloramphenicol has appeared with increasing frequency.

Resistance

In most bacterial species, large populations of chloramphenicol-susceptible cells contain occasional resistant mutants. These mutants are usually only 2–4 times more resistant than the parent populations; consequently, they emerge slowly in treated individuals. There is no cross-resistance between chloramphenicol and other drugs, but plasmids (resistance transfer factors, RTF) may transmit multiple drug resistance (chloramphenicol, tetracycline, streptomycin, etc) from one bacterium or species to another by conjugation (see Chapter 41). Such plasmid-mediated resistance to chloramphenicol results from the production of chloramphenicol acetyl transferase, a bacterial enzyme that destroys the drug. Consequently, the resistance of such plasmid-containing microorganisms is of high order.

Absorption, Metabolism, & Excretion

After oral administration, crystalline chloramphenicol is rapidly and completely absorbed. With daily doses of 2 g orally, blood levels usually reach 8 μg/mL. Chloramphenicol palmitate, administered to children in doses up to 50 mg/kg/d orally, is hydrolyzed in the intestine to yield free chloramphenicol, but the usual blood levels rarely exceed 10 μg/mL. For parenteral injection, chloramphenicol succinate, 25–50 mg/kg/d intravenously, yields free chloramphenicol by hydrolysis, giving blood levels somewhat lower than those achieved with the orally administered drug.

After absorption, chloramphenicol is widely distributed to virtually all tissues and body fluids, including the central nervous system and cerebrospinal fluid. In fact, the concentration of chloramphenicol in brain tissue may be equal to that in serum—a unique property for the treatment of central nervous system infections.

Circulating chloramphenicol is about 30% protein-bound. The drug penetrates cells readily. Most of the drug is inactivated in the body either by conjugation with glucuronic acid (principally in the liver) or by reduction to inactive aryl amines. Excretion of active chloramphenicol (about 10% of the total dose administered) and of inactive degradation products (about 90% of the total) occurs into the urine. It may be that the active drug is cleared mainly by glomerular filtration and the inactive products mainly by tubular secretion. Only small amounts of active drug are excreted into bile or feces.

Clinical Uses

Chloramphenicol is a possible drug of choice in only a few types of infections: (1) Symptomatic *Salmonella* infection, eg, typhoid fever (some strains in Central and South America are now resistant). (2) *H influenzae* meningitis, laryngotracheitis, or pneumonia not responding to ampicillin. (3) Occasional bacteremia caused by gram-negative bacteria expected (on the basis of experience) to be resistant to other drugs. (4) Infection with *Bacteroides* and other anaerobes and brain abscess attributed to a mixed flora or anaerobes. (5) Meningococcal infection in patients hypersensitive to penicillin. (6) Severe rickettsial infections.

Chloramphenicol is occasionally used topically in the treatment of eye infections but is not effective in chlamydial eye infections.

A. Salmonellosis: For *Salmonella* infections (eg, typhoid or paratyphoid fever), adults should receive chloramphenicol, 2–3 g daily orally for 14–21 days, and children 30–50 mg/kg/d orally for 14–21 days. Prolonged treatment tends to reduce the frequency of relapses. A similar program may be followed in severe rickettsial infections (eg, scrub typhus or Rocky Mountain spotted fever).

B. Haemophilus: For *H influenzae* meningitis or laryngotracheitis (in small children) or pneumonia (in the elderly), chloramphenicol, 50–100 mg/kg/d orally or intravenously, has been given for 8–14 days, depending upon clinical response and cerebrospinal fluid changes. However, ampicillin is the drug of first choice at present unless ampicillin-resistant *Haemophilus* strains have been encountered in the community. It has also been recommended that initial treatment for *Haemophilus* meningitis should consist of both chloramphenicol and ampicillin until it can be shown that the organism does not produce β-lactamase. On the other hand, chloramphenicol-resistant *Haemophilus* strains have also appeared.

C. Other Uses: In life-threatening sepsis probably originating in the lower bowel, chloramphenicol, 2 g/d, is sometimes combined with an aminoglycoside (eg, amikacin, 15 mg/kg/d). Because of the excellent penetration of chloramphenicol into all parts of the central nervous system, it is sometimes used in cerebritis, brain abscess, or meningitis of ill-defined origin. Sepsis caused by some species of *Bacteroides* and severe melioidosis may respond to chloramphenicol.

In ophthalmology, topical application of chloramphenicol to the eye has been employed because of the wide antibacterial spectrum of the drug and its penetration of ocular tissues and into the aqueous humor.

Adverse Reactions

A. Gastrointestinal Disturbances: Adults taking chloramphenicol, 1.5–2.5 g daily, occasionally develop nausea, vomiting, and diarrhea in 2–5 days. This is rare in children. After 5–10 days, the results of microbial flora alteration may become apparent, with prominent candidiasis of mucous membranes (especially of the mouth and vagina).

B. Bone Marrow Disturbances: Adults taking chloramphenicol in excess of 50 mg/kg/d regularly exhibit disturbances in red cell maturation after 1–2 weeks of blood levels above 25–30 μg/mL. These are characterized by the appearance of markedly vacuolated nucleated red cells in the marrow, anemia, and reticulocytopenia. These anomalies usually disappear when chloramphenicol is discontinued. The disturbance appears to be a maturation arrest associated with a rise in serum iron concentration and a depression of serum phenylalanine levels and is not related to the rare occurrence of aplastic anemia.

Aplastic anemia is a rare consequence of chloramphenicol administration. It probably represents a specific genetically determined idiosyncrasy of the individual. It is not related to dose or time of intake but is seen more frequently with prolonged use. It tends to be irreversible and fatal. The precise incidence of fatal aplastic anemia as a toxic reaction to chloramphenicol administration is not known, but the disease is estimated to occur 13 times more frequently after the use of the drug than it does spontaneously. Aplastic anemia probably develops once in 24,000–40,000 patients who have taken chloramphenicol. Leukemia may follow the development of hypoplastic anemia.

C. Toxicity for Newborn Infants: Newborn infants lack an effective glucuronic acid conjugation mechanism for the degradation and detoxification of chloramphenicol. Consequently, when infants are given doses of 75 mg/kg/d or more, the drug may accumulate, resulting in the "gray syndrome," with vomiting, flaccidity, hypothermia, gray color, shock, and collapse. To avoid this toxic effect, chloramphenicol should be used with caution in infants and the dosage should be limited to 50 mg/kg/d or less in full-term infants and 30 mg/kg/d or less in prematures.

D. Interaction With Other Drugs: Chloramphenicol may prolong the half-life and raise the blood concentration of phenytoin, tolbutamide, chlorpropamide, and coumadin. This is attributable to inhibition of liver microsomal enzymes by chloramphenicol. It may precipitate a variety of other drugs from solutions. Like other bacteriostatic inhibitors of microbial protein synthesis, chloramphenicol can antagonize the bactericidal action of penicillins or aminoglycosides (see Chapter 51).

Medical & Social Implications of Overuse

Because of its "broad spectrum" and its apparent lack of toxicity, chloramphenicol was used indiscriminately between 1948 and 1951 without specific indications. It has been estimated that more than 8 million people received the drug for minor complaints, respiratory (usually viral) illnesses, etc. This inappropriate use was followed by a wave of cases of aplastic anemia, which, in turn, almost resulted in the complete abandonment of an effective drug.

TETRACYCLINES

The tetracyclines are a large group of drugs with a common basic structure and activity. Chlortetracycline, isolated from *Streptomyces aureofaciens*, was introduced in 1948. Oxytetracycline, derived from *Streptomyces rimosus*, was introduced in 1950. Tetracycline (many trade names), obtained by catalytic dehalogenation of chlortetracycline, has been available since 1953. Demeclocycline (demethylchlortetracycline) was obtained by demethylation of chlortetracycline. The most recently developed tetracyclines have emphasized good absorption combined with prolonged blood levels.

Chemistry

All of the tetracyclines have the basic structure shown below.

Free tetracyclines are crystalline amphoteric substances of low solubility. They are available as hydrochlorides, which are more soluble (about 10% in water). Such solutions are acid and, with the exception of chlortetracycline, fairly stable. Chlortetracycline is very unstable in vitro, losing much of its activity in a few hours; for this reason, it is not widely used clinically at present. Tetracyclines combine firmly with divalent metal ions, and this chelation can interfere with absorption and activity of the molecule. Tetracyclines fluoresce bright yellow in ultraviolet light of 360 nm.

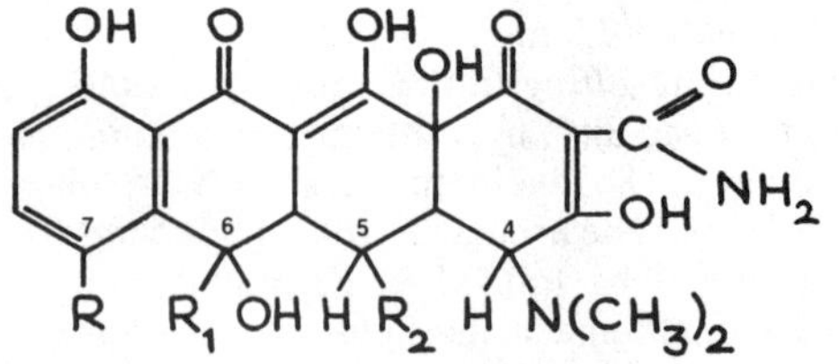

	R	R_1	R_2	Renal Clearance (mL/min)
Chlortetracycline	–Cl	$-CH_3$	–H	35
Oxytetracycline	–H	$-CH_3$	–OH	90
Tetracycline	–H	$-CH_3$	–H	65
Demeclocycline	–Cl	–H	–H	35
Methacycline	–H	$=CH_2$ *	–OH	31
Doxycycline	–H	$-CH_3$ *	–OH	16
Minocycline	$-N(CH_3)_2$	–H	–H	10

*There is no –OH at position 6 on methacycline and doxycycline.

Antimicrobial Activity

Tetracyclines are the prototype of "broad-spectrum" drugs. They are bacteriostatic for many gram-positive and gram-negative bacteria, including some anaerobes; for rickettsiae, chlamydiae, mycoplasmas, and L forms; and for some protozoa, eg, amebas. Equal amounts of tetracyclines in body fluids or tissues have approximately equal antimicrobial activity. Minocycline may have greater lipophilic properties than other congeners. Most differences in activity claimed for individual tetracycline drugs are of small magnitude and limited importance. Differences in clinical efficacy are attributable largely to features of absorption, distribution, and excretion of individual drugs. However, great differences exist in the susceptibility of different strains of a given species of microorganism. Laboratory tests on clinical isolates may therefore be important.

Tetracyclines enter microorganisms in part by passive diffusion and in part by an energy-dependent process of active transport. As a result, susceptible cells concentrate the drug so that the intracellular drug concentration is much higher than the extracellular one. Once inside the cell, tetracyclines bind reversibly to receptors on the 30S subunit of the bacterial ribosome in a position that blocks the binding of the aminoacyl-tRNA to the acceptor site on the mRNA-ribosome complex. This effectively prevents the addition of new amino acids to the growing peptide chain, inhibiting protein synthesis. The selective inhibition of protein synthesis in microorganisms may be explained largely by the lack of concentration of tetracyclines in mammalian cells.

Resistance

Susceptible microbial populations contain small numbers of mutants resistant to tetracyclines. Resistant mutants lack an active transport mechanism across cell membranes and thus do not concentrate tetracycline in their cells. Alternatively, resistant bacteria lack permeability to tetracyclines. The degree of resistance is variable, often only 2–6 times higher than that of the parent population. Among gram-negative bacterial species (especially *Pseudomonas, Proteus*, and coliforms), the selection of highly resistant types has already occurred, and tetracyclines have therefore lost some of their usefulness. Tetracycline resistance can be transmitted by plasmids (RTF). Resistance is increasing even among what were at first highly susceptible bacterial species (eg, pneumococci, *Haemophilus*, streptococci, *Bacteroides*). This is a consequence of the intense selection pressure exerted on microbial populations by the widespread use of tetracycline drugs. The incorporation of tetracyclines in animal feeds enhances the rate of growth and weight gain in animals but also results in spread of tetracycline-resistant microorganisms among farm personnel and others.

Plasmids controlling resistance may be transmitted by transduction or by conjugation. The genes for tetracycline resistance are closely associated with those for other drugs, eg, aminoglycosides, sulfonamides, and chloramphenicol. Plasmids therefore usually transmit resistance to multiple drugs rather than to tetracyclines alone.

Absorption, Metabolism, & Excretion

Tetracyclines are absorbed somewhat irregularly from the gastrointestinal tract. A portion of an orally administered dose of tetracycline remains in the gut lumen, modifies intestinal flora, and is excreted in the feces. While only 30% of chlortetracycline and 60–80% of tetracycline, oxytetracycline, and demeclocycline are absorbed in the gut, absorption is 90–100% for doxycycline and minocycline. Absorption occurs mainly in the upper small intestine and is best in the absence of food. It is impaired by chelation with divalent cations (Ca^{2+}, Mg^{2+}, Fe^{2+}) or with Al^{3+}, especially in milk and antacids, and by alkaline pH. Specially buffered tetracycline solutions can be administered intramuscularly or intravenously.

In the blood, 40–80% of various tetracyclines is protein-bound. With oral doses of 500 mg every 6 hours, tetracycline hydrochloride and oxytetracycline reach peak levels of 4–6 μg/mL. With doxycycline and minocycline, the peak levels are somewhat lower (2–4 μg/mL). Intravenously injected tetracyclines give somewhat higher levels only temporarily. The drugs are distributed widely to tissues and body fluids, except for the cerebrospinal fluid, where concentrations are low. Minocycline is unique in reaching very high concentrations in tears and saliva—a feature that permits it to eradicate the meningococcal carrier state. Tetracyclines cross the placenta to reach the fetus and are also excreted in milk. As a result of chelation with calcium, tetracyclines are bound to growing bones and teeth.

Absorbed tetracyclines are excreted mainly in bile and urine. Concentrations in bile are 10 times higher than in serum; some of the drug excreted in bile is reabsorbed from the intestine and contributes to maintenance of serum levels. Ten percent to 50% of various tetracyclines is excreted into the urine, mainly by glomerular filtration. The renal clearance of tetracyclines ranges from 10 to 90 mL/min. From 10 to 40% of tetracyclines is excreted in feces.

Doxycycline and minocycline are almost completely absorbed from the gut and are excreted more slowly, leading to persistent serum levels. Doxycycline does not require renal excretion and does not accumulate significantly in renal failure.

Clinical Uses

Tetracyclines are the most typical "broad-spectrum" antibiotics. They are effective against a variety of microorganisms and are thus used indiscriminately.

Tetracyclines are the drugs of choice in infections with *Mycoplasma pneumoniae,* chlamydiae, and rickettsiae. They are useful in mixed bacterial infections related to the respiratory tract, especially sinusitis and bronchitis. They may be employed in many gram-positive and gram-negative bacterial infections, including cholera, provided the organism is susceptible. Tetracyclines given in full doses for 5 days can eradicate acute infections with penicillin-resistant gonococci. They have been used in pneumonias and in urinary tract and skin infections, particularly acne. It is claimed that 2.5 g of tetracycline hydrochloride as a single oral dose is effective in enteritis caused by both susceptible and resistant shigellae. A single dose of doxycycline, 200 mg, may be as effective in cholera as multiple doses. However, tetracycline resistance has appeared during cholera epidemics.

Minocycline, 200 mg orally daily for 5 days—or rifampin—can eradicate the meningococcal carrier state.

A. Oral Dosage: The minimal effective oral dose for rapidly excreted tetracyclines, equivalent to tetracycline hydrochloride, is 0.25 g 4 times daily for adults and 20 mg/kg/d for children. For severe systemic infections, a dose 2–3 times larger for at least 3–5 days is indicated.

The minimal effective daily dose is 600 mg for demeclocycline or methacycline, 100 mg for doxycycline, and 200 mg for minocycline. Tetracyclines chelate with metals as noted above and thus should not be administered with milk, antacids, or ferrous sulfate. For the same reason, tetracyclines are not usually indicated for pregnant women or children under 6 years of age.

Tetracycline hydrochloride, 250–500 mg daily, is commonly taken for many months to suppress acne, especially in adolescents and young adults. This low dose presumably suppresses lipase activity of propionibacteria and inhibits inflammatory reactions.

B. Parenteral Dosage: Several tetracyclines are available for intravenous injection in doses of 0.1–0.5 g every 6–12 hours (10–15 mg/kg/d in children). Intramuscular injection is usually unsatisfactory because of pain and inflammatory reactions. There are very few instances (eg, an unconscious patient with rickettsial disease) that warrant parenteral tetracycline administration.

Adverse Reactions

Hypersensitivity reactions (drug fever, skin rashes) to tetracyclines appear to be uncommon. Most side-effects are due to direct toxicity of the drug or to alteration of microbial flora.

A. Gastrointestinal Side-Effects: Nausea, vomiting, and diarrhea are the commonest reasons for discontinuing tetracycline medication. During the first few days of administration, they appear to be attributable to direct local irritation of the intestinal tract.

After a few days of oral use, tetracyclines tend to modify the normal flora. Although some coliform organisms are suppressed, *Pseudomonas, Proteus,* staphylococci, resistant coliforms, clostridia, and *Candida* become prominent. This can result in intestinal functional disturbances, anal pruritus, vaginal or oral candidiasis, or even enterocolitis with shock and death.

Nausea, anorexia, and diarrhea can usually be controlled by administering the drug with food or carboxymethylcellulose, reducing drug dosage, or discontinuing the drug. Pseudomembranous enterocolitis associated with *Clostridium difficile* or staphylococci must be recognized promptly and treated with oral vancomycin.

B. Bony Structures and Teeth: Tetracyclines are readily bound to calcium deposited in newly formed bone or teeth in young children. When the drug is given during pregnancy, it can be deposited in the fetal teeth, leading to fluorescence, discoloration, and enamel dysplasia; it can also be deposited in bone, where it may cause deformity or growth inhibition. If the drug is given to children under 6 years of age for long periods, similar changes can result.

C. Liver Toxicity: Tetracyclines can probably impair hepatic function, especially during pregnancy, in patients with preexisting hepatic insufficiency, and when high doses are given intravenously. Hepatic necrosis has been reported with daily doses of 4 g intravenously or more.

D. Kidney Toxicity: Renal tubular acidosis and other renal injury resulting in nitrogen retention have been attributed to the administration of outdated tetracycline preparations.

Tetracyclines given together with diuretics may produce nitrogen retention. Tetracyclines, except doxycycline, may cumulate to toxic levels in patients with impaired kidney function and may aggravate the condition.

E. Local Tissue Toxicity: Intravenous injection can lead to venous thrombosis. Intramuscular injection produces painful local irritation that can lead to infiltration and should be avoided.

F. Photosensitization: Systemic tetracycline administration, especially of demeclocycline, can induce sensitivity to sunlight or ultraviolet light, particularly in blonds.

G. Vestibular Reactions: Dizziness, vertigo, nausea, and vomiting have been particularly noted with minocycline. After doses of 200–400 mg/d of minocycline, 35–70% of patients exhibited such reactions.

Medical & Social Implications of Overuse

The widespread use of tetracyclines for minor illnesses has led to the emergence of resistance even among highly susceptible species, eg, pneumococci and group A streptococci. The large-scale use of these drugs in hospitals has resulted in the selection of tetracycline-resistant organisms, particularly staphylococci and *Pseudomonas*, as superinfecting agents. In some measure, the tetracyclines (among other antibiotics) must be blamed for the rising incidence of mycotic infection in hospitalized, severely ill patients.

On the other hand, tetracyclines have been of great benefit not only for the control of existing infection but also for chemoprophylaxis in chronic bronchitis and bronchiectasis, keeping many persons well and at work.

• • •

References

Chloramphenicol

Chloramphenicol-induced bone marrow suppression. (Editorial.) *JAMA* 1970;**213:**1183.

Dajani AS, Kauffman RE: The renaissance of chloramphenicol. *Pediatr Clin North Am* 1981;**28:**195.

DuPont HL et al: Evaluation of chloramphenicol acid succinate therapy of induced typhoid fever or Rocky Mountain spotted fever. *N Engl J Med* 1970;**282:**53.

Meissner HC, Smith AL: The current status of chloramphenicol. *Pediatrics* 1979;**64:**348.

Schulkind ML et al: A comparison of ampicillin and chloramphenicol therapy in *Haemophilus influenzae* meningitis. *Pediatrics* 1971;**48:**411.

Scott JL et al: A controlled double-blind study of the hematologic toxicity of chloramphenicol. *N Engl J Med* 1965;**272:**1137.

Snyder MJ et al: Comparative efficacy of chloramphenicol, ampicillin, and co-trimoxazole in the treatment of typhoid fever. *Lancet* 1976;**2:**1155.

Wallerstein RO et al: Statewide study of chloramphenicol therapy and fatal aplastic anemia. *JAMA* 1969;**208:**2045.

Tetracyclines

Allen JC: Drugs five years later: Minocycline. *Ann Intern Med* 1976;**85:**482.

Barza M, Schiefe RT: Antimicrobial spectrum, pharmacology and therapeutic use of antibiotics. 1. Tetracyclines. *Am J Hosp Pharm* 1977;**34:**49.

Chopra I, Howe TGB: Bacterial resistance to tetracyclines. *Microbiol Rev* 1978;**42:**707.

Drew TM et al: Minocycline for prophylaxis of infection with *Neisseria meningitidis*: High rate of side effects in recipients. *J Infect Dis* 1976;**133:**194.

Hoshiwara I et al: Doxycycline treatment of chronic trachoma. *JAMA* 1973;**224:**220.

Hurwitz S: Acne vulgaris: Current concepts of pathogenesis and treatment. *Am J Dis Child* 1979;**133:**536.

Levy SB et al: Changes in intestinal flora of farm personnel after introduction of tetracycline-supplemented feed on a farm. *N Engl J Med* 1976;**295:**583.

McNeil PJ et al: Evaluation of doxycycline hyclate in the treatment of nongonococcal urethritis. *Sex Transm Dis* 1981;**8:**127.

Mhalu FS et al: Rapid emergence of El Tor *Vibrio cholerae* resistant to antimicrobials during first six months of fourth cholera epidemic in Tanzania. *Lancet* 1979;**1:**345.

Ory EM: The tetracyclines. Chap 9, pp 117–126, in: *Antimicrobial Therapy,* 3rd ed. Kagan BM (editor). Saunders, 1980.

Pickering LK et al: Single dose tetracycline therapy for shigellosis in adults. *JAMA* 1978;**239:**853.

Sack DA et al: Single-dose doxycycline for cholera. *Antimicrob Agents Chemother* 1978;**14:**462.

Sauer GC: Safety of long-term tetracycline therapy for acne. *Arch Dermatol* 1976;**112:**1603.

Siegel D: Tetracyclines: New look at old antibiotic. (2 parts.) *NY State J Med* 1978;**78:**950, 1115.

Aminoglycosides & Polymyxins | 44

Ernest Jawetz, MD, PhD

AMINOGLYCOSIDES

Aminoglycosides are a group of bactericidal drugs sharing chemical, antimicrobial, pharmacologic, and toxic characteristics. At present, the group includes streptomycin, neomycin, kanamycin, amikacin, gentamicin, tobramycin, sisomicin, netilmicin, and others. All of these agents inhibit protein synthesis in bacteria and suffer the disadvantage of multiple types of resistance.

All aminoglycosides are potentially ototoxic and nephrotoxic. All can accumulate in renal insufficiency; therefore, dosage adjustments must be made.

Aminoglycosides are used most widely against gram-negative enteric bacteria, especially in bacteremia, sepsis, or endocarditis. Streptomycin is the oldest and best-studied of the aminoglycosides. Neomycin is now limited to topical or oral use. Among the newer drugs, tobramycin, gentamicin, and amikacin are most widely employed in 1981–1982.

General Properties of Aminoglycosides

A. Physical and Chemical Properties: Aminoglycosides are water-soluble, stable in solution, and more active at alkaline than at acid pH. They have a hexose nucleus, either streptidine (in streptomycin) or deoxystreptamine (other aminoglycosides), to which amino sugars are attached by glycosidic linkages. This is why these molecules are also referred to as aminocyclitols. Each drug is characterized by the number and kind of amino sugars. Aminocyclitols may form complexes with β-lactam drugs in vitro and may lose some activity.

B. Mechanism of Action: Aminoglycosides are bactericidal for susceptible organisms by virtue of irreversible inhibition of protein synthesis. However, the precise mechanism for this bactericidal activity is not clearly evident. The initial event is penetration through the cell envelope. This is in part an active transport process, in part passive diffusion. The latter can be greatly enhanced by the presence of cell wall-active drugs, eg, penicillins. Since the active transport is an oxygen-dependent process, aminoglycosides are relatively inactive against strict anaerobes.

Once an aminoglycoside has entered the cell, it binds to receptors on the 30S subunit of the bacterial ribosome. These receptors are proteins under chromosomal control, some of which have been purified. Ribosomal protein synthesis is inhibited by aminoglycosides in at least 3 ways: (1) They interfere with the "initiation complex" of peptide formation; (2) they induce misreading of the code on the mRNA template, which causes incorporation of incorrect amino acids into the peptide; and (3) they cause a break-up of polysomes into nonfunctional monosomes.

C. Mechanisms of Resistance: Three principal mechanisms have been established: (1) Alteration in the cell surface which interferes with the permeability or active transport of aminoglycoside into the cell. This may be chromosomal or plasmid-controlled, eg, in enterococci, *Pseudomonas*. (2) The receptor (protein) on the 30S ribosomal subunit may be deleted or altered as a result of chromosomal mutation. (3) The microorganism acquires the ability to produce enzymes that destroy the aminoglycoside activity by adenylylation, acetylation, or phosphorylation. This is usually plasmid-controlled and is a prominent form of resistance among gram-negative enteric bacteria. This transmissible resistance is of great clinical and epidemiologic concern. (4) In addition, facultative organisms growing under anaerobic conditions are usually resistant to aminoglycosides because of the oxygen-dependent transport process described above.

D. Absorption, Distribution, Metabolism, and Excretion: Aminoglycosides are absorbed poorly or not at all from the intact gastrointestinal tract but may be absorbed if ulcerations are present. Virtually the entire oral dose is excreted in feces. After intramuscular injection, aminoglycosides are absorbed well, giving peak concentrations in blood within 30–90 minutes. Only about 10% of the absorbed drugs are bound to plasma proteins. Occasionally, aminoglycosides are injected intravenously.

Being highly polar compounds, aminoglycosides do not enter cells readily and are largely excluded from the central nervous system and the eye. In the presence of active inflammation, cerebrospinal fluid levels reach 20% of plasma levels, and in neonatal meningitis the levels may be higher. In order to achieve greater levels of activity in these structures, the drugs must be introduced directly. Intrathecal or intraventricular injection is required for high levels in cerebrospinal fluid. Concentrations of aminoglycosides are not high in most tissues after parenteral injection, except the renal cortex. Concentration in most secretions is also modest; in the bile, it may reach 30% of the blood level. Diffusion into pleural or synovial fluid may approach 50–90% of that of plasma with prolonged therapy. There is no significant metabolic breakdown. The half-life in serum is 2–3 hours. Excretion is mainly by glomerular filtration and is greatly reduced in impairment of renal function. Aminoglycosides are partly and irregularly removed by hemodialysis and even less effectively by peritoneal dialysis. The clearance of gentamicin by hemodialysis is in the range of 30–50%, and much less by peritoneal dialysis.

In persons with impaired renal function, there is danger of drug accumulation and toxic effects. Therefore, either the dose of drug is kept constant and the interval between doses is increased, or the interval is kept constant and the dose is reduced. Nomograms and formulas have been constructed relating serum creatinine levels to adjustments in treatment regimens. One widely used formula uses a multiplication factor (amikacin = 9, gentamicin = 8, tobramycin = 6) times the serum creatinine value (mg/dL) to give the hours of interval between doses of 1 mg/kg intramuscularly. However, there is considerable variation in aminoglycoside serum levels in different patients with similar serum creatinine values. Therefore, it is highly desirable to monitor drug levels in blood in order to avoid severe toxicity when renal functional capacity changes rapidly. Peak levels should be obtained ½–1 hour after infusion; trough levels should be obtained just prior to the next infusion.

E. Adverse Effects: Hypersensitivity occurs infrequently. All aminoglycosides can cause varying degrees of ototoxicity and nephrotoxicity. The ototoxicity can manifest itself either as hearing loss (cochlear damage) noted first with high-frequency tones or as vestibular damage evident by vertigo, ataxia, and loss of balance. Nephrotoxicity results in rising serum creatinine levels or reduced creatinine clearance. In very high doses, aminoglycosides can be neurotoxic, producing a curarelike effect with neuromuscular blockade that results in respiratory paralysis. Neostigmine can be an antidote to this neurotoxic action.

F. Clinical Uses: Aminoglycosides are used most widely against gram-negative enteric bacteria or when there is suspicion of sepsis. In the treatment of bacteremia or endocarditis caused by fecal streptococci or some gram-negative bacteria, the aminoglycoside is given together with a penicillin that enhances permeability and facilitates the entry of the aminoglycoside. Aminoglycosides are selected according to recent susceptibility patterns in a given area or hospital until susceptibility tests become available on a specific isolate. All positively charged aminoglycosides and polymyxins are inhibited in blood cultures by sodium polyanethol sulfonate and other polyanionic detergents. Some aminoglycosides (especially streptomycin) are useful as antimycobacterial drugs.

STREPTOMYCINS

Streptomycin was isolated from a strain of *Streptomyces griseus* by Waksman and his associates in 1944. Dihydrostreptomycin can be produced by catalytic reduction of streptomycin trihydrochloride. Both streptomycin compounds have similar chemical and identical antimicrobial properties. However, dihydrostreptomycin is significantly more ototoxic than streptomycin and has been abandoned.

Streptomycin is a triacidic base with the empirical formula $C_{21}H_{39}N_7O_{12}$. It consists of streptidine, streptose, and N-methyl-L-glucosamine. The latter 2 components are referred to as streptobiosamine (see formula below).

Streptomycin sulfate is a white powder, quite soluble in water and insoluble in alcohol. Neutral solutions are stable for weeks at temperatures below 25 °C. Streptomycin is more active at alkaline pH. It can be inactivated by hydroxylamine or cysteine.

The antimicrobial activity of streptomycin is typical of that of other aminoglycosides, as are the mechanisms of resistance. Resistant microorganisms have emerged in most species, severely limiting the current usefulness of streptomycin, with the exceptions listed below. Streptomycin-dependent bacteria require the drug for growth. This results from a mutation in the receptor protein (P 12).

The emergence of resistance in an apparently susceptible isolate tends to be rapid, so that treatment with streptomycin as the sole drug is usually limited to 5 days.

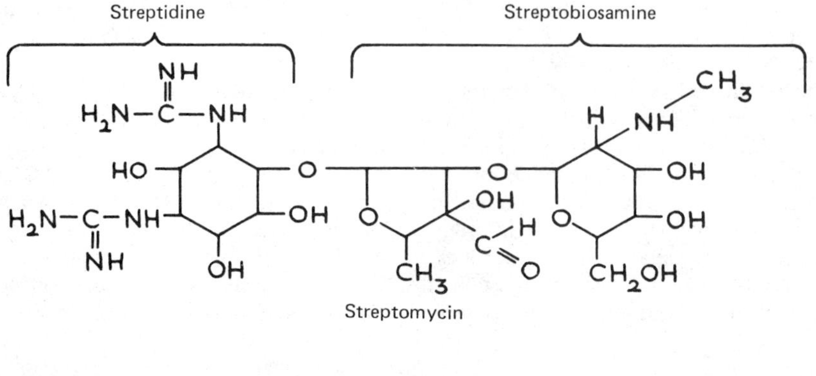

Streptomycin

Clinical Uses

A. Tuberculosis and Other Mycobacterial Infections: In pulmonary and other nondisseminated forms of tuberculosis, streptomycin, 1 g, is injected intramuscularly twice weekly or daily, as part of combined therapy. (When used in the treatment of tuberculosis, streptomycin is always combined with isoniazid, 5–10 mg/kg/d, or other drugs, for many months.) In acute tuberculous pneumonia, miliary dissemination, or meningitis in children, up to 60 mg/kg/d intramuscularly should be administered initially in combination with isoniazid or other drugs. In meningitis, streptomycin, 25 mg dissolved in 10 mL saline, may be injected intrathecally.

B. Nontuberculous Infections: In systemic infections (eg, plague, tularemia), streptomycin, 2–4 g daily intramuscularly, is given in divided doses every 4–8 hours. A second drug may be added (see below).

C. Combined Treatment: In certain infections, penicillin plus an aminoglycoside may be required for eradication of organisms even though in vitro the bacteria appear to be resistant to serum levels of the aminoglycoside alone. For example, in enterococcal endocarditis, streptomycin, 1–2 g intramuscularly daily, may be given in addition to penicillin, 12–60 g intravenously daily (or ampicillin, 4–12 g intravenously daily), to achieve bactericidal levels in serum and clinical cure.

In *Streptococcus viridans* endocarditis, the addition of an aminoglycoside may also enhance the bactericidal action of a penicillin. In tularemia and plague, streptomycin may be combined with tetracyclines.

Adverse Reactions

A. Allergy: Fever, skin rashes, and other allergic manifestations may result from hypersensitivity to streptomycin. This occurs most frequently upon prolonged contact with the drug, either in patients who receive a prolonged course of treatment (eg, for tuberculosis) or in medical personnel who handle the drug. (Nurses preparing solutions should wear gloves.) Desensitization is occasionally successful.

B. Toxicity: Pain at the injection site is common but usually not severe. The most serious toxic effect is disturbance of vestibular function—vertigo and loss of balance. The frequency and severity of this disturbance are proportionate to the age of the patient, the blood levels of the drug, and the duration of administration. Vestibular dysfunction may follow a few weeks of unusually high blood levels (eg, in individuals with impaired renal function) or months of relatively low blood levels. After the drug is discontinued, partial recovery frequently occurs.

The concurrent or sequential use of other aminoglycosides with streptomycin should be avoided to reduce the likelihood of ototoxicity. Streptomycin given during pregnancy can cause deafness in the newborn.

General Medical Problems From Overuse

Streptomycin-resistant bacteria have become prevalent as a result of widespread use of the drug, often in unnecessary combination with penicillin. Multiple drug resistance is frequent among bacteria in urinary tract infections, and the hospital transmission of such organisms aggravates treatment problems. Primary infection with streptomycin-resistant tubercle bacilli occurs in up to 15% of cases of pulmonary tuberculosis in children studied in the USA.

KANAMYCIN & NEOMYCIN

These drugs constitute a chemically and biologically closely related group. **Neomycin** was isolated by Waksman in 1949 from *Streptomyces fradiae;* **kanamycin** was isolated by Umezawa in 1957 from *Streptomyces kanamyceticus*. Other members of the group are **framycetin** and **paromomycin.** All have very similar properties.

Antimicrobial Activity

Drugs of the neomycin group are bactericidal in concentrations of 1–10 μg/mL for many gram-positive and gram-negative bacteria and mycobacteria. *Proteus* organisms are often susceptible, but *Pseudomonas* and streptococci are generally resistant. The mechanism of antibacterial action of the neomycin group is typical of the aminoglycosides. Neomycin can substitute for streptomycin in streptomycin-dependent organisms.

Resistance

Resistance mechanisms are the same as with other aminoglycosides. The widespread use of neomycin-kanamycin in bowel preparation for elective surgery of the colon has led to the selection of resistant organisms in some hospitals and outbreaks of enterocolitis. While cross-resistance between neomycin and kanamycin is complete, there is limited cross-resistance with other aminoglycosides.

Absorption, Metabolism, & Excretion

Drugs of the neomycin group are not significantly absorbed from the gastrointestinal tract. After oral administration, the intestinal flora is suppressed or modified and the drug is excreted in the feces.

After parenteral injection (0.5 g intramuscularly every 6–12 hours), serum levels reach 5–15 μg/mL. Excretion is mainly through glomerular filtration into the urine, where levels of 10–50 μg/mL may be reached. Some excretion also occurs in the bile. In the presence of renal insufficiency, the dose or the frequency of injection of these drugs must be greatly reduced.

Clinical Uses

At present, kanamycin is preferred for parenteral administration, because it is slightly less toxic than neomycin.

A. Topical: Solutions containing 1–5 mg/mL are used on infected surfaces or injected into joints, the pleural cavity, tissue spaces, or abscess cavities where infection is present. The total amount of drug given in this fashion must be restricted because much of it can be absorbed, giving rise to systemic toxicity. Ointments containing 1–5 mg/g are applied to infected skin lesions or in the nares for suppression of staphylococci. Some ointments contain polymyxin and bacitracin in addition to neomycin.

B. Oral: For preoperative reduction of gut flora, 1 g every 4–6 hours is given for 1–2 days before surgery. This is sometimes combined with oral erythromycin base. In hepatic coma, the coliform flora can be suppressed for prolonged periods by giving 1 g every 6–8 hours, together with reduced protein intake, thus reducing ammonia intoxication. Paromomycin (Humatin), 1 g every 6 hours orally for 2 weeks, has been effective in intestinal amebiasis. Kanamycin or neomycin can suppress intestinal infection with enteropathogenic *Escherichia coli,* but they are not effective in the treatment of *Shigella* or *Salmonella* infections.

C. Parenteral: Kanamycin, 0.5 g every 6–12 hours intramuscularly (15 mg/kg/d), may be effective in the treatment of bacteremia caused by gram-negative enteric organisms. It is sometimes combined with clindamycin in penetrating abdominal wounds. The use of kanamycin systemically is often limited to infants and children.

Adverse Reactions

All members of the neomycin group have nephrotoxic and ototoxic side-effects. Auditory function is affected more than vestibular. Deafness has occurred especially in adults with impaired renal function and prolonged elevated drug levels.

The sudden absorption of postoperatively instilled kanamycin from the peritoneal cavity (3–5 g) has resulted in respiratory arrest.

While hypersensitivity is not common, prolonged application of neomycin-containing ointments to skin and eyes has resulted in severe allergic dermatitis.

AMIKACIN

Amikacin is a semisynthetic derivative of kanamycin. It is relatively resistant to several of the enzymes that inactivate gentamicin and tobramycin, and it therefore can be employed against some microorganisms resistant to the latter drugs. However, bacterial resistance due to impermeability to amikacin is increasing. Many gram-negative enteric bacteria, including many strains of *Proteus, Pseudomonas,* enterobacteria, and *Serratia,* are inhibited by 1–20 μg/mL amikacin in vitro. After the injection of 500 mg amikacin every 12 hours (15 mg/kg/d) intramuscularly, peak levels in serum are 10–30 μg/mL. Some infections caused by gram-negative bacteria resistant to gentamicin respond to amikacin. Central nervous system infections require intrathecal or intraventricular injection of 1–10 mg daily.

Like all aminoglycosides, amikacin is nephro- and ototoxic (particularly for the auditory portion of the eighth nerve). Its levels should be monitored in patients with renal failure. Avoid concurrent use with diuretics, eg, furosemide, ethacrynic acid.

GENTAMICIN

Gentamicin is an aminoglycoside complex isolated from *Micromonospora purpurea*. It is effective against both gram-positive and gram-negative organisms, and many of its properties resemble those of other aminoglycosides. Sisomicin is very similar to the C_{1a} component of gentamicin.

Chemistry

The 3 active antibiotic components of gentamicin C have molecular weights of 450–475 and differ principally in methyl group content. The proposed structural formula is shown below. The sulfate is used for intramuscular injection; it is soluble in water, and such solutions are stable for weeks.

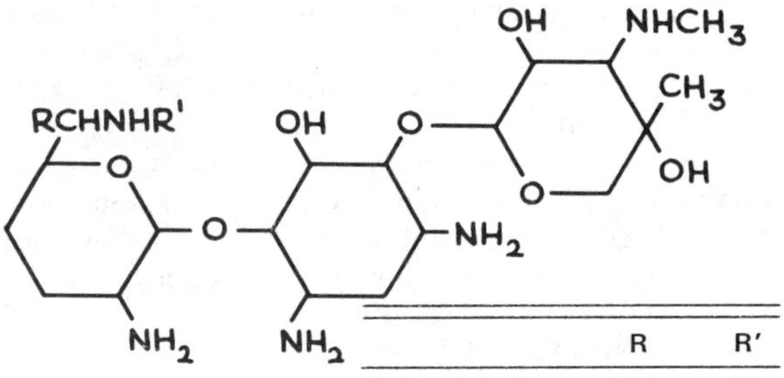

	R	R'
Gentamicin C_1	CH_3	CH_3
Gentamicin C_2	CH_3	H
Gentamicin C_{1a}	H	H

Antimicrobial Activity

In concentrations of 0.5–5 μg/mL, gentamicin is rapidly bactericidal for many gram-positive and gram-negative bacteria. Gentamicin sulfate, 10 μg/mL, inhibits in vitro many strains of staphylococci, coliform organisms (*E coli, Klebsiella, Enterobacter*), *Pseudomonas aeruginosa, Proteus,* and *Serratia*.

The simultaneous use of carbenicillin or ticarcillin and gentamicin may result in synergistic enhancement and activity against some strains of *P aeruginosa* and may permit use of smaller doses of gentamicin. However, a penicillin and gentamicin cannot be mixed in vitro.

Resistance

Most streptococci are resistant to gentamicin but can be killed by synergistic mixtures of a cell wall-inhibitory drug (eg, penicillin) with gentamicin. This resistance is based on lack of transport of gentamicin into the cell. Among gram-negative bacteria, resistance to gentamicin is increasing somewhat in proportion to the amount of drug used in a given hospital environment. This resistance is most commonly attributable to the spread of plasmids that govern gentamicin-destroying enzymes. Organisms resistant to gentamicin are often resistant to kanamycin and sometimes to tobramycin but infrequently (as yet) to amikacin.

Clinical Uses

A. Intramuscular: Gentamicin is employed in severe infections caused by gram-negative bacteria which are likely (or proved) to be resistant to other less toxic drugs. Included are sepsis, infected burns, pneumonia, and other serious infections due to coliform organisms, *Klebsiella-Enterobacter, Proteus, Pseudomonas,* and *Serratia*. In these disorders, gentamicin is employed in full systemic doses: 5–7 mg/kg/d intramuscularly (or, rarely, intravenously) in 3 equal doses for 7–10 days. Renal, auditory, and vestibular functions should be monitored, particularly in patients with preexisting nitrogen retention. Direct enzymatic or radioimmunoassays of gentamicin concentration in serum are available.

In urinary tract infections caused by these organisms, 0.8–1.2 mg/kg/d is injected intramuscularly in 2 or 3 equal divided doses for 10 days or more. Gentamicin may be employed together with a penicillin for enhanced (synergistic) action against streptococcal endocarditis or gram-negative sepsis.

B. Topical: Creams, ointments, or solutions containing 0.1–0.3% gentamicin sulfate have been used for the treatment of infected burns, wounds, or skin lesions and the prevention of intravenous catheter infections. Topical gentamicin is partly inactivated by purulent exudates. However, such topical use must be restricted in hospitals to avoid favoring the development of resistant bacteria. Ten milligrams can be injected subconjunctivally.

C. Intrathecal: Meningitis caused by gram-negative bacteria has been treated by the intrathecal injection of 1–10 mg gentamicin sulfate per day. In neonates, neither intrathecal nor intraventricular gentamicin was beneficial in meningitis, and intraventricular gentamicin was toxic. Epidural abscess has been instilled with gentamicin, 20 mg/d for 10 days.

Adverse Reactions

These are analogous to the side-effects of other aminoglycosides. Nephrotoxicity requires adjustment of regimens, especially in diminished renal function. Whenever possible, gentamicin serum levels should serve as a guide in difficult clinical situations. Ototoxicity manifests itself mainly as vestibular dysfunction, perhaps due to destruction of hair cells by prolonged elevated drug levels (more than 10 μg/mL). Loss of hearing can occur and has occasionally been extensive and irreversible. The incidence of hypersensitivity reactions to gentamicin is insufficiently defined.

TOBRAMYCIN

This aminoglycoside, available since 1975, has an antibacterial spectrum similar to that of gentamicin but is more active than the latter against *Pseudomonas* sp. While there is some cross-resistance between gentamicin and tobramycin, it is unpredictable in individual strains. Separate laboratory susceptibility tests are therefore necessary.

The pharmacologic properties of tobramycin are virtually identical to those of gentamicin. The daily dose of tobramycin is 5–7 mg/kg/d intramuscularly divided in 3 equal amounts and given every 8 hours. About 80% of the drug is excreted by glomerular filtration into the urine within 24 hours of administration. In uremia, the drug dosage must be reduced. A formula for such dosage is 1 mg/kg every (6 × serum creatinine level) hours. However, monitoring blood levels in renal insufficiency is desirable. Tobramycin can be cleared somewhat during peritoneal dialysis and about 50% during hemodialysis.

Tobramycin has the same spectrum as gentamicin, principally against aerobic gram-negative enteric bacteria. It tends to be somewhat less active against *Serratia* and more active against *Pseudomonas*. Either tobramycin or gentamicin is the aminoglycoside most often employed in combination with ticarcillin against gram-negative bacterial sepsis or in combination with penicillin G against enterococcal endocarditis.

Like other aminoglycosides, tobramycin is ototoxic and nephrotoxic. Nephrotoxicity of tobramycin may be less than that of gentamicin. It should not be used concurrently with other drugs having similar adverse effects or with diuretics, which tend to enhance aminoglycoside tissue concentrations.

SPECTINOMYCIN

Spectinomycin is an aminocyclitol antibiotic (related to aminoglycosides) dispensed as the dihydrochloride pentahydrate for intramuscular injection. While active in vitro against many gram-positive and gram-negative organisms, spectinomycin is proposed only as an alternative treatment for gonorrhea in patients who might be hypersensitive to penicillin or whose gonococci are resistant to penicillin. Most gonococci are inhibited by 6 μg/mL of spectinomycin. About 10% of gonococci may be resistant to spectinomycin, but there is no cross-resistance with other drugs used in gonorrhea.

Spectinomycin is rapidly absorbed after intramuscular injection. A dose of 2 g injected intramuscularly once results in serum levels of 100 μg/mL and is said to result in 90% cure of gonorrhea. There is pain at the injection site and occasionally fever and nausea. Nephrotoxicity and anemia have been observed rarely.

THE POLYMYXIN GROUP

The polymyxins are a group of basic polypeptides selectively active against gram-negative bacilli. Polymyxins A, B, C, D, and E were derived from a spore-forming gram-positive bacillus *(Bacillus polymyxa, Bacillus aerosporus)* in 1947. All but polymyxins B and E have been discarded because of excessive nephrotoxicity. Colistin, introduced in 1950, is identical with polymyxin E.

Chemistry

All polymyxins are cationic, basic polypeptides with molecular weights of about 1400. All contain the fatty acid D-6-methyloctan-1-oic acid and the amino acids L-threonine and L-diaminobutyric acid. In addition, polymyxins B and E contain L-leucine; B contains D-phenylalanine; and E contains D-leucine. The sulfates of polymyxins are freely soluble in water and very stable. Methanesulfonate (sulfo-methyl) complexes can be prepared which slowly release the active peptide. One microgram of pure polymyxin B sulfate equals 10 units. The relationship between micrograms and units appears to be variable in the case of methanesulfonate complexes.

Antimicrobial Activity

The activity of polymyxin B sulfate is identical with that of polymyxin E (colistin) sulfate. Similarly, the methanesulfonate complexes of polymyxins B and E have the same activity. However, it is misleading to compare quantitatively the activity of the sulfate of one polymyxin with the methanesulfonate of another. Sulfates are used in disk tests and do not reflect methanesulfonate activity.

Polymyxins are active mainly against gram-negative bacilli, particularly *Pseudomonas* and coliform organisms. They are strongly bactericidal in concentrations of 1–5 μg/mL. They act by attaching to the cell membranes of bacteria and other membranes rich in phosphatidylethanolamine and disrupting the osmotic properties and transport mechanisms of the membrane. This results in leakage of macromolecules and death of the cell. This action is inhibited by cations. The action of polymyxins is markedly inhibited by purulent exudates.

Resistance

Proteus sp, gram-positive organisms, and neisseriae are highly resistant. This is probably due to the impermeability of the outer cell wall structures to polymyxins. In susceptible bacterial populations, resistant mutants are rare. There is complete cross-resistance between polymyxin B and polymyxin E.

Absorption, Metabolism, & Excretion

Polymyxins are not absorbed from the gastrointestinal tract.

With parenterally injected polymyxins (2.5 mg/kg/d), blood levels rarely exceed 1–4 μg/mL. Tissue concentrations are even lower. Polymyxins pass the placenta but do not reach the central nervous system or cerebrospinal fluid unless injected intrathecally. They do not reach joint fluids or ocular tissues unless injected locally. Polymyxins are strongly bound by cell debris, acid phospholipids, and purulent exudates. They do not penetrate into cells, and phagocytosed or intracellular bacteria are therefore unaffected.

Excretion is mainly in the urine, where concentrations of 25–300 μg/mL may be reached during prolonged administration. Excretion is impaired in renal insufficiency.

Clinical Uses

Polymyxins were drugs of choice for the treatment of infections caused by *Pseudomonas* or coliform bacteria resistant to other antimicrobial drugs. Polymyxin treatment is now severely limited.

A. Topical: Solutions containing 1 mg/mL of polymyxin B or E sulfate can be applied to wounds, burns, sinuses, and other surfaces infected with *P aeruginosa* or other resistant microorganisms. Similar solutions (up to a total dose of 2.5 mg/kg/d) can be injected intrapleurally or intraperitoneally. Solutions of 1–10 mg/mL are inhaled as aerosols in *Pseudomonas* infections of the bronchi and lungs. Up to 20 mg of polymyxin B sulfate may be injected subconjunctivally in *Pseudomonas* infections of the eye. Ointments containing 0.5 mg/g of polymyxin B sulfate in mixture with bacitracin or neomycin (or both) are commonly applied to infected skin lesions. Solutions containing polymyxin B, 20 mg/L, and neomycin, 40 mg/L, can be employed as antiseptic for continuous irrigation of the urinary bladder through a 3-way catheter in a closed sterile system. This can delay bacterial contamination of the drainage system.

B. Intrathecal: In *Pseudomonas* meningitis, the intrathecal injection of polymyxin B or E sulfate, 2–10 mg in saline daily for 2–3 days, and then every other day for 2–3 weeks, can be curative. Polymyxin methanesulfonates are never given intrathecally.

C. Intramuscular: The intramuscular injection of polymyxin sulfates is painful and requires the simultaneous administration of a local anesthetic. For this reason, the methanesulfonate complex, which sometimes includes a local anesthetic and slowly releases active drug after intramuscular injection, is preferred. The total systemic dose can be 2.5–5 mg/kg/d. It can be used in urinary tract infections with *Pseudomonas, Enterobacter,* or other coliforms resistant to less toxic drugs. *Salmonella* infections do not respond to polymyxins in spite of in vitro susceptibility.

D. Intravenous: In serious infections, the intravenous injection of polymyxin B sulfate is preferable. The intravenous injection by slow drip of 2.5 mg/kg/d of polymyxin B sulfate in 5% dextrose in water is indicated in *Pseudomonas* bacteremia or peritonitis (eg, after peritoneal dialysis). When renal function is impaired, the drug may be administered in full doses once every 3–5 days. Hemodialysis does not remove polymyxins rapidly.

E. Oral: Polymyxins are not absorbed from the gut but have been used to suppress aerobic gram-negative members of the intestinal flora in immunosuppressed persons for "prophylaxis."

Adverse Reactions

The general toxicity of polymyxins limits both the dose and the duration of therapy. The sulfates produce intense local pain. The principal side-effects are neurotoxicity and nephrotoxicity. Hypersensitivity appears to be very rare. Very high blood levels (> 30 μg/mL) of any polymyxin can cause respiratory arrest. Respiratory paralysis caused by polymyxins can be reversed by calcium gluconate.

A. Neurotoxic Effects: Adequate systemic concentrations of any polymyxin can cause paresthesias (circumoral and stocking or glove distribution), dizziness, flushing, and incoordination. All of these disappear promptly when the drug has been discontinued and excreted.

B. Nephrotoxic Effects: Some proteinuria, hematuria, or cylindruria commonly accompanies the administration of polymyxin B or E and is evidence of tubular injury. These urinary signs usually disappear soon after the drug is discontinued. In individuals with preexisting renal disease, nitrogen retention must be monitored and the dose of polymyxin adjusted. Accidental overdosage may result in renal failure, neuromuscular paralysis, and even death.

Laboratory

The large molecules of the polymyxins diffuse poorly through agar. Consequently, disk tests reveal very narrow zones of inhibition even with fully susceptible microorganisms. Colistin disks contain sulfate, not methanesulfonate.

Use for Resistant Organisms

Polymyxins may again become important because of the increasing numbers of patients infected with *Pseudomonas* and *Enterobacter* resistant to other drugs. These are often hospitalized patients with immunosuppression and impaired renal function who require careful adjustments of a polymyxin regimen.

• • •

References

Appel JB, Neu HC: The nephrotoxicity of antimicrobial agents. (3 parts.) *N Engl J Med* 1977;**296:**663, 722, 784.

Bennett WW et al: Drug therapy in renal failure. *Ann Intern Med* 1980;**93:**62.

Brynan LE et al: Mechanism of aminoglycoside antibiotic resistance in anaerobic bacteria. *Antimicrob Agents Chemother* 1979;**15:**7.

Calderwood SB, Moellering RC: Common adverse effects of antibacterial agents on major organ systems. *Surg Clin North Am* 1980;**60:**65.

Chan RA et al: Gentamicin therapy in renal failure: A dosage nomogram. *Ann Intern Med* 1972;**76:**773.

Davis SD: Polymyxins, colistin, vancomycin and bacitracin. Chap 6, pp 77–83, in: *Antimicrobial Therapy,* 3rd ed. Kagan BM (editor). Saunders, 1980.

Egan EA et al: Prospective controlled trial of oral kanamycin in prevention of neonatal necrotizing enterocolitis. *J Pediatr* 1976;**89:**467.

Finitzohieber T et al: Ototoxicity in neonates treated with gentamicin and kanamycin. Results of a 4-year controlled follow-up study. *Pediatrics* 1979;**63:**443.

Kaiser AB, McGee ZA: Aminoglycoside therapy of gram-negative bacillary meningitis. *N Engl J Med* 1975;**293:**1215.

Klastersky J et al: Comparative clinical study of tobramycin and gentamicin. *Antimicrob Agents Chemother* 1974;**5:**133.

Krogstad DJ et al: Plasmid-mediated resistance to antibiotic synergism in enterococci. *J Clin Invest* 1978;**61:**1645.

Love LJ et al: Randomized trial of empiric antibiotic therapy with ticarcillin in combination with gentamicin, amikacin or netilmicin in febrile patients with granulocytopenia and cancer. *Am J Med* 1979;**66:**603.

McCormack WM, Finland M: Spectinomycin. *Ann Intern Med* 1976;**84:**712.

McCracken GH: Clinical pharmacology of gentamicin in infants. *Am J Dis Child* 1972;**124:**884.

McCracken GH et al: Intraventricular gentamicin therapy in gram negative bacillary meningitis or infants. *Lancet* 1980;**1:**787.

Moellering RC et al: Experience with tobramycin therapy of infections due to gentamicin-resistant organisms. *J Infect Dis* 1976;**134(Suppl):**S40.

Murillo J et al: Gentamicin and ticarcillin serum levels. *JAMA* 1979;**241:**2401.

Neu HC: Tobramycin: An overview. *J Infect Dis* 1976;**134 (Suppl):**S3.

Riff LJ, Jackson GG: Conditions for gentamicin inactivation by carbenicillin. *Arch Intern Med* 1972;**130:**887.

Sarubbi FA, Hull JH: Amikacin serum concentrations: Prediction of levels and dosage guidelines. *Ann Intern Med* 1978;**89:**612.

Smith CR et al: Double-blind comparison of the nephrotoxicity and auditory toxicity of gentamicin and tobramycin. *N Engl J Med* 1980;**302:**1106.

Tai PC et al: Streptomycin causes misreading of natural messenger by interacting with ribosomes after initiation. *Proc Natl Acad Sci USA* 1978;**75:**275.

45 | Antimycobacterial Drugs

Ernest Jawetz, MD, PhD

Mycobacterial infections may be symptomatic or asymptomatic but typically are very chronic. Therapy thus presents unusual problems. This chapter describes drugs used for tuberculosis (*Mycobacterium tuberculosis* infections), infections of clinical significance caused by various "atypical" mycobacteria, and leprosy (*Mycobacterium leprae* infections). Most of these mycobacterial infections are now controllable by specific chemotherapy, and earlier methods of rest, sunshine, and collapse therapy have been abandoned.

DRUGS USED IN TUBERCULOSIS

Streptomycin was the first antimicrobial drug to exhibit striking action against tubercle bacilli. It remains an important agent in the management of severe tuberculosis, but it is now not usually one of the initially selected drugs. First-line drugs now are isoniazid, rifampin, and ethambutol for initial treatment, with streptomycin as an alternative first-line drug. Several agents which are drugs of second choice in the treatment of tuberculosis are mentioned here only briefly.

Singular problems exist in the treatment of tuberculosis and related mycobacterial infections. The infections tend to be exceedingly chronic, but may also give rise to hyperacute, lethal complications. The organisms are frequently intracellular, exhibit long periods of metabolic inactivity, and tend to develop resistance to any one drug. All these points contribute to the complexity of antituberculosis therapy.

To delay the rapid emergence of resistance in the large mycobacterial populations that occurs in clinically active tuberculosis, combinations of first-line drugs are employed. If the organisms are susceptible to these drugs, the patient usually becomes noninfective within 2–3 weeks. While treatment in tuberculous meningitis or miliary tuberculosis is usually continued for 18–24 months, this length of treatment is no longer needed in uncomplicated pulmonary tuberculosis, the commonest clinical presentation. With the most effective "bactericidal" drug combination of isoniazid and rifampin, "short-course" schedules of 6–9 months of therapy give satisfactory results. Thus, the vast majority of patients require little hospitalization.

ISONIAZID (INH)

Isoniazid, introduced in 1952, is the most active drug for the treatment of patients whose mycobacteria are susceptible and who can tolerate isoniazid.

Chemistry

Isoniazid is the hydrazide of isonicotinic acid, often called INH. It is a white crystalline powder, freely soluble in water. The structural similarity to pyridoxine is shown below.

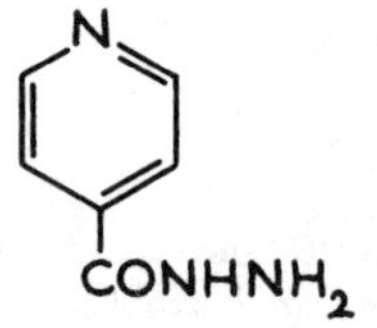

Isoniazid

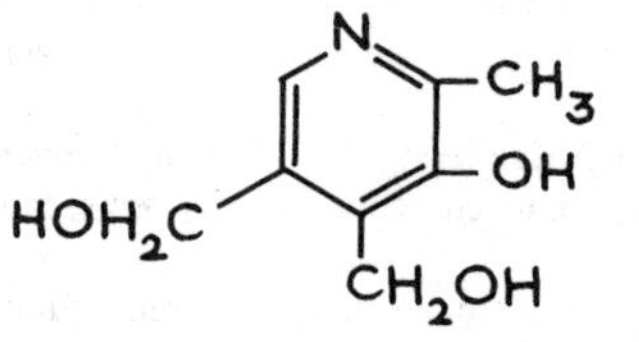

Pyridoxine

Antimycobacterial Activity

In vitro, INH inhibits most tubercle bacilli in a concentration of 0.2 μg/mL or less and is bactericidal for actively growing tubercle bacilli. INH is ineffective against many atypical mycobacteria but *Mycobacterium kansasii* is often susceptible. INH reaches similar concentrations both inside and outside animal cells and thus is able to act on intracellular mycobacteria as well as extracellular ones. Resistant mutants occur in susceptible mycobacterial populations with a frequency of about 1 in 10^6. Since tuberculous lesions often contain more than 10^7 tubercle bacilli, resistant mutants would be readily selected out if INH were to be given as the sole drug. There is no cross-resistance between INH, rifampin, and ethambutol. The simultaneous use of any 2 of these drugs markedly delays the emergence of resistance to one of them.

The mechanism of action of INH is not known. INH apparently combines with an enzyme that is peculiar to INH-susceptible strains of *M tuberculosis*, displacing a pigment precursor molecule and leading to a variety of disorders in cellular metabolism. INH may inhibit the synthesis of mycolic acids and thus interfere with the formation of mycobacterial cell walls. INH exerts competitive antagonism in pyridoxine-catalyzed reactions in *Escherichia coli*. INH and pyridoxine are structural analogs. However, this mechanism is not involved in the antituberculosis action. The administration of large doses of pyridoxine to patients receiving INH does not interfere with tuberculostatic action of INH, but it prevents neuritis.

Absorption, Metabolism, & Excretion

INH is readily absorbed from the gastrointestinal tract. The administration of usual doses (5 mg/kg/d) results in peak plasma concentrations of 3–5 μg/mL within 1–2 hours. INH diffuses readily into all body fluids and tissues. The concentration in the central nervous system and cerebrospinal fluid is about one-fifth of the plasma level. The intracellular and extracellular levels are similar.

The metabolism—particularly the acetylation—of INH is under genetic control. Two groups of people can be recognized: the "slow" and the "rapid" inactivators of the drug, through acetylation. High acetyl transferase activity results in fast INH inactivation through acetylation and is inherited as an autosomal dominant trait. The average concentration of active INH in the plasma of rapid inactivators is about one-third to one-half of that in slow inactivators. The average half-life of INH in rapid inactivators is less than 1½ hours, whereas in slow inactivators the half-life is 3 hours. It has been claimed that rapid acetylators are more prone to hepatic toxicity of INH. About half of white and black persons in the USA are slow inactivators, whereas many Eskimos, Native Americans, and Orientals are rapid inactivators. The rate of acetylation has little influence in daily dose regimens but may impair antimycobacterial activity in intermittent (2–3 times weekly) administration of INH.

INH is excreted mainly in the urine—partly as unchanged drug, partly as the acetylated form, and partly as other conjugates. The amount of unchanged, free INH in the urine is higher in the "slow" inactivators; the amount of acetylated form is higher in the "rapid" inactivators. In renal failure, normal doses of INH can be given.

Clinical Uses

Isoniazid is probably the most widely useful drug in tuberculosis. In active, clinically manifest disease, it is given in conjunction with ethambutol, rifampin, or streptomycin. The usual dose is 5 mg/kg/d (maximum for adults, 300 mg daily). Twice that dose is sometimes used in severe illness and meningitis, but there is little evidence that the higher dose (10 mg/kg/d) is more effective in adults. Children should receive 10 mg/kg/d, and for maintenance therapy after initial improvement, 15 mg/kg twice weekly is sometimes given. Pyridoxine, 10 mg per 100 mg of isoniazid, should be given to avoid neuritis.

Children or young adults converting from tuberculin negative to positive skin tests may be given INH, 5–10 mg/kg/d (maximum 300 mg/d), for 1 year as prophylaxis against the 5–15% risk of meningitis or miliary dissemination. For "prophylaxis," INH is given as the sole drug. In addition to skin test converters without active disease, "prophylactic" INH is also suggested for household and other very close contacts (especially children) of freshly recognized active cases; and for skin test-positive persons who undergo immunosuppressive or antineoplastic chemotherapy and have not received "adequate" antimycobacterial treatment in the past.

INH is usually given by mouth but can be injected parenterally in the same dosage.

Adverse Reactions

The incidence and severity of untoward reactions to INH are related to dosage and duration of administration.

A. Allergic Reactions: Fever, skin rashes, and hepatitis are occasionally seen.

B. Direct Toxicity: The most common toxic effects (10–20%) are on the peripheral and central nervous systems. These have been attributed to a relative pyridoxine deficiency, perhaps resulting from competition of INH with pyridoxal phosphate for an enzyme (apotryptophanase). These toxic reactions include peripheral neuritis, insomnia, restlessness, muscle twitching, urinary retention, and even convulsions and psychotic episodes. Most of these complications can be prevented by the administration of pyridoxine, and accidental INH overdose can be treated with pyridoxine in amounts equivalent to the INH ingested.

INH can reduce the metabolism of phenytoin, increasing its blood level and toxicity. With prolonged use on a large scale in chemoprophylaxis, isoniazid has been associated with hepatotoxicity. Abnormal liver function tests, clinical jaundice, and multilobular necrosis have been observed. In large groups, about 1% of persons develop clinical hepatitis and up to 10% subclinical abnormalities. Some fatalities have occurred. Hepatitis with progressive liver damage is age-dependent. It occurs rarely under age 20, in 1.5% of those between 30 and 50, and in 2.5% of older persons. The risk of hepatitis with permanent damage is an important determinant in the "prophylactic" use of INH.

In glucose-6-phosphate dehydrogenase deficiency, INH may cause hemolysis.

RIFAMPIN

Rifampin is a semisynthetic derivative of rifamycin, an antibiotic produced by *Streptomyces mediterranei*. It is active in vitro against some gram-positive and gram-negative cocci, some enteric bacteria, mycobacteria, chlamydiae, and poxviruses. While many meningococci and mycobacteria are inhibited by less than 1 μg/mL, highly resistant mutants occur in all microbial populations in a frequency of 1 in 10^7 or greater. The administration of rifampin as a single drug permits the emergence of these highly resistant organisms. There is no cross-resistance to other antimicrobial drugs. Rifampin resistance may be due to a permeability barrier or to a chemical modification of the microbial RNA polymerase.

Rifampin binds strongly to DNA-dependent RNA polymerase and thus inhibits RNA synthesis in bacteria and chlamydiae. Human RNA polymerase is not affected. It blocks a late stage in the assembly of poxviruses, perhaps interfering with envelope formation. Rifampin, when administered together with INH, is usually bactericidal for mycobacteria and tends to sterilize infected tissues, cavities, or sputum.

Rifampin is well absorbed after oral administration, widely distributed in tissues, and excreted mainly through the liver into bile. It then undergoes enterohepatic recirculation, with the bulk excreted in feces and a small amount in the urine. Usual doses result in serum levels of 5–7 μg/mL, and cerebrospinal fluid levels are between 10 and 40% of serum levels. Rifampin is distributed widely in body fluids and tissues.

In tuberculosis, a single oral dose of rifampin, usually 600 mg daily (10–20 mg/kg), is administered together with INH, ethambutol, or another antituberculosis drug in order to delay the emergence of rifampin-resistant mycobacteria. A similar regimen may apply to atypical mycobacteria. Rifampin is effective in leprosy.

An oral dose of 600 mg twice daily for 2 days can eliminate a majority of meningococci from carriers. Unfortunately, some highly resistant meningococcal strains are selected out by this procedure. Up to 10% of treated meningococcus carriers may exhibit rifampin-resistant organisms. Rifampin, 20 mg/kg/d for 4 days, is used as prophylaxis in contacts of children with *Haemophilus influenzae* type b disease. In urinary tract infections and in chronic bronchitis, the use of rifampin rapidly selects resistant mutants.

Rifampin imparts a harmless orange color to urine, sweat, tears, and contact lenses. Occasional adverse effects include rashes, thrombocytopenia, nephritis, and impairment of liver function. Rifampin commonly causes light chain proteinuria and may impair antibody response. If administered less often than twice weekly, rifampin causes a "flu syndrome" of uncertain nature and anemia. Rifampin increases the elimination of anticoagulants (eg, warfarin) and thus may impose a need for a higher dose of anticoagulant. Rifampin increases the urinary excretion of methadone, lowers its plasma concentration, and may thus result in "methadone withdrawal" signs.

Caution: The indiscriminate use of rifampin for minor infections may favor the widespread selection of rifampin-resistant mycobacteria and thus deprive the drug of most of its usefulness.

ETHAMBUTOL

This is a synthetic, water-soluble, heat-stable compound, the D isomer of the structure shown below, dispensed as the hydrochloride.

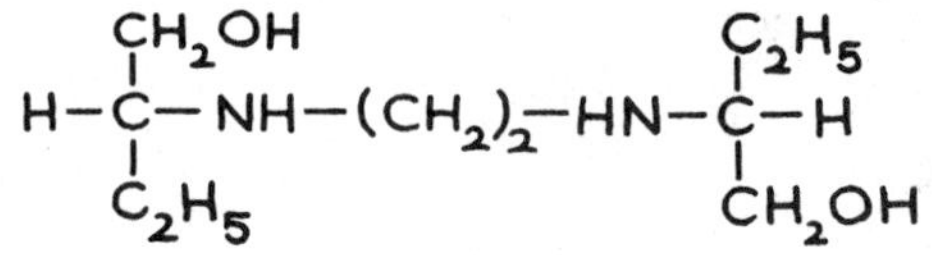

Ethambutol

Many strains of *M tuberculosis* and other mycobacteria are inhibited in vitro by ethambutol, 1–5 μg/mL. The mechanism of action is not known.

Ethambutol is well absorbed from the gut. Following ingestion of 25 mg/kg, a blood level peak of 2–5 μg/mL is reached in 2–4 hours. About 20% of the drug is excreted in feces and 50% in urine, in unchanged form. Excretion is delayed in renal failure. About 15% of absorbed drug is metabolized by oxidation and conversion to a dicarboxylic acid. In meningitis, ethambutol appears in the cerebrospinal fluid to the extent of 10–40% of serum levels.

Resistance to ethambutol emerges fairly rapidly among mycobacteria when the drug is used alone. Therefore, ethambutol is given in combination with other antituberculosis drugs.

Ethambutol hydrochloride, 15 mg/kg, is usually given as a single dose in combination with INH or rifampin. At times, the dose is 25 mg/kg/d.

Hypersensitivity to ethambutol occurs infrequently. The commonest side-effects are visual disturbances: reduction in visual acuity, optic neuritis, and perhaps retinal damage occur in some patients given 25 mg/kg/d for several months. Most of these changes apparently regress when ethambutol is discontinued. However, periodic visual acuity testing is desirable during treatment. With doses of 15 mg/kg/d, visual disturbances are very rare.

STREPTOMYCIN

The pharmacologic features of streptomycin have been discussed in Chapter 44. It is assumed that the mechanism of action of streptomycin against mycobacteria is the same as that against other microorganisms. Most tubercle bacilli are inhibited by streptomycin, 1–10 μg/mL, in vitro. Most "atypical" mycobacteria are resistant to streptomycin in pharmacologic concentrations. All large populations of tubercle bacilli contain some streptomycin-resistant mutants. On the average, 1 in 10^8 to 1 in 10^{10} tubercle bacilli can be expected to be resistant to streptomycin at levels of 10–100 μg/mL. Certain of these mutants tend to survive the in vivo exposure to therapeutic concentrations of streptomycin. This results in "treatment resistance" of clinical tuberculosis. Therefore, streptomycin is employed in combination with another drug effective against tubercle bacilli. Combined treatment can markedly delay the emergence of streptomycin-resistant mutants. It is estimated that among primary infections in children in 1970, about 15% were caused by streptomycin-resistant *M tuberculosis*.

Streptomycin exerts its action mainly on extracellular tubercle bacilli. Only about 10% of the drug penetrates into cells which harbor intracellular organisms. Thus, even if the entire microbial population were streptomycin-susceptible, at any one moment a large percentage of the tubercle bacilli would be unaffected by streptomycin. Treatment for many months is therefore required.

Streptomycin sulfate remains an important drug in the treatment of tuberculosis. It is employed principally in individuals with severe, possibly life-threatening forms of tuberculosis, particularly miliary dissemination, and extensive, active pulmonary or renal involvement. The usual dosage is 1 g intramuscularly daily for adults (20–40 mg/kg/d for children) for weeks, followed by 1 g intramuscularly 2–3 times weekly for several months. Other drugs are always given simultaneously.

Intrathecal injection of streptomycin in tuberculous meningitis has been largely abandoned, because other drugs such as INH or ethambutol appear in the cerebrospinal fluid. However, the use of streptomycin must still be considered, particularly for INH-resistant mycobacteria.

The eighth nerve toxicity of streptomycin injected intramuscularly for many weeks manifests itself principally as dysfunction of the labyrinth, resulting in inability to maintain equilibrium and in deafness. The latter is often permanent, but some compensation for the former often occurs.

ALTERNATIVE SECOND-LINE DRUGS IN TUBERCULOSIS TREATMENT

Because of their antimicrobial efficacy and their relative clinical safety, the drugs of first choice in tuberculosis in 1981–1982 are isoniazid, rifampin, ethambutol, and streptomycin. The alternative drugs listed below are usually considered only (1) in the case of resistance to the drugs of first choice, which occurs with increasing frequency; (2) in case of failure of clinical response to conventional therapy; and (3) when expert guidance is available to deal with the toxic side-effects. In most of the second choice drugs listed below, the dosage, emergence of resistance, and long-term toxicity have not been fully established.

Capreomycin

Capreomycin is a peptide antibiotic obtained from *Streptomyces capreolus*. Daily injection of 1 g intramuscularly results in blood levels of 10 μg/mL or more. Such concentrations in vitro are inhibitory for several mycobacteria. There is some cross-resistance between capreomycin, viomycin, and kanamycin. Capreomycin (20 mg/kg/d) can perhaps take the place of the latter drugs in combined antituberculosis therapy. The most serious toxicity is for the kidney, resulting in nitrogen retention, and for the eighth nerve, resulting in deafness and vestibular disturbances.

Cycloserine

Cycloserine is an antibiotic analog of D-alanine. Oral doses of 250 mg 3 times daily result in blood levels of 15–25 μg/mL. This is sufficient to inhibit many strains of tubercle bacilli. The most serious toxic reactions are various central nervous system dysfunctions and psychotic reactions. Some of these can be controlled by phenytoin, 100 mg/d orally.

The dosage of cycloserine in tuberculosis is 0.5–1 g/d. Cycloserine has been used in urinary tract infections in doses of 15–20 mg/kg/d.

Cycloserine is discussed further in Chapter 50.

Ethionamide

This yellow crystalline substance is stable and almost insoluble in water. It is a close chemical relative of isoniazid.

In spite of this similarity, there is no cross-resistance between isoniazid and ethionamide. Most tubercle bacilli are inhibited in vitro by ethionamide, 2.5 μg/mL, or less. Many photochromogenic mycobacteria are also inhibited by ethionamide, 10 μg/mL. Such concentrations in plasma and tissues are achieved by daily oral doses of 1 g. This dosage is effective in the clinical treatment of tuberculosis, but is poorly tolerated because of the intense gastric irritation and neurologic symptoms it causes. A dose of 0.5 g orally per day is better tolerated but not very effective. Resistance to ethionamide develops rapidly in vitro and in vivo. Consequently, this drug can be used only in combination with other antituberculosis drugs.

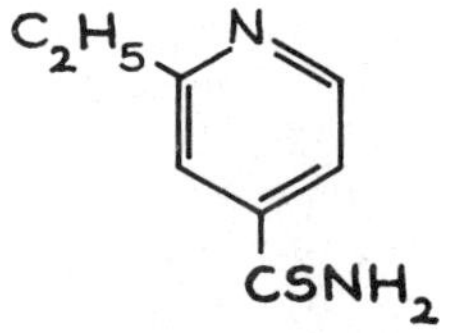

Ethionamide

Pyrazinamide (PZA)

This relative of nicotinamide is stable and sparingly soluble in water.

At neutral pH, it is inactive in vitro, but at pH 5.0 it strongly inhibits the growth of tubercle bacilli within cells in concentrations of 15 μg/mL. Such concen-

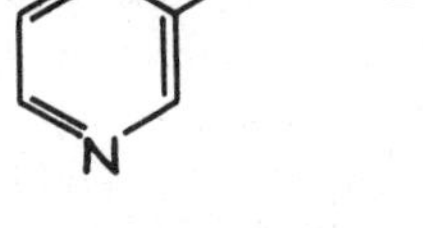

Pyrazinamide (PZA)

trations are achieved by daily oral doses of 20–30 mg/kg, given as 0.5 g 4 times daily or 0.75 g twice daily. Pyrazinamide is well absorbed from the gastrointestinal tract and widely distributed in body tissues. Tubercle bacilli develop resistance to pyrazinamide fairly readily, but there is no cross-resistance with isoniazid. Satisfactory clinical effects can be achieved with this drug, but toxicity is marked. The most serious toxic effect is the hepatic injury that frequently results. Pyrazinamide should be considered only as part of a combined drug regimen in patients harboring tubercle bacilli resistant to first choice drugs.

Aminosalicylic Acid (PAS)

Among several derivatives of salicylic and benzoic acids, *p*-aminosalicylic acid has the most marked effect on tubercle bacilli.

The structural formula of PAS reveals its close similarity to *p*-aminobenzoic acid (PABA) and to the sulfonamides (see Chapter 46).

PAS is a white crystalline powder only slightly soluble in water and rapidly destroyed by heat. The sodium salt is freely soluble in water and relatively stable at room temperature.

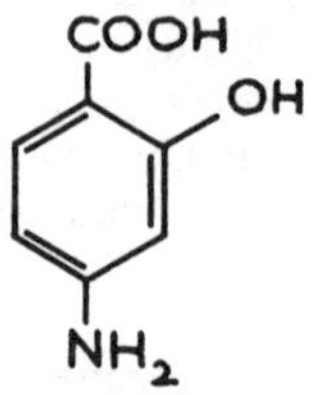

Aminosalicylic acid (PAS)

Most bacteria are not affected by PAS. Tubercle bacilli are usually inhibited in vitro by PAS, 1–5 μg/mL, but "atypical" mycobacteria are resistant. In susceptible mycobacterial populations, resistant mutants occur and tend to emerge in vitro and in vivo during exposure to PAS. The simultaneous use of a second drug with antimycobacterial activity tends to delay this emergence of resistance.

It is likely that PAS and PABA compete for the active center of an enzyme involved in converting PABA to dihydropteroic acid. The receptors for PABA attachment must be quite specific, because PAS is ineffective against most bacteria whereas sulfonamides are ineffective against tubercle bacilli.

PAS is readily absorbed from the gastrointestinal tract. Average daily doses (8–12 g) tend to give blood levels of 10 μg/mL or more. The drug is widely distributed in tissues and body fluids except the cerebrospinal fluid. PAS is rapidly excreted in the urine, in part as active PAS and in part as the acetylated compound and other metabolic products. Very high concentrations of PAS are reached in the urine. To avoid crystalluria, the urine must be kept alkaline.

Aminosalicylic acid was employed in the past together with isoniazid or streptomycin, or both, in the long-term treatment of tuberculosis. It is used infrequently now because other oral drugs are better tolerated. The dosage is 8–12 g daily orally for adults and 300 mg/kg/d for children.

Gastrointestinal symptoms often accompany full doses of PAS. Anorexia, nausea, diarrhea, and epigastric pain and burning may all be diminished by giving PAS with meals and with antacids. Peptic ulceration and hemorrhage may occur. Kidney or liver damage, thyroid gland injury (goiter with or without myxedema), and metabolic acidosis are rare.

Drug fever, joint pains, skin rashes, granulocytopenia, and a variety of neurologic symptoms—all probably due to hypersensitivity—often occur after 3–8 weeks of PAS therapy, making it necessary to stop PAS administration temporarily or permanently.

Viomycin

This antibiotic is produced by certain *Streptomyces* organisms. It is a complex basic polypeptide dispensed as a neutral sulfate that is very soluble in water. Most strains of tubercle bacilli are inhibited in vitro by viomycin, 1–10 μg/mL. Such concentrations can be achieved by the injection of 2 g intramuscularly twice weekly. Tubercle bacilli resistant to viomycin emerge fairly rapidly. There is also some cross-resistance with streptomycin, kanamycin, and capreomycin. Therefore, viomycin—if used at all—must be used in combination with other drugs to delay the emergence of resistance. The most serious toxic side-effects are damage to the kidney and to the eighth nerve, resulting in loss of equilibrium and deafness. Toxic effects are more serious than with streptomycin.

Other Antimycobacterial Drugs

Kanamycin and **tetracyclines** have been employed in combined therapy of tuberculosis. These drugs can inhibit tubercle bacilli in concentrations that may be achieved in vivo. However, they are much less effective than the drugs of first choice.

SHORT-COURSE TUBERCULOSIS CHEMOTHERAPY

Based on several recent trials, a marked change in chemotherapy for uncomplicated pulmonary tuberculosis has developed. Various schemes of drug combinations for 9–12 months, involving daily or twice weekly therapy, have achieved good success in inducing complete remissions at least on short-term follow-up.

It must be stressed that these schemes apply *only* to uncomplicated pulmonary tuberculosis and regimens that contain *both* isoniazid (INH) and rifampin (RIF) with or without other drugs. In adults, 300 mg of INH and 600 mg of RIF are given daily. Children receive INH, 10 mg/kg/d up to 300 mg/d, and RIF, 10–20 mg/kg/d up to 600 mg/d. Ethambutol, 15 mg/kg/d, should be added if the patient resides in or has come from an area with a high level of initial drug resistance. This daily regimen continues for 2–8 weeks, depending on clinical and x-ray response and speed of sputum conversion. Subsequently, INH, 15 mg/kg, can be given twice weekly (eg, INH 900 mg twice weekly for a 60-kg adult) and RIF, 600 mg twice weekly. Intermittently, patients must be monitored for thrombocytopenia. The total treatment time is 9–12 months, at least 6 months beyond conversion of sputum to culture negativity.

Other short-course treatments have been proposed.

DRUGS AGAINST ATYPICAL MYCOBACTERIA

About 10% of mycobacterial infections seen in clinical practice in the USA are not caused by *M tuberculosis* or *M leprae* but by "atypical" mycobacteria. These organisms have distinctive laboratory characteristics, occur in the environment, are generally not communicable from person to person, and are sometimes resistant to antituberculous drugs, especially streptomycin. Disease caused by these organisms is often not as severe as tuberculosis and occurs in individuals without contact with tuberculosis yet yielding acid-fast mycobacteria in smears. Chest x-rays may be negative. A few representative pathogens, with the clinical presentation and with the drugs to which they are often susceptible, are given in Table 45–1. The "Runyon grouping" depends on laboratory findings. Drug choice must be influenced by susceptibility testing, which requires weeks.

DRUGS USED IN LEPROSY

Mycobacterium leprae has never been grown in vitro, but animal models, such as growth in injected mouse footpads, have permitted laboratory evaluation of drugs. Only those drugs that have the widest clinical use are presented here.

DAPSONE & OTHER SULFONES

Several drugs closely related to the sulfonamides have been used effectively in the long-term treatment of leprosy. Dapsone, the most widely used, is diaminodiphenyl sulfone. It probably inhibits folate synthesis. Resistance can emerge in large populations of *M leprae,* eg, in lepromatous leprosy, if very low doses are given.

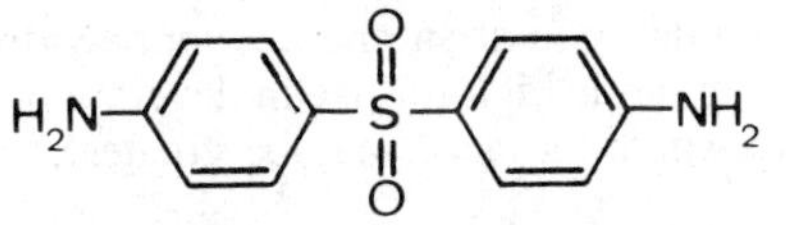

Dapsone

Sulfones are well absorbed from the gut and widely distributed throughout body fluids and tissues. The serum half-life is 1–2 days, and drug tends to be retained in skin, muscle, liver, and kidney. Skin heavily infected with *M leprae* may contain several times as much of the drug as normal skin. Sulfones are excreted into bile and reabsorbed in the intestine. Excretion into urine is variable, and most excreted drug is acetylated. In renal failure, the dose may have to be adjusted.

The usual dosage in leprosy begins with one or two 25-mg tablets of dapsone per week, increasing by one tablet weekly until a full dose of 400 mg/wk is reached. Some persons have received 600 mg/wk; others have received 200 mg/wk with apparently good results.

Untoward reactions to dapsone are common. Many patients develop some hemolysis, particularly if they have glucose-6-phosphate dehydrogenase deficiency. Methemoglobinemia is common. Gastrointestinal intolerance, fever, pruritus, and various rashes occur. During dapsone therapy of lepromatous leprosy, erythema nodosum leprosum develops often. It is sometimes difficult to distinguish reactions to dapsone from manifestations of the underlying illness. Erythema nodosum leprosum may be suppressed by corticosteroids or by thalidomide.

Acedapsone (4,4-diacetamidodiphenylsulfone) is a repository form of dapsone. A single intramuscular injection of 300 mg may maintain inhibitory dapsone levels in tissue for up to 3 months. Several other

Table 45–1. Clinical features and treatment of infections due to atypical mycobacteria.

Runyon Group	Pathogen	Frequent Clinical Features	Treatment Possibilities: Often Susceptible To—
I	*M kansasii*	Resembles tuberculous pulmonary disease.	Ethambutol + rifampin (+ INH); erythromycin, ethionamide.
	M marinum	Skin granulomas.	Minocycline, rifampin.
II	*M scrofulaceum*	Cervical adenitis in children.	Amikacin, erythromycin, rifampin, streptomycin. (Surgical excision is treatment of choice.)
III	*M avium-intracellulare*	Occasional pulmonary disease; widespread, asymptomatic.	Amikacin + rifampin, cycloserine, ethambutol.
IV	*M fortuitum*	Skin ulcers; rarely, lung disease.	Tetracycline, amikacin, ethionamide, capreomycin.
	M ulcerans	Skin ulcers.	Rifampin, streptomycin.

sulfones related to dapsone have also been used. When intolerance develops, it pertains to all sulfones.

RIFAMPIN

This drug (see above) in a dose of 600 mg daily can be strikingly effective in lepromatous leprosy. In view of the probable risk of emergence of rifampin-resistant *M leprae,* the drug is usually given in combination with dapsone or another antileprosy drug. The cost of rifampin is high for use in developing parts of the world where the need may be greatest.

CLOFAZIMINE

Clofazimine is a phenazine dye which is an alternative drug to dapsone. Its mechanism of action is unknown.

Absorption of clofazimine from the gut is variable, and a major proportion of the drug is excreted in feces. Clofazimine is stored widely in reticuloendothelial tissues and skin, and its crystals can be seen inside phagocytic reticuloendothelial cells. It is slowly released, so that the serum half-life may be 2 months. Only a small proportion of each dose is excreted into urine or bile.

Clofazimine is given for sulfone-resistant leprosy or when patients are intolerant to sulfone. A common dose is 100–300 mg/d orally. The most prominent

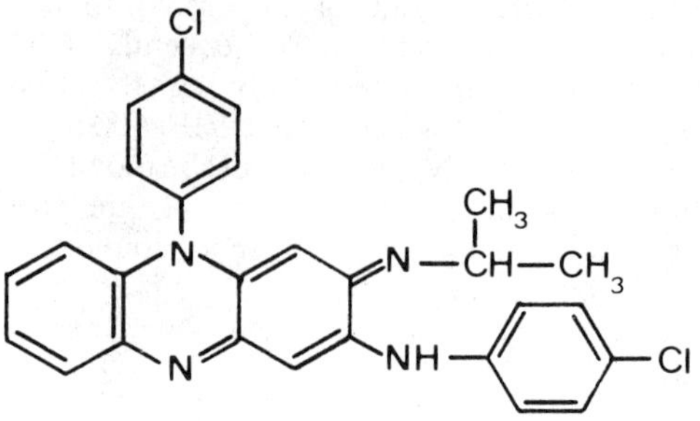

Clofazimine

untoward effect is skin discoloration ranging from red-brown to nearly black. Gastrointestinal intolerance occurs occasionally.

AMITHIOZONE

Amithiozone is a thiosemicarbazone employed as a substitute for dapsone in intolerant patients. It appears to be more effective in tuberculoid than in lepromatous leprosy. Oral administration of 150 mg daily or 450 mg twice weekly yields serum concentrations inhibitory for mycobacteria, but resistance may develop if the drug is given alone. Gastrointestinal intolerance occurs frequently and hepatic damage has been reported. The drug is currently not available in the USA.

• • •

References

Addington WW: Treatment of pulmonary tuberculosis: Current options. *Arch Intern Med* 1979;**139:**1391.

Byrd RB et al: Toxic effects of isoniazid in tuberculosis chemoprophylaxis. *JAMA* 1979;**241:**1239.

Curry FJ: Prophylactic effect of isoniazid in young tuberculin reactors. *N Engl J Med* 1967;**277:**562.

Doster B et al: Ethambutol in the initial treatment of pulmonary tuberculosis. *Am Rev Respir Dis* 1973;**107:**177.

Eickhoff TC: Studies of resistance to rifampin in meningococci. *J Infect Dis* 1971;**123:**414.

Ellard GA, Mitchison DA: The hepatic toxicity of isoniazid among rapid and slow acetylators of the drug. *Am Rev Respir Dis* 1978;**118:**628.

Graber CD et al: Light chain proteinuria and humoral immunoincompetence in tuberculous patients treated with rifampin. *Am Rev Respir Dis* 1973;**107:**713.

Johnston RF, Wildrick KH: Impact of chemotherapy on the care of patients with tuberculosis. *Am Rev Respir Dis* 1974;**109:**636.

Joint Statement by American Thoracic Society and Centers for Disease Control: Guidelines for short-course tuberculosis chemotherapy. (2 parts.) *MMWR* 1980;**29:**97, 183.

Lester TW: Drug-resistant and atypical mycobacterial disease: Bacteriology and treatment. *Arch Intern Med* 1979;**139:**1399.

Maddrey WC, Boitnott JK: Isoniazid hepatitis. *Ann Intern Med* 1973;**79:**1.

McKenzie MS et al: Drug treatment of tuberculous meningitis in childhood. *Clin Pediatr* 1979;**18:**75.

Newman R et al: Rifampin in initial treatment of pulmonary tuberculosis. *Am Rev Respir Dis* 1974;**109:**216.

Pratt TH: Rifampin induced organic brain syndrome. *JAMA* 1979;**241:**2421.

Steiner P et al: Primary isoniazid-resistant tuberculosis in children: Clinical features, strain resistance, treatment, and outcome in 26 children treated at Kings County Medical Center of Brooklyn between the years 1961 and 1972. *Am Rev Respir Dis* 1974;**110:**306.

US Leprosy Panel: Rifampin therapy of lepromatous leprosy. *Am J Trop Med Hyg* 1975;**24:**475.

Waters MF et al: Rifampicin for lepromatous leprosy: Nine years' experience. *Br Med J* 1978;**1:**133.

Wolinsky E: Nontuberculous mycobacteria and associated diseases. *Am Rev Respir Dis* 1979;**119:**107.

Sulfonamides & Trimethoprim | 46

Ernest Jawetz, MD, PhD

SULFONAMIDES

A red dye, prontosil, synthesized in Germany by Klarer and Mietzsch in 1932, was ineffective against bacteria in vitro; but Domagk reported in 1935 that it was strikingly active in vivo against hemolytic streptococcal and other infections. This was due to the conversion in the body of prontosil to sulfanilamide, the active drug. The sulfonamide molecule was chemically altered by the attachment of many different radicals, and there has been a proliferation of active compounds. Perhaps 150 different sulfonamides have been marketed at one time or another, the modifications being designed principally to achieve greater antibacterial activity, a wider antibacterial spectrum, greater solubility, or more prolonged action. In spite of the advent of the antibiotic drugs, the sulfonamides are among the most widely used antibacterial agents in the world today, chiefly because of the low cost and their relative efficacy in some common bacterial diseases. The synergistic action of sulfonamide with trimethoprim has brought about an enormous resurgence in sulfonamide use everywhere during the last decade.

Chemistry

The sulfonamides are a group of compounds whose basic formula and relationship to PABA are shown below.

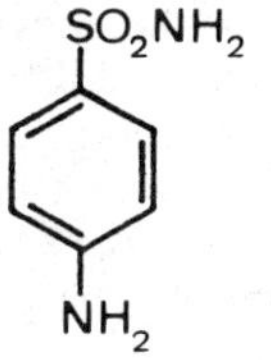

Sulfanilamide

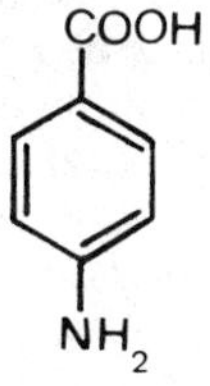

p-Aminobenzoic acid (PABA)

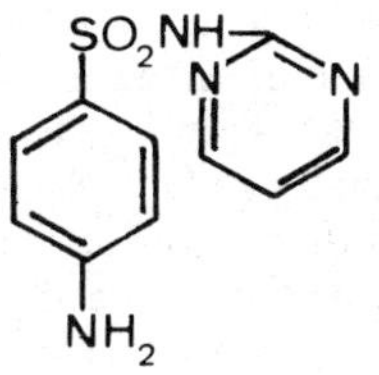

Sulfadiazine

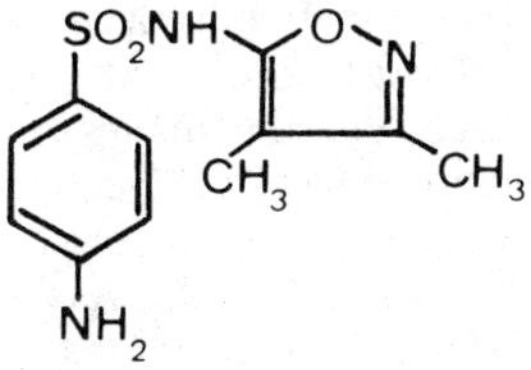

Sulfisoxazole

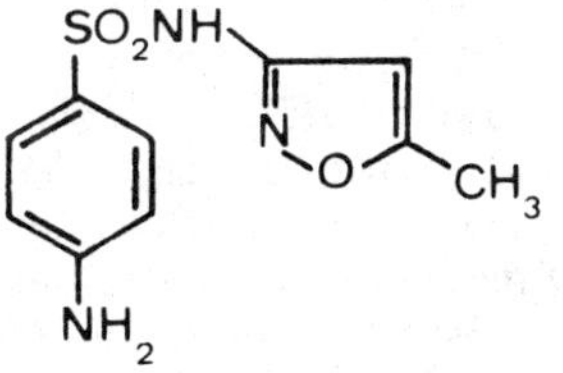

Sulfamethoxazole

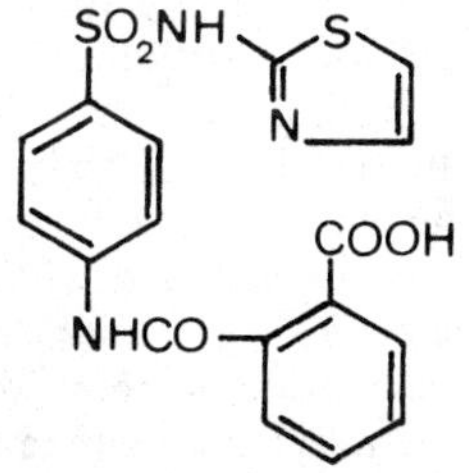

Sulfathalidine
(phthalylsulfathiazole)

All have the same nucleus to which various R radicals in the amido group ($-SO_2NHR$) have been attached or in which various substitutions of the amino group (NH_2) are made. These changes produce compounds with varying physical, chemical, pharmacologic, and antibacterial properties. In general, the sulfonamides are white, odorless, bitter tasting crystalline powders that are much more soluble at alkaline than at acid pH. In a mixture of sulfonamide drugs, each component drug exhibits its own solubility. Therefore, a mixture may be much more soluble, in terms of total sulfonamide present, than one drug used alone. This is the reason for the use of trisulfapyrimidines, a preparation that permits 3 times higher dosage than a single drug for comparable solubility in urine.

Most sulfonamides can be prepared as sodium salts that are moderately soluble, and these are used for intravenous administration. Such solutions are highly alkaline and not very stable, and may precipitate out of solution with polyionic electrolytes (eg, lactate-chloride-carbonate). Certain sulfonamide molecules are designed for low solubility (eg, phthalylsulfathiazole) so that they will stay in the lumen of the bowel for long periods.

Antimicrobial Activity

Different sulfonamides may show quantitative but not necessarily qualitative differences in activity. Sulfonamides can inhibit both gram-positive and gram-negative bacteria, *Nocardia, Chlamydia trachomatis*, and some protozoa. Some enteric bacteria are inhibited but not *Pseudomonas, Serratia, Proteus*, and other multiresistant organisms. Sulfonamides (alone or in combination with trimethoprim) are drugs of choice in previously untreated, first urinary tract infections, nocardiosis, and toxoplasmosis. Many strains of meningococci, pneumococci, streptococci, staphylococci, and gonococci are now resistant.

Sulfonamides are structural analogs of *p*-aminobenzoic acid (PABA). The action of sulfonamides is bacteriostatic and is reversible by removal of the drug or in the presence of an excess of PABA. The mode of action of the sulfonamides is a good example of **competitive inhibition.** In brief, susceptible microorganisms require extracellular PABA in order to form folic acid, an essential step in the production of purines and in the ultimate synthesis of nucleic acids. Sulfonamides can enter into the reaction in place of PABA, compete for the enzyme involved, and form nonfunctional analogs of folic acid. As a result, further growth of the microorganisms is prevented. However, growth can resume when the sulfonamide is displaced by an excess of PABA or when it dissociates from the enzyme dihydropteroate synthetase.

Resistance

Animal cells (and some bacteria) are unable to synthesize folic acid but depend upon exogenous sources and for this reason are not susceptible to sulfonamide action. Other cells that produce a large excess of PABA are resistant to sulfonamides, and still others may be relatively impermeable to the drugs. Sulfonamide-resistant cells occur in most susceptible bacterial populations and tend to emerge under suitable selection pressure. Sulfonamide resistance may occur as a result of mutation causing overproduction of PABA or a structural change in the folic acid-synthesizing enzyme with a lowered affinity for sulfonamides. Most often sulfonamide resistance is under the genetic control of a transmissible plasmid that may become rapidly and widely disseminated. Thus, the widespread therapeutic use of sulfonamides against gonococci and meningococci has resulted in the establishment of sulfonamide-resistant strains throughout the world. The widespread use of sulfonamides against beta-hemolytic streptococci similarly aided the emergence of resistant strains. Other types of microorganisms—eg, many coliform organisms—are also commonly resistant. It should be specifically mentioned that rickettsiae not only are not inhibited by sulfonamides but are actually stimulated in their growth.

Absorption, Metabolism, & Excretion

Most sulfonamides are given orally. They are rapidly absorbed from the stomach and small intestine and distributed widely to tissues and body fluids (including central nervous system and cerebrospinal fluid), placenta, and fetus. Absorbed sulfonamides become bound to serum proteins to an extent varying from 20% to over 90%. A varying proportion also becomes acetylated or inactivated by other metabolic pathways. Chemical determinations performed on serum may measure free (active) sulfonamide, the acetylated (inactive) sulfonamide, or the total of both. In order to be therapeutically effective after systemic administration, a sulfonamide must generally achieve a concentration of 8–12 mg of free drug per deciliter of blood. Peak blood levels generally occur 2–3 hours after oral intake.

Soluble sulfonamides are excreted mainly by glomerular filtration into the urine. Different compounds exhibit different degrees of reabsorption in the tubules. A portion of the drug in the urine is acetylated, but enough active drug remains for effective treatment of infections of the urinary tract (usually 10–20 times the concentration present in the blood). In significant renal failure, the dose of sulfonamide must be reduced.

Sodium salts of sulfonamides are employed for intravenous administration because of their greater solubility. Their distribution and excretion are similar to those of the orally administered drugs.

The "insoluble" sulfonamides (eg, phthalylsulfathiazole) are given orally, are absorbed only slightly in the intestinal tract, and are excreted largely in the feces. Their action is exerted mainly on the intestinal flora.

"Long-acting" sulfonamides, eg, sulfamethoxypyridazine and sulfadimethoxine, are rapidly absorbed after oral intake and are distributed widely, but urinary excretion—especially of the free form—is very slow. This results in prolonged drug levels in serum. The slow renal excretion is due in part to the high protein binding (more than 85%) and in part to the extensive tubular reabsorption of the free (unacetylated) drug. These drugs are often inadvisable because instances of severe toxicity have resulted from their use. They have been withdrawn in the USA but are still available elsewhere.

Sulfonamides of "intermediate action," eg, sulfamethoxazole, have no advantage except convenience of dosage, particularly when formulated in a mixture with trimethoprim (80 mg trimethoprim plus 400 mg sulfamethoxazole per tablet).

Laboratory Studies

In order to grow bacteria from specimens obtained from patients receiving sulfonamides, culture media should contain an excess of PABA (5 mg/dL) to overcome the inhibitory effect of the sulfonamide carried in the specimen.

Bacterial susceptibility testing with sulfonamide-containing disks is often unreliable because traces of PABA may be present in the medium or because uneven distribution of the bacterial inoculum gravely prejudices the results. Reliable susceptibility testing must be performed in well-defined liquid media that are completely free of PABA, contain all nutrients required for fastidious microorganisms (eg, meningococci), and permit the use of a small bacterial inoculum.

Clinical Uses

A. Topical: In general, the application of sulfonamides to the skin, in wounds, or on mucous membranes is undesirable because of their low activity and high risk of allergic sensitization. (An exception to the rule against topical application of sulfonamides may be the use of sodium sulfacetamide solution [30%] or ointment [10%] to the conjunctiva.) Oral administration of the "insoluble" sulfonamides, 8–15 g daily, results in a topical effect—temporary inhibition of the intestinal aerobic microbial flora—that is of value in preparing the bowel for surgery; it must be timed so that the lowest microbial levels coincide with the time of the operation (usually on the fourth, fifth, or sixth day after administration). Mafenide acetate (*p*-amino methyl benzene sulfonamide; Sulfamylon) is a sulfonamide topically applied (as 10% cream) to burned skin surfaces. The drug is absorbed in 3 hours into tissue from the vehicle. It has been effective in reducing burn sepsis but has led to an increase of burn infections by fungi and resistant bacteria.

Mafenide causes significant pain on application. Silver sulfadiazine has been applied to burn wounds with relatively little pain. The sulfadiazine is released slowly, and only low systemic levels develop. Silver sulfadiazine appears to be effective in controlling infecting flora of most burn wounds, especially if the burns are not too deep.

Sulfasalazine (salicylazosulfapyridine) is widely used in ulcerative colitis, enteritis, and other inflammatory bowel disease. There is some evidence that this drug is more effective than soluble sulfonamides or other antimicrobials taken orally—all of which may occasionally have a beneficial effect in this type of inflammatory bowel disease. Sulfasalazine is split by intestinal microflora to yield sulfapyridine and 5-aminosalicylate. The latter may be released in the colon in a high concentration and may be responsible for an anti-inflammatory effect. Comparably high concentrations of salicylate cannot be achieved in the colon by oral intake of salicylates. The sulfapyridine is absorbed and may lead to toxic symptoms if more than 4 g of sulfasalazine is taken per day, particularly in persons who are slow acetylators.

B. Oral: The highly soluble and rapidly excreted sulfonamides are most commonly employed for the following clinical indications:

1. First (previously untreated) infections of the urinary tract–Sulfisoxazole and triple sulfonamides are highly soluble in urine and therefore preferred. Sulfisoxazole, 2–4 g initially and 0.5–1 g every 4–6 hours (150 mg/kg/d for children in divided doses), gives high levels both in tissues and in urine and is effective against a large proportion of organisms producing urinary tract infections in the community.

2. Chlamydial infections–*Chlamydia trachomatis* infections of the genital tract, eye, or respiratory tract may be effectively treated with oral sulfonamides, although tetracyclines and erythromycins may be drugs of choice. Sulfonamides are ineffective in psittacosis.

3. Bacterial infections–In nocardiosis, sulfisoxazole or sulfadiazine, 6–8 g/d, is the treatment of choice. In other bacterial infections, including those caused by beta-hemolytic streptococci, meningococci, and shigellae, sulfonamides were formerly drugs of choice. However, sulfonamide resistance is now widespread among these organisms. In underdeveloped parts of the world, sulfonamides—because of their availability and low cost—are widely used for respiratory tract infections, sinusitis, bronchitis, pneumonitis, otitis media, and bacillary dysentery. Sulfonamide-trimethoprim mixtures are widely employed for these and other bacterial infections everywhere but are much more expensive. Leprosy is treated with sulfones, eg, dapsone (see Chapter 45).

4. Dermatitis herpetiformis–This is not an infectious disorder, but it often responds to sulfapyridine, 2–4 g/d, or dapsone.

C. Intravenous: Sodium salts of many sulfonamides are available for parenteral injection, but because of their marked alkalinity are injected intravenously (not intramuscularly) in 5% dextrose in water. Intravenous sulfonamides are generally reserved for comatose patients (most commonly patients with meningitis) or patients who are otherwise unable to take medication by mouth.

Adverse Reactions

The sulfonamides can produce a wide variety of side-effects that are due partly to allergy and partly to direct toxicity, and that must be considered whenever unexplained symptoms or signs occur in a patient who may have received these drugs. Up to 5% of patients may exhibit such reactions. The overall incidence of side-effects is higher with the slowly excreted "long-acting" sulfonamides than with the rapidly excreted ones.

The commonest side-effects are fever, skin rashes, photosensitivity, urticaria; nausea, vomiting, or diarrhea; and difficulties referable to the urinary tract (see below). Others include stomatitis, conjunctivitis, arthritis, hematopoietic disturbances (see below), hepatitis, exfoliative dermatitis, polyarteritis nodosa, Stevens-Johnson syndrome, psychosis, and many more.

A. Urinary Tract Disturbances: Sulfonamides may precipitate in urine, especially at neutral or acid pH, producing crystalluria, hematuria, or even obstruction. This is best prevented by using the most soluble sulfonamides (sulfisoxazole, trisulfapyrimidines), keeping the urine pH alkaline (5–15 g sodium bicarbonate daily), forcing fluids, and performing urinalysis every week.

Sulfonamides have also been implicated in various types of nephrosis and in allergic nephritis. Deterioration of renal function can occur.

In renal insufficiency, the dosage of sulfonamides must be reduced and the interval between doses prolonged.

B. Hematopoietic Disturbances: Sulfonamides can produce anemia (hemolytic or aplastic), granulocytopenia, thrombocytopenia, or leukemoid reactions. In order to prevent these reactions or to be able to withdraw the drug before the reaction has advanced to a severe or life-threatening stage, it is important to check the white blood count and hemoglobin level every 3–5 days. Sulfonamides cause hemolytic reactions, especially in patients whose erythrocytes are deficient in glucose-6-phosphate dehydrogenase. Sulfonamides taken near the end of pregnancy increase the risk of kernicterus in newborns.

Medical & Social Aspects

Sulfonamides can be made and distributed cheaply and are thus among the principal antimicrobial agents available in many developing areas of the world. They continue to be useful for the treatment of such widespread disorders as urinary tract infections and trachoma, but the emergence of drug resistance has impaired their usefulness in streptococcal, gonococcal, meningococcal, *Shigella*, and other infections. Topical use (skin) on a vast scale has contributed heavily to the sensitization of the population.

TRIMETHOPRIM & TRIMETHOPRIM-SULFAMETHOXAZOLE MIXTURES

Trimethoprim, a trimethoxybenzylpyrimidine, inhibits the dihydrofolic acid reductase of bacteria about 50,000 times more efficiently than the same enzyme of mammalian cells. **Pyrimethamine,** another benzylpyrimidine, inhibits the dihydrofolic acid reductase of protozoa more than that of mammalian cells. Dihydrofolic acid reductases are enzymes that convert dihydrofolic acid to tetrahydrofolic acid, a stage leading to the synthesis of purines and ultimately to DNA. Trimethoprim or pyrimethamine, given together with sulfonamides, produces sequential blocking in this metabolic sequence, resulting in a marked enhancement (synergism) of the activity of sulfonamides (Fig 46–1).

Microorganisms that lack the step inhibited by trimethoprim (dihydrofolate reductase) can emerge by

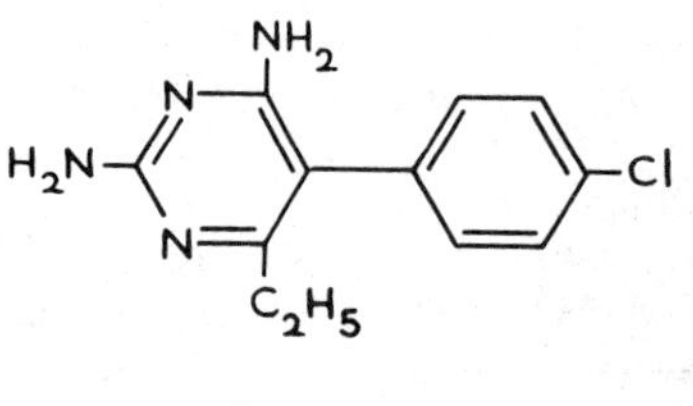

Pyrimethamine

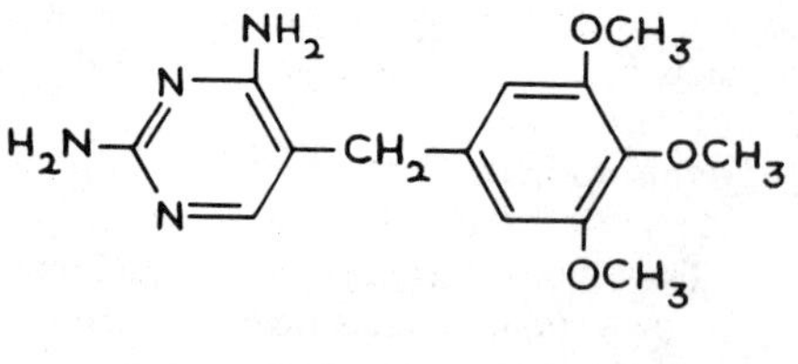

Trimethoprim

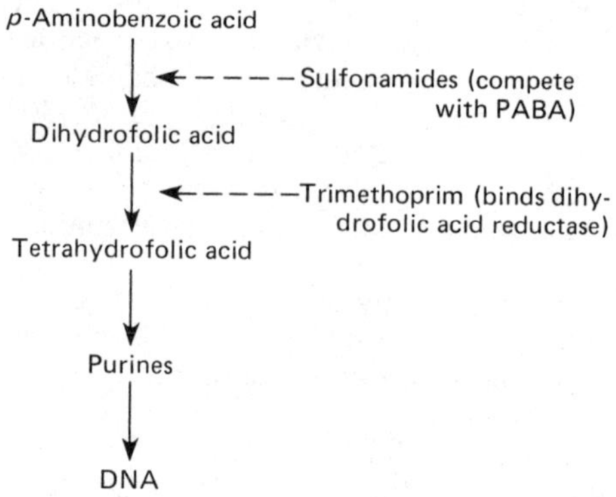

Figure 46–1. Actions of sulfonamide and trimethoprim.

mutation or by the conjugative transmission of plasmids. Such plasmids inducing trimethoprim resistance exist in coliform bacteria, *Haemophilus* sp, and others, and this resistance is increasing in frequency.

Absorption, Distribution, & Excretion

Trimethoprim is usually given orally, alone or in combination with sulfamethoxazole. The latter combination can also be given intravenously. Trimethoprim is absorbed well from the gut and distributed widely in body fluids and tissues, including cerebrospinal fluid. When 1 part trimethoprim is given with 5 parts sulfamethoxazole, close to a 1:20 ratio in tissues is achieved, which is optimal for the combined effect in vitro. About 65–70% of each participant drug is protein-bound, and 30–50% of the sulfonamide and 50–60% of the trimethoprim (or their respective metabolites) are excreted in urine within 24 hours.

Trimethoprim concentrates by nonionic diffusion in prostatic fluid (which is more acid than plasma) and probably also in vaginal fluid. Therefore, it may have more antibacterial activity in prostatic and vaginal fluids than many other antimicrobial drugs.

Clinical Uses

A. Oral Trimethoprim: Trimethoprim is used alone (100 mg every 12 hours) in acute urinary tract infections. A majority of community-acquired organisms tend to be susceptible to the high concentrations in urine (200–600 μg/mL).

B. Oral Trimethoprim-Sulfamethoxazole: This combination is dispensed in a 1:5 ratio, with tablets containing either 80 mg trimethoprim plus 400 mg sulfamethoxazole or double the amount of each drug (160 mg trimethoprim plus 800 mg sulfamethoxazole). Two tablets of the regular size given every 12 hours can be effective in recurrent infections of the lower or upper urinary tract. The same dose may be effective in prostatitis. Two tablets daily may be sufficient for prolonged suppression of chronic urinary tract infections, and one-half or 1 regular size tablet given 3 times weekly for many months may serve as prophylaxis in recurrent urinary tract infections of some women. Two tablets of the regular size every 12 hours may be effective in some *Shigella* and some *Salmonella* infections, particularly if they are resistant to ampicillin and chloramphenicol. The dose for children treated for shigellosis, urinary tract infection, or otitis media is 8 mg/kg trimethoprim and 40 mg/kg sulfamethoxazole every 12 hours.

Pneumocystis pneumonia can be treated with high doses of the combination (trimethoprim, 20 mg/kg, plus sulfamethoxazole, 100 mg/kg, daily) or can be prevented in immunosuppressed patients by 2 regular tablets twice daily. The latter seems to also prevent gram-negative bacterial sepsis in some patients. In a very few cases of *Serratia* or *Pseudomonas* sepsis, trimethoprim-sulfamethoxazole combined with polymyxin has given encouraging results.

C. Intravenous Trimethoprim-Sulfamethoxazole: A solution of the mixture containing 80 mg trimethoprim plus 400 mg sulfamethoxazole per 5 mL can be administered by intravenous infusion diluted in 125 mL of 5% dextrose in water over 60–90 minutes. It may be indicated in severe *Pneumocystis carinii* pneumonia, gram-negative bacterial sepsis, shigellosis, or urinary tract infection when patients are unable to take the drug by mouth. The recommended dose for adults is up to 5 ampules of 5 mL each per day.

D. Oral Pyrimethamine With Sulfonamide: This combination has been used in parasitic infections. In leishmaniasis and toxoplasmosis, full doses of a sulfonamide (6–8 g/d) have been given with pyrimethamine, 50 mg/d. In falciparum malaria, a combination of pyrimethamine with a sulfonamide (Fansidar) or pyrimethamine alone has been occasionally employed (see Chapter 54).

Adverse Effects

Trimethoprim produces the effects of an antifolate drug, especially megaloblastic anemia, leukopenia, and granulocytopenia. This can be prevented by the simultaneous administration of folinic acid, 6–8 mg/d. In addition, the combination trimethoprim-sulfamethoxazole may cause all of the untoward reactions associated with sulfonamides. Occasionally, there is also nausea and vomiting, drug fever, vasculitis, renal damage, or central nervous system disturbances.

• • •

References

Ballin JC: Evaluation of a new topical agent for burn therapy: Silver sulfadiazine (Silvadene). *JAMA* 1974;**230:**1884.

Bose W et al: Controlled trial of co-trimoxazole in children with urinary tract infection. *Lancet* 1974;**2:**614.

Campieri M et al: Treatment of ulcerative colitis with high-dose 5-aminosalicylic acid enemas. *Lancet* 1981;**2:**270.

Craig WA, Kunin CM: Trimethoprim-sulfamethoxazole: Effects of urinary pH and impaired renal function. *Ann Intern Med* 1973;**78:**491.

Feldman HA: Toxoplasmosis. (2 parts.) *N Engl J Med* 1968;**279:**1370, 1431.

Goldman P, Peppercorn MA: Sulfasalazine. *N Engl J Med* 1975;**293:**20.

Gurwith M et al: A prospective controlled investigation of prophylactic trimethoprim-sulfamethoxazole in hospitalized granulopenic patients. *Am J Med* 1979;**66:**248.

Hamilton HE, Sheets RF: Sulfisoxazole-induced thrombocytopenic purpura. *JAMA* 1978;**239:**2586.

Kalowski S et al: Deterioration of renal function with co-trimoxazole. *Lancet* 1973;**1:**394.

Lau WK, Young LS: Trimethoprim-sulfamethoxazole treatment of *Pneumocystis carinii* pneumonia in adults. *N Engl J Med* 1976;**295:**716.

Lawson DH, Jick H: Adverse reactions to co-trimoxazole in hospitalized medical patients. *Am J Med Sci* 1978;**275:**53.

Meares EM Jr: Long-term therapy of chronic bacterial prostatitis with trimethoprim-sulfamethoxazole. *Can Med Assoc J* 1975;**112(13):**22. [Special issue.]

Rubin RH, Swartz MN: Trimethoprim-sulfamethoxazole. *N Engl J Med* 1980;**303:**426.

Schiffman DO: Evaluation of an anti-infective combination: Trimethoprim-sulfamethoxazole. *JAMA* 1975;**231:**635.

Stamey TA, Condy M: The diffusion and concentration of trimethoprim in human vaginal fluid. *J Infect Dis* 1975;**131:**261.

Towner KJ et al: Increasing importance of plasmid-mediated trimethoprim resistance in enterobacteria. *Br Med J* 1980;**280:**517.

Yoshikawa TT, Guze LB: Concentrations of trimethoprim-sulfamethoxazole in blood after a single, large oral dose. *Antimicrob Agents Chemother* 1976;**10:**462.

47 | Antifungal Agents

Ernest Jawetz, MD, PhD

Most fungi are completely resistant to the action of antibacterial drugs. Only a few substances have been discovered that exert an inhibitory effect on the fungi pathogenic for humans, and most of these are relatively toxic. There is a great need for better antifungal drugs, made more pressing by the increased incidence of systemic dissemination of fungal infections in immunosuppressed patients.

Griseofulvin is effective in dermatophytosis. Nystatin, candicidin, and tolnaftate can only be applied topically. Miconazole is effective topically and has been used systemically on an experimental basis. Other imidazoles, especially ketoconazole, appear promising for oral therapy of some systemic mycoses.

AMPHOTERICIN B

Amphotericin B is one of 2 antibiotics produced by *Streptomyces nodosus*, purified in 1956. Amphotericin A is not used in therapy.

Chemistry

Amphotericin B is an amphoteric polyene macrolide. Amphotericin B is insoluble in water. It is unstable at 37 °C, but stable for weeks at 4 °C. Microcrystalline preparations can be applied topically but are not absorbed to a significant extent. For systemic use by intravenous injection, a colloidal preparation is employed. This is a yellow powder containing 0.8 mg of sodium deoxycholate for each milligram of amphotericin, with a phosphate buffer, to be dissolved in dextrose solution.

Antifungal Activity

Amphotericin B, 0.1–0.8 μg/mL, inhibits in vitro *Histoplasma capsulatum, Cryptococcus neoformans, Coccidioides immitis, Candida albicans, Blastomyces dermatitidis, Sporothrix schenckii*, and other organisms producing systemic mycotic disease in humans. It has no effect on bacteria.

The mode of action of the polyene antibiotics is fairly well understood. The drug apparently is bound firmly to the fungal cell membrane in the presence of certain sterols and disturbs the permeability and transport characteristics of the membrane. This results in loss of intracellular components (particularly cations) from the cell and produces irreversible damage. Bacteria are insusceptible to polyenes because they lack the sterol that is essential for attachment to the cell membrane. Amphotericin resistance may result from a decrease in membrane ergosterol or a modification in its structure so that it combines less well with the drug. Some attachment of amphotericin B to cholesterol in animal cell membranes probably accounts in part for its toxicity.

Absorption, Metabolism, & Excretion

Amphotericin is poorly absorbed from the gastrointestinal tract. Orally administered amphotericin therefore is effective only on fungi within the lumen of the tract and cannot be used for the treatment of systemic disease. The intravenous injection of 0.6 mg/kg/d amphotericin B results in average blood levels of 0.3–1 μg/mL. Amphotericin is 90% protein-bound and is removed to a very limited extent by hemodialysis. The injected amphotericin is excreted slowly in the urine over a period of several days. The drug is widely distributed in tissues, but only 2–3% of the blood level is reached in cerebrospinal fluid. Consequently, intrathecal administration is necessary in fungal meningitis.

Clinical Uses

For the treatment of systemic fungal infections, amphotericin B is available as a colloidal dry powder to be dissolved with sodium deoxycholate in 5% dextrose in water to a concentration of 0.1 mg/mL; the solution is then given by slow intravenous infusion over a period of 4–6 hours. The initial dose is 1–5 mg/d, increasing daily by 5-mg increments until a final dosage of 0.4–0.7 mg/kg/d is reached. This is usually continued for 6–12 weeks or longer, with a daily dose rarely exceeding 60 mg. Following an initial response to treatment, doses are given only 2–3 times per week.

In fungal meningitis, intrathecal injection of 0.5 mg amphotericin B may be given 3 times weekly for up to 10 weeks or longer. Continuous infusion with an Ommaya reservoir is sometimes used. Fungal meningitis relapses commonly. Combined treatment with amphotericin and flucytosine is increasingly used in *Candida* and *Cryptococcus* meningitis. This delays emergence of resistance to flucytosine and permits use of lower doses of amphotericin. The antifungal activity of amphotericin B has also been enhanced by rifampin or tetracycline given simultaneously in certain fungal infections, so that smaller doses of amphotericin may be effective.

In corneal ulcers caused by fungi, a solution (1 mg/mL) dropped onto the conjunctiva every 30 minutes can be curative. Other local administrations include injections into joints infected with coccidioidomycosis or sporotrichosis or irrigation of the bladder in *Candida* cystitis.

Adverse Reactions

The intravenous injection of amphotericin usually produces chills, fever, vomiting, and headache. This may be minimized by reducing the dosage temporarily, administering aspirin, phenothiazines, antihistamines, or corticosteroids, or stopping injections for several days.

Therapeutically active amounts of amphotericin B commonly impair renal and hepatocellular function and produce anemia. There is a fall in glomerular filtration rate and a change in tubular function. These result in a decrease in creatinine clearance and an increase in potassium clearance. Shocklike fall in blood pressure, electrolyte disturbances (especially hypokalemia), and a variety of neurologic symptoms also occur commonly. In impaired kidney function, the dose of amphotericin must be further reduced.

FLUCYTOSINE

5-Fluorocytosine (flucytosine, 5-FC) is an oral antifungal compound of the formula shown below.

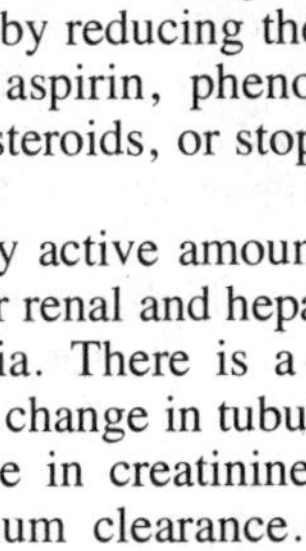

Flucytosine

Flucytosine, 5 μg/mL, inhibits in vitro many strains of *Candida, Cryptococcus*, and *Torulopsis* and some strains of *Aspergillus* and other fungi. Cells are susceptible if they convert flucytosine to fluorouracil, eventually inhibiting thymidylate synthetase and DNA synthesis. Resistant mutants emerge fairly regularly and rapidly and are selected in the presence of the drug, limiting its usefulness. For this reason, combined treatment with 5-FC and amphotericin B is being explored with some success. True synergism may occur, with enhanced antifungal effect against *Candida, Cryptococcus,* perhaps *Aspergillus,* and others.

Oral doses of 150 mg/kg/d are well absorbed and widely distributed in tissues—including the cerebrospinal fluid—where the drug concentration may be 60–80% of the serum concentration, which tends to be near 50 μg/mL. About 20% of flucytosine is protein-bound. 5-FC is largely excreted by the kidneys, and concentrations in the urine reach 10 times the concentrations in serum. In the presence of renal failure, the drug may accumulate in serum to toxic levels, but hepatic failure has no effect. Flucytosine is removed by hemodialysis.

Flucytosine appears to be relatively nontoxic for mammalian cells (perhaps because they lack a specific permease). Prolonged high serum levels often cause depression of bone marrow, loss of hair, and abnormal liver function. Uracil can inhibit the hematopoietic toxicity, manifested by bone marrow depression, but seems to have no effect on the antifungal activity of 5-FC. The untoward effects of 5-FC have been attributed to conversion to 5-fluorouracil in the body. Nausea, vomiting, and skin rashes occur occasionally. With daily amounts of 6–12 g administered in divided doses, there have been prolonged remissions of fungemia, sepsis, and meningitis caused by susceptible organisms.

ANTIFUNGAL IMIDAZOLES

These synthetic compounds inhibit fungi by blocking the biosynthesis of fungal lipids, especially the ergosterol in cell membranes, and perhaps by additional mechanisms. Clotrimazole as 10-mg troches 5 times daily can suppress oral candidiasis; as 1% cream it is effective topically in dermatophytosis. It is also available as vaginal tablets for candidiasis. It is too toxic for systemic use.

Miconazole has long been used as 2% cream in dermatophytosis and in vaginal candidiasis not responding to topical nystatin. Miconazole is also available for intravenous use. Up to 3.6 g/d (about 30 mg/kg/d) has been injected intravenously in disseminated candidiasis, coccidioidomycosis, cryptococcosis, paracoccidioidomycosis, blastomycosis, etc. The fungi causing these diseases tend to be inhibited by miconazole, 1–2 μg/mL, in vitro. Serum levels exceeding such concentrations have been achieved, and prolonged remissions have occurred. In meningitis due to these fungi, 10–20 mg/d of miconazole must be given intrathecally or intraventricularly, because little of the drug enters the cerebrospinal fluid from the serum. The relapse rate in fungal meningitis is high.

Miconazole produces many significant side-effects, including thrombophlebitis, vomiting, anemia, thrombocytosis, hyponatremia, hyperlipidemia, and, occasionally, leukopenia and hypersensitivity reactions. Miconazole markedly increases the anticoagulant effect of coumarin drugs.

Ketoconazole is the most recent addition; the formula is shown below.

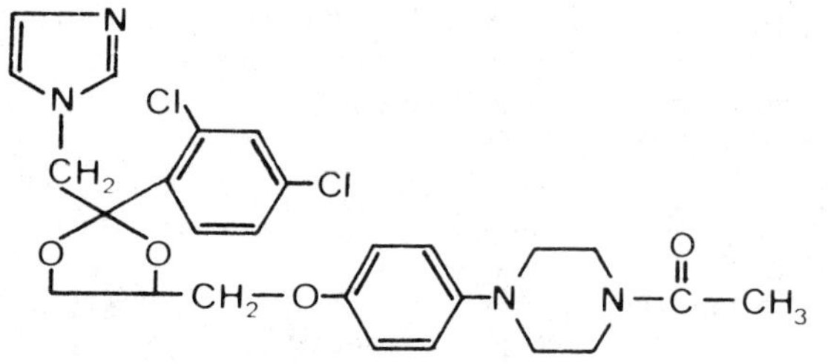

Ketoconazole

Ketoconazole is the first antifungal effective in systemic mycoses that can be given by mouth. A single daily dose of 200–400 mg is taken with food. The drug is well absorbed and widely distributed, but concentrations in the central nervous system are low. Daily dosage suppresses *Candida* infections of mouth or vagina in 1–2 weeks and dermatophytosis in 3–8 weeks. Mucocutaneous candidiasis in immunodeficient children responded in 4–10 months.

Ketoconazole is reported to suppress the clinical manifestations of systemic paracoccidioidomycosis, blastomycosis, or histoplasmosis in 2–6 months. Coccidioidomycosis may require larger doses, and *Aspergillus* or *Torulopsis* infections appear to be insusceptible. Fungal meningitis usually fails to respond.

With oral doses of 200 mg, peak levels of ketoconazole may be 2–3 μg/mL, persisting for 6 hours or more. The major toxic effects thus far are referable to the gastrointestinal tract, but some hepatic toxicity has been observed with high doses. The emergence of drug resistance has not yet been observed.

HYDROXYSTILBAMIDINE

Hydroxystilbamidine isethionate is an aromatic diamidine active against *B dermatitidis* in vitro and in vivo. It is administered intravenously in a dosage of 225 mg dissolved in 200 mL of 5% dextrose in water, infused over a 2-hour period once daily. It may be severely toxic for liver and kidneys and has been largely replaced by amphotericin B.

GRISEOFULVIN

Griseofulvin is a substance isolated from *Penicillium griseofulvum* in 1939. It was introduced clinically for the treatment of dermatophytoses in 1957.

Chemistry

The structure of griseofulvin is shown at right.

The drug is very insoluble in water but quite stable at high temperature, including autoclaving.

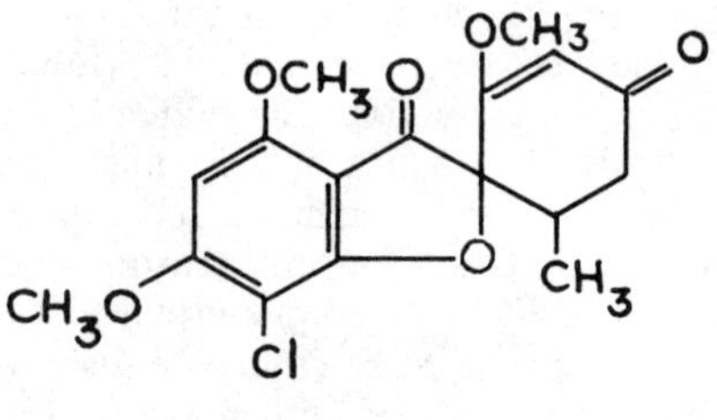

Griseofulvin

Antifungal Activity

Griseofulvin inhibits the growth of dermatophytes, including *Epidermophyton, Microsporum*, and *Trichophyton*, in concentrations of 0.5–3 μg/mL. It has no effect on bacteria, the fungi producing deep mycoses of humans, or certain fungi producing superficial lesions. Resistance can emerge among susceptible dermatophytes.

The mechanism of action has not been established, but it is probable that griseofulvin interferes with nucleic acid synthesis and polymerization. The inhibitory effect may be partially reversed by purines.

Absorption, Metabolism, & Excretion

Absorption of griseofulvin depends greatly on the physical state of the drug and is aided by high-fat foods. Preparations containing microsize particles of the drug are absorbed twice as well as those with larger particles. Microsize griseofulvin, 1 g daily, gives, in adults, blood levels of 0.5–1.5 μg/mL. Ultramicrosize griseofulvin (Gris-PEG) is absorbed twice as well. The absorbed drug has an affinity for diseased skin and is deposited there, bound to keratin. Thus it makes keratin resistant to fungal growth, and the new growth of hair or nails is freed of infection first. As the keratinized structures are shed, they tend to be replaced by uninfected ones. Little griseofulvin is present in body fluids or tissues. The bulk of ingested griseofulvin is excreted in feces and only a small part in urine.

Clinical Uses

Topical use of griseofulvin has little effect.

The microsize preparations of griseofulvin are given orally, 0.5–1 g daily, in divided doses (0.25–0.5 g for children weighing over 50 lb, or 15 mg/kg/d). An "ultramicrosize" preparation (Gris-PEG) is given in an adult dose of 0.25–0.5 g. Treatment must be continued for 3–6 weeks if only hair or skin are involved but for 3–6 months if nails are involved. Griseofulvin is indicated for severe dermatophytosis involving skin, hair, or nails, particularly if caused by *Trichophyton rubrum,* which responds poorly to other measures. Other topical antifungal drugs may have to be used with griseofulvin.

Griseofulvin may increase the metabolism of coumarin, so that higher doses of the anticoagulant are required. Experimental carcinogenicity has been reported. Phenobarbital reduces absorption of griseofulvin from the gut.

Adverse Reactions

The overall frequency of side-effects is low.

A. Allergic Reactions: Fever, skin rashes, leukopenia, and serum sickness-type reactions occur.

B. Direct Toxicity: Headache, nausea, vomiting, diarrhea, hepatotoxicity, photosensitivity, and mental confusion occur. It is teratogenic and carcinogenic in laboratory animals.

TOPICAL ANTIFUNGAL DRUGS

1. NYSTATIN

Nystatin is a product of *Streptomyces noursei*, described in 1951.

Chemistry

Nystatin is a polyene macrolide. It is slightly soluble in water but quickly decomposes in the presence of water or plasma. It is stable in dry form.

Antifungal Activity

Nystatin has no effect on bacteria or protozoa, but in vitro it inhibits many fungi, including *Candida* sp, dermatophytes, and organisms producing deep mycoses in humans. In vivo, its action is limited to surfaces where the nonabsorbed drug can be in direct contact with the yeast or mold. Resistance to nystatin does not develop in vivo, but drug-resistant strains of *Candida* sp occur.

The mode of action involves binding of nystatin to fungal membrane sterols, principally ergosterol. There it disturbs membrane permeability and transport features. This results in loss of cations and macromolecules from the cell. Resistance is due to a decrease in membrane sterols or a change in their structure and binding properties.

Absorption, Metabolism, & Excretion

Nystatin is not significantly absorbed from skin, mucous membranes, or the gastrointestinal tract. Virtually all nystatin taken orally is excreted in the feces. There are no significant blood or tissue levels after oral intake.

Clinical Uses

Nystatin can be applied topically to the skin or mucous membranes (buccal, vaginal) in the form of creams, ointments, suppositories, suspensions, or powders for the suppression of local *Candida* infections. Nystatin may be given orally for the suppression of *Candida* in the lumen of the bowel. This may be warranted in very small infants or persons with impaired host defenses (diabetes mellitus, leukemia, high doses of steroids), in whom the possibility of disseminated candidiasis exists. However, the addition of nystatin to oral tetracyclines is of dubious merit.

Nystatin preparations often contain antibacterial drugs.

2. TOLNAFTATE

Tolnaftate—2-naphthyl-N-methyl-N-(3-tolyl)-thionocarbamate—is a topical antifungal drug for use in cream, powder, or solution form in the treatment of dermatophytosis. While *Candida* is resistant, many dermatophytes are suppressed, and clinical efficacy is claimed for treatment courses of 1–10 weeks. With topical application, there appears to be no significant systemic absorption. Toxic and allergic reactions appear to be minimal.

3. CLOTRIMAZOLE & MICONAZOLE

These imidazoles are effective topical antifungals but are toxic in systemic use. They have been described above. They are used mainly in oral, vaginal, or cutaneous candidiasis, in the form of creams or tablets.

4. NATAMYCIN

This is a polyene antifungal drug active against many different fungi in vitro. Topical application of 5% ophthalmic suspension can be beneficial in the treatment of keratitis caused by *Fusarium, Cephalosporium*, or other fungi. It is approved for such use but must be combined with appropriate surgical measures.

Natamycin may be effective for oral or vaginal candidiasis. The toxicity after topical application appears to be low.

5. OTHER TOPICAL ANTIFUNGAL DRUGS

Candicidin

Candicidin is a polyene antibiotic proposed solely as a topical drug (in vaginal tablets or ointment) for the treatment of candidal vaginitis. It is not absorbed systemically and produces few toxic effects. Its efficacy is currently being tested.

Fatty Acids

Fatty acids, particularly undecylenic acid and its salts, are effective topical antifungal drugs (see Chapter 53). They are widely useful in tinea pedis and corporis as powders or creams.

Haloprogin

Haloprogin is a topical drug active in vitro against many dermatophytes and in vivo against tinea corporis. It is available as a 1% cream or solution, and 10–20% of the topically applied drug may be absorbed. It occasionally causes local irritation.

• • •

References

Bennett JE: Chemotherapy of systemic mycosis. (2 parts.) *N Engl J Med* 1974;**290:**30, 320.

Bennett JE: Flucytosine. *Ann Intern Med* 1977;**86:**319.

Bennett JE et al: A comparison of amphotericin B alone and combined with flucytosine in the treatment of cryptococcal meningitis. *N Engl J Med* 1979;**301:**126.

Block ER et al: Flucytosine and amphotericin B: Hemodialysis effects on plasma concentration in man. *Ann Intern Med* 1974;**80:**613.

Burgess JL, Birchall R: Nephrotoxicity of amphotericin B. *Am J Med* 1972;**53:**77.

Chesney PJ et al: Successful treatment of candida meningitis with amphotericin B and 5-fluorocytosine in combination. *J Pediatr* 1976;**89:**1017.

Drutz DJ, Catanzaro A: Coccidioidomycosis. *Am Rev Respir Dis* 1978;**117:**727.

Goldman L: Griseofulvin. *Med Clin North Am* 1970;**54:**1339.

Graybill JR, Drutz DJ: Ketoconazole. *Ann Intern Med* 1980;**93:**921.

Graybill JR, Levine HB: Successful treatment of cryptococcal meningitis with intraventricular miconazole. *Arch Intern Med* 1978;**138:**814.

Hamilton-Miller JMT: Chemistry and biology of polyene antibiotics. *Bacteriol Rev* 1973;**37:**166.

Hoeprich PD et al: Development of resistance to 5-fluorocytosine in *Candida parapsilosis* during therapy. *J Infect Dis* 1974;**130:**112.

Kirkpatrick CH, Alling DW: Treatment of oral candidiasis with clotrimazole troches. *N Engl J Med* 1978;**299:**1201.

Koeffler HP, Golde DW: 5-Fluorocytosine: Inhibition of hematopoiesis in vitro and reversal of inhibition by uracil. *J Infect Dis* 1979;**139:**438.

Mandy SJ, Garrott TC: Miconazole treatment for severe dermatoses. *JAMA* 1974;**230:**72.

Medoff G, Kobayashi GS: Amphotericin B. *JAMA* 1975;**232:**619.

Restrepo A, Stevens DA, Utz JP (editors): Symposium on ketoconazole. *Rev Infect Dis* 1980;**2:**519.

Stevens DA, Levine HB, Deresinski SC: Miconazole in coccidioidomycosis. 2. Therapeutic and pharmacologic studies in man. *Am J Med* 1976;**60:**191.

Utz JP et al: Therapy of cryptococcosis with a combination of flucytosine and amphotericin B. *J Infect Dis* 1975;**132:**368.

Weinstein L, Jacoby I: Successful treatment of cerebral cryptococcoma and meningitis with miconazole. *Ann Intern Med* 1980;**93:**569.

Woods RA et al: Resistance to polyene antibiotics and correlated sterol changes in isolates of *Candida tropicalis* from a patient with an amphotericin B-resistant funguria. *J Infect Dis* 1974;**129:**53.

Antiviral Chemotherapy & Prophylaxis | 48

Ernest Jawetz, MD, PhD

Fundamentally, viruses are obligate intracellular parasites. Their replication depends primarily on metabolic processes of the host cell. Consequently, many chemicals that inhibit viral replication also inhibit some host cell function and possess major toxicity. Active search is under way for chemicals that inhibit virus-specific functions, as listed below.

In many viral infections, replication of the virus reaches maximum near the time clinical symptoms first appear—or even earlier. Therefore, in order to be clinically effective, chemicals that block viral replication must be administered before the onset of disease, ie, as chemoprophylaxis. This is the case with amantadine against influenza A and methisazone against poxviruses. In some other infections, particularly those due to herpesviruses, virus replication continues for a time after symptoms and signs have manifested themselves. In those infections, inhibition of further virus replication may promote healing. This is the case with idoxuridine and other DNA inhibitors in herpetic keratitis and with vidarabine or acyclovir in disseminating herpes simplex or zoster.

Viral replication consists of the following steps: (1) adsorption to and penetration of susceptible cells; (2) synthesis of early, nonstructural proteins, eg, nucleic acid polymerases; (3) synthesis of RNA or DNA; (4) synthesis of late, structural proteins; and (5) assembly (maturation) of viral particles and their release from the cell. Antiviral drug action can be considered under these headings.

INHIBITION OF ADSORPTION & PENETRATION INTO SUSCEPTIBLE CELLS

Gamma Globulin

If gamma globulin contains specific antibodies directed against superficial antigens of a given virus, it can interfere with entry of that virus particle into a cell, probably by blocking penetration rather than adsorption. The intramuscular injection of pooled gamma globulin, 0.025–0.25 mL/kg of body weight, during the early incubation period can modify infection with the viruses of measles, hepatitis, rabies, poliomyelitis, and possibly other diseases. The protective effect of a gamma globulin injection lasts 2–3 weeks. For infections that have prolonged incubation periods, injections may have to be given every 2–3 weeks.

It often happens that viral replication is only partially inhibited, so that the development of active immunity may accompany the temporary passive protection conferred by gamma globulin.

Amantadine (Adamantanamine)

Amantadine, a tricyclic symmetric amine, inhibits the penetration into susceptible cells or the uncoating of certain myxoviruses, eg, influenza A (but not influenza B), rubella, and some tumor viruses. It therefore inhibits the replication of these viruses in vitro and in experimental animals. In humans, a daily oral dose of 200 mg of amantadine hydrochloride for 2–3 days before and 6–7 days after influenza A infection reduces the incidence and severity of symptoms and the magnitude of the serologic response. There may also be a slight therapeutic effect if amantadine is started within 18 hours of the onset of symptoms of influenza.

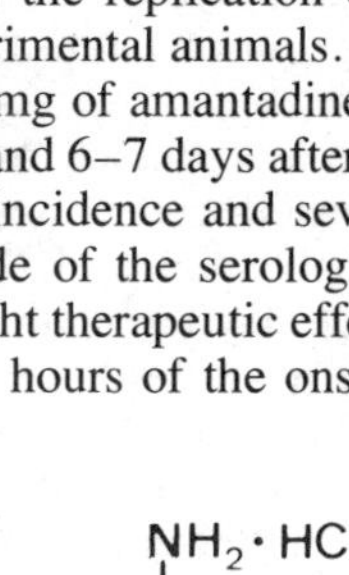

Amantadine hydrochloride

When given orally, amantadine is almost completely absorbed from the gut. The drug is largely (90%) excreted by the kidneys into the urine. In persons with renal failure, amantadine may accumulate to toxic levels unless dosage is greatly reduced in proportion to the decrease in creatinine clearance. With normal serum creatinine, the half-life is about 12 hours.

Chemoprophylaxis with amantadine can be effective in household contacts, in limiting institutional spread of infection, and in protecting adults at high risk during influenza outbreaks.

Amantadine has beneficial effects in some cases of Parkinson's disease (see Chapter 25).

The most marked untoward effects of amantadine are insomnia, slurred speech, dizziness, ataxia, and other central nervous system signs. The drug can cause release of stored catecholamines.

INHIBITION OF INTRACELLULAR SYNTHESIS

Inhibition of Early Protein Synthesis

Guanidine and hydroxybenzylbenzimidazole are both capable of inhibiting the replication of certain RNA enteroviruses but not of others. Both substances inhibit the formation of RNA polymerases at concentrations that appear to be harmless to host cells in vitro. Mutants resistant to the action of these compounds are frequent and are rapidly selected out in the presence of the drugs. Therefore, as expected, these compounds do not have significant therapeutic activity in vivo. Trials of biguanidines in RNA virus infections in humans were not encouraging.

Inhibition of Nucleic Acid Synthesis

A. Ribavarin: Ribavarin (ribofuranosyltriazole-carboxamide) can inhibit the replication of both RNA and DNA viruses in experimental models. The compound acts by interfering with guanidine monophosphate formation and subsequent nucleic acid synthesis. A therapeutic action has been noted in some experimental animal virus infections. In experimental human infections with influenza A viruses, doses of 15 mg/kg resulted in only marginal clinical benefit. Ribavarin has been employed in other countries in viral respiratory infections and hepatitis but is not approved for use in the USA.

B. Pyrimidine and Purine Analogs:

1. 5-Fluorouracil and **5-bromouracil** effectively block the replication of DNA viruses in cell culture systems, but they are relatively ineffective in vivo. **Idoxuridine** (5-iodo-2′-deoxyuridine, IDU, IUDR) can inhibit the replication of most DNA viruses in cell culture. In vivo, it inhibits the replication of herpes simplex virus in the cornea and thus aids in the healing of herpetic keratitis in humans. This is a special circumstance, since herpesvirus proliferates in the avascular corneal epithelium and the topically applied drug remains local and is not rapidly removed by the bloodstream. In the vascular conjunctiva the drug has little therapeutic effect; although adenoviruses are readily inhibited by idoxuridine in vitro, adenovirus conjunctivitis cannot be controlled by idoxuridine in vivo.

For treatment of herpetic keratitis, idoxuridine is applied to the cornea (every 2 hours around the clock) by instilling 1 drop of a 0.1% aqueous solution into the conjunctival sac. This tends to accelerate spontaneous healing. However, DNA synthesis of host cells is also affected, and some toxic effects on corneal cells are occasionally observed, especially if treatment is continued for more than 10 days. Ointments containing 0.5% idoxuridine have been prepared to provide higher drug concentrations. Idoxuridine may induce allergic contact dermatitis.

Most isolates of herpesvirus from untreated cases of herpetic keratitis are strongly inhibited in vitro by idoxuridine, 2 μg/mL. Upon prolonged exposure to idoxuridine in vitro, occasional drug-resistant mutants are selected out that are not inhibited by idoxuridine, 20 μg/mL or more. "Drug-resistant" cases of herpetic keratitis occur relatively frequently. Such patients fail to improve with prolonged idoxuridine treatment. However, many of the virus isolates from such cases appear to be intrinsically susceptible to idoxuridine inhibition in vitro. It is probable that many such strains escape the inhibitory effect of idoxuridine in vivo because they rapidly penetrate deep into the corneal stroma and thus become inaccessible to idoxuridine applied to the corneal surface.

In deep herpetic stromal keratitis there is little virus replication in the stroma. Corticosteroids help to reduce the inflammatory response. Idoxuridine is given simultaneously to prevent herpesvirus proliferation in the superficial epithelium.

Vaccinal keratitis responds irregularly to idoxuridine.

Topically applied idoxuridine has no effect on skin lesions of herpes simplex or zoster, but therapeutic claims are made for idoxuridine in dimethyl sulfoxide or injected by jet gun.

Idoxuridine is too toxic for systemic use. **Trifluorothymidine** is much more effective than idoxuridine for herpetic keratitis but is very costly.

2. Cytarabine (arabinofuranosylcytosine hydrochloride, cytosine arabinoside, ara-C), also inhibits DNA synthesis and interferes with the replication of DNA viruses. By weight it is about 10 times more effective than idoxuridine, but it is also 10 times more toxic for host cells. Idoxuridine-resistant herpesviruses can be inhibited by cytarabine. Because of its higher toxicity for the cornea, cytarabine has been employed topically only for patients with herpetic keratitis who have failed to respond to idoxuridine. Cytarabine, 0.3–2 mg/kg intravenously as a single daily dose for 5 days, has been used in severe disseminated herpes simplex and in disseminated varicella, but controlled studies have failed to support this use. The drug may inhibit immunologic responses.

3. Vidarabine (arabinofuranosyladenine, ara-A adenine arabinoside) is the least toxic and most effective of the analogs. Its structure is shown below.

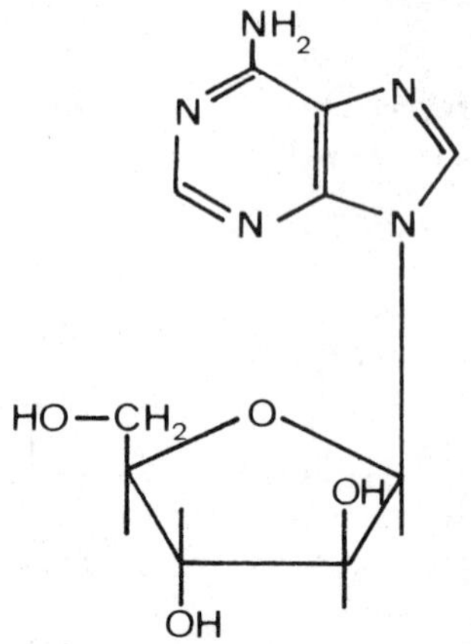

Vidarabine

Vidarabine is phosphorylated in the cell to the triphosphate derivative, which inhibits viral DNA polymerase much more effectively than mammalian DNA polymerase. In vivo, vidarabine is rapidly metabolized to hypoxanthine arabinoside, which has only slight antiviral action. Therefore, the simultaneous use of an adenosine deaminase inhibitor enhances vidarabine action—at least in experimental models.

Vidarabine as 3% ointment is significantly more active against herpesvirus type 1 than against type 2. It cannot prevent recurrences but is effective treatment for vaccinial keratitis. Topical vidarabine has no effect on skin or mucous membrane lesions (including genital lesions) of herpes simplex.

Vidarabine is also used for systemic administration because of its relatively low toxicity. There are limited effects on bone marrow and on liver and renal function, and immunosuppression appears to be minimal. Doses of 10–15 mg/kg/d intravenously over a 12-hour period result in substantial suppression of clinical systemic herpesvirus activity. In herpetic encephalitis proved by biopsy, use of this systemic treatment for 10 days resulted in a significant reduction in the mortality rate. However, only 40% of the treated survivors were able to resume normal life; the rest suffered from severe neurologic sequelae. The most encouraging results were observed in patients with herpetic encephalitis whose treatment was begun before onset of coma.

Current trials suggest that systemic vidarabine may be beneficial in neonatal disseminated herpes infection.

Systemic vidarabine can also inhibit the viremia in chronic active hepatitis and can inhibit the dissemination of herpes zoster in immunosuppressed cancer patients. However, prolonged systemic administration of vidarabine may produce more marked adverse gastrointestinal or neurologic side-effects.

C. Other Inhibitors of Nucleic Acid Synthesis:

1. Phosphonoacetic acid–Phosphonoacetic acid inhibits herpesvirus DNA polymerase. It is effective as an inhibitor of herpesvirus proliferation in vitro and in some experimental systems. Its clinical potential is unknown.

2. Acyclovir–Acyclovir (acycloguanosine) is a guanine derivative. Its structure is shown below.

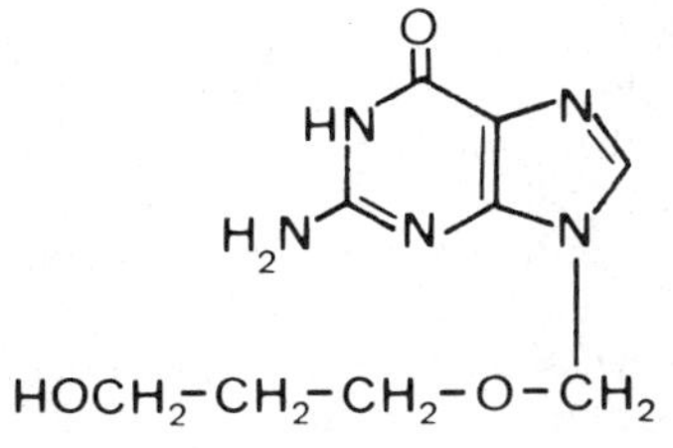

Acyclovir
(acycloguanosine)

Acyclovir is phosphorylated in herpesvirus-infected cells 30 to 100 times faster than in uninfected cells. This is due to the action of herpes-specific thymidine kinase. Acycloguanosine triphosphate inhibits herpesvirus DNA polymerase 10–30 times more effectively than cellular DNA polymerase. It may also have some other actions. Acyclovir inhibits many herpesviruses in cell culture and has some beneficial clinical effects in vivo. Given prophylactically before bone marrow transplants to seropositive individuals, acyclovir, 250 mg/m^2 every 8 hours intravenously for 18 days, significantly protected such individuals against severe herpes lesions during posttransplant immunosuppression. Given after heart transplants to prevent dissemination of herpes from existing lesions, it was effective in promoting healing of herpetic lesions but did not prevent subsequent shedding of herpesvirus. In immunocompromised patients with mucocutaneous herpetic lesions, acyclovir promoted healing of lesions and shortened viral shedding. In these trials, acyclovir, 15 mg/kg/d intravenously, produced no noticeable adverse effects in 5–18 days of administration. Acyclovir, 5% ointment applied topically, benefits mucocutaneous (especially genital) initial lesions of herpes simplex but has little effect on recurrences.

3. Photodynamic inactivation–Some viruses can be inactivated if exposed to one of several dyes and irradiated with ordinary white light. Heterotricyclic dyes, eg, neutral red or proflavine, have an affinity for the guanine base portions of DNA and are bound firmly to the DNA of some viruses. Exposure to ordinary white light then leads to inactivation of the virus by producing breaks in the viral DNA.

On this theoretic basis, photodynamic inactivation has been widely applied as topical treatment to skin and mucous membrane lesions caused by herpes simplex. Controlled clinical trials have failed to show a significant benefit from this treatment. There is experimental evidence that photodynamic inactivation can result in neoplastic transformation of cells in vitro and in some animal models. While the risk incurred by treatment of humans is not defined, there is no justification for the use of this method at present.

Interferon

Interferons are a group of proteins that exert virus-nonspecific antiviral activities, at least in homologous cells, through cellular metabolic processes involving synthesis of both RNA and protein. Interferons are produced in most animal species, but they tend to be active mainly in the species in which they are produced. Among human interferons (IFN), 3 main substances are described: IFN-α represents human leukocyte interferon (type I); IFN-β represents human fibroblast interferon (type I); and IFN-γ represents human immune interferon (type II). These groupings are tentative at present. It is important to note that interferons produced by any type of cell may have more than one kind of chemical makeup and more than one type of activity.

Interferons were initially found to be produced by cells infected by viruses (type I). It was later discovered that lymphocytes also produced interferons (type II) during the immune response. Interferons express some of their activity as lymphokines and immunomodulators. Type I interferons, which act mainly as inhibitors of viral replication in cells, do so by inducing host cell ribosomes to produce cellular enzymes that subsequently block viral reproduction by inhibiting the translation of viral messenger RNA into viral proteins.

Three known enzymes are induced by interferons: (1) a protein kinase that ultimately leads to phosphorylation of elongation factor 2, resulting in inhibition of peptide chain initiation; (2) oligoisoadenylate synthetase, which ultimately leads to activation of an RNase and degradation of viral mRNA; and (3) a phosphodiesterase that can degrade the terminal nucleotides of tRNA, inhibiting peptide elongation.

In view of the broad range of viruses that are susceptible to inhibition by interferon, this agent can be considered a potentially valuable antiviral drug. Many inducers of **endogenous** interferon (eg, double-stranded RNA, synthetic polymers, small molecules such as tilorone) have been tested as topical agents applied to mucous membranes or as systemic agents given by injection. In general, the results have been less than satisfactory: The amounts of interferon induced (or released) were small and became progressively smaller with daily inducer administration, and most inducers have exhibited some type of toxic effect. While harmless and potent inducers of endogenous interferon are still being sought, the research emphasis has been to increase production of **exogenous** human interferon on a large scale. Human interferon is now being produced in milligram quantities in pooled blood leukocytes, in fibroblasts in culture, in lymphoblastoid cells in culture, or, increasingly, by recombinant DNA technology, with bacteria acting as the producing cells.

Clinical studies have been performed mainly with human leukocyte interferon. If given early, interferon prevented dissemination of herpes zoster in cancer patients, reduced cytomegalovirus shedding after renal transplantation, and prevented reactivation of herpes after trigeminal root section. In chronic active hepatitis, interferon suppressed viremia with hepatitis B virus. Currently, the suggestion is being explored that interferon might have an adjunctive role in the management of certain neoplasms and might provide effective therapy in rabies and hemorrhagic fevers. The ultimate potential of interferons in human disease remains to be established. The doses used have been 10^6–10^9 units daily intravenously. Adverse effects include fatigue, weakness, anemia, and gastrointestinal disturbances. It has been postulated that these effects may be caused by interferon molecules rather than by contaminating proteins.

Inhibition of Late Protein Synthesis

A number of different amino acid analogs (eg, **fluorophenylalanine**) inhibit the synthesis of structural proteins for the coats of virus particles. The antibiotic **puromycin** has the same effect. However, these inhibitors of protein synthesis show no specificity for the synthesis of virus protein and impair protein synthesis of the host cell to such a degree that they are intensely toxic. Consequently, none of these substances are useful in chemotherapy at present.

In many poxviruses, various **thiosemicarbazones** inhibit virus replication by interfering with the synthesis of a "late" structural protein. As a result, the assembly of normal particles is impaired or blocked. **Methisazone** (N-methylisatin-β-thiosemicarbazone) can block replication of smallpox (variola) virus in humans if administered to contacts within 1–2 days after exposure. Methisazone, 2–4 g orally daily (100 mg/kg/d for children) for 3–4 days, gave striking protection against clinical smallpox, as shown in controlled trials. The availability of methisazone was an important consideration in abolishing smallpox vaccination.

The above application to smallpox is chemoprophylaxis rather than therapy. In addition, the replication of vaccinia virus can be inhibited by methisazone after symptoms have started, eg, in generalized vaccinia or in progressive vaccinia in immunologically deficient individuals. This is a valid form of antiviral chemotherapy restricted to poxviruses only.

Certain sugar analogs can inhibit the synthesis of virus-specific glycoproteins and glycolipids. Thus, **2-deoxy-D-glucose** is incorporated into glycoproteins of herpes simplex virus and appears to block the cellular synthesis of major glycosylated polypeptides of herpesvirus. Clinical benefit has been claimed for topical application to early lesions of genital herpes in women, but confirmation is needed.

INHIBITION OF ASSEMBLY OR RELEASE OF VIRAL PARTICLES

The assembly of intact particles can be inhibited by many agents (eg, **5-fluoro-2′-deoxyuridine** or **puromycin**) that induce the synthesis of defective viral constituents—whether nucleic acids or structural proteins.

Rifampin (see Chapter 45) inhibits DNA-dependent RNA polymerase in bacteria and mammalian cells. It also inhibits poxviruses, but by a different mechanism. Rifampin prevents the assembly of enveloped mature particles. The block apparently occurs during the stage of envelope formation and is reversible upon removal of the drug.

Rifampin has not been used in treatment of human poxvirus infections, but topical application can inhibit human vaccinia lesions.

• • •

References

Bauer DJ: Clinical experience with the antiviral drug Marboran. *Ann NY Acad Sci* 1965;**130:**110.

Blough HA et al: Successful treatment of human genital herpes infections with 2-deoxy-D-glucose. *JAMA* 1979;**241:**2798.

Cheesman SH et al: Controlled clinical trial of prophylactic human leukocyte interferon in renal transplantation: Effects on cytomegalovirus and herpes simplex virus infections. *N Engl J Med* 1979;**300:**1345.

Creasey AA, Merigan TC: Advances in interferon research. (Medical Staff Conference.) *West J Med* 1982;**136:**227.

Hirsch MS, Swartz MN: Antiviral agents. (2 parts.) *N Engl J Med* 1980;**302:**903, 949.

Hyndiuk RA et al: Trifluridine in resistant human herpetic keratitis. *Arch Ophthalmol* 1978;**96:**1839.

Jawetz E: Antiviral chemotherapy. Chap 8, pp 215–229 in: *Viral Infections: A Clinical Approach.* Drew WL (editor). Davis, 1976.

Juel-Jensen BE et al: Treatment of zoster with idoxuridine in dimethylsulfoxide. *Br Med J* 1970;**4:**776.

Kaufman RH et al: Treatment of genital herpes simplex virus infection with photodynamic inactivation. *Am J Obstet Gynecol* 1978;**132:**861.

King DH, Galasso G: Proceedings of a symposium on acyclovir. *Am J Med* 1982;**73.** [Entire issue.]

Merigan TC et al: Human leukocyte interferon for the treatment of herpes zoster in patients with cancer. *N Engl J Med* 1978;**298:**981.

Mitchell CD et al: Acyclovir therapy for mucocutaneous herpes simplex infections in immunocompromised patients. *Lancet* 1981;**1:**1389.

Myers MG et al: Failure of neutral-red photodynamic inactivation in recurrent herpes simplex virus infections. *N Engl J Med* 1975;**293:**945.

Pavan-Langston D, Buchanan RA, Alford CA Jr: *Adenine Arabinoside: An Antiviral Agent.* Raven Press, 1975.

Pazin GJ et al: Prevention of reactivated herpes simplex infection by human leukocyte interferon after operation on the trigeminal root. *N Engl J Med* 1979;**301:**225.

Pollard RB et al: Effect of vidarabine on chronic hepatitis B infection. *JAMA* 1978;**239:**1648.

Sacks SL et al: Toxicity of vidarabine. *JAMA* 1979;**241:**28.

Saral R et al: Acyclovir prophylaxis of herpes simplex virus infections: A randomized, double-blind, controlled trial in bone marrow transplant recipients. *N Engl J Med* 1981;**305:**63.

Whitley RJ et al: Adenine arabinoside therapy of biopsy-proved herpes simplex encephalitis. *N Engl J Med* 1977;**297:**289.

Whitley RJ et al: Adenine arabinoside therapy of herpes zoster in the immunosuppressed: NIAID collaborative antiviral study. *N Engl J Med* 1976;**294:**1193.

Whitley RJ et al: Herpes simplex encephalitis: Vidarabine therapy and diagnostic problems. *N Engl J Med* 1981;**304:**313.

Whitley RJ et al: Vidarabine therapy of neonatal herpes simplex virus infection. *Pediatrics* 1980;**66:**495.

49 | Drugs With Specialized Indications

Ernest Jawetz, MD, PhD

BACITRACIN

Bacitracin is a material obtained from a special strain of *Bacillus subtilis* in 1943. It is active against gram-positive microorganisms. Because of its marked toxicity when used systemically, it is now generally limited to topical use.

Chemistry

Bacitracin consists of a group of polypeptides that are water-soluble. The material is stable in the dry form or when incorporated into a petrolatum. The unit of activity is defined as the equivalent of 26 μg of a Food and Drug Administration (USA) standard.

Antibacterial Activity

Bacitracin is most active against gram-positive bacteria, including β-lactamase-producing staphylococci, in concentrations of 0.1–20 unit/mL. There is no cross-resistance between bacitracin and other antimicrobial drugs.

Bacitracin inhibits cell wall formation. It interferes with the final dephosphorylation in cycling the phospholipid carrier that transfers mucopeptide to the growing cell wall.

Absorption, Metabolism, & Excretion

Bacitracin is little absorbed from the gut, from skin, wounds, or mucous membrane surfaces, from pleura, or from synovia. Topical application thus results in local effects without significant systemic toxicity. After intramuscular injection, bacitracin is fairly well absorbed, widely distributed in the body, and excreted by glomerular filtration into the urine.

Clinical Uses

Because of its systemic toxicity, bacitracin is now used mainly for topical treatment. Bacitracin, 500 units/g in an ointment base (often combined with polymyxin or neomycin), is useful for the suppression of mixed bacterial flora in surface lesions of the skin, in wounds, or on mucous membranes. Solutions of bacitracin containing 100–200 units/mL in saline can be employed for instillation into joints, wounds, or the pleural cavity—often in conjunction with other drugs given systemically. Rarely, bacitracin, 1000 units/kg/d, is injected intramuscularly into small children with bacterial pneumonia.

Adverse Reactions

Bacitracin is markedly nephrotoxic, producing proteinuria, hematuria, and nitrogen retention. Therefore, systemic use has been virtually abandoned. Topical application only rarely causes hypersensitivity reactions (eg, skin rashes) or produces significant systemic toxicity.

VANCOMYCIN

Vancomycin is an antibiotic produced by *Streptomyces orientalis*. It is active against gram-positive bacteria, particularly staphylococci.

Chemistry

Vancomycin is a glycopeptide with a molecular weight of 1500. The hydrochloride is a white powder, soluble in water, and very stable.

Antibacterial Activity

Vancomycin is bactericidal for gram-positive bacteria in concentrations of 0.5–3 μg/mL. Most pathogenic staphylococci are killed by 10 μg/mL or less. Resistant mutants are very rare in susceptible populations, and clinical resistance emerges very slowly. There is no cross-resistance with other known antibiotics.

The mechanism of action involves inhibition of cell wall mucopeptide synthesis. Vancomycin inhibits the utilization of disaccharide(-pentapeptide)-P-phospholipid. Cell membrane function is also damaged.

Vancomycin can be synergistic with aminoglycosides against certain enterococci and other gram-positive bacteria.

Absorption, Metabolism, & Excretion

Vancomycin is not absorbed from the intestinal tract and can be given orally only for the treatment of enterocolitis. Systemic doses must be administered intravenously. After intravenous injection of 0.5 g, blood levels of 10 μg/mL are reached in 5 minutes and maintained for 1–2 hours. The drug is widely distributed in the body. Excretion is mainly through the kidneys into the urine. In the presence of renal insufficiency, striking accumulation may occur. In functionally anephric patients, the half-life of vancomycin is between 6 and 10 days. The drug is not removed by hemodialysis.

Clinical Uses

The only indication for the use of vancomycin is serious staphylococcal infection or enterococcal endocarditis not responding to other treatment. For antibiotic-associated enterocolitis, 0.5 g is given by mouth every 6 hours. For staphylococcal septicemia, 0.5 g is injected intravenously in 20–30 minutes every 6–8 hours (20–40 mg/kg/d for children). Rarely, vancomycin is given with an aminoglycoside in enterococcal endocarditis.

Adverse Reactions

A. Allergic Reactions: Skin rashes and anaphylaxis have been observed infrequently.

B. Direct Toxicity: Chills, fever, and phlebitis at the site of injection occur. Ototoxicity and nephrotoxicity were formerly common, but since 1970 vancomycin preparations have been relatively well tolerated.

ERYTHROMYCIN

This is a group of closely related compounds characterized by a macrocyclic lactone ring to which sugars are attached. The prototype drug, erythromycin, was obtained in 1952 from *Streptomyces erythreus*. Members of the group included carbomycin, oleandomycin, spiramycin, and many others.

Chemistry

The general structure is shown below with the macrolide ring and the sugars desosamine and cladinose. The molecular weight of erythromycin is 734. It is poorly soluble in water (0.1%) but dissolves readily in organic solvents. Solutions are relatively stable at 4 °C but lose activity rapidly at 20 °C and at acid pH. Erythromycins are dispensed as various esters and salts.

Antimicrobial Activity

Erythromycins are effective against gram-positive organisms, especially pneumococci, streptococci, staphylococci, and corynebacteria, in concentrations of 0.02–2 μg/mL. Neisseriae, *Bordetella, Mycoplasma, Legionella, Chlamydia trachomatis,* and certain mycobacteria *(Mycobacterium kansasii, Mycobacterium scrofulaceum)* are also susceptible.

The antibacterial action of the erythromycins is both inhibitory and bactericidal for susceptible organisms. Activity is enhanced at alkaline pH. Inhibition of protein synthesis occurs by action on the 50S unit of ribosomes. The receptor for erythromycins, lincomycins, and perhaps other drugs is a 23S rRNA on the 50S subunit. Protein synthesis is inhibited as aminoacyl translocation reactions and elongation of the peptide chain are blocked. Resistance results from methylation of the rRNA receptor, which prevents attachment of the drug to the ribosome. This mechanism is under the control of a plasmid.

Resistance

In most susceptible microbial populations, organisms occur that are highly resistant to erythromycin. Resistance is especially frequent among staphylococci, and their emergence in the course of prolonged treatment with erythromycin is highly predictable. Consequently, erythromycin should never be used as the sole drug in treating severe staphylococcal infections. Erythromycin-resistant pneumococci and streptococci are encountered occasionally.

There appears to be virtually complete cross-resistance among all members of the erythromycin group. Erythromycin resistance is based on the altered receptor on the 50S unit of the ribosome. Resistance does not involve destruction of drug. There is some cross-resistance to lincomycins.

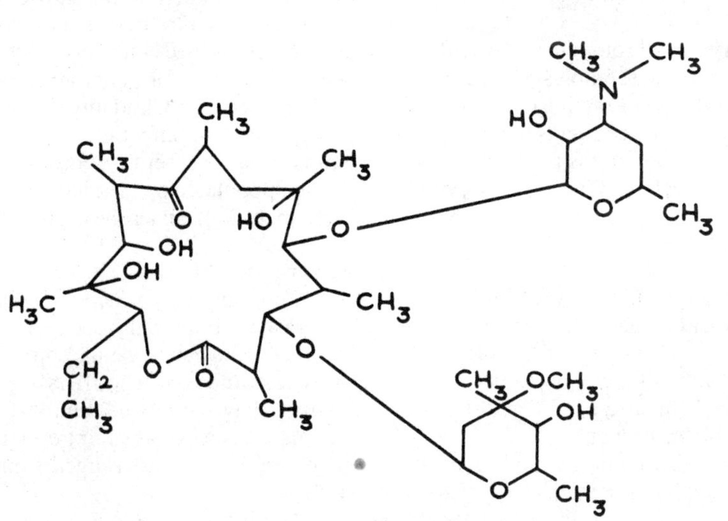

Erythromycin

Absorption, Metabolism, & Excretion

Basic erythromycins are destroyed by stomach acids and must be given in enteric-coated tablets. Erythromycin stearate is acid-resistant but not so well absorbed as esters of erythromycin. Oral doses of 2 g/d result in serum levels of up to 2 μg/mL. Large amounts are lost in feces. Absorbed drug is distributed widely *except* in the brain and cerebrospinal fluid. It traverses the placenta and reaches the fetus.

Erythromycins are excreted largely in the bile, where levels may be 50 times higher than in the blood. A portion of the drug excreted into bile is reabsorbed from the intestines. Only 5% of the administered dose is excreted in the urine.

Clinical Uses

Erythromycins are the drugs of choice in corynebacterial infections (diphtheria, diphtheroid sepsis, erythrasma); in respiratory, neonatal ocular, or genital chlamydial infections; and in pneumonias caused by *Mycoplasma* and *Legionella*. Otherwise, erythromycins are most useful as penicillin substitutes in individuals with streptococcal or pneumococcal infections who are hypersensitive to penicillin. In rheumatic individuals taking penicillin prophylaxis, erythromycin should be given prior to dental procedures as prophylaxis against endocarditis. Although erythromycin estolate is best absorbed, it also produces the greatest risk of adverse reactions. Therefore, the stearate or succinate may be preferred.

A. Oral Dosage: Adults, 0.5 g every 6 hours; children, 40 mg/kg/d. Oral erythromycin base is sometimes combined with oral neomycin or kanamycin for preoperative preparation of the colon.

B. Intravenous Dosage: (Eg, erythromycin gluceptate or lactobionate.) Adults, 0.5 g every 8–12 hours; children, 40 mg/kg/d.

Adverse Reactions

A. Gastrointestinal Effects: Anorexia, nausea, vomiting, and diarrhea occasionally accompany oral administration.

B. Liver Toxicity: Erythromycins, particularly the estolate, can produce acute cholestatic hepatitis (fever, jaundice, impaired liver function), probably as a hypersensitivity reaction. Most patients recover from this, but hepatitis recurs if the drug is readministered. Other allergic reactions include fever, eosinophilia, and rashes.

LINCOMYCIN & CLINDAMYCIN (Lincosamines)

Lincomycin is an antibiotic elaborated by *Streptomyces lincolnensis*. Clindamycin is a chlorine-substituted derivative of lincomycin.

Lincomycin resembles erythromycin in activity, but there are few if any valid indications for its use in 1982. Clindamycin is more potent and is briefly described here.

Antibacterial Activity

Many gram-positive cocci are inhibited by lincomycins, 0.5–5 μg/mL. Enterococci, *Haemophilus*, neisseriae, and *Mycoplasma* are usually resistant (in contrast to erythromycin). While lincomycins have little or no action on most gram-negative bacteria, *Bacteroides* are usually susceptible. Lincomycins inhibit protein synthesis by interfering with the formation of initiation complexes and with aminoacyl translocation reactions. The receptor for lincomycins on the 50S subunit of the bacterial ribosome is a 23S rRNA, perhaps identical with the receptor for erythromycins. Thus, these 2 drug classes may block each other's attachment and may interfere with each other. Resistance to lincomycins appears slowly, perhaps as a result of chromosomal mutation. Plasmid-mediated resistance has not been established with certainty. Resistance to lincomycin is not rare among streptococci, pneumococci, and staphylococci. *Clostridium difficile* strains appear to be regularly resistant.

Absorption, Metabolism, & Excretion

Oral doses of clindamycin, 0.15–0.3 g every 6 hours (10–20 mg/kg/d for children), yield serum levels of 2–3 μg/mL. Intravenously, 600 mg clindamycin every 6–8 hours gives levels of 5–15 μg/mL. The drug is widely distributed in the body but does not appear in the central nervous system in significant concentrations. It is about 90% protein-bound. Excretion is mainly through the liver, bile, and urine.

Clinical Uses

Probably the most important indication for clindamycin is the treatment of severe anaerobic infection caused by *Bacteroides* (especially *Bacteroides fragilis*) and other anaerobes that are often resistant to penicillin and that often participate in mixed infections.

Meningitis should *not* be treated with lincomycins. Clindamycin crosses the placenta and may reach the fetus in concentrations sufficient for the treatment of anaerobic intrauterine infections. Clindamycin, perhaps combined with an aminoglycoside, has also been considered for penetrating wounds of the abdomen and the gut. Clindamycin has found favor in the management of infections originating in the female genital tract, eg, septic abortion and pelvic abscesses that are populated by a variety of microbes, with heavy participation of anaerobes, including *B fragilis*.

Adverse Reactions

Common side-effects are diarrhea, nausea, and skin rashes. Impaired liver function (with or without jaundice) and neutropenia sometimes occur. Severe diarrhea and enterocolitis—sometimes ending fatally—have followed clindamycin administration and place a serious restraint on its use. The incidence of severe diarrhea has ranged from 2–20% in various studies.

The antibiotic-associated pseudomembranous colitis that has followed administration of clindamycin in some hospitals appears to be caused by toxigenic *C difficile*. This organism is infrequently part of the normal fecal flora but is selected out during administration of clindamycin (and occasionally other drugs). It grows to high numbers in the sigmoid colon and secretes a necrotizing toxin that produces pseudomembranous colitis. This potentially fatal complication must be recognized promptly and treated with oral vancomycin, 0.5 g 4–6 times daily (see above). Local prevalence of *C difficile* may account for the great differences in incidence of antibiotic-associated colitis.

NOVOBIOCIN

Novobiocin (also called streptonivicin, cardelmycin) is an acidic antibiotic produced by *Streptomyces niveus* and purified in 1956. It is active mainly against gram-positive bacteria.

Until the advent of β-lactamase-resistant penicillins and cephalosporins, novobiocin was useful in serious staphylococcal infections. To avoid rapid emergence of resistant variants, novobiocin had to be employed in combination with another drug. At present, there appears to be no valid indication for the use of novobiocin, especially since the incidence of adverse reactions was high.

METRONIDAZOLE

This nitroimidazole drug has found widespread use as an antiprotozoal agent. Metronidazole is well absorbed after oral intake, with peak serum levels reaching 5 μg/mL 1 hour after 250 mg orally. The serum half-life is more than 8 hours. The drug diffuses well into all tissues, including the central nervous system, and enters abscesses and empyemas with little protein binding.

In trichomonal vaginitis, both sex partners can be treated with 250 mg 3 times daily by mouth for 7 days. The same dosage applies in *Haemophilus (Gardnerella)* vaginitis. In intestinal or hepatic amebiasis, 750 mg 3 times daily is given for 7–10 days. Metronidazole is strikingly bactericidal for many anaerobes, including *B fragilis* and clostridia. In serious anaerobic infections, the oral dose is 500–750 mg 3 or 4 times daily. An intravenous preparation has become available to be used in the same dosage.

Metronidazole is also effective in eradicating giardiasis. The drug has been used for preoperative preparation of the colon, and it seems to prevent postoperative anaerobic infections. However, metronidazole has not been approved for this purpose because of laboratory evidence of its carcinogenicity.

Common adverse effects include stomatitis, nausea, diarrhea, and central nervous system disturbances, particularly vestibular reactions with ataxia, vertigo, and headaches. Metronidazole produces disulfiramlike reactions if taken with alcohol.

• • •

References

Braun P: Hepatotoxicity of erythromycin. *J Infect Dis* 1975; **119:**300.

Cook FV, Farrar WE: Vancomycin revisited. *Ann Intern Med* 1978;**88:**813.

Eichenwald HF, McCracken GH: Antimicrobial therapy in infants and children. *J Pediatr* 1978;**93:**337.

Feigen RD et al: Clindamycin treatment of osteomyelitis and septic arthritis in children. *Pediatrics* 1975;**55:**213.

Freeark RJ: Penetrating wounds of the abdomen. *N Engl J Med* 1974;**291:**185.

Ginsburg CM, Eichenwald HF: Erythromycin: Review of its uses in pediatrics. *J Pediatr* 1976;**89:**872.

Goldman P: Metronidazole. *N Engl J Med* 1980;**303:**1212.

Gorbach SL, Thadepalli H: Clindamycin in pure and mixed anaerobic infections. *Arch Intern Med* 1974;**134:**87.

Hook EW, Johnson WD: Vancomycin therapy of bacterial endocarditis. *Am J Med* 1978;**65:**411.

Keighley MRB et al: Randomised controlled trial of vancomycin for pseudomembranous and postoperative diarrhea. *Br Med J* 1978;**2:**1667.

Ledger WJ et al: Comparison of clindamycin and chloramphenicol in treatment of serious infections of the female genital tract. *J Infect Dis* 1977;**135(Suppl):**S30.

Meade RH: Antimicrobial spectrum, pharmacology and therapeutic use of erythromycin and its derivatives. *Am J Hosp Pharm* 1979;**36:**1185.

Pestka S et al: Induction of erythromycin resistance in *Staphylococcus aureus*. *Antimicrob Agents Chemother* 1975; **9:**128.

Tedesco FJ: Clindamycin and colitis: A review. *J Infect Dis* 1977;**135(Suppl):**S95.

Warner JF et al: Metronidazole therapy of anaerobic bacteremia, meningitis and brain abscess. *Arch Intern Med* 1979;**139:**167.

Willis AT et al: Metronidazole in prevention and treatment of bacteroides infections after appendicectomy. *Br Med J* 1976;**1:**318.

50 | Urinary Antiseptics*

Ernest Jawetz, MD, PhD

Urinary antiseptics are drugs that exert antibacterial activity in the urine but have little or no systemic antibacterial effect. Their usefulness is limited to urinary tract infections. Prolonged suppression of bacteriuria by means of urinary antiseptics may be desirable in chronic urinary tract infection where eradication of infection by short-term systemic therapy has not been possible.

NITROFURANTOIN

Chemistry

Many derivatives of furan possess antibacterial properties. Most of these substances are topical disinfectants (see Chapter 53). Nitrofurantoin is the main urinary antiseptic among nitrofurans.

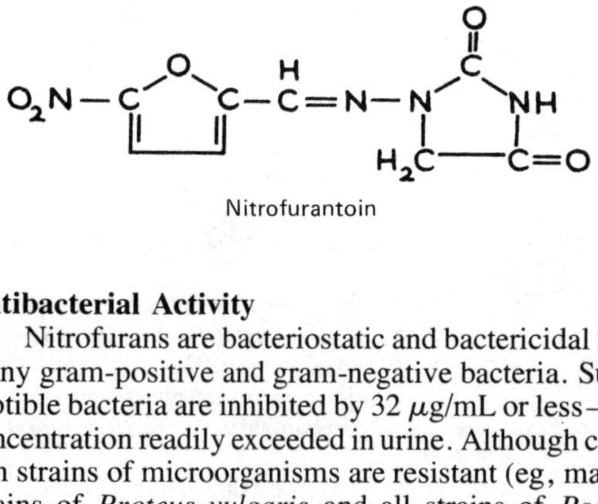

Nitrofurantoin

Antibacterial Activity

Nitrofurans are bacteriostatic and bactericidal for many gram-positive and gram-negative bacteria. Susceptible bacteria are inhibited by 32 μg/mL or less—a concentration readily exceeded in urine. Although certain strains of microorganisms are resistant (eg, many strains of *Proteus vulgaris* and all strains of *Pseudomonas aeruginosa*), resistant mutants are rare in nitrofurantoin-susceptible populations. Clinical drug resistance emerges slowly. There is no cross-resistance between nitrofurans and other antimicrobial agents.

The mechanism of action of the nitrofurans is not known. The activity of nitrofurans depends to some extent upon the size of the microbial population. With very high concentrations of bacteria in the urine or in broth, the activity of nitrofurantoin is diminished. The activity of nitrofurantoin is greatly enhanced at pH 5.5 or below.

*The sulfonamides are discussed in Chapter 46.

Absorption, Metabolism, & Excretion

Nitrofurantoin is rapidly and completely absorbed from the gastrointestinal tract, but the absorbed drug is distributed and excreted so rapidly that no antibacterial effect can be detected in the blood. Nitrofurantoin has no systemic antibacterial activity. In the kidneys, the drug is separated from the carrier protein and excreted in the urine by both glomerular filtration and tubular secretion. Tubular reabsorption occurs, and concentration in hilar lymph is high. Significant nitrofurantoin levels may also be found in renal interstitial tissue. With average daily doses, concentrations of 200 μg/mL are reached in urine. In renal failure, urine levels are insufficient for antibacterial action, but high blood levels may cause toxicity.

Clinical Uses

The average daily dose for urinary tract infection in adults is 400 mg orally in divided doses (5–8 mg/kg/d for children) taken with meals or after eating. Some persons can tolerate up to 600 mg/d, but this higher dose often results in nausea or vomiting. Gastrointestinal disturbance due to nitrofurantoin can be reduced if the drug is taken with food or milk. Nitrofurantoin must never be given to patients with severe renal insufficiency. Oral nitrofurantoin can be given for weeks, months, or even years for the suppression of chronic urinary tract infection. It is desirable to keep urinary pH below 5.5 (see Acidifying Agents, below). Some women are subject to recurrent urinary tract infection as a result of sexual activity. In many of these cases, daily administration of nitrofurantoin, 100 mg, for months may result in freedom from symptoms and infection.

It is possible to administer the soluble sodium salt of nitrofurantoin intravenously. From 360 to 540 mg is injected daily by continuous infusion for a few days. Even the intravenously injected drug has no systemic antimicrobial activity, but this route reduces severe gastrointestinal disturbances.

Another nitrofuran, furazolidone, 400 mg (5–8 mg/kg in children) daily orally, may reduce diarrhea in cholera and perhaps shorten vibrio excretion. It usually fails in shigellosis.

Adverse Reactions

A. Direct Toxicity: Anorexia, nausea, and vomiting are the principal (and frequent) side-effects of orally administered nitrofurantoin. They occur rarely with intravenous administration. Neuropathies and hemolytic anemias (in glucose-6-phosphate dehydrogenase deficiency) are rare.

B. Allergic Reactions: Various skin rashes, pulmonary infiltration, and other hypersensitivity reactions have been reported.

NALIDIXIC ACID & OXOLINIC ACID

These are urinary antiseptics for use in the management of urinary tract infections with gram-negative bacteria. They are effective when taken orally and have no significant systemic activity. Nalidixic acid is the older and better-studied drug.

Chemistry

Nalidixic and oxolinic acids are synthetic chemicals with the formulas shown below. They are stable in dry form and poorly soluble in water.

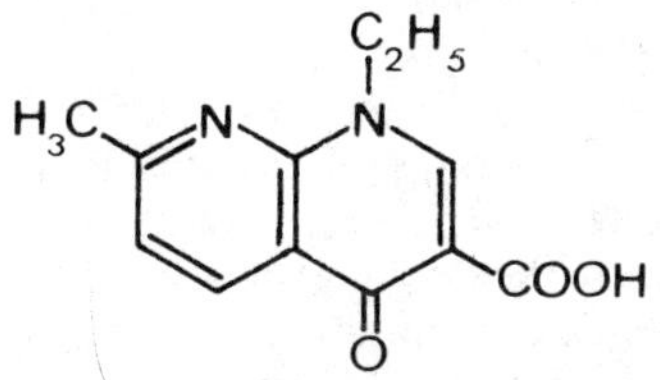

Nalidixic acid

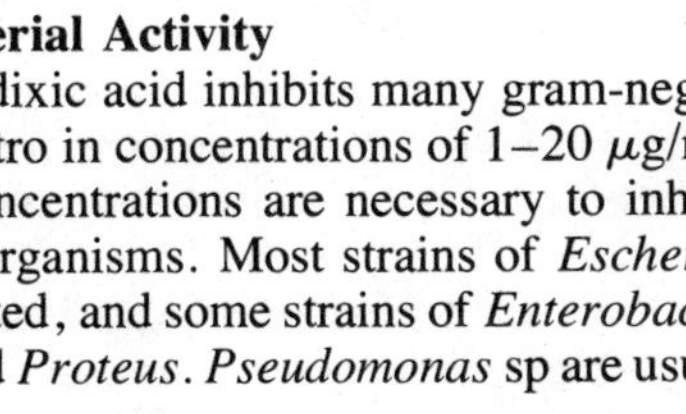

Oxolinic acid

Antibacterial Activity

Nalidixic acid inhibits many gram-negative bacteria in vitro in concentrations of 1–20 μg/mL. Much higher concentrations are necessary to inhibit gram-positive organisms. Most strains of *Escherichia coli* are inhibited, and some strains of *Enterobacter, Klebsiella*, and *Proteus*. *Pseudomonas* sp are usually resistant.

The mechanism of the chemotherapeutic effect is not clear. These drugs may lower the pH of the urine sufficiently to result in inhibition of bacteria. These acids are powerful inhibitors of DNA synthesis in *E coli* (they inhibit DNA gyrase), but it is not certain that this effect is the sole basis of their therapeutic action.

Resistant microorganisms emerge rapidly during therapy, both by selection of drug-resistant mutants in the population and by superinfection with drug-resistant microorganisms of another strain or species. Plasmid-mediated resistance to nalidixic acid has not been demonstrated. There is no cross-resistance with other antimicrobial drugs.

Oxolinic acid is 2–4 times more active in vitro than nalidixic acid.

Absorption, Metabolism, & Excretion

After oral administration, the drugs are readily absorbed from the gut. In the blood they are firmly bound to protein. Thus, there is no significant systemic antibacterial action. About 20% of the absorbed drug is excreted in the urine in the active form and 80% in an inactive form as a glucuronide conjugate. Levels of active drug in the urine reach 20–50 μg/mL.

Clinical Uses

The only indication for these agents is urinary tract infection with coliform organisms. The dose of nalidixic acid for adults is 1 g orally 4 times a day for 1–2 weeks (children, 30–60 mg/kg/d). The dose of oxolinic acid is 0.75 g twice a day. Cinoxacin (1 g/d), a drug related to nalidixic acid, can also be used in urinary tract infections.

Adverse Reactions

Nalidixic acid excreted in the urine may give rise to false-positive tests for glucose, but true hyperglycemia and glycosuria may also be produced. There are occasional gastrointestinal disturbances, skin rashes, sensitization to sunlight, visual disturbances, and central nervous system stimulation. Convulsions have been reported following overdosage. The central nervous system toxicity of oxolinic acid is probably higher; consequently, nalidixic acid may be preferred.

METHENAMINE MANDELATE & METHENAMINE HIPPURATE

Methenamine mandelate is the salt of mandelic acid and methenamine and possesses to some extent the properties of both of these urinary antiseptics. Methenamine hippurate is the salt of hippuric acid and methenamine. Mandelic acid ($C_6H_5CHOHCOOH$) or hippuric acid taken orally is excreted unchanged in the urine, where these drugs are bactericidal for some gram-negative bacteria if the pH can be kept below 5.5. Methenamine is absorbed readily after oral intake and excreted in the urine. If the urine is strongly acid (pH below 5.5), methenamine releases formaldehyde, which is antibacterial.

Methenamine mandelate, 1 g 4 times daily, or methenamine hippurate, 1 g twice daily by mouth (children, 50 mg/kg/d or 30 mg/kg/d), is used only as a urinary antiseptic. If necessary, acidifying agents (eg, ascorbic acid, 4–12 g daily) may be given to lower urinary pH below 5.5. Sulfonamides cannot be given at the same time because they may form an insoluble compound with the formaldehyde released by methenamine. Persons taking methenamine may exhibit falsely elevated tests for catecholamines.

The action of methenamine mandelate or hippurate is nonspecific against many different microorganisms and consists of the simultaneous effects of formaldehyde and acidity. Microorganisms such as *Proteus* that make a strongly alkaline urine through release of ammonia from urea usually are insusceptible.

ACIDIFYING AGENTS

In chronic urinary tract infections, eradication of the organisms often fails. It is then important to suppress bacteria for as long as possible.

Any substance that will produce a urine pH below 5.5 usually inhibits bacterial growth in urine. Ketogenic diets, ammonium chloride, ascorbic acid, mandelic acid, methionine, and hippuric acid (eg, from ingestion of cranberry juice) all can be employed to that end. It is important to check urinary pH frequently and to ascertain by direct microscopic examination that the bacteriuria is actually suppressed. Prolonged suppression (6–18 months) occasionally permits healing of the infection, probably because it blocks the frequent ascending reinfection of the kidneys from the lower tract.

SYSTEMICALLY ACTIVE DRUGS IN URINARY TRACT INFECTION

Many antimicrobial drugs are excreted in the urine in active form. The concentration in urine is often many times higher than the concentration in body fluids or tissues. Effective antibacterial concentrations can therefore be attained in urine with doses too low to be effective in systemic infections. This permits the use of drugs that are relatively toxic. Drugs such as gentamicin, kanamycin, amikacin, or the polymyxins can be administered in doses sufficient to achieve high urine levels without risking significant adverse effects. Even more toxic drugs such as cycloserine (see below) can be administered in a dose that produces urine levels sufficient to suppress highly resistant organisms, eg, *Proteus*, with only a moderate risk of serious toxicity. Penicillins in systemic doses are excreted in the urine to yield concentrations of 100–5000 units/mL. This may be sufficient to suppress not only gram-positive but also many gram-negative bacteria. Ampicillin and carbenicillin are particularly effective against many gram-negative bacteria in the urinary tract unless they are inactivated by high concentrations of β-lactamase in bladder urine. A single 3-g dose of amoxicillin orally may be effective in uncomplicated first urinary tract infections.

Soluble sulfonamides (eg, sulfisoxazole, trisulfapyrimidines USP) constitute perhaps the prime choice for initial treatment of urinary tract infection. The dosage (0.5 g 4–6 times daily orally) is substantially smaller than the systemically active amount, yet concentrations in the urine are high. Even better may be the simultaneous use of sulfamethoxazole, 400 mg, with trimethoprim, 80 mg. Four such tablets daily is an adequate urinary dose. One tablet daily may be useful as a prophylactic drug to be taken by some sexually active women who are subject to recurrent urinary tract infections or the urethral syndrome.

Cycloserine

Cycloserine is an antibiotic produced by *Streptomyces orchidaceus* in 1955 and later synthesized.

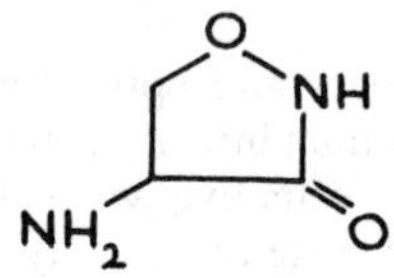

Cycloserine

The substance is water-soluble and very unstable at acid pH. Cycloserine inhibits many microorganisms, including coliforms, *Proteus*, and mycobacteria. The mode of action involves the inhibition of incorporation of D-alanine into mucopeptide of the bacterial cell wall by inhibiting the enzyme alanine racemase. After ingestion of cycloserine, 0.25 g every 6 hours, blood levels reach 20–30 μg/mL—sufficient to inhibit many strains of mycobacteria and gram-negative bacteria. The drug is widely distributed in tissues. Most of the drug is excreted in active form into the urine, where concentrations are sufficiently high to inhibit many organisms causing urinary tract infections. The urinary tract dose is 10–15 mg/kg/d.

Cycloserine may produce serious central nervous system toxicity manifested by headaches, tremor, vertigo, acute psychosis, and convulsions. With careful management of oral dosage (below 0.75 g/d), these symptoms can usually be avoided. Cycloserine is occasionally employed for the treatment of tuberculosis or urinary tract infections. The dosage is usually 0.25 g 2–3 times daily by mouth (for children, 20 mg/kg/d). In nocardiosis, cycloserine, 0.25 g 4 times daily with full systemic doses of a sulfonamide, has been occasionally curative.

TOPICAL USE OF ANTIMICROBIAL DRUGS IN THE URINARY TRACT

Indwelling catheterization of the urinary bladder has a high risk of producing urinary tract infection. This risk can be markedly reduced if a closed, sterile collection system is employed with strictest asepsis. This is often combined with the use of an irrigating solution that contains 0.25% acetic acid or bactericidal concentrations of polymyxins and neomycins, administered by 3-way catheter. Such systems may delay infection with indwelling catheterization for several weeks. They have no place in the treatment of urinary tract infections. Occasionally, amphotericin B, 20 μg/mL, is instilled into the urinary bladder for control of *Candida* infection.

• • •

References

Bose W et al: Controlled trial of co-trimoxazole in children with urinary tract infection. *Lancet* 1974;**2:**614.

Crumplin GC, Smith JT: Nalidixic acid: An antibacterial paradox. *Antimicrob Agents Chemother* 1974;**8:**251.

Fang LST et al: Efficacy of single dose and conventional amoxicillin therapy in urinary tract infections localized by the antibody-coated bacteria technic. *N Engl J Med* 1978; **298:**413.

Freeman RB et al: Long-term therapy for chronic bacteriuria in men. *Ann Intern Med* 1974;**83:**133.

Hamilton-Miller JM, Brumfitt W: Methenamine and its salts as urinary antiseptics. *Invest Urol* 1977;**14:**287.

Kunin CM: *Detection, Prevention, and Management of Urinary Tract Infections,* 3rd ed. Lea & Febiger, 1979.

Lohr JA et al: Prevention of recurrent urinary tract infections in girls. *Pediatrics* 1977;**59:**562.

Matthew AD et al: Prevention of bacteriuria after transurethral prostatectomy with nitrofurantoin. *J Urol* 1978;**120:**442.

Shapera RM, Matsen JM: Oxolinic acid therapy for urinary tract infections in children. *Am J Dis Child* 1977;**131:**34.

Strauss WG, Griffin LM: Nitrofurantoin pneumonia. *JAMA* 1967;**199:**765.

Turck M, Anderson KN, Petersdorf RG: Relapse and reinfection in chronic bacteriuria. *N Engl J Med* 1966;**275:**70.

Vosti KL: Recurrent urinary tract infections: Prevention by prophylactic antibiotics after sexual intercourse. *JAMA* 1975;**231:**934.

51 | Clinical Use of Antimicrobials

John Mills, MD, & Ernest Jawetz, MD, PhD

The development of antimicrobial drugs represents one of the most important advances in therapeutics, since the effective treatment of serious infections has improved the quality of life and has permitted advances in many other areas of medicine. For example, cancer chemotherapy, organ transplantation, and major surgery (especially involving insertion of prosthetic devices) are almost entirely dependent on the availability of antimicrobials. It is fortunate that most antimicrobials are relatively nontoxic; however, all have side-effects (eg, allergic reactions or effects on the normal bacterial flora) that may be troublesome or even life-threatening. Thus, as with all forms of drug therapy, good clinical judgment and overall management are important to optimal patient care.

EMPIRIC ANTIMICROBIAL THERAPY

In many clinical situations in which antimicrobials are used, the pathogen causing the disease is not known at the time therapy is initiated—or, if the pathogen is known, its susceptibility to specific antimicrobials is unknown. This use of antimicrobials constitutes **empiric therapy** (also called **presumptive therapy**)—ie, therapy initiated on the presumption of infection based on broad experience with similar clinical situations rather than on specific information about a given patient's disease. The principal justification for empiric therapy is that infections are best treated early. To withhold antimicrobials until the results of cultures and susceptibility testing are available (generally 1–3 days) may expose the patient to serious morbidity or death. There are many clinical circumstances in which this is true—eg, a severely neutropenic patient who develops evidence of infection may die within a few hours if effective therapy is not begun. On the other hand, clinicians must also be cognizant of the many circumstances in which empiric therapy is unnecessary, so that antimicrobials can be withheld pending culture and susceptibility testing. For example, antimicrobial therapy of streptococcal pharyngitis does not significantly shorten the clinical course and will prevent rheumatic fever even if delayed for as long as 7–9 days—more than enough time to obtain microbiologic confirmation of the clinical diagnosis. Empiric therapy has 2 main disadvantages: (1) If the patient proves not to have an infection, the expense and possible toxicity of antimicrobial drug administration are not justified; and (2) if proper specimens for diagnosis are not obtained initially, the patient may improve but the diagnosis may be obscured, thus complicating later decisions about definitive therapy.

Initiation of empiric therapy (and, to a certain extent, all antimicrobial therapy) should conform to a well-defined protocol:

(1) Formulate a clinical diagnosis of microbial infection. Using all available data, the clinician should conclude that there is evidence of infection and should then formulate as specific a clinical diagnosis as possible—eg, pneumonia, cellulitis, septicemia.

(2) Obtain specimens for laboratory examination. Examination of specimens by microscopy (Gram's stain or other methods) may provide reliable information within an hour or so about the microbial pathogen. Culture or other specialized examinations (eg, antigen detection by immunofluorescence or other methods) will provide an etiologic diagnosis within 1 or 2 days in most cases. Blood and material from the site of infection (eg, urine from patients with suspected urinary tract infection; sputum from patients with pneumonia) are commonly obtained.

Specimens for microbiologic diagnosis are best collected *before* administration of antimicrobials, because properly selected antimicrobials should eliminate or suppress the causative organisms and make specific diagnosis impossible. Identification of the causative agent permits refining antimicrobial therapy with reduction of toxicity and cost.

(3) Formulate the microbiologic diagnosis. Based on the history, physical examination, and immediately available laboratory results (eg, Gram-stained smear of sputum), the clinician should formulate as specific a microbiologic diagnosis as possible. In some instances, this may be quite specific and accurate (eg, a patient with lobar pneumonia with organisms resembling pneumococci in a Gram-stained smear of sputum); in other cases, there may be no clues to a specific bacteriologic diagnosis.

(4) Determine the necessity for empiric therapy. This is a clinical decision based partly on experience. Empiric therapy is indicated when there is a significant risk of serious morbidity if the infection is allowed to continue untreated for the time required for the laboratory to identify the causative agent and to determine its antimicrobial susceptibility pattern (usually 1–3 days).

(5) Institute treatment. Selection of empiric therapy may be based on **microbiologic diagnosis,** where antimicrobial susceptibilty data are lacking (eg, based on a Gram-stained smear or preliminary culture result); on a **clinical diagnosis** without further microbiologic information (eg, cellulitis, meningitis, pneumonia); or on a combination of the two. If no microbiologic information is available, the antimicrobial spectrum of the drugs chosen must necessarily be broader than if some information about the pathogen is known.

Selection of antimicrobial drugs based on presumed site of infection or microbiologic diagnosis is not an exact science, and selection from among 2 or 3 effective agents is often based on the physician's personal preference. Brief guides to empiric therapy based on presumptive microbial diagnosis and site of infection are given in Tables 51–1 and 51–2.

A number of clinical situations may warrant further modification of empiric therapeutic regimens. For example, in the severely leukopenic patient, 2 or 3 drugs (usually a broad-spectrum penicillin such as carbenicillin with an aminoglycoside, with or without a cephalosporin) are always used in combination. Serious gram-negative infections in these patients often respond poorly, even when 2 drugs are used; in addition, the variety of pathogens observed is great enough to warrant broad-spectrum coverage.

ANTIMICROBIAL THERAPY OF ESTABLISHED INFECTIONS

INTERPRETATION OF CULTURE RESULTS

Properly obtained and processed specimens for culture frequently yield important information about the cause of infection. Reports may be **false-negative** for a number of reasons, including sampling of the wrong sites or materials, sampling after initiation of antimicrobial therapy, overgrowth of pathogens by normal flora, and infections due to fastidious or noncultivable pathogens for which the proper tests were not performed (eg, *Rickettsia, Mycoplasma,* many viruses, *Bordetella pertussis*). **False-positive** reports may occur as a result of contamination of bacteriologic media or because the pathogen is merely colonizing the host but not causing the infection (eg, recovery of *Staphylococcus aureus* or coliforms from sputum specimens contaminated by oropharyngeal secretions). Performing semiquantitative cultures may be helpful in this latter instance, because finding large numbers of the pathogen (especially with little of the normal flora) is evidence against the organism being a commensal. Likewise, microscopic examination of stained specimens will be helpful because the presence of leukocytes and a single type of organism favors its role as a pathogen.

GUIDING ANTIMICROBIAL THERAPY OF ESTABLISHED INFECTION

Susceptibility Testing

Testing pathogens for their susceptibility to antimicrobials is now a commonplace clinical procedure. Tests measure the concentration of drug required to inhibit growth of the organism (minimum inhibitory concentration, MIC) or to kill the organism (minimum lethal concentration, MLC; often also called minimum bactericidal concentration, MBC). The results of these tests may then be compared with known drug concentrations in various body compartments and with studies correlating clinical outcome with MIC or MLC to determine whether the organism should be considered sensitive or resistant. Only MICs are routinely measured in most laboratories, as this is adequate for treatment of most infections.

Some organisms, such as group A streptococci, have such reproducible susceptibility patterns that routine testing is not required. For other organisms, only beta-lactamase assays need be done (see below). Other organisms (fungi, fastidious anaerobes) have growth characteristics that make routine susceptibility testing impractical. On the other hand, with many common pathogens (aerobic gram-negative bacilli, staphylococci), antimicrobial susceptibility patterns are variable, and the results of susceptibility testing correlate well with clinical efficacy.

Two methods of susceptibility testing in common use are the disk (agar) diffusion or Kirby-Bauer method and broth dilution method. In the **disk diffusion method,** a disk containing a standardized amount of the test antimicrobial is placed on an agar plate lightly seeded with the test bacteria. The bacteria are then allowed to grow under carefully controlled conditions while the antibiotic diffuses out into the agar. The diameter of the zone of inhibition correlates with MIC, although zone sizes are not comparable from one drug to another. In the **broth dilution method,** the bacteria are inoculated into liquid medium containing graduated concentrations of the test antimicrobial for direct determination of the MIC. This latter assay has recently been miniaturized and automated, so that it is suitable for widespread clinical use. With both methods, determining whether an organism with a given MIC is susceptible or resistant must be based on knowledge of the human pharmacology of the drug. In general, if the MIC is one-half or less of the peak serum levels obtained routinely, the organism is considered susceptible.

Disk diffusion methods are satisfactory for determining susceptibility of many antimicrobial-organism combinations, and they are really all that is

Table 51–1. Empiric antimicrobial therapy based on microbiologic etiology.

Suspected or Proved Disease or Pathogen	Drug(s) of First Choice	Alternative Drug(s)
Gram-negative cocci (aerobic)		
Gonococcus	Penicillin (parenteral only),[1] ampicillin,[2] tetracycline[3]	Spectinomycin,[4] cefoxitin[4]
Meningococcus	Penicillin[1]	Chloramphenicol
Gram-positive cocci (aerobic)		
Pneumococcus	Penicillin[1]	Erythromycin, cephalosporin[5]
Streptococcus, hemolytic groups A, B, C, G	Penicillin[1]	Erythromycin, cephalosporin[5]
Viridans streptococci	Penicillin[1] (?) plus aminoglycoside	Cephalosporin,[5] vancomycin
Staphylococcus, nonpenicillinase-producing	Penicillin[1]	Cephalosporin,[5] vancomycin
Staphylococcus, penicillinase-producing	Penicillinase-resistant penicillin[6]	Vancomycin, cephalosporin[5]
Streptococcus faecalis (enterococcus)	Ampicillin or penicillin plus aminoglycoside[7]	Vancomycin
Gram-negative rods (aerobic)		
Coliforms (*Escherichia coli, Klebsiella, Enterobacter, Serratia, Proteus, Providencia, Arizona,* etc)	Aminoglycoside[7] or third-generation cephalosporin[8]	
Shigella	Trimethoprim-sulfamethoxazole[9]	Chloramphenicol, ampicillin
Salmonella	Chloramphenicol	Trimethoprim-sulfamethoxazole,[9] ampicillin
Haemophilus sp	Chloramphenicol[4]	Trimethoprim-sulfamethoxazole,[4,9] ampicillin, cefamandole,[4] or third-generation cephalosporin[4,8]
Brucella	Tetracycline[3]	Streptomycin plus sulfonamide[10]
Yersinia pestis (plague) and *Franciscella tularensis* (tularemia)	Tetracycline	Chloramphenicol or streptomycin
Vibrio sp	Tetracycline or trimethoprim-sulfamethoxazole	
Pseudomonas aeruginosa	Aminoglycoside[7] plus antipseudomonal penicillin[11]	Third-generation cephalosporin[8] or aminoglycoside[7] or both
Pseudomonas pseudomallei (melioidosis) or *Pseudomonas mallei* (glanders)	Tetracycline	Chloramphenicol
Gram-positive rods (aerobic)		
Bacillus sp (eg, anthrax)	Penicillin[1]	Erythromycin
Listeria monocytogenes	Ampicillin (? plus aminoglycoside)	Chloramphenicol
Nocardia	Sulfonamide[10]	Minocycline
Anaerobes		
Gram-positive (peptococci, peptostreptococci, clostridia, etc)	Penicillin[1]	Clindamycin, tetracycline,[3] cephalosporins, cefoxitin
Bacteroides fragilis	Clindamycin or metronidazole	Chloramphenicol, cefoxitin, third-generation cephalosporin[8]
Gram-negatives other than *B fragilis (Bacteroides, Fusobacterium)*	Penicillin[1]	Clindamycin, tetracycline,[3] cephalosporin,[5] cefoxitin
Mycobacteria		
Mycobacterium tuberculosis	Isoniazid (INH) plus ethambutol or rifampin[10] or both	Other antituberculosis drugs
Mycobacterium leprae	Dapsone or sulfoxone	Rifampin, amithiozone
Spirochetes		
Borrelia (relapsing fever)	Tetracycline[3]	Penicillin
Leptospira	Penicillin[1]	Tetracycline
Treponema (syphilis, yaws)	Penicillin[1]	Erythromycin, tetracycline
Mycoplasma pneumoniae	Tetracycline[3]	Erythromycin
Chlamydia trachomatis, Chlamydia psittaci	Tetracycline[3]	Erythromycin, chloramphenicol
Rickettsiae	Tetracycline[3]	Chloramphenicol
Fungi		
Candida sp, *Torulopsis*	Ketoconazole[12]	Amphotericin B, flucytosine
Cryptococcus neoformans	Amphotericin B plus flucytosine	Ketoconazole[12]
Coccidioidomycosis	Ketoconazole[12]	Amphotericin B
Histoplasmosis	Ketoconazole[12]	Amphotericin B
Blastomycosis	Ketoconazole[12]	Amphotericin B
Paracoccidioidomycosis	Ketoconazole[12]	Amphotericin B
Sporotrichosis	Ketoconazole[12]	Amphotericin B

required when the susceptibility pattern of the organism is bimodal (ie, very susceptible or very resistant, with few intermediate cases), as is seen with the susceptibility of *S aureus* to penicillin G. However, when there is no sharp dividing line between susceptible and resistant, determination of the MIC may be very helpful for guiding therapy.

The results of laboratory susceptibility testing generally correlate well with clinical response. When there is a discrepancy, the various possibilities for drug failure must be considered as outlined below. (See section on failure of antimicrobial therapy and Table 51–3.) Susceptibility testing procedures have been standardized to minimize false reports of susceptibility, although they may occur 1–2% of the time. False susceptibility is usually found because the protocol for susceptibility testing was not properly adhered to. False reports of resistance are more common, especially with the disk diffusion method, and can usually be resolved by determination of the MIC or serum bactericidal titers (see below).

Infected patients given antimicrobials shown to be ineffective by in vitro tests may still recover satisfactorily. Host defense mechanisms may be sufficient to permit recovery in many cases, and there is ample evidence that subinhibitory concentrations of antimicrobials may have beneficial effects—eg, enhancing ingestion and killing of bacteria by phagocytes.

Drug Concentrations in Body Fluids

For most antimicrobials, the relationship of dose to body fluid concentrations is well established, and the therapeutic index of most antimicrobials is high enough so that measurement of antimicrobial concentrations in body fluids is rarely necessary. Exceptions are antimicrobials with a low therapeutic index (vancomycin, aminoglycosides), administration of the antimicrobial by an unreliable route for a serious infection (oral therapy), investigation of clinical failure of apparently adequate antimicrobial therapy, and determination of drug concentrations in unusual sites (eg, central nervous system).

There are several ways in which antimicrobial concentrations can be determined. The most generally applicable method is bioassay, because it can be modified for use with any antimicrobial drug. In this method, the degree of growth inhibition of a standard organism by the clinical specimen is compared with that produced by several known concentrations of drug, and the concentration in the clinical specimen is determined by interpolation. This method is sufficiently accurate for most clinical purposes, although somewhat slow, and becomes technically difficult and potentially inaccurate only when the patient is receiving multiple antimicrobials.

For antimicrobials such as the aminoglycosides, where drug concentrations are determined frequently, a variety of automated assay methods have been developed that are not different in principle from those used to measure other drugs. Immunologic, enzymatic, and chromatographic methods have all been employed, and all are sufficiently specific and precise for clinical use. Kits for these assays are widely available commercially.

Serum Bactericidal Titers

In many infectious disorders (eg, soft tissue infections, pneumonias, enteritis), host defenses contribute materially to cure. Thus, inhibitory drug concentrations are sufficient for treatment. In other disorders (infective endocarditis, bacteremia in the immunosuppressed host, bacterial meningitis), host defenses may contribute minimally to cure. Consequently, bactericidal drug concentrations must be achieved in the infected tissue. An assay of the titer of inhibitory as well as bactericidal activity in body fluids may be performed and will establish susceptibility and adequacy of drug dosage and absorption in one simple test procedure. Serum is obtained from the patient at the appropriate time after the last dose of drug, and serial dilutions of serum are incubated with a standardized amount of the pathogen obtained from the patient. Growth inhibition and killing at a serum dilution (titer) of 1:8 is generally considered to be satisfactory, al-

[1] Penicillin G is preferred for parenteral injection; penicillin V for oral administration. Only very susceptible microorganisms should be treated with oral penicillin.

[2] Ampicillin, ampicillin esters (eg, hetacillin, bacampicillin), or amoxicillin.

[3] All tetracyclines have similar activity against microorganisms (with rare exceptions) and comparable therapeutic activity and toxicity. Dosage is determined by the rates of absorption and excretion of different preparations. Doxycycline is generally easier to administer parenterally.

[4] Effective against beta-lactamase–producing strains.

[5] First-generation cephalosporin: cephalothin, cephapirin, or cefazolin for parenteral administration; cephalexin or cephradine for oral administration.

[6] Parenteral nafcillin, oxacillin, or methicillin. Oral dicloxacillin, cloxacillin, or oxacillin.

[7] Gentamicin, tobramycin, or amikacin. Kanamycin is satisfactory in some cases; streptomycin should be used only for drug-susceptible strains of *M tuberculosis* and streptococci (with penicillin or ampicillin).

[8] Moxalactam, cefotaxime, or cefoperazone.

[9] Trimethoprim-sulfamethoxazole is a mixture of 1 part trimethoprim plus 5 parts sulfamethoxazole.

[10] Trisulfapyrimidines have the advantage over sulfadiazine of greater solubility in urine for oral administration; sodium sulfadiazine is suitable for intravenous injection in severely ill persons.

[11] Carbenicillin, ticarcillin, mezlocillin, or piperacillin.

[12] Ketoconazole does not penetrate the central nervous system and is unsatisfactory for meningitis.

Table 51–2. Empiric antimicrobial therapy based on site of infection.*

Presumed Site of Infection	Common Pathogens	Drug(s) of First Choice	Alternative Drug(s)
Bacterial endocarditis			
Acute	Staphylococci, streptococci, aerobic gram-negative rods	Penicillin plus nafcillin[1] plus aminoglycoside[2]	Vancomycin plus aminoglycoside[2]
Subacute	Viridans streptococci, enterococci	Penicillin plus gentamicin	Vancomycin plus gentamicin
Hematogenous osteomyelitis	*Staphylococcus aureus*	Nafcillin[1]	Clindamycin, vancomycin
Septic arthritis			
Child	*Haemophilus influenzae, S aureus,* streptococci	Cefamandole or third-generation cephalosporin[3]	Clindamycin plus chloramphenicol
Adult	*Neisseria gonorrhoeae, S aureus,* streptococci	Cephalosporin[4]	
Cystitis	*Escherichia coli, Proteus mirabilis, Staphylococcus saprophyticus*	Sulfonamide or ampicillin or tetracycline	Nitrofurantoin or trimethoprim-sulfamethoxazole
Pyelonephritis	Coliforms	Cefamandole or trimethoprim-sulfamethoxazole	Third-generation cephalosporin[3] or aminoglycoside[2]
Otitis media and sinusitis	*H influenzae,* streptococci	Ampicillin or amoxicillin	Erythromycin plus sulfa or trimethoprim-sulfamethoxazole or cefaclor
Bronchitis (bacterial)	*H influenzae,* pneumococci	Tetracycline	Ampicillin or trimethoprim-sulfamethoxazole or cefaclor
Pneumonia (bacterial)[5]			
Neonate	Group B streptococci, *E coli, Listeria*	Ampicillin plus aminoglycoside[2]	Chloramphenicol; penicillin plus third-generation cephalosporin[3]
Child	Pneumococci, *S aureus, H influenzae*	Cefamandole or nafcillin plus trimethoprim-sulfamethoxazole	Clindamycin plus either chloramphenicol or trimethoprim-sulfamethoxazole
Adult	Pneumococci, *Klebsiella, S aureus*	Cephalosporin[4]	Clindamycin plus aminoglycoside[2]
Cellulitis	Group A streptococci	Penicillin	Erythromycin
Abscess with cellulitis	Staphylococci	Nafcillin[1]	Clindamycin
Meningitis			
Neonate	Group B streptococci, *E coli, Listeria*	Ampicillin plus aminoglycoside[2]	Chloramphenicol; penicillin plus third-generation cephalosporin[3]
Child	*H influenzae,* pneumococci, meningococci	Chloramphenicol	Penicillin plus either moxalactam or trimethoprim-sulfamethoxazole
Adult	Pneumococci, meningococci	Penicillin	Chloramphenicol
Peritonitis due to ruptured viscus	Coliforms, *Bacteroides fragilis,* streptococci	Penicillin[6] plus clindamycin plus cefamandole or third-generation cephalosporin[3] or aminoglycoside[2]	Either clindamycin or penicillin plus metronidazole plus aminoglycoside[2]
Septicemia	Any	Third-generation cephalosporin[3] (? with aminoglycoside[2])	Clindamycin plus aminoglycoside[2]

*Adapted, with permission, from Conte JE Jr, Barriere SL: *Manual of Antibiotics and Infectious Diseases,* 4th ed. Lea & Febiger, 1981.

[1] Nafcillin, oxacillin, or methacillin.

[2] Gentamicin, tobramycin, or amikacin.

[3] Moxalactam, cefotaxime, or cefoperazone.

[4] First-generation cephalosporins: cephalothin, cephapirin, or cefazolin (for parenteral therapy).

[5] Pneumonia may be caused by many different agents, and selection of empiric therapy is complex. Consult more specialized texts for specifics (see References).

[6] Penicillin may be omitted if patient is allergic.

though the data supporting this figure are conflicting. Although this assay is not fully standardized, it is simple to perform and is useful for confirming choice of antimicrobial and dosage. It is also helpful where *bactericidal* antimicrobials are needed and where antimicrobial combinations are being studied for possible synergism (see below).

Specialized Assay Methods

A. Beta-Lactamase Assay: For some bacteria (eg, gonococci, *Haemophilus influenzae*), the susceptibility patterns of all strains are virtually identical except for production of beta-lactamase, which confers resistance to various beta-lactam antimicrobials. In these cases, extensive susceptibility testing may be omitted and a direct test for beta-lactamase done utilizing a chromogenic beta-lactam substrate. This test is sensitive, specific, rapid, and reliable.

B. Synergy Studies: These in vitro tests attempt to measure synergistic, additive, indifferent, or antagonistic drug interactions in vitro. The methods are not standardized and in general have not been correlated with clinical outcome. See section on combination chemotherapy for details.

Selection of Route of Administration

Parenteral therapy is generally preferred for acutely ill patients. The choice of intravenous over intramuscular administration is primarily determined by the drug preparations available. A few agents have such reliable oral absorption that parenteral therapy is seldom required (eg, chloramphenicol, rifampin, trimethoprim-sulfamethoxazole); however, for other agents, oral therapy is best reserved for mild to moderate infections or for definitive treatment of serious infections in situations where absorption is documented (eg, by drug levels or serum bactericidal titers).

Monitoring Therapeutic Response; Duration of Therapy

The therapeutic response should be monitored both microbiologically and clinically. Cultures of specimens taken from infected sites should show progressively smaller numbers of the pathogen during therapy and should eventually become sterile. Monitoring of cultures is also useful for detecting superinfections or the development of resistance (see below). Clinically, the patient's general manifestations of infection (malaise, fever, leukocytosis, etc) should improve and the specific findings also should abate (eg, clearing of x-ray infiltrates in pneumonia). The speed of clinical response to antimicrobial therapy is generally inversely proportionate to the duration of the illness prior to therapy.

The duration of therapy required for cure depends on the pathogen, the site of infection, and host factors; precise data on duration of therapy are available for a few infections, eg, streptococcal pharyngitis, cystitis, syphilis, gonorrhea, and tuberculosis. In many other situations, duration of therapy is determined empirically. For serious infections, continuing therapy for 7–10 days after the patient has become afebrile or cultures have become negative is a useful general rule.

Management of Antimicrobial Drug Toxicity

Because of the large number of antimicrobials available, when drug toxicity occurs it can often be managed by substitution of another drug with equivalent efficacy (Table 51–1). In the rare cases where this is not possible, continuing the drug while simultaneously treating the adverse reaction may be possible, although it is associated with some risk. For example, *Clostridium difficile* colitis induced by antimicrobials may be managed by oral administration of vancomycin without discontinuing the inducing drug. In addition, some types of drug toxicity (eg, drug fever) may be confused with manifestations of the infection.

Clinical Failure of Antimicrobial Drug Therapy

When the patient has an inadequate clinical or microbiologic response to antimicrobial therapy selected by in vitro susceptibility testing, a systematic investigation should be undertaken to determine the cause of the problem (Table 51–3). Errors in susceptibility testing are rare, but the original results should be confirmed by repeated testing. Drug dosing and absorption should be scrutinized and tested directly with serum drug concentrations or a serum bactericidal titer. However, drug pharmacology problems rarely account for clinical failures.

The clinical data should be reviewed to make certain the patient's host defenses are adequate (adequate numbers of granulocytes, etc) and that there are no abscesses requiring drainage or infected foreign bodies that need to be removed. If the patient has responded well to therapy except for persistence of fever, drug fever should be considered. Lastly, repeat cultures and susceptibility testing should be performed

Table 51–3. Common causes of failure of antimicrobial therapy.

Drug
Inappropriate drug.
Inadequate dose.
Improper route of administration.
Malabsorption.
Accelerated drug excretion or inactivation.
Poor penetration of drug into a privileged site of infection (eg, brain, eye, prostate).
Host
Poor host defenses (leukopenia, etc).
Undrained pus (eg, abscess).
Retained infected foreign body.
Pathogen
Development of drug resistance.
Superinfection by other pathogens.
Dual infection initially—only one of the pathogens detected and treated.
Susceptibility Testing
Erroneous report of susceptible pathogen.

to determine if superinfection has occurred with another organism or if the original pathogen has developed drug resistance.

Adjunctive Measures in the Treatment of Infection

A. Surgery: It is often necessary to drain abscesses, remove foreign bodies, and close persistent sources of contamination (eg, perforated bowel). Although one is often tempted to delay surgery until the patient's systemic symptoms ("toxicity") have abated, in many cases the patient will remain ill until essential surgery is performed. On the other hand, if the patient is improving and particularly if diagnostic tests (eg, ultrasonography, CT scanning) show shrinkage of an abscess, then surgery may be postponed. Likewise, some abscesses can be drained by percutaneous needle or catheter under sonographic or CT guidance, thus avoiding an extensive surgical procedure.

B. Management of Fever: Antipyretic drugs (eg, aspirin) should be used to keep the temperature below dangerous levels (40.5 °C [105 °F] in most adults; 39.5 °C [103.2 °F] in children, especially those with a history of febrile seizures) and to make the patient comfortable. If fever is not troublesome and is below dangerous levels, antipyretics are not indicated. Do not be concerned about "masking" the infection with antipyretics. In most cases of infection, antipyretic agents will lower the temperature, but some degree of fever will persist as long as the infection is active.

Antipyretics should be administered on a regular basis (usually every 4 hours), *not* given only for an elevated temperature. Intermittent administration produces wide swings in body temperature, making the patient more uncomfortable than if antipyretic drugs were not given.

C. General Supportive Measures: Rest and proper diet will improve the patient's sense of well-being. Aside from correction of obvious malnutrition, however, there is little evidence that such measures are important to recovery from a short illness if adequate antimicrobial therapy has been given.

Correction of host abnormalities associated with

Table 51–4. Antimicrobial pharmacokinetics in renal failure and dialysis.

Drug	Principal Mode of Excretion or Detoxification	Approximate Half-Life in Serum: Normal	Approximate Half-Life in Serum: Renal Failure*	Proposed Dosage Regimen in Renal Failure: Initial Dose†	Proposed Dosage Regimen in Renal Failure: Give Half of Initial Dose at Interval Of	Significant Removal of Drug by Dialysis (H = Hemodialysis; P = Peritoneal Dialysis)	Nephrotoxicity
Penicillin G	Tubular secretion	0.5 h	6 h	6 g IV	8–12 h	H, P no	Very rare
Ampicillin	Tubular secretion	1 h	8–12 h	6 g IV	8–12 h	H yes, P no	Very rare
Carbenicillin, ticarcillin	Tubular secretion	1 h	16 h	4 g IV	12–18 h	H yes, P no	Very rare
Methicillin, oxacillin	Tubular secretion	0.5 h	6 h	6 g IV	8–12 h	H, P no	Very rare
Nafcillin	Mainly liver	0.5 h	1.5 h	No change		No data	Very rare
Cephalothin, cephapirin	Tubular secretion	0.5 h	2–3 h	4 g IV	8–12 h	H, P yes	Very rare
Cephalexin, cephradine	Tubular secretion and glomerular	1 h	15 h	2 g orally	8–12 h	H, P yes	Very rare
Cefazolin	filtration	2 h	30–60 h	2 g IM or IV	24 h	H, P no	Very rare
Cefotaxime, cefamandole	Tubular secretion and liver	1 h	16–20 h	2 g IV	12–18 h	H, P yes	Very rare
Cefoxitin	Tubular secretion	1 h	20 h	2 g IV	18–24 h	H, P yes	Very rare
Moxalactam	Tubular secretion and liver	2 h	30 h	2 g IM or IV	24 h	H, P yes	Very rare
Kanamycin, amikacin	Glomerular filtration	2.5 h	3 d	15 mg/kg IM	3 d	H, P yes	Common
Tobramycin, gentamicin	Glomerular filtration	2.5 h	2–4 d	3 mg/kg IM	2–3 d	H, P yes‡	Common
Vancomycin	Glomerular filtration	6 h	6–9 d	1 g IV	5–8 d	H, P no	Probably yes
Polymyxin B	Glomerular filtration	5 h	2–3 d	2.5 mg/kg IV	3–4 d	H no, P yes	Very common
Tetracycline	Glomerular filtration	8 h	3 d	1 g orally or 0.5 g IV	3 d	H, P no	Very rare
Chloramphenicol	Mainly liver	3 h	4 h	1 g orally or IV	8 h	H, P poorly	No
Erythromycin	Mainly liver	1.5 h	5 h	1 g orally or IV	8 h	H, P poorly	No
Clindamycin	Glomerular filtration and liver	2.5 h	4 h	600 mg IV or IM	8 h	H, P no	No

*Considered here to be marked by creatinine clearance of 10 mL/min or less.

†For a 60-kg adult with a serious systemic infection. The "initial dose" listed is administered as an intravenous infusion over a period of 1–8 hours, or as 2 intramuscular injections during an 8-hour period, or as 2–3 oral doses during the same period.

‡Aminoglycosides are removed irregularly in peritoneal dialysis. Gentamicin is removed 60% in hemodialysis.

infection is an essential component of therapy of infectious diseases. Respiration (oxygen uptake and carbon dioxide excretion) and circulation must be supported, if inadequate. Electrolyte and acid-base disturbances should be corrected. Antitoxins to the core glycolipid (endotoxin) of gram-negative bacteria reduce shock and mortality rates in gram-negative bacterial infections. Antibodies to other bacterial components (eg, *Pseudomonas* toxins) may be beneficial as well. These approaches will doubtless be of increasing importance in the future.

CONDITIONS ALTERING ANTIMICROBIAL PHARMACOLOGY

Diseases of the major excretory organs as well as physiologic states such as infancy or pregnancy alter the disposition of antimicrobials along with other drugs. Some of these changes are shown in Tables 51–4 and 51–5. A variety of other clinical states (puerperium, burns, cystic fibrosis) are known to alter antimicrobial pharmacokinetics; thus, measures of adequate dosing (drug concentrations or serum bactericidal titers) are advisable in patients with serious infections and significant underlying disease.

ANTIMICROBIAL DRUG INTERACTIONS

Like other classes of drugs, antimicrobials may interact with other medication being given to the patient, with possible adverse results. Some antimicrobial drug interactions of clinical importance are shown in Table 51–6. In addition to the interactions listed in the earlier chapter, virtually all broad-spectrum antimicrobials (other than rifampin) enhance the effect of coumarin anticoagulants, presumably by inhibiting production of vitamin K by the intestinal flora. Likewise, inhibition of bacterial sterol biotransformation by antimicrobial agents may decrease blood levels of contraceptive medication following oral administration (eg, pregnancy occurring in women taking birth control pills).

ANTIMICROBIAL DRUG COMBINATIONS

Possible Indications for Therapy With Multiple Antimicrobials

(1) In certain desperately ill patients with suspected infections of unknown origin, it may be desirable to administer more than one antimicrobial drug empirically in an effort to suppress all of the most

Table 51–5. Antimicrobial pharmacology in pregnancy and the neonatal period.*

Drug Group	Pregnancy		Neonatal Period		Antibiotic Found in Breast Milk
	Pharmacology	Fetal Toxicity	Pharmacology	Toxicity	
Sulfonamides	No change.	Slight possibility of teratogenesis.	No change.	Kernicterus–displaces bilirubin from serum albumin. Hemolysis (G6PD deficiency).	Yes. Use with caution.
Penicillins	Accelerated excretion.	None.	No change.	Same as adult.	Small amounts. Safe.
Cephalosporins	Accelerated excretion.	None.	No change.	Same as adult.	Small amounts. Safe.
Aminoglycosides	Accelerated excretion.	Eighth nerve toxicity (especially streptomycin).	Accelerated excretion; higher dose required.	Same as adult–probably occurs less often.	Probably yes. Use if indicated, as gastrointestinal absorption is low.
Vancomycin	No change.	None known.	Probably no change.	Same as adult.	Unknown.
Tetracyclines	Do not use.	1. Tooth discoloration and dysplasia. 2. Inhibition of bone growth.	Do not use.	Same as fetal.	Yes. Do not use. (Risk probably low due to malabsorption by infant.)
Chloramphenicol	No change.	None known.	Diminished hepatic conjugation–lower dose required.	Gray baby syndrome.	Yes. Do not use.
Trimethoprim	No change.	Teratogenic.	Not recommended.	Same as adult.	Probably yes. Use with caution.
Erythromycins	No change.	None.	No change.	Same as adult. Very safe.	Some. Safe.
Lincomycins	No change.	None known.	Probably no change.	Little experience–probably safe.	Small amounts. Safe.

*Modified and reproduced, with permission, from Conte JE Jr, Sweet RW: *Infectious Diseases in Clinical Practice.* University of California, San Francisco, 1982. [Course syllabus.]

Table 51–6. Interactions between antimicrobials and other drugs of clinical significance.

Antimicrobial	Other Agent(s)	Results of Interaction
Aminoglycosides	Neuromuscular blocking drugs.	Increased neuromuscular blockade.
	Other nephrotoxins or ototoxins.	Increased nephrotoxicity or ototoxicity.
Sulfonamides	Sulfonylureas.	Hypoglycemia.
	Methenamine.	Precipitates in urine.
	Phenytoin.	Increased blood concentration of other agents.
Chloramphenicol	Phenytoin, tolbutamide, ethanol.	Increased blood concentration of other agents.
Metronidazole (also cefamandole, moxalactam)	Ethanol.	Disulfiramlike reaction.
Erythromycin	Theophylline.	Increased blood theophylline concentration.
Rifampin	Coumarin anticoagulants.	Decreased anticoagulant effect (increased metabolism of drug).
	Quinidine.	Decreased effect of quinidine.
	Digoxin.	Decreased effect of digoxin.
Tetracyclines	Antacids, iron, calcium.	Inhibit intestinal absorption of tetracycline.
Penicillins and cephalosporins	Uricosuric agents (probenecid, high-dose aspirin, etc).	Block excretion of beta-lactams, causing higher serum levels.

likely pathogens. Thus, in suspected septicemia, an antistaphylococcal drug (eg, nafcillin) might be combined with a drug having activity against aerobic gram-negative bacilli (gentamicin, tobramycin, or amikacin) until blood cultures yield a specific microorganism (Table 51–2).

(2) In mixed infections, it is possible that 2 or 3 drugs may be required to "cover" all of the potential or known pathogens. For example, in peritonitis following perforation of the colon, a drug active against anaerobes and gram-positive bacteria (clindamycin) may be combined with one active against coliforms (an aminoglycoside).

(3) In some clinical situations, the rapid emergence of bacteria resistant to one drug may impair the chances for cure. The addition of a second drug may delay or prevent the emergence of resistant strains. This effect has been demonstrated unequivocally in tuberculosis and is the basis for the frequent use of combinations of isoniazid, ethambutol, rifampin, or other drugs in this disease.

(4) The simultaneous use of 2 drugs may in some situations achieve an effect not obtainable by either drug alone. One drug enhances the antibacterial activity of the second drug against a specific microorganism. Such an effect can be considered a manifestation of drug synergism. Unfortunately, such synergism is unpredictable: A given combination of drugs must be specifically tailored by laboratory tests to fit a certain strain of a given microorganism. A synopsis of the dynamics of combined antibiotic action is given below. One of the best-established examples of synergism is the cure of bacterial endocarditis caused by enterococci *(Streptococcus faecalis)* by a combination of a penicillin with an aminoglycoside, as compared to the frequent failure of treatment with a penicillin alone.

(5) Drug combinations may occasionally reduce the dosage required, and therefore the incidence or intensity of adverse reactions to single agents. A given microorganism may be susceptible to each of 2 drugs but only in doses likely to cause severe adverse reactions. If the drugs are used simultaneously, each can be used in half the dosage—perhaps below the threshold of adverse reaction. The availability of newer, more efficacious antimicrobials has made combination therapy based on this justification much less common.

DYNAMICS OF COMBINED ANTIMICROBIAL DRUG ACTION IN VITRO

Problems in Measuring Antimicrobial Drug Effects

Even when technically feasible, chemical measures of antimicrobial drug concentration may not accurately reflect antibacterial activity. Direct evaluation of bacteriostasis or bactericidal activity is the only useful way of measuring the effects of these drugs. Several methods can be employed, and all may be applicable to the measurement of combined drug action. The results of any one type of examination need not coincide with those of any other type, because the different methods may measure different events in the test system.

A. Bacteriostatic Effect: End points are expressed as the minimum amount of drug necessary to suppress visible growth for a given time.

B. Bactericidal Effect as Shown by Rate of Killing: Results are expressed as the bactericidal rate, ie, the slope of the plot of viable survivors at various time intervals after addition of drug. This is the "time-kill curve" method (Fig 51–1).

C. Bactericidal Effect as Shown by Completeness of Killing: The results are expressed as the smallest concentration of drug resulting in a given number of viable survivors (eg, $< 0.1\%$) in a given time, ie, a bactericidal end point.

D. Curative Effect as Shown in Therapeutic Trials in Vivo: The results are expressed as the smallest drug concentrations measured in patients whose infections are eradicated.

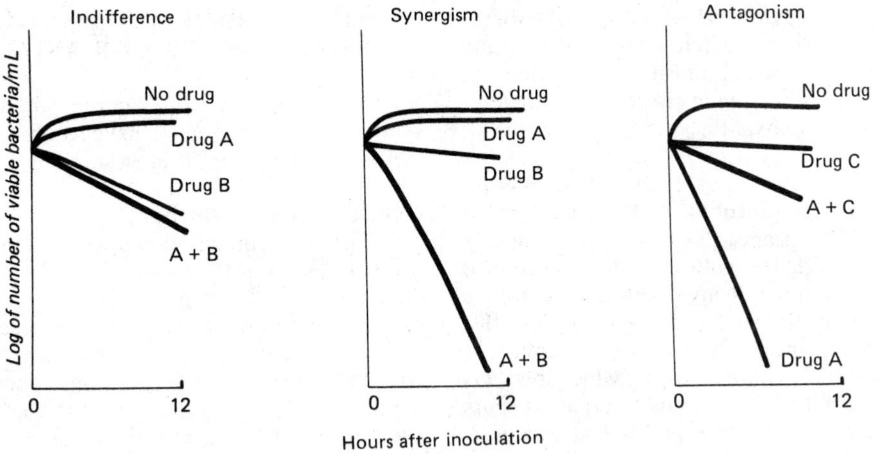

Figure 51–1. Types of combined action of antimicrobial drugs, measuring bactericidal activity by the "time-kill curve" method.

Outcomes of Combined Antimicrobial Action

The nature of the interaction of 2 antimicrobial drugs can be judged from the plot of drug activity in an isobologram (Fig 51–2). From the results of measurements (according to any of the methods described in paragraphs A–D, above) with different doses of each drug alone and in combination acting on a given microbial population, it can be determined whether the drugs are additive, synergistic, or antagonistic. These terms can be applied to any specified intensity (the criterion) of bacteriostatic or curative effects as well as to bactericidal effects. Bactericidal action in vitro and in vivo is important, and the 3 main results that are observed are (1) indifference or additive effect, (2) synergism, and (3) antagonism (Fig 51–1).

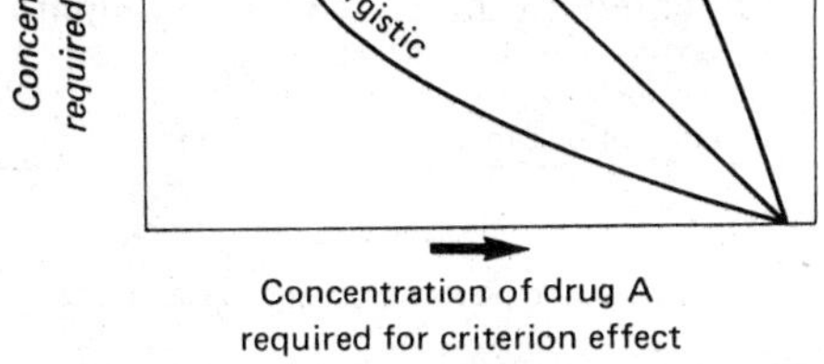

Figure 51–2. Isobologram showing possible interactions between 2 antimicrobials. The criterion effect is defined in setting up the assay and may be a specific bacteriostatic or bactericidal end point. The lines cross the ordinate at the concentration of drug B that is required to achieve the criterion effect when drug B is used alone. Similarly, the lines cross the abscissa at the concentration required for drug A alone to achieve the same effect.

Indifference or Additive Effect

The most common result is indifference. The combined effect of drugs A and B is equal to that of the single more active component of the mixture A + B or is equal to the arithmetic sum of the effects of the individual drugs in their chosen doses. The same total effect could be obtained by the use of a single drug in a dose equivalent to that of the mixture.

Synergism

At times, the simultaneous action of 2 drugs results in an effect (A + B) far greater than that of either A alone or B alone in much larger dosages and also greater than could be expected from simple addition of individual drug effects.

In at least 3 types of antimicrobial synergism, the mechanism is fairly well understood (see also Chapter 41):

A. Blocking Successive Steps in a Metabolic Sequence: The best example is the combination of a sulfonamide and trimethoprim. Sulfonamides compete with *p*-aminobenzoic acid, which is required by some bacteria for the synthesis of dihydrofolate. Folate antagonists such as trimethoprim inhibit the enzyme (dihydrofolic acid reductase) that reduces dihydrofolate to tetrahydrofolate. The simultaneous presence of a sulfonamide and trimethoprim results in the simultaneous block of sequential steps leading to the synthesis of purines and nucleic acid and can result in a much more complete inhibition of growth than either component of the mixture alone.

B. One Drug Inhibits an Enzyme That Can Destroy the Second Drug: The best example of this mechanism is the noncompetitive inhibition of beta-lactamase by clavulanic acid or other substances. Organisms that produce beta-lactamase are resistant to the action of penicillin G because the drug is hydrolyzed by the enzyme. However, if the beta-lactamase is inhibited, the penicillin G is protected and can inhibit or kill the microorganism. This mechanism is an attractive one just beginning to be used clinically. A combination of amoxicillin and clavulanic acid, Augmentin, has recently been introduced.

C. One Drug Promotes Entry of a Second Drug Through the Microbial Cell Wall or Cell Membrane: This appears to be a widely applicable mechanism of synergism, with considerable clinical importance. For example, many streptococci exhibit a partial permeability barrier to aminoglycosides. If a cell wall-inhibitory drug is also present, it enhances the penetration of the aminoglycoside, which then acts on ribosomes and kills the cell. This effect also occurs with some viridans streptococci, group B streptococci, and group D enterococci. Combined therapy permits cure of sepsis or endocarditis caused by these organisms, whereas either drug alone often fails.

Antagonism

At times the addition of a second drug actually diminishes the antibacterial effectiveness of the first drug, as shown by the interaction of drugs A and C in Fig 51–1. This "antagonism" can be manifested by a decrease in the inhibitory activity or in the early bactericidal rate of a drug mixture below that of one or both of its components. Antagonism can be demonstrated only when the drugs act on organisms capable of multiplication and is most marked when a barely active amount of bacteriostatic drug is added to a minimal bactericidal amount of a second drug. The bacteriostatic drug (tetracycline, chloramphenicol, erythromycin, etc) acts as an inhibitor of protein synthesis; the bactericidal drug (a penicillin, cephalosporin, or aminoglycoside) requires active protein synthesis for killing. In the case of cell wall-active drugs, it has been suggested that the inhibition of protein synthesis by chloramphenicol or tetracycline interferes with the production of some autolytic enzyme system postulated to be an important final step in cell lysis.

CLINICAL EVIDENCE FOR ANTIMICROBIAL DRUG SYNERGISM OR ANTAGONISM

Multiple in vitro examples of antimicrobial synergism and antagonism have resulted in only a few well-substantiated clinical examples.

Clinical Evidence for Synergism

The best clinical evidence for antibiotic synergism comes from the treatment of bacterial endocarditis, a disease that can be cured only if the infecting organisms are eradicated by bactericidal drugs. Endocarditis caused by enterococci *(S faecalis)* can usually not be cured by penicillin alone, since penicillin is inhibitory but not bactericidal for enterococci. The addition of an aminoglycoside is strikingly bactericidal for many strains of enterococci, and the cure of many such patients with a combination of penicillin or ampicillin with an aminoglycoside is an accepted example of clinical synergism. Beta-lactam antibiotics combined with aminoglycosides also appear to be synergistic in the treatment of endocarditis due to other streptococci and staphylococci, although the evidence is weaker. Likewise, there is some evidence that drug combinations (usually a beta-lactam plus an aminoglycoside) selected for synergy on the basis of in vitro studies have synergistic activity in the treatment of aerobic gram-negative rod infections, especially in the immunocompromised host.

There is good clinical evidence from controlled trials that in cryptococcal meningitis, amphotericin B plus flucytosine is superior to either drug alone. This combination was selected because of in vitro evidence of synergism.

Clinical Evidence of Antimicrobial Drug Antagonism

Antagonism is sharply limited by time-dose relationships both in vitro and in vivo. It is readily demonstrated with single-dose treatment of animal infections but only with difficulty in multiple-dose treatment. In clinical practice, it is usual to give a large excess of antimicrobial drug in multiple doses. Consequently, antagonism cannot be expected to be a frequent outcome of clinical antimicrobial therapy, and there are few documented examples. The combination of

Table 51–7. Some examples of clinically used antimicrobial combinations and their justification.

Indication	Drug Combination	Justification
Empiric therapy of various conditions (see Table 51–2)	Various.	Expanded spectrum compared with single agent.
Pseudomonas aeruginosa infections	Beta-lactam plus aminoglycoside.	Increased activity (additive or synergistic). Decreased toxicity. Inhibits development of resistance.
Enterococcal endocarditis	Penicillin or vancomycin plus aminoglycoside.	Synergy: converts bacteriostatic drug to bactericidal.
Tuberculosis	Various—especially isoniazid (INH) plus rifampin.	Inhibits development of resistance. Accelerated bacterial killing (not clearly synergistic), permitting shorter treatment course.
Cryptococcal meningitis	Amphotericin B plus flucytosine.	Probably synergy as well as decreased toxicity.
Severely leukopenic patients	Beta-lactam plus aminoglycoside.	Increased activity (additive or synergistic). Possibly decreased toxicity.

Table 51–8. Nonsurgical antimicrobial prophylaxis of documented benefit or in common use.*

Disease or Infection to Be Prevented	Appropriate Subjects for Prophylaxis	Drugs and Adult Doses	Duration of Prophylaxis	Evidence for Efficacy	Comments
Group A streptococcal infection	1. Previous rheumatic fever or known rheumatic heart disease. 2. Epidemic of streptococcal impetigo.	1. Benzathine penicillin, 1.2 million units IM monthly. 2. Penicillin G, 125 mg twice a day. 3. Sulfadiazine, 1 g daily.	1. For rheumatic fever, prophylaxis should continue well into adult life. 2. For impetigo, until epidemic has abated.	Excellent (about 100%).	Does not prevent endocarditis.
Meningococcosis	Close contacts (household, sex partners, day care center, etc) of index case.	1. Rifampin, 20 mg/kg once a day. 2. Minocycline, 100 mg twice a day. 3. Sulfisoxazole, 1 g twice a day (if organism is susceptible).	Rifampin and sulfonamide: 2 days. Minocycline: 5 days.	Excellent (about 80–90%).	Problems: 1. Rifampin resistance with widespread usage. 2. Vertiginous reactions with minocycline.
Haemophilus influenzae infection	Same as meningococci, but of susceptible age (< 5–7 years old).	Rifampin, 20 mg/kg once a day.	Four days.	Good.	Agreement on clinical use is not uniform. Emergence of resistance has occurred.
Tuberculosis	1. Close contacts of index case (pending tuberculin testing). 2. Tuberculin converters. 3. Positive tuberculin test in high-risk groups (children, etc).	Isoniazid (INH), 300 mg/d.	One year.	Excellent (about 80%).	Definition of high-risk groups is variable. See American Thoracic Society guidelines for details.
Plague	Close contacts.	Tetracycline, 500 mg twice daily.	One week after exposure has ended.	Good.	
Gonorrhea	1. Contacts of index case. 2. All newborns.	1. As for treatment of gonorrhea. 2. Topical eye drops—silver nitrate or antimicrobial.	One dose. One dose.	Excellent. Excellent.	Required by law in USA.
Syphilis	Contacts of index case.	Benzathine penicillin, 2.4 million units IM.	Once.	Excellent (about 100%).	
Toxigenic *Escherichia coli* infection (traveler's diarrhea)	Persons traveling from nonendemic areas to endemic areas.	Many drugs effective. Doxycycline, 100 mg daily, most popular.	Duration of exposure.	Good.	Agreement on clinical use is not uniform. Not effective for antimicrobial-resistant strains.
Rickettsiosis	Exposure in endemic area (eg, scrub typhus).	Tetracycline (or chloramphenicol), 1 g/d.	Duration of exposure.	Good.	Recrudescence may occur when prophylaxis is discontinued.
Malaria	Exposure in endemic area.	Chloroquine phosphate, 500 mg weekly.	Duration of exposure.	Excellent.	1. Not effective for chloroquine-resistant *Plasmodium falciparum*. 2. Recrudescence may occur when prophylaxis is stopped.
Influenza A	Exposure in epidemic or to index case with documented infection.	Amantadine, 100 mg twice a day.	Duration of exposure.	Good (about 80%).	Agreement on clinical use is not uniform. Dose of 100 mg daily may be satisfactory.
Mycoplasmal pneumonia	Exposure to index case.	Tetracycline, 500 mg 4 times a day.	One week.	Poor.	Agreement on clinical use is not uniform.
Pneumocystis carinii infection	High-risk individual (high-dose corticosteroids, etc).	Trimethoprim, 10 mg/kg/d (with fixed ratio of sulfamethoxazole).	Uncertain. Probably duration of risk period.	Excellent.	Agreement on clinical use is not uniform.

*Modified, with permission, from Conte JE Jr, Sweet RW: *Infectious Diseases in Clinical Practice.* University of California, San Francisco, 1982. [Course syllabus.]

Table 51–8 (cont'd). Nonsurgical antimicrobial prophylaxis of documented benefit or in common use.*

Disease or Infection to Be Prevented	Appropriate Subjects for Prophylaxis	Drugs and Adult Doses	Duration of Prophylaxis	Evidence for Efficacy	Comments
African trypanosomiasis	Living in endemic area.	Pentamidine, 3 mg/kg IM every 3–6 months.	Duration of exposure.	Good.	
Endocarditis (endovasculitis)	Individuals with abnormal heart valves (increased susceptibility to endocarditis) or intravascular devices, undergoing a procedure known to cause bacteremia and increased risk of endocarditis (eg, dental extractions).	Penicillin or vancomycin; streptomycin or gentamicin added for gastrointestinal or genitourinary procedures.	Once for each exposure.	None.	See American Heart Association guidelines for details.
Otitis media	Individuals with recurrent otitis media.	Ampicillin or sulfonamides or trimethoprim-sulfamethoxazole.	Approximately 1 year.	Good.	
Bite wounds	Individuals bitten by humans, cats, occasionally other animals (eg, camels, gorillas).	Ampicillin or tetracycline, 0.5 g 4 times daily.	Three to 5 days.	Fair.	Close observation required even with prophylaxis.
Urinary tract infections	Individuals with a history of recurrent UTI.	Trimethoprim-sulfamethoxazole, 1 tablet twice weekly. Nitrofurantoin, 50 mg daily.	1. Continuously for uncertain duration. 2. After coitus (if a clear history of postcoital UTI).	Excellent.	Can substitute prompt, empiric treatment of each recurrence for continuous prophylaxis.
Exacerbations of chronic bronchitis	Individuals with established chronic bronchitis and frequent wintertime exacerbations.	Tetracycline, 0.5 g twice daily.	During the winter.	Good.	Not generally recommended—empiric treatment of each recurrence less toxic, equally efficacious.
Infection in the compromised host	Severely leukopenic patients (circulating granulocytes < 500/μL).	1. Oral, nonabsorbable antimicrobials (various regimens). 2. Trimethoprim-sulfamethoxazole by mouth.	Duration of leukopenia.	Variable.	Not generally recommended. Adjunctive measures required: laminar air flow, sterile hospital environment, sterilization of food, etc.

*Modified with permission, from Conte JE Jr, Sweet RW: *Infectious Diseases in Clinical Practice.* University of California, San Francisco, 1982. [Course syllabus.]

penicillin and chlortetracycline cured fewer patients with pneumococcal meningitis than did the same dose of penicillin alone. Similarly, the addition of chloramphenicol to ampicillin resulted in more treatment failures in bacterial meningitis than did ampicillin alone.

SELECTION OF ANTIMICROBIAL COMBINATIONS IN CLINICAL PRACTICE

Antimicrobial combinations are used commonly in clinical practice, often with good justification (Tables 51–1, 51–2, and 51–7). Although the evidence for synergism is not clear in many cases, there is good evidence for clinical benefit for some combinations. On the other hand, the use of antimicrobial combinations that have not been validated by clinical trials—or at least by in vitro or animal testing—is to be deplored. The cost and toxicity of antimicrobials increase in direct proportion to the number of drugs used. Whenever drug combinations are employed and a clinical microbial isolate is available, it is desirable to establish the rationale for the choice by in vitro studies and to estimate the clinical effect with serum bactericidal titers.

ANTIMICROBIAL CHEMOPROPHYLAXIS

Anti-infective chemoprophylaxis is the administration of drugs to prevent the acquisition and establishment of pathogenic microorganisms. In a broader sense, it also includes the use of drugs soon after the acquisition of pathogenic microorganisms but before the development of symptoms and signs of disease.

Table 51–9. Surgical prophylaxis of documented benefit or in common use.*

Disease or Operation	Usual Antimicrobial Employed	Evidence for Efficacy	Comments
Esophagus and stomach	Penicillin G parenterally, cephalosporin[1]	Good	Needed primarily if bacterial flora (normally scanty) is increased by cancer, obstruction, or other disease.
Colon and rectum			
Elective	Oral, poorly absorbed antimicrobials (eg, erythromycin plus kanamycin) with mechanical bowel preparation.	Good	Example of short-term "sterilization" of normal flora to prevent infection. Addition of systemic antimicrobials probably not helpful.
Perforation	Cefoxitin alone. Clindamycin plus gentamicin (see Table 51–2).	Good	Perhaps should not be considered true prophylaxis, as gross fecal soilage of peritoneum has occurred.
Biliary tract	Ampicillin or cephalosporin[1]	Good	Need only for high-risk patients.
Hysterectomy			
Vaginal	Cephalosporin,[1] ampicillin, tetracycline	Good	Indicated.
Routine abdominal	Cephalosporin[1]	Fair	
Radical	Various	Fair	Probably indicated.
Cesarean section	Cephalosporin[1]	Good	Give after cord has been clamped.
Joint replacement	Cephalosporin[1]	Good	Benefit greater in group *not* using laminar flow operating room.
Open fractures	Cephalosporin[1]	Good	Perhaps should not be considered true prophylaxis as wound is often grossly contaminated.
Cardiac valve replacement	Cephalosporin,[1] oxacillin, or nafcillin	Fair to poor	Has become the standard of practice—controlled study no longer possible.

*Modified, with permission, from Conte JE Jr, Sweet RW: *Infectious Diseases in Clinical Practice.* University of California, San Francisco, 1982. [Course syllabus.]

[1] First-generation cephalosporins such as cephapirin, cephalothin, or cefazolin. Cefazolin is generally preferred. Its long serum half-life and the feasibility of intramuscular administration make this drug generally the least expensive of the group.

Some general principles have emerged from human and animal studies of antimicrobial prophylaxis:

(1) Prophylaxis should be directed against a specific pathogen or condition. Administration of antimicrobials cannot remove all microorganisms colonizing the host and cannot prevent all types of infections.

(2) The shorter the duration of prophylaxis, the broader the range of pathogens that may be prevented. Thus, prevention of "all" infections in severely leukopenic patients by broad-spectrum antimicrobial prophylaxis is successful only over the short term (resistance developing with long-term usage), whereas lifetime prophylaxis against group A streptococcal infections is possible.

(3) Prophylaxis is more effective and may be more widely used against pathogens that are unable to develop resistance to the drug used. The continued efficacy of penicillin prophylaxis against group A streptococcal infection contrasts with its rapidly dwindling efficacy against gonococcal infection.

(4) Prophylactic administration of antimicrobials generally requires doses equal to those used for therapy. In fact, since the host response to colonization or early infection may be different than to disease, drugs effective for therapy may be relatively ineffective for prophylaxis and vice versa. For example, penicillin is highly effective treatment for meningococcal disease but is clinically ineffective for prophylaxis, because it does not prevent colonization of the nasopharynx. Rifampin, highly effective for prophylaxis of meningococcal disease, is not recommended for therapy.

(5) As antimicrobial chemoprophylaxis entails risks (cost, drug toxicity, superinfection, and development of resistant organisms), it should be used only in situations where its efficacy has been documented.

Commonly used prophylactic regimens for nonsurgical infections are shown in Table 51–8. With the exception of the prevention of endocarditis following certain surgical procedures, the efficacy of these measures has been documented by adequate clinical trials. Prevention of endocarditis is now so widely practiced that adequately controlled studies are not possible. Not dealt with in this table are a multiplicity of clinical situations in which antimicrobial chemoprophylaxis was shown to be *ineffective:* heart failure, viral upper respiratory infections, comatose patients, etc.

In surgery, antimicrobials are given in the perioperative period to prevent postsurgical infectious complications. The general principles outlined above also apply to surgical prophylaxis, although there are some additional important principles:

(1) The antimicrobial agent must be active against the majority of organisms causing infections after the operation under consideration.

(2) Prophylaxis should be started immediately (not more than 6 hours) before surgery and should not be continued for more than 12–48 hours after surgery.

Antimicrobial drug activity must be present in the surgical wound at the time of closure.

(3) The antimicrobial should be nontoxic and inexpensive and should not be essential for therapy of serious infections.

(4) Prophylaxis is indicated for surgical procedures in which the wound infection rate (under optimal conditions) is 5% or more except in procedures involving implantation of a foreign body, in which general usage is warranted.

Common indications for surgical prophylaxis are shown in Table 51–9.

• • •

References

Conte JE, Barriere SL: *Manual of Antibiotics and Infectious Diseases,* 4th ed. Lea & Febiger, 1981.

Garrod LP, Lambert HP, O'Grady F: *Antibiotic and Chemotherapy,* 5th ed. Churchill Livingstone, 1981.

Kucers A, Bennett N McK: *The Use of Antibiotics,* 3rd ed. Heinemann, 1979.

Mandell GL, Sande MA: Chemotherapy of microbial disease. Section 12 in: *Goodman and Gilman's The Pharmacological Basis of Therapeutics,* 6th ed. Gilman AG, Goodman LS, Gilman A (editors). Macmillan, 1980.

Mandell GL, Douglas RG Jr, Bennett JE: *Principles and Practice of Infectious Diseases.* Vols 1 and 2. Wiley, 1979.

Rahal JJ: Antibiotic combinations: The clinical relevance of synergy and antagonism. *Medicine* 1978;**57:**179.

Wilson JT et al: Drug excretion in human breast milk: Principles, pharmacokinetics and projected consequences. *Clin Pharmacokinet* 1980;**5:**1.

Vaccines, Immune Globulins, & Other Complex Biologic Products | 52

John Mills, MD

Active immunization against infectious agents, begun in the distant past with variolation for smallpox, is one of the earliest proved methods for prevention of disease. Development of antitoxins at the turn of the century permitted treatment and prevention of disease through passive immunization. Recent developments in science presage improvements in both active and passive immunization. Antigens from many infectious agents are already being produced in bacteria or yeasts using recombinant DNA technology, and within a few years it may be possible to produce large amounts of specific human immunoglobulins using the hybridoma technique. Additionally, other complex biologic products such as interferon, transfer factor, and lymphokines are being used experimentally for treatment and prevention of certain diseases; some of them (eg, interferon) show considerable promise of efficacy with minimal toxicity. Recombinant DNA technology is already permitting simplified, large-scale production of some of these materials.

PASSIVE IMMUNIZATION

Passive immunization means transfer of immunity to a host using preformed immunologic effectors. From a practical standpoint, only immunoglobulins have been utilized for passive immunization, since passive administration of immune effector cells is technically difficult and has been associated with graft-versus-host reactions. Note, however, that nonimmune effector cells (eg, granulocytes) are being administered to humans with success, and cellular immunity has been transferred or augmented by other means (interferon, transfer factor).

Passive immunization with antibodies may be accomplished with either animal or human immunoglobulins in varying degrees of purity. These may contain relatively high titers of antibodies directed against a specific antigen or, as is true for pooled immune globulin, may simply contain antibodies found in most of the population. Standard immune globulin preparations must be given intramuscularly; however, a preparation of pooled gamma globulin has recently become available that can be given intravenously.

Passive immunization is useful (1) for individuals unable to form antibodies (eg, congenital agammaglobulinemia); (2) for prevention of disease when time does not permit active immunization (eg, postexposure); (3) for treatment of certain diseases (eg, tetanus); and (4) for treatment of conditions for which active immunization is unavailable or impractical (eg, snake bite).

Complications from administration of *human* immunoglobulins are rare. The injections may be moderately painful, and, rarely, sterile abscesses occur. Individuals with certain immunoglobulin deficiency states (IgA deficiency, etc) may occasionally develop hypersensitivity reactions to immune globulin that may limit therapy. Immune globulin contains aggregates of IgG; it will cause severe reactions if given intravenously.

However, if the passively administered antibodies are derived from *animal* sera, hypersensitivity reactions ranging from anaphylaxis to serum sickness are common. To avoid anaphylactic reactions, tests for hypersensitivity to the animal serum must be performed. If the tests give evidence of hypersensitivity, it is best to avoid that specific type of foreign protein (eg, horse serum) and obtain antibodies made in another animal (eg, human, goat, rabbit). If an alternative preparation is not available and administration of the specific antibody is deemed essential, desensitization can be carried out. A summary of tests for hypersensitivity and a desensitization protocol for antibody-containing proteins are presented below.

Antibodies derived from human serum not only avoid the risk of hypersensitivity reactions but also have a much longer half-life in humans (about 23 days for IgG antibodies) than those from animal sources (5–7 days or less). Consequently, much smaller doses of human antibody can be administered to provide therapeutic concentrations for several weeks. These advantages point to the desirability of using human antibodies for passive protection whenever possible. Materials available for passive immunization are summarized in Tables 52–1 and 52–3.

Table 52–1. Materials available for passive immunization.*

Indication	Product	Dosage	Comments
Black widow spider bite	Black widow spider antivenin, equine.	One vial (6000 units) IM or IV.	Use should be limited to children < 15 kg, the only group with significant morbidity or mortality. Available from Merck Sharp & Dohme.
Botulism	ABE polyvalent antitoxin, equine. (Hexavalent ABCDEF, bivalent AB, and monovalent E antitoxins are also available.)	One vial IV and 1 vial IM; repeat after 2–4 hours if symptoms worsen, and after 12–24 hours.	For treatment of botulism. Available from CDC.† Twenty percent incidence of serum reactions. Only type E antitoxin has been shown to affect outcome of illness. Prophylaxis is not routinely recommended but may be given to asymptomatic persons with unequivocal exposure.
Diphtheria	Diphtheria antitoxin, equine.	20,000 (1 vial)–120,000 units IM depending on severity and duration of illness.	For treatment of diphtheria. Active immunization and (perhaps) erythromycin prophylaxis should be given to nonimmune contacts of active cases rather than antitoxin prophylaxis. Contacts should be observed for signs of illness so that antitoxin may be administered if needed. Also available from CDC.†
Gas gangrene	Gas gangrene antitoxin, polyvalent, equine.		Clinically ineffective; no longer manufactured. Not recommended for use.
Hepatitis A ("infectious")	Immune globulin.	0.02 mL/kg IM as soon as possible after exposure up to 6 weeks. A protective effect lasts about 2 months.	Modifies but does not prevent infection. Recommended for household contacts and other contacts of similar intensity. Not office or school contacts unless an epidemic appears to be in progress. Also recommended for travel to endemic areas.
		For chronic exposure, a dose of 0.1 mL/kg is recommended every 6 months.	Personnel of mental institutions, facilities for retarded children, and prisons appear to be at chronic risk of acquiring hepatitis A, as are those who work with nonhuman primates.
Hepatitis B ("serum")	Hepatitis B immune globulin (regular immune globulin may be effective as well).	0.06 mL/kg IM as soon as possible after exposure, preferably within 7 days. A second injection should be given 25–30 days after exposure. (Dose of immune globulin uncertain; 0.1–0.2 mL/kg suggested.)	Administer to nonimmune individuals as postexposure prophylaxis following either parenteral exposure to or direct mucous membrane contact with HBsAg-positive materials. Should not be given to persons already demonstrating anti-HBsAg antibody. Administration of various live virus vaccines should be delayed for at least a couple of months after this concentrated immune globulin has been given. Some experts also advise administration of a single dose of 0.13 mL/kg to newborns of mothers who develop hepatitis B in the third trimester and who are seropositive at time of delivery.
Hepatitis non-A non-B	Immune globulin.	0.02–0.04 mL/kg IM as soon as possible after exposure.	Give to individuals with parenteral exposure to sera from patients with hepatitis, or other close contacts.
Hypogammaglobulinemia	Immune globulin.	0.6 mL/kg IM every 3–4 weeks.	Give double dose at onset of therapy. Immune globulin is of no value in prevention of frequent infections in the absence of demonstrable hypogammaglobulinemia.
Measles	Immune globulin (measles immune globulin no longer available).	0.25 mL/kg IM as soon as possible after exposure. This dose may be ineffective in immunoincompetent patients, who should receive 20–30 mL.	Live measles vaccine will usually prevent natural infection if given within 48 hours following exposure. If immunoglobulin is administered, delay immunization with live virus for 3 months.
Mumps	Mumps immune globulin, human.	1.5 mL IM for child; 4.5 mL for > 12 years old.	Efficacy doubtful; no longer manufactured. Possibly useful in nonimmune boys to prevent orchitis after development of parotitis. Not indicated for postexposure prophylaxis, for which mumps vaccine is effective.
Organ transplant	Antilymphocyte or antithymocyte serum or globulin (ALG).	Variable. See manufacturer's guidelines.	Used as adjunctive immunosuppressive agent in patients undergoing organ transplantation.
Pertussis	Pertussis immune globulin.	1.5 mL IM (child).	Efficacy doubtful, both for treatment as well as prophylaxis. Available from Cutter Laboratories.

*Modified, with permission, from Cohen SN: Immunization. Chapter 39 in: *Basic & Clinical Immunology,* 4th ed. Stites DP et al (editors). Lange, 1982.

†Centers for Disease Control, (404) 329–3670 during the day, (404) 329–2888 nights, weekends, and holidays.

Note: Passive immunotherapy or immunoprophylaxis should always be administered as soon as possible after exposure to the offending agent. Immune antisera and globulin are always given intramuscularly unless otherwise noted. Always question carefully and test for hypersensitivity before administering animal sera (see text).

Table 52–1 (cont'd). Materials available for passive immunization.*

Indication	Product	Dosage	Comments
Poliomyelitis	Immune globulin.	0.15 mL/kg IM.	Indicated only for exposed, unimmunized subject. Immunize with live or inactivated vaccine after 2–3 months, with subsequent boosters.
Rabies	Rabies immune globulin. (Equine antirabies serum is available but is much less desirable and requires a higher dose.)	20 IU/kg, up to half of which is infiltrated locally at the wound site, and the remainder given IM.	Give as soon as possible after exposure. Recommended for all bite or scratch exposure to carnivores, especially bat, skunk, fox, coyote, or raccoon, despite animal's apparent health, if the brain cannot be immediately examined and found rabies-free. Not recommended for individuals with demonstrated antibody response from preexposure prophylaxis. Must be combined with rabies immunization. Also available through CDC.†
Rubella	Immune globulin.	20–40 mL IM at time of exposure.	Prevents disease in recipient but *not* in fetus of exposed mother—hence not recommended.
Rh isoimmunization (erythroblastosis fetalis)	Rh_0 (D) immune globulin.	One dose IM within 72 hours of abortion, amniocentesis, obstetric delivery of an Rh-positive infant, or transfusion of Rh-positive blood in an Rh_0 (D)-negative woman.	For nonimmune females only. May be effective at much greater postexposure interval; therefore, give even if more than 72 hours have elapsed. One vial contains 300 μg antibody and can reliably inhibit the immune response to a fetomaternal bleed of 7.5–8 mL as estimated by the Betke-Kleihauer smear technique.
Snakebite	Coral snake antivenin, equine. Crotalid (pit viper) antivenin, polyvalent, equine.	At least 3–5 vials IV (preferred) or IM.	Dose should be sufficient to reverse symptoms of envenomation. Consider antitetanus measures as well. Available from Wyeth Laboratories ([215] 688–4400) or CDC.†
Tetanus	Tetanus immune globulin. (Bovine and equine antitoxins are available but are not recommended. They are used at 10 times the dose of tetanus immune globulin.)	Prophylaxis: 250–500 units IM. Therapy: 3000–6000 units IM.	Give in separate syringe at separate site from simultaneously administered toxoid. Recommended only for major or contaminated wounds in individuals who have had fewer than 2 doses of toxoid at any time in the past (fewer than 3 doses if wound is more than 24 hours old or otherwise highly tetanus-prone).
Vaccinia	Vaccinia immune globulin.	Prophylaxis: 0.3 mL/kg IM. Therapy: 0.6 mL/kg IM. May be repeated as necessary for treatment and at intervals of 1 week for prophylaxis.	May be useful in treatment of vaccinia of the eye, eczema vaccinatum, generalized vaccinia, and vaccinia necrosum and in the prevention of such complications in exposed patients with skin disorders. Available from CDC.†
Varicella	Varicella-zoster immune globulin or zoster immune globulin.	3–5 mL IM within 96 hours of exposure.	Available for nonimmune immunosuppressed or immunoincompetent children under 15 years of age and with household, hospital (same 2- or 4-bed room or adjacent beds in large ward), or playmate (>1 hour play indoors) contact with a known case of varicella-zoster, and for neonates whose mothers have developed varicella within 4 days before or 48 hours after delivery. The products modify natural disease but may not prevent the development of immunity. Convalescent plasma collected 1–5 weeks after onset of varicella or zoster may be available at local blood banks and is also effective in dosage of 7–10 mL/kg IV. If neither globulin product nor convalescent plasma is available, immune globulin, 0.6–1.2 mL/kg IM, may modify the illness. Available from local American Red Cross chapters. For information, contact main office, (617) 731–2130.

*Modified, with permission, from Cohen SN: Immunization. Chapter 39 in: *Basic & Clinical Immunology,* 4th ed. Stites DP et al (editors). Lange, 1982.

†Centers for Disease Control, (404) 329–3670 during the day, (404) 329–2888 nights, weekends, and holidays.

Note: Passive immunotherapy or immunoprophylaxis should always be administered as soon as possible after exposure to the offending agent. Immune antisera and globulin are always given intramuscularly unless otherwise noted. Always question carefully and test for hypersensitivity before administering animal sera (see text).

Table 52–2. Materials commonly used for active immunization. (DTP = diphtheria and tetanus toxoids and pertussis vaccine; DT = diphtheria and tetanus toxoids; Td = tetanus and diphtheria toxoids, adult type; and T = tetanus toxoid.)*†

Disease	Product (Source)	Type of Agent	Route of Administration	Primary Immunization	Duration of Effect	Comments
Cholera	Cholera vaccine.	Killed bacteria	Subcut, IM	Two doses 1 week or more apart.	6 months‡	Fifty percent protective.
Diphtheria	DTP, DT (adsorbed) for child under 6; Td (adsorbed) for all others. Also available as diphtheria toxoid alone.	Toxoid	IM	Three doses 4 weeks or more apart, with an additional dose 1 year later for a child under 6. (Can be given at the same time as polio vaccine if doses at least 8 weeks apart.)	10 years§	Use DT if convulsions follow use of DTP. Give school children and adults third dose 6–12 months after second.
Hepatitis B	Hepatitis B virus and surface antigen, inactivated (human plasma from carriers).	Killed virus and virus coat protein	IM	Three doses at monthly intervals.	Years	Greater than 90% protective. Give preexposure to individuals who are not immune (ie, lack HBs antibody) and who are at high risk of acquiring disease (medical personnel, spouses of carriers, etc). May be difficult to obtain (released first in 1982).
Influenza	Influenza virus vaccine, monovalent or bivalent (chick embryo). Composition of the vaccine is varied depending upon epidemiologic circumstances.	Killed whole or split virus; types A and B	IM	One dose. (Two doses 4 weeks or more apart are preferable when a major new antigenic component is first incorporated into the vaccine. Two doses of the split virus products should be used in persons under 26 years because of a lower incidence of side-effects.) Give annually.	1–3 years	Give immunization by November. Recommended annually for patients with cardiorespiratory disease, diabetes, other chronic diseases, and the elderly. Patients receiving chemotherapy for malignant disease are likely to respond better if immunized between or before courses of treatment.
Measles	Measles virus vaccine, live attenuated (chick embryo).	Live virus	Subcut	One dose at age 15 months.	Permanent	Reimmunize if given before 15 months of age; may prevent natural disease if given less than 48 hours after exposure.
Meningococcal meningitis	Meningococcal polysaccharide vaccine, group A or group C. (Preparations are available containing the Y and W serotypes in addition.)	Polysaccharide	Subcut	One dose. Since primary antibody response requires at least 5 days, antibiotic prophylaxis with rifampin (600 mg or 10 mg/kg every 12 hours for 4 doses) should be given to household contacts.	?Permanent	Recommended in epidemic situations, for use by the military to prevent outbreaks in recruits, and possibly as an adjunct to antibiotic prophylaxis in preventing secondary cases in family contacts. Not reliably effective in infants. A combination A and C vaccine is also available.
Mumps	Mumps virus vaccine, live, Jeryl Lynn strain (chick embryo).	Live virus	Subcut	One dose.	Permanent	Reimmunize if given before 1 year of age.
Pertussis	DTP; also pertussis vaccine alone.	Killed bacteria	IM	As for DTP.	See§	Not generally recommended after age 6.
Pneumococcal pneumonia	Pneumococcal polysaccharide vaccine, polyvalent (12–14 of the most common serotypes).	Polysaccharide	Subcut, IM	0.5 mL.	Uncertain; probably at least 5 years	Recommended for individuals at high risk of serious pneumococcal disease: asplenia, sickling hemoglobinopathies, chronic cardiorespiratory ailments, etc.
Poliomyelitis	Poliovirus vaccine, live, oral, trivalent (monkey kidney, human diploid). (Monovalent vaccines also available.)	Live virus types I, II, and III	Oral	Two doses 6–8 weeks or more apart, followed a third dose 8–12 months later. (Can be given at the same time as primary DTP immunization.) A fourth dose before entering school is recommended for children immunized in the first 1–2 years of life.	Permanent	Recommended for adults only if at increased risk by travel to epidemic or highly endemic areas or occupational contact. (Inactivated vaccine may be preferable in this circumstance). Individuals who have completed a primary series may take a single booster dose if the risk of exposure is high.

	Poliomyelitis vaccine.	Killed virus types I, II, and III	IM	Three doses 1–2 months apart, followed by a fourth dose 6–12 months later and a fifth dose before entering school.§	2–5 years, perhaps longer	Killed virus vaccines are licensed but not readily available and are no longer recommended except for immunologically deficient patients or possibly for unimmunized adults who are at risk of exposure to poliomyelitis by reason of travel or immunization of their children.
Rabies	Rabies vaccine (duck embryo).	Killed virus	Subcut	**Preexposure:** Two doses 1 month apart followed by a third dose 6–7 months later, **or** Three doses 1 week apart, followed by a fourth dose 3 months later.	2 years§	Preexposure immunization only for occupational or avocational risk or residence in hyperendemic area. Antibody response should be measured 3–4 weeks after last injection to ensure successful immunization, and repeat injection should be given if no response.
	Effective rabies vaccines derived from other animal sources (eg, rabbit brain, mouse brain) are available in some foreign countries. See manufacturer's guidelines for use.			**Postexposure:** Always give rabies immune globulin as well. (See Table 52–1.) If not previously immunized, give a total of 23 doses. Give 2 injections per day for the first 7 days, then 7 daily doses, and boosters on days 24 and 34 following start of treatment. Alternatively, give 21 daily doses and boosters on days 24 and 34. If previously immunized and an antibody response demonstrated, do not give serum therapy. For nonbite exposure, give one booster dose. For the bite of a rabid animal, give 5 daily boosters followed by one dose on day 25. If an antibody response was not previously demonstrated, treat as unimmunized.		Wounds should be copiously swabbed and flushed with soap and water. (See Table 52–1 regarding use of hyperimmune serum or immune globulin.) For animal bite, consider antitetanus measures as well.
	Rabies vaccine (human diploid cell-derived).	Killed virus	IM	**Preexposure:** Two doses 1 week apart, followed by third dose 2–3 weeks later. **Postexposure:** Five doses on days 0, 1, 3, 7, and 21.	Unknown; probably > 2 years	Indications the same as for duck embryo vaccine. Diploid vaccine preferable: higher efficacy, lower toxicity.
Rubella	Rubella virus vaccine, live (human diploid).	Live virus	Subcut	One dose.	Permanent	Give after 15 months of age. Do not give during pregnancy. Women must prevent pregnancy for 3 months after immunization. Prevents disease but not infection.
Smallpox	Smallpox vaccine (calf lymph, chick embryo).	Live vaccinia virus	Intradermal	One dose.	3 years‡	Not recommended and no longer required for international travel, as smallpox has been eradicated. ***Vaccine has no indications for use at this time.***

*Adapted, with permission, from Cohen SN: Immunization. Chapter 39 in: *Basic & Clinical Immunology,* 4th ed. Stites DP et al (editors). Lange, 1982.

†Dosages for the specific product, including variations for age, are best obtained from the manufacturer's package insert. Immunizations should be given by the route suggested for the product.

‡Revaccination interval required by international regulations.

§A single dose is a sufficient booster at any time after the effective duration of primary immunization has passed.

**For contaminated or severe wounds, give booster if more than 5 years has elapsed since full immunization or last booster.

††Test for PPD conversion 2 months later and reimmunize if there is no conversion.

Table 52–2 (cont'd). Materials commonly used for active immunization. (DTP = diphtheria and tetanus toxoids and pertussis vaccine; DT = diphtheria and tetanus toxoids; Td = tetanus and diphtheria toxoids, adult type; and T = tetanus toxoid.)*†

Disease	Product (Source)	Type of Agent	Route of Administration	Primary Immunization	Duration of Effect	Comments
Tetanus	DTP, DT (adsorbed) for children under age 6; Td or T (adsorbed) for all others.	Toxoid	IM	Three doses 4 weeks or more apart.	10 years§**	Give school children and adults a fourth dose 6–12 months after initial series of injections.
Tuberculosis	BCG vaccine (bacille Calmette-Guérin).	Live attenuated *Mycobacterium bovis*	Intradermal or subcut (per manufacturer's recommendation)	One dose.	?Permanent	Not recommended for use in USA. Has shown highly variable efficacy.
Typhoid	Typhoid vaccine.	Killed bacteria	Subcut or intradermal	Two doses 4 weeks or more apart or 3 doses 1 week apart (less desirable).	3 years§	Seventy percent protective. Recommended only for exposure from travel, epidemic, or household carrier and not, eg, because of floods.
Yellow fever	Yellow fever vaccine (chick embryo) (17-D strain).	Live virus	Subcut	One dose.	10 years‡	Recommended for residence in or travel to endemic areas of Africa and South America.

*Adapted, with permission, from Cohen SN: Immunization. Chapter 39 in: *Basic & Clinical Immunology,* 4th ed. Stites DP et al (editors). Lange, 1982.

†Dosages for the specific product, including variations for age, are best obtained from the manufacturer's package insert. Immunizations should be given by the route suggested for the product.

‡Revaccination interval required by international regulations.

§A single dose is a sufficient booster at any time after the effective duration of primary immunization has passed.

**For contaminated or severe wounds, give booster if more than 5 years has elapsed since full immunization or last booster.

††Test for PPD conversion 2 months later and reimmunize if there is no conversion.

HUMAN GAMMA GLOBULIN
(Immune Globulin USP)

Immune globulin USP is a commercial preparation of gamma globulin derived from large pools of human plasma (> 1000 donors) by low-temperature ethanol fractionation. This procedure was developed by Cohn during World War II—hence the alternative name for this product, Cohn fraction II. The fractionation procedure removes most other serum proteins and infectious hepatitis viruses, thus providing a safe product for intramuscular injection. The preparation contains about 165 mg of gamma globulin per milliliter of solution (representing a 25-fold concentration of antibody-containing immunoglobulins of plasma). About 95% of the gamma globulin is IgG, with only trace amounts of IgM and IgA. Glycine is present as a stabilizing agent and thimerosal as a preservative. Immune globulin costs $1–3/mL from commercial sources.

In addition to its use in the prevention of hepatitis, measles, poliomyelitis, chickenpox, and possibly rubella, as shown in Table 52–1, immune globulin is also given in a dose of 0.7 mL/kg every 2–4 weeks to individuals with antibody immunodeficiencies. Although immune globulin has been used to prevent some other conditions (allergies, viral upper respiratory infections, and others), it is not effective for these conditions and should not be so used.

Recently, immune globulin has been altered so that it is suitable for intravenous administration. Immune globulin intravenous (Gamimune) contains 5% immune globulin in 10% maltose. This product may be useful for patients who need high levels of antibodies immediately and for those who cannot be given intramuscular injections (eg, patients with bleeding diatheses). Its toxicity appears equivalent to immune globulin intramuscular, but without the local side-effects.

ACTIVE IMMUNIZATION

Active immunization means the administration of antigens to the host to induce formation of antibodies and cell-mediated immunity. Immunization is practiced to induce protection against many infectious agents and may utilize either inactivated (killed) material or live attenuated agents (Tables 52–2 and 52–3). Desirable features of the ideal immunogen include complete prevention of disease, prevention of the carrier state, production of prolonged immunity with a minimum of immunizations, absence of toxicity, and suitability for mass immunization (ie, cheap and easy to administer). Active immunization is generally preferable to passive immunization, because host resistance is better (higher levels of antibody present at the time of exposure; coexisting cellular immunity in some cases) and the procedure need not be repeated as frequently. However, active immunization is associated with complications that do not occur with passive immunization, largely related to administering foreign proteins (eg, allergy, nonspecific toxic reactions). The advantages and disadvantages of active immunization with live attenuated and inactivated immunogens are compared in Table 52–4.

Current recommendations for routine active immunization of children are given in Table 52–5.

Legal Liability for Untoward Reactions

It is the physician's responsibility to inform the patient of the risk of immunization and to employ vaccines and antisera in an appropriate manner. Some of the risks described above are, however, currently unavoidable; on balance, the patient and society are better off for accepting the risks for routinely administered immunogens (eg, poliomyelitis and tetanus vaccines).

Manufacturers should be held legally accountable for failure to adhere to known production safeguards. However, in the present litigious atmosphere in the US, the filing of large liability claims by the statistically inevitable victims of good public health practice has caused manufacturers to abandon efforts to develop and produce low-profit but medically valuable therapeutic agents such as vaccines. Since the use and sale of these products are subject to careful review and approval by government bodies such as the Surgeon General's Advisory Committee on Immunization Practices and the Food and Drug Administration, "strict product liability" (liability without fault) may be an inappropriate legal standard to apply when rare immunologic reactions are involved.

RECOMMENDED IMMUNIZATION OF ADULTS FOR TRAVEL

Every adult, whether traveling or not, must be immunized with tetanus toxoid and should also be fully immunized against poliomyelitis and diphtheria. In addition, every traveler must fulfill the immunization requirements of the health authorities of the countries visited. These are listed in *Health Information for International Travel 1976,* HEW Publication No. (CDC) 76-8280, available from the Director, Quarantine Division, Centers for Disease Control, Atlanta 30333. The immunizations received should be recorded on the International Certificate of Immunization. ***Note:*** Smallpox immunization is not recommended or required for travel anywhere.

Table 52–3. Vaccines and other biological products of restricted availability or usage.

Material	Product	Use	Tested and Widely Used in Humans	Undergoing Extensive Human Trials	Highly Experimental
Adenovirus vaccine	Live enteric-coated vaccine against types 4, 7, and 21.	Prevents pneumonitis. Used primarily in military.	X		
Anthrax vaccine*	Protein antigen from culture filtrates, absorbed.	Occupational exposure.	X		
Arbovirus antibodies (human)*	Immune (convalescent) plasma for Ebola, Lassa, Marburg, Junin, and Machup viruses; EEE, WEE, VEE, SLE, and California encephalitis viruses; and Russian spring-summer encephalitis virus.	Treatment of suspected or documented cases; prophylaxis of exposure to active case.			X
Arbovirus vaccines*	Inactivated vaccines–equine encephalitides.	Occupational exposure (virologists).	X		
Botulism vaccine*	Pentavalent (ABCDE) botulinum toxoid.	Occupational exposure (laboratory personnel).	X		
Cholera vaccine	Experimental antitoxins.	Prevents cholera.		X	
Cytomegalovirus vaccine	Live attenuated virus.	Immunocompromised, susceptible hosts.		X	
Eastern equine encephalitis (EEE) vaccine*	Inactivated virus.	Occupational exposure. Epidemics.	X		
Escherichia coli enterotoxin	Purified *E coli* enterotoxin.	Prevents reaction to toxin.			X
Gonococcal vaccine	Purified gonococcal pili.	Prevents gonorrhea.			X
Haemophilus influenzae B vaccine	Purified polysaccharide.	Works in adults but not immunogenic in target population–young children.		X	
Herpes B (monkey B encephalitis) virus antibody (human)*	Immune (convalescent) plasma from patients.	Treatment of herpes B infection; prophylaxis of documented exposure to virus.			X
Influenza vaccine	Subunit vaccines. Live virus vaccines.	Prevents influenza.			X
Leprosy vaccine	Killed bacteria.	Efficacy uncertain.			X
Endotoxin antibody (human)	Human hyperimmune serum against endotoxin.	Highly effective in improving outcome of serious gram-negative infection. Appears to be IgM antibody.		X	
Malaria vaccine	Killed merozoites.	Prevents malaria.			X
Meningococcus group B vaccine	Various experimental vaccines.	Prevents meningitis.		X	
Mycoplasma pneumoniae vaccine	Killed vaccines. Live attenuated vaccine.	Prevents infection.			X
Plague vaccine	Inactivated (USA). Live attenuated (not available in the USA).	Occupational exposure; travel to epidemic areas.	X		
Pseudomonas aeruginosa vaccine	Polyvalent vaccines.	For high-risk populations, eg, burn patients.		X	
Q fever vaccine	Inactivated *Rickettsia*.	Epidemics; occupational exposure.	X		
Respiratory syncytial virus vaccine	Live attenuated virus.	Prevents bronchiolitis and pneumonia in infants.			X
Rocky Mountain spotted fever vaccine	Inactivated *Rickettsia*.	Occupational exposure.	X		
Shigella	Live attenuated vaccines.	High-risk groups.			X
Group A streptococcus vaccine	Purified M proteins.	High-risk groups.		X	
Group B streptococcus vaccine	Polysaccharide capsule.	Infants do not respond; may need to give to mother before delivery.		X	

*Available through CDC. Telephone (404) 329–3356 during the day, (404) 329–2888 nights, weekends, and holidays.

Table 52–3 (cont'd). Vaccines and other biological products of restricted availability or usage.

Material	Product	Use	Tested and Widely Used in Humans	Undergoing Extensive Human Trials	Highly Experimental
Typhus vaccine	Inactivated *Rickettsia.*	High-risk groups and travel to epidemic areas.	X		
Tularemia vaccine*	Live attenuated. (Inactivated vaccines available in some countries.)	Occupational exposure.	X		
Typhoid vaccine	Live attenuated virus.	Prevents infection.		X	
Varicella vaccine	Live attenuated virus.	For immunocompromised patients without antibody.		X	
Venezuelan equine encephalitis (VEE) vaccine*	Live attenuated virus.	Occupational exposure.	X		
Interferon	Leukocyte- and fibroblast-derived; also produced by recombinant DNA technology.	Antiviral—effective for zoster, hepatitis B, perhaps other viruses.		X	
		Cancer chemotherapy—enhanced cytotoxic responses; inhibition of tumor growth.		X	
Transfer factor	Derived from leukocytes of immune donors.	Restores delayed hypersensitivity.		X	
Thymic hormones (eg, thymosin)	Derived from thymic tissue.	Enhanced maturation of T lymphocytes.			X

*Available through CDC. Telephone (404) 329–3356 during the day, (404) 329–2888 nights, weekends, and holidays.

HYPERSENSITIVITY TO ANIMAL PROTEINS & DESENSITIZATION

Many persons are hypersensitive to animal proteins or drugs. If they are given such material by injection, there is a chance that anaphylaxis may develop. Therefore, tests for hypersensitivity are indicated prior to any such injection. Serum sickness can develop in anyone, independently of prior sensitization. The following steps are desirable as a safeguard against anaphylactic reactions and must be observed with biologic products administered for prophylaxis or therapy, particularly with animal sera.

Evaluation & Testing

A. Past History: Has the patient received a similar material before? Does the patient have known allergy, eg, to egg protein, which would increase the likelihood of allergy to other animal proteins?

B. Materials Available for Desensitization: Have ready the following: epinephrine, 1:1000 solution, in sterile syringe; airway; soluble corticosteroids; tourniquet; antihistamine drug (eg, diphenhydramine) for injection; oxygen; and suction. A cardiopulmonary resuscitation cart will have all of the necessary materials. An intravenous catheter should be inserted before beginning desensitization.

C. Intradermal Test: About 0.02 mL of dilute

Table 52–4. Advantages and disadvantages of live versus dead immunogens.

Type of Immunization	Advantages	Disadvantages
Inactivated (killed) product	1. No risk of disease from infection. 2. May be highly purified (eg, toxoids). 3. Often easy to ship and store (ie, stable).	1. Immunity may be short-lived—reimmunization often required. 2. May not stimulate protective factors (eg, inactivated measles vaccine). 3. May not eliminate reinfections (without disease) or carrier state. 4. Inherent toxicity of immunogen (eg, pertussis, influenza). 5. Parenteral administration usually required.
Live attenuated product	1. Long-lasting immunity. 2. Simulate resistance induced by natural infection. 3. May not need to be given parenterally.	1. Risk of disease due to reversion to virulence (eg, polio) or failure of host restriction (eg, immunosuppressed host). 2. Mild disease often required to induce immunity. 3. Risk of carrying contaminants higher than with inactivated vaccines. 4. Attenuated agent may cause new kind of disease. 5. Generally more labile and difficult to store.

Table 52–5. Recommended schedule for active immunization and skin testing of children.

Age	Product Administered	Test Recommended
2 months	DTP[1] Oral poliovaccine[2], trivalent	
4 months	DTP Oral poliovaccine, trivalent	
6 months	DTP Oral poliovaccine, trivalent	
15–19 months	DTP Measles vaccine[3] Oral poliovaccine, trivalent Mumps vaccine[4]	
4–6 years	DTP Oral poliovaccine, trivalent	Tuberculin test[5]
12–14 years	Rubella vaccine[6] Td[7]	Tuberculin test[5]

[1] **DTP:** Toxoids of diphtheria and tetanus, alum-precipitated or aluminum hydroxide adsorbed, combined with pertussis bacterial antigen. Suitable for young children. Three doses of 0.5 mL intramuscularly at intervals of 4–8 weeks. Fourth injection of 0.5 mL intramuscularly given about 1 year later.

[2] **Oral live poliomyelitis virus vaccine:** Trivalent (types 1, 2, and 3 combined) given 3 times at intervals of 6–8 weeks and then as a booster 1 year later. Monovalent vaccine is rarely used now; it can be given at 6-week intervals, followed by a booster of trivalent vaccine 1 year later. Inactive (Salk type) trivalent vaccine is available but not recommended. ***Note:*** One sequence of monovalent vaccines (type 2, then 1, then 3) is in accord with the recommendations of the US Public Health Service Advisory Committee on Immunization Practices. The American Academy of Pediatrics recommends the sequence 1, 3, 2.

[3] **Live measles virus vaccine,** 0.5 mL intramuscularly. When using attenuated (Edmonston) strain, give human gamma globulin, 0.01 mL/lb, injected into the opposite arm at the same time, to lessen the reaction to the vaccine. This is not advised with "further attenuated" (Schwarz) strain vaccine. Inactivated measles vaccine should not be used.

[4] **Live mumps virus vaccine (attenuated),** 0.5 mL intramuscularly.

[5] The frequency with which **tuberculin tests** are administered depends on the risk of exposure, ie, the prevalence of tuberculosis in the population group. The intervals indicated are the recommended minimum.

[6] **Rubella live virus vaccine (attenuated)** can be given between age 1 year and puberty. Some physicians recommend rubella vaccine only for prepubertal girls. The entire contents of a single dose vaccine vial, reconstituted from the lyophilized state, are injected subcutaneously. The vaccine must *not* be given to women who are pregnant or are liable to become pregnant within 3 months of vaccination. Women must be warned that there is a possibility of developing arthralgias or arthritis after vaccination. The cell culture-grown RA 27/3 rubella virus vaccine was licensed in USA in 1979. No live vaccine should be given to immunodeficient patients.

[7] **Tetanus toxoid and diphtheria toxoid,** purified, suitable for adults, given every 7–10 years.

(at least 1:100) test material is injected intradermally, and the site is observed for 15 minutes. The appearance of erythema and edema with wheal formation suggests specific hypersensitivity. Normal saline solution should be injected into a comparable (eg, contralateral) skin site as a control.

D. Conjunctival Test: This is a less sensitive alternative to the intradermal test. Instillation of 1 drop of 1:10 dilution of test material into a normal conjunctiva results in itching, lacrimation, and redness within 5 minutes if the person is hypersensitive. One drop of physiologic saline solution instilled into the other eye serves as a control.

A negative conjunctival or intradermal test is a reliable (but not conclusive) indication that the patient is not allergic to the test material. When the skin test or conjunctival test indicates hypersensitivity, it is preferable to avoid injection of the material in question and substitute another product. Thus, in place of diphtheria horse serum antitoxin, diphtheria antitoxin raised in goats might be administered. If an alternative product is not available and the material is essential to the patient's welfare, desensitization may be attempted as described in the following paragraphs.

Desensitization Procedure

Collect materials listed above and insert an intravenous catheter (keep open with normal saline). Inject gradually increasing doses of the product subcutaneously in an extremity every 30–60 minutes, observing for possible significant reactions. Begin with 0.1 mL of product diluted 1:100 or more. If there is no reaction, give 0.1 mL undiluted. If a significant local reaction occurs, inject the same dose, or a smaller dose together with 0.5 mL of aqueous epinephrine, 1:1000. Increase the doses of the product gradually but steadily until 2 or 3 mL of undiluted product has been administered without significant reaction. Repeat this dose every 30–60 minutes until the full prophylactic or therapeutic dose has been given.

Desensitization often permits the administration of an animal protein to which the person exhibits moderate hypersensitivity. However, if major reactions occur during the procedure, desensitization attempts generally should be abandoned.

SKIN TEST REAGENTS

Skin tests are widely employed to determine the presence of allergy (immediate hypersensitivity), to diagnose infection, or to determine if cell-mediated immunity is intact. Skin tests commonly used for determining cell-mediated immunity or the presence of past or present infection with certain pathogens are presented in Table 52–6. Skin test materials for determining the presence of allergy (immediate hypersensitivity) are less standardized and are not discussed here.

OTHER BIOLOGIC PRODUCTS

A number of biologic products are being used on a limited basis for treatment or prevention of infectious diseases (Table 52–3). These include **interferon** (an antiviral of proved efficacy but not yet commercially available; may also be useful as a cancer chemotherapeutic agent), **transfer factor** (transfers cell-mediated immunity without a graft-versus-host reaction; is undergoing clinical trials), and **antiendotoxic antiserum.** As our understanding of lymphokines increases and the ability to produce human proteins by tissue culture and recombinant DNA technology improves, immunotherapy with other human products will doubtless become more common.

Table 52–6. Some commonly used materials for assessing cell-mediated immunity.

Material	Description and Major Manufacturer	Usual Intradermal Dose	(+) Response at 24–72 Hours	Interpretation and Comments
PPD-S	Purified protein derivative of *Mycobacterium tuberculosis,* stabilized with Tween-80. Potency tested by comparison with US standard tuberculin (many manufacturers).	0.1 mL, intermediate, strength (5 TU)	≥ 10 mm induration (≥ 5 mm in some circumstances)	Positive reaction indicates previous infection with *M tuberculosis* or other mycobacteria. Does not indicate whether disease is present. Response to lower or higher doses (1 and 250 TU) difficult to interpret.
Candida	Partially purified and inactivated suspension of *Candida albicans.* (Iatric Corp.)	0.1 mL of 1:500 dilution	≥ 5 mm induration	Indicates presence of intact cellular immunity. Not useful for diagnosing *Candida* infection.
Diphtheria toxin (Shick test)	Diphtheria toxin. (Massachusetts Public Health Labs.)	. . .	Erythema and edema	*Positive* reaction indicates *lack* of circulating diphtheria antitoxin. A positive reaction after full immunization with diphtheria toxoid suggests an antibody immunodeficiency.
SK-SD	Mixture of streptokinase (SK) and streptodornase (SD).	0.1 mL (4 units SK and 1 unit SD)	≥ 5 mm induration	Indicates presence of intact cellular immunity. Not useful for diagnosis of streptococcal infection. Not specifically FDA-approved as a skin testing antigen.
Trichophyton	Culture filtrate of trichophyton. (Iatric Corp.)	0.1 mL of 1:500	≥ 5 mm induration	Indicates presence of intact cellular immunity; not useful for diagnosis of infection.
Mumps	Suspension of mumps virus. (Eli Lilly.)	0.1 mL (20 CF units)	≥ 1.5 cm of erythema, with induration	Not a reliable indicator of past mumps infection (many false-negatives). Indicates presence of intact cellular immunity.
Coccidioidin and spherulin	Purified culture filtrate of *Coccidioides immitis* mycelia or spherules, respectively. (Berkeley Biological and Iatric Corp.)	0.1 mL of 1:10 or 1:100 dilution (use 1:100 first; use 1:10 if 1:100 negative)	≥ 5 mm induration	Indicates past infection with *C immitis.* Not useful for determining if infection is active or whether disease is present. Does not alter antibody titers. Spherulin may be more sensitive; most authorities recommend using both antigens.
Histoplasmin	Culture filtrate of *Histoplasma capsulatum.* Standardized by comparison with histoplasmin reference standard. (Parke-Davis.)	0.1 mL of solution	≥ 5 mm induration	Indicates past infection with *H capsulatum;* does not indicate if disease is present. Raises antibody titers that may confuse diagnosis; improved skin test reagents under development.

• • •

References

*Centers for Disease Control: *Collected Recommendations of the Advisory Committee on Immunization Practices* (''ACIP Recommendations''). [Updated at regular intervals.]

*Centers for Disease Control: *Health Information for International Travelers*. [Updated annually with supplemental information in *Morbidity and Mortality Weekly Report* as needed.]

*Centers for Disease Control: *Immunobiologic Agents and Drugs Available from the Centers for Disease Control: Descriptions, Recommendations and Adverse Reactions*, 3rd ed. 1982.

Cohen SN: Immunization. Chapter 39 in: *Basic & Clinical Immunology*, 4th ed. Stites DP et al (editors). Lange, 1982.

Conte JE, Barriere S: *Manual of Antibiotics and Infectious Diseases*. Lea & Febiger, 1981.

Fulginiti VA: Immunization. Chapter 5 in: *Current Pediatric Diagnosis & Treatment*, 7th ed. Kempe CH, Silver HK, O'Brien D (editors). Lange, 1982.

Fulginiti VA (editor): *Immunization in Clinical Practice*. Lippincott, 1982.

Rimland D, McGowan JE Jr, Shulman JA: Immunization for the internist. *Ann Intern Med* 1976;**85**:622.

Stiehm ER: Standard and special human immune serum globulins as therapeutic agents. *Pediatrics* 1979;**63**:301.

*May be obtained from the CDC, Building 1, Room SB 253, Atlanta 30333.

Disinfectants & Antiseptics | 53

Ernest Jawetz, MD, PhD

The antiseptics and disinfectants differ fundamentally from systemically active chemotherapeutic agents in that they possess little or no selective toxicity. Most of these substances are toxic not only for microbial parasites but for host cells as well. Therefore, they may be used to reduce the microbial population in the inanimate environment, but they can usually be applied only topically, not systemically, to humans.

The terms disinfectants, antiseptics, or germicides have been used interchangeably by some, and the definitions overlap greatly in the literature. The term **disinfectant** often denotes a substance that kills microorganisms in the inanimate environment. The term **antiseptic** often is applied to substances that inhibit bacterial growth both in vitro and in vivo when applied to the surface of living tissue under suitable conditions of contact.

The antibacterial action of antiseptics and disinfectants is largely dependent on concentration, temperature, and time. Very low concentrations may stimulate bacterial growth, higher concentrations may be inhibitory, and still higher concentrations may be bactericidal for certain organisms.

Evaluation of the antiseptics and disinfectants is difficult. Methods of testing are controversial and results are subject to different interpretations. There is a need for effective, nontoxic compounds to neutralize disinfectants in vitro. Ideally, disinfectants should be lethal for microorganisms in high dilution, noninjurious to tissues or inanimate substances, inexpensive, stable, nonstaining, odorless, and rapid-acting even in the presence of foreign proteins, exudates, or fibers. No preparation now available combines these characteristics to a high degree.

Many antiseptics and disinfectants were at one time used in medical and surgical practice. Most have now been displaced by chemotherapeutic substances. The 2 remaining areas of use are urinary antiseptics (see Chapter 50) and topical antiseptics. Most topical antiseptics do not aid wound healing but, on the contrary, often impair healing. In general, cleansing of abrasions and superficial wounds by washing with soap and water is far more effective and less damaging than the application of topical antiseptics. Substances applied topically to skin or mucous membranes are absorbed irregularly and often unpredictably. Occlusive dressings with plastic films often greatly enhance absorption. Penetration of drugs through skin epithelium is also greatly influenced by relative humidity and temperature.

A few chemical classes of disinfectants and antiseptics are briefly characterized in the following paragraphs.

Alcohols

Aliphatic alcohols are antimicrobial in varying degree by precipitating protein. Ethanol (ethyl alcohol) in 70% concentration is bactericidal in 1–2 minutes at 30 °C but less effective at lower and higher concentrations. Ethyl alcohol, 70%, and isopropyl alcohol, 70–90%, are at present the most satisfactory general disinfectants for skin surfaces. They may be useful for sterilizing instruments but have no effect on spores, and better agents are available for this purpose. Aerosols of 70% alcohol with 1-μm size droplets may be the best disinfectants for mechanical respirators.

Propylene glycol and other glycols have been used as vapors to disinfect air. Precise control of humidity is necessary for good antimicrobial action. Glycol vapors are rarely employed at present.

Aldehydes

Formaldehyde in a concentration of 1–10% effectively kills microorganisms and their spores in 1–6 hours. It acts by combining with and precipitating protein. It is too irritating for use on tissues, but it is widely employed as a disinfectant for instruments. Formaldehyde solution USP contains 37% formaldehyde by weight, with methyl alcohol added to prevent polymerization.

Glutaraldehyde as a 2% alkaline solution in 70% isopropanol (pH 7.5–8.5) serves as a liquid disinfectant for some optical and other instruments and for some prosthetic materials. It kills viable microorganisms in 10 minutes and spores in 3–10 hours. Contact with tissue must be avoided.

Methenamine taken orally can release formaldehyde into acid urine. It is employed as a urinary antiseptic (see Chapter 50).

Acids

Several inorganic acids have been used for cauterization of tissue. Although they are effective antimicrobial agents, the tissue destruction they cause precludes their use. Benzoic acid, 0.1%, is employed as a food preservative. Esters of benzoic acid (parabens) are used as antimicrobial preservatives of certain other drugs. Acetic acid, 1%, can be used in surgical dressings as a topical antimicrobial agent; 0.25% acetic acid is a useful antibacterial agent for irrigation of the lower urinary tract. This can also be used with an indwelling catheter and a closed system for urinary drainage. It is particularly active against *Pseudomonas aeruginosa*. Boric acid, 5% in water, or as powder, can be applied to a variety of skin lesions as an antimicrobial agent. However, the toxicity of absorbed boric acid is high, particularly for small children, and its use is not advisable. Salicylic and undecylenic and other fatty acids can serve as fungicides on skin.

Mandelic acid is excreted unchanged in the urine after oral intake; 12 g daily taken orally can lower the pH of urine to 5.0, sufficient to be antibacterial. (See Urinary Antiseptics, Chapter 50.)

Halogens & Halogen-Containing Compounds

A. Iodine: Elemental iodine is an effective germicide. Its mode of action is not definitely known. A 1:20,000 solution of iodine kills bacteria in 1 minute and spores in 15 minutes, and its tissue toxicity is relatively low. Iodine tincture USP contains 2% iodine and 2.4% sodium iodide in alcohol. It is the most effective disinfectant available for intact skin and should be used to disinfect skin when obtaining blood cultures by venipuncture. Its principal disadvantage is the occasional dermatitis that can occur in hypersensitive individuals. This can be avoided by promptly removing the tincture of iodine with alcohol.

Iodine can be complexed with polyvinylpyrrolidone to yield povidone-iodine USP. This is a water-soluble complex that liberates free iodine in solution (eg, 1% free iodine in 10% solution). It is widely employed as a skin disinfectant, particularly for preoperative skin preparation. It is an effective local antibacterial substance, killing not only vegetative forms but also clostridial spores. Hypersensitivity reactions are infrequent. Povidone-iodine (Betadine, Isodine) is available in many forms: solution, ointment, aerosol, surgical scrub, shampoo, skin cleanser, vaginal gel, vaginal douche, and individual cotton swabs. Povidone-iodine solutions can become contaminated with *Pseudomonas* sp.

B. Chlorine: Chlorine exerts its antimicrobial action in the form of undissociated hypochlorous acid (HOCl), which is formed when chlorine is dissolved in water at neutral or acid pH. Chlorine concentrations of 0.25 ppm are effectively bactericidal for many microorganisms except mycobacteria, which are 500 times more resistant. Organic matter greatly reduces the antimicrobial activity of chlorine. The amount of chlorine bound by organic matter in an environment (eg, water) and thus not available for antimicrobial activity is called the "chlorine demand." The chlorine demand of relatively pure water is low, so that the addition of 0.5 ppm chlorine is sufficient for disinfection. The chlorine demand of grossly polluted water may be very high, so that 20 ppm or more of chlorine may have to be added for effective bactericidal action.

Chlorine gas causes severe poisoning in concentrations of 1:100,000 or less. It was one of the earliest agents employed in chemical warfare and acts as an intense lung irritant.

Chlorine is used mainly for the disinfection of inanimate objects and particularly for the purification of water. Chlorinated lime forms hypochlorite solution when dissolved. It is a cheap (but unstable) form of chlorine used mainly for disinfection of excreta in the field. Halazone USP is a chloramine employed in tablet form for the sterilization of drinking water. The addition of 4–8 mg halazone per liter will sterilize water in 15–60 minutes unless a large quantity of organic material is present. It may not inactivate cysts of *Entamoeba histolytica*.

Sodium hypochlorite solution USP, 0.5% NaOCl (diluted sodium hypochlorite [modified Dakin's] solution), contains about 0.1 g of available chlorine per 100 mL and can be used as an irrigating fluid for the cleansing and disinfecting of contaminated wounds. Household bleaches containing chlorine can serve as disinfectants for inanimate objects.

Oxidizing Agents

Some antiseptics exert an antimicrobial action because they are oxidizing agents. Most are of no practical importance, and only hydrogen peroxide, sodium perborate, and potassium permanganate are occasionally used.

Hydrogen peroxide solution USP contains 3% H_2O_2 in water. Contact with tissues releases molecular oxygen and there is a brief period of antimicrobial action. There is no penetration of tissues, and the main applications of hydrogen peroxide are as a mouthwash and for the cleansing of wounds. Hydrogen peroxide can probably be used to disinfect smooth contact lenses that are subsequently applied to the eye. Hydrous benzoyl peroxide USP can be bactericidal to microorganisms. When applied to the skin as a lotion, it is also keratolytic, antiseborrheic, and irritant. It has been used in treating acne and seborrhea, but it bleaches clothing and may produce contact dermatitis.

Potassium permanganate USP consists of purple crystals that dissolve in water to give deep purple solutions that stain tissues and clothing brown. A 1:10,000 dilution of potassium permanganate kills many microorganisms in one hour. Higher concentrations are irritating to tissues. The principal use of potassium permanganate solution is in the treatment of weeping skin lesions.

Heavy Metals

A. Mercury: Mercuric ion precipitates protein and inhibits sulfhydryl enzymes. Microorganisms inactivated by mercury can be reactivated by thiols (sulfhydryl compounds). Mercurial antiseptics inhibit the sulfhydryl enzymes of tissue cells as well as those of bacteria. Therefore, most mercury preparations are highly toxic if ingested. Mercury bichloride NF

(1:100) can be used as a disinfectant for instruments or unabraded skin.

Ammoniated mercury ointment USP contains 5% of the active insoluble compound ($HgNH_2Cl$). It is a skin disinfectant in impetigo.

Some organic mercury compounds are less toxic than the inorganic salts and somewhat more antibacterial. Nitromersol USP, thimerosal USP (merthiolate), and phenylmercuric acetate or nitrate are marketed in many different liquid and solid forms as bacteriostatic antiseptics. They are also used as "preservatives" in various biologic products to reduce the chance of accidental contamination. Merbromin (Mercurochrome) is used as a 2% solution that is a feeble antiseptic but stains tissue a brilliant red color. The psychologic effect of this stain has lent support to the (otherwise almost negligible) antiseptic properties of this material.

B. Silver: Silver ion precipitates protein and also interferes with essential metabolic activities of microbial cells. Inorganic silver salts in solution are strongly bactericidal. Silver nitrate, 1:1000, destroys most microorganisms rapidly upon contact. Silver nitrate ophthalmic solution USP contains 1% of the salt, to be instilled into the eyes of newborns to prevent gonococcal ophthalmia. It is effective for this purpose but may cause chemical conjunctivitis by being quite acid; therefore, antibiotic ointment has been used instead at times. Other inorganic silver salts are rarely used for their antimicrobial properties because they are strongly irritating to tissues. In burns, compresses of 0.5% silver nitrate can reduce infection of the burn wound, aid rapid eschar formation, and reduce mortality. If silver nitrate is reduced to nitrite by bacteria in the burn, methemoglobinemia may result. Silver sulfadiazine 1% cream slowly releases sulfadiazine and also silver (see Chapter 46) and effectively suppresses microbial flora in burns. It may have some advantages and causes less pain than mafenide acetate (Sulfamylon) in the treatment of burns, but it has occasionally produced leukopenia.

Colloidal preparations of silver are less injurious to superficial tissues and have significant bacteriostatic properties. Mild silver protein contains about 20% silver and can be applied as an antiseptic to mucous membranes. Prolonged use of any silver preparation may result in argyria.

Other Metals

Other metal salts (eg, zinc sulfate, copper sulfate) have significant antimicrobial properties but are rarely employed in medicine for this purpose.

Soaps

Soaps are anionic surface-active agents, usually sodium or potassium salts of various fatty acids. They vary in composition depending on the specific fats or oils and on the particular alkali from which they are made. Since NaOH and KOH are strong bases, whereas most fatty acids are weak acids, most soaps when dissolved in water are strongly alkaline (pH 8.0–10.0). Thus, they may irritate skin, which has a pH of 5.5–6.5. Special soaps (eg, Neutrogena) use triethanolamine as a base and, when dissolved, are near pH 7.0. While most common soaps are well tolerated, excessive use will dry normal skin. Admixed synthetic fragrances may cause irritation or photosensitization of skin.

Most common soaps remove dirt as well as surface secretions, desquamated epithelium, and bacteria contained in them. The physical action of thorough handwashing with plain soaps is quite effective in removing transient bacteria and other contaminating microorganisms from skin surfaces. For additional antibacterial action, certain disinfectant chemicals (hexachlorophene, phenols, carbanilides, etc) have been added to certain soaps. These chemicals may be both beneficial and potentially harmful and are discussed below.

Phenols & Related Compounds

Phenol denatures protein. It was the first antiseptic employed, as a spray, during surgical procedures by Lister in 1867. Concentrations of at least 1–2% are required for antimicrobial activity, whereas a 5% concentration is strongly irritating to tissues. Therefore, phenol is used mainly for the disinfection of inanimate objects and excreta. Substituted phenols are more effective (and more expensive) as environmental disinfectants. Among them are many proprietary preparations containing cresol and other alkyl-substituted phenols.

Other phenol derivatives such as resorcinol, thymol, and hexylresorcinol have enjoyed some popularity in the past as antiseptics. Several chlorinated phenols are much more active antimicrobial agents.

Hexachlorophene USP is a white crystalline powder that is insoluble in water but soluble in organic solvents, dilute alkalies, and soaps and is an effective bacteriostatic agent. Hexachlorophene liquid soap USP and many proprietary preparations are used widely in surgical scrub routines and as deodorant soaps. Single applications of such preparations are no more effective than plain soaps, but daily use results in a deposit of hexachlorophene on the skin that exerts a prolonged bacteriostatic action. Thus, the number of resident skin bacteria is lower on the surgeon's hands if hexachlorophene soap is used daily and if other soaps, which promptly remove the residual hexachlorophene film, are not employed.

Soaps or detergents containing 3% hexachlorophene are effective in delaying or preventing colonization of the newborn's skin with pathogenic staphylococci in hospital nurseries. However, repeated bathing of newborns (and particularly premature infants) with such preparations may permit sufficient absorption of hexachlorophene to result in toxic effects to the nervous system, especially a spongiform degeneration of the white matter in the brain. For this reason, the "routine prophylactic use" of 3% hexachlorophene preparations was discouraged. Stopping the use of hexachlorophene-containing preparations for bathing of newborns has been accompanied by a resurgence of staphylococcal infections in nursery populations.

Other antiseptics have been added to soaps and detergents, eg, carbanilides or salicylanilides. Trichlorocarbanilide now takes the place of hexachlorophenes in several "antiseptic soaps." Regular use of such antiseptic soaps may reduce body odor by preventing bacterial decomposition of organic material in apocrine sweat. All antiseptic soaps may induce allergic reactions or photosensitization.

Chlorhexidine is a bisdiguanide antiseptic that disrupts the cytoplasmic membrane, especially of gram-positive organisms. It is employed as a skin cleanser and as a constituent of disinfectant soaps. A 4% solution of chlorhexidine gluconate can be used to cleanse wounds. When incorporated into soaps it is used as an antiseptic handwashing preparation, especially in hospitals, and for surgical scrub and preparation of skin sites for operative procedures. Repeated application of chlorhexidine-containing soap results in persistence of the chemical on the skin to give a cumulative antibacterial effect. Chlorhexidine is somewhat less effective against *Pseudomonas* and *Serratia* strains than against coliform and gram-positive organisms.

Gamma benzene hexachloride (Gamene, Kwell) is employed as a 1% lotion, shampoo, or cream to treat scabies, mites, or lice. Usually it is used just twice: It is applied after the skin or hairy areas have been washed with soap and water, and the treatment is repeated one week later. Up to 10% of the chemical may be absorbed from application to the skin, and it may produce toxic effects (skin rashes, blood dyscrasias, or convulsions), especially if ingested accidentally by infants. To prevent reinfestation with mites and lice it is necessary to treat all contacts and wash all clothes of the afflicted individual. When employed in agriculture as lindane, it has given rise to poisoning after inhalation of spray or liquid.

Cationic Surface-Active Agents

Surface-active compounds are widely used as wetting agents and detergents in industry and in the home. They act by altering the energy relationship at interfaces. Cationic surface-active agents are bactericidal, probably by altering the permeability characteristics of the cell membrane. Cationic agents are antagonized by anionic surface-active agents and thus are incompatible with soaps. Cationic agents are also strongly adsorbed onto porous or fibrous materials, eg, rubber or cotton, and are effectively removed by them from solutions.

A variety of cationic surface-active agents are employed as antiseptics for the disinfection of instruments, mucous membranes, and skin, eg, benzalkonium chloride USP (Zephiran) and cetylpyridinium chloride USP. Aqueous solutions of 1:1000–1:10,000 exhibit good antimicrobial activity but have some disadvantages. These quaternary ammonium disinfectants are antagonized by soaps, and soaps should not be used on surfaces where the antibacterial activity of quaternary ammonium disinfectants is desired. They are adsorbed onto cotton and thereby removed from solution. When applied to skin, they form a film under which microorganisms can survive. Because of these properties, these substances have given rise to outbreaks of serious infections due to *Pseudomonas* and other gram-negative bacteria. They cannot be employed safely as skin disinfectants and can only rarely be used as disinfectants of instruments.

Nitrofurans

Many derivatives of furan have antimicrobial properties, especially if a nitro group is in the 5 position of the furan ring. Such compounds are markedly bactericidal for many bacteria in concentrations of 1:20,000 or less. The mechanism of action is not known. Strains of *Pseudomonas* and *Proteus* are often resistant.

Nitrofurantoin USP (Furadantin) is a urinary antiseptic (see Chapter 50). Nitrofurazone USP (Furacin) is used as a topical antimicrobial agent on superficial wounds or skin lesions and as a surgical dressing. The preparations contain about 0.2% of the active drug and do not interfere with wound healing. However, about 2% of patients may become sensitized and may develop reactions, eg, allergic pneumonitis.

Miscellaneous Antiseptics

Lysostaphin, a peptide enzyme, prepared for topical application, can eliminate staphylococci from the nostrils of carriers, but it is not marketed.

Many synthetic organic dyes have antimicrobial properties. Gentian violet USP is bacteriostatic and inhibits yeast growth, but it is aesthetically unappealing. Acridine dyes have been used as topical antiseptics in 1:2000 concentration. Methylene blue was formerly used as a urinary antiseptic. Pyridium, an azo dye, was used as a urinary antiseptic although it acts primarily as an analgesic in the bladder. Local anesthetics (eg, procaine, lidocaine) have some inhibitory effect on the growth of bacteria and fungi. Thus, they may interfere with culture of an etiologic agent in specimens from tissues or surfaces exposed to these agents.

Sulfur, in various preparations, is employed as a fungicide and parasiticide for topical use. Many fatty acids, especially propionic and undecylenic acids, are important topical antifungal drugs. Undecylenic acid NF, 5%, and zinc undecylenate NF, 20%, are among the least irritating and most fungistatic drugs available for treatment of dermatophytosis.

STERILIZATION PROCEDURES

It is the purpose of sterilization to make materials free from viable microorganisms, spores, or viruses. This is accomplished commonly by the application of heat under controlled conditions.

Incineration, using controlled burning, is used to dispose of infectious materials. Dry heat (160–170 °C for more than 1 hour) is employed to sterilize dry glassware, ceramics, and other materials. Moist heat or autoclaving (121 °C for 15 minutes or more at 15 lb/in^2) is used for many instruments, dressings, linens, and bacteriologic media. All of these procedures must be carefully controlled with respect to time, temperature, size of materials, air circulation, displacement of cold air by steam, permeability of packaging materials, and other features that determine the efficacy of the application of heat.

Many materials that must be sterilized do not tolerate high heat, eg, plastics, optical devices, pump oxygenators, and extracorporeal circulation devices. These materials are "gas sterilized" by exposure to **ethylene oxide**, because irradiation is not readily controllable. Ethylene oxide can destroy the viability of microorganisms, probably by the alkylation of sulfhydryl groups of proteins.

Since ethylene oxide is a highly flammable gas, it is usually employed in combination with either 90% CO_2 or fluorinated hydrocarbons. With such a mixture at a temperature of about 40 °C and a relative humidity of 40%, about 4 hours are required for sterilization. Ethylene oxide rapidly penetrates many types of materials exposed to it in a vacuum, and sterilization is accomplished in 4 hours; it then must be removed because it leaves toxic residues, eg, ethylene glycol and ethylene chlorohydrin. For proper ethylene oxide sterilization, materials must be wrapped in cloth, paper, or polyethylene; exposed to the gas for a proper period under controlled temperature; and then evacuated to remove gas and toxic residues and aerated for a prescribed time (often 12–120 hours) before being used.

In most sterilization procedures, indicators of adequate time and temperature exposure and of sterility ("spore strips") must be employed. Careful records are essential and must be kept for years. Chemical indicators for ethylene oxide exposure must be employed.

• • •

References

Aly R, Maibach HI: Comparative study on the antimicrobial effect of 0.5% chlorhexidine gluconate and 70% isopropyl alcohol on the normal flora of hands. *Appl Environ Microbiol* 1979;**37:**610.

Ballin JC: Evaluation of a new topical agent for burn therapy. *JAMA* 1974;**230:**1184.

Beck WC: Handwashing substitute for degerming. *Am J Surg* 1978;**135:**728.

Block SS: *Disinfection, Sterilization and Preservation,* 2nd ed. Lea & Febiger, 1977.

Cason JS, Lowbury EJL: Mortality and infection in extensively burned patients treated with silver-nitrate compresses. *Lancet* 1968;**1:**651.

Dixon RE et al: Aqueous quaternary ammonium antiseptics and disinfectants: Use and misuse. *JAMA* 1976;**236:**2415.

Drewett SE et al: Skin distribution of *Clostridium welchii:* Use of iodophor as sporicidal agent. *Lancet* 1972;**1:**1172.

Fraser GL, Beaulieu JT: Leukopenia secondary to sulfadiazine silver. *JAMA* 1979;**241:**1928.

Gezon HM et al: Control of staphylococcal infections in the newborn through the use of hexachlorophene bathing. *Pediatrics* 1973;**51:**331.

Kaslow RA et al: Nosocomial pseudobacteremia: Positive blood cultures due to contaminated benzalkonium antiseptic. *JAMA* 1976;**236:**2407.

Kimbrough RD: Review of evidence of toxic effects of hexachlorophene. *Pediatrics* 1973;**51:**391.

Kundsin RB, Walter CW: The surgical scrub: Practical considerations. *Arch Surg* 1973;**107:**75.

Orkin M et al: Treatment of today's scabies and pediculosis. *JAMA* 1976;**236:**1136.

Perkins JJ: *Principles and Methods of Sterilization in Health Sciences,* 2nd ed. Thomas, 1969.

Reddish GF (editor): *Antiseptics, Disinfectants, Fungicides, and Chemical and Physical Sterilization.* Lea & Febiger, 1957.

54 | Antiprotozoal Drugs

John F. Catchpool, MB, BS (Lond), LRCP, MRCS, MD

THE CHEMOTHERAPY & CHEMOSUPPRESSION OF MALARIA

The choice of a drug or combinations of drugs for the chemotherapy or chemosuppression of malaria depends on the following factors:

The Species of the Infecting Parasite

Human malaria can be caused by 4 species of protozoal parasites. Three of the 4, *Plasmodium vivax, Plasmodium malariae,* and *Plasmodium ovale,* are classified as "relapsing malarias" because they have a secondary or persisting stage of their life cycle. This secondary exoerythrocytic stage of development provides a reservoir of parasites for the reinfection of the erythrocytes that can give rise to a recrudescence of symptoms months or even years after a clinical cure has been obtained by the destruction of the asexual forms in the blood.

Plasmodium falciparum, the most lethal form of malaria, has no exoerythrocytic stages. Prompt diagnosis and treatment are essential. An average of 4 deaths a year from malaria are reported in the USA; most are due to *P falciparum.* If the strain is not resistant, it readily responds to treatment and a radical cure can be achieved. Malaria caused by this parasite is sometimes called "malignant tertian malaria" because it produces a fulminating infection in nonimmune victims, with spikes of fever every third day corresponding to the bursting of the erythrocytes and the release of the merozoites. Untreated falciparum malaria in nonimmune individuals may rapidly progress to a fatal conclusion.

The disease caused by *P malariae* is sometimes called "quartan malaria" because the spikes of fever come every fourth day. In West Africa, quartan malaria is associated with a high incidence of nephrotic syndrome. *P malariae* is unique because infection can remain dormant for many years.

A rare form of relapsing malaria is caused by *P ovale* (common in West Africa). Its periodicity is similar to that of *P vivax* (3 days), but it runs a milder course and is more easily treated.

Chemosuppression for the relapsing malarias must be continued for several weeks after the last exposure to infection.

The Prevalence of Drug-Resistant Strains of Plasmodia

During the 1960s, strains of malaria resistant to chloroquine and other antimalarials spread rapidly through Southeast Asia and Latin America. The emergence of chloroquine-resistant strains was caused by a combination of heavy drug pressure, the introduction of large numbers of nonimmune military personnel, and the partial eradication of the disease, which had destabilized the ecology of malaria. However, in Africa, where much of the black population is still exposed to malaria from birth and has acquired a considerable degree of immunity and where the use of antimalarial drugs is not so widespread, chloroquine-resistant strains of malaria are still rare. Chloroquine-resistant strains are now frequently encountered in Southeast Asia, New Guinea, South America, Central America, and all of the Indian subcontinent, but they have not yet become established in Africa or the Middle East. All symptomatic *P falciparum* infections occurring in immigrants from Southeast Asia should be assumed to be chloroquine-resistant and therefore should be treated with oral or parenteral quinine. The best available country-by-country information listing the prevalence of malaria and the risk of chloroquine-resistant *P falciparum* infections is contained in USPHS Publication 79-8280, *Health Information for International Travel 1981,* published by the Centers for Disease Control (CDC), Atlanta 30333.

In emergencies, information may be obtained by telephoning (404) 329–3670 (days) or (404) 329–2888 (nights, weekends, and holidays). CDC keeps stocks of parenteral chloroquine and quinine.

The Stage of Parasitization

Different antimalarials exert their effects at different stages of the parasite's life cycle. Chemoprophylaxis or therapy of acute attacks by chemosuppression of the clinical manifestations of the disease—or the elimination of all parasites at all stages (a radical cure)—may be achieved by drugs attacking at (1) the pre-erythrocytic stages (sometimes called "primary exoerythrocytic" or "tissue" stages), which take place in the liver; (2) the erythrocytic stages, in which the parasites multiply rapidly in erythrocytes; or (3) the exoerythrocytic or secondary tissue stages of the relapsing malarias *(P vivax, P malariae,* and *P ovale),* which also take place in the liver. In addition, some drugs may have a selectively toxic effect on the gametocytes that form in the erythrocytes and are responsible for transferring the infection to the mosquito. Other drugs, when ingested in the blood by the mosquito, may prevent the transmission of malaria to another victim by preventing multiplication (sporogony) in the mosquito gut and salivary glands.

Antimalarial drugs are sometimes classified as follows:

(1) Primary tissue schizonticides: Drugs that destroy the primary (pre-erythrocytic) tissue schizonts in the liver soon after infection (eg, primaquine).

(2) Blood schizonticides: ("Chemosuppressive" or "clinically curative" drugs.) Drugs that suppress the symptoms of malaria by destroying the schizonts and merozoites in the erythrocytes (eg, quinine, quinacrine, chloroquine, and amodiaquine).

(3) Gametocides: Drugs that prevent infection of mosquitoes and therefore the spread of infection by mosquitoes by destroying gametocytes in the blood (eg, primaquine).

(4) Sporonticides: Drugs that help to eradicate the disease by preventing sporogony and multiplication of the parasites in the mosquito when ingested with the blood of the human host (eg, chloroguanide and pyrimethamine).

(5) Secondary tissue schizonticides: ("Radically curative" drugs.) Drugs used to cure the chronic relapsing fevers due to infection by *P vivax, P malariae,* and *P ovale* by destroying the secondary (exoerythrocytic) tissue schizonts developing in the liver (eg, primaquine).

The Frequency of Administration

The antimalarial drugs presently available offer a range in speed and duration of drug action. Rapid-acting drugs are needed for therapy of acute attacks. For suppressive therapy (see Table 54–1), drugs taken once a week or once a month are convenient, but drugs taken daily may have advantages. It is usually easier to form a daily habit than to remember a weekly or biweekly drug dose. The dangers of double dosage or of dose omission are fewer, and a more constant blood level is likely to be obtained.

The Race of the Recipient

Certain otherwise unfavorable genetic polymorphisms have been maintained in populations living in malarial areas by conferring a greater tolerance to *P falciparum* malaria. For example, heterozygosity for the sickle cell gene provides a measure of protection against *P falciparum* infection, and it is likely that glucose-6-phosphate dehydrogenase deficiency, hemoglobin C disease, hemoglobin E disease, and β-thalassemia do so also.

US blacks not previously exposed to malaria are notably less susceptible to *P vivax* malaria than US whites. However, because of glucose-6-phosphate dehydrogenase deficiency, 15% of US blacks are liable to suffer an acute self-limiting hemolysis when treated with primaquine.

Table 54–1. Indications for malaria chemoprophylaxis* and suppression. (Modified from: *MMWR [Morbidity and Mortality Weekly Report]* [March 10] 1978;**27[Suppl]**:81.)

Purpose	Drugs of Choice	Alternative Drugs
To prevent acquisition of malaria in areas without known chloroquine resistant malaria	Chloroquine phosphate Amodiaquine Hydroxychloroquine Chloroquine sulfate	Pyrimethamine Chlorguanide†
To prevent acquisition of malaria in areas with known chloroquine resistant strains *P falciparum*	Pyrimethamine-sulfadoxine	
To prevent relapses of *P vivax* and *P ovale*	Primaquine‡	

*Malaria chemoprophylaxis in pregnant women: Pregnancy is not a contraindication for malaria chemoprophylaxis. The most suitable agent for use during pregnancy is chloroquine or one of the other 4-aminoquinolines, because they have not been associated with teratogenic effects when administered for malaria suppression. Neither pyrimethamine nor pyrimethamine-sulfadoxine should be used in pregnant women because of reports of congenital defects associated with the administration of pyrimethamine to animals. To avoid excessive use of drugs during pregnancy, prophylaxis with primaquine, if indicated, should be withheld until after delivery.

†Not available in the USA.

‡Not recommended for all travelers to malarious areas.

The Degree of Host Immunity

In many parts of the world, the malaria death rate of children under age 4 is as high as 15%. Chronic malarial infection may significantly impair the growth and development of the survivors. However, neonates born to immune mothers are partially immune by virtue of transplacentally acquired antibodies. This protection decreases in the first few months of life, and a partial immunity is acquired by repeated mild attacks of malaria. By age 5, this ability to acquire immunity largely disappears. Chemosuppression of malaria during these first few years may deprive a child of the ability to form active immunity. Nevertheless, epidemiologic studies show that continuous regular chemosuppression in children born in malarious areas will not only reduce the high morbidity and mortality rates due to malaria but will also enhance their physical development.

Epidemiologic Factors

Mass chemosuppression of malaria must also take into account the danger of resistant strain emergence. Intermittent and inadequate chemosuppression of nonimmune and partially immune populations who are constantly being reinfected from indigenous reservoirs of parasites greatly favors the emergence and spread of drug-resistant strains of malaria.

Immune populations should not be given chemosuppressive drugs unless the dosage regimens are adequate and strictly adhered to. Areas now cleared of

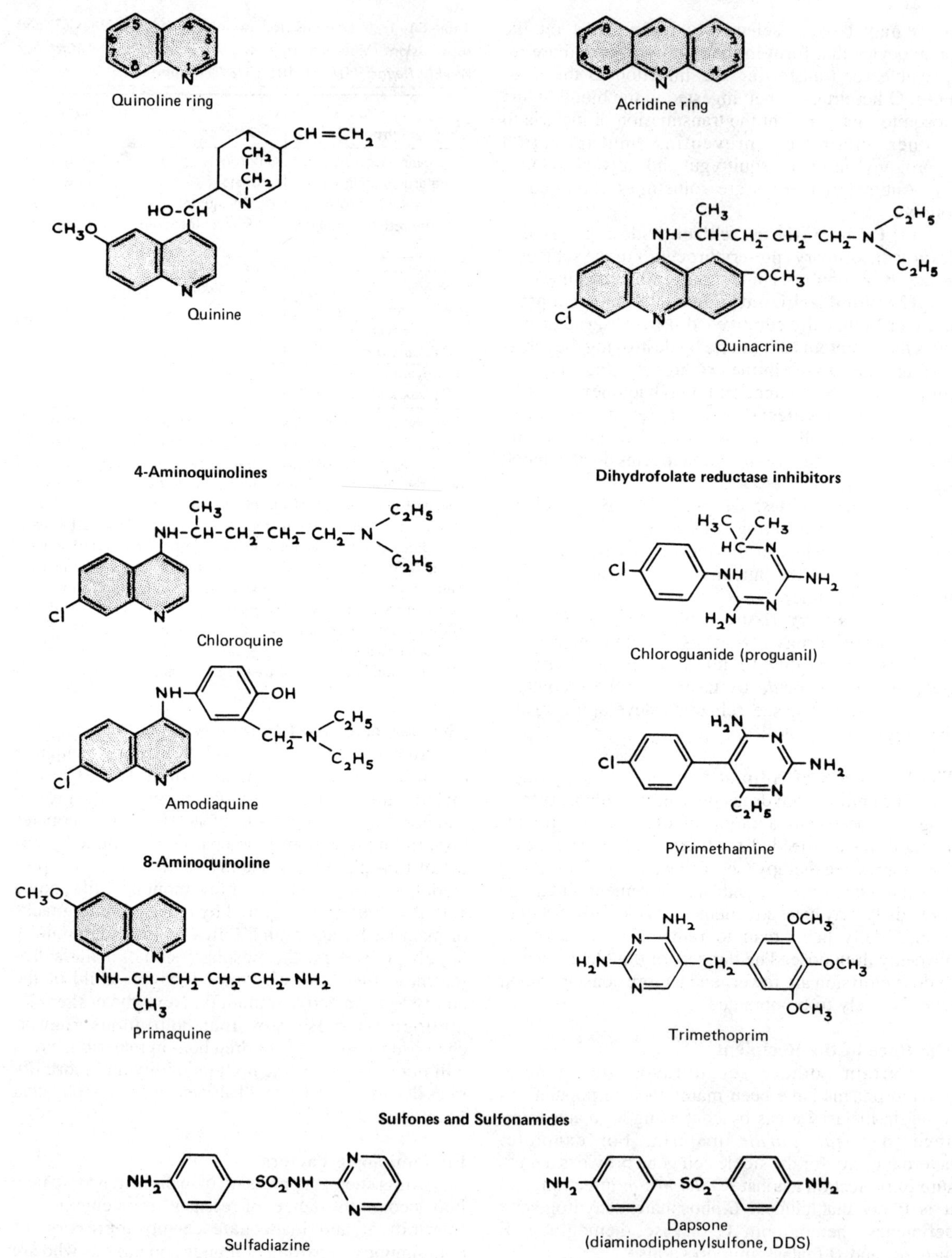

Figure 54–1. Structural formulas of antimalarial drugs, arranged to show structural relationships and historical development of the compounds.

malaria but having suitable anopheline mosquitoes may become reinfected by individuals carrying inadequately treated resistant strains of relapsing malaria. Therefore, travelers leaving areas in which malaria is common should be adequately treated with a tissue schizonticide (such as primaquine) for 4 weeks to obtain a radical cure of the relapsing malarias. In areas with (as yet) only rare cases of chloroquine-resistant malaria, most epidemiologists recommend that chloroquine be reserved for therapy and that it not be used for mass chemoprophylaxis.

Malaria Following Blood Transfusion

A number of cases of malaria (some fatal) have resulted from transfusions of infected blood. In most cases, a donor is incriminated by the presence in the serum of fluorescent antibodies to malaria, but often no parasites can be found in the donor's blood. Subsequent inquiry always reveals that the infected donor once lived in a malarious area. Most of these infections are due to *P vivax* malaria, but infections with *P malariae* and *P ovale,* and even *P falciparum,* have been reported.

QUININE

History

Quinine is the principal alkaloid found in the bark of the South American cinchona tree. Its introduction into Europe in the 17th century is usually credited to the Jesuits. Without quinine, the European colonization of tropical Africa would have been impossible. For 300 years, until World War II intensified the search for synthetic antimalarial drugs, the powdered bark was the only drug that could effectively suppress the symptoms of malaria. Although quinine can now be synthesized, it and the other cinchona alkaloids are still extracted from cinchona bark.

Of the more than 20 alkaloids found in cinchona bark, only quinine and quinidine are now in use. Both have schizonticidal activity, but because of its superior absorption, only quinine is used for the treatment of malaria. Quinidine is the D-isomer of quinine (see Chapter 12).

Absorption, Metabolism, & Excretion

Quinine is rapidly absorbed from the small intestine, and peak plasma concentrations are obtained 1–3 hours after ingestion. Excretion reaches a maximum after 4 hours, tapers off after another 4 hours, and is almost complete in 24 hours. Only 10% of the oral dose is excreted unchanged in the urine; the rest is metabolized. Subcutaneous or intramuscular quinine is poorly absorbed, and inflammation and sloughing may occur at the site of injection.

Pharmacologic Effects

A. Mechanism of Action: The exact mechanism of quinine's antimalarial action is uncertain. Quinine can form a hydrogen-bonded complex with double-stranded DNA that inhibits protein synthesis by preventing strand separation and therefore DNA replication and transcription to RNA. Quinine has been observed to depress so many enzyme systems that it has in the past been described as a "general protoplasmic poison."

B. Effects on Malaria: Quinine, along with quinacrine, chloroquine, and amodiaquine, is classed as a "blood schizonticide." It has no effect on the primary or secondary exoerythrocytic "tissue" forms of the parasites and therefore cannot bring about a radical cure of malaria caused by *P vivax, P malariae,* or *P ovale;* neither is it effectively gametocidal or sporonticidal to *P falciparum.* Although quinine cannot prevent infection, it can suppress the symptoms of malaria and also bring about rapid control of an acute attack. Quinine by intravenous drip is now once again the treatment of choice for acute attacks of chloroquine-resistant falciparum malaria.

C. Other Effects: The actions of quinine on the cardiovascular system are similar to those of quinidine (see Adverse Reactions, below). Quinine has little effect on smooth muscle other than a slight oxytocic action on the gravid uterus, especially during the third trimester of pregnancy. Clinically, it has no effect until labor has started, although dangerously toxic amounts may cause abortion.

In skeletal muscle, quinine has a curarelike effect on the motor end-plate and causes a lengthening of the refractory period. Tetanic contractions associated with various conditions may be diminished by quinine, and the drug has been used to lessen the contractions of myotonia congenita and to provide a diagnostic test for myasthenia gravis by aggravating the symptoms. Quinine was used for centuries to abate fevers due to any cause; its antipyretic action was due mostly to peripheral vasodilation.

Clinical Uses

A. Use in Acute Malaria: For 300 years, quinine was the drug of choice for the treatment and chemosuppression of malaria. By 1959, quinine as an antimalarial had been totally superseded by synthetic antimalarials. However, 3 years later, chloroquine-resistant strains of *P falciparum* were being reported from Colombia and Brazil, and later from Southeast Asia.

By 1965, 80% of US servicemen treated in Vietnam for malaria with chloroquine showed a persisting parasitemia that could only be brought under control with intravenous quinine. Relapses were frequent until, in 1969, quinine therapy was combined with use of pyrimethamine. Unfortunately, in 1968 a strain of *P falciparum* (the Smith strain) appeared that does not respond to quinine-pyrimethamine treatment. Infections with the Smith strain induced in volunteers in US prisons either relapsed after or were completely refractory to treatment with combinations of quinine, chloroquine, pyrimethamine, proguanil, and trimethoprim but were sensitive to a combination of quinine and sulfametopyrazine (sulfalene). Cerebral malaria occurs in about 2% of cases of *P falciparum* malaria in nonimmune individuals. Contrary to previous belief, corticosteroids such as dexamethasone are of *no value* in reducing the mortality rate and may actually prolong coma (*N Engl J Med* 1982;**306:**313).

B. Other Uses: Quinine (Quinam) is used to relieve leg cramps occurring during recumbency at night. In many parts of the world, quinine is still used as an all-purpose antipyretic. Many tonic waters and cocktail mixes contain quinine in trace amounts.

Adverse Reactions

A. Side-Effects:

1. Cinchonism–This term denotes the mild toxic state that usually develops when the plasma level of quinine exceeds 10–12 mg/L. Symptoms include flushed and sweaty skin, tinnitus, blurred vision, impaired hearing, dizziness, nausea and vomiting, and diarrhea. With severe cinchonism, there may be papular or urticarial skin rashes, deafness, somnolence, diminished visual acuity or blindness (toxic amblyopia) due to ischemia of the retinal vessels, abdominal pain, and disturbances in cardiac rhythm or conduction. Marked hypotension is common, especially with intravenous therapy, and on the ECG, lengthening of the P–R and Q–T intervals and the QRS complex is frequently observed.

2. Local irritant effect–Quinine is an irritant to the gastric mucosa, causing nausea and pain. Painful sterile abscesses frequently result from intramuscular injections. Intravenous injections may cause thrombophlebitis.

3. Hematologic effects–Hemolysis directly attributable to quinine occurs in 0.05% of people treated for acute malaria. Quinine inhibits phagocytosis and may rarely cause leukopenia, agranulocytosis, thrombocytopenic purpura, and Schönlein-Henoch purpura.

4. Blackwater fever–Blackwater fever is the syndrome of massive intravascular hemolysis, hemoglobinuria, azotemia, intravascular sludging and coagulation, renal failure, uremia, and death in 25–50% of cases. It is seldom seen in immune populations unless they have been treated with quinine. Hemoglobinuria occurs most often in patients who are also glucose-6-phosphate dehydrogenase-deficient. However, irregular or heavy therapy with any antimalarial, repeated and inadequately treated infections, sensitization to the parasite, fatigue, chilling, and perhaps idiosyncrasy to quinine may all be predisposing factors. It is at times necessary to continue quinine therapy in spite of the hemolytic reaction if the infection is due to a resistant strain that cannot be treated with another drug.

B. Overdosage Toxicity: The lethal dose of quinine for adults is about 8 g, but survival has been reported after much larger doses. After overdosage, prompt gastric lavage is imperative because the drug is rapidly absorbed and death may ensue within a few hours. There is usually a profound fall of blood pressure owing to peripheral vasodilatation and myocardial depression. Respiration becomes slow and shallow, and cyanosis develops. The quinidinelike action produces the expected electrocardiographic changes and arrhythmias. Doses greater than 4 g in 24 hours usually lead to visual impairment, which may be reversed by discontinuing the drug.

Preparations & Dosages for Chloroquine-Resistant Malaria*

Because of the high proportion of chloroquine-resistant *P falciparum* in Southeast Asia, all falciparum infections originating in that area should be assumed resistant, and one of the following regimens should be used:

(1) Quinine sulfate, 650 mg, 3 times a day for 3 days plus pyrimethamine, 25 mg, 2 times a day for 3 days plus sulfadiazine, 500 mg, 4 times a day for 5 days; these 3 drugs must be administered concurrently.

(2) Quinine sulfate, 650 mg, 3 times a day for 3 days plus Bactrim Double Strength (160 mg trimethoprim and 800 mg sulfamethoxazole), 2 tablets, 2 times a day for 5 days, administered concurrently.

(3) Quinine sulfate, 650 mg, 3 times a day for 3 days plus tetracycline, 250 mg, 4 times a day for 10 days, administered concurrently.

Several points about the above therapy should be noted. Sulfonamides are used in combination with a folic acid antagonist (eg, pyrimethamine or trimethoprim) because they are synergistic. The type of sulfonamide used is not critical provided that a sufficient blood level is maintained for at least 5 days. While combinations of sulfonamide, a folic acid antagonist, and a tetracycline are effective schizonticides, their rate of action is slow. Thus, at least 3 days of quinine therapy is important to rapidly reduce the parasite density to safe levels. Treatment of *P falciparum* malaria is effective in up to 95% of cases; however, such patients should be carefully followed for at least 90 days to detect recurrent symptoms or parasitemia. Recurrences are usually within the first 30 days but may occur later. Re-treatment may be with the same or another drug combination.

THE 4-AMINOQUINOLINE DERIVATIVES

1. CHLOROQUINE

History

Originally synthesized in 1934 in Germany, chloroquine was tested for antimalarial activity, but in 1935 it was reported to be too toxic for human use. In April 1942, following the fall of the Javanese cinchona plantations to the Japanese, the US War Production Board instigated a crash program of research for synthetic antimalarial drugs. By late 1944, US workers had synthesized 25 different 4-aminoquinoline derivatives, finally selecting a compound designated SN 7618 (later named chloroquine) as the most promising—only to discover a few months later that it

*Reproduced from *MMWR* (Aug 24) 1972;**28:**389.

was identical with the compound patented in Germany and the USA under the name of Resochine. From 1946 to 1966, chloroquine was the drug of choice for the treatment of malaria the world over. In 1966, chloroquine-resistant malaria began to appear in Southeast Asia.

Chemistry & Nomenclature

Chloroquine (Aralen) is 7-chloro-4-(4′-diethylamino-1′-methylbutylamino)quinoline. Trade names are as follows: **chloroquine diphosphate:** Aralen, Avloclor, Resochin; **chloroquine sulfate:** Nivaquine; **hydroxychloroquine sulfate:** Plaquenil.

Chloroquine diphosphate is a bitter, colorless, dimorphic crystalline powder soluble in water at pH 4.5 but with diminishing solubility at more neutral or alkaline pH. The D and L isomers are equally potent, but the D isomer is slightly less toxic. Chloroquine has a quinoline ring like that of quinine with a side chain identical to that of quinacrine. The chlorine atom in the seventh position appears to be crucial to the antimalarial activity of the 4-aminoquinolines and quinacrine.

Absorption, Metabolism, & Excretion

Absorption from the gastrointestinal tract is rapid and complete; maximum plasma concentrations are reached in 1–2 hours. The half-life of chloroquine in the body is about 5 days. Chloroquine is rapidly removed from the plasma and concentrated in those tissues where active protein synthesis and cell multiplication are greatest. The liver, spleen, kidneys, lungs, and leukocytes often contain 200–700 times the plasma concentration (whereas the brain and spinal cord contain only 10–30 times the plasma concentration). As a result, the apparent volume of distribution is very large (5–10 L/kg). For this reason, whenever an effectively schizonticidal plasma level is urgently needed, a loading dose should be given. The concentration of chloroquine in the erythrocytes is about 10–20 times greater than in the plasma and in parasitized erythrocytes about 25 times greater than in normal erythrocytes. Only 10–25% of the oral dose is excreted unchanged in the urine. The rate of excretion may be increased by acidification or decreased by alkalinization of the urine. Concomitant administration of other 4-aminoquinolines or 8-aminoquinolines prolongs and potentiates plasma levels of chloroquine.

Pharmacologic Effects

A. Mechanism of Action: Chloroquine and its congeners block the enzymatic synthesis of DNA and RNA in both mammalian and protozoal cells. The selective toxicity for the malarial parasites must therefore depend on a chloroquine-concentrating mechanism in parasitized cells. These drugs form a complex with DNA that prevents DNA from acting as a template for its own replication or transcription to RNA. It has been postulated that the quinoline ring of chloroquine is inserted between the base pairs of the DNA double helix so that the chlorine atom in position 7 of the quinoline ring lies in close proximity to the 2-amino group of guanine in a guanine-cytosine base pair. The diaminoaliphatic side chain of chloroquine lying across the minor groove of the DNA helix ties the 2 strands together by interacting ionically with the phosphoric acid groups of both strands. The electronegativity of the substituent at position 7 of the quinoline ring appears to be critical to the stability of the complex. The length of the side chain bridging the minor groove of the DNA helix is also critical; antimalarial activity is maximal when there are 4 carbon atoms between the 2 nitrogen atoms in the side chain, whereas a side chain with 3 or 5 carbon atoms instead of 4 has only two-thirds of the antimalarial activity of chloroquine, and a chain with 2 or 6 carbon atoms instead of 4 exhibits only one-third the activity.

B. Effects:

1. In malaria–Chloroquine is an excellent blood schizonticidal drug for all 4 types of malaria. The fever and parasitemia produced by non-drug-resistant strains of plasmodia are usually controlled within 24–48 hours, and in *P falciparum* infections a complete cure can be obtained. However, the drug has no effect on secondary tissue schizonts of relapsing malarias and thus cannot effect a "radical" cure of malaria caused by *P vivax, P malariae,* or *P ovale.*

Chloroquine, like quinine, is not lethal to the gametocytes or sporozoites of *P falciparum,* so that the blood of falciparum-infected chloroquine-treated humans can remain infective to mosquitoes for months. This may favor the emergence of drug-resistant strains of *P falciparum* in endemic areas.

Mechanism of chloroquine resistance. Parasites grown for many months in the presence of steadily increasing but sublethal doses of chloroquine will eventually become partially or totally resistant to the drug, and no concentration of chloroquine in the parasitized red cells can be demonstrated.

Plasmodial resistance to chloroquine is probably due to an impaired mechanism of drug transport across the parasite cell wall, so that the concentration of chloroquine in resistant schizonts never reaches a level sufficient to arrest nucleic acid synthesis.

2. On cardiovascular system–Chloroquine has a slight quinidinelike effect on the cardiovascular system, and changes in the T wave of the ECG may be noticeable during therapy. Chloroquine depresses myocardial excitability to approximately the same extent as quinidine, but it has hardly any effect on the conduction velocity. It has on occasion been used in place of quinidine. Toxic doses depress vasomotor function and induce circulatory collapse, shock, respiratory paralysis, and death.

3. Anti-inflammatory effects–Chloroquine has anti-inflammatory effects that have been useful in the treatment of rheumatoid arthritis and discoid lupus erythematosus. The mechanism is not understood.

Clinical Uses

A. Malaria, Acute Attacks: Chloroquine usually terminates the fever and parasitemia of acute attacks of nonresistant strains of falciparum malaria within 24–48 hours, and complete cures are usually obtained because *P falciparum* has no secondary tissue stage. Severe malaria with more than 100,000 parasites per microliter of blood or with cerebral, renal, or pulmonary complications requires immediate treatment with slow intravenous infusions of quinine. If an acute attack does not respond to chloroquine within 24 hours, a resistant strain may be involved and other antimalarial drugs must be tried (see below). For acute attacks of *P vivax* malaria, chloroquine is the drug of choice; however, because it has no effect on the exoerythrocytic stages, radical cure is not possible.

The recommended treatment for *P vivax* infections (*MMWR* [Aug 24] 1979;**28:**389) is a total dose of 1.5 g of chloroquine (base) over a 2-day period (600 mg initial dose, followed by 300 mg at 6, 24, and 48 hours). There have been no reports of resistance of this species to chloroquine, and this regimen should eliminate the parasitemia and symptoms within 24–72 hours. Radical curative therapy is administered to eliminate the exoerythrocytic schizonts in the liver; the 2 accepted regimens are as follows: (1) Primaquine, 15 mg (base) daily for 14 days. The initial dose should be in association with chloroquine, either with the normal therapeutic course or, if administered later, with a single dose of 600 mg (base) of chloroquine. (2) Primaquine, 45 mg (base) weekly for 8 weeks.

For a closely supervised patient, the 14-day regimen may be preferable because regular drug-taking would be assured and the likelihood of missing doses during the 8-week course would be avoided.

Primaquine or chloroquine-primaquine mixtures may cause gastrointestinal symptoms in some patients. Patients with glucose-6-phosphate dehydrogenase deficiency may experience mild to severe hemolysis during primaquine therapy. It is recommended that all patients be screened for glucose-6-phosphate dehydrogenase deficiency before primaquine treatment is begun and that periodic determinations of hematocrit be done during therapy. Those with a glucose-6-phosphate dehydrogenase deficiency should be placed on the once-weekly dosage schedule rather than the daily regimen. The hemolysis is reversible upon cessation of the drug, and a significant and persistent fall in hematocrit should dictate cessation of treatment.

Most authorities believe that *P malariae* is not a relapsing species of malaria. There are no reports of *P malariae* resistance to chloroquine. Therefore, this species may be treated with chloroquine as outlined above for *P vivax;* no primaquine is indicated.

B. Suppression of Malaria: Chloroquine effectively suppresses all types of malaria except the resistant strains of *P falciparum* (see Table 54–1). If the drug is discontinued too soon after *P vivax* infections, parasitemia may recur after several days. Chloroquine is more potent, less toxic, better tolerated, and more easily administered than quinine or quinacrine. Complete suppression may be obtained with a plasma level of 5–8 μg/L. The prophylactic use of chloroquine or other 4-aminoquinolines involves the risk of the development of resistant strains. Perhaps chloroquine should be used only for the treatment of acute disease and chloroguanide or pyrimethamine for routine prophylaxis except in areas where resistance to these drugs has been reported.

Note: Increasingly frequent reports of treatment failures with chloroquine and *P falciparum* infections in nonimmune travelers to East Africa following chloroquine prophylaxis have prompted the CDC to revise their recommendations for Tanzania, Kenya, Uganda, Madagascar, and Comoros (*MMWR* [June 25] 1982;**31:**328). Experts now recommend a weekly dose of one tablet of Fansidar *plus* one tablet of chloroquine (300 mg base). Both tablets may be taken at the same time. Because of the teratogenic potential of the pyrimethamine component of Fansidar, nonimmune pregnant women should try to avoid travel in East Africa or take only chloroquine. Those allergic to sulfonamides may have to use maloprim instead of Fansidar. Children under age 2 months should not be given Fansidar because of the risk of inducing neonatal jaundice. The concurrent effects of long-term Fansidar plus chloroquine prophylaxis are not yet known. Therefore, hemograms should be checked every 6 months. The recommendations for West Africa have not changed: chloroquine, 300 mg base once weekly.

C. Amebiasis: Chloroquine can bring about rapid and complete clinical cures of hepatic amebiasis, although it is slightly less effective than emetine, which is directly toxic to the myocardium (see p 585).

D. Fluke Infections: See Chapter 55.

Adverse Reactions

A. Side-Effects: When used in the very low doses required for the chemosuppression of malaria, chloroquine has essentially no toxic effects. During chloroquine therapy of active malaria, vertigo, malaise, anorexia, diarrhea, headache, blurring of vision, pruritus, and urticaria may occur.

After high dosage there may be macropapular eruptions, desquamation, or exfoliative lesions of the skin, and alopecia or graying of the hair. Lupus erythematosus, lichenoid skin eruptions, and leukopenia induced by chloroquine have been reported.

Toxic psychoses with hallucinations and agitation and peripheral neuropathies with loss of reflexes and muscle power in the lower limbs can occur. Electrocardiographic changes, particularly flattening or inversion of the T waves, are frequent with high doses.

Congenital deafness and mental retardation have been reported in children born to mothers who were taking large doses of chloroquine during pregnancy. Permanent nerve deafness in adults has followed high-dose chloroquine therapy.

B. Ocular Toxicity: Severe and often permanent eye damage may be caused by the prolonged administration of chloroquine in high dosage.

1. Corneal changes–Chloroquine, secreted in tears, is absorbed by the corneal epithelium. The cornea at first becomes insensitive, and diffuse white granules appear in the epithelium. These granules later aggregate into curved lines just below the center of the cornea. Between 10 and 33% of patients taking large doses of chloroquine develop these symptomless corneal deposits, which always regress when the drug is discontinued.

2. Retinal changes–These are nearly always permanent and often progress after withdrawal of the drug. Early symptoms include halos around lights and ill-defined blurring of vision. Ophthalmoscopic examination at this time may reveal a slight edema with fine degrees of pigment clumping, and frequently small pericentral scotomas causing reading discomfort. These scotomas later coalesce into ring scotomas causing large visual field defects. A characteristic ophthalmoscopic picture consists of a granular or stippled hyperpigmentation of the macula, surrounded by a clear zone of depigmentation encircled by another ring of pigment, much like a bull's-eye. Most cases occur after more than 300 mg has been given daily for more than a year. Retinal thresholds have been abnormal in all patients given a total of more than 100 g of chloroquine. More than 13% of patients with rheumatoid arthritis treated with chloroquine have retinal changes. All patients on prolonged, high-dose chloroquine must have vision tested and retinas examined at least every 3 months.

C. Overdosage Toxicity: After a toxic dose, there are visual disturbances, hyperexcitability, convulsions, atrioventricular block, and death within 2 hours. At autopsy, no abnormalities can be demonstrated except (sometimes) the presence of undissolved tablets in the stomach and tissue levels of chloroquine that are 20 times as high as the prophylactic tissue levels.

There is no antidote. Because chloroquine is rapidly absorbed, gastric lavage must be done before symptoms occur if it is to be of any value. Peritoneal dialysis or hemodialysis is usually unsuccessful.

Contraindications & Cautions

Chloroquine crosses the placenta and may damage the fetus when large doses have been taken during pregnancy. Patients with porphyria and psoriasis should not use chloroquine because it may precipitate an acute attack, and chloroquine should not be combined with other drugs known to cause dermatitis. Gold or phenylbutazone therapy should be discontinued during chloroquine therapy.

Chloroquine should be used with caution in patients with a history of liver damage, or neurologic or hematologic disorders.

Many malariologists condemn the use of chloroquine for mass chemotherapy because of the danger of resistant strain selection. Resistance to chloroquine always extends to the other 4-aminoquinolines and quinacrine, and often to chlorguanide and pyrimethamine as well.

Therapy of acute attacks should never be attempted with combined chloroquine-primaquine tablets, because an adequate therapeutic dose of chloroquine cannot be achieved without also giving toxic amounts of primaquine.

2. THE CHLOROQUINE CONGENERS

None of the 200 known derivatives of 4-aminoquinoline with proved schizonticidal activity have been conclusively shown to be superior to chloroquine; therefore, chloroquine, whose potency and side-effects have been abundantly documented, is the preferred preparation.

The 1972 WHO scientific group on the chemotherapy of malaria lists only 3 other 4-aminoquinolines "in common use": (1) **amodiaquine dihydrochloride (Basoquin, Camoquin, Flavoquine)** (for the prophylactic dose of amodiaquine, see Table 54–2); (2) **cycloquine (Ciklochin, Halochin)**; and (3) **amopyroquin (Propoquin)**.

THE 8-AMINOQUINOLINES

History & Chemical Characteristics

Guttmann and Ehrlich observed in 1891 that methylene blue had a weak activity against vivax malaria. German workers in 1926 replaced the acridine ring of methylene blue with a quinoline ring similar to that of quinine to create an 8-aminoquinoline (pamaquine) that was 60 times more potent than quinine but too toxic for prophylactic use. Later, Atabrine (quinacrine USP, mepacrine BP) was synthesized by combining the side chain of pamaquine with the acridine ring of methylene blue. During World War II, Atabrine became the first synthetic to be used for the mass chemosuppression of malaria.

In the search for an effective cure of the relapsing malarias, the 8-aminoquinolines were restudied. Primaquine was found to have the highest therapeutic index of the 8-aminoquinolines synthesized and tested. It is the only antimalarial now in use that is able to accomplish a radical cure of malaria due to *P vivax*.

1. PRIMAQUINE

Chemistry, Absorption, Metabolism, & Excretion (See Fig 54–1.)

Absorption from intestine is essentially complete, and peak plasma levels are reached in 6 hours. Only trace amounts are in the plasma 24 hours later, and only about 1% is excreted in the urine unchanged.

Effective clearance of tissue schizonts does not begin until primaquine has undergone biodegradation by demethylation and oxidation to quinoline-quinone derivatives, the active antimalarial and hemolytic agents. Tissue concentrations of primaquine are highest in liver and lungs, but primaquine is also concentrated in brain, heart, and skeletal muscle.

Pharmacologic Action

A. Mechanism of Action: Unlike the 4-aminoquinolines, the 8-aminoquinolines do not inhibit DNA replication and transcription.

Primaquine undergoes biotransformation to

Table 54–2. Drugs and doses for malaria chemoprophylaxis (modified from: *MMWR* [March 10] 1978;**27[Suppl]**:81).

Generic Name	Brand Names	Adult Dose	Pediatric Dose
Amodiaquine	Camoquin Flavoquine Basoquin	520 mg (400 mg base) once weekly and continued for 6 weeks after last exposure in a malarious area	< 1 year: 65 mg (50 mg base) 1–3 years: 130 mg (100 mg base) 4–6 years: 195 mg (150 mg base) 7–10 years: 260 mg (200 mg base) 11–16 years: 390 mg (300 mg base)
Chloroquanide (Proguanil)	Paludrine	100–200 mg daily and continued for 6 weeks after last exposure in a malarious area	2 years and under: 25–50 mg 3–6 years: 50–75 mg 7–10 years: 100 mg
Chloroquine phosphate	Aralen Avloclor Resochin	500 mg (300 mg base) weekly and continued for 6 weeks after last exposure in a malarious area	< 1 year: 62 mg (37.5 mg base) 1–3 years: 125 mg (75 mg base) 4–6 years: 165 mg (100 mg base) 7–10 years: 250 mg (150 mg base) 11–16 years: 375 mg (225 mg base) or 5 mg/kg base
Chloroquine sulfate	Nivaquine	500 mg (300 mg base) weekly and continued for 6 weeks after last exposure in a malarious area	< 1 year: 62 mg (37.5 mg base) 1–3 years: 125 mg (75 mg base) 4–6 years: 165 mg (100 mg base) 7–10 years: 250 mg (150 mg base) 11–16 years: 375 mg (225 mg base) or 5 mg/kg base
Hydroxychloroquine	Plaquenil	400 mg (310 mg base) weekly and continued for 6 weeks after last exposure in a malarious area	< 1 year: 50 mg (37.5 mg base) 1–3 years: 100 mg (75 mg base) 4–6 years: 130 mg (100 mg base) 7–10 years: 200 mg (150 mg base) 11–16 years: 290 mg (225 mg base) or 5 mg/kg base
Primaquine	None	26.3 mg (15 mg base) daily for 14 days or 79 mg (45 mg base) once weekly for 8 weeks; start during the last 2 weeks of or following a course of suppression with chloroquine or a comparable drug	0.3 mg/kg base/d for 14 days or 0.9 mg/kg base/d weekly for 8 weeks
Pyrimethamine	Daraprim	25 mg weekly and continued for 6 weeks after last exposure in a malarious area	2 years and under: 6.25 mg 3–10 years: 12.5 mg Over 10 years: Adult dosage
Pyrimethamine-sulfadoxine*	Fansidar Falcidar Antemal Methipox	25 mg pyrimethamine and 500 mg sulfadoxine weekly and continued for 6 weeks after last exposure in a malarious area	In terms of sulfadoxine: 6–11 months: 125 mg 1–3 years: 250 mg 4–8 years: 500 mg 9–14 years: 750 mg

*Countries where pyrimethamine-sulfadoxine can be obtained: Belgium, Brazil, Burma, Cambodia, Germany, Hong Kong, Indonesia, Laos, Malaysia, Philippines, Singapore, Switzerland, Thailand, USA, Venezuela, Vietnam.

quinoline-quinone intermediates that are electron-carrying redox compounds capable of acting as oxidants. The intermediate metabolites probably account for the hemolysis and methemoglobinemia as well as the schizonticidal action of the drug.

B. Effects: Although the 8-aminoquinolines structurally resemble the 4-aminoquinolines, their actions on malaria parasites are quite different. The 8-aminoquinolines act on the exoerythrocytic stages and have practically no effect on the erythrocytic stages. Their mode of action is probably related to the mechanism by which they produce an acute self-limiting intravascular hemolysis in individuals with an inherited glucose-6-phosphate dehydrogenase deficiency.

It is postulated that, in contrast to the erythrocytic schizonts, both the tissue schizonts and the glucose-6-phosphate dehydrogenase-deficient erythrocytes have a deficiency of an enzyme or cofactor involved in the pentose phosphate pathway, making them especially susceptible to oxidative damage.

Primaquine also has an effect on the gametocytes; some are destroyed in the blood, and others cannot later mature in the mosquito gut. Primaquine is therefore a "tissue schizonticide" and the only antimalarial able to bring about "radical cures" of the relapsing malarias. Its gametocidal activity also makes it the best available drug to interrupt the transmission of malaria.

Primaquine given orally in therapeutic doses has no pharmacologic effects other than its antimalarial action and its toxic effect on erythrocyte metabolism. It is never given parenterally because it can produce electrocardiographic changes and a profound fall of blood pressure.

Clinical Uses

Primaquine is highly active against the primary exoerythrocytic stages of falciparum and vivax malaria and the secondary exoerythrocytic forms of the relapsing malarias (*P vivax, P malariae,* and *P ovale*). It is also highly active against the gametocytes of all 4 species causing human malaria and is therefore used to limit the transmission of malaria. It has only a slight effect on the blood schizonts and cannot be used to relieve the fever and parasitemia of acute attacks. Primaquine is at the moment the only drug able to attack the late tissue stages of *P vivax, P malariae,* or *P ovale* and therefore able to effect a radical cure. Unfortunately, strains of *P vivax* have now appeared in Southeast Asia that are partially resistant to primaquine.

Several programs of mass chemoprophylaxis with primaquine have been carried out in areas of heavy malaria endemicity by WHO and other public health authorities.

Adverse Reactions

A. Primaquine Sensitivity: Glucose-6-phosphate dehydrogenase deficiency, sometimes called primaquine sensitivity, is an inherited error of metabolism transmitted by a gene of partial dominance located on the X chromosome. It is estimated that over 100 million people are affected. Red cells deficient in glucose-6-phosphate dehydrogenase are sensitive in various degrees to the 8-aminoquinolines and many other drugs, eg, sulfonamides, PAS, aspirin, certain vitamin K derivatives, nitrofurans, and fava beans.

Normal red cells require glucose for survival. Of the glucose metabolized by red cells, 90% is broken down via the Embden-Meyerhof pathway and the other 10% is metabolized by the pentose phosphate pathway. The enzyme glucose-6-phosphate dehydrogenase is necessary for the regeneration of NADPH, which in turn is required for the reduction of oxidized glutathione. One of the functions of reduced glutathione is to protect sulfhydryl-dependent enzymes and other cellular proteins against oxidation. The level of reduced glutathione in the red cells of glucose-6-phosphate dehydrogenase-deficient individuals fluctuates and is usually lower than normal. Cells with a low level of reduced glutathione and an impaired mechanism for the regeneration of NADPH are particularly vulnerable to the oxidizing effects of substances such as the quinoline-quinones derived from primaquine. When primaquine brings about a further reduction of the level of reduced glutathione in cells that already have an impaired mechanism for the regeneration of NADPH, glucose metabolism may be so deranged that the red cells undergo hemolysis.

The amount of hemolysis occurring with primaquine therapy is therefore dependent on the following 3 factors:

1. The degree of glucose-6-phosphate dehydrogenase deficiency–Because the disease is carried on the X chromosome, affected males and the rare females who are homozygous for the trait have the full expression of the disease. Female carriers of the disease are heterozygous for the trait and have a variable expression of the disease. For some reason not yet fully understood, affected whites (especially those whose ancestors inhabited the Mediterranean littoral) have a much more severe expression of primaquine sensitivity than glucose-6-phosphate dehydrogenase-deficient blacks.

2. Age of the erythrocyte population–The older erythrocytes have a lower level of glucose-6-phosphate dehydrogenase than younger cells and will be the first to hemolyze. Therefore, if aging susceptible cells have already been removed by hemolysis, the remaining younger population of red cells, which are relatively more resistant, will suffer less hemolysis. For this reason, the hemolysis produced by small doses, eg, 15 mg of primaquine per day, is usually self-limiting. Hemolysis occurring at the inception of primaquine therapy can cause a flulike febrile episode consisting of malaise, weakness, and chills lasting 2–3 days.

3. Dose size–The amount of primaquine-induced hemolysis is dose-dependent. Daily doses of 15 mg of primaquine are well tolerated by young glucose-6-phosphate dehydrogenase-deficient blacks, and only minor hemolytic disturbances are encountered; with a daily dose of 30 mg, the incidence and severity of the reactions increase sharply.

In some populations, over 20% of those who live in (or whose ancestors came from) areas of endemic falciparum malaria carry the glucose-6-phosphate dehydrogenase deficiency trait. The distribution of this potentially lethal gene can be explained by the fact that it confers a small degree of protection against falciparum malaria.

Other less common types of inherited enzyme deficiencies involving erythrocyte metabolism (eg, glutathione reductase deficiency) may also be expressed as primaquine sensitivity.

B. Side-Effects: Toxic reactions, often seen when large doses (60–240 mg) are given, include nausea, headache, disturbances of visual accommodation, pruritus, and abdominal cramps (which may be relieved with antacids). Severe reactions associated with high-dose therapy include leukopenia and methemoglobinemia usually presenting as cyanosis. All patients receiving primaquine should be told to report any signs of hemolysis, such as reddening or darkening of the urine.

Contraindications & Cautions

Blacks, Greeks, Sephardic Jews, Sardinians, and Iranians, who are known to have a high incidence of glucose-6-phosphate dehydrogenase deficiency, should be watched for signs of hemolysis during primaquine therapy. Before initiating treatment with primaquine, it is recommended that all patients be screened for erythrocyte glucose-6-phosphate dehydrogenase deficiency. Periodic determinations of the hematocrit or hemoglobin are essential during therapy. Patients with active rheumatoid arthritis, lupus erythematosus, or any grave systemic disease should not receive primaquine therapy. Primaquine should not be given at the same time as quinacrine or other drugs known to have depressant effects on the bone marrow.

When primaquine was used for mass chemosuppression, drug resistance of *P falciparum* was induced. In the laboratory, strains of *Plasmodium berghei* made resistant to primaquine show significant cross-resistance to cycloguanil, pyrimethamine, and dapsone.

Dosages

For primaquine malaria chemoprophylaxis for adults and for children, see Table 54–2.

There are no indications or preparations for intravenous or intramuscular primaquine therapy.

QUINACRINE
(Mepacrine)

Quinacrine, also known as Atabrine and mepacrine, was the first effective synthetic antimalarial of low toxicity. Until the introduction of chloroquine, it was the principal synthetic drug used for antimalarial prophylaxis.

The standard malaria suppressive dose of quinacrine is 100 mg orally. It is readily absorbed from the intestinal tract, and peak plasma levels are reached 8 hours later. Four to 6 weeks after discontinuing therapy, quinacrine can still be detected in the pancreas, lungs, bone marrow, liver, and erythrocytes. Quinacrine crosses the placenta, and fetal tissue levels are nearly the same as the maternal levels.

Quinacrine, like quinine and the 4-aminoquinolines, is a blood schizonticide. Continuous therapy can effectively suppress all 4 types of human malaria and can effect a radical cure of nonresistant strains of *P falciparum*. Malaria due to *P vivax, P malariae,* and *P ovale* will relapse a few weeks or months after discontinuing the drug because quinacrine has no effect on the exoerythrocytic schizonts. There is cross-resistance between chloroquine and quinacrine.

Quinacrine can be a cerebrocortical stimulant, producing heightened awareness, increased physical activity, restlessness, and insomnia.

Clinical Uses

A. Treatment and Chemosuppression of Malaria: Quinacrine as an antimalarial agent was superseded in 1945 by the far more potent and less toxic 4-aminoquinolines.

B. Other Uses: See Chapters 55 and 56.

Adverse Reactions

When quinacrine was used in low dosages as an antimalarial, it produced yellow staining of the skin and infrequent incidence of psychotic reactions. A grayish-blue discoloration of the ears, nasal cartilages, and fingernail beds that can be mistaken for cyanosis was sometimes seen.

THE ANTIFOLS (DIHYDROFOLATE REDUCTASE INHIBITORS): CHLOROGUANIDE (PROGUANIL), PYRIMETHAMINE, & TRIMETHOPRIM

History

Research for a completely nontoxic antimalarial for mass chemoprophylaxis resulted, in 1946, in chloroguanide (proguanil); however, its effectiveness was soon compromised by the emergence of resistant strains. In 1948, a number of 2,4-diaminopyrimidines had been shown, like guanidine, to antagonize folic acid metabolism. Pyrimethamine was tested and found to be a highly effective antimalarial. Trimethoprim, an antifolic originally developed as an antibacterial agent, was not tested for antimalarial activity until the desperate search in 1968 and 1969 for drugs effective against the Southeast Asian strains of *P falciparum* resistant to chloroguanide, chloroquine, and pyrimethamine. The discovery of the synergistic potentiation of the antimalarial activity of the antifols when combined with sulfonamides such as sulfamethoxypyridazine and sulfamethoxazole and with sulfones such as dapsone (DDS) opened a whole new field of antimalarial therapy. However, because of the rapid development of resistance, with cross-resistance to other combinations of antifols and sulfonamides, it is now recommended that these combinations be used only for the treatment of chloroquine-resistant strains.

Chemistry & Nomenclature

A. Chloroguanide (Proguanil) Hydrochloride: The structure of chloroguanide is shown in Fig 54–1. It is also known as Balusil, bigumal, biguanide, chlorguanide, Chloroguanil, Diguanyl, Drinupal, Guanatol, Lepadina, Paludrine, Palusil, Plasin, Proguanide, and Tirian. For prophylaxis, see Table 54–2.

B. Pyrimethamine: The structure of pyrimethamine is shown in Fig 54–1. It is also known by the proprietary names Chloridin, Darapram, Daraprim, Erbaprelina, and Malocide.

C. Trimethoprim: The structure of trimethoprim is shown in Fig 54–1 (see also Chapter 46). It is available as a combination of one part trimethoprim and 5 parts sulfamethoxazole, known as Bactrim or Septra.

D. Pyrimethamine-Sulfadoxine (Fansidar, Falcidar, Antemal, Methipox): This preparation is the recommended chemoprophylactic antimalarial (by WHO and CDC) for use in parts of the world where chloroquine-resistant *P falciparum* malaria is now endemic. It is a fixed-combination tablet of a long-acting sulfonamide (sulfadoxine, 1000 mg) combined with pyrimethamine, 50 mg.

Pediatric dose (in terms of sulfadoxine): 6–11 months, 125 mg; 1–3 years, 250 mg; 4–8 years, 500 mg; 9–14 years, 750 mg. See Table 54–2.

Fansidar, now available in the USA, should replace chloroquine prophylaxis when the traveler enters areas reported to be harboring chloroquine-resistant strains of *P falciparum* (see Table 54–2.) Fansidar is principally effective against the erythrocytic stages of the malarial parasite. It can procure adequate suppression of most *P falciparum, P ovale,* and *P vivax* malarias, but not if they are also pyrimethamine-resistant. For these cases, chloroquine must be added. It is also possible that the "relapsing malarias" will relapse after Fansidar therapy is discontinued. Therefore, it is advisable to follow Fansidar prophylaxis with several weeks of primaquine prophylaxis.

Absorption, Metabolism, & Excretion

Chloroguanide, pyrimethamine, and trimethoprim are slowly but adequately absorbed from the gastrointestinal tract. Peak plasma levels are reached in 3–7 hours after an oral dose, and loading doses are not necessary. Chloroguanide is so rapidly eliminated from the body that it must be administered daily; pyrimethamine is excreted more slowly. Trimethoprim is excreted more slowly than sulfamethoxazole, with which it is combined.

Unlike the quinoline drugs, chloroguanide, pyrimethamine, and trimethoprim do not accumulate in the tissues. Only very low levels of chloroguanide can be detected in the plasma 24 hours after an oral dose, but significant quantities of pyrimethamine and its metabolites—and of trimethoprim—can be found in the tissues 9 days after an oral dose. Between 40 and 60% of the oral dose of chloroguanide is excreted in the urine; 60% of that is excreted unchanged and 30% as the triazine metabolite. Sufficient pyrimethamine is excreted in maternal milk so that chemosuppressive levels of the drug may be reached in wholly breast-fed infants.

Pharmacologic Effects

When the antifols are given in therapeutic doses, no effects are seen other than the intended antiprotozoal or antibacterial effects. In excessive doses, abdominal pain, diarrhea, hematuria, and a macrocytic anemia like that of folic acid deficiency may occur.

Antimalarial Effects

All 3 of these drugs are strongly sporonticidal. Pyrimethamine, the most potent of the 3, has been calculated to be 2000 times as toxic to the malarial parasite as to the host. These drugs can also prevent sporogony in the mosquito gut, and a single dose of pyrimethamine given to a nonimmune person can interrupt transmission for several weeks. All 3 can provide effective and nontoxic antimalarial chemoprophylaxis provided they are continued for at least 10 weeks after the last infected mosquito bite and that there are no resistant strains in the area. They should not be used for the treatment of acute attacks because their blood schizonticide action is too slow. *P falciparum* malaria resistant to pyrimethamine is increasing and has been found not only in Southeast Asia and East Africa but also in West Africa. Pyrimethamine-resistant strains are usually also resistant to proguanil.

Mode of Action of the Antifols

Chloroguanide itself is not active; only its triazine metabolite, which is rapidly excreted, is active. The selective toxicity of all 3 antifols depends on the fact that plasmodia, unlike humans and many other animals, have not lost the enzymes needed for the synthesis of folic acid from *p*-aminobenzoic acid (PABA), glutamic acid, and pteridine but yet cannot make use of preformed folic acid. The plasmodicidal effects of these 3 antimalarials are due to a deficiency of tetrahydrofolate that results in the inhibition of cell division and schizogony. This interference with folic acid metabolism therefore explains the marked synergistic enhancement of potency that occurs when any of these drugs are combined with sulfonamides or sulfones, causing a sequential blockade of folic acid synthesis at 2 different stages along the metabolic pathway (see Chapter 46).

Clinical Uses

A. Malaria Chemosuppression: Chloroguanide must be taken in daily 100-mg doses because of its rapid excretion. Pyrimethamine is the most potent chemoprophylactic available (requiring only 25 mg weekly), but, like chloroguanide, it must be taken for 10 weeks after leaving the endemic area. Cures of acute attacks of malaria in nonimmune patients should not be attempted with these drugs because their ability to reduce fever and parasitemia is much too slow.

B. Combination Therapy of Chloroquine-Resistant Falciparum Malaria: In 1969, 12 cases of agranulocytosis occurred among 200,000 soldiers in Vietnam who were taking the standard CP (chloroquine, 300 mg base; primaquine, 45 mg base) tablet once a week plus 25 mg of dapsone weekly. Various other combinations such as pyrimethamine plus quinine and pyrimethamine plus sulfadoxine are advocated and have been found to be effective, but malaria resistance to these new combinations soon develops. For this reason, combinations of antifols and sulfonamides should only be used for chloroquine-resistant malaria.

C. Endemic Malaria: Pyrimethamine has been used to interrupt the transmission of malaria in communities of partially immune patients. Such eradication programs should always follow a course of a quick-acting blood schizonticide to minimize the risk of resistant strain emergence. Endemic malaria control has been attempted by the addition of pyrimethamine to cooking salt supplies. However, when this is done, the dosage levels in children under 6 are extremely variable and the emergence of resistant strains is practically assured.

D. Toxoplasmosis: Pyrimethamine, 25 mg, combined with trisulfapyrimidines, 1 g, given orally 4 times a day for 6 weeks, can be used for the treatment of toxoplasmosis. However, if toxoplasmic chorioretinitis is present or if there is a danger of congenital toxoplasmosis, corticosteroids should also be given.

Adverse Reactions

Chloroguanide occasionally induces anorexia but is the least toxic of all the antimalarials.

Pyrimethamine is also well tolerated. Large doses of pyrimethamine given for long periods sometimes lead to folic acid deficiency. Supplementary folic acid can correct the hematologic defect without impairing the drug's therapeutic effect.

Contraindications & Cautions

Cross-resistance to chloroguanide and pyrimethamine may develop when these drugs are given singly in low doses and for long periods of chemosuppression.

Preparations & Dosages

Chloroguanide hydrochloride (proguanil, Paludrine) is available as tablets of 25, 50, 100, and 300 mg containing 87% of the base. For the chemosuppression of malaria, 100–200 mg daily is usually sufficient.

Pyrimethamine is available as 25-mg tablets. For the chemosuppression of malaria, the dosage is 1 or 2 tablets per week. For children under 14, give pyrimethamine elixir (6.25 mg/mL), 2 mL weekly. The first dose should be taken before entering endemic areas, and suppressive therapy must be continued for 10 weeks after leaving the area.

For the treatment of drug-resistant falciparum malaria, 25 mg of pyrimethamine can be given every 8 hours for the first 3 days of a 14-day course of quinine (650 mg every 8 hours). One gram of sulfadoxine, a long-acting sulfonamide, has been combined with 50 mg of pyrimethamine to produce a single-dose cure of chloroquine-resistant malaria. Because of the true synergism between these 2 drugs, one-tenth of the curative dose of pyrimethamine plus one-fourth of the curative dose of sulfadiazine add up to one curative dose for the treatment of *P falciparum* malaria.

OTHER DRUGS WITH ANTIMALARIAL ACTIVITY

For chloroquine-sensitive falciparum malaria, chloroquine therapy remains the treatment of choice. Therapy should always be followed by a 6-week course of primaquine to prevent relapses due to possible concomitant *P vivax* infections.

For chloroquine-resistant malaria, quinine by intravenous infusion followed by a single dose of sulfadoxine and pyrimethamine is highly effective.

Maloprim is a fixed-combination tablet containing 100 mg dapsone with 12.5 mg pyrimethamine. The recommended prophylactic dose is 2 tablets for the week preceding exposure, followed by 1 tablet per week.

Cycloguanil embonate (Camolar), the active metabolite of proguanil, is so poorly soluble in the embonate form that it can be used as an intramuscular repository drug. A single injection provides protection for up to 3 months. However, resistance to cycloguanil has been reported.

Tetracycline, 250 mg orally every 6 hours for 7 days, can clear asexual forms of the parasites of chloroquine-resistant *P falciparum* infections, but tetracycline has no effect against the gametocytes. Tetracycline may have value as an adjunctive agent to achieve radical cures of drug-resistant infections.

Minocycline is a tetracycline analog. Administration of 540 mg quinine base plus 100 mg minocycline 3 times orally daily for 3 days, followed by minocycline, 100 mg orally for 7 days, has produced radical cures in 97% of patients with *P falciparum* infections.

Clindamycin and **lincomycin** are drugs that have also proved effective against resistant *P falciparium.*

THE TREATMENT OF AMEBIASIS

Robert S. Goldsmith, MD, DTM&H

Amebiasis may present as a severe intestinal infection (dysentery), a mild to moderate symptomatic intestinal infection, an asymptomatic intestinal infection, an ameboma or liver abscess, or in the form of other extraintestinal infections.

Drugs available for therapy can be classified according to their site of antiamebic action. Luminal amebicides such as diiodohydroxyquin and diloxanide furoate are active against luminal organisms but are ineffective against parasites in the bowel wall or tissues. The parenterally administered tissue amebicides dehydroemetine and emetine are effective against parasites in the bowel wall and tissues but not against luminal organisms. Chloroquine acts only against organisms in the liver. Antibiotics taken orally are indirect-acting luminal amebicides that exert their effects against bacterial associates of *Entamoeba histolytica* in the bowel lumen and in the bowel wall but not in other tissues. Given parenterally, antibiotics have little antiamebic activity at any site. Paromomycin, however, has a direct effect on amebas. Metronidazole is uniquely effective against organisms at 3 sites: the bowel lumen, bowel wall, and tissues. However, metronidazole used alone is not sufficient as a luminal amebicide.

The following is a partial list of useful antiamebic drugs:

(1) Tissue amebicides (drugs that act primarily in the bowel wall, liver, and other extraintestinal tissues):

(a) Dehydroemetine, emetine.

(b) Chloroquine (site of action principally in the liver).

(2) Luminal amebicides (drugs that act primarily in the bowel lumen):

(a) Halogenated hydroxyquinolines: Diiodohydroxyquin (iodoquinol), iodochlorhydroxyquin

Table 54–3. Treatment of amebiasis.

	Drug(s) of Choice	Alternative Drug(s)
Asymptomatic intestinal infection	Diloxanide furoate[1,2]	Diiodohydroxyquin (iodoquinol)[3]
Mild to moderate intestinal infection (nondysenteric colitis)	(1) Metronidazole[4] **plus** (2) Diloxanide furoate[2] or diiodohydroxyquin[3]	(1) Diloxanide[2] or diiodohydroxyquin[3] **plus** (2) A tetracycline[5] **followed by** (3) Chloroquine[6] **or** (1) Paromomycin[7] **followed by** (2) Chloroquine[6]
Severe intestinal infection (dysentery)	(1) Metronidazole[8] **plus** (2) Diloxanide furoate[2] or diiodohydroxyquin[3] **If parenteral therapy is needed initially** (1) Intravenous metronidazole[9] until oral therapy can be started (2) Then give oral metronidazole[8] plus diloxanide furoate[2] or diiodohydroxyquin[3]	(1) A tetracycline[5] **plus** (2) Diloxanide furoate[2] or diiodohydroxyquin[3] **followed by** (3) Chloroquine[10] **or** (1) Dehydroemetine[1,11] or emetine (see text for dosage) **followed by** (2) A tetracycline[5] plus diloxanide furoate[2] or diiodohydroxyquin[3] **followed by** (3) Chloroquine[10]
Hepatic abscess	(1) Metronidazole[8,9] **followed by** (2) Diloxanide furoate[2] or diiodohydroxyquin[3] **plus** (3) Chloroquine[10]	(1) Dehydroemetine[1,12] or emetine (see text for dosage) **plus** (2) Chloroquine[13] **plus** (3) Diloxanide furoate[2] or diiodohydroxyquin[3]
Ameboma or extraintestinal infection	As for hepatic abscess, but not including chloroquine	As for hepatic abscess, but not including chloroquine

[1] Available in the USA only from the Parasitic Disease Drug Service, Centers for Disease Control, Atlanta 30333. Telephone requests may be made by calling (404) 329–3670 days; (404) 329–2888 nights, weekends, and holidays.
[2] Diloxanide furoate, 500 mg 3 times daily for 10 days.
[3] Diiodohydroxyquin (iodoquinol), 650 mg 3 times daily for 21 days.
[4] Metronidazole, 750 mg 3 times daily for 10 days.
[5] A tetracycline, 250 mg 4 times daily for 10 days; in severe dysentery, give 500 mg 4 times daily for the first 5 days, then 250 mg 4 times daily for 5 days.
[6] Chloroquine, 250 mg (salt) twice daily for 7 days.
[7] Paromomycin, 25–30 mg/kg (maximum 3 g) daily in 3 divided doses for 5–10 days.
[8] Metronidazole, 750 mg 3 times daily for 5–10 days.
[9] An intravenous metronidazole is available; change to oral medication as soon as possible. See manufacturer's recommendation for dosage.
[10] Chloroquine, 250 mg (salt) twice daily for 14 days.
[11] Dehydroemetine, 1 mg/kg IM or subcut daily for the least number of days necessary to control severe symptoms (usually 3–5 days) (maximum daily dose 0.1 g).
[12] Dehydroemetine, 1 mg/kg IM or subcut daily for 8–10 days (maximum daily dose 0.1 g) or emetine (see text for dosage).
[13] Chloroquine, 500 mg (salt) twice daily for 2 days and then 250 mg twice daily for 21 days.

(clioquinol, Entero-Vioform), dibromohydroxyquinoline (broxyquinoline).

(b) Dichloroacetamides: Diloxanide furoate (Furamide), clefamide (Mebinol), teclozan, etofamide.

(c) Antibiotics: Tetracyclines, paromomycin (Humatin), erythromycin.

(3) Tissue and luminal amebicides: Nitroimidazoles: Metronidazole (Flagyl), tinidazole (Fasigyn), ornidazole, seconidazole.

(4) Other compounds: Niridazole is also a luminal and tissue amebicide, but its neurotoxicity has markedly limited its usefulness. The pentavalent arsenicals, glycobiarsol, carbarsone, difetarsone, and acetarsone, should no longer be used because of their potential arsenical toxicity. Emetine-bismuth-iodine (EBI), an oral luminal amebicide, is little used at present because of its side-effects, which include nausea, vomiting, and rare instances of emetine toxicity. Iodochlorohydroxyquin has been withdrawn in many countries because of its neurotoxicity.

Treatment may require the concurrent or sequential use of several drugs. Table 54–3 outlines a preferred and an alternative method of treatment for each clinical type of amebiasis. No drugs are recommended as safe or effective for chemoprophylaxis.

In the past few years, the increasing association of several of the most useful antiamebic drugs with serious or potentially serious adverse reactions has required the reevaluation and reassignment of the drugs of choice and alternative drugs. Metronidazole has been found to induce neoplasms in rodents and to be mutagenic for certain bacteria; thus, it is potentially hazardous for humans. In addition, the halogenated hydroxyquinolines have been increasingly implicated in the production of neurotoxicity. The tetracyclines should not be used for children under age 8 years. Such findings reinforce the need for accurate identification of *E histolytica* before drug therapy is initiated.

Asymptomatic Intestinal Infection

When infection is confined to the bowel lumen, cure may often be obtained by use of luminal amebicides alone; but of the drugs in use, none is completely reliable in eradicating the infection. When available, diloxanide furoate is recommended as the most effective and least toxic. The alternative drug is diiodohydroxyquin (iodoquinol). Other alternatives for treatment or re-treatment are paromomycin, paromomycin plus diiodohydroxyquin, or metronidazole plus diiodohydroxyquin or diloxanide furoate. Usually in asymptomatic infection drugs are not given to prevent liver infection.

Mild to Moderate Intestinal Infection

Metronidazole plus a luminal amebicide is the treatment of choice. Although metronidazole is highly effective against tissue parasites, a course of diiodohydroxyquin or diloxanide must also be given to achieve a high likelihood of intestinal cure. The alternative treatment is to combine a luminal amebicide with tetracycline and then follow with a short course of chloroquine. When diiodohydroxyquin is used, concomitant use of a tetracycline probably increases intestinal cure rates. It is less well established that adding a tetracycline to diloxanide furoate also increases effectiveness. Chloroquine is used to destroy trophozoites in the liver or to eradicate an undetected, early stage of amebic liver abscess; the minimum dose needed to accomplish this is not known. In settings where intestinal infection and reinfection are common yet hepatic abscess is extremely rare, as in urban homosexual communities, it is probably unnecessary to use chloroquine in mild intestinal disease. A second alternative treatment is a course of paromomycin (some workers include diiodohydroxyquin) followed by chloroquine.

Severe Intestinal Infection

The treatment of choice is metronidazole plus a concurrent course of diloxanide furoate or diiodohydroxyquin. For patients requiring initial parenteral therapy, an intravenous preparation of metronidazole is available.

A tetracycline plus diloxanide furoate or diiodohydroxyquin usually provides an excellent alternative form of treatment. An additional alternative method, particularly for patients requiring initial parenteral therapy, is to give dehydroemetine (or emetine) intramuscularly or subcutaneously for the minimum number of days (usually 3–5; significant toxicity usually does not occur in this period) needed to control severe symptoms. Then start an oral course of a tetracycline plus diloxanide furoate or diiodohydroxyquin; follow these with a course of chloroquine.

Fluid and electrolyte therapy and opiates to control bowel motility are necessary adjuncts in severe amebic dysentery.

Hepatic Abscess

When metronidazole, the drug of choice, is given for 10 days, early or late treatment failure occurs rarely. If a satisfactory clinical response has not occurred within 2–3 days, especially if the abscess has been adequately drained, therapy should be changed to the alternative mode of treatment: dehydroemetine (or emetine) plus chloroquine. When the clinical response to metronidazole is adequate, it is suggested that a 2-week course of chloroquine follow to prevent late failures. The need for adding this course of chloroquine remains to be evaluated.

Since a comparative trial of metronidazole with and without aspiration has not been reported, the indications for therapeutic aspiration are still controversial. Aspiration is clearly indicated, however, when the diagnosis is in doubt, if rupture of a large abscess is impending, or if there is a lack of response to therapy.

Concurrent with either mode of abscess treatment, a course of diloxanide fuorate or diiodohydroxyquin should be given to eradicate intestinal infection.

Ameboma or Extraintestinal Disease

Metronidazole is the drug of choice. Dehydroemetine (or emetine) is an alternative drug; chloroquine is not included because it does not reach sufficiently high tissue concentrations (except in the liver) to be effective. A simultaneous course of a luminal amebicide should also be given.

CHLOROQUINE

The pharmacology, cautions, contraindications, and side-effects of chloroquine are described under malaria. In the treatment of amebiasis the drug is used both to eradicate and to prevent amebic liver abscess. Because chloroquine reaches high liver concentrations, it is highly effective in conjunction with dehydroemetine (or emetine) in the treatment of amebic liver abscess. In the prevention of liver abscess, chloroquine is used during the treatment of moderate to severe intestinal amebiasis (and in selected mild cases) to eradicate trophozoites carried to the liver or to treat undetected early abscesses there. The minimal dose needed to prevent an abscess is not well established, nor is the minimal indication for using chloroquine in abscess prevention, although invasive amebiasis as evidenced by mucosal ulceration would be a specific indication. Chloroquine is not used, however, in the treatment of the intestinal phase of amebiasis, because the drug is not active against luminal organisms and shows only moderate activity in amebic dysentery. Chloroquine is given in a loading dose of 500 mg (salt) twice daily for 2 days, which is followed by 250 mg twice daily for 1–3 weeks. When chloroquine is used in prophylaxis of liver abscess, a 1-week course is recommended during the treatment of mild to moderate intestinal infection, but a 2-week course is used for dysenteric cases. In the treatment of liver abscess, the drug is used for 3 weeks in conjunction with dehydroemetine (or emetine). At these dosage levels, the retinopathy sometimes associated with long-term use of chloroquine does not occur.

DEHYDROEMETINE

Racemic 2-dehydroemetine dihydrochloride, available since 1964, is a synthetic substance that can substitute for emetine as an equally effective and probably less toxic drug. Nevertheless, marked myocardial toxicity has been reported following use of the drug. In the USA, the drug is only available from the Parasitic Disease Drug Service, Centers for Disease Control, Atlanta 30333.

In laboratory animals, dehydroemetine is less toxic on an equal weight basis than emetine, although qualitatively their toxicities are alike. In humans, the therapeutic action of dehydroemetine is equal to that of emetine.

In experimental animals, dehydroemetine disappears more rapidly from the heart (but not from the liver) than emetine and is excreted more rapidly. If this also occurs in humans, it could account for the fewer electrocardiographic changes that dehydroemetine causes when identical doses of the 2 drugs are given as reported in some studies. However, Sharad and Vakil reported comparable cardiovascular toxicity for the 2 drugs. Thus, greater comparative clinical experience is needed to establish that dehydroemetine is indeed less toxic.

The clinical uses of dehydroemetine are similar to those of emetine: treatment of severe intestinal amebiasis, amebic liver abscess in conjunction with chloroquine, and extraintestinal amebic infections.

The adverse reactions, cautions, and contraindications are the same as for emetine.

Dehydroemetine is available for injection in 1- and 2-mL ampules containing 30 mg/mL. The dosage for severe intestinal disease is 1 mg/kg intramuscularly or subcutaneously daily for the least number of days necessary to control symptoms (usually 3–5 days). The maximum daily dose is 0.1 g. A tetracycline and diiodohydroxyquine or diloxanide furoate should be given in conjunction with or after dehydroemetine, and chloroquine should follow.

For liver abscess, dehydroemetine is given in conjunction with chloroquine; a course of a luminal amebicide should follow. The dosage of dehydroemetine is 1 mg/kg/d intramuscularly or subcutaneously for 8–10 days. The maximum daily dose is 0.1 g. For children and some adults, the daily dose is divided into 2 parts.

EMETINE HYDROCHLORIDE

Emetine hydrochloride, used for more than 70 years for the treatment of *Entamoeba histolytica* infection, remains one of the principal drugs used for the treatment of severe intestinal infection (amebic dysentery), liver abscess, and other forms of extraintestinal amebiasis. Emetine should not be used to treat asymptomatic or mild intestinal infections.

When available, use dehydroemetine rather than emetine, since the former is equally effective and may be less toxic.

Chemistry

Emetine can be derived from ipecac or synthesized. Since emetine has 4 asymmetric centers, several stereoisomers are possible, but the structure below is generally accepted as the configuration of the natural (−) alkaloid.

Emetine is usually prepared as the hydrochloride. To prevent deterioration, it should be protected from light.

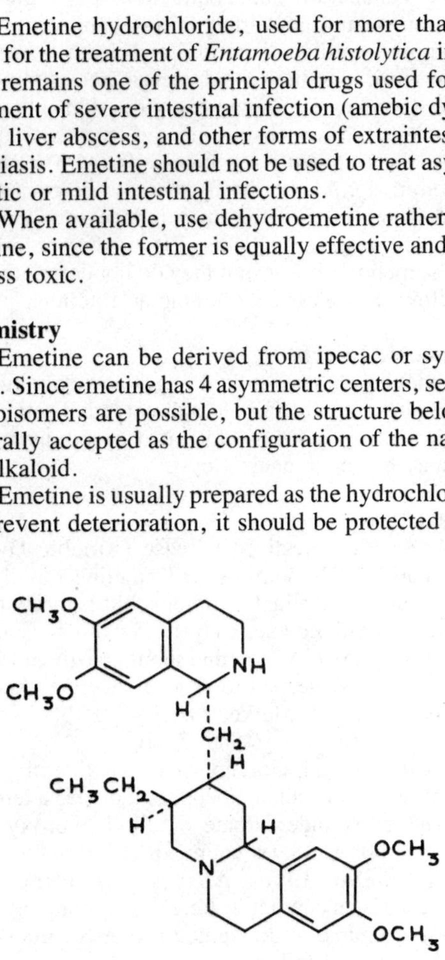

Emetine

Absorption, Metabolism, & Excretion

Emetine is administered parenterally, not orally, because it is absorbed erratically from the gastrointestinal tract and may induce emesis. When given parenterally, it is stored primarily in the liver, lungs, spleen, and kidneys; only a small amount is found in other tissues, including cardiac, striated, and intestinal muscle. Because emetine is eliminated slowly via the kidney, the drug is cumulative; trace amounts are detectable in the urine 1–2 months after stopping therapy.

Pharmacologic Effects

Emetine affects almost all tissues. It irreversibly blocks the synthesis of protein in eukaryotes by inhibiting the movement of the ribosome along messenger RNA; DNA synthesis is blocked secondarily. In experimental animals, emetine given parenterally in toxic doses causes cellular damage in the liver, kidneys, and skeletal and cardiac muscle. In the myocardium, cloudy swelling and necrosis of myocardial fibers occurs, with focal areas of cellular infiltration and interstitial proliferation resembling Aschoff bodies. Cardiac conduction and contraction are depressed, which may result in a variety of atrial and ventricular arrhythmias, cardiac dilatation, and death.

In vitro, emetine has adrenergic and cholinergic blocking actions. The antiadrenergic action of the drug in vivo may be responsible for the hypotension and diarrhea that frequently accompany its use. The nausea and vomiting common during therapy are considered central in origin. Emetine may reduce serum potassium levels in some patients. Elevated transaminase levels sometimes occur, but they do not correlate well with clinical or electrocardiographic findings.

Antiamebic Effects

Emetine in therapeutic dosages acts only against trophozoites, on which it has a direct lethal action. At high doses (beyond those tolerated by humans), the drug may be active against cysts.

Clinical Uses

A. Severe Intestinal Disease (Amebic Dysentery): Parenterally administered emetine rapidly alleviates severe intestinal symptoms but is rarely curative even if a full course is given. For this reason and because of its toxicity, emetine should be given for the minimum period needed to relieve severe symptoms (usually 3–5 days). Marked toxicity is unlikely when the drug is used for less than 7 days.

In addition to a short course of emetine, the regimen for severe intestinal amebiasis includes a tetracycline and diloxanide furoate or diiodohydroxyquin. These are followed by a course of chloroquine.

B. Amebic Liver Abscess: Emetine plus chloroquine is an alternative treatment for amebic liver abscess. A course of diloxanide furoate or diiodohydroxyquin should follow.

C. Amebomas and Extraintestinal Amebiasis: Emetine is effective in treating other forms of extraintestinal amebiasis and amebomas.

D. Other Parasites: Emetine has occasionally been useful in the treatment of infections with *Balantidium coli, Fasciola hepatica,* and *Paragonimus westermani,* but safer drugs should be used first.

Adverse Reactions

Emetine is cumulative in its toxic action. Few and (usually) mild side-effects appear if the drug is given for 3–5 days; additional mild to severe side-effects appear if the drug is given for up to 10 days; serious toxicity is common if it is given for more than 10 days. Therefore, use of emetine for more than 10 days is contraindicated. No fatalities have been reported after a single dose. Of the small number of deaths that have resulted from repeated doses, most were in patients given total doses of over 1200 mg; however, a few occurred when the total dose did not exceed the recommended limit of 650 mg over 10 days.

A. Local Reactions: Pain, tenderness, and muscle weakness in the area of the injection are frequent, often starting 24–48 hours after the injection, and may persist for 1–2 weeks. Occasionally, eczematous or purpuric lesions or sterile abscesses develop.

B. Gastrointestinal Effects: Transient nausea occurs in about 30% of patients; vomiting is infrequent. Diarrhea is induced or exacerbated in many patients, generally beginning several days after the onset of therapy. A course of treatment can usually be completed in spite of gastrointestinal symptoms, but if these are too severe, therapy must be discontinued.

C. Cardiovascular Effects: Minor electrocardiographic changes occur frequently, but severe cardiac toxicity with significant conduction defects is rare. The most serious symptoms and findings are tachycardia and other arrhythmias, precordial pain, and congestive heart failure with dyspnea and hypotension. Electrocardiographic changes induced in more than 50% of patients include flattening and inversion of P and T waves, lengthening of the P–R and Q–T intervals, ST elevation, premature beats, and transient atrial fibrillation. These changes usually appear about 7 days after the onset of treatment but occasionally not until 2–3 weeks after the last injection. They are generally reversible, requiring about 6 weeks to return to normal. In rare instances, emetine-induced abnormalities have persisted for several years.

D. Neuromuscular Effects: Generalized muscular weakness—sometimes associated with tenderness, stiffness, aching, or tremors—is reported by many patients. At therapeutic doses, the weakness is usually mild and reversible, but it may persist for several weeks after treatment is stopped. These symptoms are attributed to a direct action of emetine on the muscles and not to neuritis. Although mild paresthesias are reported by patients, a true polyneuritis with objective signs of nerve damage occurs rarely, if ever.

E. Other Side-Effects: Many other mild and often transient side-effects may occur, including fatigue, headache, dizziness, and urticarial, eczematous, or purpuric skin lesions. Proteinuria may also be present.

Contraindications & Cautions

Since emetine is a potentially dangerous drug, careful hospital supervision is essential. Considerable caution should be observed to avoid dangerous inadvertent intravenous administration.

Patients should be kept at bed rest with bathroom privileges during treatment and for several days afterward. They should be examined daily for cardiovascular, neuromuscular, and gastrointestinal signs or symptoms. Pulse and blood pressure should be recorded 3 times a day and electrocardiograms taken prior to the first injection, on the fifth and tenth days of therapy, and weekly for 2 weeks after the last injection.

The drug should be discontinued if the resting pulse (or, particularly, the sleeping pulse) exceeds 110/min (correct for fever) or if marked hypotension, precordial pain, marked gastrointestinal symptoms (especially bloody diarrhea), prostration, or marked neuromuscular symptoms develop. Generalized weakness and muscular aching (to be distinguished from local reactions due to injections) tend to develop before more serious toxic symptoms and thus can be used as a guide for avoiding overdosage.

Electrocardiographic criteria for discontinuing therapy have not been established. Some clinicians believe that prolongation of the P–R, QRS, or Q–T interval is an indication for stopping treatment; ectopic rhythms, although rare, clearly require cessation of therapy.

Patients should remain sedentary for about 4 weeks after completion of therapy, and surgery is inadvisable for at least 6 weeks after administration of emetine.

Great care should be exercised in administering the drug to aged or debilitated people; dosage is usually reduced by half for such patients.

Emetine should not be used in patients with cardiac or renal disease, in those with a recent history of polyneuritis, or in young children, unless alternative drugs have not been effective in controlling severe dysentery or liver abscess. Emetine should not be used during pregnancy.

Preparations & Dosages

Aqueous solutions of emetine hydrochloride are supplied in ampules containing 32 or 65 mg.

The daily dose of emetine for adults and children is 1 mg/kg subcutaneously (preferred) or intramuscularly. The maximum daily dose for adults is 65 mg; for children under 8 years, 10 mg. For children and some adults, the daily dose is divided into 2 parts.

For the treatment of severe intestinal disease, injections are generally given for the minimum number of days needed to control severe symptoms, generally 3–5 days. See under Clinical Uses for additional drugs needed to complete the course of therapy.

For the treatment of hepatic abscess, other extraintestinal disease, and ameboma, the same doses of emetine are used but for a total of 8–10 days.

If a second course of therapy is needed, an intervening period of 6–8 weeks is required.

DILOXANIDE FUROATE (Furamide)

Diloxanide furoate was introduced in 1957 and has since been extensively used outside the USA for the treatment of intestinal amebiasis. The drug is not effective in the treatment of extraintestinal amebiasis. In the USA, diloxanide furoate is only available from the Parasitic Disease Drug Service, Centers for Disease Control, Atlanta 30333, (404) 329–3670.

Chemistry

Diloxanide furoate (Furamide), a substituted acetanilide, is the furoic acid ester of diloxanide (Entamide). It is nearly insoluble in water. For stability, it should be protected from light.

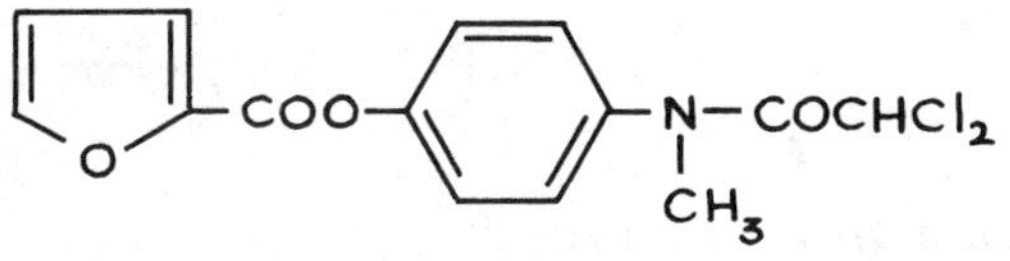

Diloxanide furoate

Pharmacology & Anthelmintic Action

Diloxanide furoate is directly amebicidal, but its mode of action is not known. The acute oral toxicity in rats is a function of age and sex; the LD50 ranges from 0.5 to 9.6 g/kg. A dose of 0.75 g/kg to pregnant rats or rabbits resulted, for some animals, in abortion or death. No teratogenic effects were observed.

Absorption, Metabolism, & Excretion

In the gut, diloxanide furoate is split into diloxanide and furoic acid; about 90% of the diloxanide is rapidly absorbed and then conjugated to form the glucuronide. The glucuronide reaches a peak blood level within about 1 hour, drops to low levels within 6 hours, and is rapidly excreted in the urine. The unabsorbed diloxanide is the active antiamebic substance and is not attacked by gut bacteria.

Clinical Uses

Diloxanide furoate is only effective in the treatment of intestinal amebiasis. Although sufficient comparative studies are not available, the drug's effectiveness is apparently not appreciably different from the other luminal amebicides, diiodohydroxyquin (iodoquinol) and paromomycin, but it is probably the least toxic of the three.

Diloxanide furoate is most effective in asymptomatic to mild intestinal infection and is less effective in moderate to severe intestinal disease. It is used alone as a drug of choice in the treatment of asymptomatic infections. For patients having intestinal symptoms, diloxanide furoate is used in conjunction with other drugs as shown in Table 54–3. It is not yet clear if diloxanide furoate combined with a tetracycline is more effective than when it is used alone. Chloroquine is given with diloxanide furoate to prevent the development of amebic liver abscess. In the treatment of liver abscess, diloxanide is added to the regimen in order to eradicate intestinal infection.

When diloxanide furoate was used alone in the treatment of asymptomatic and mildly symptomatic cyst-passers at a dosage of 20 mg/kg for 5–10 days, reported cure rates were 90–100% for studies conducted in temperate areas and 80–90% for studies in tropical areas. In studies of patients with moderate to severe intestinal disease, cure rates were 75–90%; however, when diloxanide furoate and metronidazole were combined, cure rates of 98% have been reported.

Adverse Reactions, Contraindications, & Cautions

Diloxanide furoate is free of serious side-effects. Flatulence is common. Nausea and abdominal cramps are infrequent. Esophagitis, dryness of the mouth, vomiting, persistent diarrhea, pruritus, urticaria, proteinuria, and a vague tingling sensation are rarely reported.

The drug should not be used in pregnancy or administered to children under 2 years of age.

Preparations & Dosages

Diloxanide furoate (Furamide) is given orally with meals, 500 mg 3 times daily for 10 days. The drug is supplied as 500-mg tablets. The dosage for children is 20 mg/kg orally divided into 3 doses and given for 10 days. A course of treatment may be repeated in several weeks if necessary.

THE HALOGENATED HYDROXYQUINOLINES
Diiodohydroxyquin (Iodoquinol), Iodochlorhydroxyquin (Clioquinol)

The halogenated hydroxyquinolines were among the first synthetic drugs active in amebiasis. Iodochlorhydroxyquin (introduced in 1931) and diiodohydroxyquin (introduced in 1936) are effective against organisms in the bowel lumen but not against trophozoites in the intestinal wall or extraintestinal tissues.

Chemistry

Three synthetic halogen-substituted 8-hydroxyquinolines have had extensive clinical use—chiniofon (8-hydroxy-7-iodoquinoline-5-sulfonic acid), iodochlorhydroxyquin (clioquinol) (5-chloro-8-hydroxy-7-iodoquinoline), and diiodohydroxyquin (iodoquinol) (8-hydroxy-5,7-diiodoquinoline). Iodochlorhydroxyquin contains approximately 40% iodine and 12% chlorine, and diiodohydroxyquin contains approximately 64% iodine.

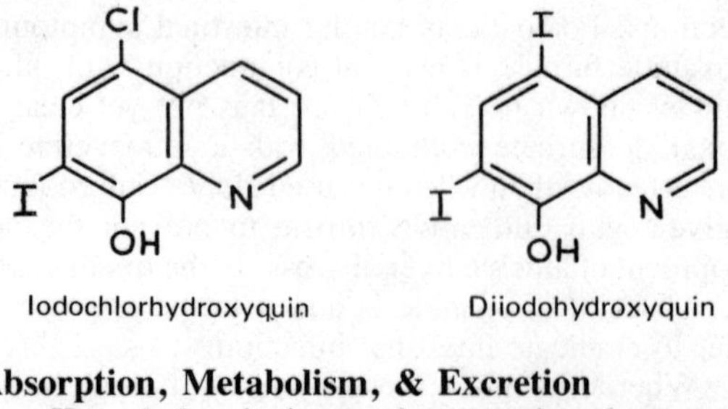

Iodochlorhydroxyquin   Diiodohydroxyquin

Absorption, Metabolism, & Excretion

Knowledge is incomplete on the pharmacokinetics of the hydroxyquinolines. Iodochlorhydroxyquin is more readily absorbed than diiodohydroxyquin. Metabolic studies in humans using ^{14}C-iodochlorhydroxyquin indicated that maximal plasma concentrations were reached at 4 hours after administration of a single dose and then decreased, with an apparent half-life of between 11 and 14 hours. Approximately 25% of a single 750-mg oral dose was excreted in the urine over 72 hours. Use of radioactive iodochlorhydroxyquin in animals showed high uptake of the drug in visceral tissues.

The drugs may interfere with certain thyroid function tests by increasing protein-bound serum iodine levels, leading to a decrease in ^{131}I uptake.

Antiamebic Effects

The mechanism of action of diiodohydroxyquin and iodochlorhydroxyquin against amebas is not known. Opinions vary on whether the drugs act only against trophozoites or against cysts as well.

Clinical Uses

A. Intestinal Amebiasis: Diiodohydroxyquin and iodochlorhydroxyquin are alternative drugs for the treatment of asymptomatic or mild to moderate intestinal amebiasis. However, until the question of the association of iodochlorhydroxyquin with the SMON syndrome (see below) is resolved, only diiodohydroxyquin should be used in therapy. The drugs are not effective in the initial treatment of severe intestinal disease but are used in the subsequent eradication of the infection. They are not effective against amebomas or extraintestinal forms of the disease, including hepatic amebiasis, but are used in the eradication of concurrent intestinal infection. Reported cure rates for each of the 2 compounds are as high as 80%. Diiodohydroxyquin may cause less diarrhea and gastric irritation than iodochlorhydroxyquin.

B. *Trichomonas vaginalis* Vaginitis: Iodochlorhydroxyquin, given in vaginal inserts or insufflation powders, has been used for the topical treatment of this infection.

C. Other Intestinal Parasites: Diiodohydroxyquin (650 mg 3 times daily for 10 days) when used alone or in conjunction with a tetracycline (250 mg 4 times daily for 7 days) provides adequate treatment for *Dientamoeba fragilis* infections. Diiodohydroxyquin has been reported also to be effective in the treatment of some cases of *Giardia lamblia* and *Balantidium coli* infection.

D. Travelers' Diarrhea and Nonspecific Diarrhea: Neither drug should be used in the prophylaxis or treatment of travelers' diarrhea or for the treatment of chronic nonspecific diarrhea in children and adults.

Adverse Reactions

Evidence is increasing that certain halogenated hydroxyquinolines can produce neurotoxicity, particularly if the drugs are given at greater than recommended doses and for long periods of time. The principal findings associated with this level of use are optic atrophy, visual loss, and peripheral neuropathy. Although these adverse reactions usually improve when the drug is discontinued, some patients have experienced irreversible neurologic damage.

Diiodohydroxyquin has not been implicated in producing neurotoxic side-effects when used at the standard dosage of 650 mg 3 times daily for 21 days.

Mild and infrequent side-effects at the standard dosage include diarrhea, which usually stops after several days, and nausea and vomiting, gastritis, abdominal discomfort, constipation, pruritus ani, headache, malaise, and slight enlargement of the thyroid gland. Rarely reported side-effects have been agranulocytosis, discoloration of hair or nails, hair loss, and iodine sensitivity characterized by furunculosis, chills, fever, and a variety of mild to severe skin reactions. Diiodohydroxyquin may be more toxic for infants and young children.

Formerly, when diiodohydroxyquin was given at high doses and for long periods of time to young children with acrodermatitis enteropathica (1200–3300 mg daily for 2–24 months), at least 7 cases of optic atrophy occurred, with decreased visual acuity or blindness.

Iodochlorhydroxyquin was considered nearly free of significant side-effects at the standard dosage (250 mg 3 times daily for 10 days) until the question arose—as yet unresolved—about the drug's etiologic relationship to the SMON syndrome (described below). Infrequent side-effects from iodochlorhydroxyquin are the same as described for diiodohydroxyquin. The risk of neurotoxicity, however, appears to be greater and to increase with increasing dosage. At dosages of 750–1500 mg/d for less than 2 weeks, about 1% of patients had neurotoxic symptoms; at the same dosages given for over 2 weeks, symptoms appeared in approximately 35% of patients.

Controversy continues about whether a serious new neurologic disease reported from Japan was due to the widespread use there of iodochlorhydroxyquin, to a newly isolated virus, or to other factors. The syndrome is subacute myelo-optic neuropathy (SMON), characterized by chronic abdominal symptoms, peripheral polyneuritis with dysesthesia and weakness in the lower extremities, optic atrophy, and disturbances of vision. Evidence for the association of the drug with the disease included retrospective studies, animal experimental studies, the improvement of symptoms in individual patients when use of the drug was stopped, and the abrupt cessation of the epidemic with withdrawal of hydroxyquinoline drugs from the market. It is not yet possible to reach a conclusion about the cause of SMON syndrome or the risk to be attributed to the use of iodochlorhydroxyquin.

Contraindications & Cautions

The halogenated hydroxyquinolines should no longer be used for the prophylaxis or treatment of travelers' diarrhea or nonspecific diarrhea, and worldwide the drugs should be made available only on a prescription basis. When used for the treatment of amebiasis, they should be taken for the prescribed period of time and dosage.

The drugs should be discontinued when they produce a persistent diarrhea or signs of iodine reactions. They are contraindicated in patients with known intolerance to iodine, in renal and thyroid disease, and probably in severe liver disease not due to amebiasis.

When the drugs are used for young children, careful ophthalmologic assessment should be made before and during the course of therapy.

Preparations & Dosages

The drugs are taken orally after meals. A course should not be repeated without an intervening period of 2–3 weeks.

A. Diiodohydroxyquin, Iodoquinol (Embequin, Lanodoxin, Savorquin, Sebaquin, Yodoxin): Diiodohydroxyquin is available as uncoated tablets containing 210 mg and 650 mg. The adult dosage is 650 mg orally 3 times a day for 21 days. The pediatric dosage is 10 mg/kg 3 times a day for 21 days. The medication is well accepted by young children when it is crushed and mixed with applesauce or chocolate syrup.

B. Iodochlorhydroxyquin, Clioquinol (Entero-Vioform, Nioform, Vioform): Iodochlorhydroxyquin is available as enteric-coated tablets or vaginal inserts containing 250 mg and as a powder for vaginal insufflation. The oral dosage is 250 mg 3 times a day for 10 days. In the USA and many other countries, the drug has been withdrawn from the market pending further study of its toxicity.

THE ARSENICALS

The pentavalent arsenical drugs carbarsone and glycobiarsol have been used for many years for the treatment of amebiasis, but their potential toxicity no longer warrants their inclusion as alternative drugs for the treatment of intestinal infections.

The side-effects of glycobiarsol and carbarsone are due to arsenical reactions. Although infrequent, the most common signs and symptoms are nausea and vomiting, diarrhea, epigastric distress, and skin rashes, which start after several days of therapy. More severe toxicity includes weight loss and polyuria. Exfoliative dermatitis, agranulocytosis, encephalitis, and hepatitis are very rare; a few fatalities have been reported.

METRONIDAZOLE (Flagyl)

Metronidazole, introduced in 1959 for the treatment of trichomoniasis, was approved in the USA in 1971 for the treatment of amebiasis. Metronidazole is an excellent drug for the eradication of amebic tissue infections (liver abscess, intestinal wall and extraintestinal infections), but it requires the concomitant use of a luminal amebicide to achieve satisfactory cure rates for luminal infections. In vitro studies show that metronidazole kills trophozoites but does not kill cysts of *Entamoeba histolytica*.

Metronidazole has been reported to increase the incidence of certain naturally occurring tumors in mice and rats given high doses over long periods of time and to induce mutagenic changes in bacterial test systems (see p 594). Metronidazole has not been shown to be teratogenic in animals or humans, but the data are not sufficient to rule this out. Overall, it appears prudent to judge metronidazole as a potentially hazardous drug.

The chemistry, pharmacokinetics, adverse reactions, and contraindications and cautions of this drug are described on pp 593–594.

Clinical Uses

A. Severe Intestinal Disease (Amebic Dysentery): The suggested dosage is 750 mg 3 times daily for 10 days, plus a course of a luminal amebicide.

B. Liver Abscess: For the treatment of hepatic abscess, a standard regimen of metronidazole is 750 mg 3 times daily for 10 days; however, the 5-day course is also highly effective. A course of a luminal amebicide should be added to enhance eradication of luminal organisms. Metronidazole has 2 advantages over emetine, dehydroemetine, and chloroquine for the treatment of liver abscess. It has less short-term toxicity than emetine or dehydroemetine and, unlike them, is moderately effective against luminal organisms. In one report on amebic liver abscess therapy, 58 of 60 patients were cured by the combination of metronidazole treatment plus aspiration. Subsequent case reports by others suggest occasional metronidazole failures within a few days of starting treatment or weeks later—whether or not the abscess was aspirated.

C. Ameboma and Extraintestinal Infections: Treat as for intestinal disease. However, cure rates for these conditions using metronidazole have not been well determined.

Preparations & Dosage

Metronidazole (Flagyl) is marketed as 250-mg tablets for oral use. The dosage for children is 35–50 mg/kg of body weight divided into 3 doses and given orally for 10 days. The tablets have a bitter taste and are often difficult for children to accept. A tasteless oral suspension of benzoyl metronidazole appears to be equally effective. An intravenous preparation is available (see the manufacturer's recommendations for dosage), but it should be used only until the patient can resume taking the medication orally. The effectiveness of metronidazole administered by rectal suppository remains to be determined.

OTHER NITROIMIDAZOLES

Other nitroimidazole derivatives include tinidazole, nimorazole, secondizole, and ornidazole. They have similar side-effects and the same mutagenic action in the *Salmonella* test systems as metronidazole. Because of its short half-life, metronidazole must be administered every 8 hours; other drugs such as tinidazole and secondizole can be administered at longer intervals. However, with the exception of tinidazole, the other nitroimidazoles have given poorer results than metronidazole.

PAROMOMYCIN SULFATE

Paromomycin sulfate, a broad-spectrum antibiotic, is also used in the treatment of intestinal amebiasis and tapeworm infections. It is an aminoglycoside derived from *Streptomyces rimosus* and is closely related to neomycin, kanamycin, and streptomycin in properties and structure. Paromomycin is directly amebicidal in addition to its indirect effect through the inhibition of normal bacteria.

Because paromycin is not significantly absorbed from the gastrointestinal tract, it can only be used as a luminal amebicide and has no effect in extraintestinal amebic infections. The small amount absorbed is excreted slowly and unchanged, mainly by glomerular filtration; some excretion also occurs in the bile. In the presence of ulcerative lesions of the bowel, however, and perhaps with impaired gastrointestinal motility, increased absorption may occur. In renal insufficiency, the drug may accumulate and reach a toxic level.

Mild gastrointestinal side-effects are not uncommon. The number of stools increase; diarrhea, sometimes intense, has been reported in up to 16% of patients. Less frequent are anorexia, nausea and vomiting, epigastric pain, abdominal cramps, and pruritus ani. Other occasional side-effects are headache, dizziness, rashes, and arthralgia. Paromomycin can cause malabsorption as well as overgrowth of nonsusceptible organisms, particularly fungi. The aminoglycosides as a group can be ototoxic (auditory and vestibular) and nephrotoxic as a result of unexpected absorption; theoretically, paromomycin has similar potential, but such reactions have apparently not been reported.

Paromomycin is an alternative drug used in the treatment of asymptomatic and mild intestinal infection. Some workers combine it with a course of diiodohydroxyquine. It has also been used, with variable success, in more severe intestinal disease. The drug is contraindicated in patients with impaired renal function, ulcerative bowel lesions, and intestinal obstruction. In intestinal amebiasis with severe ulceration, paromomycin should not be used because of the risk of increased absorption.

Paromomycin sulfate (Humatin) is administered orally, after meals, at 25–30 mg/kg of body weight (maximum 3 g); the daily dose is divided into 3 parts and given for 5–10 days. The pediatric dose is the same as the adult dose. The drug is supplied in 250-mg capsules and as syrup containing 125 mg/5 mL. The above doses are expressed as the base.

OTHER ANTIBIOTICS

Although the tetracyclines have very weak direct amebicidal action, through their effects on the gut flora they (especially oxytetracycline) are useful in conjunction with a luminal amebicide in the eradication of mild to severe intestinal disease. However, because of their potential toxicity, the tetracyclines should not be used during pregnancy or in the treatment of children under 8 years of age; when an antibiotic is needed in the treatment of amebiasis for these patients, erythromycin stearate, although somewhat less effective, can be used instead.

THE TREATMENT OF LEISHMANIASIS

Leishmaniasis includes a variety of diseases produced by protozoal parasites of the genus *Leishmania* of the family Trypanosomidae. They are transmitted to humans by the bite of several different species of phlebotomine (flesh-eating) flies, which carry the parasites directly from human to human or from infected rodents or canines to humans. Different varieties of *Leishmania* produce different lesions and require different treatments. The diseases produced by *Leishmania tropica* and *Leishmania mexicana* are characterized by cutaneous lesions only, which usually undergo a spontaneous cure. Infection with *Leishmania braziliensis* (mucocutaneous leishmaniasis) causes large destructive ulcers of the mucous membranes that rarely undergo spontaneous cure. *Leishmania donovani* (visceral leishmaniasis, dumdum fever, tropical splenomegaly, black sickness, ponos) produces a small primary sore, often ignored, followed by hematogenous spread, causing massive enlargement of the spleen and often of the liver and recurring bouts of fever resembling brucellosis. Disease caused by *L donovani* requires hospitalization, correction of the accompanying malnutrition, and specific drug therapy (the choice of drug depending on the geographic location where the disease was encountered) with one or a combination of pentavalent antimonials and one of the aromatic diamidines. The pentavalent antimonial drugs are discussed in Chapter 55.

OTHER DRUGS USED FOR THE TREATMENT OF LEISHMANIASIS

Amphotericin B (Fungizone), 25–50 mg in 500 mL of 5% glucose-saline solution, given by slow intravenous drip on alternate days for periods of weeks and even months, has led to complete healing of lesions of mucocutaneous leishmaniasis that were resistant to antimony therapy.

The suggested daily dose of amphotericin B is 0.25–1 mg/kg. (For toxicity, see Chapter 47.) Amphotericin B may be more potent as a leishmanicide than the antimonials.

Cures of *L braziliensis* and *L tropica* infections have also been obtained with intramuscular injections of the antimalarial repository drug **cycloguanil embonate** (cycloguanil pamoate), an insoluble salt of the dihydrotriazine metabolite of chloroguanide (proguanil). One or 2 intramuscular injections of 350 mg (2.5 mL) of the base have given cure rates of up to 85%.

Oral **dehydroemetine resinate (Mebadin)** in doses of 1.5 mg/kg orally after meals (to a total dose of 0.85–7 g) gave a 70% cure rate of *L tropica* infections in a study carried out in Iraq.

Metronidazole (Flagyl), 250 mg twice daily orally for 15 days, produced an excellent cure rate of Mexican cutaneous leishmaniasis.

Local injection of mepacrine or antimony compounds into the edges of mucocutaneous ulcers, accompanied by 10 injections of neostibosan on alternate days, is often used.

Nifurtimox (Lampit),* a nitrofurazone derivative now used to destroy the extracellular trypanosomes in trypanosomiasis, has also been successfully used to treat mucocutaneous leishmaniasis in doses of 8–10 mg/kg daily for 3–5 weeks.

THE TREATMENT OF TRYPANOSOMIASIS

THE AROMATIC DIAMIDINES: PENTAMIDINE, STILBAMIDINE, & PROPAMIDINE

History

Pentamidine, stilbamidine, and propamidine are the only aromatic diamidine derivatives that are sufficiently potent as trypanosomicides and have toxicities low enough to be used for the treatment of trypanosomiasis (sleeping sickness). Pentamidine is now the drug of choice for the treatment and prevention of *Trypanosoma rhodesiense* and *Trypanosoma gambiense* infection and is an alternative to sodium stibogluconate for the treatment of leishmaniasis. Propamidine and the dihydroxyl derivative of stilbamidine are occasionally used.

Chemistry

Pentamidine isethionate (Lomidine, M&B 800) is a 4,4′-diamidinophenoxypentane. It is a white, hydroscopic, crystalline powder soluble 1:10 in water.

*In the USA, nifurtimox is called Bayer 2502 and is available only from the Centers for Disease Control, Atlanta 30333.

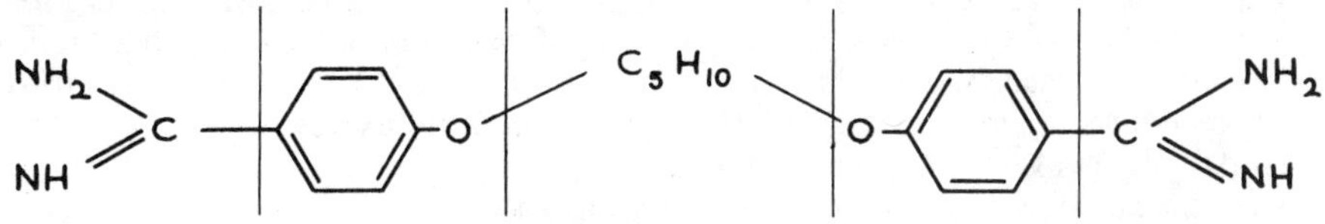

Pentamidine

The in vitro trypanosomicidal activity of the guanidine derivatives is associated with the terminal amidine and guanidine groups, and the activity is maximal when the amidine groups are connected by an undecane methylene chain.

Absorption, Metabolism, & Excretion

Diamidine compounds are not well absorbed from the gastrointestinal tract, but absorption after parenteral administration is satisfactory. Following intravenous injection, the drug rapidly leaves the circulation and only small amounts appear in the urine. The liver, spleen, kidneys, and adrenals maintain high levels of the diamidines for months after treatment. Single injections of pentamidine can prevent infection by *T gambiense* for up to 6 months. A portion of the drug is metabolized in the body, and part is excreted in the urine. Intermediary metabolic products are not known.

Diamidine compounds cross the placenta but are not excreted in milk. Only trace amounts appear in the central nervous system, so that other trypanosomicides such as tryparsamide or one of the melanyl arsenicals must be used for the treatment of late stages of African trypanosomiasis with central nervous system involvement.

Pharmacologic Effects

The aromatic diamidines are highly toxic to certain species of protozoa and only slightly toxic to others. *T rhodesiense* and *T gambiense* infections in humans can be cured with pentamidine, but the drug has no effect on *Trypanosoma cruzi* infection in mice. The diamidines have some plasmocidal, bactericidal, and fungicidal activity and have been used for the treatment of systemic blastomycosis.

Intravenous injections of the diamidines produce a sharp fall of blood pressure that can be only partially blocked by atropine. The peripheral vasodilatation is probably due to a release of tissue-bound histamine and peripheral adrenergic blockade.

After injection of a diamidine drug, the trypanosomes quickly take up the drug to a concentration about 1400 times that of the surrounding tissues. Trypanosomicidal effects appear only after a long latent period. The trypanosomicidal action of the diamidines is antagonized by glucose, and the addition of insulin to cultures slows trypanosome multiplication. Diamidines may interfere with glycolysis in a susceptible protozoon.

Clinical Uses

Pentamidine is the drug of choice for the prevention and treatment of *T gambiense* infections. In the early stages, pentamidine can clear the organisms from the blood and lymph nodes. Diamidines cannot be given intrathecally and do not reach the central nervous system in sufficient quantities to have any therapeutic effect. Thus, other drugs such as melarsoprol or suramin must be used. In early trypanosomiasis, propamidine and stilbamidine can also be employed.

The diamidines are also used for visceral leishmaniasis (kala-azar) in patients who do not respond to or cannot tolerate antimonials.

Adverse Reactions

The diamidines may result in initial respiratory stimulation followed by respiratory depression. Intravenous injections usually produce a fall in blood pressure, dizziness, and headache together with breathlessness, tachycardia, and vomiting. Respiratory failure and death occur rarely.

The diamidines are nephrotoxic and occasionally neurotoxic, causing nystagmus, ataxia, convulsions, and death.

Delayed toxicity of stilbamidine (but not pentamidine) consists of paralysis of the trigeminal nerve and other peripheral neuropathies.

Preparations & Dosages

Pentamidine isethionate (Lomidine) is not licensed in the USA, although it is available in countries where trypanosomiasis is still endemic. Both pentamidine and nifurtimox may be obtained from the Centers for Disease Control (CDC), Atlanta 30333, for use on an investigational basis, with CDC acting as the "investigator."

For the early stages of *T rhodesiense* and *T gambiense* infections, pentamidine, 4 mg/kg intramuscularly, is given every 1–2 days for 10 doses. For chemoprophylaxis, give 3 mg/kg intramuscularly every 3–6 months.

For *L donovani* infections (kala-azar, visceral leishmaniasis), give pentamidine, 2–4 mg/kg intravenously or intramuscularly daily for up to 15 days.

For the late central nervous system stages of *T rhodesiense* and *T gambiense* infections, melarsoprol must be given.

MELARSOPROL

Melarsoprol (Mel B), an organic arsenical, is a 2-*p*-(4,6-diamino-1,3,5-triazin-2-ylamino)phenyl-4-hydroxymethyl-1,3,2-dithoarsolan.

Pharmacologic Effects

Melarsoprol is formed by condensing a toxic trivalent arsenical trypanosomicide (melarsen oxide) with an arsenic antagonist (BAL [dimercaprol]). In the product, the trypanosomicidal activity is retained while the toxicity of arsenic is mitigated. Its mode of action is probably related to an interaction with the sulfhydryl groups of enzymes essential to trypanosome metabolism.

Absorption, Metabolism, & Excretion

Melarsoprol is well absorbed from the gastrointestinal tract, but it is given only intravenously. The drug is quickly excreted.

Clinical Uses

Melarsoprol has now replaced tryparsamide (a

pentavalent arsenical) as the drug of choice for the treatment of *T gambiense* infection (African sleeping sickness). Tryparsamide, used for 50 years to control epidemics of trypanosomiasis, had an unfortunate tendency to cause optic atrophy.

Unlike pentamidine, melarsoprol appears in the cerebrospinal fluid in sufficient amounts to exert a trypanosomicidal effect on the late meningoencephalitic stages of human trypanosomiasis. It is also effective in the earlier stages of the disease, but it is used only for the rare pentamidine-refractory cases.

Adverse Effects

The most serious side-effect of melarsoprol therapy, usually occurring at the end of the first week of therapy, is a reactive encephalopathy that may be fatal. Patients in the most advanced stages of the disease are most severely affected.

If the intravenous injections are given too fast, vomiting and colicky abdominal pains occur.

Hypersensitivity reactions can be relieved with corticosteroids.

Preparations & Dosages

Melarsoprol (Mel B) is available for intravenous injection as a solution containing 3.6% (w/v) in propylene glycol. For the therapy of the late stages of *T rhodesiense* and *T gambiense* infections, three 3-day courses are given with an interval of 7 days between courses. Daily injections of 90 mg are given very slowly for the first 3 days; 90–180 mg for the second 3-day course; and 180 mg for the last 3-day course.

Leakage at injection sites causes intense pain and sometimes sloughing.

In the USA, melarsoprol is available only from the Centers for Disease Control, Atlanta 30333.

OTHER TRYPANOSOMICIDAL DRUGS

NIFURTIMOX
(Bayer 2502, Lampit)

Nifurtimox, a nitrofurazone derivative, is the drug of choice for acute Chagas' disease *(T cruzi)*. However, serious allergic skin reactions, gastrointestinal disturbances, and neurologic toxicities are frequently noted. In chronic forms of Chagas' disease, the toxicity may outweigh the drug's usefulness.

SURAMIN
(Bayer 205, Belganyl, Germanin, Naphuride)

Suramin sodium, an organic urea compound available in the USA only from the Centers for Disease Control, is the drug of choice for the early stages of African trypanosomiasis before there is any central nervous system involvement. It is also the drug of choice for the adult forms of the filarial parasite *Onchocerca volvulus* (see Chapter 55). It is of no value in the treatment of Chagas' disease.

TREATMENT OF TRICHOMONIASIS & GIARDIASIS

METRONIDAZOLE
(Flagyl)

Metronidazole is the result of a search for an effective trichomonicidal agent by French workers in the 1950s. It was not approved for use in the USA until 1963, but since then it has become the drug of choice for *Trichomonas vaginalis* infection in females and for the asymptomatic carrier state in males. It is also the drug of choice for treatment of intestinal infections with *Giardia lamblia,* another motile protozoon.

Chemistry & Pharmacokinetics

Metronidazole is 1-(2-hydroxyethyl)-2-methyl-5-nitroimidazole, a crystalline nonhygroscopic powder only slightly soluble in water or ethanol.

Metronidazole is a low-molecular-weight compound that is un-ionized at physiologic pH. Eighty percent of the oral dose is absorbed within 1 hour. Food intake does not influence its bioavailability, and the half-life of the unchanged drug is 7½ hours. Impaired renal function does not prolong the half-life, but impaired hepatic function may do so. Peak plasma concentrations are not achieved until 5–12 hours after administration by rectal suppository. Protein binding is minimal.

Because of its small molecular size, metronidazole permeates all the tissues and fluids of the body, including cerebrospinal fluid and alveolar bone, and the intracellular concentration rapidly approaches extracellular concentrations. Entry into the cell is by simple diffusion and not by active transport.

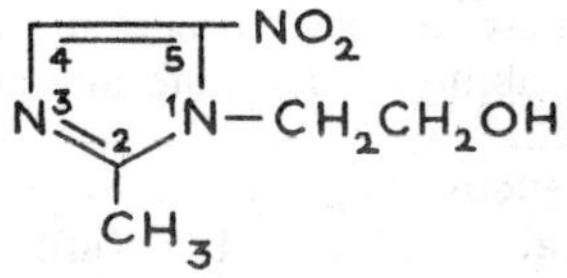

Metronidazole

Mechanism of Action

Within anaerobic bacteria and sensitive protozoal cells, the nitro group of metronidazole is chemically reduced by ferredoxin (or ferredoxin-linked metabolic processes), and the reduction products appear to be responsible for killing the cell by reacting with various intracellular macromolecules. Thus, reduction is the driving force for the selective toxicity in anaerobic cells. Metronidazole is actively bactericidal (not bacteriostatic) in susceptible organisms. Metronidazole's narrow spectrum of activity, largely limited to anaerobic bacteria and certain protozoa, does not encourage the overgrowth of antibiotic-resistant aerobes or facultative anaerobes and should not facilitate the transmission of drug-resistance factors. However, there is some evidence for an additional aerobic antibacterial effect in mixed anaerobic/aerobic infections. Severe vaginitis caused by *Gardnerella (Haemophilus) vaginalis* (an aerobic bacterium) is clinically improved by treatment with metronidazole when other antibiotics have failed.

Metronidazole also has a radiosensitizing effect on tumor cells. This effect has been demonstrated in vitro and in rodents in vivo. As with its antibacterial action, the mechanism of action appears to be dependent on relative hypoxia in the target cells and may involve interaction with free radicals.

Clinical Uses

A. Urogenital Trichomoniasis: The treatment of choice is metronidazole, 250 mg orally 3 times a day for 7 days. A single dose of 2 g (8 tablets) is also effective. The sexual partner should be treated simultaneously. In pregnancy, treatment with metronidazole should be delayed until after the first trimester. Metronidazole-resistant strains of *T vaginalis* have been described.

B. Giardiasis: The adult dosage of metronidazole is 250 mg orally 3 times a day for 7 days. Children should receive 5 mg/kg 3 times a day for 5 days.

C. Amebiasis: See p 589.

D. Balantidiasis: If tetracycline is ineffective, give metronidazole, 750 mg 3 times a day for 7 days.

E. *Gardnerella (Haemophilus) Vaginalis:* In refractory infections only, give metronidazole, 500 mg orally twice a day for 5 days.

F. Anaerobic Infections: Metronidazole has been reported to reduce postoperative anaerobic infections following procedures such as appendectomy, colorectal surgery, and abdominal hysterectomy. Furthermore, serious anaerobic infections involving *Bacillus fragilis* and clostridia that are refractory to other agents may respond to metronidazole, in part because of its ability to penetrate into abscesses and necrotic tissue.

G. Phagedenic Leg Ulcers, Acute Ulcerative Gingivitis, Cancrum Oris, Decubitus Ulcers, and Other Indolent Lesions: Metronidazole, 250 mg orally 4 times a day, together with a penicillin or sulfonamide and appropriate topical treatment, promotes healing and provides rapid relief of pain, inflammatory edema, and purulent discharge. Anaerobic cultures of pus from these lesions often reveal fusobacteria and gram-positive cocci in addition to *B fragilis*.

Toxicity

Minor side-effects of metronidazole include a metallic taste, glossitis, oral candidiasis, nausea and vomiting, and headache. The urine may be dark or reddish-brown in color.

Serious toxic effects are very uncommon. However, neurotoxic effects—including dizziness and ataxia—and leukopenia have been reported. Both effects are fully reversible when the drug is withdrawn. Metronidazole also has a disulfiramlike effect, so that nausea and vomiting occur if alcohol is consumed while the drug is still in the body.

Mutagenicity & Carcinogenicity

Metronidazole and its metabolites recovered from the urine of patients taking the drug have been proved by in vitro assays to be mutagenic in certain strains of *Salmonella typhimurium* (Ames test). Chronic oral administration of very large doses to mice has produced a statistically significant increase in the number of lung and liver tumors. This effect has not been found in any nonrodent species. In humans, despite millions of doses that have been given during pregnancy for the distressing symptoms of *T vaginalis* infections, no adverse effects on the fetus have been reported. Although the drug has been used for 20 years, no increase of congenital abnormalities, stillbirths, or low birth weight has been reported. Culture of human lymphocytes with metronidazole, up to 10,000 μg/mL, has revealed no toxic activity. No increase in frequency of chromosomal aberration was found in patients receiving large doses for the treatment of amebic hepatitis.

Contraindications & Cautions

Although tumorigenicity and mutagenic activity in in vivo assays are well documented, no genetic damage or irreversible toxicity has been reported after 20 years of clinical use. Prudence dictates that metronidazole should be used in pregnant or nursing women only on clear indications.

Drug Interactions

Metronidazole has been reported to potentiate the anticoagulant effect of coumarin-type anticoagulants. Its disulfiramlike effect requires that all patients receiving it should be specifically warned not to use alcohol. The SGOT test of liver function may be depressed, and patients with severe liver disease may accumulate the drug and its metabolites in the plasma.

Preparations & Dosages

Metronidazole is available in 250-mg and 500-mg tablets for oral administration. Rectal suppositories are available outside the USA. The daily dose and the duration of treatment vary with the disease being treated (see above). Should re-treatment be needed, 4–6 weeks should be allowed between courses. Metronidazole hydrochloride for intravenous injection (Flagyl IV) is available in single-dose lyophilized vials containing 500 mg. The powder is reconstituted to produce an acidic solution with a pH of 0.5–2.0. The reconstituted solution should not be given by direct injection but must be further diluted and neutralized according to the manufacturer's instructions.

References

Malaria

General

Chemoprophylaxis of malaria. *MMWR* (March 10) 1978; **27[Suppl]:**81.

Clyde DF et al: Treatment of falciparum malaria caused by strain resistant to quinine. *JAMA* 1970;**213:**2041.

Hall AP: The treatment of malaria. *Br Med J* 1976;**1:**323.

Revised recommendations for malaria chemoprophylaxis. *MMWR* (June 25) 1982;**31:**328.

Peters W: Chemotherapy of malaria. Pages 145–283 in: *Malaria*. Vol 1: *Epidemiology, Chemotherapy, Morphology and Metabolism*. Kreier JP (editor). Academic Press, 1980.

Trenholme G, Carson PE: Therapy and prophylaxis of malaria. *JAMA* 1978;**240:**2293.

Warrell DA et al: Dexamethasone proves deleterious in cerebral malaria. *N Engl J Med* 1982;**306:**313.

World Health Organization: *Chemotherapy of Malaria and Resistance to Malarials*. Report of a WHO Scientific Group. Technical Report Series No. 529, 1973.

Quinine

Hall AP et al: Human plasma and urine quinine levels following tablets, capsules, and intravenous infusion. *Clin Pharmacol Ther* 1973;**14:**580.

Powell RD: Treatment of malaria. *Ration Drug Ther* (April) 1972;**6:**1.

Sheehy TW, Reba RC: Complications of falciparum malaria and their treatment. *Ann Intern Med* 1976;**66:**807.

Chloroquine

Blount RD: Chloroquine-resistant falciparum malaria. *JAMA* 1967;**200:**886.

Burns RP: Delayed onset of chloroquine retinopathy. *N Engl J Med* 1966;**275:**693.

Carson JW, Barringer ML, Jones RE Jr: Fatal chloroquine ingestion: An increasing hazard. *Pediatrics* 1967;**40:**449.

Ciak J, Hahn FE: Chloroquine: Mode of action. *Science* 1966;**151:**347.

McCann WP, Permisohn R, Palmisano PA: Fatal chloroquine poisoning in a child: Experience with peritoneal dialysis. *Pediatrics* 1975;**55:**536.

Congeners of Chloroquine

Booth K, Larkin K, Maddocks I: Agranulocytosis coincident with amodiaquine therapy. *Br Med J* 1967;**3:**32.

Lucasse C: Single-dose treatment of acute malaria. *J Trop Med Hyg* 1963;**66:**280.

8-Aminoquinolines

Cahn MM, Levy EJ: The tolerance to large weekly doses of primaquine and amodiaquine in primaquine-sensitive and non-sensitive subjects. *Am J Trop Med Hyg* 1962;**11:**605.

Peters W: The possible role of primaquine in inducing multiple drug resistance in *Plasmodium falciparum*. *Trans R Soc Trop Med Hyg* 1966;**60:**140.

Quinacrine

Sapp OL III: Toxic psychosis due to quinacrine and chloroquine. *JAMA* 1964;**187:**373.

Proguanil, Pyrimethamine, & Trimethoprim

Bushby SRM, Hitchings GH: Trimethoprim, a sulphonamide potentiator. *Br J Pharmacol* 1968;**33:**72.

Laing ABG: Treatment of acute falciparum malaria with sulphorthodimethoxine (Fanasil). *Br Med J* 1965;**1:**905.

McGregor IA, Williams K, Goodwin LG: Pyrimethamine and sulphadiazine in treatment of malaria. *Br Med J* 1963; **2:**728.

Pearlman EJ, Hall AP: Prevention of chloroquine-resistant falciparum malaria. (Correspondence.) *Ann Intern Med* 1975;**82:**590.

Amebiasis

General

Adams EB, MacLeod IN: Invasive amebiasis. 1. Amebic dysentery and its complications. *Medicine* 1977;**56:**315.

Adams EB, MacLeod IN: Invasive amebiasis. 2. Amebic liver abscess and its complications. *Medicine* 1977;**56:**325.

Juniper K: Amoebiasis. *Clin Gastroenterol* 1978;**7:**3.

Knight R: The chemotherapy of amebiasis. *J Antimicrob Chemother* 1980;**6:**577.

Masters DK, Hopkins AD: Therapeutic trial of four amoebicide regimes in rural Zaire. *J Trop Med Hyg* 1979; **82:**99.

Wilmot AJ: *Clinical Amoebiasis*. Blackwell, 1962.

World Health Organization Expert Committee: Amoebiasis. Technical Report Series No. 421, 1969.

Emetine & Dehydroemetine

Klatskin G, Friedman H: Emetine toxicity in man: Studies on the nature of early toxic manifestations, their relation to the dose level, and their significance in determining safe dosage. *Ann Intern Med* 1948;**28:**892.

Lister GD: Delayed myocardial intoxication following the administration of dehydroemetine hydrochloride. *J Trop Med Hyg* 1968;**71:**219.

Pain A, Wingfield A: Electrocardiographic changes due to emetine therapy. *Trans R Soc Trop Med Hyg* 1968;**62:**221.

Sharad CS, Vakil BJ: Cardiovascular toxicity of emetine and dehydroemetine. *Indian Pract* 1971;**24:**237.

Wilmot AJ, Powell SJ, Adams EB: Chloroquine compared with chloroquine and emetine combined in amebic liver abscess. *Am J Trop Med Hyg* 1959;**8:**623.

Yang WCT, Dubick M: Mechanism of emetine cardiotoxicity. *Pharmacol Ther* 1980;**10:**15.

Diloxanide Furoate

Bell S: An investigation of carriers of *Entamoeba histolytica*. *Trans R Soc Trop Med Hyg* 1967;**61:**506.

Botero RD: Treatment of intestinal amoebiasis with diloxanide furoate, tetracycline and chloroquine. *Trans R Soc Trop Med Hyg* 1967;**61:**769.

Gubey MP, Gupta PS, Chuttani HK: Entamide furoate in the treatment of intestinal amoebiasis. *J Trop Med Hyg* 1965; **68:**63.

Wolfe MS: Nondysenteric intestinal amebiasis: Treatment with diloxanide furoate. *JAMA* 1973;**224:**1601.

Halogenated Hydroxyquinolines & Arsenicals

Committee on Drugs: Blindness and neuropathy from diiodohydroxyquin-like drugs. *Pediatrics* 1974;**54:**378.

Inoue YK: An avian-related new herpesvirus infection in man—subacute myelo-optico-neuropathy (SMON). *Prog Med Virol* 1976;**21:**35.

Jack DB, Riess W: Pharmacokinetics of iodochlorhydroxyquin in man. *J Pharm Sci* 1973;**62:**1929.

Kono R: The S.M.O.N. virus theory. (Correspondence.) *Lancet* 1975;**2:**370.

Oakley GP Jr: The neurotoxicity of the halogenated hydroxyquinolines. *JAMA* 1973;**225:**395.

Worden AN, Heywood R: Clioquinol toxicity. (Correspondence.) *Lancet* 1978;**1:**212.

Metronidazole

Beard CM et al: Lack of evidence for cancer due to use of metronidazole. *N Engl J Med* 1979;**301:**519.

Brogden R et al: Metronidazole in anaerobic infections: A review of its activity, pharmacokinetics and therapeutic use. *Drugs* 1978;**16:**387.

Finegold SM: Metronidazole. *Ann Intern Med* 1980;**93:**585.

Finegold SM, McFadzean JA, Roe FJC (editors): Metronidazole. Proceedings of the International Metronidazole Conference, Montreal, Quebec, 26–28 May, 1976.

Fisher LS et al: Failure of metronidazole in amebic liver abscess. *Am J Med Sci* 1976;**271:**65.

Friedman GD: Cancer after metronidazole. (Letter.) *N Engl J Med* 1980;**302:**519.

Goldman P: Metronidazole. *N Engl J Med* 1980;**303:**1212.

Kanani SR, Knight R: Experiences with the use of metronidazole in the treatment of non dysenteric intestinal amoebiasis. *Trans R Soc Trop Med Hyg* 1972;**66:**244.

Metronidazole (Flagyl). *Med Lett Drugs Ther* 1979;**21:**89.

Metronidazole: Proceedings of the Second International Symposium on Anaerobic Infections. Geneva, 25–27 April, 1979. Royal Society of Medicine, Series 18, 1979.

Metronidazole: Unanswered questions. (Editorial.) *Lancet* 1981;**1:**818.

Muller M: *Metronidazole: Its Action on Anaerobes*. Rockefeller Univ Press, 1980.

Powell SJ: Metronidazole in the treatment of amoebic dysentery. *Medicine Today* 1969;**3:**48.

Powell SJ, Stewart-Wynne EJ, Elsdon-Dew R: Metronidazole combined with diloxanide furoate in amoebic liver abscess. *Ann Trop Med Parasitol* 1973;**67:**367.

Scragg JN, Proctor EM: Tinidazole treatment of acute amebic dysentery in children. *Am J Trop Med Hyg* 1977; **26:**824.

Paromomycin Sulfate

Courtney KO et al: Paromomycin as a therapeutic substance for intestinal amoebiasis and bacterial enteritis. *Ann Biochem Exper Med* 1960;**20(S):**449.

Keusch GT, Troncale FJ, Buchanan RD: Malabsorption due to paromomycin. *Arch Intern Med* 1970;**125:**273.

Simon M et al: Paromomycin in the treatment of intestinal amebiasis: A short course of therapy. *Am J Gastroenterol* 1967;**48:**504.

Woolfe G: The chemotherapy of amoebiasis. *Prog Drug Res* 1965;**8:**13.

Leishmaniasis

Beltran HF, Gutierrez FM, Biagi FF: [Treatment of Mexican cutaneous leishmaniasis with metronidazole.] *Bull Soc Pathol Exot* 1967;**60:**61.

Chavarria AP, Kotcher E: Preliminary evaluation of cycloguanil pamoate in dermal leishmaniasis. *JAMA* 1965; **194:**1142.

Hassan Abd-Rabbo: Dehydroemetine in leishmaniasis (Oriental sore). *J Trop Med Hyg* 1966;**69:**171.

Prata A: Treatment of kala-azar with amphotericin B. *Trans R Soc Trop Med Hyg* 1963;**57:**266.

Reinhard M, Wacker H: [Treatment of cutaneous leishmaniasis with cycloguanil pamoate.] *Dtsch Med Wochenschr* 1970;**95:**2380.

Salem HH et al: The treatment of cutaneous leishmaniasis with oral dehydroemetine. *Trans R Soc Trop Med Hyg* 1967; **61:**776.

Trypanosomiasis

Gutteridge WE: Chemotherapy of Chagas' disease: The present situation. *Trop Dis Bull* 1976;**73:**699.

Williamson J: Chemotherapy of African trypanosomiasis. *Trop Dis Bull* 1976;**73:**531.

Trichomoniasis

Metronidazole

Baker RM, Kennan AL: Therapy of trichomoniasis. *Wis Med J* 1967;**66:**370.

Diddle AW: *Trichomonas vaginalis:* Resistance to metronidazole. *Am J Obstet Gynecol* 1967;**98:**583.

Is Flagyl dangerous? *Med Lett Drugs Ther* 1975;**17:**53.

McLoughlin DK: Drug tolerance by *Trichomonas foetus*. *J Parasitol* 1967;**53:**646.

Minnesota Department of Health: *Communicable Disease Newsletter* 2(9), (Nov) 1975.

Anthelmintic Drugs | 55

Robert S. Goldsmith, MD, DTM&H

CHEMOTHERAPY OF HELMINTHIC INFECTIONS

Anthelmintic drugs are a group of compounds used to eradicate or reduce in numbers helminthic parasites in the intestinal tract or tissues of humans. Table 55–1 lists the major helminthic infections and provides a guide to the drug of choice and alternative drugs for each infection. In the text that follows, these drugs are arranged alphabetically, with the exception of several drugs that are used in the treatment of schistosomiasis and are presented under antimonial compounds.

Most anthelmintics in use today are active against specific parasites, and some are toxic. Therefore, parasites must be identified before treatment is started, usually by finding the parasite, ova, or larvae in the feces, urine, blood, sputum, or tissues of the host.

Administration of Anthelmintic Drugs

Unless otherwise indicated, oral drugs should be taken with water during or after meals. If pre- or posttreatment purges are necessary in conjunction with a specific drug, magnesium or sodium sulfate may be used. The usual dose, 15–30 g for an adult and 0.2–0.4 g/kg of body weight for children, is dissolved in a glass of water. The intensely bitter taste may be partially masked by giving the salts in lemon juice. Magnesium sulfate must not be given to individuals with impaired renal function, and sodium sulfate may be contraindicated in patients with congestive heart failure. Other contraindications to severe purgation are signs of intestinal obstruction, debilitation, and pregnancy.

Dosages for Children

Dosages for infants and children are on a less secure basis than for adults; when not shown in milligrams per kilogram of body weight (or otherwise specified), the dosage may be calculated as a fraction of the adult dose based on Clark's rule or Young's rule (see Chapter 10).

Contraindications

Pregnancy and ulcers of the gastrointestinal tract are contraindications for most of the drugs listed. Specific contraindications are given in the discussions that follow.

ANTIMONY COMPOUNDS

The trivalent antimony compounds were for many years the principal drugs for the treatment of schistosomiasis (bilharziasis) but, because of their toxicity, should be considered alternative drugs, to be used when the preferred drugs are not available or when the infection is resistant to the preferred drugs.

Research efforts over 50 years to combine high cure rates with safety have resulted in the synthesis and screening of thousands of antimonial compounds. The successful antischistosomal agents all have trivalent antimony chelated to oxygen or sulfur. The drugs currently used are antimony potassium tartrate (tartar emetic), introduced in 1918, and antimony sodium dimercaptosuccinate (stibocaptate), in 1954. Other trivalent preparations include antimony sodium tartrate, antimony lithium thiomalate (anthiomaline), antimony thioglycollamide, antimony pyrocatechol sodium disulfonate (stibophen), and antimony sodium gluconate (triostam).

Each of the antimony drugs has one or more major defects, including severe toxicity, difficulty with administration, the necessity for prolonged treatment, or low effectiveness. Tartar emetic is superior to the other antimonials for the treatment of *Schistosoma japonicum* infection but is the most toxic drug of the group, is unstable in solution, requires intravenous administration, and requires that patients be hospitalized. Stibocaptate is the preferred antimonial for the treatment of *Schistosoma mansoni* and *Schistosoma haematobium* infections because it is stable, is moderately effective, can be given intramuscularly, is less toxic than comparably effective doses of tartar emetic, and can be given on an outpatient basis.

Although standardization of methodology for clinical trials and the number of comparative drug studies are increasing, it continues to be difficult to compare the effectiveness and safety of antischistosomal drugs (antimonial and nonantimonial agents) given in different parts of the world. Discrepancies reflect varying criteria of cure, differences in the drug susceptibility of parasitic strains from widely sepa-

Table 55–1. Drugs for the treatment of helminthic infections.

Infecting Organism	Drug of Choice	Alternative Drugs
Roundworms (nematodes)		
Ascaris lumbricoides (roundworm)	Pyrantel pamoate	Piperazine, mebendazole, levamisole,[1] or bephenium[1]
Trichuris trichiura (whipworm)	Mebendazole	Oxantel pamoate[1,2] or hexylresorcinol[1] by retention enema
Necator americanus (hookworm) *Ancylostoma duodenale* (hookworm)	Pyrantel pamoate[2] or mebendazole	Bephenium,[1] tetrachloroethylene, or thiabendazole
Strongyloides stercoralis (threadworm)	Thiabendazole	Mebendazole,[3,4] niridazole,[4] pyrvinium pamoate,[3,4] or levamisole[1,4]
Enterobius vermicularis (pinworm)	Mebendazole or pyrantel pamoate	Pyrvinium pamoate
Trichinella spiralis (trichinosis)	ACTH, corticosteroids, and thiabendazole[4] or mebendazole[3,4]	None
Trichostrongylus species	Pyrantel pamoate[3] or mebendazole[2]	Bephenium,[1] levamisole,[1] or thiabendazole[3]
Cutaneous larva migrans (creeping eruption)	Thiabendazole	Diethylcarbamazine[4,5]
Visceral larva migrans	Thiabendazole[4]	Diethylcarbamazine[4,5]
Angiostrongylus cantonensis	Levamisole[1,4]	None
Wuchereria bancrofti (filariasis) *Brugia malayi* (filariasis) Tropical eosinophilia *Loa loa* (loiasis)	Diethylcarbamazine[5]	None
Onchocerca volvulus (onchocerciasis)	Suramin[6] plus diethylcarbamazine[5]	None
Dracunculus medinensis (guinea worm)	Niridazole[6] or metronidazole[3]	Thiabendazole[3]
Intestinal capillariasis	Mebendazole	Thiabendazole
Flukes (trematodes)		
Schistosoma haematobium (bilharziasis)	Metrifonate[6] or praziquantel[7]	Niridazole[6] or stibocaptate[6] (see antimony compounds)
Schistosoma mansoni	Oxamniquine or praziquantel[7]	Niridazole[6] or stibocaptate[6] (see antimony compounds)
Schistosoma japonicum	Praziquantel[7]	Niridazole,[6] tartar emetic, or stibocaptate[6] (see antimony compounds)
Clonorchis sinensis (liver fluke) *Opisthorchis* species	Praziquantel[2,7]	None
Paragonimus westermani (lung fluke)	Bithionol[6]	Praziquantel[2,7]
Fasciola hepatica (sheep liver fluke)	Bithionol[6]	Emetine, dehydroemetine,[6] or metronidazole[3,4]
Fasciolopsis buski (large intestinal fluke)	Tetrachloroethylene, niclosamide, or praziquantel[4,7]	Hexylresorcinol[1] or dichlorophen[1,4]
Heterophyes heterophyes, Metagonimus yokogawai (small intestinal flukes)	Tetrachloroethylene or niclosamide	Hexylresorcinol,[1] bephenium,[1] or praziquantel[2,4,7]
Tapeworm (cestodes)		
Taenia saginata (beef tapeworm)	Niclosamide	Praziquantel,[2,7] dichlorophen,[1] paromomycin,[3] or mebendazole[3,4]
Diphyllobothrium latum (fish tapeworm)	Niclosamide	Praziquantel[2,7] or dichlorophen[1]
Taenia solium (pork tapeworm)	Niclosamide	Praziquantel[2,7] or mebendazole[3,4]
Cysticercosis (pork tapeworm larval stage)	Praziquantel[2,4,7]	None
Hymenolepis nana (dwarf tapeworm)	Praziquantel[7]	Niclosamide or paromomycin[3]
Hymenolepis diminuta (rat tapeworm) *Dipylidium caninum*	Niclosamide	Praziquantel[4,7]
Echinococcus granulosus (hydatid disease) *Echinococcus multilocularis*	Mebendazole[2,3,4]	None

[1] Not available in the USA.
[2] Undergoing clinical investigation.
[3] Available in the USA but not approved for this indication.
[4] Effectiveness not established.
[5] Available in the USA only from Lederle Laboratories, telephone (914) 753–5000.
[6] Available in the USA only from the Parasitic Disease Drug Service, Parasitic Diseases Branch, Centers for Disease Control, Atlanta 30333. Telephone (404) 329–3670 during the day, (404) 329–2888 nights, weekends, and holidays.
[7] Expected to become available shortly in the USA.

rated regions, and host factors such as sex, race, intensity and duration of infection, and immunity and nutritional status. Quantitative methods such as multiple ovum counts and tests for ovum viability are essential. Therapeutic results become significant only after long follow-up periods (12 months) and when reinfection does not occur, but these objectives are difficult to accomplish.

Pharmacologic Effects

A. Action in Humans: Relatively little information is available on the physiologic and biochemical effects of the trivalent antimonials or the mechanisms of their toxicity, which affect many tissues. When the drugs are given parenterally, the intense vomiting and coughing that may occur are thought to be due both to central effects and to local irritation of antimony excreted on the gastrointestinal and bronchial mucosa.

B. Anthelmintic Action: Trivalent antimony compounds inhibit phosphofructokinase in schistosomes, an enzyme necessary for glycolysis, which is a major source of energy for the parasite. Within minutes to several hours after administration, worm paralysis occurs, followed by relaxation of the suckers that hold the helminth in place in terminal veins. As a result, the schistosomes are carried by the venous flow to the liver or to the lungs, depending upon their original location (bladder or bowel wall) and whether portal bypass occurs via extrahepatic collaterals in advanced liver disease. After the initial injections, the enzyme inhibition and paralysis are reversible and the worms may return to the terminal venules, but repeated administration of the drugs will ultimately result in the death of many of the parasites. Still undetermined is whether significant liver or lung damage occurs when dead worms accumulate in these tissues. Antimony compounds also both affect the reproductive organs of schistosomes, impairing deposition of eggs, and produce morphologic changes in eggs before and after deposition.

Absorption, Distribution, & Excretion

Trivalent antimonials must be given parenterally because of their strong emetic action and slow absorption when given orally. Parenteral administration results in high but transient blood levels because these agents have a high affinity for blood cells and for thyroid, liver, renal, and other tissues. The return of antimony to the blood plasma is slow, thus permitting accumulation. In humans, antimony is excreted mainly via the kidneys; a small amount appears in the feces. Excretion is slow and varies according to the drug, dosages, and the individual responsiveness of the patient. After a single parenteral dose of tartar emetic (2.5 mg/kg), 49% of the antimony was excreted in the urine in 24 hours and 56% in 1 week. After a single injection of stibocaptate (3.1 mg/kg), 14% of the antimony was excreted in 24 hours and 27% in 1 week. Following a full course of tartar emetic, antimony was detected in the urine after 100 days.

Adverse Reactions

Under physiologic conditions the trivalent antimonials dissociate, releasing a small amount of antimonial ions; the frequency and intensity of toxic reactions appear to be associated with the degree of this dissociation. Side-effects occur in most patients, but the drugs are often better tolerated by children than by adults. Most side-effects are mild and disappear within 1–2 days after the last injection; however, many are so severe that up to 50% of patients will be unwilling to complete a course of treatment. The most frequent adverse reactions are pain at the site of injection (for the intramuscular compounds), anorexia, nausea and vomiting, diarrhea, abdominal pain, coughing (less frequent for stibocaptate), myalgia, arthralgia, dizziness, headache, and fatigue.

Frequent cardiovascular side-effects include bradycardia appearing shortly after injections, and hypotension. Electrocardiographic changes occur in most patients; they usually return to normal within 4 weeks after therapy is stopped but may persist longer. These changes include increased amplitude of P waves, prolonged Q–T intervals, depressed ST segments, inverted T waves, and fusion of the ST segment with the T wave. There is no evidence that these changes correlate with abnormal cardiac function or that they are precursors of serious toxicity. The exception is the appearance of extrasystoles and other arrhythmias or symptoms suggesting a Stokes-Adams attack.

Less common side-effects are skin rash, substernal pain, pyrexia, prostration, conjunctivitis, pruritus, depression, and a metallic taste. Rare side-effects include hepatomegaly with laboratory evidence of liver dysfunction, peripheral neuritis, herpes zoster, retrobulbar neuritis with central scotomas, hematuria, thrombocytopenia, and hemolytic anemia (of the autoimmune type).

Pain at the injection site when stibocaptate is used can be reduced by prior administration of 1% lidocaine through the same needle used for giving the drug. Vomiting tends to start late in the course of treatment and usually 2–4 hours after injection. Mild nausea and vomiting may sometimes be reduced by giving 6–10 mL of aluminum hydroxide gel orally before the injection or 15–20 drops of tincture of belladonna orally 3 times a day before meals. Hypotension responds to subcutaneous injections of epinephrine.

Mild muscle or joint pains and nausea are not indications to stop or modify treatment. However, if pain or nausea and vomiting are increasing, the interval between injections should be increased or the dosage reduced. Treatment should be suspended temporarily if skin rashes, marked fatigue, or temperature elevation appears. Urine and blood should be examined at frequent intervals. Therapy should be discontinued in the event of severe and persistent vomiting, substernal pain, continued fever, hematuria, progressive proteinuria, thrombocytopenia, falling hematocrit, signs of hemolytic anemia, or electrocardiographic evidence of arrhythmias. The electrocardiographic changes described above are not an indication to stop treatment.

Among the millions of patients treated with antimonial compounds, sudden and unpredictable deaths have occurred with all of the agents but are considered to be most frequent with tartar emetic and least frequent with stibocaptate. Two mechanisms of death have been recognized: cardiac arrhythmias and shock.

Contraindications & Cautions

Intestinal helminth infections, particularly ascarids, should be eradicated before starting treatment. For stibocaptate, inadvertent intravenous administration may intensify side-effects; therefore, the needle and syringe should be observed carefully and their position changed if blood appears on aspiration.

Antimonial drugs should be used with caution or not at all in debilitated and malnourished individuals. They are contraindicated in the presence of tuberculosis; acute febrile conditions; herpes simplex and zoster; severe anemia; cardiac, renal, and hepatic insufficiency (except that due to schistosomiasis); terminal forms of schistosomiasis; and for patients treated with antimonials within the previous 2 months. Medication containing iron salts should not be given concurrently with antimonial compounds.

1. STIBOCAPTATE (Antimony Sodium Dimercaptosuccinate, Astiban)

Chemistry

Stibocaptate is antimony sodium dimercaptosuccinate (antimony III sodium meso 2,3-dimercaptosuccinate; TWSb; Astiban). It is a trivalent antimonial that differs from antimony tartrate in that the oxygen atoms of the hydroxyl groups are replaced by sulfur. Stibocaptate contains 25–26% antimony and is provided as a powder, which is stable. It is readily soluble but unstable in water and should be used shortly after being placed in solution.

Clinical Uses

Stibocaptate is an alternative drug for the treatment of schistosomiasis. Most patients can be treated on an outpatient basis.

A wide range of effectiveness has been reported for stibocaptate in different clinical trials. Reported cure rates for *S mansoni* infection are 29–91%; for *S haematobium* infection, 12–100%; usually there has been a significant drop in the ovum count in those not cured. There have been relatively few studies on the use of stibocaptate for *S japonicum* infections, but cure rates of 50–87% have been reported.

Adverse Reactions, Contraindications, & Cautions

As described above under Antimony Compounds.

Preparations & Dosages

Stibocaptate (Astiban) is supplied in vials containing 0.5 g of the lyophilized drug, to be dissolved in 5 mL of sterile water or normal saline. The resultant 10% solution should be refrigerated and used within 24 hours. Cloudy or discolored solutions should be discarded. The drug is not marketed in the USA but can be obtained from the Parasitic Disease Drug Service, Centers for Disease Control, Atlanta 30333.

The total dose for treatment of *S haematobium* or *S mansoni* infections is 40 mg/kg (maximum total 2.5 g) and for *S japonicum* infection 50 mg/kg (maximum total 2.5 g). The total dose is divided into 5 equal intramuscular injections given once a week for 5 weeks. After each injection, the patient should rest for half an hour. If necessary, a course of treatment may be repeated in 2 months. If individual doses are given at shorter intervals, such as twice weekly, side-effects are often more severe.

2. TARTAR EMETIC (Antimony Potassium Tartrate)

Chemistry

Antimony potassium tartrate (tartar emetic) contains 36.5% of trivalent antimony. It is soluble 1:12 in water. The sodium salt may be more stable and less toxic than the potassium preparation but requires the same precautions in its use.

Clinical Uses

A. *S japonicum*: Tartar emetic is an alternative drug for treatment of *S japonicum* infection. Most et al reported 13 failures among 79 patients treated with a total of 1.8 g and 2 failures among 50 patients treated with 2.08 g during a course of 25–33 days. Ata and Mousa reported the use of a longer course of 12–16 injections given at weekly intervals; the drug was well tolerated and the therapeutic results were similar to those of the standard course. A WHO Expert Committee (1972) summarized the efficacy of tartar emetic as resulting in 40–75% cure rates, with a comparable reduction in ovum count in the uncured.

B. *S mansoni* and *S haematobium*: Although tartar emetic is effective for the treatment of *S mansoni* and *S haematobium* infections, other less toxic drugs should be used. Most et al reported that a total of 1.8 g of tartar emetic would cure more than 90% of infections with *S mansoni* and that 1.5–1.7 g would cure more than 90% of *S haematobium* infections.

Adverse Reactions

Each injection must be given intravenously with scrupulous care, since leakage of even small amounts into the perivascular tissues causes severe necrosis. Phlebitis is a frequent complication of subcutaneous administration. The speed of injection should be very slow to reduce the incidence of immediate side-effects: cough, dyspnea, a sense of chest constriction, tachycardia, dizziness, vomiting, and hypotension.

Paroxysms of coughing occur in most patients but usually subside within a few minutes after the injection. Hypotension responds promptly to stopping the injection and giving epinephrine subcutaneously. Acute vascular collapse is rare. Many other side-effects occur as described above under Antimony Compounds.

Contraindications & Cautions

The drug must be given very slowly by the intravenous route, taking care to avoid leakage into the perivascular tissues. Patients should be hospitalized and kept under continuous observation during administration. A syringe containing epinephrine (1:1000) should be immediately available during each injection.

For other essential comments regarding cautions and contraindications, see above under Antimony Compounds.

Preparations & Dosages

Antimony potassium tartrate (tartar emetic) is available as a granular powder. A 0.5% solution that contains 1.8 mg of metallic antimony or 5 mg of tartar emetic per milliliter should be freshly prepared in 5% glucose, physiologic saline solution, or distilled water and sterilized by filtration or by gentle boiling for 5 minutes. Boiling for more than 5 minutes and autoclaving should be avoided. The resultant solution should be used within 2 hours and should be crystal clear and free of sediment.

Patients should refrain from vigorous exercise during the course of treatment. The drug is best given 2–3 hours after a light meal, and the patient should remain recumbent for several hours afterward.

The drug is administered intravenously very slowly through a fine needle over a 10-minute period. The initial dose is 8 mL of the 0.5% solution. Subsequent doses of 12, 16, 20, 24, and 28 mL are given on alternate days. Thereafter, continue 28 mL on alternate days for 9 additional doses until a total of 360 mL (1.8 g of the drug) has been given. If a second course is required, a few months should elapse before resuming treatment.

ASPIDIUM OLEORESIN (Extract of Male Fern)

One dose of aspidium oleoresin, formerly the major drug for the treatment of tapeworm infections, will eradicate *Taenia saginata, Taenia solium,* and *Diphyllobothrium latum* in more than 80% of patients. However, because of its unpredictable and often severe toxicity (including death rarely), the drug was superseded first by quinacrine and, more recently, by niclosamide, praziquantel, and dichlorophen. Aspidium should no longer be used.

BEPHENIUM HYDROXYNAPHTHOATE (Alcopar, Alcopara)

Bephenium hydroxynaphthoate, synthesized in 1958, is an alternative drug for the treatment of hookworm infections but is less effective against necatoriasis than against ancylostomiasis. The drug is moderately effective for treating ascariasis and trichostrongyliasis, has a low order of activity in trichuriasis, and is ineffective in strongyloidiasis. The drug is not marketed in the USA.

Chemistry

The bephenium salts are quaternary ammonium compounds. Bephenium hydroxynaphthoate (benzyldimethyl[2-phenoxyethyl]ammonium 3-hydroxy-2-naphthoate) has an aqueous solubility of 0.02–0.03%. It must be stored in an airtight container.

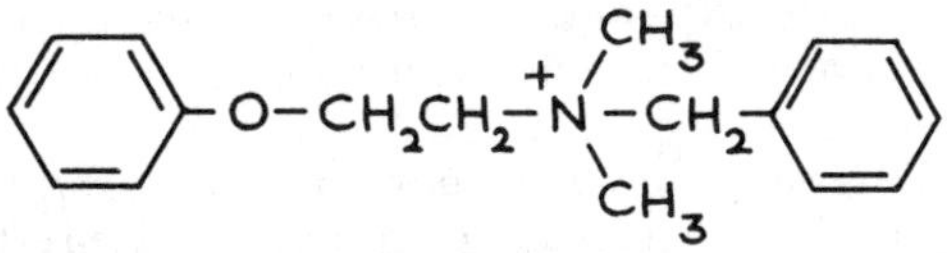

Bephenium base

Absorption, Metabolism, & Excretion

Bephenium hydroxynaphthoate is poorly absorbed after oral administration. In humans, less than 0.5% of an oral dose of 1 g (of base) was recovered in the urine within 24 hours.

Pharmacologic Effects

Embryopathy was observed when 250–500 mg/kg was given to pregnant rabbits. The water-soluble chloride salt, when inoculated parenterally into dogs and cats, had ganglion-blocking properties and caused a brief fall in blood pressure. In humans, no abnormal effects on the liver or kidney have been noted.

Anthelmintic Actions

The effects of bephenium hydroxynaphthoate on ascarid musculature are those of excitation followed by paralysis, associated with a loss of muscular reactivity to acetylcholine. These effects are not reversible.

Clinical Uses

Bephenium hydroxynaphthoate is a safe, moderately well tolerated drug. It may be used in the very young and also in the presence of diarrhea or marked anemia, either of which may accompany severe hookworm disease. The drug's deficiencies are its bitter taste, a high incidence of vomiting after its use, and a higher frequency of side-effects than for other drugs used in the treatment of ascariasis and hookworm infection.

A. *Ancylostoma duodenale:* Bephenium hydroxynaphthoate is an alternative drug for the treatment of hookworm infections due to *A duodenale.*

Many studies indicate that a single course of treatment results in a cure rate of 76–98% and that the worm burden in the remaining patients is markedly reduced.

B. *Necator americanus:* Hookworm infections due to *N americanus* are more resistant than those due to *A duodenale* and therefore require treatment on 3 successive days to achieve about 80% reduction in worm loads.

C. *Ascaris lumbricoides:* Bephenium hydroxynaphthoate is moderately effective against roundworms. The reported cure rate after one dose varies from 30 to 82%, which is less satisfactory than the results obtained with piperazine.

D. Mixed *Ascaris* and Hookworm Infections: Bephenium hydroxynaphthoate paralyzes roundworms. Therefore, it can be used to treat mixed infestations of hookworms and roundworms without stimulating ascarid migration as reported for tetrachloroethylene, mebendazole, and thiabendazole.

E. *Trichostrongylus orientalis:* Single treatments have resulted in the eradication of the infection from 75–82% of patients.

F. *Heterophyes heterophyes* and *Metagonimus yokogawai:* A single course of treatment is often effective.

Adverse Reactions

Bephenium hydroxynaphthoate has a very low toxicity at therapeutic doses. Nausea and vomiting, the common side-effects, are mild and short-lasting and occur more frequently in young children. Other symptoms—dizziness, headache, cramping abdominal pain, and diarrhea—are less frequent. Variations in tolerance by ethnic groups have been described.

Contraindications & Cautions

Patients with marked anemia, diarrhea, or dehydration should have the condition partially corrected before the drug is given. In the presence of severe diarrhea due to hookworm disease, it may be necessary to use smaller daily doses and to continue daily treatments for 4–7 days.

The drug should not be used in pregnancy, hypertension, or ulcerative conditions of the gastrointestinal tract not due to hookworms.

Preparations & Dosages

Bephenium hydroxynaphthoate (Alcopar, Alcopara) is prepared as granules in 5-g packets (5 g of the granules contain 4.3 g of bephenium hydroxynaphthoate, equivalent to 2.5 g of bephenium base).

The drug should be given orally on an empty stomach and food then withheld for 2 hours. Since it is bitter when mixed with water, it can be made more palatable (and less vomiting occurs) when mixed in chocolate milk, orange juice, flavored syrups, or milk. No purgatives should be used.

The dosage for adults and older children is 5 g of the granules (one packet), mixed with water or other liquid, taken twice a day; children weighing less than 22 kg take half of the adult dosage. One day of treatment results in a high cure rate for *A duodenale* and *T orientalis* infections. The same daily dosage should be repeated for 3 days if the drug is used for *N americanus* infections or if the species of hookworm is not known. Two weeks later, reexamine the stools and re-treat if necessary. It is not always possible or essential to completely eradicate hookworm infection. If iron deficiency anemia accompanies severe hookworm disease, it should be treated with iron medication and a high-protein diet.

BITHIONOL
(Bitin)

Bithionol is the drug of choice for the treatment of fascioliasis (liver fluke), pulmonary paragonimiasis (lung fluke), and acute cerebral paragonimiasis. The drug has been used in some countries in the treatment of large tapeworm infections, and it needs further evaluation in the treatment of clonorchiasis and opisthorchiasis.

Bithionol (Actamer, Lorothidol) is not marketed in the USA but can be obtained for use in treatment of parasitic diseases from the Parasitic Disease Drug Service, Centers for Disease Control, Atlanta 30333 (telephone [404] 329–3670).

Chemistry, Absorption, Metabolism, Excretion, & Anthelmintic Actions

Bithionol, 2,2′-thiobis(4,6-dichlorophenol), reaches peak blood levels in humans in 4–8 hours. At a daily dosage of 50 mg/kg orally in 3 divided doses for 5 days, a serum level of 50–200 μg/mL is maintained. Excretion appears to be mainly via the kidney. The mode of action of bithionol against *Paragonimus westermani* has not been established, but the drug does inhibit oxidative phosphorylation.

Clinical Uses

A. Pulmonary Paragonimiasis: A series of clinical reports from 1961 to 1967 indicated that 97% of 420 patients were cured using a dosage schedule ranging from 10 to 50 mg/kg in divided doses on alternate days for a total of 5–15 doses. Kim reported a cure rate of 91% among 1113 treated patients.

B. Cerebral Paragonimiasis: Bithionol may be useful in acute cerebral paragonimiasis but more than one course of treatment is sometimes required. The drug has little effectiveness in chronic cerebral infections.

C. Subcutaneous Paragonimiasis: Information on the effectiveness of bithionol in subcutaneous paragonimiasis is limited. The recommended dosage is 1 g 3 times daily every other day for 10 doses.

D. *Fasciola hepatica:* D'Sa and Grados and Berrocal each reported the cure of 4 patients with fascioliasis infections.

Adverse Reactions

Side-effects occur in up to 40% of patients. They

are generally mild and transient, but occasionally their severity requires interruption of therapy. Diarrhea and abdominal cramps are most common; these may diminish or stop after several days of treatment. Anorexia, nausea, vomiting, dizziness, and headache may also occur. Pruritic, urticarial, or papular skin rashes are less frequent and usually begin after a latent period of a week or more of therapy; they are probably allergic in nature and result from release of antigens from dying worms. Other infrequent reactions are lassitude, pyrexia, tinnitus, insomnia, and proteinuria. Isolated instances of leukopenia, hepatitis, hypertension, and first-degree heart block have been described.

Contraindications & Cautions

The drug should be used with caution in children under 8 years of age because of limited experience with that age group.

Serial liver function and hematologic tests should be done to observe for possible development of toxic hepatitis and leukopenia. Treatment apparently does not worsen the neurologic condition of patients with cerebral paragonimiasis, but this possibility should be kept in mind.

Preparations & Dosages

For treatment of paragonimiasis and fascioliasis, the dosage of bithionol (Bitin) is 30–50 mg/kg of body weight, given orally after meals on alternate days for 10–15 days. The total daily dosage should be given in 2–3 divided doses. Three negative sputum and stool specimens obtained 3 months after completion of treatment indicate eradication of the parasite. Within 4–6 months, chest film abnormalities will clear in up to 75% of cases; however, this is less likely to occur in chronic cases. Surgery is indicated in selected cases of cerebral paragonimiasis.

DICHLOROPHEN
(Anthiphen)

Dichlorophen (bis[5-chloro-2-hydroxyphenyl]-methane) is effective and safe for the treatment of several tapeworm infections. Reported cure rates for *Taenia saginata* infection range from 36 to 90% for doses greater than 5 g. Cure rates for *Taenia solium* infection are probably similar, but few reports are available. One investigator reported 64% of 73 patients cured of *Diphyllobothrium latum* infection using 6 g daily for 2 days. The drug has low efficacy in the treatment of *Hymenolepis nana* infections.

Dichlorophen has a consistent laxative effect; colic and mild nausea and vomiting may also occur. Lassitude and rash are rare, and jaundice has been reported.

The same cautions should be observed for the treatment of *T solium* infection with dichlorophen, especially the posttreatment purge, as are described for niclosamide with respect to the theoretic risk of cysticercosis after release of ova from disintegrating tapeworm segments. Because of the risk of drug-induced vomiting, in *T solium* infection it is preferable to use niclosamide. Dichlorophen is contraindicated in the presence of liver disease. Alcoholic beverages should be avoided during treatment.

Dichlorophen (Anthiphen) is prepared as 0.5-g tablets. The dosage is 75 mg/kg (maximum 6 g) taken on an empty stomach in the morning, without prior dietary restrictions or purgatives. Breakfast may follow in 2 hours. Repeat the dose the following morning. Except for *T solium* infection, no posttreatment purge is necessary even if a search for the scolex is intended, because the drug itself has a laxative action. Since the disintegrated scolex can rarely be identified, the results of treatment are not known with certainty until stools are reexamined 3–4 months later, when worms, if not expelled, will have regenerated and begun to shed new segments.

Dichlorophen is not marketed in the USA.

DIETHYLCARBAMAZINE CITRATE
(Banocide, Caricide, Hetrazan, Notézine)

Diethylcarbamazine, discovered in 1947, is the drug of choice for the treatment of filariasis infections.

Chemistry

Diethylcarbamazine citrate, 1-diethylcarbamyl-4-methylpiperazine dihydrogen citrate, is a piperazine derivative. The citrate salt contains 51% of the active base.

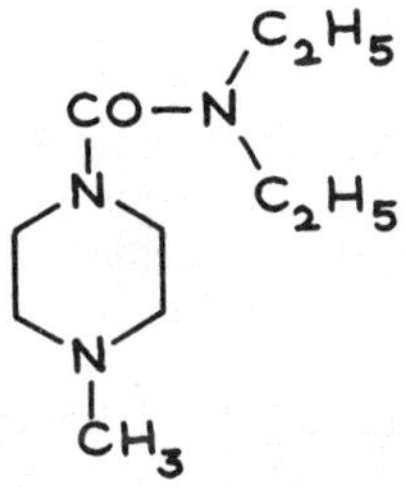

Diethylcarbamazine base

Absorption, Metabolism, & Excretion

When given orally, diethylcarbamazine is rapidly absorbed from the gastrointestinal tract. A single oral dose of 200 mg of base produces a peak blood level of 1.6 μg/mL in 1–2 hours. The minimum effective blood concentration appears to be 0.8–1.0 μg/mL.

Distribution studies indicate that the drug rapidly equilibrates with all tissues (including blood cells) except fat. It is excreted within 30 hours in the urine, either as unchanged drug or as a variety of degradation products. There is no tendency to accumulation with repeated doses. When the urine is alkaline, urinary excretion of the drug slows.

Pharmacologic Effects

A. Actions on Humans: The headache, sleepiness, and vomiting that may accompany administration of the drug are probably due to stimulating effects of the compound on the central nervous system. In high concentrations, diethylcarbamazine has anti-inflammatory or blocking action in some anaphylactic reactions; the mechanism is imperfectly understood. Oral doses of 100–200 mg/kg to pregnant rats and rabbits had no teratogenetic effects. Diethylcarbamazine is absorbed when applied to the conjunctiva and has a microfilaricidal effect in the aqueous humor. However, in heavily infected patients, a severe anterior uveitis may follow. Ocular inserts with varying concentrations of diethylcarbamazine are undergoing clinical trials. The drug is also absorbed topically when applied as a 1% lotion. However, reports vary on its effectiveness and freedom from significant side-effects.

B. Anthelmintic Actions: Diethylcarbamazine does not kill microfilariae in vitro. In vivo, microfilariae disappear from the blood when a therapeutic course is administered to patients infected with *Wuchereria bancrofti, Brugia malayi, Loa loa,* or *Onchocerca volvulus*. Microfilariae also disappear from the skin of patients infected with *Dipetalonema streptocerca,* but the drug is less effective or inactive against microfilariae of *Dipetalonema perstans* or *Mansonella ozzardi*. In the course of treatment, many microfilariae are killed on the first day, but others die in subsequent days. Thus, antigen may be released from dying worms over several days.

Diethylcarbamazine causes a shift in location of microfilariae. In nocturnally periodic *W bancrofti* infection, if the drug is given in the daytime, the microfilariae apparently lose their position in the lung and appear in increased numbers in the peripheral circulation. In onchocerciasis, the drug flushes microfilariae from the dermis into the epidermis within 2 hours of treatment; and in some patients microfilariae may then be found in blood, urine, sputum, aqueous humor, and cerebrospinal fluid.

Diethylcarbamazine kills adult worms of *W bancrofti, B malayi, L loa,* and *D streptocerca* but not of *O volvulus* or *Dirofilaria immitis*. The drug may have some lethal or sterilizing effect on *D perstans* and *M ozzardi* and is highly effective against adult worms of *L loa*. However, the extent to which adult worms of *W bancrofti* and *B malayi* are killed in humans is not known. If therapy is adequate, microfilariae do not reappear in the majority of patients, which suggests that the adult worms are killed or at least permanently sterilized. The death of adult worms has been confirmed by experimental studies on *B malayi* infection in cats, by direct observation of *L loa* infection in humans, and by biopsies of *W bancrofti* infections in humans. No conclusion can be drawn, however, about the mode of action of diethylcarbamazine against adult worms, and it is not known if the drug can kill either third-stage or fourth-stage larvae.

Clinical Uses

A. *W bancrofti, B malayi, L loa:* Diethylcarbamazine is the drug of choice for treatment of these parasites, given its high order of therapeutic efficacy and relative lack of serious toxicity. Microfilariae are rapidly killed by diethylcarbamazine. Adults are killed more slowly, often requiring several courses of treatment.

B. *O volvulus:* Treatment must be individualized for each patient to determine if clinical findings indicate the necessity for treatment and if the patient can tolerate drug side-effects. Although diethylcarbamazine kills microfilariae, it causes severe, sometimes violent reactions. Furthermore, the reduction in microfilariae is only temporary, since diethylcarbamazine does not kill adult worms.

The preferred treatment of onchocerciasis consists of surgical removal of accessible nodules (particularly those on the head), the use of suramin in selected patients to kill adult worms, and use of a course of diethylcarbamazine both before and after suramin treatment to kill microfilariae (see p 605).

If it is elected not to use suramin, a standard course of diethylcarbamazine followed by weekly doses of 200 mg of diethylcarbamazine may be useful in keeping infected persons symptom-free and preventing microfilariae from invading the eye.

C. Other Parasites: Diethylcarbamazine is effective against tropical eosinophilia when given orally in a variety of dosage schedules. As much as 6 mg/kg 3 times daily, for 5–10 days or longer, may be necessary. If microfilariae are present in the blood, smaller doses (3–4 mg/kg) should be given.

Diethylcarbamazine may have some effect against *D perstans* and *M ozzardi* infections, but it is not effective against *D immitis*. It has been used in the treatment of *Ascaris* infections and cutaneous larva migrans, but other drugs are superior.

D. Mass Therapy: One important application of diethylcarbamazine therapy has been its use for mass treatment of *W bancrofti* infections to reduce transmission and, it is hoped, to achieve eradication in some areas. Various regimens have been used, a common one being 5–6 mg/kg orally 1 day each week or month for 6–12 doses. Often, because of side-effects, patients will not return for repeated doses.

E. Prevention of *L loa* Infection: For the prevention of *L loa* infections, a regimen of 2.5 mg/kg twice daily for 3 consecutive days once a month may be tried.

Adverse Reactions

Diethylcarbamazine is a safe drug at therapeutic levels. Only a few mild, occasional side-effects that start in 2–4 hours can be attributed directly to the drug: headache, malaise, anorexia, and weakness. Nausea, vomiting, and sleepiness occur less often. Side-effects also occur as a result of the release of foreign proteins from dying microfilariae or adult worms in sensitized patients. The immunologic mechanism underlying these reactions has not been elucidated.

A. Reactions in Onchocerciasis: In onchocerciasis, a cluster of symptoms known as the "Mazzotti reaction'' occurs in most patients and is often severe, especially in heavily infected patients. The Mazzotti reaction is usually localized in the skin but may also be systemic. Symptoms may start within 30 minutes to 24 hours after the initial dose of diethylcarbamazine, persist for 3–7 days, and then subside, after which high doses can be tolerated without further symptoms. Pruritus, which may be intense, may be accompanied by edema of the skin and a papular rash. The skin reactions may be localized or generalized, and the lymph glands draining the affected areas may become swollen, tender, and painful. Systemic findings include pyrexia (up to 39 °C), malaise or prostration, nausea and vomiting, cough, joint and muscle pains, vertigo, tachycardia, respiratory distress, and hypotension. Proteinuria has been reported, and some deaths have occurred in patients debilitated by malnutrition or tuberculosis.

Patients with many microfilariae in the cornea and conjunctiva may experience a rapid exacerbation of lacrimation and photophobia. The rapid death of microfilariae in the anterior uveal tissues may result in red eye and by flare and cells in the anterior chamber—signs of iridocyclitis. With the latter, there is serious danger of synechiae unless appropriate treatment is given; oral diethylcarbamazine treatment under expert supervision is generally considered to be beneficial for anterior chamber infection. However, diethylcarbamazine therapy has recently been implicated as a cause of posterior segment changes.

B. Reactions in *W bancrofti, B malayi,* and *L loa* Infections: Reactions to dying microfilariae are usually mild or absent for *W bancrofti,* more intense for *B malayi,* and occasionally severe for *L loa* infections. Nevertheless, even in *W bancrofti* infection, about 25% of patients experience generalized reactions including headache, gastrointestinal symptoms, cough, chest pains, muscle or joint pain, malaise, fever, and papular rash. In *W bancrofti* and *B malayi* infections, symptoms are most likely to occur in patients with heavy loads of microfilariae but may also occur even if the patient is apparently amicrofilaremic.

Local reactions may occur around dying adult or immature worms. These reactions are commonest from the third day of treatment onward and may last as long as 10 days. In *W bancrofti* infections, focal reactions of lymphangitis, lymphadenitis, and lymph abscess can occur. In *L loa* infections, small wheals can appear in the skin at the site of dying worms; and in *D streptocerca* infection, flat papules can appear. Except for an allergic encephalitis that occurs rarely in loiasis, these symptoms are never life-threatening.

Contraindications & Cautions

Severe reactions due to death of microfilariae may occur when diethylcarbamazine is used in the treatment of onchocerciasis, particularly in heavy infections (skin concentrations of microfilariae over 100/mg), if microfilariae are producing symptoms in the skin, or if they are found in or near the eyes. Such patients should be hospitalized and treated by physicians with adequate ophthalmologic knowledge and the necessary equipment for eye examination, including a slit lamp.

Patients with attacks of lymphangitis due to *W bancrofti* or *B malayi* infection should be treated in a quiescent period between attacks.

In loiasis, reactions are more likely in patients with pretreatment microfilariae counts greater than 50/μL of blood; exchange transfusion has been suggested to reduce such counts.

Patients suspected of having malaria should be treated with chloroquine before they are given diethylcarbamazine, since the latter drug may provoke a relapse in nonsymptomatic malaria infections.

There are no absolute contraindications to the use of diethylcarbamazine, but caution is advised in patients with hypertension.

Preparations & Dosages

Diethylcarbamazine citrate (Banocide, Caricide, Hetrazan, Notézine) is available as 50-mg tablets or as a syrup containing 24 mg/mL. It is available in the USA only from Lederle Laboratories; telephone (914) 735–5000.

A. *W bancrofti, B malayi, L loa:* These infections are treated with 2 mg of the citrate salt per kilogram of body weight given orally 3 times a day after meals for 12 days to a total of 72 mg/kg. To reduce the incidence of allergic reactions from dying microfilariae, a single dose (2 mg/kg) is administered on the first day, 2 doses on the second day, and 3 doses on the third day and thereafter. For *B malayi* or for loiasis (with its risk of encephalopathy), the same schedule should be used, but individual doses should start at 1 mg/kg once on the first day and gradually increase to 2 mg/kg 3 times daily by the fourth to fifth day.

Antihistamines may be given for the first 4–5 days of diethylcarbamazine therapy to reduce the incidence of ''allergic'' reactions. Corticosteroids should be started and doses of diethylcarbamazine temporarily lowered or interrupted if severe reactions occur.

Blood should be checked for microfilariae several weeks after treatment is completed; if any are still present, a course may be repeated at intervals of 3–4 weeks. However, since the initial treatment does not kill all adult worms, microfilariae may reappear in 3–12 months. Cure may require subsequent courses of treatment over 1–2 years.

B. *O volvulus:* If possible, treatment should be started in the hospital, using low doses initially and increasing progressively depending upon progress. The following is one type of dosage schedule for heavy infections, with the drug to be given after meals: initially, give 25 mg once and wait several days for the reaction to subside; then give 25 mg twice daily for 1 day; then 50 mg twice daily for 1 day; then 100 mg twice daily for 1 day; thereafter, continue 200 mg once daily until the microfilarial load in the skin has been reduced to near zero, a process that takes about 7–14 days. Suramin treatment is then started to kill the adult worms (see p 620). During the course of suramin, continue diethylcarbamazine, 200 mg twice daily, for 3–5 days and repeat every 2–4 weeks. At the end of the suramin treatment, repeat diethylcarbamazine, 200 mg twice daily for 3–5 days at 3- to 4-week intervals until pruritic skin reactions no longer occur.

If suramin is *not* used, diethylcarbamazine may be used as a microfilarial suppressive by initially giving the standard course of therapy and then continuing the drug indefinitely at weekly intervals in a dosage of 50–200 mg; in these weekly treatments, allergic reactions will usually be insignificant if they occur at all.

In mild infections, symptomatic relief of pain, fever, and headache is sometimes possible with aspirin and codeine, but use of corticosteroids may become necessary. Antihistamines have not been useful. However, all patients with heavy infections should receive betamethasone, 1–2 mg 3 times daily starting 1–2 days before the first dose of diethylcarbamazine, continued through the major part of the reaction, and then tapered off over 4 days. If keratoconjunctivitis occurs, administer betamethasone eye drops; if iridocyclitis occurs, administer both eye drops and atropine, with appropriate caution to avoid precipitating acute glaucoma.

EMETINE HYDROCHLORIDE

Emetine and dehydroemetine are alternative drugs for the treatment of *Fasciola hepatica* infection. Both drugs may be effective in removing the parasite, but they are more toxic than bithionol, the drug of choice. Dehydroemetine is probably less toxic than emetine; general pharmacologic information, dosage, and precautions in their usage are presented in Chapter 54.

HEXYLRESORCINOL
(Crystoids)

Chemistry, Absorption, Metabolism, & Excretion

Hexylresorcinol (1,3-dihydroxy-4-hexylbenzene), a phenol derivative, was used for many years as a broad-spectrum anthelmintic but has been superseded for most indications by drugs that are more effective and easier to use. It continues to be an alternative drug for trichuriasis and for several intestinal fluke infections. The drug is not available in the USA.

After ingestion, approximately one-third of hexylresorcinol is absorbed from the gastrointestinal tract and then eliminated rapidly in the urine. Since the drug is soluble in fat and combines with protein, food should not be present in the upper gastrointestinal tract.

Adverse Reactions

Hexylresorcinol is nearly devoid of systemic toxicity at therapeutic levels, but used topically it is corrosive to the oral mucosa and perianal skin. When given orally, mucosal ulceration may occur in the mouth unless the crystals are incorporated into hard gelatin-coated pills. Although the mucosa of the intestinal tract is protected by its mucous secretions, the drug may cause epigastric discomfort, vomiting, or diarrhea in a few individuals.

Contraindications & Cautions

To protect the oral mucosa, considerable care must be taken to ensure that pills are swallowed immediately and not chewed. Children should be supervised to be certain that the pills are not retained between the teeth and cheeks or under the tongue. For uncooperative children, hexylresorcinol crystals dissolved in 20 mL of water may be delivered through a duodenal tube. Hexylresorcinol is contraindicated in the presence of peptic ulcers, ulcerative colitis, and intestinal obstruction.

Clinical Uses, Preparations, & Dosages

Hexylresorcinol is prepared as gelatin-coated pills (Crystoids) for oral use or in bulk form for preparation of enemas. The pills contain 0.2 g of the drug. Hexylresorcinal is no longer marketed in the USA.

A. Trichuriasis (Whipworm, Trichocephaliasis): Hexylresorcinol by retention enema is an alternative drug in the treatment of trichuriasis. However, it is recommended only for patients with significant symptoms and if the preferred drugs, mebendazole or oxantel pamoate, are not available.

In the evening, a warm soapsuds enema is followed by a 0.2% hexylresorcinol enema (volume, 20–30 mL/kg of body weight up to 1200 mL). The enema should be retained for 30 minutes; retention is facilitated by taping the buttocks together. If necessary, a small saline enema may be used to initiate expulsion. Two or more treatments at weekly intervals may be necessary to reduce worm loads and stop symptoms, but removal of all the parasites is not necessary and should not be attempted. ***Caution:*** Perianal skin irritation that develops when hexylresorcinol is used as a retention enema is preventable by the application of a film of petrolatum.

B. *Fasciolopsis buski, Heterophyes heterophyes,* and *Metagonimus yokogawai:* Alcohol should be avoided for 24 hours before and after treatment. Pretreatment purges are generally omitted except in the treatment of fasciolopsiasis. The day before treatment, the total diet should be reduced and the evening meal limited to soft, fat-free foods. Breakfast should be omitted on the morning of treatment and the drug administered with water. No food should be taken for 5 hours, but water is permissible. A saline purge (for adults use 30 g magnesium sulfate) should be given 2 hours after treatment. An additional course of treatment can be given a week later.

Adults and children over age 12 years receive 1 g; children age 8–12 years, 0.8 g; children age 6–8 years, 0.6 g; and infants and children up to age 6 years, 0.1 g per year of age. A minimum dose of 0.4 g is usually necessary for small children, who tolerate it well.

HYCANTHONE METHANESULFONATE (Etrenol)

Hycanthone has been undergoing clinical trials since 1968 for the treatment of schistosomiasis. It is effective against *Schistosoma mansoni* and *Schistosoma haematobium* but not *Schistosoma japonicum*. The drug's important contribution is its high effectiveness with only a single intramuscular injection. However, its hepatotoxicity in some patients and accumulating data on its potential for teratogenicity and carcinogenicity have led to its deletion in this text for treatment of schistosomiasis. In spite of the adoption of contraindications, at least 72 deaths have been attributed to the drug; the deaths occurred within 2–5 days after treatment and were characterized by acute hepatic necrosis.

Hycanthone is not available in the USA.

LEVAMISOLE (Decaris, Ketrax)

Levamisole hydrochloride and tetramisole hydrochloride are synthetic imidazothiazole derivatives, levamisole being the L isomer of DL-tetramisole. Since most of the anthelmintic activity of the compounds is limited to the L isomer, use of levamisole rather than tetramisole permits a reduction in dosage and hence in side-effects. Tetramisole, introduced in 1966, has been extensively studied in humans. Levamisole was introduced subsequently and continues under active clinical investigation for its anthelmintic and immunologic properties. Neither drug is marketed in the USA.

Levamisole is highly effective in eradicating *Ascaris* and *Trichostrongylus* from most patients with a single course of treatment. It is only moderately effective in hookworm infections due to *A duodenale* and has a low effectiveness in *N americanus, Trichuris trichiura,* and pinworm infections. Its usefulness in strongyloidiasis remains to be determined.

Chemistry

Levamisole hydrochloride (L-tetramisole HCl), (−)-2,3,5,6-tetrahydro-6-phenylimidazo[2,1-*b*]-thiazole hydrochloride, is highly soluble in water at physiologic pH. It is normally given orally but may be injected subcutaneously.

Absorption, Metabolism, & Excretion

Levamisole is rapidly and extensively absorbed. In humans, a single tritium-labeled oral dose of 150 mg produces a peak plasma level of 0.5 μg/mL in 2–4 hours. (This is the same order of concentration needed in vitro to restore depressed phagocyte and T cell function to normal.) Levamisole is widely distributed to the tissues, with a high concentration in the liver, where it is extensively metabolized. Although blood levels fall rapidly—the plasma half-life is 4 hours—the pharmacologic and immunologic effects are prolonged. Within 24 hours, 60% of the oral dose is found in the urine, mostly as metabolites, and by 72 hours an additional 11% appears. Only 4% of the administered radioactivity is excreted in the feces. Apparently levamisole crosses the blood-brain barrier, for it is effective against *Angiostrongylus cantonensis* in rats.

Pharmacologic Effects & Anthelmintic Actions

At relatively high concentrations, levamisole has a reversible ganglion-stimulating effect on mammalian tissue at both parasympathetic and sympathetic sites. In general, this results in stimulation of the central and autonomic nervous systems and skeletal muscle. Levamisole also has a positive inotropic and chronotropic effect on the fatigued heart muscle and is a strong inhibitor of mammalian alkaline phosphatases, except for intestinal and placental isoenzymes. Toxicologic studies in pregnant animals did not indicate any teratogenic or embryotoxic effects.

Levamisole is an immunomodulating, immunostimulating agent (see Chapter 57). It affects host defenses by modulating cell-mediated immune responses, including polymorphonuclear leukocyte, macrophage, and T cell functions. In theory, the drug is useful only when cell-mediated immunity is depressed; it has little effect on normal immune mechanisms except at dosages that greatly exceed therapeutic concentrations. The immune reactivity increases promptly after only a single dose and is thought to persist from days to months. However, the responses to levamisole are not always predictable. The drug is under intensive clinical investigation to determine its mechanism of action and effectiveness in a variety of clinical conditions.

In nematodes, levamisole stimulates ganglionlike structures, causing contraction of muscle and then neuromuscular inhibition of the depolarizing type, resulting in paralysis. The worms are then eliminated by peristalsis. There is some indication that the anthelmintic action of levamisole may also stem from its inhibiting action on fumarate reductase. Levamisole has little ovicidal action on *Trichuris* and none on *Ascaris*.

Adverse Reactions

When levamisole is used in a single dose for the treatment of *Ascaris* and hookworm infections, side-effects are mild and transient. They include nausea and vomiting, mild abdominal cramping pain, headache, dizziness, weakness, and skin rash. In Moens' report on 1734 patients tested in 10 studies, 12% had one or more of these symptoms, yet 15% of the group receiving placebos also had these symptoms. In other studies, reported side-effects ranged from none to 23%; workers were in agreement that the symptoms were mild. Transient optic neuritis after a single dose and an anaphylactic reaction in a patient receiving the third of 3 doses given at intervals of 2–4 weeks have recently been reported.

When levamisole is used for its immunologic properties in long-term treatment at dosages of 150 mg/d 3–7 times a week for several months, side-effects, which are sometimes severe, occur in about 20% of patients. The adverse reactions include an influenzalike syndrome with fever, gastrointestinal symptoms, central nervous system stimulation (headache, dizziness, nervousness, irritability, insomnia, sensory stimulation, and vertigo), skin rash, thrombocytopenia, renal medullary damage, iridocyclitis, and nonfatal and fatal agranulocytosis. Single-dose treatment of parasites does not seem to carry the risk of these side-effects.

Clinical Uses, Preparations, & Dosages

Levamisole (Decaris, Ethnor, Ketrax, Solaskil) is available in 50- and 150-mg tablets and as a syrup. Adults receive a single dose of 150 mg and children a single dose of 3 mg/kg. Stools should be checked 2 weeks later.

A. Ascariasis: In a multicenter study involving 10 centers and 768 patients, 91% of cases were cured with a single treatment and there was a marked (85%) reduction in ovum count in those not cured. Other studies confirm cure rates in the range of 86–100%.

B. Hookworm Infection: In the few studies available, single doses of levamisole produced cure rates of 64–100% in the treatment of *Ancylostoma* infections. However, cure rates reported for *Necator* infections, after 1–2 doses, ranged from 0 to 32% in 6 studies and were 80–84% in 3 studies. Studies are needed to evaluate efficacy and side-effects of higher doses or longer courses of treatment.

C. Other Infections: In *Trichostrongylus* infections, a single dose is curative in over 95% of patients. In **strongyloidiasis** the results are promising but need confirmation after standard treatment is given weekly for 3 weeks. In **filariasis** studies in animals and humans, levamisole has microfilaricidal effects but is not macrofilaricidal at doses that can be tolerated.

MEBENDAZOLE
(Vermox)

Mebendazole, introduced in 1972, has a wide spectrum of anthelmintic activity and is nearly free of side-effects. It is a drug of choice in trichuriasis, pinworm infection, trichostrongyliasis, and infections with both species of hookworm, and is particularly useful in mixed infections with trichurids, ascarids, and hookworms, but it does not produce satisfactory cure rates in strongyloidiasis. Mebendazole is also highly effective in capillariasis and has shown promise in the treatment of trichinosis. Clinical trials suggest that mebendazole may be the first drug useful in the treatment of some cases of echinococcosis. Flubendazole, the parafluoro analog of mebendazole, is undergoing early clinical trials. It is similar to mebendazole in its anthelmintic spectrum and few side-effects, but in addition it appears to be active in the treatment of strongyloidiasis and had no teratogenic effect in rats or rabbits.

Chemistry

Mebendazole (methyl 5-benzoylbenzimidazole-2-carbamate) is a synthetic benzimidazole. Unlike the benzimidazole anthelmintic thiabendazole, mebendazole is substituted in position 5 and has a carbamate function. It is slightly soluble in water and is not unpleasant in taste.

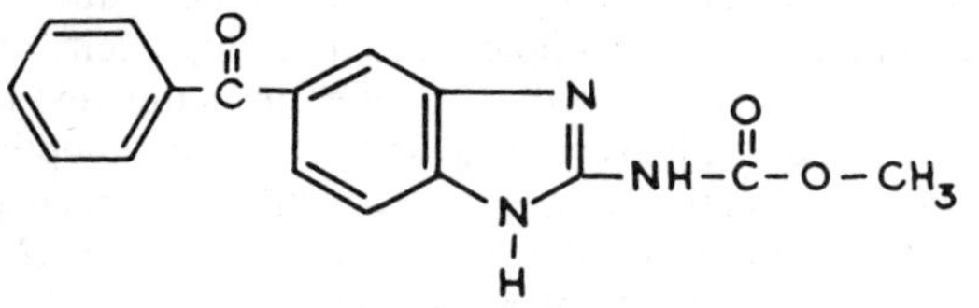

Mebendazole

Absorption, Metabolism, & Excretion

Mebendazole is poorly absorbed. Following oral administration, peak plasma levels are reached in 2–4 hours. After ingestion of 0.1 mg of ^{14}C-labeled mebendazole per kilogram of body weight, 6–10% of radioactivity was recovered in the urine, of which 2.5% was unconjugated mebendazole, 20% was the decarbamate metabolite, and 75% was of undetermined identity. Sensitive methods for determining plasma levels of the drug have become available only recently. With administration of 100 mg of mebendazole twice daily for 3 days, plasma levels of the drug and its principal metabolite, the 2-amine, never exceeded 0.03 μg/mL and 0.09 μg/mL, respectively. These studies led to the estimation that less than 10% of the administered dose was absorbed.

Pharmacologic Effects & Anthelmintic Actions

Mebendazole irreversibly blocks uptake of exogenous glucose by nematodes, leading to glycogen depletion and reduced generation of ATP required for survival. As a result, the parasites die or are immobilized only slowly, and their clearance from the gastrointestinal tract may not be complete until several days after treatment. Mebendazole does not affect blood glucose levels in animals or humans. Efficacy of the drug varies with gastrointestinal transit time and intensity of infection and possibly with the strain of parasite and whether or not the drug is chewed. The drug also kills hookworm, *Ascaris*, and *Trichuris* eggs.

Acute and chronic toxicologic studies in animals indicate a wide range between therapeutic and toxic doses. The LD50 (mg/kg orally) was more than 640 in rabbits and dogs and more than 1280 in mice and rats. Significant hematologic, biochemical, or pathologic abnormalities were not found in animals given 40 mg/kg daily for 13 weeks but were noted in rats given a daily dosage of 130 mg/kg. In pregnant rats the drug had embryotoxic and teratogenic activity at single oral doses as low as 10 mg/kg.

Clinical Uses

A. *Trichuris trichiura* (Whipworm): Most studies indicate that when mebendazole is given at a dosage schedule of 100 mg twice daily for 3–4 days, cure rates are 60–90%, with marked reduction in ovum counts in those not cured. However, lower cure rates have also been reported. The heavier the infection, the more difficult it becomes to eradicate with only one course of treatment.

B. *Enterobius vermicularis* (Pinworm): Reports from various studies indicate cure rates of 90–100%. Thus, mebendazole compares favorably with the single-dose regimen of pyrvinium pamoate and pyrantel pamoate but has the advantages of fewer side-effects and the absence of staining properties.

C. *Ascaris lumbricoides,* Hookworm, and *Trichostrongylus:* A 3-day course produces cure rates of 90-100% for ascariasis and *Trichostrongylus* infections and 70–95% for hookworm infections by both species, with a marked reduction in the worm burden in those not cured.

D. Tapeworms: Mebendazole at a dosage of 300 mg twice daily for 3 days has been tested in the treatment of taeniasis. Reports on its effectiveness have varied. In the treatment of *T solium* infection, mebendazole has one theoretic advantage over niclosamide—proglottids are expelled intact after therapy. The standard 3-day course of mebendazole treatment is not effective in *Hymenolepis nana* infections; possibly extended treatment might be useful.

E. Hydatid Disease: The results of treatment of *Echinococcus granulosus* infections with high doses of mebendazole for long periods of time are unpredictable. Reports have varied from no change in the expected course of the disease (although the natural history of hydatid disease is not well established); to no progression while under treatment, with recurrence when the drug is stopped; to apparent cure as documented by regression or obliteration of cysts on sequential roentgenographic examinations or by the rare opportunities to examine tissues histologically. However, regression of cysts is not proof of cure, since subsequent recurrences have been described. In nonresponsive cases, it is possible that plasma levels of mebendazole were insufficient, since large variations in plasma concentrations have been reported in different individuals and even in the same patients monitored at different times.

Clinical studies continue in order to determine efficacy, indications, and optimal dosages. For patients with hydatid disease who are unable to undergo surgery or whose cysts have ruptured and disseminated, a recommended dose is 50 mg/kg in 3 divided doses daily for 3 months. For patients who do undergo surgery, many surgeons provide mebendazole coverage in the perioperative period. For *Echinococcus multilocularis* infections, daily treatments up to 5 years have provided stabilization in some cases, but the long-term prognosis is still uncertain.

Occasional side-effects are pruritus, rash, eosinophilia, fever, and acute pain in the cyst area, associated with tenderness; some of these findings may be due to cyst rupture with release of antigen. In studies with mice, cyst necrosis and rupture were followed by death of some animals; however, in humans, no deaths or cases of anaphylaxis or dissemination have been described in instances of presumed cyst rupture. Gastric irritation, cough, and transient liver function abnormalities have also been described. In addition, at least 6 cases of histologically confirmed glomerulonephritis have been reported, as well as 3 cases of drug-induced agranulocytosis, with death of one of the latter patients. Mebendazole should be taken with meals, preferably with food containing fat, which enhances absorption. In the USA, the drug is not approved for use in treatment of *Echinococcus* infections.

F. Other Infections: For treatment of **intestinal capillariasis,** mebendazole is the drug of choice at a dosage of 400 mg daily in divided doses for 21 or more days.

In **trichinosis,** initial reports suggest therapeutic efficacy against adult worms in the intestinal tract, migrating larvae, and larvae in muscle. The suggested dosage for adult patients is 1 g daily in divided doses for 14 days.

In a few studies there are reported cures of **strongyloidiasis** with a standard 3-day course of therapy; a longer course and higher dosages may be more effective and should be tested. The efficacy of mebendazole in **dracontiasis** needs further study. The combined usage of mebendazole plus levamisole in **filariasis** continues under study. Mebendazole may be the first drug available for the treatment of ***Dipetalonema perstans* infection.**

Adverse Reactions

Mebendazole therapy has been remarkably free of side-effects even in debilitated patients. Mild nausea and vomiting, diarrhea, and abdominal pain have been reported infrequently. In children heavily parasitized by *Ascaris,* abdominal cramps are not uncommon; oral passage of ascarids in those under age 5 years has been reported from some countries.

Contraindications & Cautions

The drug is contraindicated in pregnant women. It should be used with caution in children under age 2 years because of limited experience.

Preparations & Dosages

Mebendazole (Vermox) is prepared as tablets containing 100 mg of the drug. They can be taken before or after meals. It may be therapeutically advantageous to advise that the tablets be *chewed* before swallowing.

The same dosage is used for adults and for children over age 2 years. For the treatment of ascariasis, trichuriasis, and hookworm infections, give 100 mg twice daily for 3 days. In severe trichuriasis infections, a longer course (up to 6 days) or a repeat course will often be necessary. No pretreatment or posttreatment purging is used. Reexamine stools for ova in 2–3 weeks to determine if a second course of treatment is necessary.

For the treatment of pinworms, give 100 mg once only. Repeat the dose at 2 and 4 weeks.

In the USA, mebendazole has been approved for use only in ascariasis, trichuriasis, and hookworm and pinworm infections.

METRIFONATE
(Bilarcil)

Metrifonate was introduced in 1952 as the insecticide trichlorfon (Dipterex) and then in 1960 as an oral drug for the treatment of *Schistosoma haematobium* infections, for which it has become a drug of choice because of its effectiveness, safety, and ease of administration. It is not effective against *Schistosoma mansoni* or *Schistosoma japonicum*.

Chemistry, Absorption, Metabolism, & Excretion

Metrifonate, an organophosphorus compound, is O,O-dimethyl-[1-hydroxy-2,2,2-trichloroethyl]-phosphonate.

In humans, metrifonate is rapidly absorbed after oral administration and rapidly broken down, although the metabolic pathway is not yet understood. In various animal species, a peak of radioactive ^{32}P-labeled substance is found in plasma, kidneys, lungs, liver, and adrenals 2 hours after administration; the drug is no longer detectable after 24–48 hours.

Pharmacologic Effects & Anthelmintic Actions

Metrifonate is a cholinesterase inhibitor and appears to act indirectly as a result of its being transformed into the active metabolite dichlorvos (2,2-dichlorovinyl dimethyl phosphate). Dichlorvos was formerly used in the treatment of humans with hookworm infections and ascariasis.

The mode of action of metrifonate against schistosomes is not established, but it is assumed to act on both the immature and mature stages of the parasites by cholinesterase inhibition, causing temporary paralysis. This results in a shift of adult schistosomes from the bladder venous plexus to small arterioles of the lungs, where they are trapped and encased and then die.

In acute toxicity studies in experimental animals, the oral LD50 was between 400 and 674 mg/kg. In chronic toxicity studies, unresolved discrepancies regarding toxicity of the compound for specific organs may be caused by differences in the purity of the test material. Some studies show no abnormalities; others indicate potential for hepatotoxicity and hematologic toxicity.

Some organophosphorus compounds are known to have mutagenic properties. Metrifonate showed mutagenicity in the *Salmonella typhimurium* direct test system and in the host-mediated assay system in mice. It induced gene mutations in *Escherichia coli* but caused no chromosomal abnormalities in animals or humans. Reproduction toxicity studies showed negative results except for suggestions of impaired spermatogenesis.

Studies using therapeutic dosages in humans or comparable doses in animals produced no untoward physiologic or chemical abnormalities except for cholinesterase inhibition, which results in the accumulation of acetylcholine at nerve synapses and may produce some short-lasting signs and symptoms. Following oral ingestion of 7.5–12.5 mg/kg of metrifonate by infected persons, there is an almost complete inhibition of plasma cholinesterase and a marked reduction (about 50%) of erythrocytic cholinesterase. Plasma recovery is usually 70% or more by 2 weeks and is completed by 4 weeks, but erythrocyte recovery may take up to 15 weeks.

Clinical Uses

In the treatment of *S haematobium* infections, cure rates in various clinical trials ranged from 44 to 93% when 3 doses of 7.5–10 mg/kg were given orally at 14- to 28-day intervals. Those not cured showed a marked reduction in ovum counts. Metrifonate was also effective as a prophylactic when given monthly to children in a highly endemic area.

Adverse Reactions

In clinical trials, tolerance has been excellent. Some studies report no side-effects; others note mild and transient findings including nausea and vomiting, diarrhea, abdominal pain, bronchospasm, headache, weakness, and vertigo. These symptoms may begin within 30 minutes and persist up to 12 hours. The drug was well tolerated by patients in advanced stages of the disease.

One case of organophosphate poisoning following a standard dose has been reported; the patient responded well to the use of atropine. The polyneuropathy reported from the Soviet Union and eastern Europe has been attributed to an unknown contaminant or to excessive doses.

Contraindications & Cautions

Metrifonate should not be used after recent exposure to insecticides or drugs that might potentiate cholinesterase inhibition. The use of muscle relaxants, particularly as part of general anesthesia, should be avoided for 48 hours after administration of the drug. The drug is contraindicated in pregnancy. In the USA, it is required that plasma cholinesterase levels be determined before each dose of the drug.

Preparations & Dosages

Metrifonate (Bilarcil) is supplied in 100-mg divided tablets and is taken orally at a dosage of 7.5–10 mg/kg once, and then repeated twice at 2-week intervals. The drug is not marketed in the USA but can be obtained from the Parasitic Disease Drug Service, Centers for Disease Control, Atlanta 30333 (telephone number [404] 329–3670).

NICLOSAMIDE
(Nicloside, Yomesan)

Niclosamide, introduced in 1960, has been for many years the drug of choice for the treatment of most tapeworm infections.

Chemistry

Niclosamide is N-(2′-chloro-4′-nitrophenyl)-5-chlorosalicylamide.

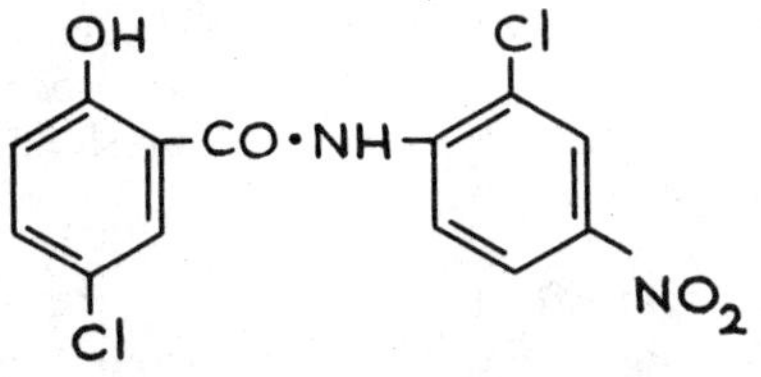

Niclosamide

Absorption & Metabolism

Niclosamide is apparently not absorbed from the gastrointestinal tract. The unaltered drug has not been recovered from the blood or urine.

Pharmacologic Effects & Anthelmintic Actions

Following oral administration in animals and humans, no hematologic, renal, or hepatic abnormalities have been noted.

The scoleces and segments of cestodes, but not the ova, are rapidly killed on contact with niclosamide. This may be due to the drug's inhibition of oxidative phosphorylation or to its ATPase stimulating property. Associated with the death of the parasite is release of the scolex from the intestinal wall. Even if a purge is used to expel the tapeworm, the scolex and proglottids may be partially digested and difficult to identify.

Clinical Uses

Niclosamide has far fewer and less severe side-effects than quinacrine or aspidium oleoresin and is equally or more effective. Dichlorophen, another taeniacide, is also highly effective but has given variable results. Its side-effects are also mild but may be more frequent than those of niclosamide.

A. *Taenia saginata* (Beef Tapeworm): With a single dose of niclosamide, cure rates of 90–95% can be expected.

B. *Taenia solium* (Pork Tapeworm): Niclosamide is considered equally effective for *T solium* infection.

C. *Diphyllobothrium latum* (Fish Tapeworm): In a group of 297 adult patients receiving 2 g in a single dose, the cure rate was 73% when the tablets were swallowed whole and 87% when they were chewed.

D. *Hymenolepis nana* (Dwarf Tapeworm): Niclosamide is effective against the adult parasites in the lumen of the intestine but not against cysticercoids embedded in the villi. For the drug to be successful, it must be given until all of the cysticercoids have emerged (about 4 days). Thus, the minimum course of treatment must be 5–7 days; some workers repeat the course of treatment 5 days later. In a series of approximately 350 cases, the overall cure rate for niclosamide was 75%.

E. Other Tapeworms: Results have been promising in patients treated for *Hymenolepis diminuta* and *Dipylidium caninum* infections. Theoretically the prolonged treatment required for *H nana* infection should not be necessary for *H diminuta* infections, since the latter infection in humans has no tissue phase. In one study of *H diminuta* infections, 17 of 19 patients were cured with the 5–7 day course and 2 required a second course of treatment. Niclosamide is not effective against cysticercosis or hydatid disease.

F. Other Parasites: Niclosamide can be used as an alternative drug for the treatment of *Fasciolopsis buski* infection, although it is not as effective as tetrachloroethylene or hexylresorcinol.

Adverse Reactions

The drug rarely produces side-effects. Nausea, vomiting, and intestinal colic have been reported.

Contraindications & Cautions

The consumption of alcohol should be avoided on the day of treatment and for 1 day afterward.

There are no contraindications to the use of niclosamide. The drug can probably be given safely after the first 3 months of pregnancy.

Preparations & Dosages

Niclosamide (Nicloside, Yomesan) is prepared as chewable tablets, each containing 0.5 g of the drug. Tablets are flavored with saccharin and vanilla. The adult dosage is 4 tablets (2 g). Children weighing more than 34 kg are given 3 tablets; children 11–34 kg, 2 tablets.

Pre- and posttreatment purges are not necessary, except for an occasional patient with chronic constipation. Niclosamide should be given in the morning on an empty stomach. The tablets *must be chewed thoroughly* and then swallowed with water. For small children, pulverize the tablets and then mix with water. The patient may eat 2 hours later. In the treatment of infections with the large tapeworms, segments may continue to pass for several days with normal peristalsis.

A. *T saginata, D latum,* and *D caninum:* Treatment requires only a single dose. Although not usually necessary, a purge may be given 2 hours after treatment in an attempt to recover and identify the scolex before it disintegrates to confirm that the entire worm has passed and will not regenerate. If the scolex is not found or is not searched for, cure can be presumed only if regenerated segments have not reappeared 3–5 months after treatment.

B. *T solium:* Treatment requires only a single dose. However, 2 hours after treatment, an effective purge (such as 15–30 g of magnesium or sodium sulfate) must be given to eliminate all mature segments before ova can be released. The patient should be monitored closely to ensure that prompt evacuation occurs. Since niclosamide does not kill ova released from disintegrating tapeworm segments, cysticercosis is theoretically possible after treatment of *T solium* infections. It is unknown whether larvae are released from ova in the large bowel. If so, they could penetrate the intestinal wall and reach the tissues. However, no cases of cysticercosis have been reported after use of niclosamide.

C. *H nana:* A variety of dosage schedules have been proposed. A recommendation for adults is 2 g daily for 5–7 days. The dosage for children weighing over 34 kg is 1.5 g as a single dose on the first day and then 1 g daily for the next 4–6 days; for children 11–34 kg, the dosage is 1 g on the first day and then 0.5 g daily for 4–6 days. Some workers repeat the course of treatment after 5 days.

D. *H diminuta:* Treat as for *H nana*.

E. *Fasciolopsis buski, Heterophyes heterophyes,* and *Metagonimus yokogawai:* The standard dosage is given every other day for 3 doses.

NIRIDAZOLE

Niridazole has been used for 20 years in the oral treatment of schistosomiasis. Most persons experience side-effects, sometimes severe. Mutagenic and carcinogenic properties have been reported. For these reasons, niridazole is considered an alternative drug, to be used when the preferred drugs are not available. Niridazole is also effective in the treatment of dracontiasis. The drug is not marketed in the USA but may be obtained from the Parasitic Disease Drug Service, Centers for Disease Control, Atlanta 30333.

Chemistry

Niridazole is 1-(5-nitro-2-thiazolyl)-2-imidazolidinone, a nitrothiazole derivative.

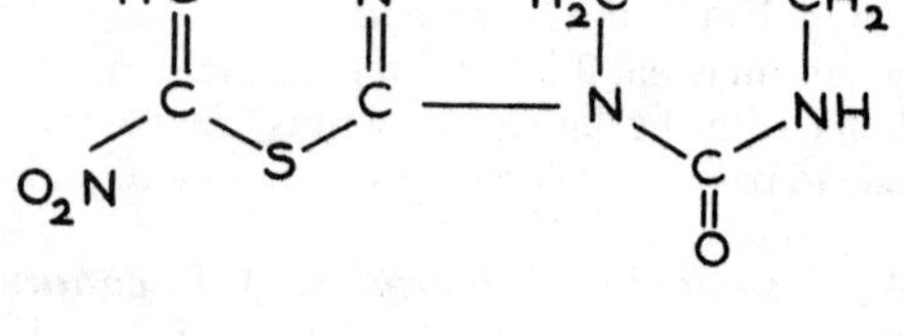

Niridazole

Absorption, Metabolism, & Excretion

Following oral administration, niridazole is absorbed slowly; the maximum blood concentration is reached in 6 hours. Greater blood levels are reached if the drug is given in 2 divided doses 12 hours apart rather than in one single larger dose. The concentration of the unmetabolized drug (the active agent against the parasite) is 5 times higher in the portal blood than in the peripheral circulation because most of the drug is metabolized in the first cycle through the liver. Elimination is mostly through urine and through bile into feces. Niridazole itself completely disappears from human plasma 15 hours after a single dose of 25 mg/kg, whereas the drug metabolites, which are largely bound to serum albumin, have a half-life of about 40 hours.

High blood concentrations of the unmetabolized drug are found in the peripheral circulation in patients with hepatic dysfunction (because metabolic degradation is impaired) and in the presence of portal-systemic shunts (because the drug bypasses the liver). The many side-effects of niridazole are thought to occur when this unmetabolized drug reaches a threshold level in the peripheral circulation.

Pharmacologic Effects

A. Actions in Experimental Animals and Humans: Niridazole produces temporary inhibition of spermatogenesis in experimental animals, but inhibition is reversible, with no subsequent interference with fertility and no posttreatment teratogenic effect. Present evidence indicates that the drug does not have permanent effects on spermatogenesis in humans. Niridazole has been shown to have a glycogen-lowering effect in monkey muscle; such glycogen depletion may be responsible for some of the side-effects in humans. Niridazole also has uricosuric effects.

In addition to its antiparasitic actions, niridazole has antibacterial and anti-inflammatory properties and suppresses delayed hypersensitivity. Manifestations of the latter have included depression of skin test reactivity and lymphocyte transformation in humans, and retardation of allograft rejection and granuloma formation in mice. Thus, niridazole is potentially useful as an immunosuppressant drug.

In animals, signs of damage to the hematopoietic system have been noted following several weeks of niridazole therapy, but in humans there have been no reports of adverse effects on peripheral blood counts or bone marrow, nor have there been reports of increased susceptibility to infection.

B. Anthelmintic Actions: In experimental animals infected with *Schistosoma mansoni,* adequate oral doses of niridazole cause a "liver shift" of adult worms that is followed by their death. Niridazole is rapidly concentrated in adult worms, resulting in the inhibition of phosphorylase inactivation followed by glycogen depletion of the parasite. Niridazole also inhibits or interrupts egg production.

In dracontiasis, animal studies suggest that the drug's action is anti-inflammatory rather than parasiticidal.

Clinical Uses

A. *Schistosoma haematobium, Schistosoma mansoni,* and *Schistosoma japonicum:* Of the 3 species, *S haematobium* is the easiest to eradicate with niridazole treatment and *S japonicum* the most difficult. Since it is not uncommon for live ova to be undetectable for 2–6 months after treatment and then to reappear at 6–12 months, cure rates are best based on the longer follow-up period. In clinical trials based on a 12-month follow-up, cure rates of 78–82% have been reported for *S haematobium,* 38–80% for *S mansoni,* and 26–48% for *S japonicum.* Among patients not cured, marked reduction in ovum counts (80–90%) usually occurs.

In the treatment of *S mansoni* infections, relatively recent infections appear to be more difficult to treat than older infections; perhaps for this reason, children with this infection sometimes appear to be more refractory to treatment than adults. Despite niridazole's moderate effectiveness against *S japonicum,* the drug is often so poorly tolerated that alternative drugs must be used.

Efforts to reduce side-effects but retain effectiveness by giving niridazole over longer periods than the standard course and at reduced daily doses have had variable success. In the treatment of *S haematobium* infections, evidence suggests that short courses of standard doses given for only 3 days result in cure rates of two-thirds or more of patients and marked reduction in ovum counts in the others. Further studies with long-term follow-up are needed to establish the effectiveness of this approach.

B. *Dracunculus medinensis:* Niridazole may provide effective treatment for dracontiasis (guinea worm infection). Reduction of swelling and rapid relief of pain follow treatment, often facilitating spontaneous expulsion or retraction of the worm as well as increasing the rate of healing.

Adverse Reactions

Side-effects are transient and occur in more than 70% of patients. They are often more intense in the first 3–5 days and then diminish as therapy continues. Children generally tolerate the drug better than adults; patients with *S japonicum* infections are most likely and patients infected with *S haematobium* least likely to have significant side-effects.

The most common adverse reactions are anorexia, nausea and vomiting, diarrhea, abdominal pain, fatigue, headache, dizziness, myalgia, arthralgia, sweating, palpitation, and skin rashes. The urine may become dark brown or dark red, with an unpleasant musty odor. Liver function tests may become abnormal. Cough, pulmonary infiltrates, and marked eosinophilia may occur. Niridazole can provoke hemolysis in persons with red cells deficient in glucose-6-phosphate dehydrogenase. In animal experiments, damage to the hematopoietic system has been observed. In humans, the drug has not been incriminated as a cause of bleeding tendencies, yet epistaxis and gastrointestinal hemorrhage have rarely been reported during niridazole therapy, and Stevens-Johnson syndrome has been described.

Niridazole also produces temporary inhibition of spermatogenesis in some men. Concern has been expressed about possible teratogenic effects, but none have been observed in limited follow-ups of patients. Tachycardia and minor electrocardiographic changes (flattening or inversion of T waves and ST depression) occur frequently but have not been associated with impairment of cardiac function.

Headache and myalgia may be relieved by aspirin. Antispasmodics may relieve gastrointestinal symptoms. Antihistamines may be helpful in controlling allergic reactions caused by release of foreign proteins from disintegrating worms.

Neuropsychiatric symptoms in patients who appear to be free of hepatic dysfunction have been reported in 1–2% of those infected with *S haematobium* and in up to 5% of those infected with *S mansoni;* however, in advanced schistosomal liver disease, up to 60% may have symptoms. Central nervous system symptoms tend to reach a maximum about the third day and may decrease after that. Initial central nervous system symptoms may include mild headache, paresthesias, insomnia, and anxiety. Electroencephalographic changes are also common but have not been useful in predicting more serious side-effects. If headache persists for more than 24 hours, treatment should be stopped for 12–48 hours, and then it may be possible to resume at the same dosage or a reduced dosage. If the following symptoms occur, the drug should be discontinued: marked mood changes (agitation, anxiety, depression), slurred speech, confusion, psychosis (auditory or visual hallucinations, violent behavior), and convulsions. These symptoms will usually subside within 48 hours after discontinuation of medication. However, in rare instances a normal mental state may not be reached for about 3 weeks. Administration of phenobarbital throughout niridazole therapy may diminish the central nervous system reactions.

Liver function tests and blood counts should be followed during the course of therapy.

Niridazole has recently been shown to have both mutagenic and carcinogenic properties. Niridazole itself, and metabolic derivatives in the urine of patients treated with the drug, have been shown to have mutagenic activity in *Salmonella* test systems. In addition, niridazole has been reported to induce malignant tumors in mice, hamsters, and rats. Although in the 20 years of its use in human infections there have been no reports implicating niridazole in causing cancer, the agent must be considered potentially hazardous for humans.

Contraindications & Cautions

Niridazole should always be used under close daily medical supervision. The drug is generally given on an outpatient basis, but hospitalization is required in the USA. The following patients should always be hospitalized for treatment: debilitated patients, the elderly and very young, and patients with any degree of impairment of hepatic function. In advanced cases of schistosomal liver disease there is some evidence to support the use of much smaller doses given over an extended period of time. Patients should be tested for glucose-6-phosphate dehydrogenase deficiency; if positive, observe carefully for hemolysis during the course of treatment.

Patients with the following conditions generally should not receive the drug: history of liver disease; impaired liver function; the hepatosplenic form of schistosomiasis; cardiac or renal disease; hypertension; age over 50; or a history of psychiatric disorders, epilepsy, or gastrointestinal hemorrhage or ulcer. Patients with severe malnutrition, anemia, infections, and other debilitating conditions should have these problems corrected before therapy is begun. Niridazole should not be administered concurrently with isoniazid.

Preparations & Dosages

Niridazole (Ambilhar) is prepared as 100- and 500-mg tablets. The dosage for schistosomiasis and dracontiasis is 25 mg/kg (maximum 1.5 g) daily for 7 days, divided into 2–3 fractions and given with meals. Although the evidence for its effectiveness is not fully convincing, some workers recommend that adult patients receive phenobarbital, 100–150 mg daily in divided doses, to reduce the incidence of central nervous system side-effects. For the treatment of *S japonicum* infections, it is currently recommended that the course of treatment be stopped in 5 days.

Children infected with *S mansoni* receive the above dosage. However, for children infected with *S haematobium,* the duration of treatment can be reduced to 5 days if daily doses of 30–35 mg/kg are administered in divided doses.

OXAMNIQUINE
(Mansil, Vansil)

Oxamniquine has been undergoing clinical trials for about 10 years. It is a drug of choice for the treatment of individual cases of *Schistosoma mansoni* infection and for mass treatment because of its high level of effectiveness, ease of administration, and freedom from significant side-effects. It is not effective against *Schistosoma haematobium* or *Schistosoma japonicum.*

Chemistry, Absorption, Metabolism, & Excretion

Oxamniquine, a synthetic tetrahydroquinoline derivative, is 6-hydroxymethyl-2-isopropylaminomethyl-7-nitro-1,2,3,4-tetrahydroquinoline. It is structurally related to hycanthone.

Although oxamniquine is effective when given intramuscularly, this is no longer done because it causes severe local pain. Oxamniquine is readily absorbed after oral administration. Following oral doses of 15 mg/kg in 17 adult patients, maximum serum concentrations ranging from 70 to 2600 ng/mL were reached within 1½–3 hours; most of the drug was cleared from the serum after 10 hours. Oxamniquine is converted into inactive metabolites that are largely excreted in the urine.

Several studies have shown that some *S mansoni* strains which infect humans have true resistance to oxamniquine. In addition, intersubject variations in serum concentrations have been noted, which could explain some treatment failures. Although the drug is taken with food to decrease side-effects, food does delay its absorption.

Pharmacologic Effects & Anthelmintic Actions

Oxamniquine is active against both the mature and immature stages of *S mansoni,* male schistosomes being more susceptible than females. Although the exact mechanism of action is not known, the drug induces a shift of the worms from the mesentery to the liver, where many die; residual females returning to the liver cease to lay eggs.

Instances of mild to moderate liver enzyme elevations, eosinophilia, transient pulmonary infiltrates, and urticaria occurring several days after treatment have been ascribed to the death of parasites rather than a direct toxic effect of the drug. When liver biopsy specimens were examined before and at 48 hours following intramuscular injection of the drug, there was no evidence of a toxic effect on the liver cells. This contrasts with damage to the hepatic endoplasmic reticulum in all patients studied following hycanthone administration.

Clinical Uses

Oxamniquine is effective only against *S mansoni.* It can be used in the acute, subacute, and chronic stages of the disease and, unlike niridazole, is both safe and effective in the advanced (hepatosplenic) form of the disease. Following a single dose of 15–20 mg/kg in adults, cure rates of 80–95% were reported in Brazil; in those not cured, a 90–95% reduction in egg excretion was observed. In Egypt and some other parts of Africa, however, a larger dose—about 60 mg/kg given over 2–3 days—was needed to achieve similar cure rates. The drug is generally less effective in children than in adults.

In mixed infections with *S mansoni* and *S haematobium,* oxamniquine has been successfully used in combination with metrifonate.

Adverse Reactions

The drug is safe and free of significant side-effects, but mild symptoms, lasting for several hours, can occur in up to one-third of patients. Dizziness is not uncommon. Drowsiness, nausea and vomiting, diarrhea, abdominal colic, headache, and pruritus are less frequent. A low-grade fever starting on the second day of treatment or several days later is frequently reported in Egypt but occurs less often in Brazil. An orange to red discoloration of the urine may appear. A transient decrease of leukocytes and lymphocytes or eosinophilia may be seen, and liver function abnormalities, particularly transaminase elevations, may appear as late as 1 week after treatment. Central nervous system stimulation may occur; at least 11 cases of behavioral changes, 6 episodes of seizures, and several episodes of hallucinations have been reported. Urticaria is rare.

Oxamniquine has shown mutagenicity in the *S typhimurium* test system and in the host-mediated assay system in mice, but chromosomal abnormalities were not found in animals or humans. Oxamniquine has also been shown to have an embryocidal effect in rabbits and mice when given in doses 10 times the equivalent human dose.

Contraindications & Cautions

It appears prudent to observe patients for 2 hours after ingestion of the drug for signs of central nervous system disturbances. Patients with a history of epilepsy should be hospitalized for treatment; further experience with the drug in such patients may show that an alternative drug should be used. Since the drug makes many patients dizzy or drowsy, it should be used with caution in patients whose work or activity requires mental alertness.

Oxamniquine is contraindicated in pregnancy.

Preparations & Dosages

Oxamniquine (Mansil, Vansil) is prepared for oral use as 250-mg capsules and as a syrup containing 50 mg/mL. The drug is better tolerated if given after food. Optimal dosage schedules vary for different regions of the world.

The recommended dosage for strains of *S mansoni* in the western hemisphere is 12–15 mg/kg given once; for children under 30 kg, 20 mg/kg given in 2 divided doses of 10 mg/kg in 1 day, with an interval of 2–8 hours between doses. For African strains, the total dosage for adults and children varies by region from 40 to 60 mg/kg; Egyptian and Sudanese strains require 15 mg/kg twice daily for 2 days.

OXANTEL PAMOATE
(Quantrel)

Oxantel pamoate, an *m*-oxyphenol analog of pyrantel pamoate, is undergoing clinical evaluation for the treatment of trichuriasis. It is not effective in the treatment of ascariasis, strongyloidiasis, hookworm, or *Trichostrongylus* infection. The pamoate salt is nearly insoluble in water and is very poorly absorbed after oral administration.

For patients with light to moderate trichuriasis, the following cure rates were obtained using only a single dose of oxantel: at 10 mg/kg, 57–75% were cured; at 15 mg/kg, 88%; and at 20 mg/kg, 100%. A dosage of 15 mg/kg daily for 2 days is suggested for moderate and heavy infections. The drug is free of significant side-effects; rarely, nausea and vomiting and abdominal cramps were noted.

Therapeutic trials have recently been reported for the preparation combining oxantel and pyrantel. Because pyrantel is effective against *Ascaris* and hookworm, the combination has shown such a level of effectiveness in mixed infections with *Ascaris,* hookworm, and trichurids that it rivals mebendazole as a broad-spectrum anthelmintic. Unfortunately, neither drug is effective in strongyloidiasis.

Using only a single dose of oxantel-pyrantel pamoate, 10 mg/kg of each component, plus 100 mg of mebendazole, Sinniah et al have reported a 100% cure rate for ascariasis and cure rates and egg reduction rates of 81% and 94% for trichuriasis and 67% and 86% for necatoriasis respectively.

PAROMOMYCIN SULFATE
(Humatin)

Paromomycin, a member of the kanamycin-neomycin group of antibiotics (see Chapter 44), is effective in the treatment of infection with the large tapeworms and of *Hymenolepis nana* infections. It is also used in the treatment of amebiasis and to reduce the number of intestinal bacteria. Although the drug is poorly absorbed from the gastrointestinal tract, side-effects, especially diarrhea, are not uncommon, but they may be reduced by giving the drug after meals. Although nephrotoxicity, ototoxicity, and central nervous system toxicity are theoretically possible with paromomycin as with other members of the neomycin group, such complications apparently have not been reported.

One-day and 5-day courses of paromomycin have been used in the treatment of infection with the large tapeworms. A recommended dosage for adults is 1 g every 15 minutes for 4 doses; for children, 11 mg/kg every 15 minutes for 4 doses. Botero cured 14 of 15 patients with *Taenia saginata* or *Taenia solium* infections, and Wittner and Tanowitz cured all of 15 patients with *T saginata, T solium,* and *Diphyllobothrium latum* infections. Paromomycin, however, should not be used for *T solium* infections, because drug-induced vomiting may result in regurgitation of proglottids into the stomach, which could be followed by cysticercosis.

In the treatment of *H nana* infections, the dosage of paromomycin is 45 mg/kg (maximum 4 g) daily; treatment must be continued for 5–7 days to effect high cure rates. However, there are relatively few reports to substantiate the drug's effectiveness in this condition.

Paromomycin sulfate (Humatin) is available as 250-mg capsules and as a pediatric syrup containing 125 mg/5 mL. It should be administered after meals. Although the drug is marketed in the USA for other indications, its use here for tapeworm infections is considered investigational.

PIPERAZINE

Piperazine salts, introduced in 1949, continue to be alternative drugs in the treatment of roundworms. Piperazine is not useful for treatment of hookworm infection, trichuriasis, or strongyloidiasis and is no longer recommended in this text for the treatment of pinworms.

Chemistry

Piperazine is available as a hexahydrate (which contains about 44% of the base) and as a variety of neutral salts: citrate, phosphate, adipate, tartrate, and others.

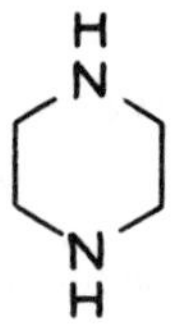

Piperazine base

Absorption, Metabolism, & Excretion

A portion of the absorbed salt is metabolized in the body. The remainder is excreted in the urine, but the rate of excretion varies widely for different persons.

Orally administered piperazine is almost free of pharmacologic action.

Anthelmintic Actions

In vivo studies indicate that piperazine causes a paralysis of *Ascaris* by blocking the stimulating effects of acetylcholine at the myoneural junction. Piperazine has a similar myoneural blocking action on mammalian skeletal muscle, but of a low order. When the drug is used in humans, the paralyzed roundworms are unable to maintain their position in the host and are expelled by normal peristalsis. The worms passed are alive.

Clinical Uses

Several properties of the piperazine salts combine to make these drugs nearly ideal for the treatment of *Ascaris* infections: palatability, a high order of effectiveness, low cost, a low toxicity at therapeutic levels, and the lack of need for pretreatment or posttreatment purges.

A. *Ascaris lumbricoides:* Piperazine is an alternative drug for roundworm infections. When patients are treated once daily for 2 days, cure rates are over 90%. Longer courses are needed for equivalent cure rates in patients with heavy infections. Piperazine syrup, administered via an intestinal drainage tube, is used in the nonsurgical management of intestinal obstruction due to heavy *Ascaris* infection.

B. *Enterobius (Oxyuris) vermicularis:* Piperazine is no longer recommended here for pinworm infections. Although 95% cure rates are achieved by the 7-day course of treatment, equivalent cure rates are possible with only a single dose of pyrvinium pamoate, pyrantel pamoate, or mebendazole.

Adverse Reactions

There is a wide range between the therapeutic and toxic doses of piperazine. Mild side-effects occur occasionally, including nausea and vomiting, diarrhea, abdominal pain, and headache. Neurotoxic side-effects, including vertigo, incoordination, difficulty in focusing, muscular weakness, tremors, paresthesias, hyperreflexia, lethargy, and confusional states, are rarely reported. Patients with a predisposition to grand mal or petit mal epilepsy may have an exacerbation of seizures. Although piperazine is potentially allergenic, only rarely have the following allergic symptoms been attributed to it: urticaria, erythema multiforme, purpura, fever, hepatitis, hemolysis, and arthralgia. Serum sickness-like syndromes have been reported 2–14 days after the initial dose of piperazine.

Contraindications & Cautions

Piperazine compounds should not be given to patients with impaired renal or hepatic function or with a history of epilepsy or chronic neurologic disease. Piperazine may be used during the last trimester of pregnancy. Piperazine and phenothiazines should not be given together. Caution should be exercised in patients with severe malnutrition or anemia.

Preparations & Dosages

The therapeutic effectiveness of the various piperazine salts is about the same; in solution, all form piperazine hexahydrate. Among the many preparations available as tablets, wafers, or syrups are piperazine citrate (Antepar, Anthecole, Multifuge, Pipizan, Vermago, Vermidol), piperazine phosphate (Antepar wafers, Pripsen), piperazine calcium edetate (Perin), piperazine tartrate (Piperat, Veroxil), piperazine adipate (Entacyl, Oxurasin, Oxyzin), and piperazine hexahydrate (Arpezine, Dispermin).

Piperazine citrate (Antepar) is prepared as a syrup containing 110 mg/mL (the equivalent of 100 mg of piperazine hexahydrate) or as tablets containing 550 mg (the equivalent of 500 mg of piperazine hexahydrate).

A. Ascariasis: The dosage of piperazine (as the hexahydrate) is 75 mg/kg of body weight (to a maximum dose of 3.5 g) for 2 days in succession, giving the drug orally before or after breakfast. For heavy infestations, treatment should be continued for 4 days in succession or the 2-day course repeated after 1 week. No pre- or posttreatment cathartics are used. In most cases, cure is obtained, but stools should be reexamined at 2-week intervals and treatment repeated until ova are no longer found.

B. Enterobiasis: The daily oral dose of piperazine (as the hexahydrate) is 65 mg/kg up to a maximum dose of 2.5 g. This dosage should be given daily for 7 days, before or after breakfast. Cathartics are not used. The course of treatment should be repeated after 2 weeks. Because of its long course of treatment, piperazine is no longer recommended in this text for enterobiasis if the drugs of choice are available.

PRAZIQUANTEL
(Biltricide, Ceneride, Cesol)

Praziquantel is a recently introduced drug that has the unique characteristic of being effective in the treatment of infections with all schistosome species pathogenic to humans and many human trematode and cestode infections. It shows promise of being the first drug to be useful in the treatment of cysticercosis. It is not effective against *Fasciola hepatica* or in hydatid disease.

Chemistry

Praziquantel, a synthetic isoquinoline compound, is 2-cyclohexylcarbonyl-1,2,3,6,7,11b-hexahydro-4*H*-pyrazino[2,1*a*]isoquinolin-4-one. It is a crystalline powder that is slightly soluble in water and has a bitter taste.

Absorption, Metabolism, & Excretion

Praziquantel is rapidly absorbed after an oral dose, reaching a maximum serum concentration of the unchanged drug in 1–2 hours. Most of the drug is rapidly metabolized to mono- and polyhydroxylated products after a first pass in the liver. The elimination half-life from the serum is 1–1½ hours and that of praziquantel plus its metabolites is 4–5 hours using ^{14}C-labeled praziquantel. Excretion of the drug and its metabolites is for the most part via the kidneys—approximately 70% in the first day and 80% in 4 days.

Pharmacologic Effects

In experimental animals, neither single oral doses equivalent to human therapeutic doses nor long-term administration produced significant toxic effects, except that following single high doses, signs of cerebral intoxication were noted.

In humans, no important alterations in biochemical or hematologic laboratory test results have been described, and there were no signs of toxic damage to vital organs or systems. Transient elevations in liver function tests may occur and, rarely, minor electrocardiographic changes have been noted.

In a wide variety of mutagenicity studies using in vitro and in vivo test systems, no abnormalities were found. Carcinogenicity studies to date and reproductive studies for embryotoxicity and teratogenicity have also shown negative results. However, 3 recent reports that appeared in abstract form only presented findings suggesting that praziquantel acts as a co-mutagen in *S typhimurium* and mammalian cell test systems. The significance of these findings is yet to be determined.

Anthelmintic Actions

Information on the anthelmintic action of praziquantel is limited. The serum concentration of praziquantel in animals and humans who have received therapeutically effective doses is above the threshold level of about 0.3 μg/mg of plasma. Praziquantel's action on all platyhelminths appears to be the same—the drug causes vacuolization of the surface, leading to death of the parasites. In cestodes, the sites of vacuolization are restricted to the neck of the strobila, but in trematodes, vacuoles occur in numerous areas over the entire surface. No reaction occurs in *Fasciola hepatica* and only a slight one in *Paragonimus westermani*. In addition, in vitro studies with *Hymenolepis diminuta* and with schistosomes have shown that praziquantel inhibits glucose uptake under anaerobic and aerobic conditions; however, this effect is thought to be secondary.

In schistosome infections of animals, praziquantel was effective against adult worms of both sexes and against the immature stages; adult worms were found to be rapidly immobilized and shifted to the liver. In addition, when a single high dose of praziquantel was given concurrently with the infecting dose of cercariae, all immature forms were killed; thus, praziquantel had a prophylactic effect.

Clinical Uses

A. Schistosomiasis: Because of its high efficacy, low toxicity, and ease of administration as a single oral dose, praziquantel will probably replace oxamniquine and metrifonate as the drug of choice in the treatment of both *Schistosoma haematobium* and *Schistosoma mansoni* infections. In addition, praziquantel's 2-day course of treatment of *Schistosoma japonicum* has an efficacy and freedom from side-effects found with no other drug. Praziquantel was effective in adults and children and was well tolerated by patients in the hepatosplenic stage of advanced schistosomiasis.

The above characteristics and praziquantel's environmental stability appear to make the drug uniquely satisfactory for use in mass treatment.

More than 10,000 patients were treated initially in 31 study groups. At various dosage schedules high cure rates were achieved at 3–6 months, with marked reduction in ova counts in those not cured. For *S haematobium* infections, the cure rate for persons given 20–50 mg/kg one time was 83%. For *S mansoni* in Africa, the cure rate for patients who received 40 mg/kg once was 84%; for *S mansoni* in Brazil, the cure rate for patients who received 20 mg/kg three times daily for one day was 96%. For *S japonicum*, the cure rate for persons given 20 mg/kg three times daily was 86%.

B. Clonorchiasis and Opisthorchiasis: A dosage of 25 mg/kg 3 times daily for 1 day cured 92% of patients with *Clonorchis* and 100% of those infected with *Opisthorchis* spp. A 2-day course cured 100% of *Clonorchis* infections.

C. Paragonimiasis: When treated with one

course of 25 mg/kg 3 times daily for 1 day, 73% of patients with pulmonary paragonimasis were cured; 89% were cured when treated for 2 days.

D. Taeniasis and Diphyllobothriasis: In 9 studies of 498 patients infected with *Taenia saginata* or *Taenia solium* and treated with a single dose of praziquantel, 10 mg/kg, 97–100% were cured.

In 2 studies of patients infected with *Diphyllobothrium latum,* 95% of 213 patients were cured with a single dose of 25 mg/kg. In addition, all of 52 patients infected with *Diphyllobothrium pacificum* were cured with a single dose of 10 mg/kg.

E. Cysticercosis: Praziquantel is undergoing clinical investigation for this use and appears to be the first drug to be effective against cysticercosis. Treatment has ranged in duration from 4 to 16 days at a variety of dosage schedules. Steroids must be administered concurrently to block possible inflammatory reactions around cysticerci, which may cause intracranial edema. The results of treatment have been promising in many cases—reduction in cerebral hypertension, amelioration of seizures, or disappearance of lesions on cerebral tomograms.

F. *Hymenolepsis nana:* Praziquantel is the drug of choice and the first drug to be highly effective. In 5 studies of 473 persons treated with one dose of 15 mg/kg, 86% were cured; of an additional 521 persons treated wth 25 mg/kg, 94% were cured.

G. Other Parasites: There have been limited reports that praziquantel is effective in the treatment of *Metagonimus yokogawai* and *Dicrocoelium dendriticum.*

Adverse Reactions

Mild and transient side-effects directly attributable to the drug are not uncommon. They begin within several hours after ingestion and may persist for hours to 1 day. The most common symptoms are headache, dizziness, and anorexia. Other side-effects are fatigue, drowsiness, nausea and vomiting, generalized abdominal pain, loose to mushy stools, pruritus, urticaria, arthralgia and myalgia, and low-grade fever. Low-grade fever and skin rashes (macular and urticarial), sometimes associated with augmented eosinophilia, may also appear several days after starting the medication and are more likely to be due to the release of foreign proteins from dying worms than to a direct reaction to the drug.

Praziquantel appears to be better tolerated in children than in adults. Side-effects may be more frequent in heavily infected patients. The intensity and frequency of side-effects also increase with dosage, being mild and infrequent at dosages of 10 mg/kg given once but occurring in up to 50% of patients receiving 20 mg/kg 3 times daily.

Contraindications & Cautions

There are no specific contraindications.

In areas where cysticercosis is known to exist, special precautions should be taken to avoid concurrent treatment of cysticercosis, which requires treatment in hospital by a specialist. Because the drug induces dizziness, patients whose work or activities require physical coordination and alertness should be warned of this effect.

The drug should not be taken during the first 3 months of pregnancy. Lactating women may be given praziquantel provided the infant is not nursed on the day of treatment and for 3 subsequent days.

Preparations & Dosages

Praziquantel (Biltricide, Ceneride, Cesol) is prepared as 600-mg tablets, which should be taken with a liquid after a meal. If the drug is taken more than once on the same day, the interval between doses should be no less than 4 and no more than 6 hours. Although optimal dosage schedules are still being determined, the following dosages are currently recommended:

A. Schistosomiasis: For *Schistosoma mansoni* infections in Africa and *Schistosoma haematobium* and *Schistosoma intercalatum* infections, give a single dose of 40 mg/kg, or give 20 mg/kg and repeat in 4–6 hours. *S mansoni* infections in South America may require a dosage of 25 mg/kg initially and repeated in 4–6 hours. The dosage for *S japonicum* is 30 mg/kg initially and repeated in 4–6 hours.

B. *Clonorchis sinensis, Opisthorchis* Species, and *Paragonimus* Species: *Clonorchis* and *Opisthorchis* infections have been treated with 25 mg/kg given 3 times in 1 day, with intervals of 4–6 hours between doses. For paragonimiasis, a 2-day course of treatment is recommended.

C. *Taenia saginata* and *Diphyllobothrium latum:* Only a single dose is necessary; 10 mg/kg has been used successfully for *T saginata* infections and will probably be satisfactory for *D latum* infections, although in reports to date a dosage of 25 mg/kg has been used for the latter. Within 24–48 hours after treatment, a disintegrating worm is usually passed with normal peristalsis. Pre- and posttreatment purges are not necessary. If the scolex is not found or is not searched for, cure can be presumed only if regenerated segments have not reappeared 3–5 months after treatment.

D. *Taenia solium:* Give a single dose of 10 mg/kg. At present, it is recommended that an effective purge (such as magnesium or sodium sulfate, 15–30 g) be given 2 hours after treatment to eliminate all mature segments before ova can be released from disintegrating segments. Since praziquantel does not kill the ova, it is theoretically possible that larvae released from ova in the large bowel could penetrate the intestinal wall, giving rise to cysticercosis. As with niclosamide, this hazard is probably minimal, but the precaution of a posttreatment purge is advised.

E. *Hymenolepis nana:* *H nana* infections are treated with a single dose of praziquantel, 15–25 mg/kg.

PYRANTEL PAMOATE
(Antiminth, Combantrin)

Pyrantel pamoate is a highly effective drug for the treatment of pinworm, ascarid, and *Trichostrongylus orientalis* infections. It is moderately effective against both species of hookworm, but less so against *N americanus*. It is not effective in trichuriasis or strongyloidiasis. Oxantel, an analog of pyrantel, has been used successfully in the treatment of trichuriasis (see p 615).

Chemistry

Pyrantel pamoate, a tetrahydropyrimidine, is *trans*-1,4,5,6-tetrahydro-1-methyl-2-(2-[2-thienyl]-vinyl)-pyrimidine hydrogen pamoate.

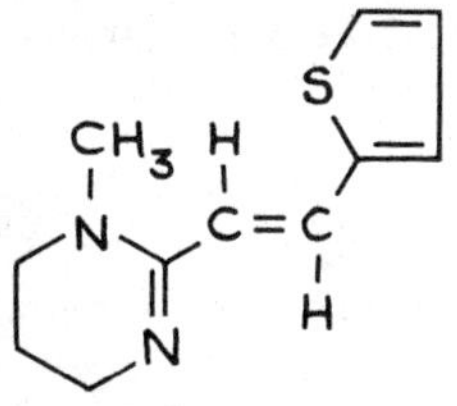

Pyrantel base

Absorption, Metabolism, & Excretion

Pyrantel is poorly absorbed from the gastrointestinal tract. Peak plasma levels (0.05–0.13 μg/mL) of unchanged drug are reached in 1–3 hours. Over half of the administered dose is recovered unchanged in the feces, and only 7% or less of the dose is found in the urine unchanged or as a metabolite of the drug.

Pharmacologic Effects & Anthelmintic Actions

The anthelmintic action of pyrantel is probably due to an inhibitory action on neuromuscular transmission. In the helminth, a spastic neuromuscular paralysis occurs and the worm is subsequently expelled from the host's intestinal tract. In both vertebrate neuromuscular preparations and strip preparations of *Ascaris*, pyrantel shows the activity typical of depolarizing neuromuscular blocking agents. Pyrantel also inhibits cholinesterases.

Clinical Uses

A. *Enterobius vermicularis:* In most reports, pyrantel given as a single dose and repeated in 2 weeks is effective in curing pinworms in over 95% of patients. In 3 comparative studies of pyrantel and pyrvinium pamoate, both drugs were equally effective, but pyrantel may have produced fewer side-effects. Unlike pyrvinium, pyrantel does not stain stool or clothing red. Mebendazole is equally effective and is without significant side-effects. Piperazine, which is effective and safe, has the disadvantage of requiring a 7-day course of treatment.

B. *Ascaris lumbricoides:* Pyrantel given only once in a dosage of 11 mg/kg has been reported in different studies to be curative in 85–100% of patients.

C. Hookworm and *T orientalis:* Pyrantel has a high order of effectiveness against *T orientalis*. In *Ancylostoma duodenale* infections, pyrantel given as a single dose produces cures in over 90% of cases and a marked reduction in the worm burden in the remainder. However, for *N americanus* infections, the cure rate depends on the intensity of infection. A single dose may give a satisfactory cure rate in light infections, but for moderate or heavy infections (over 2000 ova per gram of feces) a 3-day course is necessary to give cure rates in the range of 90%.

Adverse Reactions, Contraindications, & Cautions

Side-effects are infrequent, mild, and transient. Reports vary on their incidence; 4–20% of adults and children may experience one or more of the following: nausea and vomiting, diarrhea, abdominal cramps, dizziness, drowsiness, and headache. Less frequently reported are insomnia, rash, fever, and weakness. No important effects on hematologic, renal, or hepatic function have been recorded.

There are no contraindications to pyrantel, but it should be used with caution in patients with liver dysfunction, since low, transient SGOT elevations have been noted in a small number of patients. Experience with the drug in children under age 2 years is limited.

Preparations & Dosages

Pyrantel pamoate (Antiminth, Combantrin) is prepared as a suspension containing 50 mg of pyrantel base per milliliter and as tablets containing 125 mg of the base.

For the treatment of pinworm infections and ascariasis, give a single oral dose of 10 mg of pyrantel base per kilogram of body weight (maximum 1 g). Treatment may be given before or after meals; purges are not used. For pinworm infections, repeat the dose at 2 and 4 weeks; for ascariasis, repeat only if ova are still found 2 weeks after treatment.

For hookworm infections due to *A duodenale*, give a single oral dose of 10 mg of pyrantel base per kilogram of body weight (maximum 1 g). For infections due to *N americanus* or when the species is unknown, a single dose may be sufficient for light infections, but for moderate or heavy infections repeat the dose daily for 3 days. Recheck stools in 2 weeks. In the USA, pyrantel is considered an investigational drug when used for hookworm and *T orientalis* infections.

PYRVINIUM PAMOATE
(Povan)

Pyrvinium pamoate, a cyanine dye, is a highly effective drug for the treatment of pinworm infections; however, because of its side-effects it is recommended only as an alternative drug. Although the drug may be useful for the treatment of *Strongyloides stercoralis* infection, it has only a low order of anthelmintic action against *Trichuris trichiura* and hookworm infections and is not effective against *Ascaris lumbricoides* infection.

Chemistry, Absorption, Metabolism, & Excretion

Pyrvinium pamoate (viprynium embonate, pyrvinium embonate) is the bis-6-dimethylamino-2(2-[2, 5-dimethyl-1-phenyl-3-pyrrolyl]vinyl)-1-methylquinolinium salt of pamoic acid.

Pyrvinium pamoate is not appreciably absorbed from the gastrointestinal tract when taken orally.

Anthelmintic Actions

As a group, the cyanine dyes contain the amidinium ion system, which may be responsible for their anthelmintic activity. Pyrvinium pamoate is highly effective against *Enterobius vermicularis;* it appears to exert its effect by preventing the parasite from using exogenous carbohydrates. The parasite dies when its endogenous reserves are depleted. The drug does not kill *Enterobius* ova.

Clinical Uses

A. *Enterobius vermicularis* (Pinworm): Pyrvinium is an alternative drug for pinworm infections. Reported cure rates after a single dose range from 90 to 100%. Thus, it is as effective as pyrantel and mebendazole; each of the drugs requires only one treatment (followed by repeat doses at 2 and 4 weeks), but pyrvinium produces more side-effects. Although piperazine is equally effective and causes few side-effects, it requires a 7-day course of treatment.

When one member of a household is treated for pinworms, diagnosis and treatment of all other members may be considered. However, reinfection from the outside occurs so frequently in families with young children that a pragmatic approach to therapy for such families may be to offer treatment only to symptomatic persons and to eradicate infections in all members of the household only when children are older.

B. *Strongyloides stercoralis* (Dwarf Threadworm): There are few reports of the use of pyrvinium pamoate for the treatment of strongyloidiasis. Wang and Galli reported clearing larvae from the stools of 11 of 12 patients using 2–6.4 mg of pyrvinium pamoate suspension per kilogram of body weight for 7 days. The safety and effectiveness of this extended treatment have yet to be confirmed, and the drug is not approved for this indication in the USA.

Adverse Reactions

Pyrvinium pamoate is well tolerated, but it may cause nausea and vomiting, diarrhea, or dizziness in some persons, particularly older children and adults. Emesis occurs more often with the suspension than the tablet formulation. Photosensitization and other allergic reactions have been reported. Parents and patients should be told that posttreatment stools are often stained red for several days and the suspension, if spilled, will stain most materials red.

Relatively recently, pyrvinium pamoate was found to contain a promutagen capable of being converted by mammalian metabolic processes to a mutagenic metabolite. Further testing of the compound is needed. In similar testing of pyrantel pamoate, test results were negative.

Contraindications & Cautions

Tablets should be swallowed intact to avoid transient staining of the teeth. The drug should be used cautiously in children weighing less than 10 kg (22 lb), for experience with the drug is limited in young children.

There are no contraindications to the use of pyrvinium pamoate. However, it is preferable not to use the drug in the presence of inflammatory conditions of the gastrointestinal tract that theoretically might facilitate absorption.

Dosage

For the treatment of pinworm infections, a single dose is administered orally before or after meals. The dosage is 5 mg of pyrvinium base per kilogram of body weight up to a maximum of 350 mg. No pre- or posttreatment purges are used. Treatment should be repeated at 2 and 4 weeks.

Preparations Available

Pyrvinium pamoate (Povan) is available in tablets containing 50 mg of pyrvinium base and as a suspension (Povan Suspension) containing 10 mg of base per milliliter.

QUINACRINE HYDROCHLORIDE
(Atabrine, Mepacrine)

Quinacrine was formerly an alternative drug for the treatment of tapeworm infections. Because of its toxicity, it should no longer be used unless the drug of choice (niclosamide) or alternative drugs (praziquantel, mebendazole, paromomycin, or dichlorophen) are not available.

Quinacrine commonly causes nausea and vomiting in the high dosage used for tapeworm therapy. Additional side-effects include dizziness, mild diarrhea, colic, headache, urticaria, and central nervous system stimulation. The latter may be manifested by restlessness, confusion, anxiety, euphoria, aggressive behavior, or psychotic reactions.

SURAMIN
(Antrypol, Bayer-205, Belganyl, Germanin, Naphuride)

Suramin, introduced in 1921 for the treatment of African trypanosomiasis, is the drug of choice to eradicate adult parasites of *Onchocerca volvulus* infections and the drug of choice in the treatment of the hemolymphatic stage of African trypanosomiasis due to *Trypanosoma gambiense* and *Trypanosoma rhodesiense*. The drug is not marketed in the USA but can be obtained from the Parasitic Disease Drug Service, Centers for Disease Control, Atlanta 30333.

Chemistry, Absorption, Metabolism, & Excretion

Suramin, a complex derivative of urea, is freely soluble in water. Because it is poorly absorbed from the gastrointestinal tract and causes intense local irritation when given subcutaneously or intramuscularly, it should be given intravenously. Suramin persists in the plasma firmly bound to plasma proteins and accumulates in the reticuloendothelial cells throughout the body, especially in the Kupfer cells of the liver and in the epithelium of the renal proximal convoluted tubules. The plasma concentration falls during the first few hours to become constant for several days; this is followed by a low concentration for up to 6 months. Sequential doses have a cumulative effect, but there is considerable variation in the extent to which accumulation occurs in different patients. The drug appears to be relatively resistant to catabolism, and active metabolites are not known. After a single dose a small amount is excreted in the urine in the first few days, but thereafter most of the dose cannot be recovered. Because suramin does not cross the blood-brain barrier, it is effective only in the early stage of African trypanosomiasis.

Pharmacologic & Anthelmintic Actions

Suramin's general tendency to firmly bind to serum proteins results in nonspecific inhibition of many enzymes. As a result, it is a potent ATP inhibitor, and it has multiple actions on clotting through its effects on complement, on fibrinolysis, and on kinin formation.

The drug's specific action on enzymes concerned with DNA and RNA metabolism may be the basis for its antiparasitic action. In onchocerciasis, the drug acts principally on adult female worms, causing them to die and degenerate after the fifth week of treatment; male worms live much longer. Some microfilariae (but not all) are also killed. However, unlike diethylcarbamazine, suramin kills microfilariae slowly during its 6-week course of treatment.

Although suramin has an abortive action on pregnant rats and is teratogenic, no cases of abortion or fetal malformation have been noted following its use in pregnant women.

Clinical Uses

A. *Onchocerca volvulus:* Suramin and Mel W (melarsonyl potassium) are the only effective drugs against adult *Onchocerca* worms. Unpredictable deaths have occurred with both compounds, but suramin is the safer of the two and the only drug that should be considered for treatment. An effective therapeutic program for individual patients consists of nodulectomy for accessible *Onchocerca* nodules (particularly those on the head) plus drug therapy in the form of suramin against adult worms and diethylcarbamazine to kill the microfilariae. Before starting suramin, all patients should receive a course of diethylcarbamazine to eliminate most microfilariae. However, treatment must be individualized to determine whether the patient can tolerate the side-effects of suramin and whether clinical findings warrant the risk of using the drug. Hawking concluded, "Probably suramin should be given to all heavily infected patients with considerable pruritus or with danger of ocular complications, eg, microfilariae in the skin of the head." If the eyes are not endangered, many authorities limit treatment to nodulectomy and an initial intensive course of diethylcarbamazine, followed by weekly doses of 200 mg indefinitely. Scharlau discusses risk factors and indications for chemotherapy.

B. *Trypanosoma gambiense* and *Trypanosoma rhodesiense:* See Chapter 54.

Adverse Reactions

Side-effects of suramin during treatment of onchocerciasis are attributable to pharmacologic reactions to the drug itself and to allergic reactions resulting from release of antigen following death of adult worms or microfilariae.

A. Drug-Induced Reactions: The drug-induced reactions are both immediate and delayed. The immediate reactions, which occur in about 0.2–0.4% of patients, are characterized by nausea and vomiting, colic, urticaria, and, rarely, circulatory collapse and loss of consciousness. A test dose is given very slowly over 3 minutes to detect patients subject to this immediate reaction.

Delayed drug-induced reactions are fever; renal irritation manifested by albumin, red blood cells, and casts in the urine; polyuria and increased thirst; anorexia and tiredness; and hyperesthesia of the palms and soles, sometimes accompanied by desquamation. Rarely, one or more of the following severe reactions may occur: nephrotoxicity leading to renal shutdown, agranulocytosis, hemolytic anemia, jaundice, prolonged high fever, prostration, arthritis, diarrhea lasting more than 3 days, exfoliative dermatitis (which must be differentiated from the inconsequential desquamation due to microfilariae dying in the skin), and severe ulcerations of the mouth and pharynx, sometimes extending to the trachea. The mortality rate following use of suramin has varied in different parts of the world, but no deaths were reported among 27,000 persons treated in Venezuela.

B. Reactions Due to Dying Parasites: Allergic reactions due to dying parasites tend to occur after the fourth or fifth week but may start with the first dose and increase as the course of treatment proceeds.

Within an hour of the first injection, urticaria and swelling can occur over parts of the body where adult parasites are located. Later, superficial and deep abscesses can develop around the worms; if these abscesses are near the hip joint, they may be accompanied by painful immobilization of the joint.

Reactions due to dying microfilariae include fever and itching, inflammation, and edema of the skin that may be followed by papular and vesicular eruptions with subsequent desquamation. Although these reactions are similar to those provoked by diethylcarbamazine, they appear later and are more prolonged and less severe than those due to diethylcarbamazine.

The drug's effects on intraocular microfilariae include an aggravation of punctate and sclerosing keratitis accompanied by photophobia, lacrimation, burning, and itching; the development of iridocyclitis, with the risk of formation of anterior and posterior synechiae; and possible excitation of optic neuritis or choroidoretinal lesions leading to postneuritic optic atrophy and associated loss of peripheral vision. Optic atrophy following suramin therapy has only recently been noted; its pathogenesis is postulated to be similar to that following diethylcarbamazine treatment. The development of iridocyclitis requires prompt treatment with topical steroid drops.

Most reactions are not severe, but they can be so annoying that the patient may refuse to complete the course of treatment. Minor symptoms may be partially relieved by aspirin; severe systemic reactions require betamethasone, 1 mg 3 times daily for several days, after which this drug is tapered off.

Contraindications & Cautions

Patients receiving suramin must be closely watched, preferably in the hospital. Those with heavy loads of microfilariae in the ocular tissues should be treated under the supervision of a physician with adequate ophthalmologic experience and the necessary equipment for eye examination, including a slit lamp. The drug is contraindicated for those intolerant to a test dose, for pregnant patients, and for patients with hypertension or preexisting hepatic and renal insufficiency; it should be used with caution in children under age 10 years, in those with a history of allergy, and in the aged or debilitated. Malnutrition and severe anemia should be corrected before initiating therapy.

Urine should be examined for protein, red cells, and casts before each treatment. Slight proteinuria is not an indication to stop therapy, as it usually clears within 2 months and there is no residual damage to the kidneys. However, the presence of considerable protein (equivalent to 20 mg or more per deciliter) or formed elements in the urine calls for skipping a dose, reducing subsequent doses, or ceasing therapy. Other indications for discontinuation of treatment are prolonged high fever, severe prostration, marked arthritis, exfoliative dermatitis, ulceration of the buccal mucosa, and persistent diarrhea.

Preparations & Dosages

Suramin (Antrypol, Bayer-205, Belganyl, Germanin, Naphuride) is marketed in ampules containing 0.5 and 1 g dry powder that must be kept dry, cool, and sealed in dark bottles during storage. A 10% solution should be prepared for injection in cold, pyrogen-free distilled water or saline and must be used within 30 minutes.

A. Onchocerciasis: To reduce reactions due to the slow death of microfilariae during suramin therapy, it is advisable before starting suramin to treat all cases, whether lightly or heavily infected, with a course of diethylcarbamazine to eliminate most of the microfilariae (see p 603).

An initial dose of suramin, 0.1 g, is given intravenously very slowly over 3 minutes to test for rare intolerance to the drug—recognized by the immediate reactions noted above. If the drug is tolerated, the course for adults weighing over 60 kg is 1 g (10–15 mg/kg in children) weekly for 5–6 weeks. Light infections may require only 1 g weekly for 4 weeks, heavy infections 1 g weekly for 7 weeks. Injections must be given intravenously and *slowly* over a period of 1 minute, with great care to avoid leakage outside the vein, which is very painful, but the drug can be tolerated and is effective by deep intramuscular injection if no vein can be found. A second course of treatment cannot be given earlier than 3 months after the first course.

About 3–4 weeks after completing the course of suramin, remaining microfilariae in the skin are killed by giving a course of diethylcarbamazine, 200 mg twice daily for 3–5 days, and repeating the course at 3- to 4-week intervals until pruritic skin reactions no longer occur.

Small, gradually increasing doses of suramin have been tested recently in West Africa in mass treatment of heavily infected persons. Tolerance and therapeutic results were favorable.

B. African Trypanosomiasis: See Chapter 54.

TETRACHLOROETHYLENE

Tetrachloroethylene was introduced in 1925 for the treatment of hookworm infections due to *Necator americanus* or *Ancylostoma duodenale* and remains an effective alternative drug.

Chemistry

Tetrachloroethylene (perchloroethylene; $Cl_2C{=}CCl_2$), an unsaturated halogenated hydrocarbon, is a colorless, volatile liquid that is slowly decomposed by light and by various metals. A major problem with tetrachloroethylene, and one that may have affected its efficacy in clinical trials, is its deterioration in tropical climates. To preserve its potency, it should be stored in a cool dark place.

Although the drug is nearly insoluble in water, its solubility is increased by the presence of alcohol or lipids in the gastrointestinal tract.

Absorption, Metabolism, & Excretion

Absorption of tetrachloroethylene is minimal in a

normal gastrointestinal tract if the drug is taken in the absence of lipids or alcohol. The small amount absorbed is excreted in the expired air.

Anthelmintic Actions

Tetrachloroethylene is more effective against *N americanus* than against *A duodenale*. Its mode of action has not been clearly established; it may depress muscle cells or neighboring nerve structures. Paralysis results, causing the hookworms to release their attachment to the intestinal mucosa.

Tetrachloroethylene does not paralyze or kill *Ascaris lumbricoides* but is thought to stimulate them, causing their migration; this effect has not been established.

Clinical Uses

A. *N americanus:* Up to 80% of patients infected with this hookworm species will be cured after a single treatment with tetrachloroethylene; the worm load in the remaining patients is reduced.

B. *A duodenale:* The reported cure rates for *Ancylostoma* infection after a single treatment with tetrachloroethylene are 25–65%. Several additional treatments at 4- to 7-day intervals are usually required to achieve higher cure rates.

C. Intestinal Flukes: Tetrachloroethylene is often effective in the eradication of the small intestinal flukes *Heterophyes heterophyes* and *Metagonimus yokogawai;* the large intestinal fluke, *Fasciolopsis buski; Echinostoma* spp; and *Gastrodiscoides hominis*. The drug is used in the same dosages and in the same manner as for hookworm infections.

Adverse Reactions

Tetrachloroethylene has had extensive use without serious side-effects. However, mild gastrointestinal symptoms (nausea and vomiting, epigastric burning, and abdominal cramps) and central nervous system symptoms (dizziness, vertigo, headache, and drowsiness) occur frequently. Transient loss of consciousness has been reported, and hypotensive episodes have occurred in severely anemic patients. Therefore, when feasible, the patient should be kept at bed rest and under observation for 4 hours after administration of the drug.

Contraindications & Cautions

It is not well established whether the presence of *Ascaris* infection contraindicates the use of tetrachloroethylene. Therefore, in mixed infections with both roundworms and hookworms, the roundworms should be eliminated first or, preferably, a drug should be used that is effective against both parasites.

The drug is contraindicated in the treatment of small, severely ill children. It should be avoided in pregnancy, hepatic diseases, gastroenteritis, alcoholism, severe constipation, and patients undergoing heavy metal therapy.

Patients with severe anemia should have this partially corrected before administration of the drug.

Preparations & Dosages

Tetrachloroethylene USP, while approved for human use, is available in the USA only as a veterinary preparation (Nema worm capsules); however, this preparation is safe and effective for use in humans. It is available in a liquid form or in soft gelatin capsules containing 0.2, 1, and 5 mL. The gelatin capsules prevent irritation of the oral mucous membranes.

The patient should be told to avoid alcohol and fatty foods for 24 hours before and 3 days after medication. Food, but not water, is withheld the morning the drug is administered. The dosage is 0.12 mL/kg up to a maximum of 5 mL and is taken orally in capsule form. The patient should be kept at bed rest for 4 hours following treatment, and then food may be started. Purgation following treatment is no longer advised, for it may increase side-effects and decrease the effectiveness of the drug. An alternative (and probably preferable) time to give the drug is at bedtime, but 6 hours after the last meal. Stool specimens should be examined at the end of 2 weeks. One treatment may be sufficient for necatoriasis, but for ancylostomiasis 2 or more treatments at intervals of 4–7 days may be required to clear the infection or reduce the worm burden to levels at which the remaining parasites cause no significant blood loss. If iron deficiency anemia is present, it should be treated with ferrous sulfate and a high-protein diet.

THIABENDAZOLE
(Mintezol)

Thiabendazole is the drug of choice for the treatment of strongyloidiasis and cutaneous larva migrans infections. Given the absence of known effective drugs, it may also be tried in trichinosis and visceral larva migrans infections. Although it has a broad spectrum of anthelmintic activity, because of its frequent and sometimes severe toxicity it is no longer recommended in this text for the treatment of pinworm, ascarid, or hookworm infection unless the safer alternative drugs are not available. Thiabendazole has only a low level of effectiveness in trichuriasis.

Chemistry

Thiabendazole (2-[4-thiazolyl]-1*H*-benzimidazole) is a benzimidazole compound. It is tasteless and nearly insoluble in water. Although a chelating agent that forms stable complexes with a number of metals, including iron, it does not bind calcium.

Absorption, Metabolism, & Excretion

Studies in humans have shown that thiabendazole is rapidly absorbed after an oral dose. Drug concentrations in plasma peak within 1 hour and are barely detectable after 8 hours. Excretion is mainly via the urine, 90% appearing in 1 hour. The drug is almost completely metabolized to the 5-hydroxy form, which appears in the urine largely as the glucuronide or sulfate conjugate. Thiabendazole can also be absorbed from the skin.

In some clinical situations it may be useful to monitor serum drug concentrations.

Pharmacologic Effects & Toxicity

Thiabendazole given to cats and dogs in large doses orally (4 g/kg) and intravenously (40 mg/kg) did not produce significant effects on the cardiovascular or respiratory system. Thiabendazole has anti-inflammatory properties, which may be an important factor in its ability to relieve symptoms in some parasitic diseases. It also has immunomodulating effects on T cell function: It appears to be an immunorestorative agent, demonstrating maximum immunopotentiation in the immunosuppressed host.

Clinical Uses

A. *Strongyloides stercoralis:* Thiabendazole is the drug of choice for the treatment of strongyloidiasis. Of 134 patients treated in 9 studies, 125 (93%) were cured with a dosage of 25 mg/kg twice daily for 2–3 days.

B. Cutaneous Larva Migrans (Creeping Eruption): Thiabendazole is the first effective systemic drug for the treatment of cutaneous larva migrans, an infection caused by *Ancylostoma braziliense* or *Ancylostoma caninum*.

C. *Enterobius vermicularis* (Pinworm): Thiabendazole eradicates pinworms in over 95% of patients treated. However, because of its potential toxicity, the equally effective drugs pyrantel pamoate or mebendazole should be used instead.

D. Trichinosis: Information is limited on the effect of thiabendazole on the intestinal phase of trichinosis in humans. During the invasive stage, biopsy evidence suggests that the drug destroys some (though not all) larvae in muscle during the first 2 months of the disease. Amelioration or remission of signs and symptoms is usual without equivalent improvement in abnormal laboratory findings.

ACTH and corticosteroids are also effective in controlling the clinical manifestations of trichinosis and may be lifesaving in severe infections.

E. *Ascaris lumbricoides:* When a dosage of 25 mg/kg is used twice daily for 2–3 days, the mean cure rate as reported by various investigators is 75%. Pyrantel will clear over 90% of *Ascaris* infections when used for 1 day and causes fewer side-effects than thiabendazole.

F. Other Infections: Reported cure rates for *Trichuris trichiura* infections range from 5 to 35% when thiabendazole is used for 2 days. In those not cured, the worm load is reduced. Cure rates increase when the drug is continued for 3–5 days, but side-effects also increase.

When 25 mg/kg of thiabendazole was used twice daily for 2–3 days for the treatment of **hookworm infections** of both species, the mean cure rate among 488 patients in 14 trials was 77% (range 30–100%).

Intestinal capillariasis has been successfully treated with thiabendazole at a dosage of 12 mg/kg given twice daily for 30 days.

For the treatment of **dracunculiasis,** Sastry et al report high effectiveness when the drug is used at a dosage of 50–75 mg/kg in divided doses for 1 day. Local inflammation subsides rapidly, followed by death of the worms in 4–6 days. Most worms are then spontaneously extruded or can be extracted manually. Re-treatment is occasionally needed.

The effectiveness of thiabendazole in **visceral larva migrans** has not been established. Several reports have indicated the usefulness of topical thiabendazole for the treatment of **scabies** and **tinea nigra palmaris.**

Adverse Reactions

Side-effects from thiabendazole are common but generally mild and transient. They tend to occur 3–4 hours after ingestion of the drug and last 2–8 hours. Reports on their incidence vary from 7% to more than 50% of patients treated with 25 mg/kg twice daily for 2 days. Higher doses or extension of treatment beyond 2 days increases symptoms.

The most common side-effects are dizziness, anorexia, and nausea and vomiting. Less frequent are epigastric pain, abdominal cramping pain, diarrhea, headache, drowsiness, giddiness, lethargy, and pruritus. Perianal rashes, tinnitus, paresthesias, bradycardia, hypotension, and visual disturbances are rare.

Other side-effects have been reported, but some may represent manifestations of the disease or reactions to dying parasites rather than drug reaction. They include fever, chills, conjunctival injection, angioneurotic edema, lymphadenopathy, skin rashes, toxic epidermal necrolysis, and anaphylaxis.

Occasionally reported during thiabendazole treatment have been leukopenia, crystalluria, and hematuria, all of which subsided when therapy was discontinued.

Some patients may excrete a metabolite that imparts an asparaginelike odor to the urine during therapy and for 24 hours thereafter.

Rarely seen are hyperglycemia, jaundice, and liver function abnormalities. Severe intrahepatic cholestasis due to thiabendazole hypersensitivity has been reported.

Seven cases of erythema multiforme have been associated with thiabendazole therapy in children; in 2 severe cases (Stevens-Johnson syndrome), fatalities occurred.

Contraindications & Cautions

Experience with thiabendazole is limited in children weighing less than 15 kg. It may be best to use alternative drugs in patients with hepatic or renal dysfunction. The drug should be used with caution where drug-induced vomiting may be dangerous. There are a few reports of ascarids becoming hypermotile after treatment and appearing at the nose or mouth.

Since the drug makes some patients dizzy or

drowsy, it should not be used during the day for patients whose work or activity requires mental alertness.

Ideally, supportive therapy is indicated for anemic, dehydrated, or malnourished patients prior to starting thiabendazole therapy.

Discontinue the drug immediately if hypersensitivity symptoms appear—including fever, chills, conjunctival injection, skin rashes, and lymphadenopathy.

Preparations & Dosages

Thiabendazole (Mintezol) is available as a suspension containing 100 mg of the drug per milliliter and as tablets containing 500 mg of the drug. It should be given after meals, and the tablet formulation *should be chewed well.* Pre- and posttreatment purges and dietary restrictions are not necessary.

In the treatment of strongyloidiasis, the dosage is 25 mg/kg twice daily for 2 days. The maximum single dose should not exceed 1.5 g, and the total daily dose should not exceed 3 g. The same dosage may be used for ascariasis or hookworm infection if the preferred drugs are not available. A second course may be given 1 week later if indicated.

In systemic strongyloidiasis, thiabendazole should be continued for 5–7 days, by which time the intestinal infection has usually cleared; however, a longer course may be necessary.

In the treatment of cutaneous larva migrans, the dosage is 25 mg/kg twice daily for 2–5 days (maximum daily dose 3 g). If active lesions are still present 2 days after completion of therapy, a second course should be given. Excellent results have also followed daily application for about 5 days of a cream containing 15% thiabendazole in a hygroscopic base. An easily prepared cream can also be made from a ground 0.5-g tablet mixed with 5 g of petroleum jelly.

The current recommendation for the treatment of trichinosis is 25 mg/kg twice daily for 5 days. However, as experience is gained, longer courses of therapy may be shown to be necessary. The total daily dose should not exceed 3 g.

Thiabendazole is no longer recommended in this text for pinworms or trichuriasis.

• • •

References

Antischistosomal Compounds

Friedheim E: Chemotherapy of schistosomiasis. Pages 29–144 in: *Chemotherapy of Helminthiasis.* Vol 1 in: *International Encyclopedia of Pharmacology and Therapeutics.* Pergamon, 1973.

Frohberg H, Schencking MS: Toxicological profile of praziquantel, a new drug against cestode and schistosome infections, as compared to some other schistosomicides. *Arzneim Forsch* 1981;**31:**555.

Katz N: Current results in the clinical therapy of schistosomiasis mansoni. *Rev Inst Med Trop Sao Paulo* 1980;**22:**8.

Long-term toxicity of antischistosomal drugs. *J Toxicol Environ Health* 1975;**1:**173. [Entire issue.]

McMahon JE: Treatment of schistosomiasis: Factors affecting chemotherapy and reflections on ideal drug treatment. *Trop Geog Med* 1978;**30:**161.

WHO reports on schistosomicidal drugs. *Bol of Sanit Panam* 1972;**6:**82.

Woolhouse N: Biochemical and pharmacological effects in relation to the mode of action of antischistosomal drugs. *Biochem Pharmacol* 1979;**28:**2413.

Antimony Compounds

Ata A-H, Mousa AH: Treatment of bilharziasis by the slow method. *J Egypt Med Assoc* 1960;**43:**746.

Davis A: Comparative trials of antimonial drugs in urinary schistosomiasis. *Bull WHO* 1968;**38:**197.

El-Shabrawy M et al: Intestinal schistosomiasis: A comparative therapeutic trial. *J Egypt Med Assoc* 1972;**55:**69.

Most H et al: Schistosomiasis japonicum in American military personnel: Clinical studies of 600 cases during the first year after infection. *Am J Trop Med Hyg* 1950;**30:**239.

Rugemalila JB: Fatal stibocaptate toxicity. *East Afr Med J* 1980;**57:**720.

Also see references under Antischistosomal Compounds.

Bephenium

Cavier R: Chemotherapy of intestinal nematodes. Chap 4, pp 215–436, in: *Chemotherapy of Helminthiasis.* Vol 1 in: *International Encyclopedia of Pharmacology and Therapeutics.* Pergamon, 1973.

Davis A: *Drug Treatment in Intestinal Helminthiases.* World Health Organization, 1973.

Senewiratne B et al: A comparative study of the relative efficacy of pyrantel pamoate, bephenium hydroxynaphthoate and tetrachlorethylene in the treatment of *Necator americanus* infection in Ceylon. *Ann Trop Med Parasitol* 1975;**69:**233.

Bithionol

Cabrera BD: The treatment of taeniasis saginata with bithionol (Bitin) in Jaro, Leyte. *Acta Med Philippinensis* 1973;**9:**139.

D'Sa CJ: Human fascioliasis. *Proc R Soc Med* 1970;**63:**285.

Grados O, Berrocal LA: Chemotherapy of fascioliasis with bithionol. *Rev Inst Med Trop Sao Paulo* 1977;**19:**425. [English summary.]

Kim JS: Treatment of *Paragonimus westermani* infections with bithionol. *Am J Trop Med Hyg* 1970;**19:**940.

Miyazaki I, Nishimura K: Cerebral paragonomiasis. Pages 109–132 in: *Topics on Tropical Neurology.* Hornabrook R (editor). Davis, 1975.

Yokogawa M: *Paragonimus* and paragonimiasis. Pages 99–158 in: *Advances in Parasitology.* Vol 3. Dawes B (editor). Academic Press, 1965.

Yokogawa M: *Paragonimus* and paragonimiasis. Pages 375–387 in: *Advances in Parasitology.* Vol 7. Dawes B (editor). Academic Press, 1969.

Dichlorophen

Gemmell MA, Johnstone PD: Cestodes. Pages 54–114 in: *Antibiotics and Chemotherapy.* Vol 30. Schonfeld H (editor). Karger, 1981.

Seaton DR: On the use of dichlorophen as a taenifuge for *Taenia saginata. Ann Trop Med Parasitol* 1960;**54:** 338.

Turner PP: The treatment of tapeworm infestation with "Anthiphen." *J Trop Med Hyg* 1963;**66:**259.

Diethylcarbamazine

Anderson J, Fuglsang H: Further studies on the treatment of ocular onchocerciasis with diethylcarbamazine and suramin. *Br J Ophthalmol* 1978;**62:**450.

Bird AC et al: Visual loss during oral diethylcarbamazine treatment for onchocerciasis. (Correspondence.) *Lancet* 1979;**2:**46.

Bryceson ADM, Warrell DA, Pope HM: Dangerous reactions to treatment of onchocerciasis with diethylcarbamazine. *Br Med J* 1977;**1:**742.

Duke BOL: Treatment of onchocerciasis. Pages 46–53 in: *Research and Control of Onchocerciasis in the Western Hemisphere: Proceedings of an International Symposium, Washington, D.C., 18–21 November, 1974.* Pan American Health Organization Scientific Publication No. 298, 1974.

Hawking F: Diethylcarbamazine and new compounds for the treatment of filariasis. *Adv Pharmacol Chemother* 1979; **16:**129.

Emetine

Hadden JW, Pascarelli EF: Diagnosis and treatment of human fascioliasis. *JAMA* 1967;**202:**149.

Hexylresorcinol

Jung RC: Use of a hexylresorcinol tablet in the enema treatment of whipworm infection. *Am J Trop Med Hyg* 1954; **3:**918.

Levamisole

Amery WK, Gough DA: Levamisole and immunotherapy: Some theoretic and practical considerations and their relevance to human disease. *Oncology* 1981;**38:**168.

Levamisole: A cautionary note. (Editorial.) *Lancet* 1979; **2:**291.

Miller JM: Use of levamisole in parasitic infections. *Drugs* 1980;**19:**122.

Moens J et al: Levamisole in ascariasis: A multicenter controlled evaluation. *Am J Trop Med Hyg* 1978;**27:**897.

Multicentre Study Group: Levamisole in rheumatoid arthritis: A randomised double-blind study comparing two dosage regimens of levamisole with placebo. *Lancet* 1978;**2:** 1007.

Symoens J et al: Levamisole. Pages 407–464 in: *Pharmacological and Biochemical Properties of Drug Substances.* Vol 2. Goldberg ME (editor). American Pharmaceutical Association, 1979.

Mebendazole

Bekhti A et al: Chemotherapy of human hydatid disease with mebendazole: Follow-up of 16 cases. *Acta Gastroenterol Belg* 1980;**43:**48.

Braithwaite PA: Long-term high-dose mebendazole for cystic hydatid disease of liver: Failure in two cases. *Aust NZ J Surg* 1981;**51:**23.

Chongsuphajaisiddhi T et al: Treatment of soil-transmitted nematode infections in children with mebendazole. *Ann Trop Med Parasitol* 1978;**72:**59.

Keystone JS, Murdoch JK: Diagnosis and treatment. Drugs five years later: Mebendazole. *Ann Intern Med* 1979;**91:**582.

Scragg JN, Proctor EM: Further experience with mebendazole in the treatment of symptomatic trichuriasis in children. *Am J Trop Med Hyg* 1978;**27:**255.

Sonnett JJ, Thienpont D: The treatment of trichinosis with mebendazole. *Acta Clin Belg* 1977;**32:**297.

Wilson JF, Davidson M, Rausch RL: A clinical trial of mebendazole in the treatment of alveolar hydatid disease. *Am Rev Respir Dis* 1978;**118:**747.

Wolfe AS, Wershing JM: Mebendazole: Treatment of trichuriasis and ascariasis in Bahamian children. *JAMA* 1974;**230:**1408.

Metrifonate

Holmstedt B et al: Metrifonate: Summary of toxicological and pharmacological information available. *Arch Toxicol* 1978;**41:**3.

Jewsbury JM, Cooke MJ, Weber MC: Field trial of metrifonate in the treatment and prevention of schistosomiasis infection in man. *Ann Trop Med Parasitol* 1977;**71:**67.

Omer AHS, Teesdale CH: Metrifonate trial in the treatment of various presentations of *Schistosoma haematobium* and *S mansoni* infections in the Sudan. *Ann Trop Med Parasitol* 1976;**72:**174.

Plestina R, Davis A, Bailey DR: Effect of metrifonate on blood cholinesterases in children during the treatment of schistosomiasis. *Bull WHO* 1972;**46:**747.

Metronidazole

Nik-Akhtar B, Tabibi V: Metronidazole in fascioliasis: Report of four cases. *J Trop Med Hyg* 1977;**80:**179.

Niclosamide

Jones WE: Niclosamide as a treatment for *Hymenolepis diminuta* and *Dipylidium caninum* infection in man. *Am J Trop Med Hyg* 1979;**28:**300.

Kahra A, Veharanta T: [Expelling the broad tapeworm with Yomesan.] *Suom Laak* 1963;**8:**325. [Finnish.]

Most H et al: Yomesan (niclosamide) therapy of *Hymenolepis nana* infections. *Am J Trop Med Hyg* 1971;**20:**206.

Perera DR et al: Niclosamide treatment of cestodiasis: Clinical trials in the United States. *Am J Trop Med Hyg* 1970; **19:**610.

Niridazole

Bassily S et al: Low-dose niridazole in the treatment of *Schistosoma mansoni. Ann Trop Med Parasitol* 1979;**73:**295.

Kale OO: A controlled field trial of the treatment of dracontiasis with metronidazole and niridazole. *Ann Trop Med Parasitol* 1974;**68:**91.

The pharmacological and chemotherapeutic properties of niridazole and other antischistosomal compounds. (Conference.) *Ann NY Acad Sci* 1969;**160:**426.

Saif M et al: On the treatment of urinary bilharziasis with niridazole. *J Egypt Med Assoc* 1974;**57:**83.

Sy FS: Niridazole in the treatment of schistosomiasis japonica. *J Philippine Med Assoc* 1977;**53:**151.

Also see references under Antischistosomal Compounds.

Oxamniquine

Clarke V de V et al: Dose-finding trials of oral oxamniquine in Rhodesia. *S Afr Med J* 1976;**50:**1867.

Farid Z et al: Treatment of advanced hepatosplenic schistosomiasis with oxamniquine. *Trans R Soc Trop Med Hyg* 1980;**74:**400.

Katz N et al: Field trials with oxamniquine in a schistosomiasis mansoni-endemic area. *Am J Trop Med Hyg* 1977;**26:** 234.

Omer AHS: Oxamniquine for treating *Schistosoma mansoni* infection in Sudan. *Br Med J* 1978;**2:**163.

Oxamniquine symposium. *Rev Inst Med Trop Sao Paulo.* 1980;**22(Suppl 4):**1. [Entire issue.]

Oxantel Pamoate

Dissanaike AS: A comparative trial of oxantel-pyrantel and mebendazole in multiple helminth infection in school children. *Drugs* 1978;**15(Suppl 1):**11.

Farahmandian I et al: Comparison of the effect of oxantel-pyrantel and mebendazole on soil-transmitted nematodes in Iran. *Curr Ther Res* 1979;**26:**114.

Garcia EG: Treatment for trichuriasis with oxantel. *Am J Trop Med Hyg* 1976;**25:**914.

Sinniah B et al: Single dose treatment of intestinal nematodes with oxantel-pyrantel pamoate plus mebendazole. *Ann Trop Med Parasitol* 1980;**74:**619.

Paromomycin

Botero D: Paromomycin as effective treatment of *Taenia* infections. *Am J Trop Med Hyg* 1970;**19:**234.

Pawlowski Z, Schultz AG: Taeniasis and cysticercosis *(Taenia saginata). Adv Parasitol* 1972;**10:**292.

Tanowitz HB, Wittner M: Paromomycin in the treatment of *Diphyllobothrium latum* infection. *Am J Trop Med Hyg* 1973;**76:**151.

Ulivelli A: Paromomycin and taeniasis. *Lancet* 1968;**1:**696.

Wittner M, Tanowitz H: Paromomycin therapy of human cestodiasis with special reference to hymenolepiasis. *Am J Trop Med Hyg* 1971;**20:**433.

Piperazine

Berger JR et al: Acute transitory cerebellar dysfunction associated with piperazine adipate. *Arch Neurol* 1979;**36:**180.

Brown HW, Chan KF, Hussey KL: Treatment of enterobiasis and ascariasis with piperazine. *JAMA* 1956;**161:**515.

Bumbalo TS, Plummer LJ: Piperazine (Antepar) in the treatment of pinworm and roundworm infections. *Med Clin North Am* 1957;**41:**575.

Farid Z et al: Single-dose treatment for *Ascaris* infection with piperazine citrate: With a study of the egg-parasite ratio. *Am J Trop Med Hyg* 1966;**15:**516.

Fernando MA, Balasuriya S: Control of ascariasis by mass treatment with piperazine citrate. *Ceylon Med J* 1977;**22:**120.

Hamlyn AN et al: Piperazine hepatitis. *Gastroenterology* 1976;**70:**1114.

Praziquantel

Botero RD, Castano MS: Cisticercosis: Tratamiento con praziquantel. *Tribuna Medica* 1981;**741:**31.

Bunnag D, Harinasuta T: Studies in the chemotherapy of human opisthorchiasis in Thailand. 1. Clinical trial of praziquantel. *Southeast Asian J Trop Med Public Health* 1980;**11:**528.

Classen HG, Schramm V (editors): Praziquantel (Embay 8440, Biltricide). Given at the Biltricide Symposium on African Schistosomiasis, Nairobi, 24–26, February 1980. *Drug Res* 1981;**31:**535.

Groll E: Praziquantel for cestode infections in man. *Acta Trop* 1980;**37:**293.

Praziquantel: A new hope for schistosomiasis. (Editorial.) *Lancet* 1980;**1:**635.

Rim H-J et al: Clinical evaluation of the therapeutic efficacy of praziquantel (Embay 8440) against *Clonorchis sinensis* infection in man. *Ann Trop Med Parasitol* 1981;**75:** 27.

Schenone H: Praziquantel in the treatment of *Hymenolepis nana* infections in children. *Am J Trop Med Hyg* 1980; **29:**320.

Seed JL, Feng Z, Bueding E: Mutagenic and comutagenic activity of the antischistosomal drug, praziquantel, in *Salmonella typhimurium.* (Abstract.) *Fed Proc* 1981;**40:** 668.

World Health Organization: Multicentre trials of praziquantel in human schistosomiasis. *Bull WHO* 1979;**57:**767.

Zhejiang Clinical Cooperative Research Group for Praziquantel: Clinical evaluation of praziquantel in treatment of *Schistosomiasis japonicum. Chin Med J* 1980; **93:**375.

Pyrantel Pamoate

Bell WJ, Nassif S: Comparison of pyrantel pamoate and piperazine phosphate in the treatment of ascariasis. *Am J Trop Med Hyg* 1971;**20:**584.

Botero D, Castanõ A: Comparative study of pyrantel pamoate, bephenium hydroxynaphthoate, and tetrachlorethylene in the treatment of *Necator americanus* infections. *Am J Trop Med Hyg* 1973;**22:**45.

Carney DE, O'Reilly BJ, Tweddell ED: Pyrantel embonate in the treatment of enterobiasis. *Med J Aust* 1971;**2:**254.

Davis A: *Drug Treatment in Intestinal Helminthiases.* World Health Organization, 1973.

Pitts NE, Migliardi JR: Antiminth (pyrantel pamoate): The clinical evaluation of a new broad-spectrum anthelmintic. *Clin Pediatr* 1974;**13:**87.

Pyrvinium Pamoate

Buchanan RA et al: Pyrvinium pamoate. *Clin Pharmacol Ther* 1974;**16:**716.

Macphee DG, Podger DM: Mutagenicity tests on anthelmintics: Microsomal activation of viprynium embonate to a mutagen. *Mutat Res* 1977;**48:**307.

Turner JA, Johnson PE Jr: Pyrvinium pamoate in the treatment of pinworm infection (enterobiasis) in the home. *J Pediatr* 1962;**60:**243.

Wang CC, Galli GA: Strongyloidiasis treated with pyrvinium pamoate. *JAMA* 1965;**193:**847.

Suramin

Anderson J, Fuglsang H: Further studies on the treatment of ocular onchocerciasis with diethylcarbamazine and suramin. *Br J Ophthalmol* 1978;**62:**450.

Hawking F: Suramin: With special reference to onchocerciasis. *Adv Pharmacol Chemother* 1978;**15:**289.

Research and Control of Onchocerciasis in the Western Hemisphere: Proceedings of an International Symposium, Washington, D.C., 18–21 November, 1974. Pan American Health Organization Scientific Publication No. 298, 1974.

Scharlau G: Onchocerciasis-chemotherapy: A risk-approach. *Trop Doct* 1981;**11:**8.

Thylefors B, Rolland A: The risk of optic atrophy following suramin treatment of ocular onchocerciasis. *Bull WHO* 1979;**57:**479.

Tetrachloroethylene

Bueding E, Swartzwelder C: Anthelmintics. *Pharmacol Rev* 1957;**9:**329.

Carr HP, Sardá MEP, Nuñez NA: Anthelmintic treatment of uncinariasis. *Am J Trop Med Hyg* 1954;**3:**495.

Senewiratne B et al: A comparative study of the relative efficacy of pyrantel pamoate, bephenium hydroxynaphthoate and tetrachlorethylene in the treatment of *Necator americanus* infection in Ceylon. *Ann Trop Med Parasitol* 1975;**69:**233.

Thiabendazole

Casali AJ, Costa EA: Investigacion clinica y anatomopatologica del tratamiento de la triquinosis aguda con tiabendazol. *Bol Chil Parasitol* 1977;**32:**66.

Fink AI, MacKay CJ, Cutler SS: Sicca complex and cholestatic jaundice in two members of a family caused by thiabendazole. *Trans Am Ophthalmol Soc* 1978;**76:** 108.

Harland PSEG, Meakins RH, Harland RH: Treatment of cutaneous larva migrans with local thiabendazole. (Correspondence.) *Br Med J* 1977;**2:**772.

Perrin J et al: Thiabendazole treatment of presumptive visceral larva migrans. *Clin Pediatr* 1975;**14:**147.

Sastry SC, Kumar KJ, Lakshminarayana V: The treatment of dracontiasis with thiabendazole. *J Trop Med Hyg* 1978;**81:**32.

Scowden EB et al: Overwhelming strongyloidiasis: An unappreciated opportunistic infection. *Medicine* 1978;**57:**527.

Thiabendazole. *Tex Rep Biol Med* 1969;**27(Suppl 2):**1.

Cancer Chemotherapy | 56

Sydney E. Salmon, MD, & Alan C. Sartorelli, PhD

Cancer is a group of neoplastic diseases that occur in humans of all age groups and races as well as in all animal species. The incidence, geographic distribution, and behavior of specific types of cancer are related to multiple factors including sex, age, race, genetic predisposition, and exposure to environmental carcinogens. Of these factors, the last is probably most important. Chemical carcinogens (particularly those in tobacco smoke) as well as agents such as azo dyes, aflatoxins, and benzene have been clearly implicated in cancer induction in humans as well as in animals. Identification of potential carcinogens in the environment has been greatly simplified by the widespread use of the "Ames test" for mutagenic agents. Ninety percent of carcinogens can be shown to be mutagenic on the basis of this assay. Ultimate identification of potential human carcinogens requires, however, testing in 2 animal species. Certain herpes group DNA viruses and type C RNA viruses have also been implicated as causative agents in animal cancers and might be responsible for some human cancers as well. Oncogenic RNA viruses all appear to contain a "reverse transcriptase" enzyme that permits translation of the RNA message of the tumor virus into the DNA code of the infected cell. Thus, the information governing transformation can become a stable part of the genome of the host cell. Expression of virus-induced neoplasia probably also depends on additional host and environmental factors that modulate the transformation process.

Whatever the cause, cancer is basically a disease of cells characterized by a shift in the control mechanisms that govern cell proliferation and differentiation. Cells that have undergone neoplastic transformation usually express cell surface antigens that appear to be of normal fetal type and have other signs of apparent "immaturity." Such cells proliferate excessively and form local tumors that can compress or invade adjacent normal structures. A small subpopulation of cells within the tumor can be described as **tumor stem cells.** They retain the ability to undergo repeated cycles of proliferation as well as to migrate to distant sites in the body to colonize various organs in the process called **metastasis.** Such tumor stem cells thus can express **clonogenic** or colony-forming capability. Maintenance of the clonogenic potential of tumor stem cells can be demonstrated in animals or in vitro by recovering tumor colonies and reseeding the cells that comprise them, thus showing that the cells can renew themselves and give rise to secondary colonies. Fig 56–1 depicts a typical human tumor colony cloned from a tumor stem cell in vitro. Tumor stem cells often have chromosome abnormalities reflecting their genetic instability, which leads to progressive selection of subclones that can survive more readily in the multicellular environment of the host. Quantitative abnormalities in various metabolic pathways and cellular components accompany this neoplastic progression. The invasive and metastatic processes as well as a series of metabolic abnormalities resulting from the cancer cause illness and eventual death of the patient unless the neoplasm can be eradicated with treatment.

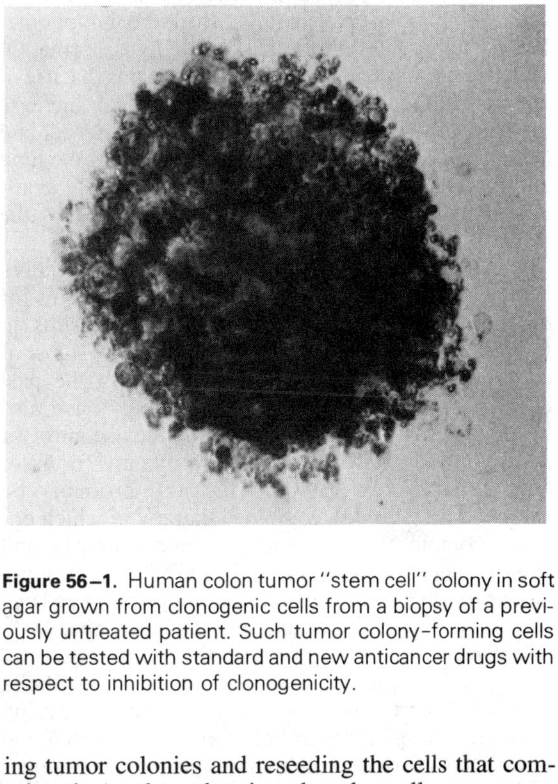

Figure 56–1. Human colon tumor "stem cell" colony in soft agar grown from clonogenic cells from a biopsy of a previously untreated patient. Such tumor colony-forming cells can be tested with standard and new anticancer drugs with respect to inhibition of clonogenicity.

Next to heart disease, cancer is the major cause of death in the USA, causing over 400,000 fatalities annually. With present methods of treatment, one-third of patients are cured with local measures (surgery or radiation therapy), which are quite effective when the tumor has not metastasized by the time of treatment. Earlier diagnosis might lead to cure of 50% of patients with such local treatment; however, in the remaining cases, early micrometastasis is a characteristic feature of the neoplasm, indicating that a systemic approach such as can be attained with chemotherapy will be required (often along with surgery or radiation) for effective cancer management.

Cancer chemotherapy as currently employed can be curative in disseminated neoplasms that have undergone either gross or microscopic spread by the time of diagnosis. These include testicular cancer, diffuse histiocytic lymphoma, Hodgkin's disease, and choriocarcinoma as well as childhood tumors such as acute lymphoblastic leukemia, Burkitt's lymphoma, Wilms' tumor, and embryonal rhabdomyosarcoma. Of major importance are recent demonstrations that use of chemotherapy along with initial surgery can increase the cure rate in relatively early stage breast cancer and osteogenic sarcoma. Common carcinomas of the lung and colon are generally refractory to currently available treatment and have usually disseminated by the time of diagnosis.

At present, chemotherapy provides palliative rather than curative therapy for many forms of disseminated cancer. Effective palliation results in temporary clearing of the symptoms and signs of cancer and prolongation of useful life. In the past decade, advances in cancer chemotherapy have also begun to provide evidence that chemical control of neoplasia may become a reality for many forms of cancer during the 1980s. This will probably be achieved first through combined therapy in which optimal combinations of surgery, radiotherapy, and chemotherapy are used to eradicate both the primary and its occult micrometastases before gross spread can be detected on physical or x-ray examinations.

Drug research may provide the ultimate cure for cancer, although many of the currently available agents fall short of this goal. A major effort to develop anticancer drugs through both empiric screening and rational design of new compounds has now been under way for 3 decades. This program has employed testing in a few well-characterized transplantable animal tumor systems. The development of a simple in vitro colony assay for measuring drug sensitivity of human tumor stem cells may augment and shorten the testing program in the near future. An example of such an in vitro assay for standard anticancer drugs is presented in Fig 56–2. Once new drugs with potential anticancer activity are identified, they are subjected to preclinical toxicologic and limited pharmacologic studies in animals. Promising agents that do not have excessive toxicity are then advanced to phase I clinical trials wherein their pharmacologic and toxic effects are tested in patients with advanced cancer. Phase II clinical trials are then used to establish the tumor types for which the drug is useful, followed by phase III trials to compare the new agent with the best standard therapy. Subsequently, the drug may be licensed by the FDA for use in practice. This development program for a single new drug frequently requires 10 years of testing at the various steps before a drug is ready for general use.

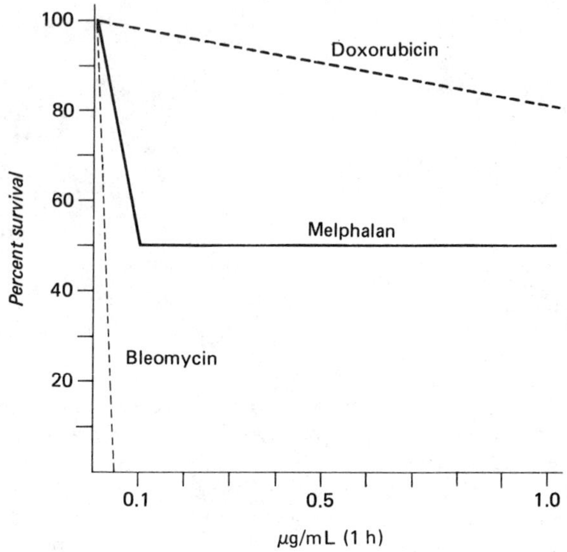

Figure 56–2. Example of an in vitro sensitivity assay with pharmacologically achievable doses of cytotoxic anticancer drugs tested against tumor colony-forming stem cells from a patient's tumor biopsy sample. The cells were incubated in various concentrations of the drugs for 1 hour prior to plating in soft agar and then cultured for 1 week prior to counting the survival of tumor colony-forming units. The results demonstrate sensitivity to bleomycin, resistance to doxorubicin, and heterogeneity in response to melphalan. Fifty percent of the colony-forming cells showed sensitivity to melphalan at the lowest dose tested, while the remaining 50% were resistant to the highest dose.

Ideal anticancer drugs would theoretically be those that eradicate cancer cells without harming normal tissues. Unfortunately, few currently available agents meet this criterion, and clinical use of these drugs involves a weighing of benefits against toxicity in a search for a favorable therapeutic index.

Information on cell and population kinetics of cancer cells in part explains the limited effectiveness of most available anticancer drugs. A schematic summary of cell cycle kinetics is presented in Fig 56–3. This information is relevant to the mode of action, indications, and scheduling of cell cycle-specific (CCS) and cell cycle-nonspecific (CCNS) drugs. Agents falling in these 2 major classes are summarized in Table 56–1. Other classes of drugs have recently also entered development, including the following: inducers of differentiation, intended to force neoplastic cells past a maturation block to form end stage cells with little or no neoplastic potential; antimetastatic drugs, designed to perturb surface properties of malignant cells and thus alter their invasive and metastatic potential; hypoxic tumor stem cell-specific agents, designed to exploit the greater capacity for reductive reactions in these therapeutically resistant cells created

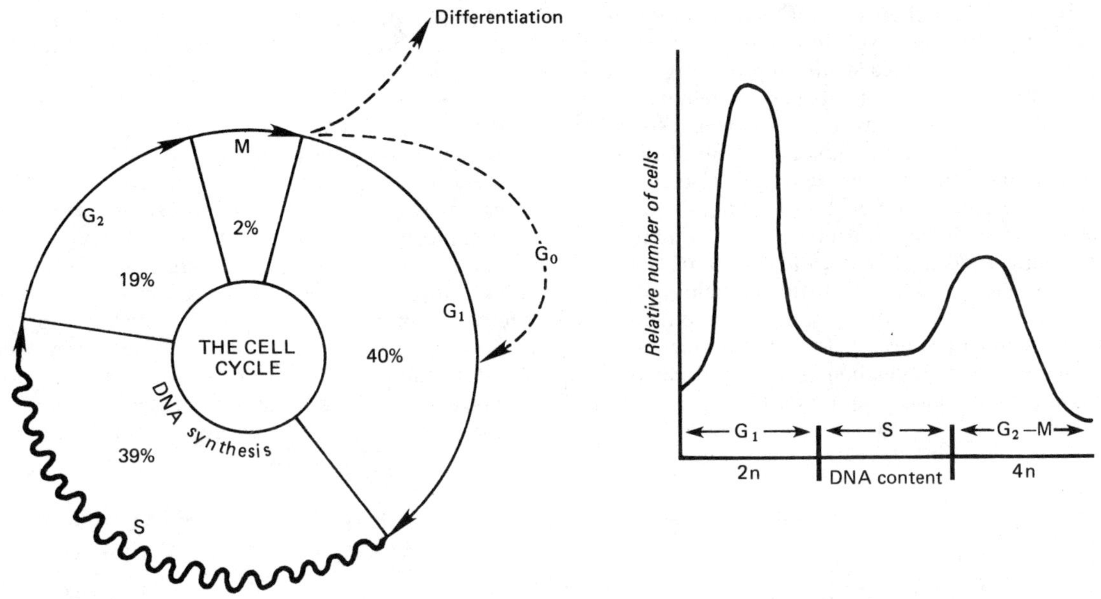

Figure 56–3. The cell cycle and cancer. The illustration at left is a conceptual depiction of the cell cycle phases that all cells—normal and neoplastic—must traverse prior to cell division. The relative durations of the various phases of the cycle are given in approximate percentages spent in each phase by a typical malignant cell; the duration of G_1, however, can vary markedly. At right is a histogram of DNA content of an unperturbed population of tumor cells as determined by flow microfluorimetry (FMF), a technique that permits quantitation of the proportion of cells in the major phases of the cell cycle. Many of the effective anticancer drugs exert their action on cells traversing the cell cycle and are called cell cycle-specific (CCS) drugs (Table 56–1). A second group of agents called cell cycle-nonspecific (CCNS) drugs can sterilize tumor cells irrespective of whether they are cycling or resting in the G_0 compartment. G_1 is the initial phase of the cell cycle of a cell committed to proliferation and is associated with synthesis of enzymes required for function and for DNA synthesis. The S (synthesis) phase is the time during which the DNA genome is duplicated. The G_2 phase is associated with synthesis of cellular components required for mitosis followed by the brief M (mitotic) phase of cell division. CCNS drugs are capable of killing both G_0 and cycling cells (although cycling cells are more sensitive). The damage induced by CCNS drugs is often manifested as a lengthening of the S phase and an irreversible G_2 block. An FMF curve of cells treated with a CCNS drug would be reduced in size in comparison to that seen above, and with a shift in DNA content of intact cells to a 4n accumulation.

by oxygen deficiency of solid tumors; tumor radiosensitizing and normal tissue radioprotecting drugs, aimed at increasing therapeutic effectiveness of radiation therapy; and "biologic response modifiers," which alter tumor-host metabolic and immunologic relationships. Patients with widespread cancer (eg, acute leukemia) may have 10^{12} (1 trillion) tumor cells throughout the body at the time of diagnosis. If tolerable dosing of an effective drug is capable of killing 99.9% of clonogenic tumor cells, this would induce a clinical remission of the neoplasm associated with symptomatic improvement. However, there would still be many logs (10^9) of tumor stem cells remaining in the body, including some that may be inherently resistant to the drug because of heterogeneity, while others might reside in pharmacologic sanctuaries (eg, the central nervous system) where effective drug concentrations may be difficult to achieve. When CCS drugs are used, the tumor stem cells must also be in the sensitive phase of the cell cycle (and not in G_0), so scheduling of these agents is of particular importance. In common bacterial infections, a 3-log reduction in microorganisms might be curative, because host resistance factors can eliminate residual bacteria through immunologic and microbicidal mechanisms; however, host mechanisms for eliminating moderate numbers of cancer cells appear to be generally ineffective. To overcome the limited "log kill" of individual anticancer drugs, combinations of agents with differing

Table 56–1. Cell cycle relationships of major classes of drugs.

Cell Cycle-Specific (CCS) Agents	Cell Cycle-Nonspecific (CCNS) Agents
Antimetabolites (azacytidine, cytarabine, fluorouracil, mercaptopurine, methotrexate, thioguanine)	Alkylating agents (busulfan, cyclophosphamide, mechlorethamine, melphalan, thiotepa)
Bleomycin peptide antibiotics	Antibiotics (dactinomycin, daunorubicin, doxorubicin, mithramycin, mitomycin)
Podophyllin alkaloids (VP16-213, VM26)	Cisplatin
Vinca alkaloids (vincristine, vinblastine, vindesine)	Nitrosoureas (BCNU, CCNU, methyl-CCNU)

toxicities and mechanisms of action have been employed. If the drugs do not have too much overlap in toxicity, they can be used at almost full dosage, and at least additive cytotoxic effects can be achieved with combination chemotherapy; and subclones resistant to only one of the agents can potentially be eradicated. Some combinations of anticancer drugs also appear to exert true synergism wherein the effect of the 2 drugs is greater than additive. The efficacy of combination chemotherapy has now been validated in many forms of human cancer, and the scientific rationale appears to be sound. As a result, combination chemotherapy is now the standard approach to curative treatment of testicular cancer and lymphomas and improved palliative treatment of many other tumor types. This important therapeutic approach was first formulated by Skipper and Schabel and described as the "log-kill hypothesis." It is depicted in Fig 56–4.

In general, CCS drugs have proved most effective in hematologic malignancies and other tumors in which a relatively large proportion of the cells are proliferating or are in the **growth fraction.** CCNS drugs (many of which bind to DNA and damage these macromolecules) are useful in low-growth-fraction "solid tumors" as well as in high-growth-fraction tumors. In all instances, effective agents sterilize or inactivate tumor stem cells, which are often only a small fraction of the cells within a tumor. Non-stem cells (eg, those that have irreversibly differentiated) are considered sterile by definition and are not a significant component of the cancer problem.

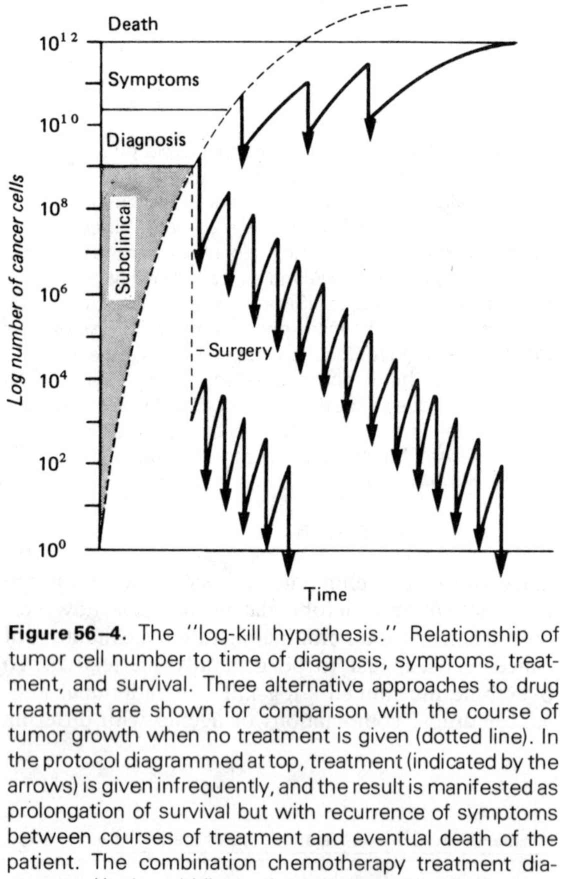

Figure 56–4. The "log-kill hypothesis." Relationship of tumor cell number to time of diagnosis, symptoms, treatment, and survival. Three alternative approaches to drug treatment are shown for comparison with the course of tumor growth when no treatment is given (dotted line). In the protocol diagrammed at top, treatment (indicated by the arrows) is given infrequently, and the result is manifested as prolongation of survival but with recurrence of symptoms between courses of treatment and eventual death of the patient. The combination chemotherapy treatment diagrammed in the middle section is begun earlier and is more intensive. Tumor cell kill exceeds regrowth, drug resistance does not develop, and "cure" results. In this example, treatment has been continued long after all clinical evidence of cancer has disappeared (1–3 years). This approach has been established as effective in the treatment of childhood acute leukemia, testicular cancers, and Hodgkin's disease. In the treatment diagrammed near the bottom of the graph, early surgery has been employed to remove the primary tumor, and intensive adjuvant chemotherapy has been administered long enough (up to 1 year) to eradicate the remaining 10^3 tumor stem cells that comprise the remaining occult micrometastases.

POLYFUNCTIONAL ALKYLATING AGENTS

History

This group of agents evolved from the sulfur mustard vesicant gas dichloroethyl sulfide used in World War I. During World War II, the nitrogen mustards were developed for use as chemical warfare agents. In addition to their vesicant effect upon the skin, these compounds produced atrophy of lymphoid tissue and bone marrow. Because of these latter effects, they were introduced for the treatment of malignant lymphomas and leukemias and were later found to be effective against bronchogenic carcinoma and carcinoma of the ovary as well. Since the introduction of the parent nitrogen mustard "HN2"—methyl-bis(β-chloroethyl)amine, mechlorethamine, Mustargen—new and more stable polyfunctional alkylating drugs have been developed in the search for more effective and less toxic agents. It is now recognized that different alkylating agents have some specificity for selected neoplasms, largely because of differences in reactivity that alter patterns of absorption, distribution, and excretion.

Chemistry

The major clinically useful alkylating agents (Fig 56–5) have a structure containing a bis(chloroethyl)-amine, ethyleneimine, or nitrosourea moiety. Among the bis(chloroethyl)amines, cyclophosphamide, mechlorethamine, melphalan, and chlorambucil have the greatest utility. The aziridine thiotepa and the alkylsulfonate busulfan are used for specialized purposes for ovarian cancer and chronic myeloid leukemia, respectively. The major nitrosoureas are BCNU (carmustine), CCNU (lomustine), and methyl-CCNU (semustine). A variety of investigational alkylating agents have been synthesized that link various carrier molecules such as amino acids, nucleic acid bases, hormones, or sugar moieties to a group capable of alkylation; however, successful "site-directed" alkylation has not to date been achieved.

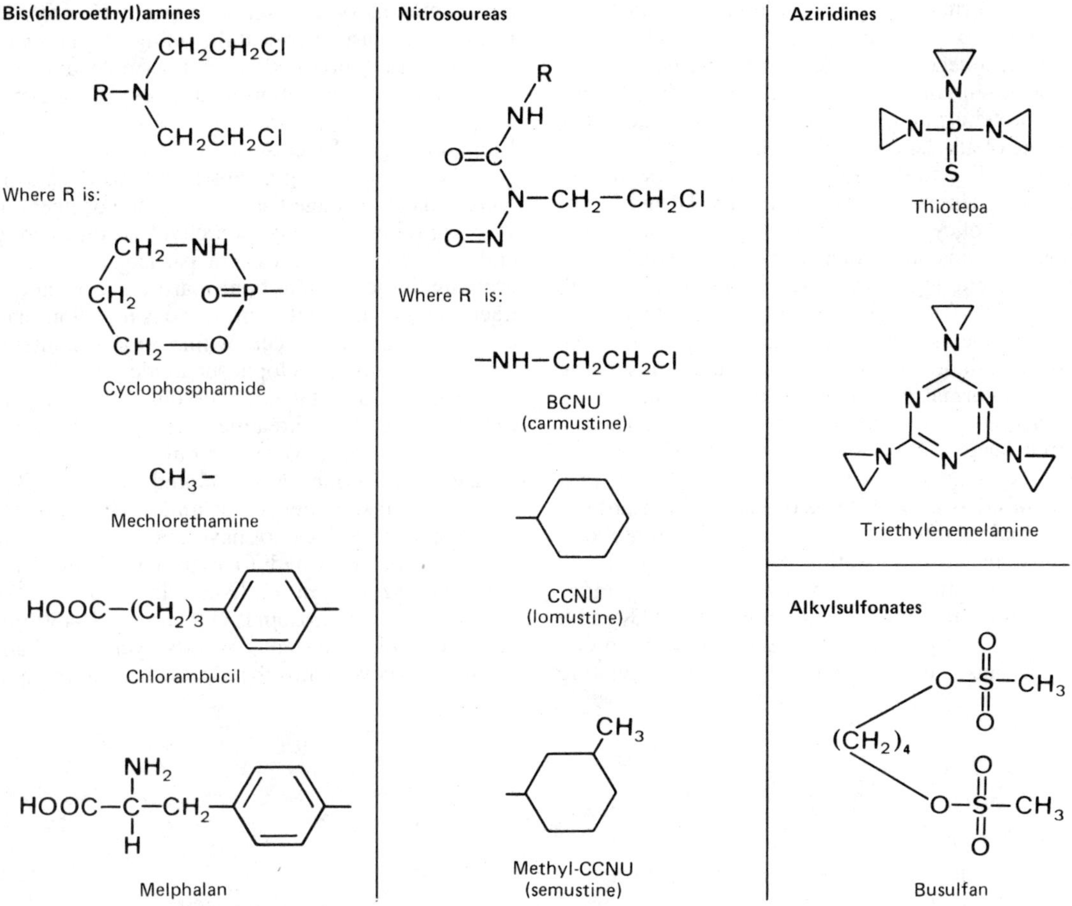

Figure 56–5. Structures of major classes of alkylating agents.

As a class, the alkylating agents act by exerting cytotoxic effects via transfer of their alkyl groups to various cellular constituents. Alkylations of DNA within the nucleus probably represent the major interactions that lead to cellular lethality. However, these drugs react chemically with sulfhydryl, amino, hydroxyl, carboxyl, and phosphate groups of all cellular nucleophiles as well. The general mechanism of action of these drugs involves intramolecular cyclization to form an ethyleneimonium ion that may directly

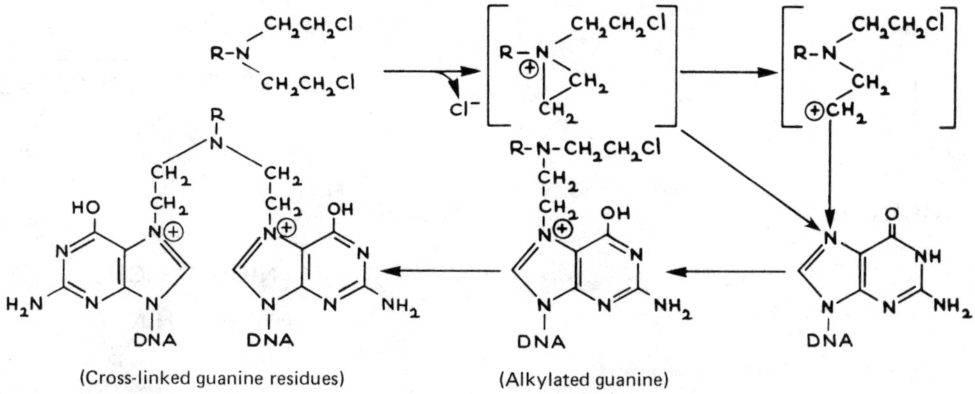

Figure 56–6. Mechanism of alkylation of DNA guanine. A bis(chloroethyl)amine forms an ethyleneimonium ion and a carbonium ion that react with a base such as N7 of guanine in DNA, producing an alkylated purine. Alkylation of a second guanine residue, through the illustrated mechanism, results in cross-linking of DNA strands.

or through formation of a carbonium ion transfer an alkyl group to a cellular constituent. In addition to alkylation, a secondary mechanism that occurs with nitrosoureas involves carbamoylation of lysine residues of proteins through formation of isocyanates. The major site of alkylation within DNA is the N7 position of guanine (Fig 56–6); however, other bases are also alkylated to lesser degrees, including N1 and N3 of adenine, N3 of cytosine, and O6 of guanine, as well as phosphate atoms and proteins associated with DNA. These interactions can occur on a single strand or both strands of DNA through cross-linking, as most major alkylating agents are bifunctional, with 2 reactive groups. Alkylation of guanine can result in miscoding through abnormal base pairing with thymine, or in depurination by excision of guanine residues. The latter effect leads to DNA strand breakage through scission of the sugar-phosphate backbone of DNA. Cross-linking of DNA appears to be of major importance to the cytotoxic action of alkylating agents, and replicating cells are most susceptible to these drugs. Thus, although alkylating agents are not cell cycle-specific, cells are most susceptible to alkylation in late G_1 and S phases of the cell cycle and express blockage in G_2. The mechanism of acquired resistance to alkylating agents may involve increased capacity to repair DNA lesions, decreased permeability of the alkylating drug, and increased production of low-molecular-weight thiols that serve as a trap for the alkylating agents.

Pharmacologic Effects

Active alkylating agents have direct vesicant effects and can damage tissues at the site of injection as well as produce systemic toxicity. Toxicities are generally dose-related and occur particularly on rapidly growing tissues such as bone marrow, gastrointestinal tract, and gonads. After intravenous injection, nausea and vomiting usually occur within 30–60 minutes with mechlorethamine, cyclophosphamide, or BCNU. The emetic effects are of central nervous system origin and can be reduced by pretreatment with phenothiazines or cannabinoids (tetrahydrocannibinol, nabilone). Subcutaneous injection of mechlorethamine or BCNU leads to tissue necrosis and sloughing. Cyclophosphamide does not have direct vesicant effects and must be activated to cytotoxic forms by microsomal enzymes in the liver (Fig 56–7).

The liver microsomal cytochrome P-450 mixed function oxidase system converts cyclophosphamide to 4-hydroxycyclophosphamide, which is in equilib-

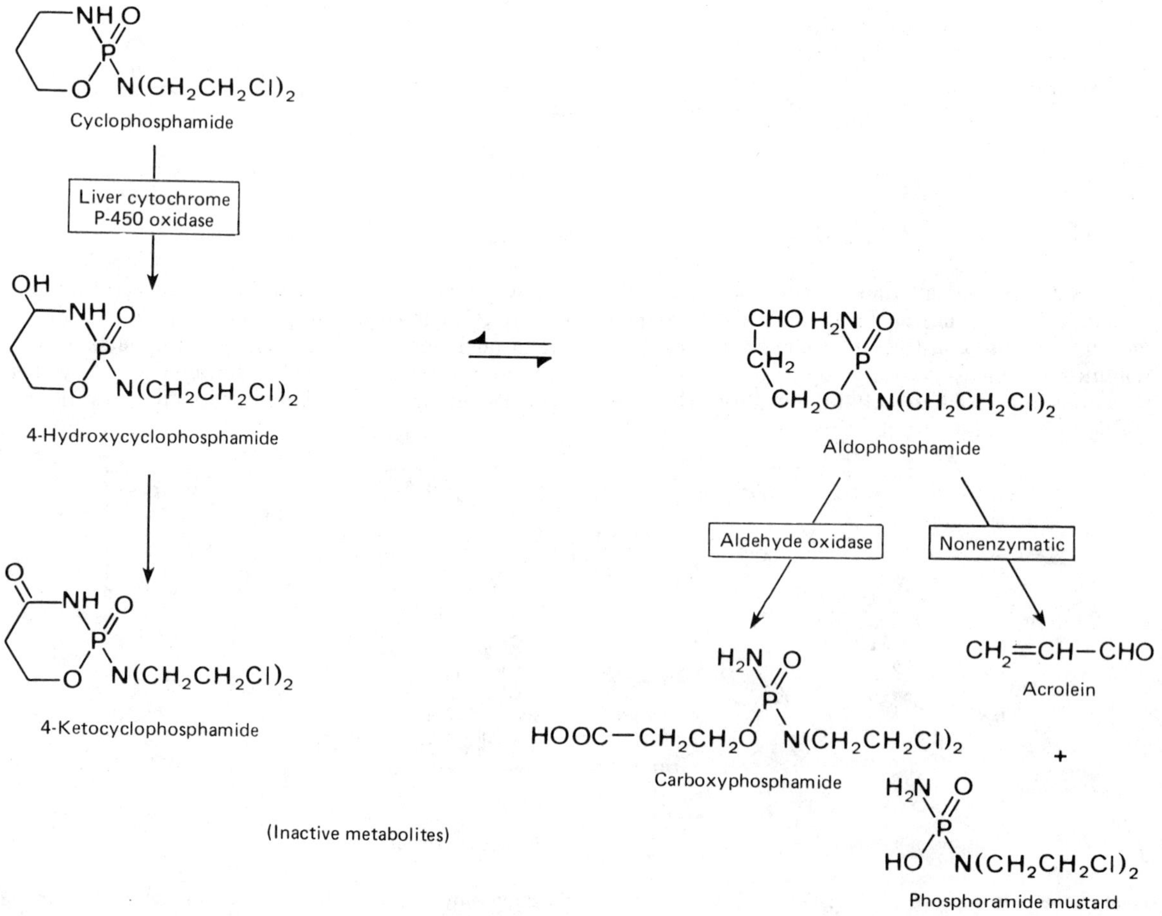

Figure 56–7. Cyclophosphamide metabolism.

rium with aldophosphamide. These active metabolites are believed to be carried by the bloodstream to tumor and normal tissue, where nonenzymatic cleavage of aldophosphamide to the cytotoxic forms—phosphoramide mustard and acrolein—occurs. The liver appears to be protected through the enzymatic formation of the inactive metabolites 4-ketocyclophosphamide and carboxyphosphamide. The major toxicity of alkylating agents is on the bone marrow and results in dose-related suppression of myelopoiesis. The white blood count and absolute granulocyte count reach their low point 10–12 days after injection of mechlorethamine or cyclophosphamide, with subsequent recovery within 21 days (cyclophosphamide) to 42 days (mechlorethamine). The white count nadir with nitrosoureas is delayed to 28 days, with recovery by 42 days. Effects on megakaryocytes and platelets parallel those on granulocytes. Because of the long life span of the erythrocyte, effects on erythropoiesis are minor, and the red cell count is usually only mildly reduced. Side-effects on the bone marrow may be more severe when an alkylating agent is given along with other myelosuppressive drugs or radiation therapy, and dose reductions are often required in such circumstances to avoid excessive toxicity.

Following hematopoietic recovery, these agents may be given again on an intermittent dosage schedule at sufficient intervals to permit blood count recovery. Ovarian or testicular failure is a common late sequela of alkylating agent therapy, while acute leukemia is a relatively rare complication of use of these mutagenic agents.

Oral dosage forms of alkylating agents have been of great value and have been developed using relatively less reactive alkylating drugs. Oral administration of cyclophosphamide, melphalan, chlorambucil, busulfan, and CCNU represents the most common route of administration of these agents and produces effects similar to those observed with parenteral administration. In general, if a tumor is resistant to one alkylating agent, it will be relatively resistant to other agents of this class (although not necessarily to nitrosoureas); however, there are distinct exceptions to this rule for specific tumor types. Overall, cyclophosphamide is the most useful alkylating agent currently available. The oral drug busulfan has a major degree of specificity for the granulocyte series and therefore is of particular value in therapy of chronic myelogenous leukemia. Busulfan does not cause nausea or vomiting despite uniform absorption. Increased skin pigmentation is common with this drug, and rarer syndromes of pulmonary fibrosis or adrenal insufficiency or wasting have been reported often enough so that they can be attributed to busulfan. With all oral alkylating agents, some degree of leukopenia is necessary to provide evidence that the drug has been absorbed adequately. Repeated blood counts are essential during administration of these agents, as the development of severe leukopenia or thrombocytopenia necessitates interruption of therapy.

NITROSOUREAS

Carmustine (BCNU), lomustine (CCNU), and semustine (methyl-CCNU) appear to be non-cross-reactive (as regards tumor resistance) with other alkylating agents; all appear to require biotransformation for antitumor activity, which occurs by nonenzymatic decomposition to liberate derivatives with both alkylating and carbamoylating activities. The nitrosoureas are highly lipid-soluble and cross the blood-brain barrier, making them of use in the treatment of brain tumors. The nitrosoureas appear to function by cross-linking through alkylation of DNA. The drugs may be more effective against plateau phase cells than exponentially growing cells, although within a cycling cell population the drugs appear to slow cell progression through the DNA synthetic phase. After oral administration of lomustine or semustine, plasma metabolites account for virtually all the administered drug, with peak plasma levels of metabolites appearing within 1–4 hours, and prompt central nervous system appearance of 30–40% of the activity present in the plasma. While the initial plasma $t_{1/2}$ is in the range of 6 hours, a second $t_{1/2}$ is in the range of 1–2 days, and 15–20% of the metabolites are still in the body at 5 days. Urinary excretion appears to be the major route of elimination from the body. One naturally occurring sugar-containing nitrosourea, streptozocin (Zanosar), is interesting because it has minimal bone marrow toxicity but is frequently effective in the treatment of insulin-secreting islet cell carcinoma of the pancreas and occasionally in non-Hodgkin lymphomas. Chlorozotocin, a related synthetic nitrosourea, which also lacks marrow toxicity, is now in clinical investigation.

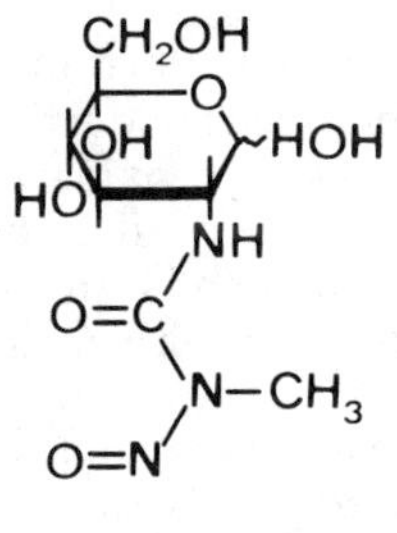

Streptozocin

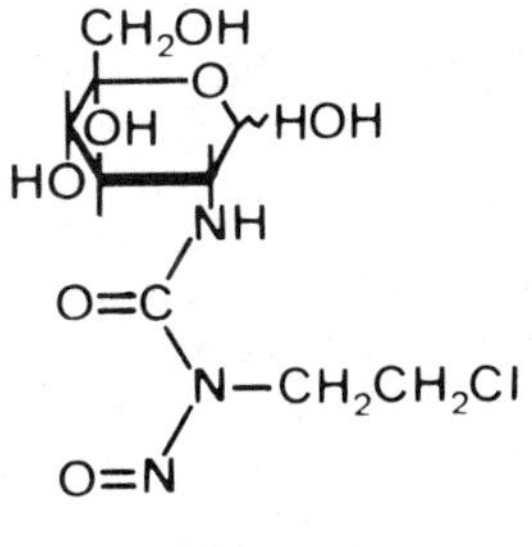

Chlorozotocin

RELATED DRUGS POSSIBLY ACTING AS ALKYLATING AGENTS

A variety of other compounds have mechanisms of action that involve alkylation. These include procarbazine, dacarbazine, hexamethylmelamine, and cisplatin.

1. PROCARBAZINE

The oral agent procarbazine (Matulane) is a methylhydrazine derivative with chemotherapeutic ac-

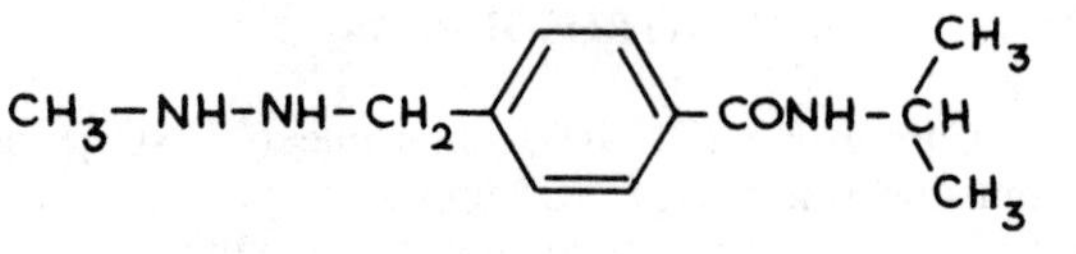

N-Isopropyl-α-(2-methylhydrazino)-
p-toluamide (procarbazine)

tivity (particularly in Hodgkin's disease). The drug is also leukemogenic and has teratogenic and mutagenic properties.

The mechanism of action of procarbazine is uncertain; however, the drug inhibits the syntheses of DNA, RNA, and protein, prolongs interphase, and produces chromosome breaks. Oxidative metabolism of this drug by microsomal enzymes generates azoprocarbazine and H_2O_2, which may be responsible for DNA strand scission. A variety of other metabolites of the drug are formed that may be cytotoxic. One metabolite is a monoamine oxidase (MAO) inhibitor, and adverse side-effects can occur when procarbazine is given with other MAO inhibitors. In addition to predictable nausea, vomiting, and myelosuppression, hemolytic anemia, pulmonary reactions, and adverse responses with alcohol (disulfiramlike) have also been reported, as have skin rashes when procarbazine is given with phenytoin.

Procarbazine has had major use in combination chemotherapy of Hodgkin's disease, as it is not cross-resistant with *Vinca* alkaloids or conventional alkylating agents. However, its leukemogenic properties may eventually lead to its replacement with drugs that have lesser carcinogenic potential.

2. DACARBAZINE

Dacarbazine is a synthetic compound that functions as an alkylating agent following metabolic activation by liver microsomal enzymes by oxidative N-demethylation to the monomethyl derivative that spontaneously decomposes to 5-aminoimidazole-4-carboxamide, which is excreted in the urine, and diazomethane. The diazomethane generates a methyl carbonium ion that is believed to be the likely cytotoxic species. Dacarbazine is administered parenterally and is not schedule-dependent. It produces marked nausea, vomiting, and myelosuppression. Its major applications are in melanoma, Hodgkin's disease, and some soft tissue sarcomas. In the latter 2 tumors, its activity is potentiated by doxorubicin.

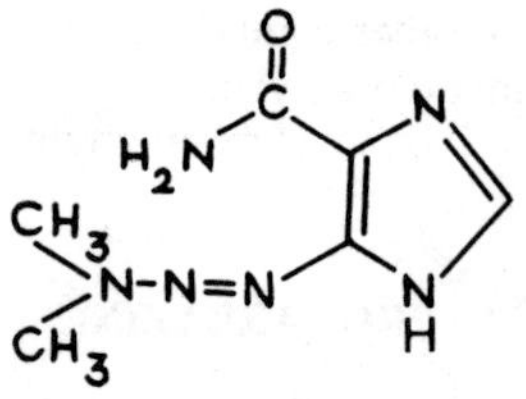

Dacarbazine
(dimethyl imidazole carboxamide)

3. HEXAMETHYLMELAMINE

Hexamethylmelamine is an investigational drug structurally similar to triethylenemelamine. It is relatively insoluble and available only in oral form. A related compound, pentamethylmelamine, which is a major metabolite of hexamethylmelamine, is more soluble and is now in clinical trial in an intravenous form. Both agents are rapidly biotransformed by demethylation, presumably to active intermediates. These agents cause nausea, vomiting, and central and peripheral nervous system neuropathies but relatively mild myelosuppression. They are currently classed as investigational. Hexamethylmelamine is useful in alkylating agent-resistant ovarian carcinoma and will probably be approved by the FDA for use in that disorder in the near future.

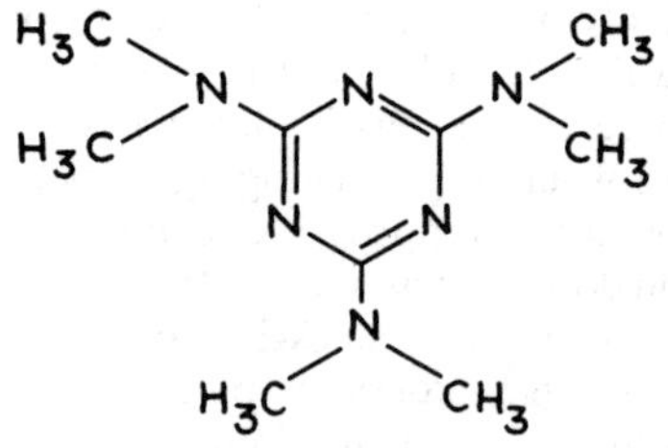

Hexamethylmelamine

4. CISPLATIN

Cisplatin (cis-diamminedichloroplatinum [II], Platinol) is an inorganic metal complex discovered by Rosenberg and his colleagues, who made the serendipitous observation that neutral platinum complexes inhibit division and induce filamentous growth of *Escherichia coli*. A whole series of platinum analogs have been synthesized, but cisplatin is the only one currently in clinical use. While the precise mechanism of action of cisplatin is still to be defined, it is thought to act analogously to alkylating agents. It kills cells in all stages of the cell cycle, produces inhibition of DNA biosynthesis, and binds DNA through the formation of interstrand cross-links. The primary binding site is the N7 of guanine, but covalent interaction with adenine and cytosine also occurs. The platinum complexes appear to synergize with certain other anticancer drugs. After intravenous administration, the major acute toxicity is nausea and vomiting. Cisplatin has relatively little effect on the bone marrow, but it can induce significant renal dysfunction and occasional acoustic nerve dysfunction. Hydration with saline

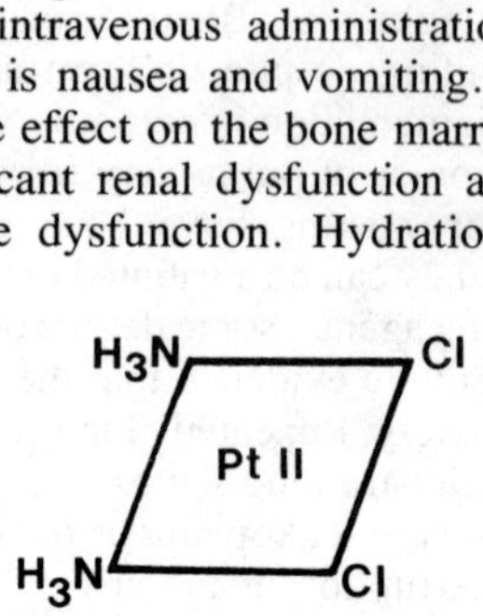

Cisplatin

infusion—alone or with mannitol or other diuretics—appears to minimize nephrotoxicity.

Cisplatin has major antitumor activity in genitourinary cancers, particularly testicular, ovarian, and bladder cancer. Its use along with vinblastine and bleomycin has been a major advance in the development of curative therapy for nonseminomatous testicular cancers.

CLINICAL USES OF POLYFUNCTIONAL ALKYLATING AGENTS

The alkylating agents are used in the treatment of a wide variety of hematologic and solid cancers, generally as components of combination chemotherapy. These are summarized in Table 56–2 and discussed under various specific tumors.

ADVERSE REACTIONS TO POLYFUNCTIONAL ALKYLATING AGENTS

Nausea and vomiting are almost universally reported with intravenously administered mechlorethamine, cyclophosphamide, and carmustine and occur with moderate frequency with oral cyclophosphamide.

The important toxic effect of therapeutic doses of virtually all the alkylating drugs is depression of bone marrow and subsequent leukopenia and thrombocytopenia. Severe infections and septicemia may result, with granulocytopenia below 600 PMNs/μL. Platelet depression below 40,000/μL may be accompanied by induced hemorrhagic phenomena. Cyclophosphamide may produce slight to severe alopecia in up to 30% of patients. It may also cause hemorrhagic cystitis. The cystitis can often be averted with adequate hydration.

The hematopoietic effects of toxic doses of alkylating drugs are treated by discontinuing the agent. Red cell and platelet transfusions and antibiotics to control infections are employed as needed until the marrow has regenerated.

ANTIMETABOLITES (Structural Analogs)

The development of drugs with actions on intermediary metabolism of proliferating cells has been important both clinically and conceptually. While biochemical properties unique to all cancer cells have yet to be discovered, neoplastic cells do have a number of quantitative differences in metabolism from normal cells that render them more susceptible to a number of antimetabolites or structural analogs. Many of these

Table 56–2. Polyfunctional alkylating agents and probable alkylating agents: Dosages and toxicity.

Alkylating Agent	Single Agent Dose	Acute Toxicity	Delayed Toxicity
Nitrogen mustard (HN2, mechlorethamine, Mustargen)	0.4 mg/kg IV in single or divided doses	Nausea and vomiting	Moderate depression of peripheral blood count. Excessive doses produce severe bone marrow depression with leukopenia, thrombocytopenia, and bleeding. Alopecia and hemorrhagic cystitis occasionally occur with cyclophosphamide. Cystitis can be prevented with adequate hydration.
Chlorambucil (Leukeran)	0.1–0.2 mg/kg/d orally; 6–12 mg/d	None	
Cyclophosphamide (Cytoxan)	3.5–5 mg/kg/d orally for 10 days; 1 g/m² IV as single dose	Nausea and vomiting	
Melphalan (Alkeran)	0.25 mg/kg/d orally for 4 days every 4–6 weeks	None	
Thiotepa (triethylenethiophosphoramide)	0.2 mg/kg IV for 5 days	None	
Busulfan (Myleran)	2–8 mg/d orally; 150–250 mg/course	None	
Carmustine (BCNU)	200 mg/m² IV every 6 weeks	Nausea and vomiting	Leukopenia and thrombocytopenia. Rarely hepatitis.
Lomustine (CCNU)	150 mg/m² orally every 6 weeks	Nausea and vomiting	
Semustine (methyl-CCNU)	150 mg/m² orally every 6 weeks	Nausea and vomiting	
Hexamethylmelamine	10 mg/kg/d for 21 days	Nausea and vomiting	Leukopenia, thrombocytopenia, and peripheral neuropathy.
Procarbazine	50–200 mg/d orally	Nausea and vomiting	Bone marrow depression, central nervous system depression.
Dacarbazine	300 mg/m² daily IV for 5 days	Nausea and vomiting	Bone marrow depression.
Cisplatin (Platinol)	20 mg/m²/d IV for 5 days or 50–70 mg/m² as single dose every 3 weeks	Nausea and vomiting	Renal dysfunction. Acoustic nerve dysfunction.

agents have been rationally designed and synthesized, based on knowledge of cellular processes, although a few have been discovered as antibiotics. The prototype for inhibiting malignant growth is the folic acid antagonist methotrexate, which acts directly as a substitute for a normal metabolite.

Biochemical Mechanisms

Antimetabolites or their active products (after biotransformation) can work by any of a number of different mechanisms to inhibit cell proliferation. For example, the antimetabolite may be metabolized instead of the normal substrate for a biosynthetic pathway, so that the antimetabolite is incorporated into a critical macromolecule which then cannot function properly. A second mechanism involves competition with a normal metabolite that acts at either the catalytic site of an enzyme or at an allosteric (regulatory) site. Binding to either of these sites on the enzyme may be reversible or irreversible depending on the specific structure and function of the antimetabolite. One form of antimetabolite that binds to the catalytic site of an enzyme will strongly inhibit it when the enzyme is in a transition state with respect to the substrate. In some instances, inhibition of an enzyme will cause cell death by causing toxic products to accumulate; however, this mechanism appears to be relatively uncommon.

The biochemical pathways that have thus far proved to be most exploitable with antimetabolites have been those relating to nucleotide and nucleic acid synthesis. In a number of instances, when an enzyme is known to have a major effect on pathways leading to cell replication, inhibitors of the reaction it catalyzes have proved to be useful anticancer drugs. A summary of sites of action of some of the antimetabolites affecting DNA synthesis is depicted in Fig 56–8.

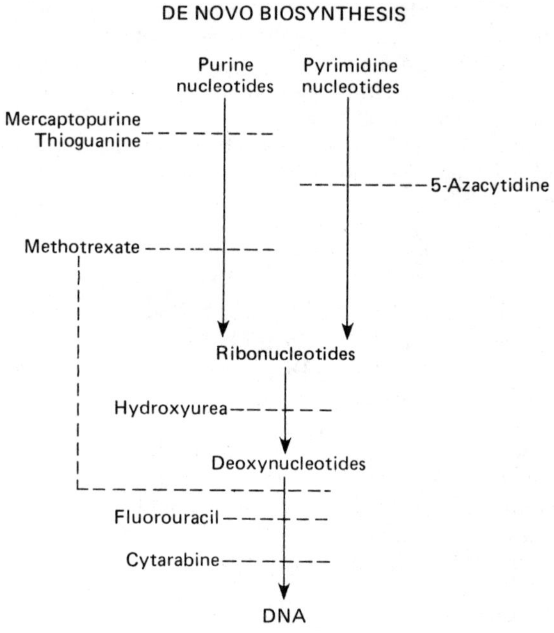

Figure 56–8. Sites of action of antimetabolites on DNA synthetic pathways.

These drugs and their doses and toxicities are shown in Table 56–3. The principal drugs are discussed below.

METHOTREXATE

Methotrexate (4-amino-N[10]-methylpteroylglutamate, MTX) is a folic acid antagonist that binds to

Table 56–3. Structural analogs: Dosages and toxicity.

Chemotherapeutic Agent	Single Agent Dose	Delayed Toxicity*
Methotrexate (amethopterin, MTX)	2.5–5 mg/d orally; 10 mg intrathecally 1–2 times weekly	Oral and gastrointestinal tract ulceration, bone marrow depression, leukopenia, thrombocytopenia.
Mercaptopurine (Purinethol, 6-MP)	2.5 mg/kg/d orally	Usually well tolerated. Larger dosages may cause bone marrow depression.
Thioguanine (6-TG)	2 mg/kg/d orally	Usually well tolerated. Larger dosages may cause bone marrow depression.
Fluorouracil (5-FU)	15 mg/kg/d IV for 5 days by 24-hour infusion; 15 mg/kg weekly IV	Nausea, oral and gastrointestinal ulceration, bone marrow depression.
Cytarabine (ara-C, Cytosar)	100 mg/m^2/d for 5–10 days, either by continuous IV infusion or subcutaneously every 8 hours	Nausea and vomiting, bone marrow depression, megaloblastosis, leukopenia, thrombocytopenia.
5-Azacytidine	200 mg/m^2/d IV for 5 days	Nausea and vomiting, diarrhea, fever, hypotension, prolonged marrow hypoplasia.
Supportive Agent With All Drugs	**Dose**	**Delayed Toxicity**
Allopurinol (Zyloprim)	300–800 mg/d orally for prevention or relief of hyperuricemia	Usually none. Enhances effects and toxicity of 6-MP when used in combination.

*These drugs do not cause acute toxicity.

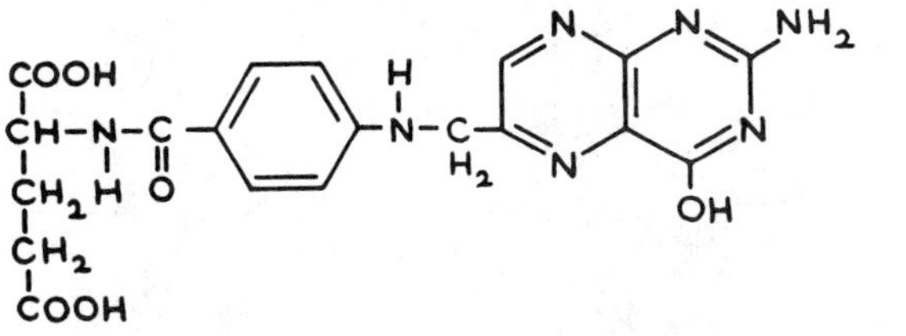

Folic acid

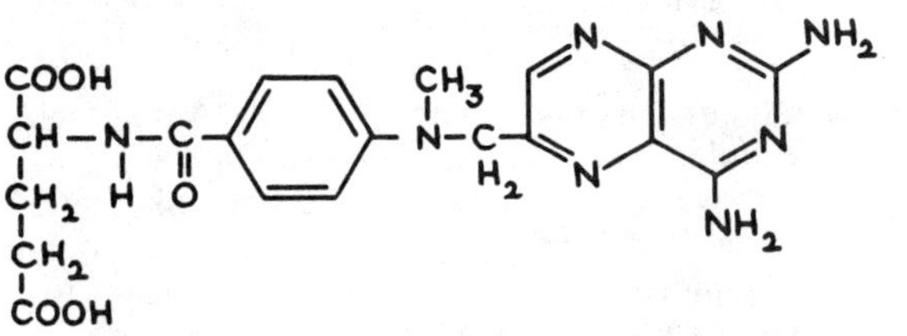

Methotrexate

the active catalytic site of dihydrofolate reductase (DHFR), interfering with the synthesis of the reduced form that accepts one-carbon units. Lack of this cofactor interrupts the synthesis of thymidylate, purine nucleotides, and the amino acids serine and methionine, thereby interfering with the formation of DNA, RNA, and protein. The enzyme binds methotrexate extremely tightly, and at pH 6 virtually no dissociation of the enzyme-inhibitor complex occurs (inhibition constant about 1 nM). At physiologic pH, reversible competitive kinetics occur (inhibition constant about 1 μM). Tumor cell resistance to methotrexate has been attributed to (1) decreased drug transport, (2) altered DHFR with lower affinity for methotrexate, and (3) synthesis of increased levels of DHFR. This occurs through gene amplification and results in a marked increase in DHFR messenger RNA. It remains to be established whether this genetic resistance mechanism is relevant for other drugs or for resistant tumors in patients receiving methotrexate.

Methotrexate is administered clinically by the intravenous or oral route. Up to 90% of an oral dose is excreted in the urine within 12 hours. The drug is not subject to metabolism, and serum levels are therefore proportionate to dose as long as renal function and hydration status are adequate. Toxic side-effects to proliferating tissues are usually observed on the bone marrow and to a lesser extent on the skin and gastrointestinal mucosa. The effects of methotrexate can be reversed by administration of leucovorin (citrovorum factor). Leucovorin "rescue" has been used with accidental overdose or experimentally along with high-dose methotrexate therapy in a protocol intended to rescue normal cells while still leaving the tumor cells subject to its cytotoxic action.

PURINE ANTAGONISTS

Mercaptopurine (Purinethol, 6-MP) was the first of the thiopurine series found useful as an anticancer drug. Like other thiopurines, it must be anabolized by hypoxanthine-guanine phosphoribosyltransferase (HGPRT) to the nucleotide form (6-thioinosinic acid), which in turn inhibits a number of the enzymes of purine interconversion. Significant amounts of thioguanylic acid and 6-methylmercaptopurine ribotide (MMPR) also are formed from 6-MP. These metabolites may also contribute to the action of the mercaptopurine. 6-MP is used primarily in the treatment of childhood acute leukemia, and a closely related analog, azathioprine, is used as an immunosuppressive agent (Chapter 57).

Thioguanine (6-TG) inhibits several enzymes in the purine nucleotide pathway. Resistance to both 6-MP and 6-TG occurs most commonly by decrease in HGPRT activity; an alternative mechanism in acute leukemia involves elevation of levels of alkaline phosphatase, which results in dephosphorylation of thiopurine nucleotide and cellular loss of the resulting ribonucleoside. A variety of metabolic lesions are associated with the cytotoxic action of the purinethiols. These include inhibition of purine nucleotide interconversion; decrease in intracellular levels of guanine nucleotides, which leads to inhibition of glycoprotein synthesis; interference with the formation of DNA and RNA; and incorporation of purinethiols into both DNA and RNA. 6-TG has a synergistic action when used together with cytarabine in the treatment of adult acute leukemia.

Mercaptopurine and thioguanine are both absorbed rapidly from the gut and excreted mainly in the urine. However, 6-MP is converted to an inactive metabolite (6-thiouric acid) by an oxidation catalyzed by xanthine oxidase, whereas 6-TG requires deamination before metabolism by this enzyme. This factor is important because the purine analog allopurinol (Zyloprim), a potent xanthine oxidase inhibitor, is frequently used along with chemotherapy in hematologic cancers. Simultaneous therapy with allopurinol and 6-MP results in excessive mercaptopurine toxicity unless the dose of mercaptopurine is reduced to 25–30% of the usual level. This effect does not occur with 6-TG, which can be used in full dosage despite administration of allopurinol. Allopurinol

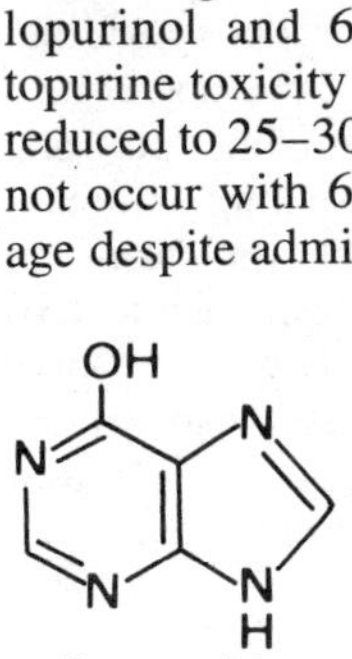

Hypoxanthine

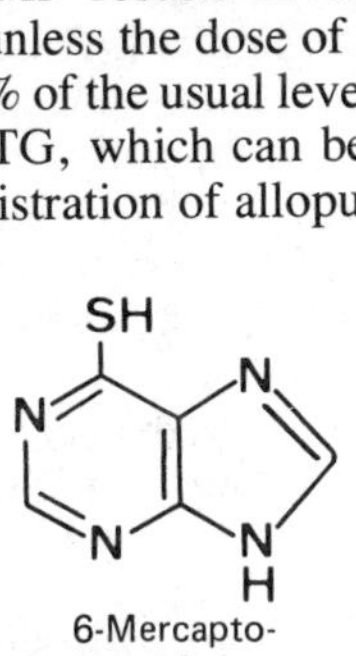

6-Mercapto-purine

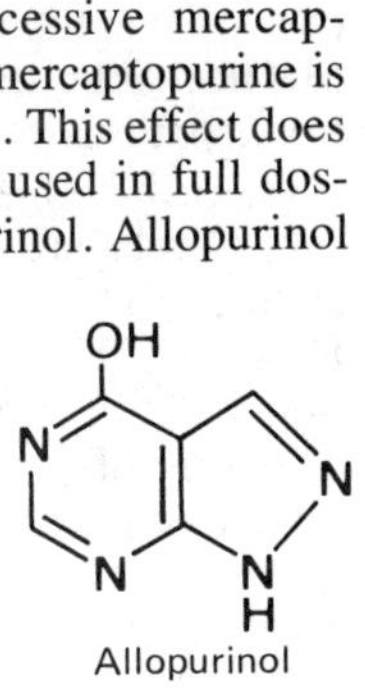

Allopurinol

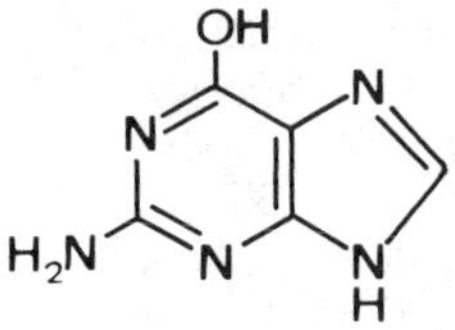

Guanine

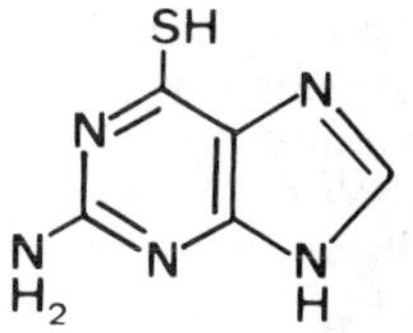

6-Thioguanine

plays an important supportive role in chemotherapy of the leukemias and lymphomas. Even though it is noncytotoxic, it prevents toxicity from purine bases released through tumor lysis by inhibition of xanthine oxidase activity. This allows excretion of cellular purines relatively more soluble than uric acid. Nephrotoxicity and acute gout produced by excessive uric acid is thereby prevented.

PYRIMIDINE ANTAGONISTS

1. FLUOROURACIL

Fluorouracil (5-FU) undergoes anabolic biotransformation to ribosyl and deoxyribosyl nucleotide metabolites. One of these metabolites, 5-fluoro-2′-deoxyuridine 5′-phosphate (FdUMP), forms a covalently bound ternary complex with the enzyme thymidylate synthetase and its cofactor $N^{5,10}$-methylenetetrahydrofolate, a reaction critical for the synthesis of thymine nucleotides. This results in inhibition of DNA synthesis through "thymineless death."

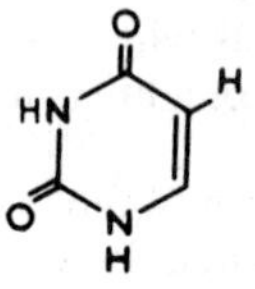
Uracil

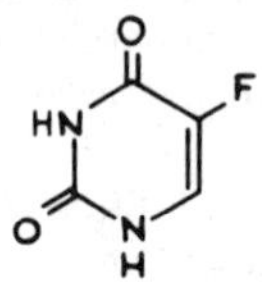
5-FU

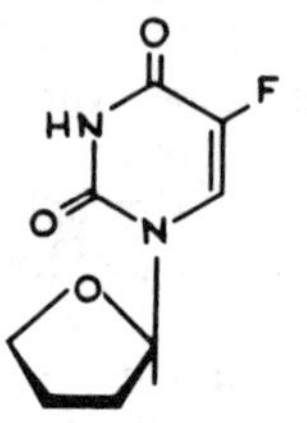
Ftorafur

5-FU is normally given intravenously and has a short metabolic half-life. Although it is active when given orally, its bioavailability is erratic by that route of administration. Floxuridine (5-fluorodeoxyuridine, FUDR) has an action similar to that of 5-FU and is used for hepatic artery infusions. A cream incorporating 5-FU (Efudex) is used topically for treating skin cancers. A related investigational drug, tegafur (ftorafur), appears to release 5-FU slowly after it is injected. However, this new agent has neurotoxicity that may limit its utility. Fluorouracil is used systemically in the treatment of a variety of adenocarcinomas. Its major toxicities are myelosuppression and mucositis.

2. CYTARABINE

Cytarabine (cytosine arabinoside, ara-C, Cytosar) is an S phase-specific antimetabolite that is converted by deoxycytidine kinase to the 5′-mononucleotide (AraCMP). AraCMP is further anabolized to the triphosphate (AraCTP), which competitively inhibits DNA polymerase. This results in blockage of DNA synthesis while RNA and protein formation continues and leads to unbalanced growth.

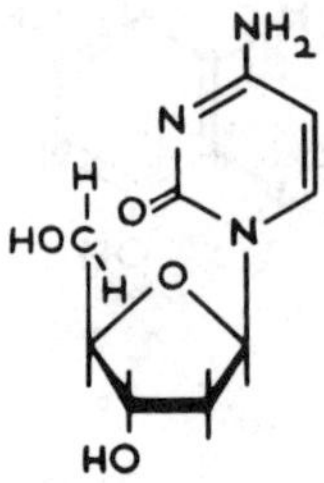
Cytosine deoxyriboside

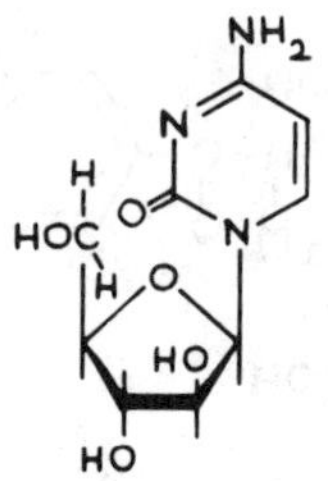
Cytosine arabinoside

Cytarabine is also incorporated into RNA and DNA. The cellular retention time for AraCTP appears to correlate with its lethality to malignant cells.

After intravenous administration, the drug is cleared rapidly, with most of it being deaminated to an inactive form. The ratio of the anabolic enzyme deoxycytidine kinase to the inactivating catalyst cytidine deaminase is important to the cytotoxicity of cytarabine.

In view of cytarabine's S phase specificity, the drug is highly schedule-dependent and must be given either by continuous infusion or every 8–12 hours for 5–7 days. Its activity is limited almost entirely to treatment of acute myelogenous leukemia, for which it is a major drug. Side-effects include nausea, severe myelosuppression, and varying degrees of stomatitis or alopecia.

3. AZACYTIDINE

Azacytidine (5-azacytidine) produces multiple effects associated with its cytotoxicity. It is phosphorylated to the mononucleotide form by uridine-cytidine kinase. Azacytidine 5′-phosphate then inhibits orotidylate decarboxylase, which reduces production of pyrimidine nucleotides. Further metabolism results in incorporation of azacytidine into DNA and RNA as well as inhibition of DNA, RNA, and protein synthesis.

Azacytidine is administered intravenously and must be shielded from light and kept at slightly acid pH, as it is unstable and can undergo ring opening. Nausea and fever are observed during drug administration. The half-life is 3–6 hours, with most of the drug excreted either unchanged or in deaminated form.

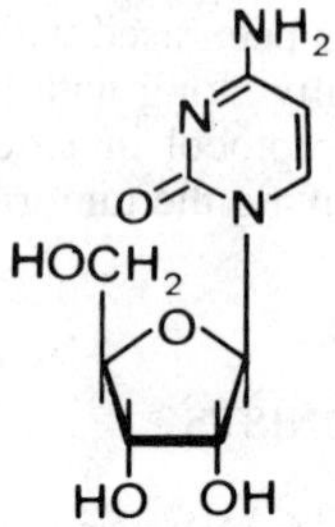
Cytidine

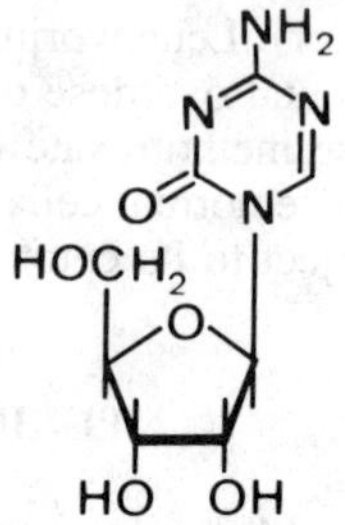
5-Azacytidine

Azacytidine is currently an investigational agent in the USA, but it is a recognized "second-line agent" in the treatment of acute leukemia. Optimal dosage schedules have yet to be developed. The drug can produce profound myelosuppressive toxicity of long duration.

PLANT ALKALOIDS

VINBLASTINE

Vinblastine (Velban) is an alkaloid derived from *Vinca rosea,* the periwinkle plant (see below). Its mechanism of action involves depolymerization of microtubules, which are an important part of the cyto-

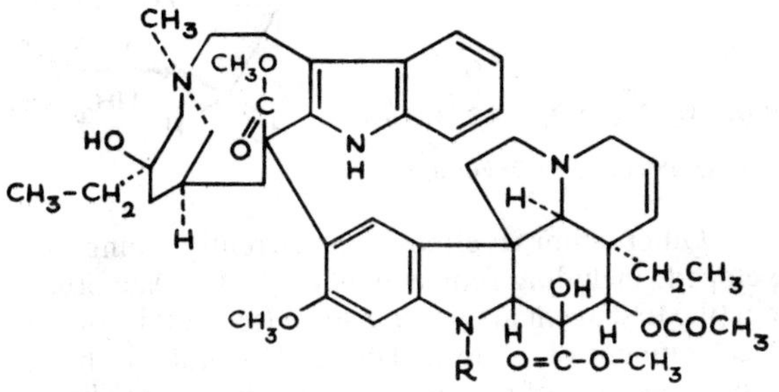

R is: O=C–H
Vincristine

R is: CH_3
Vinblastine

skeleton and the mitotic spindle. It binds specifically to the microtubular protein tubulin in dimeric form; the drug-tubulin complex adds to the forming end of the microtubules to terminate assembly, and depolymerization of the microtubules then occurs. This results in mitotic arrest at metaphase, dissolution of the mitotic spindle, and interference with chromosome segregation. It produces nausea and vomiting and marrow depression as well as alopecia. It has value in the treatment of systemic Hodgkin's disease and other lymphomas. See clinical section below and Table 56–4. A related agent, desacetylvinblastine (Vindesine), is currently in clinical trial as an investigational drug.

VINCRISTINE

Vincristine (Oncovin), also an alkaloid derivative of *Vinca rosea,* is closely related in structure to vinblastine. Its mechanism of action is considered to be identical to that of vinblastine, and it also appears to be a "spindle poison" and to cause arrest of the mitotic cycle. Despite these marked similarities to vinblastine, vincristine has a strikingly different spectrum of clinical activity and qualitatively different toxicities.

Vincristine has been used with considerable success in combination with prednisone for remission induction in acute leukemia in children. It is also useful in certain other rapidly proliferating neoplasms. It causes a significant incidence of neurotoxicity, which limits its use to short courses. The principal serious toxic effects are areflexia, peripheral neuritis, and paralytic ileus. It occasionally produces bone marrow depression.

Table 56–4. Natural product cancer chemotherapy drugs: Dosages and toxicity.

Drug	Single Agent Dose	Acute Toxicity	Delayed Toxicity
Vinblastine (Velban)	0.1–0.2 mg/kg IV weekly	Nausea and vomiting	Alopecia, loss of reflexes, bone marrow depression.
Vincristine (Oncovin)	1.5 mg/m^2 IV (maximum: 2 mg weekly)	None	Areflexia, muscle weakness, peripheral neuritis, paralytic ileus, mild bone marrow depression, alopecia.
Dactinomycin (actinomycin D, Cosmegen)	0.04 mg/kg IV weekly	Nausea and vomiting	Stomatitis, gastrointestinal tract upset, alopecia, bone marrow depression.
Daunorubicin (daunomycin)	30–60 mg/m^2 daily IV for 3 days, or 30–60 mg/m^2 IV weekly	Nausea, fever, red urine (not hematuria)	Cardiotoxicity, bone marrow depression, alopecia.
Doxorubicin (Adriamycin)	60 mg/m^2 IV every 3 weeks to a maximum total dose of 550 mg/m^2	Nausea, red urine (not hematuria)	Cardiotoxicity, alopecia, bone marrow depression, stomatitis.
Mithramycin (Mithracin)	25–50 μg/kg IV every other day for up to 8 doses	Nausea and vomiting	Thrombocytopenia, hepatotoxicity.
Mitomycin (Mutamycin)	20 mg/m^2 every 6 weeks	Nausea	Thrombocytopenia, leukopenia.
Bleomycin (Blenoxane)	Up to 15 mg/m^2 twice weekly to a total dose of 200 mg/m^2	Allergic reactions, fever, hypotension	Edema of hands, pulmonary fibrosis, stomatitis, alopecia.
Asparaginase	20,000 IU/m^2 daily IV for 5–10 days	Nausea and fever	Hepatotoxicity, mental depression, pancreatitis.

PODOPHYLLOTOXINS

Two compounds, VP16 and a related drug, VM26, are promising semisynthetic derivatives of podophyllotoxin, which is extracted from the root of the May apple or mandrake *(Podophyllum peltatum)*. Both drugs are currently on clinical trial in the USA and Europe. VP16 and VM26 are quite similar, both chemically, in their block of cells in the late S–G_2 phase of the cell cycle, and clinically. The mode of action is felt to involve degradation of DNA, inhibition of nucleoside transport, and inhibition of mitochondrial electron transport. The drugs are water-insoluble and require a lipid-solubilizing vehicle for clinical formulation. They are protein-bound and evenly distributed throughout the body, except for the brain. Excretion is predominantly in the urine, with a lesser amount excreted in bile. In addition to nausea, vomiting, and alopecia, significant toxicity occurs to the hematopoietic and lymphoid systems. Thus far, VP16 has shown activity in monocytic leukemia and oat cell carcinomas of the lung, and VM26 has activity in various lymphomas. The activity of VP16 in oat cell carcinoma is significant and clinically useful.

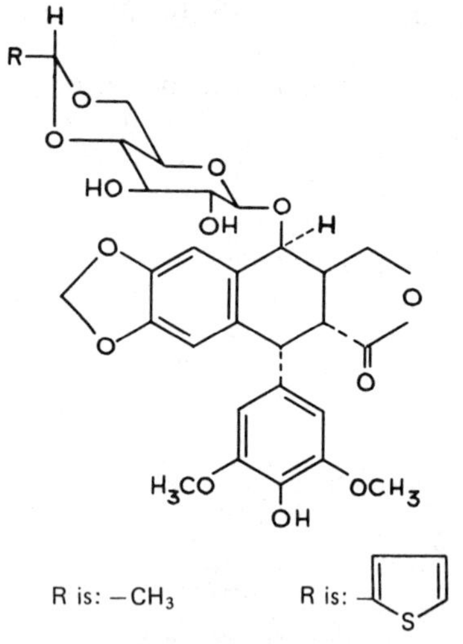

VP16-213, Etoposide (4′-demethyl-epipodophyllotoxin-β-D-ethylidene glucoside) VM26

ANTIBIOTICS

Screening of microbial products has led to the discovery of a number of growth inhibitors that have proved to be clinically useful in cancer chemotherapy. Many of these antibiotics bind to DNA through intercalation between specific bases and block the synthesis of new RNA or DNA (or both), cause DNA strand scission, and interfere with cell replication. All of the clinically useful antibiotics are products of various strains of the soil fungus *Streptomyces*. These include the anthracyclines, actinomycin, bleomycin, mitomycin, and mithramycin.

ANTHRACYCLINES

The anthracycline antibiotics, isolated from *Streptomyces peucetius* var *caesius*, are among the most useful cytotoxic anticancer drugs. Two congeners—doxorubicin (Adriamycin) and daunorubicin (Cerubidine)—are FDA-approved and in general use. Their structures are shown below.

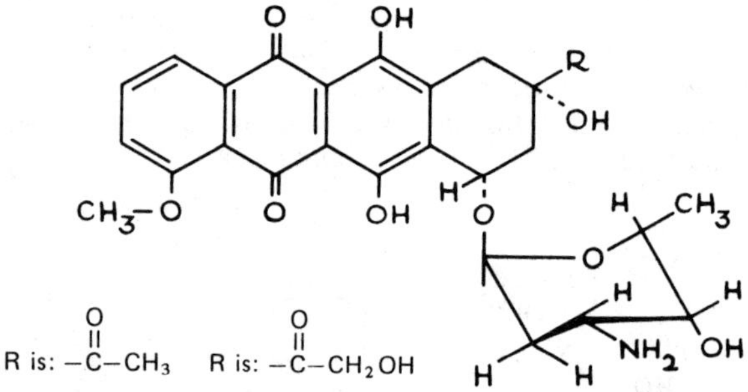

Daunorubicin Doxorubicin

Other anthracyclines are currently being developed, including semisynthetic agents. Daunorubicin (the first agent in this class to be isolated) is used in the treatment of acute leukemia. Doxorubicin has a broad spectrum of potent activity against many different types of cancers.

Mechanism of Action

Three major actions have been documented for the organ and tumor toxicities of the anthracyclines. These include (1) high-affinity binding to DNA through intercalation with consequent blockade of the synthesis of DNA and RNA, and DNA strand scission; (2) binding to membranes, to alter fluidity and ion transport; and (3) generation of the semiquinone free radical and oxygen radicals through a cytochrome P-450-mediated reductive process. This latter action may be responsible for cardiac toxicity through oxygen radical-mediated damage to membranes, since the free radical scavenger α-tocopherol (vitamin E) lessens cardiac damage of doxorubicin in experimental systems without decreasing anticancer activity.

Absorption, Metabolism, & Excretion

Clinically used anthracyclines are administered only by the intravenous route. Peak blood concentration halves within the first 30 minutes after injection, but significant levels persist for up to 20 hours. The anthracyclines are metabolized by the liver, with reduction and hydrolysis of the ring substituents. An alcohol form is an active metabolite, whereas the aglycone is inactive. Most of the drug and its metabolites are excreted in bile, and about one-sixth is excreted in urine. Some metabolites retain antitumor activity. The biliary route of excretion includes enterohepatic recirculation of cytotoxic moieties. Therefore, the initial dose of anthracyclines must be reduced by 75% in patients with significant elevations of serum bilirubin (greater than 2.5 mg/dL).

Clinical Uses

Doxorubicin is one of the most important anticancer drugs, with major clinical application in carcinomas of the breast, endometrium, ovary, testicle, thyroid, and lung and in treatment of many sarcomas, including neuroblastoma, Ewing's sarcoma, osteosarcoma, and rhabdomyosarcoma. It is useful also in hematologic cancers, including acute leukemia, multiple myeloma, Hodgkin's disease, and the diffuse non-Hodgkin lymphomas. It is used in adjuvant therapy in osteogenic sarcoma and breast cancer. It is generally used in combination with other agents (eg, cyclophosphamide, cisplatin, and nitrosoureas), with which it often synergizes, yielding longer remissions than are observed when used as a single agent. This approach can also minimize some of the toxicities that would otherwise be associated with use of higher dosages of doxorubicin. The major use of daunorubicin is in acute leukemia, and for this purpose the drug may have slightly greater activity than doxorubicin. However, daunorubicin appears to have a far narrower spectrum of utility, as its efficacy in solid tumors appears to be limited.

A series of new anthracycline analogs has recently entered clinical trial as investigational agents. These include aclacynomycin A (Japan), 4-epiadriamycin (Italy), carminomycin (USSR), and N-trifluoroacetyl adriamycin-14-valerate (AD-32) (USA). These new agents may have differing spectrums of action and somewhat less toxicity. For example, initial reports indicate that aclacynomycin A causes far less alopecia and cardiac toxicity than other anthracyclines. Antitumor activity is only now being defined for these new agents.

Adverse Reactions

In common with many other cytotoxic drugs, the anthracyclines cause bone marrow depression, which is of short duration with rapid recovery. Toxicities more pronounced with anthracyclines (doxorubicin and daunorubicin) than with other agents include a potentially irreversible, cumulative dose-related cardiac toxicity. This is rarely seen at doxorubicin dosages below 500 mg/m^2. Tachycardia is a common clinical sign; however, abnormalities in cardiac scintiscans appear to correlate closely with myocardial fibrosis on endomyocardial biopsies. Other noninvasive tests (echocardiography) appear to be less sensitive. Such studies should probably be obtained on all patients for whom administration of more than 400 mg/m^2 is contemplated. Patients with prior thoracic irradiation (including the heart), significant hypertension, or other intrinsic cardiovascular disease or increased age (over 70) are thought to be at greater risk of anthracycline-induced cardiac toxicity at lower total dosages.

A second toxicity of doxorubicin and daunorubicin is the almost universal occurrence of severe or total alopecia at standard dosages. A technique recently devised to minimize doxorubicin-induced alopecia is local scalp hypothermia with cold packs (ice or other coolants) 10 minutes prior to intravenous drug administration, with maintenance for at least an additional 30 minutes. This procedure is not recommended for patients with circulating tumor stem cells (eg, acute leukemia) but appears to be quite satisfactory for a variety of other neoplasms. Hypothermia limits circulation of the drug to the scalp as well as energy-dependent uptake of the drug by the hair follicles.

DACTINOMYCIN

Dactinomycin (actinomycin D, Cosmegen) is an antitumor antibiotic isolated from a *Streptomyces*. The drug is composed of 2 identical cyclic polypeptides linked to an aromatic planar phenoxazone ring system. A number of analogs have been devised naturally and semisynthetically, but most have not been tested carefully for antitumor activity.

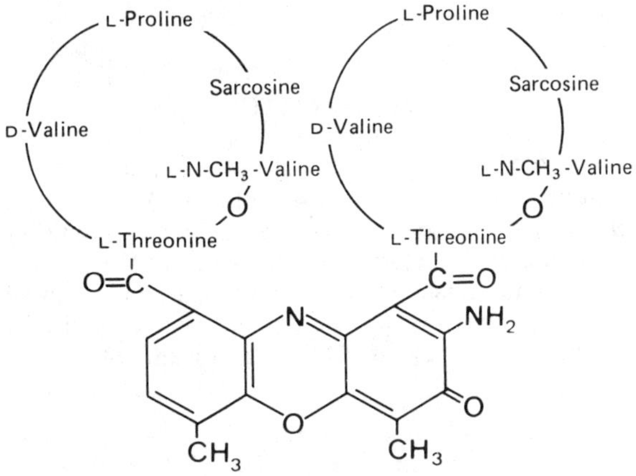

Dactinomycin

Mechanism of Action

Dactinomycin binds tightly to double-stranded DNA through intercalation between adjacent guanine-cytosine base pairs. Dactinomycin inhibits the synthesis of all forms of DNA-dependent RNA synthesis, with ribosomal RNA formation being most sensitive to drug action. The degree of responsiveness to dactinomycin appears to be dependent on the cellular capacity for accumulation and retention of the antibiotic.

Absorption, Metabolism, & Excretion

Approximately half of the intravenous dose of dactinomycin remains unmetabolized and is excreted in the bile; a small amount is lost by urinary excretion. The plasma half-life is short. Because the drug is irritating to tissues, it is usually administered with caution to avoid extravasation and with "flushing" with normal saline to wash out the vein.

Clinical Uses

Dactinomycin is used in combination with surgery and vincristine (with or without radiotherapy) in the adjuvant treatment of Wilms' tumor. It is also used along with methotrexate to provide potentially curative treatment for patients with localized or disseminated gestational choriocarcinoma.

Adverse Reactions

Bone marrow depression, the major dose-limiting toxicity of this agent, is usually evident within 7–10 days. All blood elements are affected, but platelets and leukocytes are affected most profoundly, and severe thrombocytopenia sometimes occurs. Nausea and vomiting, diarrhea, oral ulcers, and skin eruptions may also be noted. The agent is also immunosuppressive, and patients receiving this drug should not receive live virus vaccines during that time. Alopecia and various skin abnormalities occur occasionally. As with anthracyclines, dactinomycin can interact with radiation, producing a "radiation recall" skin abnormality associated with inflammation at sites of prior radiation therapy.

MITHRAMYCIN

Mithramycin (Mithracin) is one of the chromomycin antibiotics isolated from *Streptomyces plicatus*. It has a high molecular weight and a complex structure that includes a polycyclic chromophoric group with 2 attached sugar chains. The mechanism of action of mithramycin is thought to involve binding of the drug to DNA, possibly through an antibiotic-Mg^{2+} complex; this interaction interrupts DNA-directed RNA synthesis. Additionally, the drug causes a calcium-lowering effect, apparently through an action on osteoclasts that is independent of its action on tumor cells. The drug has some usefulness in testicular cancers refractory to standard treatment, but it is of greater utility in reversing severe hypercalcemia associated with malignant disease.

Toxic side-effects of mithramycin include nausea and vomiting, thrombocytopenia, leukopenia, hypocalcemia, bleeding disorders, and liver toxicity. Aside from its use in management of hypercalcemia, mithramycin currently has few other indications.

Other chromomycin antibiotics (eg, toyomycin) have also been studied in Japan but appear to be of limited utility.

MITOMYCIN

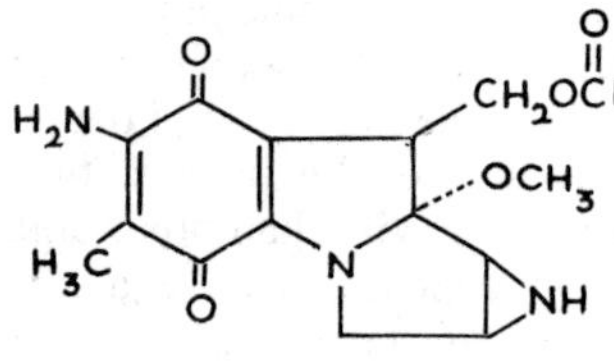

Mitomycin

Mitomycin (mitomycin C, Mitocin-C, Mutamycin) is an antibiotic isolated from *Streptomyces caespitosus*. It contains quinone, carbamate, and aziridine groups, all of which may have activity. The drug is a "bioreductive" alkylating agent which undergoes metabolic activation through a cytochrome P-450–reductase mediated reduction to generate an alkylating agent that cross-links DNA. Hypoxic tumor stem

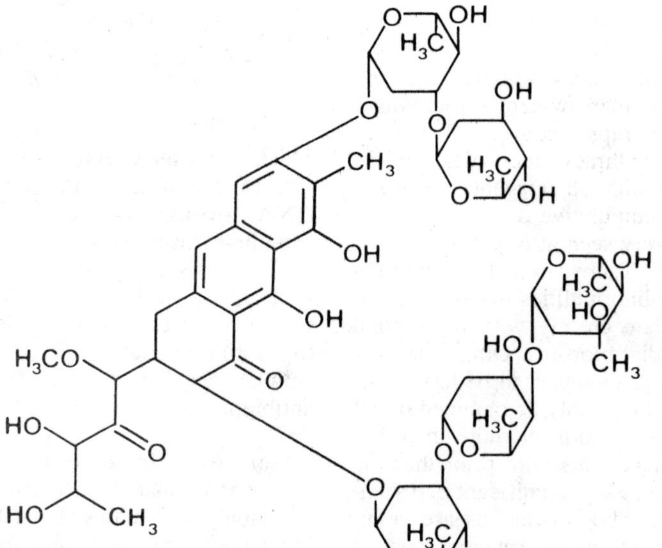

Mithramycin

cells of solid tumors exist in an environment conducive to reductive reactions and are more sensitive to the cytotoxic actions of mitomycin than oxygenated normal and tumor cells. Mitomycin is thought to be a CCNS alkylating agent. While this agent is one of the more toxic drugs available for clinical use, it is the best available drug for use against hypoxic tumor cells and appears to have increasing usefulness in combination chemotherapy (with bleomycin and vincristine) for squamous cell carcinoma of the cervix and for adenocarcinomas of the stomach, pancreas, and lung (along with doxorubicin and fluorouracil). The drug also has some usefulness as a second-line agent for metastatic colon cancer. A special application of the use of mitomycin has been in topical intravesical treatment of small bladder papillomas. Topical instillations of the agent in distilled water are usually held in the bladder for 3 hours, and the procedure is repeated over a course of weeks. Very little of the agent is absorbed systemically, and it can be quite effective at reducing the frequency of such bladder tumors.

Mitomycin is administered intravenously, is cleared rapidly from the vascular compartment, and appears to be eliminated primarily by liver metabolism. Mitomycin causes severe myelosuppression with relatively late toxicity against all 3 formed elements from the bone marrow, with increasingly profound toxicity after repeated doses. This late form of toxicity suggests an action on hematopoietic stem cells as opposed to later progenitors. Nausea, vomiting, and anorexia commonly occur shortly after injection, and occasional instances of renal toxicity and interstitial pneumonitis have also been reported.

BLEOMYCIN

The bleomycins are a series of antineoplastic antibiotics produced by *Streptomyces verticillus*. The clinically used material is a mixture of 11 different glycopeptides with the major components being bleomycin A_2 and bleomycin B_2. Bleomycin appears to act through binding to DNA, which results in single- and double-strand breaks following free radical formation, and inhibition of DNA biosynthesis. The fragmentation of DNA seems to be due to oxidation of a DNA-bleomycin-Fe(II) complex and leads to chromosomal aberrations. Bleomycin is a CSS drug that causes accumulation of cells in G_2. It appears to be schedule-dependent, and chronic low-dose administration by repeated injection or continuous infusion seems to be the most effective schedule. The drug synergizes with other drugs such as vinblastine and cisplatin, thus comprising one-third of the curative regimen used for testicular cancers. It is also used in squamous cell carcinomas of the head and neck, cervix, skin, penis, and rectum, and has utility in combination chemotherapy for the lymphomas. A special use has been for intracavitary therapy of malignant effusions in ovarian and breast cancer. Its efficacy in this latter setting may be associated with intrinsic sensitivity of the tumor stem cells in these effusions, as opposed to a nonspecific vesicant effect. The drug can be given subcutaneously, intramuscularly, or intravenously as well as by the intracavitary route. Peak blood levels of bleomycin after intramuscular injection appear within 30–60 minutes. Intravenous injection of similar dosages yields higher peak concentrations and a terminal half-life of about 2½ hours. Although there is some metabolic inactivation of this agent through an aminopeptidase B-like activity in tumor and normal tissues, approximately 50% can be recovered as the active drug in the urine within 24 hours.

A number of toxic side-effects have been described, including lethal anaphylactoid reactions and a high incidence of fever, with or without chills, particularly in patients with lymphoma. Fever may result in dehydration and hypotension in susceptible patients, and small test doses of the drug are commonly used to anticipate this potentially serious toxicity. More common toxic side-effects include blistering and hyperkeratosis of the palms and anorexia. A form of

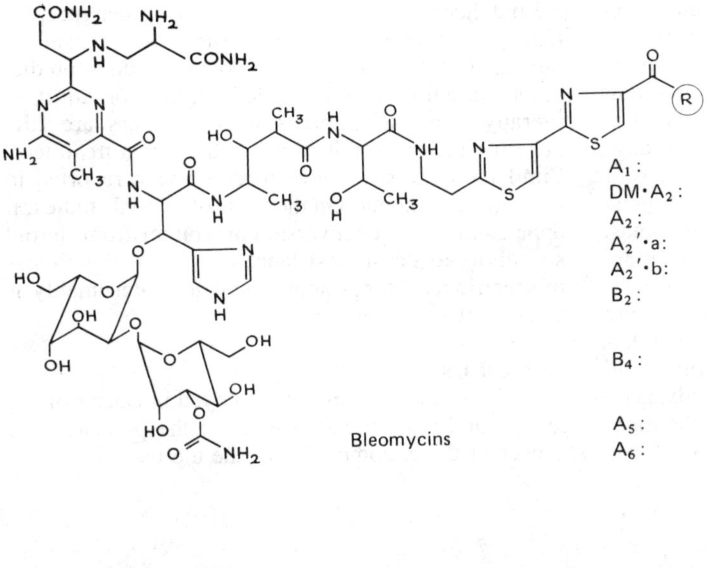

Bleomycins

Bleomycin components (R is):

A_1:	$-NH-CH_2-CH_2-CH_2-SO-CH_3$
$DM \cdot A_2$:	$-NH-CH_2-CH_2-CH_2-S-CH_3$
A_2:	$-NH-CH_2-CH_2-CH_2-S^+(CH_3)_2$
$A_2' \cdot a$:	$-NH-CH_2-CH_2-CH_2-CH_2-NH_2$
$A_2' \cdot b$:	$-NH-CH_2-CH_2-CH_2-NH_2$
B_2:	$-NH-CH_2-CH_2-CH_2-CH_2-NH-C(=NH)-NH_2$
B_4:	$-NH-(CH_2)_4-NH-C(=NH)-NH-(CH_2)_4-NH-C(=NH)-NH_2$
A_5:	$-NH-(CH_2)_3-NH-(CH_2)_4-NH_2$
A_6:	$-NH-(CH_2)_3-NH-(CH_2)_4-NH-(CH_2)_3-NH_2$

pulmonary fibrosis is an uncommon but sometimes fatal adverse effect seen particularly in older patients who have received a total dose over 200 mg/m^2 and develop a reduced diffusion capacity for oxygen. Patients receiving large doses should undergo serial pulmonary function studies, so that the drug can be discontinued before severe pulmonary toxicity develops. Cough and pulmonary infiltrates are additional indications for discontinuing bleomycin and initiating therapy with antibiotics and corticosteroids. The drug does not have significant myelosuppressive effects, which means that it may be incorporated into a number of different combination chemotherapy programs with no significant addition to bone marrow toxicity.

MISCELLANEOUS AGENTS

ASPARAGINASE

Asparaginase (L-asparagine amidohydrolase) is an enzyme that is isolated for clinical use from various bacteria (eg, *E coli, Erwinia carotovora*). The active enzyme has a molecular weight of 133,000 and a tetrameric structure containing 4 identical subunits. The drug is used in childhood acute leukemia. Asparaginase acts indirectly by catabolic depletion of serum asparagine to aspartic acid and ammonia. Blood glutamine levels are also reduced. This results in inhibition of protein synthesis in neoplastic cells, requiring an external source of asparagine because of low or deficient levels of asparagine synthetase, and cell proliferation is blocked. Most normal cells are capable of synthesizing asparagine and thus are less susceptible to its action.

STEROID HORMONES

Sex hormones and adrenocortical hormones are employed in the management of several types of neoplastic disease. The sex hormones are concerned with the stimulation and control of proliferation and function of certain tissues, including the mammary and prostate glands. Cancer arising from and retaining properties of these tissues may be inhibited or stimulated by appropriate changes in hormone balance. Cancer of the breast and cancer of the prostate have been effectually palliated with sex hormone therapy or ablation of certain endocrine organs. Recently, antiestrogens have assumed an important role in breast cancer. While such agents are nonsteroidal, they are best discussed in the context of steroid hormones.

The adrenal corticosteroids (particularly the glucocorticoid analogs) have been useful in the treatment of acute leukemia, lymphomas, myeloma, and other hematologic cancers as well as in advanced breast cancer, and as supportive therapy in the management of hypercalcemia resulting from many types of cancer. These steroids produce dissolution of lymphocytes, regression of lymph nodes, and inhibition of growth of certain mesenchymal tissues.

The most useful steroid hormones are as follows:

(1) Androgens: Testosterone propionate, fluoxymesterone.

(2) Estrogens: Diethylstilbestrol, ethinyl estradiol.

(3) Antiestrogens: Tamoxifen, nafoxidine, clomiphene.

(4) Progestins: Hydroxyprogesterone caproate, medroxyprogesterone, megestrol acetate.

(5) Adrenocortical compounds: Hydrocortisone acetate, prednisone, prednisolone, dexamethasone.

Absorption, Metabolism, & Excretion

With the exception of testosterone propionate and hydroxyprogesterone caproate, the steroids are administered orally and are readily absorbed. Testosterone and hydroxyprogesterone are oil-soluble and must be administered intramuscularly. The mechanisms of their metabolism and excretion are described in Chapter 38.

Pharmacologic Effects

The mechanism of action of steroid hormones on lymphoid, mammary, or prostatic cancer has been clarified. Recent observations indicate that steroid hormones bind to receptor proteins in cancer cells and that high levels of receptor proteins are predictive for responsiveness to endocrine therapy. Highly specific receptor proteins have been identified for estrogens, progesterone, corticosteroids, and androgens in neoplastic cells. Data indicate that steroid hormones form a mobile steroid-receptor complex which ultimately binds directly to nuclear nonhistone protein of DNA to activate transcription of associated clusters of genes.

Prednisone-sensitive lymphomas and estrogen-sensitive breast and prostatic cancers contain, respectively, specific receptors for prednisone, estrogens, and androgens. Most steroid-sensitive cancers have specific receptors. It is now possible to assay biopsy specimens for steroid receptor content and to predict which individual patients are likely to benefit from steroid therapy. Measurement of the estrogen receptor (ER) protein in breast cancer tissue is now a standard clinical test (Fig 56–9). ER positivity does predict responsiveness to endocrine ablation or additive therapy, whereas patients whose tumors are ER-negative generally fail to respond to such treatment. Similar observations have recently been reported in prostatic carcinoma. On the basis of animal studies, it appears likely that conversion of a tumor from steroid sensitivity to steroid resistance is associated with loss of specific receptor protein production, presumably as a result of selection.

Clinical Uses

The sex hormones are employed in cancer of the female and male breast, cancer of the prostate, and cancer of the endometrium of the uterus.

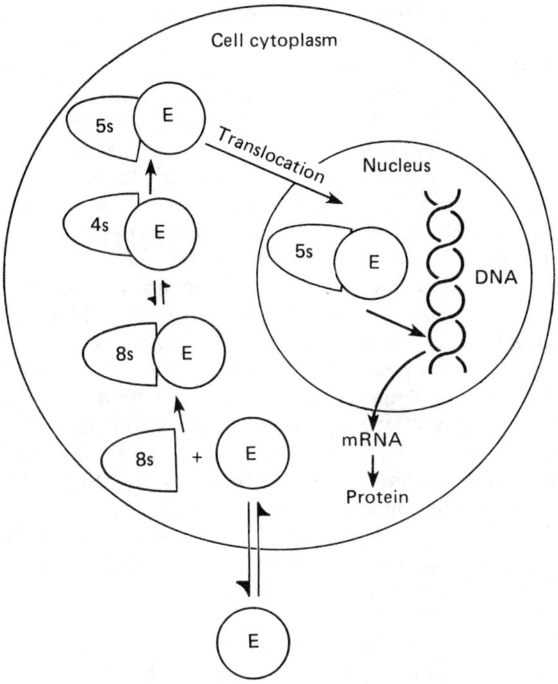

Figure 56–9. Prototype cancer cell that is estrogen receptor-"positive." Estrogen (E) binds to an 8s receptor, which then undergoes metabolic transformations, with reduction in molecular weight, after which it is translocated to the cell nucleus. The complex is then bound to chromatin, and RNA synthesis and protein synthesis are initiated. A similar process appears to apply for progesterone or androgen receptors. Cells bearing such steroid hormone receptors often respond to endocrine therapy.

The relationship between hormones and hormone-dependent tumors was initially demonstrated by Beatson in 1896 when it was shown that oophorectomy produced improvement in women with advanced breast cancer. Extensive studies with the androgenic, estrogenic, and progestational sex hormones have demonstrated their value in advanced inoperable mammary cancer, cancer of the prostate, and cancer of the endometrium (see pp 649 and 656–659).

Adverse Reactions

Androgens, estrogens, and adrenocortical hormones all can produce fluid retention through their sodium-retaining effect. Prolonged use of androgens and estrogens will cause masculinization and feminization, respectively. Extended use of the adrenocortical steroids may result in hypertension, diabetes, increased susceptibility to infection, and the development of cushingoid appearance ("moon facies") (see Chapter 37 and Table 56–5).

ANTIESTROGEN

The antiestrogenic compound tamoxifen has proved to be extremely useful for the treatment of breast cancer. As an antiestrogen, it inhibits estrogen-stimulated increases in uterine weight and vaginal cornification. Tamoxifen functions as a competitive inhibitor of estrogen and binds to the cytoplasmic estrogen receptor (ER) protein of estrogen-sensitive tissues and tumors. Translocation of the receptor complex to the nucleus appears to occur normally, suggesting that the antiestrogen acts at the nuclear level. Studies in

Table 56–5. Steroid hormones and antagonists: Dosages and toxicity.

	Usual Adult Dose	Acute Toxicity	Delayed Toxicity
Androgens			
Testosterone propionate	100 mg IM 3 times weekly	None	Fluid retention, masculinization.
Fluoxymesterone (Halotestin)	10–20 mg/d orally	None	Cholestatic jaundice in some patients receiving fluoxymesterone.
Calusterone	200 mg/d orally in divided doses	None	None.
Estrogens			
Diethylstilbestrol	1–5 mg 3 times a day orally	Occasional nausea and vomiting	Fluid retention, feminization, uterine bleeding.
Ethinyl estradiol (Estinyl)	3 mg/d orally		
Antiestrogen			
Tamoxifen (Nolvadex)	10 mg twice daily orally	None	None.
Progestins			
Hydroxyprogesterone caproate (Delalutin)	1 g IM twice weekly	None	None.
Medroxyprogesterone (Provera)	100–200 mg/d orally; 200–600 mg orally twice weekly	None	None.
Megestrol acetate (Megace)	40 mg 4 times daily orally	None	Fluid retention.
Adrenocorticosteroids			
Hydrocortisone	50–200 mg/d orally	None	Fluid retention, hypertension, diabetes, increased susceptibility to infection, "moon facies."
Prednisone	20–100 mg/d orally or, when effective, 50–100 mg every other day orally as single dose	None	

tissue culture have shown that in the absence of estrogen, tamoxifen is cytotoxic to ER-positive breast cancer cells. This provides evidence that the antiestrogen has a potent direct effect. However, tamoxifen has a 100- to 1000-fold lower affinity constant for ER than does estradiol, indicating the importance of ablation of endogenous estrogen for optimal antiestrogen effect.

Excellent plasma levels of the drug are obtained after oral administration, and the agent has a much longer biologic half-life than estradiol. The usual dosages in breast cancer treatment are in the range of 10 mg twice daily, although doses up to 100 mg/m^2 have been administered without major toxicity. Because it may take several weeks to achieve a steady-state level of the active metabolite (monohydroxytamoxifen) with the dosage of 10 mg twice daily, it is advisable to give an 80-mg "loading course" on the first day to achieve good blood levels rapidly.

Side-effects in the usual dose range are quite mild. Hot flashes are the most frequent side-effect. Nausea is observed occasionally, as is fluid retention and mild hematologic toxicity. Occasional "flares" of breast cancer are observed, but it is uncertain if this is a side-effect or a manifestation of preexisting rapid tumor growth.

Tamoxifen has recently proved to have significant antitumor activity in estrogen-resistant prostatic cancer and progesterone-resistant endometrial cancer. A lesser degree of activity has also been observed in metastatic melanoma, and a variety of tumor types are now being studied for their content of estrogen receptor to determine whether they might also be amenable to growth inhibition with tamoxifen.

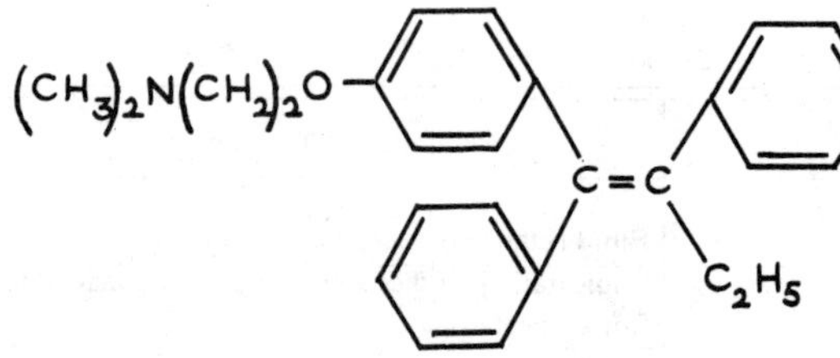

Tamoxifen

In advanced breast cancer, clinical improvement is observed in 40–50% of patients who receive tamoxifen. Patients who show objective benefit with treatment are largely those who (1) lack endogenous estrogens (oophorectomy or postmenopausal state) and (2) have breast cancers in which the cytoplasmic ER protein is demonstrable on radioreceptor assay. Thus, it is not rational therapy to use tamoxifen in patients who are known to be ER-negative or have endogenous estrogen production. Oophorectomy is often indicated in premenopausal women with ER-positive tumors, as this procedure enhances the utility of tamoxifen.

OTHER ANTICANCER DRUGS

Hydroxyurea

Hydroxyurea is an analog of urea whose mechanism of action is through inhibition of DNA synthesis, exerting its lethal effect on cells in S phase. This action is through inhibition of the enzyme ribonucleotide reductase, with resulting depletion of deoxynucleoside triphosphate pools. The drug is administered orally and is available in capsules (0.5 g). Its major uses are in melanoma and chronic myelogenous leukemia; however, it plays a secondary role in both of these circumstances. Its role in combination chemotherapy has yet to be defined. The major side-effect of this agent is bone marrow depression. At high dosages (greater than 40 mg/kg/d), megaloblastosis unresponsive to vitamin B_{12} or folic acid may appear. Gastrointestinal symptoms, including nausea, vomiting, and diarrhea, are common in patients receiving high dosages of the drug. Less common reactions include skin reactions and mucositis and occasional renal dysfunction or central nervous system abnormality.

Mitotane (*o,p'*-DDD, Lysodren)

This drug (1,1-dichloro-2-[*o*-chlorophenyl]-2-[*p*-chlorophenyl]ethane) is a DDT congener that was first found to be adrenolytic in dogs. Subsequently, it was found to be of use in the treatment of adrenal carcinoma. The drug produces tumor regression and relief of the excessive adrenal steroid secretion that often occurs with this malignancy. Toxicities include skin eruptions, diarrhea, and mental depression.

About 40% of an oral dose is absorbed, and 60% is excreted in stool. Of the amount reaching the tissues, most is stored in fat for several weeks. About 25% of an absorbed dose is excreted as a urinary metabolite. It produces anorexia, nausea, somnolence, and dermatitis.

The utility of mitotane appears to be limited to adrenal carcinoma, and it is marketed for that one indication.

Quinacrine

This antimalarial drug has been found to be of occasional use in the control of malignant pleural, pericardial, and abdominal effusions. It is instilled

Table 56–6. Miscellaneous anticancer drugs: Dosages and toxicity.

Drug	Usual Dose	Acute Toxicity	Delayed Toxicity
Hydroxyurea	300 mg/m^2 orally for 5 days	Nausea and vomiting	Bone marrow depression.
Mitotane	6–15 g/d orally	Nausea and vomiting	Dermatitis, diarrhea, mental depression.
Quinacrine	100–300 mg/d by intracavitary injection for 5 days	Local pain and fever	None.

Table 56–7. Malignancies responsive to chemotherapy.*

Diagnosis	Current Treatment of Choice	Other Valuable Agents
Acute lymphocytic leukemia	Induction: vincristine plus prednisone. Remission maintenance: mercaptopurine, methotrexate, and cyclophosphamide in various combinations.	Asparaginase, daunorubicin, carmustine, doxorubicin, cytarabine, allopurinol,† craniospinal radiation therapy
Acute myelocytic and myelomonocytic leukemia	Combination chemotherapy: doxorubicin, vincristine, cytarabine, prednisone or thioguanine, cytarabine, and daunorubicin	Methotrexate, thioguanine, mercaptopurine, allopurinol,† BCG,‡ azacytidine,‡ AMSA‡
Chronic myelogenous leukemia	Busulfan	Vincristine, mercaptopurine, hydroxyurea, vindesine,‡ melphalan, cytarabine, allopurinol†
Chronic lymphocytic leukemia	Chlorambucil and prednisone (if indicated)	Vincristine, androgens,† allopurinol,† doxorubicin
Hodgkin's disease (stages III and IV)	Combination chemotherapy: mechlorethamine, vincristine, procarbazine, prednisone ("MOPP")	Vinblastine, doxorubicin, lomustine, dacarbazine, VM26,‡ bleomycin
Non-Hodgkin lymphomas	Combination chemotherapy: cyclophosphamide, doxorubicin, vincristine, prednisone	Bleomycin, lomustine, carmustine, VM26,‡ BCG,‡ AMSA,‡ interferon‡
Multiple myeloma	Melphalan plus prednisone or multiagent combination chemotherapy	Cyclophosphamide, vincristine, carmustine, bisantrene,‡ interferon,‡ vindesine,‡ doxorubicin, androgens,† aminoglutethimide,‡ levamisole‡
Macroglobulinemia	Chlorambucil	Melphalan
Polycythemia vera	Busulfan, chlorambucil, or cyclophosphamide	
Carcinoma of lung	Cyclophosphamide plus doxorubicin, methotrexate, and lomustine	Cisplatin, quinacrine,† hexamethylmelamine,‡ vindesine,‡ vincristine, BCG,‡ VP16‡
Carcinomas of the head and neck	Methotrexate, bleomycin, and cisplatin	Hydroxyurea, fluorouracil, doxorubicin, vinblastine
Carcinoma of endometrium	Doxorubicin plus cyclophosphamide	Progestins, fluorouracil
Carcinoma of ovary	Doxorubicin, cyclophosphamide, and cisplatin	Melphalan, fluorouracil, vincristine, hexamethylmelamine,‡ bleomycin, BCG‡
Carcinoma of the cervix	Mitomycin plus bleomycin, vincristine, and cisplatin	Lomustine, cyclophosphamide, doxorubicin, methotrexate
Breast carcinoma	(1) Combination chemotherapy alone or plus tamoxifen (see text) if lymph nodes are positive at mastectomy. (2) Combination chemotherapy ("D/C" or "CMF"); hormonal manipulation for late recurrence (eg, tamoxifen).	Cyclophosphamide, doxorubicin, vincristine, methotrexate, fluorouracil, mitoxantrone,‡ bisantrene,‡ quinacrine,† prednisone,† megestrol, androgens
Choriocarcinoma (trophoblastic neoplasms)	Methotrexate, alone or in combination with vincristine, dactinomycin, and cyclophosphamide	Vinblastine, mercaptopurine, chlorambucil, doxorubicin
Carcinoma of testis	Combination therapy: cisplatin, vinblastine, bleomycin	Methotrexate, dactinomycin, mithramycin, doxorubicin, cyclophosphamide, VP16‡
Carcinoma of prostate	Estrogens	Doxorubicin plus cyclophosphamide, prednisone,† estramustine, fluorouracil, progestins
Wilms' tumor	Vincristine plus dactinomycin after surgery and radiation therapy	Methotrexate, cyclophosphamide, doxorubicin
Neuroblastoma	Cyclophosphamide plus doxorubicin and vincristine	Dactinomycin, daunorubicin, cisplatin
Carcinoma of thyroid	Radioiodine (^{131}I), doxorubicin	Bleomycin, fluorouracil, melphalan
Carcinoma of adrenal	Mitotane	Doxorubicin
Carcinoma of stomach or pancreas	Fluorouracil plus doxorubicin and mitomycin	Hydroxyurea, lomustine, cisplatin
Carcinoma of colon	Fluorouracil	Cyclophosphamide, mitomycin, nitrosoureas
Carcinoid	Doxorubicin plus cyclophosphamide	Dactinomycin, methysergide,† streptozocin
Insulinoma	Streptozocin	Doxorubicin, fluorouracil, mitomycin, streptozocin
Osteogenic sarcoma	Doxorubicin, or methotrexate with citrovorum rescue initiated after surgery	Cyclophosphamide, dacarbazine, interferon‡
Miscellaneous sarcomas	Doxorubicin plus dacarbazine	Methotrexate, dactinomycin, cyclophosphamide, vincristine, vinblastine
Melanoma	Dacarbazine, dactinomycin, and BCG‡	Lomustine, hydroxyurea, mitomycin, bisantrene‡

*Modified from Krupp MA, Chatton MJ (editors): *Current Medical Diagnosis & Treatment 1982.* Lange, 1982.
†Supportive agent, not oncolytic.
‡Investigational agent. Treatment available through qualified investigators and centers authorized by National Cancer Institute and Cooperative Oncology Groups.

directly into the fluid-containing cavity. Although its exact mechanism of action is uncertain, it is a local irritant and leads to the production of local fibrous adhesions.

INVESTIGATIONAL AGENTS

Several of the drugs mentioned in the text remain in an investigational status in the USA until their efficacy and safety for cancer chemotherapy can be established. In specific instances where treatment with one of these agents seems warranted, it usually can be arranged through a university hospital or cancer center or by contacting the Division of Cancer Treatment of the National Cancer Institute, which can provide further information and identify investigators who are authorized to administer these drugs.

This status applies to rubidazone, deoxycoformycin, and AMSA, useful in acute leukemia. Chemical compounds and other natural products to which this designation also applies include semustine, mitoxantrone, bisantrene, hexamethylmelamine, azacytidine, tegafur (ftorafur), desacetylvinblastine, and epipodophyllotoxins (VM26, VP16). All of these drugs have substantial toxicities. Until their pharmacology is more completely understood and their net effects have proved to be beneficial, their use will be restricted to clinical research. New inhibitors of nucleoside metabolism include the adenosine deaminase inhibitor deoxycoformycin. Of the biologic response modifiers, 13-*cis* retinoic acid and all-*trans* retinoic acid (Etretinate) (vitamin A analogs), levamisole, and human interferon appear to be particularly promising. It appears likely that VP16, AMSA, mitoxantrone, bisantrene, interferon (natural and recombinant DNA), and hexamethylmelamine will have major uses in cancer chemotherapy and will be added to the practicing oncologist's list of effective anticancer drugs.

CLINICAL PHARMACOLOGY OF CANCER CHEMOTHERAPEUTIC DRUGS

(See Table 56–7.)

Knowledge of the kinetics of tumor cell proliferation and total body tumor cell number, as well as information on the pharmacology and mechanism of action of cancer chemotherapeutic agents, has become important in designing optimal chemotherapeutic regimens for patients with advanced cancer. The strategy for developing drug regimens requires a knowledge of the particular characteristics of specific tumors—eg, Is there a high growth fraction? Is there a high spontaneous cell death rate? Are most of the cells in G_0? Is a significant fraction of the tumor composed of hypoxic stem cells? Are their normal counterparts under hormonal control? Similarly, knowledge of the pharmacology of specific drugs is equally important—eg, Does the drug have a particular affinity for uptake by the tumor cells (streptozocin)? Are the tumor cells sensitive to the drug? Is the drug cycle-phase specific?

Drugs that affect cycling cells can often be used most effectively after treatment with a cycle-nonspecific agent (eg, alkylating agents); this principle has been tested in only a few human tumors, but with increasing success. Similarly, recognition of true drug synergism (tumor cell kill by the drug combination greater than the additive effects of the individual drugs) or antagonism is important in the design of combination chemotherapeutic programs. The combination of cytarabine with 6-thioguanine in the treatment of acute myelogenous leukemia, the use of doxorubicin and cyclophosphamide in breast cancer, and the use of vinblastine, cisplatin, and bleomycin in testicular tumors are some of the best examples of true drug synergism against cancer cells but not against normal tissues.

In general, it is preferable to use cytotoxic chemotherapeutic agents in intensive "pulse" courses every 3–4 weeks rather than to give continuous daily dosage schedules. This allows for maximum effects against neoplastic cell populations with complete hematologic and immunologic recovery between courses rather than leaving the patient continuously suppressed with cytotoxic therapy. This approach reduces side-effects and does not reduce therapeutic efficacy.

The application of these principles is well illustrated in the current approach to the treatment of acute leukemia, lymphomas, Wilms' tumor, and testicular neoplasms.

ADJUVANT CHEMOTHERAPY FOR MICROMETASTASES: MULTIMODALITY THERAPY

The most important role for effective cancer chemotherapy is undoubtedly as an "adjuvant" to initial or "primary field" treatment with other methods of treatment such as surgery or radiation therapy. Failures with primary field therapy are due principally to occult micrometastases outside the primary field. With the currently available treatment modalities, this form of multimodality therapy appears to offer the greatest chance of curing the highest percentage of patients with solid tumors.

Distant micrometastases are usually present in patients with one or more positive lymph nodes at the time of surgery (eg, in breast cancer) and in patients with tumors having a known propensity for early hematogenous spread (eg, osteogenic sarcoma, Wilms' tumor). The risk of recurrent or metastatic disease in such patients can be extremely high (80%). Only systemic therapy can adequately attack micrometastases. Chemotherapy regimens that are at least moderately effective against advanced cancer may have curative potential (at the right dosage and schedule) when combined with primary therapy such as surgery. Recent studies show prolongation of disease-free survival in patients with osteogenic sarcoma, rhabdomyosarcoma, or breast cancer who receive adjuvant chemotherapy. In osteogenic sarcoma, methotrexate with leucovorin (folinic acid) rescue, doxorubicin alone, and doxorubicin in combination with other drugs have proved effective. Similar comments apply to the use of 3 cycles of combination chemotherapy (MOPP) prior to total nodal radiation in stage IIB Hodgkin's disease.

In breast cancer, women with positive lymph nodes at the time of mastectomy have benefited from combination chemotherapy alone or with the addition of tamoxifen. Useful combination chemotherapy regimens for adjuvant therapy for breast cancer include CMF (cyclophosphamide-methotrexate-fluorouracil) or the same combination plus vincristine and prednisone (CMFVP), and D/C (doxorubicin-cyclophosphamide). The end results obtained with combination chemotherapy have already proved superior to results obtained with single agents, because combination chemotherapy can cope with tumor cell heterogeneity and produces a greater tumor cell log kill. Full protocol doses of cytotoxic agents are required to maximize the likelihood of efficacy. The D/C and CMFVP regimens appear to be effective in both pre- and postmenopausal women, perhaps because of the greater potency of these combinations against breast cancer. Early results of ongoing clinical trials of tamoxifen alone or in combination with chemotherapy have yielded encouraging results in women with positive estrogen receptor tests on the primary tumor. Whether tamoxifen suppresses or eradicates micrometastases remains to be established. Adjuvant chemotherapy should definitely be considered as part of standard and indicated therapy in the patient groups discussed above. Other areas of current investigation include adjuvant chemotherapy for "Dukes C" colorectal cancer (fluorouracil in combination with semustine or radiotherapy) and in testicular (vinblastine, bleomycin, and cisplatin), head and neck, and gynecologic neoplasms (various drugs). Thus, adjuvant chemotherapy (with curative intent) should now be given serious consideration for patients who undergo primary surgical staging and therapy and are found to have a stage and histologic type of cancer known to be associated with a high risk of micrometastasis. This policy is particularly germane to those tumor types for which palliative chemotherapy has already been developed and been shown to include complete remissions in advanced stages of the disease.

ACUTE LEUKEMIA

Acute leukemia is a general term for a group of malignant disorders of blood leukocytes. Age at onset of disease and certain morphologic characteristics have significant implications for patient survival and responsiveness to chemotherapy. With current agents, childhood acute leukemia is more treatable than that which occurs later in life. In all leukemic patients, major emphasis must be given to intensive support of the patient with necessary red cell and platelet transfusions, and prevention of hyperuricemia and infection.

A useful distinction can be drawn between remission induction and maintenance chemotherapy, because the therapeutic agents used, dosage schedules, and objectives are somewhat different. Remission induction is in general a more intensive type of chemotherapy and often uses multiple agents administered simultaneously. The objective of induction therapy is to clear the body of all detectable leukemic leukocytes, ie, to reduce the leukemic cell number by many logs. This objective can sometimes be obtained using drugs that would have prohibitive toxicities if used on a chronic basis. The objective of maintenance therapy is to keep the population of residual leukemic cells in check so that they do not repopulate the blood and bone marrow and lead to the return of symptoms. In general, drugs used for remission maintenance are those that have relatively little delayed or cumulative toxicity and can be taken for months or years on an outpatient basis. Current schemes of chemotherapy often use courses of "reinduction" medications between remission treatments even though the patient has remained in complete remission. This is intended to further reduce the body's burden of leukemic cells. Thus, the objective today is not remission maintenance but complete cure of acute leukemia.

Leukemia of Childhood

Acute lymphoblastic leukemia (ALL) is the predominant form of leukemia in childhood and the most common form of cancer in children. The usual cell of origin appears to be a "null" lymphocyte. These children now have a relatively good prognosis. A subset of patients with a poor prognosis have neoplastic lymphocytes expressing surface antigenic features of T lymphocytes (see Chapter 57). A cytoplasmic enzyme expressed by normal thymocytes, terminal deoxycytidyl transferase (terminal transferase), is also expressed in many cases of ALL. T cell ALLs also express high levels of the enzyme adenosine deaminase (ADA). (This led to interest in the use of the ADA-inhibitor deoxycoformycin for treatment of such T cell cases.) Until 1948, the median survival in ALL was 3 months. With the advent of the folic acid antagonists, a major increase in survival was attained. Subsequently, corticosteroids, mercaptopurine, cyclophosphamide, vincristine, daunorubicin, and asparaginase were all found to have activity in this disease. In general, current practice is to employ a combination of vincristine and prednisone for initial induction of remission. Over 85% of children enter complete remission with this therapy, with only minimal toxicity. Because circulating tumor stem cells often lodge in the brain, such cells are not killed by these drugs, as they do not cross the blood-brain barrier. The value of "prophylactic" intrathecal methotrexate therapy for prevention of central nervous system leukemia (a major mechanism of relapse) has been clearly demonstrated. Intrathecal therapy with methotrexate should therefore be considered as a standard component of the induction regimen for children with ALL. Alternative approaches for prevention of central nervous system leukemia that also appear to be efficacious are intrathecal cytarabine and craniospinal irradiation. Radiation therapy to the neuraxis can cause skeletal growth retardation as a side-effect. Once a complete remission has been induced (greater than a 3-log cell kill), "maintenance" or "consolidation" therapy is always indicated. This usually consists of a combination of oral methotrexate, mercaptopurine, and cyclophosphamide, administered either in pulses, simultaneously, or in various sequences. Some centers employ periodic "reinforcements," with repeated courses of the inducing agents (vincristine and prednisone) several times each year. Such efforts at "total therapy" should be considered as the standard approach to treatment, because they have resulted in a substantial increase in the cure rate of children with acute leukemia. Although many of the clinical trials are still under way, such therapy appears to offer the best hope of cure for an increasing percentage of patients. The median survival in childhood acute leukemia is now approaching 4 years. Many centers discontinue intensive chemotherapy in patients who have shown no sign of relapse after 3 years of intensive chemotherapy. Such children are markedly immunosuppressed during therapy; however, both humoral and cell-mediated immunity usually return to normal within 6 months after cessation of chemotherapy. Cell-mediated immunity to ALL can definitely be demonstrated—more readily when the patient enters complete remission. Children who survive for 5 years in complete remission have a greater than 50% chance of having a permanent remission or cure.

If leukemia does recur in a patient in remission, an attempt is made to reinduce the remission with the same drugs used initially. If resistance is observed, reinduction is attempted with different agents (daunorubicin, vincristine, asparaginase, methotrexate, etc) in various combinations. The possibility of cure of this dread disease of young patients has imparted great impetus to current investigations of intensive combination chemotherapy with proved agents plus asparaginase, daunorubicin, and other experimental agents and has led to increased interest in combination chemotherapy of other kinds of neoplastic diseases.

Leukemia in Adults

Acute leukemia in adults is predominantly of the myelocytic variety, although some cases of lymphoblastic leukemia are also seen. Acute myelogenous leukemia (AML) has been quite difficult to treat, and until recently the median survival was in the range of 3 months. Unlike ALL, induction therapy in AML requires the use of drugs toxic to normal bone marrow cells. The single most active agent for AML is cytarabine; however, it is best used in combination. Combinations of thioguanine, cytarabine, and daunorubicin (TAD) or of cytarabine, vincristine, and prednisone are capable of inducing remissions in over 50% of previously untreated cases. Doxorubicin has had similar activity to daunorubicin and may act synergistically when used in combination with prolonged cytarabine infusions. Recent trials with combinations of doxorubicin with cytarabine and thioguanine have induced complete remissions in about 70% of patients. Currently, cytarabine is being tested at doses 10 times those used conventionally in the treatment of leukemia. The patient often requires intensive supportive care during the toxic period of induction chemotherapy before remission is achieved. Such supportive care includes platelet transfusions to prevent bleeding due to thrombocytopenia and combinations of bactericidal antibiotics plus granulocyte transfusions to combat infections. Patients over 60 respond less well to chemotherapy, primarily because their resistance is weaker. Remission maintenance is usually with thioguanine and cytarabine courses. Azacytidine and AMSA are utilized as secondary agents for patients who develop resistance to standard therapy. The median life expectancy of patients with AML who enter complete remission is now in excess of 1 year, and some patients are in remission for over 3 years. About 20% of adult patients who achieve complete remission with current standard chemotherapy appear to remain free of recurrent leukemia and are probably cured.

CHRONIC MYELOGENOUS LEUKEMIA

Chronic myelogenous leukemia (CML) arises from a chromosomally abnormal hematopoietic stem cell. An abnormal chromosome 22 with deletion of a short arm or translocation to the long arm of chromosome 9 is present in 90% of cases. The clinical symptoms and course are related to the leukocyte level and its rate of increase. Most patients with leukocyte counts over 50,000/μL should be treated. The goal of treatment is to reduce the granulocytes to normal levels, to raise the hemoglobin concentration to normal, and to relieve metabolic symptoms. The most useful form of treatment is chemotherapy with busulfan, although other oral alkylating agents can also be used. Local splenic x-ray therapy is occasionally used. In the early stages of the disease, treatment produces a prompt decrease in spleen size and a fall in the leukocyte count associated with subjective well-being. Current therapy does not prolong survival, but it markedly relieves symptoms. Efforts to achieve better results with combination chemotherapy plus splenectomy have thus far been unsuccessful.

Initial chemotherapy consists of giving busulfan, 4 mg daily orally, until the number of leukocytes falls to 12,000/μL. If the initial white count is higher than 100,000/μL, allopurinol should be used prophylactically to prevent the development of hyperuricemia. Maintenance therapy is advisable if the leukocyte count doubles within 1 month after discontinuance of the initial course of treatment. A maintenance dose of 2 mg of busulfan daily is usually sufficient, but as the disease progresses it may be necessary to increase the dose to 6 or 8 mg daily.

Resistance to busulfan eventually develops. The hemoglobin falls, the spleen enlarges, and the differential count shows increasing cellular immaturity, with large numbers of blast cells. At this point, busulfan is discontinued and agents such as hydroxyurea or mercaptopurine may be of some value, but only partial and temporary success can be anticipated. This blastic transformation, or "blast crisis," generally occurs 3–4 years after diagnosis, and the disease converts to acute leukemia. Therapy at that point is still investigational, but combination chemotherapy, including cytarabine, vincristine, vindesine, or hydroxyurea with or without prednisone, and asparaginase, may have some benefit in a subset of patients. In some instances of "blast crisis," the malignant cell population is quite undifferentiated and has a "lymphoblastic" appearance. The enzyme terminal transferase appears in many such cell populations, suggesting a possible relationship to thymocytes. With treatment, the leukocyte count falls, but there is often little or no effect on bone marrow infiltration. True remissions rarely occur in patients who have undergone blast crisis. Bone marrow transplantation is now showing promise for CML patients who have an HLA-matched donor.

CHRONIC LYMPHOCYTIC LEUKEMIA

Treatment of chronic lymphocytic leukemia is markedly different from that of chronic myelogenous leukemia. Whereas chronic myelogenous leukemia is a proliferative neoplasm requiring chemotherapy for symptomatic control, chronic lymphocytic leukemia appears to result from a gradual accumulation of monoclonal B lymphocytes rather than from rapid neoplastic cell proliferation. Chronic lymphocytic leukemia is often detected accidentally long before the development of symptoms. Although the average life expectancy is only 3 years, the disease occurs frequently in elderly patients, which skews the survival data. Many patients who are asymptomatic may have prolonged survival (eg, 5–15 years) without any therapy. In patients whose disease is restricted to lymphocytosis in the peripheral blood, it is reasonable to withhold treatment because in chronic lymphocytic leukemia one does not "treat the lymphocyte count" unless it is well above 150,000/μL. When anemia, immunodeficiency, weight loss, fever, and generalized organ and bone marrow involvement do occur, treatment is indicated.

The therapeutic resources available for the treatment of chronic lymphocytic leukemia include corticosteroids and low-dose total body irradiation or alkylating agent chemotherapy. Prednisone is often quite effective, and after an initial course of 80 mg/d for several weeks the dose can be tapered to low levels or switched to an intermittent (every other day) schedule, which virtually eliminates side-effects. Hemolytic anemia may respond dramatically to prednisone, although thrombocytopenia is often more refractory. Alkylating agents will also decrease the number of lymphocytes and organ enlargement in most patients, and the choice between corticosteroids and alkylating agents is frequently based on relative contraindications of one drug or the other.

Chlorambucil (Leukeran) is probably the most easily administered oral alkylating agent and has fewest side-effects. The dose is usually 0.1 mg/kg/d, with monitoring of blood counts at weekly intervals. Alternatively, melphalan can be given in "pulse courses" of 1 mg/kg orally over 4 days every 4–6 weeks. More aggressive therapy, eg, with cyclophosphamide, vincristine, and prednisone, is indicated in instances of severe hemolytic anemia and rapidly progressive disease. The goal of therapy is to eliminate the systemic manifestations of the disease, and complete normalization of the lymphocyte count is not necessary. Therapy can be discontinued once the patient's condition has stabilized, but maintenance therapy should be considered if symptoms reappear quickly. Local x-ray therapy is useful for shrinking symptomatic enlarged lymph nodes but is only occasionally indicated. It is important not to overtreat these patients, because of the poor host resistance of elderly patients.

THE LYMPHOMAS

1. HODGKIN'S DISEASE

Although remarkably little is known about the cause of Hodgkin's disease, its therapy has undergone revolutionary improvement. Hodgkin's disease is a lymphoma with certain unique characteristics in its natural history: its apparent tendency to progress from a single involved node to anatomically adjacent nodes in a somewhat "orderly" fashion, and its tendency to appear confined to the lymphoid system for a long period of time, with progression to involve retroperitoneal nodes and spleen. Extranodal involvement may also occur, and involvement of the liver, bone marrow, lungs, or other sites is taken as evidence of more "malignant" behavior of the tumor. A concerted attempt at adequate staging of the extent of disease is essential to effective treatment of this disorder, and newly diagnosed cases must be adequately studied with x-rays, lymphography, and exploratory laparotomy and splenectomy (looking for occult disease) in order to prepare a rational treatment plan. Widespread involvement is manifested by symptoms such as sweats, fever, anorexia, and weight loss and infiltration of other organs, including the lungs, liver, and bone marrow.

Intensive x-ray therapy with supervoltage equipment is curative in most cases of early Hodgkin's disease confined to one lymph node area or several adjacent areas above the diaphragm (stages I and II). Radiation therapy is also of some use in asymptomatic patients with more generalized Hodgkin's disease limited to the lymphoid system above and below the diaphragm (stage III), and occasionally in stage IV for palliation of symptoms due to enlarging lymph nodes. As can be seen in Table 56–7, a variety of chemotherapeutic agents are active in Hodgkin's disease; however, as of the past few years, it is clear that optimal treatment is with combination chemotherapy.

Combination chemotherapy is now indicated in patients presenting with stage III or stage IV Hodgkin's disease. The results have been sufficiently promising to lead to present trials of combination chemotherapy along with x-ray therapy in stage I and stage II disease. Results in stage IIIA Hodgkin's disease with 3 cycles of chemotherapy (see below) followed by total nodal radiotherapy are clearly superior to those achieved with radiotherapy alone. The most effective form of chemotherapy at present is with a 4-drug combination known as MOPP, consisting of mechlorethamine (HN2, Mustargen), Oncovin (vincristine), procarbazine (Matulane), and prednisone. This form of treatment, developed by DeVita and his associates at the National Cancer Institute, is given repeatedly for at least 6 months and sometimes for as long as a year. Over 80% of previously untreated patients with advanced Hodgkin's disease (stages III and IV) go into complete remission, with disappearance of all symptoms and objective evidences of tumor.

A current schedule for use of MOPP includes repeated courses every 2 months with M (mechlorethamine), 6 mg/m^2 intravenously on days 1 and 8; O (vincristine), 1.4 mg/m^2 intravenously on days 1 and 8; P (procarbazine), 50 mg orally on day 1, 100 mg orally on day 2, and 100 mg/m^2 on days 3–10; and P (prednisone), 40 mg/m^2 orally on days 1–10. A "non-cross-resistant" alternative to the MOPP regimen developed by Bonadonna consists of doxorubicin (Adriamycin), bleomycin, vinblastine, and dacarbazine (ABVD). The ABVD program appears to be similar in efficacy to MOPP and, more importantly, has been of value in treatment of MOPP failures. Studies employing the 2 regimens alternatively are currently under way, and results to date suggest that use of these "alternating, non-cross-resistant combinations" may yield better results than either combination alone. Complex treatment regimens such as these should be under the direction of a medical oncologist who is familiar with the individual and synergistic toxicities and contraindications for each of the drugs involved. Frequent blood counts are obtained, and treatment is modified or suspended temporarily in the event of severe depression of the white cell or platelet count. With this form of remission induction with at least 6 courses of MOPP or ABVD, approximately 50% of patients will remain free of all signs of Hodgkin's disease for over 2 years. The ABVD combination has thus far been free from association with late complications of acute leukemia, perhaps because of the lack of alkylating agents and procarbazine from this combination.

Theoretic calculations based on the number of logs of tumor cells likely to be killed with this type of intensive therapy suggest that a cellular cure of Hodgkin's disease may be accomplished in some of these cases, but follow-ups of 5–15 years after cessation of all chemotherapy are required for confirmation. Thus far, about half of patients who have achieved complete remission with MOPP appear to remain disease-free at 10 years. This form of chemotherapy therefore represents a major improvement in the management of advanced Hodgkin's disease, and patients should be afforded every chance to achieve complete remission.

Some of the reasons for the success of MOPP and ABVD chemotherapy were the previously demonstrated antineoplastic activity of each of the individual drugs used in Hodgkin's disease, the differing modes of action of the drugs in these combinations, and the lack of cross-resistance of tumors to these different drugs. Even better results than those obtained with MOPP or ABVD have been achieved by alternating cycles of MOPP and ABVD with more than 90% of advanced Hodgkin's disease patients achieving complete remission. This is the first clinical combination of the "Goldie-Goldman hypothesis" for use of alternating non-cross-resistant combination chemotherapy.

Nitrosoureas such as lomustine are also effective in Hodgkin's disease and have been combined with other drugs for reinduction of remission in patients who relapse from the standard regimens.

2. NON-HODGKIN LYMPHOMAS

The characteristics of non-Hodgkin lymphomas are related to major histopathologic features present in the neoplasm and the immunologic origin of the neoplastic cells. The most useful pathologic classification is one based on cell type plus the presence or absence of nodularity in the lymphomatous tissues. Thus, a non-Hodgkin lymphoma may be any one of 9 different cell types (nodular histiocytic, diffuse histiocytic, nodular mixed histiocytic-lymphocytic, diffuse mixed, nodular lymphocytic, diffuse lymphocytic, undifferentiated, etc). This histopathologic classification has great prognostic significance in terms of clinical features, sites of involvement, response to irradiation or chemotherapy, and overall survival. In general, the nodular lymphomas have a far better prognosis (median survival up to 7 years) than do the diffuse ones (median survival about 1–2 years). The term histiocyte is probably inappropriate also in the current classification, inasmuch as these cells are probably transformed lymphocytes. Immunologic classifications are still being worked out, but it is already clear that 80–90% of non-Hodgkin lymphomas (and all nodular lymphomas) are B cell neoplasms. T cell lymphomas that have been identified are a convoluted T cell lymphoma arising in the mediastinum and mycosis fungoides.

Careful clinical, radiographic, laboratory, and surgical evaluation of patients with non-Hodgkin lymphoma prior to treatment appears justified, since as many as one-third are still localized (stages I and II). Modern megavoltage irradiation is curative in some cases of localized diffuse lymphoma. In a recent study, addition of combination chemotherapy (see below) to radiotherapy further increased the cure rate. Liver and bone marrow core biopsy techniques are useful during initial staging to define the extent of spread. Liver, bone marrow, gastrointestinal, and localized extralymphatic involvement are all observed more commonly in these tumors than in Hodgkin's disease, and, accordingly, a higher fraction of patients (about a third) have stage IV disease at presentation—in contrast to 15% of patients with Hodgkin's disease.

Alkylating agents, doxorubicin, vincristine, and prednisone all have a place in the management of the advanced stages of these lymphomas. Combination chemotherapy is clearly preferred to single agent therapy; nodular lymphomas respond much better to conventional agents than do the diffuse lymphomas; however, some of the diffuse lymphomas are curable with available drugs, whereas nodular lymphomas are not. Attainment of complete remission with combination therapy is a major objective, since it not only leads to relief of all symptoms but also significantly lengthens useful life expectancy. One approach includes cyclophosphamide, vincristine (Oncovin), and prednisone in combination (COP). With COP therapy, complete remissions occur in 60% of patients with nodular lymphomas and 30% of patients with diffuse lymphomas. These results are clearly superior to those that can be achieved with single agent therapy. Once complete remission is attained with COP, it appears desirable to continue the same form of chemotherapy. However, in diffuse histiocytic lymphomas, early relapse is quite common, and some other form of chemotherapy is needed to handle the subclinical phase of this tumor (less than 10^9 tumor cells).

Doxorubicin has been found to be extremely active in the treatment of non-Hodgkin lymphomas. Doxorubicin has been combined with cyclophosphamide, vincristine, prednisone, and other agents with excellent results in "poor-prognosis" large cell or diffuse histiocytic lymphomas. These doxorubicin-containing combinations induce complete remissions in excess of 60% of cases of non-Hodgkin lymphomas, irrespective of the histologic appearance, and are more effective than COP in the diffuse lymphomas. Based on currently available data, it appears likely that one-third of patients with diffuse histiocytic lymphoma will remain in permanent remission after intensive combination chemotherapy has been discontinued. For patients with nodular lymphomas, adding doxorubicin has not improved results over those obtained with COP. Another active regimen combines carmustine with COP. Bleomycin has also been combined with COP with some improvement in results; however, the bleomycin dosage employed in early studies now appears excessive, and serious pulmonary toxicity was observed in some cases. Human interferon has been observed to cause tumor regression in nodular lymphoma, and this will undoubtedly be an area of future investigation, particularly with the introduction of highly purified interferon prepared synthetically with recombinant DNA technique. Monoclonal antisera directed against T cell antigens have recently been tested in a few patients with T cell leukemias or lymphomas, with encouraging results.

Thus, our concepts of the non-Hodgkin lymphomas are rapidly changing: The importance of histology, clinical staging, and immunology is just being realized. A whole series of useful drugs have been identified, and major trials are under way to develop treatment that has curative potential. In view of the multiplicity of agents that are active—and modern radiotherapy—this objective does not appear to be unreasonable for the diffuse lymphomas.

MULTIPLE MYELOMA

This plasma cell tumor is now one of the "models" of neoplastic disease in humans because the tumor arises from a single tumor stem cell, and the tumor cells all produce a marker protein (myeloma immunoglobulin) that allows for quantitation of the total body burden of tumor cells. The tumor grows principally in the bone marrow and the surrounding bone, causing anemia, bone pain, lytic lesions, bone fractures, and anemia as well as increased susceptibility to infection. It has been clear for about 10 years that patients do improve if treated with oral alkylating agents such as melphalan or cyclophosphamide and that intermittent high doses of prednisone also have an oncolytic effect. Relatively simple combination chemotherapy was therefore developed by combining melphalan and prednisone, administering both drugs for courses of 4 days every 4–6 weeks. More recently, better results have been obtained in advanced-stage cases with the use of more intensive regimens containing alkylating agents, doxorubicin, a nitrosourea, and a *Vinca* alkaloid. About 75% of myeloma patients improve with this treatment, and patients who have the greatest reduction in total body tumor cell number (generally only 1–2 logs) have significant relief of symptoms and prolongation of survival with this treatment and return to a more active life. Such therapy, although beneficial, is far from optimal, because between 10^{10} and 10^{11} myeloma cells persist in a "plateau," and resistance to chemotherapy usually occurs after 2–3 years of treatment in most responding cases.

It has recently become clear that vincristine is also active if given when the population has been reduced in size by one or more logs (in which case more cells are cycling), and new efforts at developing combination chemotherapy must have as their objective the maximum degree of reduction in total body tumor cell number rather than just prolongation of survival. This objective can be followed serially, and intensified treatment can be administered during the "plateau."

Other drugs with definite activity in myeloma now being evaluated in combination are doxorubicin and carmustine. This latter combination has proved useful for reinduction of remission for patients who initially respond to melphalan and subsequently relapse. Approximately 50% of such cases can be brought back into remission (at least briefly) with this treatment. The new *Vinca* alkaloid, vindesine, has also been useful. It is of interest that addition of the immunomodulating agent levamisole appears to prolong remissions. Human interferon has been observed to induce remissions in 30% of myeloma patients in relapse from cytotoxic drugs. With the advent of gene-cloning techniques, large-scale production of human interferons has become feasible, and such interferons are now in clinical trial in multiple myeloma.

Treatment of complications of myeloma is another important aspect of comprehensive therapy, and this effort is most important shortly after diagnosis, when they are most likely to be present.

The anemia of myeloma often responds well to androgen therapy, eg, testosterone enanthate (Delatestryl), 600 mg intramuscularly every 6 weeks for 2 or 3 doses. Hypercalcemia should be treated with fluids, corticosteroids, and calcium restriction; if this is not sufficient, mithramycin (Mithracin), 25 μg/kg intravenously, should be given every second or third day for 2 or 3 doses. The initial induction course of chemotherapy with alkylating agents and prednisone will often correct the hypercalcemia, but this complication is potentially lethal and should be viewed as a medical emergency and treated promptly. Painful bone lesions should be treated with x-ray therapy (if the area is not too extensive), as this will help ready the patient for ambulation and thereby minimize the possibility of hypercalcemia. Myeloma patients are often subject to recurrent infection because of a functional hypogammaglobulinemia. Prophylactic administration of gamma globulin does not correct the susceptibility to infection, but induction of remission with chemotherapy often does. Sodium fluoride may increase the density of osteoporotic bone in some instances; however, this approach remains investigational and unproved despite many years of effort. The degree of reduction of myeloma globulin in the serum or urine is the most useful objective measure of the effectiveness of chemotherapy. A myeloma stem cell assay has been developed to detect differences in sensitivity of myeloma stem cells to anticancer drugs. The technique is analogous to that used for drug sensitivity testing in the management of bacterial infections.

Similar comments apply to Waldenström's macroglobulinemia, which is a related plasma cell neoplasm. The growth characteristics of this tumor are more analogous to those of chronic lymphocytic leukemia; treatment need not be quite so aggressive, because the macroglobulin-producing cells rarely attack the skeleton. In most instances, low-dosage chlorambucil therapy proves adequate, and the patients have a relatively long life expectancy. Plasmapheresis using a blood cell separator can also be utilized to remove the excessive amounts of macroglobulin that produce many of the symptoms and signs of the disorder.

CARCINOMA OF THE BREAST

Stage I & Stage II Neoplasms

The management of primary carcinoma of the breast is currently undergoing remarkable change as a result of major efforts at early diagnosis (through encouragement of self-examination as well as through the use of cancer detection centers) and the implementation of multimodality clinical trials incorporating systemic chemotherapy as an adjuvant to surgery. Women with stage I lateral lesions at the time of breast surgery (small primaries and negative axillary lymph node dissections) are currently treated with surgery and have an 80% chance of cure with surgery alone. A current trend is toward more conservative surgery. The mutilating radical and extended radical mastectomies have largely been abandoned. While the standard surgical procedure is now the modified radical mastectomy, recent studies suggest that segmental mastectomy (lumpectomy) plus an axillary lymph node sampling may prove to be of equivalent value.

Women with one or more positive lymph nodes have a very high risk of systemic recurrence and death from breast cancer (approaching 90% at 10 years) if treated with surgery alone, and 80% of cases with 4 or more positive lymph nodes will recur within 5 years. Thus, lymph node status can be taken as a direct indication of the risk of occult distant micrometastasis of a few (10^0–10^1) or a moderate number (10^1–10^4) of tumor stem cells. In this setting, postoperative use of cycles of combination chemotherapy sufficient to eradicate this order of magnitude of tumor stem cells is warranted. Such clinical trials have now reached the 5-year mark; the results observed by Bonadonna and associates from Milan, who have used monthly cycles of cyclophosphamide-methotrexate-fluorouracil (CMF), show a low relapse rate in the treated group (over 150 women) as compared to a 65% relapse rate in a similar number of patients randomized to a control group. A recent update (median follow-up of 5 years) of the CMF trial indicates that overall survival (not just delay in recurrence) is improved in women who received CMF. As a result of this study and other clinical tests, much fewer women are now being treated with surgery alone when they have lymph node involvement. An effective combination currently under study at the University of Arizona is the use of cycles of doxorubicin and cyclophosphamide (D/C) every 3 weeks for 8 cycles (6 months) after mastectomy. Thus far (at a median follow-up of 4 years), the effects of D/C appear to be as potent in postmenopausal as in premenopausal women. Both the D/C and the CMF combinations were developed in earlier studies of women with advanced metastatic breast cancer. The CMFVP program also appears quite effective in both pre- and postmenopausal women. The antiestrogen tamoxifen may also prove very useful in combination with chemotherapy; 2-year results in the National Surgical Adjuvant Breast Project (which has utilized this approach) are encouraging. In elderly women with ER-positive tumors, long-term use of tamoxifen as an adjuvant also appears reasonable and lacks significant toxicity. At present, the optimal adjuvant combination cannot be specified, since long-term effects (5 and 10 years) on overall survival and the potential delayed toxicity of chemotherapy have yet to be assessed. It is not established whether local radiotherapy (in addition to surgery and chemotherapy) will play any role.

Advanced Breast Cancer (Stage III & Stage IV)

Until such multimodality programs as those discussed above are fully effective in the population at risk, the treatment of women with advanced breast cancer remains a major problem. Indeed, some women still present with inoperable "local" lesions with suspected metastases (stage III) or overt distant metastases (stage IV). Currently, most women with local or distant recurrence have had prior breast cancer surgery or surgery plus radiotherapy.

Efforts at treatment of advanced breast cancer are entirely palliative inasmuch as the available treatment modalities are not capable of eliminating the overt 10^{10}–10^{12} tumor cells in the body. In addition to local radiotherapy for stage III lesions, 2 major (and complementary) systemic approaches are available: hormonal manipulation and combination chemotherapy. When compared directly in an unselected population, combination chemotherapy was more effective than hormonal management. Consideration of hormonal procedures (ablation or addition) can now potentially be made on a rational basis through the direct measurement of estrogen (and progesterone) receptors in breast cancer tissue. While a spectrum of receptor levels has been observed, the presence of such receptor proteins appears to reflect the more biochemically differentiated tumors that appear to be present in about half of women with breast cancer. Biochemically differentiated breast cancers (as determined with this test) retain many of the intrinsic hormonal sensitivities of the normal breast—including the growth stimulatory response to ovarian, adrenal, and pituitary hormones. While oophorectomy and perhaps other hormonal ablation procedures seem most reasonable in premenopausal women with skin, lymph node, pleural, or bone metastases, only two-thirds of women with positive hormone receptor assays show subjective and objective benefit from such procedures. Patients who show improvement with ablative procedures also respond to the addition of the antiestrogen drug tamoxifen. Patients with moderate to severe lung, liver, brain, or visceral involvement generally have biochemically undifferentiated metastases and rarely benefit to any great extent from hormonal maneuvers, which means that initial systemic chemotherapy is indicated in such cases. Irrespective of sites of involvement, if the estrogen receptor is absent, the likelihood of observing a response to hormonal therapy is less than 5%. Premenopausal patients who respond objectively to oophorectomy may have remissions of 1–2 years' duration and constitute the group that responds best also to adrenalectomy or hypophysectomy and to antiestrogens. The rare male patients with breast cancer show similar therapeutic responses to castration at almost any age.

Androgenic Hormones

Androgens are used as palliative agents predominantly in premenopausal women who have responded to oophorectomy, but they are also useful beyond the menopause. Testosterone propionate, 100 mg intramuscularly 3 times weekly, results in subjective improvement characterized by euphoria and relief of pain from bone metastases within 1–2 weeks after therapy is started. Soft tissue metastases are less responsive to androgens, and lesions in the liver or brain rarely respond. Oral halogenated androgens such as fluoxymesterone produce similar results but carry a risk of cholestatic jaundice.

Unpleasant side-effects of androgens include virilism, hirsutism, deepening of the voice, acne, flushing, sodium retention, and increased libido. The oral androgen derivative calusterone appears to be less virilizing than other preparations and of similar therapeutic efficacy. Hypercalcemia, which occurs in about 10% of patients with extensive osteolytic metastases, may increase with androgen treatment, and in such patients androgens should be discontinued.

Estrogenic Hormones

Estrogens (as well as antiestrogens) are useful in both men and women with widespread breast cancer. In women, estrogens are rarely used until several years after the menopause. It is likely that only those patients whose primary tumors arose in an estrogen-free environment and also possess the estrogen receptor will respond to estrogen therapy. In responsive patients, large doses may produce tumor regression lasting for many months. It generally takes a 3-month trial to determine if estrogens will be effective, and, as in the case of androgen, it is unreasonable to expect a response in rapidly progressive disease, particularly in patients with extensive visceral involvement. Side-effects of estrogens include sodium retention and edema, anorexia, uterine bleeding, occasional depression, nausea and vomiting, breast tenderness, hypercalcemia, and tumor growth.

Antiestrogens

The antiestrogen tamoxifen has proved to be a virtually nontoxic alternative to conventional endocrine therapy of breast cancer and has already supplanted the use of other agents in many settings. "Flare" of disease is observed occasionally with tamoxifen and can herald the subsequent achievement of an excellent remission, but meticulous supportive care (eg, for bone pain or hypercalcemia) is required. Tamoxifen is effective in both pre- and postmenopausal women who are ER-positive. However, oophorectomy may be preferable in premenopausal ER-positive patients.

Systemic Chemotherapy

Use of cytotoxic drugs and hormones has become a highly specialized and increasingly effective means of treating cancer. Combination chemotherapy has improved considerably for patients with visceral involvement from advanced breast cancer. Doxorubicin is the most active single agent, with an average response rate of 40%. The use of combination chemotherapy has been found to induce much more durable remissions in 50–80% of patients. For example, in a study at the University of Arizona of 55 women with advanced breast cancer who had received no prior chemotherapy, the use every 3–4 weeks of the 2-drug combination of doxorubicin (40 mg/m^2 intravenously) and cyclophosphamide (800 mg/m^2 orally in divided doses over 4 days) (D/C) induced an 80% response rate, with 18% of patients achieving complete remission. The addition of vincristine to this combination did not increase the remission rate significantly but did improve remission duration and survival. A similar schedule employed at M.D. Anderson Hospital (which also adds fluorouracil) has virtually identical results, but with slightly greater hematologic toxicity. Both regimens are effective against involvement of liver and lung as well as other visceral sites. The 3-drug combination of cyclophosphamide, methotrexate, and fluorouracil (CMF) developed by the National Cancer Institute has a 50–60% response rate with a complete response rate similar to those reported from the Arizona and Texas programs. In each of these programs, partial remissions have a median duration of about 10 months and complete remissions a duration of about 15 months. Addition of the antiestrogen tamoxifen to such programs yields only modest additional improvement. When doxorubicin is used in such combinations, it is generally discontinued before the patient reaches cardiotoxic limits. At that point, other drugs are generally substituted. A somewhat more complex 5-drug regimen originally reported by Cooper (cyclophosphamide, fluorouracil, methotrexate, vincristine, and prednisone) has been variously observed to induce remissions in 50–80% of women, but with a greater degree of toxicity.

Suffice it to say that the field is currently in a stage of transition, with various combination protocols available most of which are clearly superior to single agents. It is now established that combination chemotherapy can prolong the survival of women with advanced metastatic breast cancer. The overall objective of this work is to develop a combination regimen with a higher complete remission rate and thereby increase the probability that there may be some long-term disease-free survivors. Thus far, the latter objective is still elusive, and introduction of other new agents (eg, mitoxantrone, bisantrene, and interferon) is eagerly awaited.

It is because of these results in patients with many logs of tumor stem cells that combination chemotherapy has been brought into the multimodality setting for control of micrometastases in stage II breast cancer cases.

Management of Complications of Breast Cancer

Several common complications of metastatic breast cancer deserve particular mention. These are hypercalcemia, cerebral metastases, and bone pain. While hypercalcemia may respond well to remission induction chemotherapy, it is important to treat this complication vigorously with ancillary measures because it can be rapidly lethal. Symptoms of hypercalcemia include mental confusion, constipation, and somnolence. When the serum calcium is less than 15 mg/dL, liberal use of intravenous fluids, diuretics, oral phosphates, and prednisone usually suffices to normalize the calcium within a day or two. When the calcium is in excess of 15 mg/dL, more vigorous measures, including the intravenous use of mithramycin (25 μg/kg every few days) and high-dose prednisone therapy, should be initiated immediately. If hypercalcemia appears during estrogen or androgen therapy, the hormone should be discontinued immediately. For that reason, sex hormone preparations with long durations of action should not be employed until the response to a short-acting agent can be assessed and the lack of induction of hypercalcemia assured. Cerebral metastases may present with seizures, headache, or other central nervous system signs. Brain involvement may occur in patients in "peripheral remission" receiving chemotherapeutic agents that do not cross the blood-brain barrier. If central nervous system involvement occurs, high doses of prednisone or dexamethasone should be administered until whole brain radiotherapy (4000 R) can be administered. Because such lesions are usually multiple, surgery is not warranted. Bone pain generally responds well to androgen therapy or systemic chemotherapy. In cases where these systemic approaches or analgesics are inadequate, use of local palliative radiotherapy is usually of benefit.

CARCINOMA OF THE CERVIX

The incidence of invasive squamous carcinoma of the cervix has decreased markedly as a result of improved early diagnosis with cervical cytologic surveillance by Papanicolaou smear. Invasive lesions that do occur are still difficult to treat. Stage II (and stage III) lesions are generally treated with surgery and radiotherapy. Until recently, there was virtually no systemic chemotherapy of value, although occasional responses to nitrosoureas or bleomycin were observed. Now, a useful 4-drug regimen (mitomycin-vincristine-bleomycin plus cisplatin) has been developed with a high objective response rate (including some complete responses). Some of the patients appear to have prolonged complete remissions, so this regimen can be recommended as initial therapy for patients with stage III and stage IV metastatic cervical carcinomas.

CARCINOMA OF THE ENDOMETRIUM OF THE UTERUS

The incidence of endometrial carcinoma appears to be increased approximately 5-fold in women who have had prolonged conjugated estrogen therapy.

Progesterone derivatives cause dramatic objective tumor regression and symptomatic improvement lasting for several years in about 30% of patients with stage IV metastatic endometrial carcinoma. Those tumors that regress on progesterone probably have cytoplasmic progesterone receptors expressed, with prognostic significance similar to that of the estrogen receptor in breast cancer. Tamoxifen has also proved useful in this patient population and is nontoxic. Remissions can also be achieved with the combination of doxorubicin and cyclophosphamide. It therefore appears reasonable to combine hormones with chemotherapy in such patients and to consider this combination along with local radiotherapy in multimodality approach to patients with stage II endometrial carcinoma (endocervical extension), since such patients may have distant micrometastases at the time of primary therapy.

CHORIOCARCINOMA OF THE UTERUS

This is a rare tumor of women arising from fetal trophoblastic tissue and was the first metastatic cancer cured with chemotherapy. It has been found that massive doses of methotrexate—25 mg daily for 4–5 days—will produce a high percentage of cures associated with complete regression of metastatic lesions and disappearance of chorionic gonadotropic hormones in the urine. Therapy should be given repeatedly until some months after all evidence of the disease has disappeared. In some cases, combination or sequential chemotherapy with methotrexate, chlorambucil, vincristine, dactinomycin, and mercaptopurine is required to achieve cure if methotrexate alone is not adequate.

CARCINOMA OF THE OVARY

This neoplasm often remains occult until it has metastasized to the peritoneal cavity; it may present with malignant ascites. It is important to stage such patients accurately, using laparoscopy, ultrasound, lymphangiography, or ^{57}cobalt-bleomycin scanning. Stage I patients appear to benefit from pelvic radiotherapy and might receive additional benefit from combination chemotherapy. Radiotherapy (including whole abdomen radiotherapy) does not improve the survival of patients with higher stages of involvement and is generally not indicated. Combination chemotherapy is now the standard approach to stage III and stage IV disease. The most useful combinations include doxorubicin, cyclophosphamide, and cisplatin, often with hexamethylmelamine, wherein 70–80% of patients achieve remission, with approximately 40% complete remissions. Multimodality therapy utilizing surgery, radiotherapy, and combination chemotherapy in adjuvant fashion in stage I and stage II patients appears rational and has shown promising signs of efficacy in current clinical trials. Assays of tumor stem cells are being utilized increasingly to aid in tailoring treatment regimens for individual patients with ovarian cancer.

TESTICULAR NEOPLASMS

Single agent chemotherapy has produced some impressive tumor regressions in advanced nonseminomatous testicular neoplasms but few complete responses lasting more than 1 year. The introduction of combination chemotherapy with cisplatin, vinblastine, and bleomycin (PVB) by Einhorn at Indiana University has made an impressive change in these statistics. Ninety-five percent of patients respond to chemotherapy, with approximately 90% entering complete remission. It now seems likely that over half of patients achieving complete remission are cured with chemotherapy. Alternative regimens combining VP16 are also being tested in hope of reducing toxicity. Because of the effectiveness of this treatment in advanced disease, its use in the adjuvant setting for patients who have positive lymph nodes is currently under investigation. Use of PVB in an adjuvant setting is quite controversial, inasmuch as not all patients relapse after primary treatment and the apparent salvage rate in advanced disease has been quite good.

CARCINOMA OF THE PROSTATE

Carcinoma of the prostate was one of the first forms of cancer shown to be responsive to hormonal manipulation. Orchiectomy or low-dose estrogen therapy (or both) has resulted in prolonged improvement in patients with bone lesions. Hormonal treatment produces symptomatic benefit in 70–80% of patients and a significant degree of regression of established metastases. Subjective relief of bone pain, objective evidence of normalization of involved bones, and reduction of the prostatic fraction of alkaline phosphatase are common criteria of response to therapy for this disorder. Responsive patients are treated indefinitely until relapse occurs. At that point, use of progestins, doxorubicin, fluorouracil, or other agents is warranted. Because many patients with carcinoma of the prostate are in their seventh or eighth decades at the time of presentation, the use of initial hormonal management is clearly preferable to chemotherapy, and further therapy is often not required in such cases.

CARCINOMA OF THE THYROID

Until recently, only radioactive iodine (^{131}I) had therapeutic activity in metabolic thyroid cancer, and its effects were limited to well-differentiated tumors that could concentrate iodine. It is now clear that doxorubicin has significant activity in thyroid cancer of a variety of histologic types (particularly anaplastic lesions), induces excellent regressions of tumor, and prolongs survival. Bleomycin also has some activity, although of lesser magnitude. The use of combination chemotherapy in thyroid cancer appears promising in conjunction with ^{131}I therapy for high-risk patients who have anaplastic cell pictures on histologic examination or vascular invasion of the thyroid gland.

GASTROINTESTINAL CARCINOMAS

This group of neoplasms has only limited sensitivity to available chemotherapeutic agents. It is of interest that all of these lesions release carcinoembryonic antigen (CEA), and radioimmunoassay can be used to detect recurrence after surgery as well as response (or relapse) with systemic chemotherapy. Colorectal adenocarcinoma is the most common type, and only 43% of cases are curable with surgery. Fluorouracil is the most active single agent for patients with metastatic disease, but it induces only a 21% patient remission rate and virtually no complete remissions. Semustine, mitomycin, and cyclophosphamide all have definite but lesser degrees of activity. Mitomycin or carmustine also has activity in combination with fluorouracil. All of these regimens induce substantial hematologic toxicity. Because these combinations (1) do not induce complete remission, (2) do not prolong survival as yet, and (3) are rather toxic, their use should be limited to patients with symptomatic metastatic disease. Their use in the adjuvant setting with postoperative patients with Dukes stage C colon cancer is currently a matter for investigation, and routine application should be discouraged because of the substantial risk of major or life-threatening toxicity. Fluorouracil alone has been extensively tried as a surgical adjuvant and has produced only a minor reduction in the relapse rate observed with surgery alone.

Gastric carcinoma and pancreatic carcinoma are less common but far more aggressive lesions that usually cannot be completely resected surgically and are generally grossly metastatic at the time of surgery. The combination of fluorouracil, doxorubicin, and mitomycin has a 50% response rate in advanced stomach cancer, with definite prolongation of survival in at least 20% of patients, and the use of this regimen is therefore indicated in such cases. Responses are less frequent in pancreatic cancer.

Islet cell carcinoma of the pancreas arising from B cells and secreting insulin has been found to be exquisitely sensitive to the antibiotic streptozocin. The results have been exceedingly good in this rare tumor, and this therapy may be curative in some patients.

BRONCHOGENIC CARCINOMA

The management of epidermoid cancers, large cell cancers, and adenocarcinomas of the lung is very unsatisfactory, and prevention (primarily through avoidance of cigarette smoking) remains the most important means of control. The average life expectancy after diagnosis has been 8 months. The tumor can rarely be cured by surgery, and x-ray therapy is used primarily for palliation of pain, obstruction, or bleeding. Intrapleural BCG may play a modest adjunctive role in operable stage I lung cancer and appears to reduce the early recurrence rate. However, in most cases of lung cancer, distant metastases (including spread to the bone marrow) have often occurred by the time of diagnosis, and chemotherapy therefore appears to be the most feasible approach.

Although lung cancer had been notoriously resistant to all conventional forms of cancer chemotherapy, several novel approaches now show promise. Histologic examination of tumor tissue has been found to be important in identifying subgroups of patients who will respond to chemotherapy. For adenocarcinomas of the lung, the combination of fluorouracil, vincristine, and mitomycin induces remissions in 40% of patients. Patients with oat cell lung cancer (the most rapidly growing type) show the best responses to cyclophosphamide as well as to combination chemotherapy with agents such as doxorubicin, cyclophosphamide, VP16, methotrexate, and nitrosoureas.

Oat cell carcinoma patients with limited extent of disease respond best to such regimens. They also require whole brain irradiation to sterilize occult central nervous system metastases, which are usually present in such patients.

Several local complications also deserve mention, as they can be improved with chemotherapy. Mechlorethamine treatment of patients with superior vena caval compression often relieves this acute and frequently fatal complication of bronchogenic carcinoma. Pleural effusion due to carcinomatous metastasis may be controlled by intrapleural injection of mechlorethamine, quinacrine, or tetracycline (see below).

MALIGNANT MELANOMA & MISCELLANEOUS SARCOMAS

Metastatic melanoma is one of the most difficult neoplasms to treat. Most chemotherapeutic agents are reported to induce regression in at least 10% of melanoma patients; however, spontaneous regressions also occur, especially in skin metastases, and regressions of cutaneous lesions thus may not necessarily imply sensitivity to chemotherapy. Immunologic reactivity to the tumor by host lymphocytes may partially explain the evanescent changes in skin lesions, but "spontaneous regression" of visceral disease is rare, and metastases occur in virtually every organ in the body. Alkylating agents such as melphalan and hydroxyurea occasionally cause visceral regressions. Dacarbazine is the most active single drug and may be useful in combinations. Combinations of carmustine and vincristine have been tried with limited success. The addition of nonspecific immunotherapy with BCG (to chemotherapy or surgery or both) remains controversial and has not yet been shown to improve therapy significantly. Tamoxifen is also active occasionally, but is not clearly related to ER-like activity in the tumor.

Osteogenic sarcoma and Ewing's sarcoma respond to doxorubicin, and a combination of doxorubicin and dacarbazine may induce substantial regressions in about 40% of cases of rhabdomyosarcoma, fibrosarcoma, osteogenic sarcoma, and related tumors. The use of doxorubicin as part of adjuvant therapy after primary surgery for osteosarcoma has already increased the median survival time and now appears likely to increase the long-term salvage rate for this otherwise almost uniformly fatal neoplasm. While high-dose methotrexate therapy followed by leucovorin rescue can produce similar results, it has a greater likelihood of serious toxicity.

BRAIN TUMORS

Stage III and stage IV astrocytomas (predominantly glioblastoma multiforme) are the most common primary brain tumors, and they have been extraordinarily refractory to surgical therapy. Although advances in diagnostic methods such as CT scan have better delineated the site of primary involvement for surgical therapy, the median survival time with surgery alone is still in the range of 20 weeks. As shown by the National Brain Tumor Study Group, the addition of whole brain radiotherapy (approximately 5500 R) or carmustine alone (220 mg/m^2 every 6–8 weeks) increases the median survival time to 36 weeks, whereas the use of multimodality therapy (surgery plus radiotherapy plus carmustine) increases it to 50 weeks, with approximately 25% of patients still alive at 18 months. This multimodality approach, although still limited in efficacy, can be recommended as palliation for patients with such tumors until more effective regimens are developed by investigative teams particularly interested in research on the treatment of brain tumors.

CONTROL OF MALIGNANT EFFUSIONS & ASCITES

The direct injection of mechlorethamine or other anticancer drugs into the involved cavity will eliminate or suppress an effusion in about two-thirds of patients with ascites and effusions due to carcinoma. The method is useful irrespective of the types of primary tumor.

The procedure is as follows: Most of the pleural or ascitic fluid is withdrawn, and the drug is injected into the cavity. The dose of mechlorethamine employed intrapleurally is 0.4 mg/kg, or a total dose of 20–30 mg in the usual patient. The solution is prepared immediately before administration so as to avoid loss of potency through hydrolysis. A free flow of fluid from the cavity must be established before the drug is injected to avoid injection into the tissues. Pleural or peritoneal effusions due to ovarian or breast carcinoma are frequently responsive to an intracavitary dose of 60 mg/m^2 of bleomycin. After the drug is injected, the patient is placed in a variety of positions in order to distribute the drug throughout the pleural cavity. On the following day, the remaining fluid is withdrawn.

Pain, nausea, and vomiting sometimes occur following injection of mechlorethamine into the pleural cavity. Nausea and vomiting usually occur within a few hours after administration but can be controlled with chlorpromazine, 25 mg intramuscularly given immediately before the procedure and at intervals following the injection. Bone marrow depression is mild with this method of administration, except in patients who have received extensive radiation therapy. Agents such as bleomycin or thiotepa are preferable to mechlorethamine for intraperitoneal use, since they cause significantly less peritoneal irritation and pain.

Quinacrine and tetracycline have been employed intrapleurally with similar therapeutic benefit. Local pain and fever are commonly noted. There is no systemic hematopoietic depression.

EVALUATION OF TUMOR RESPONSE

Inasmuch as cancer chemotherapy can induce clinical improvement, significant toxicity, or both, it is extremely important to assess critically the beneficial effects of treatment to determine that the net effect is favorable. Preliminary evidence regarding predictive selection of chemotherapy with the tumor stem cell assay is quite encouraging, particularly with respect to rejecting drugs that would probably cause toxicity without compensating clinical benefit. The assay also appears to be relatively accurate (70%) in identifying drugs that will prove useful in the patient. The most valuable signs to follow after initiation of therapy include the following:

A. Tumor Size: Demonstration of significant shrinkage in tumor size on physical examination, chest film or other x-ray, or special scanning procedure such as bone scanning (breast, prostate cancer), CT scan, or ultrasonography.

B. Marker Substances: Significant decrease in the quantity of a tumor product or marker substance that reflects the amount of tumor in the body. Examples of such markers include paraproteins in the serum or urine in multiple myeloma and macroglobulinemia, chorionic gonadotropin in choriocarcinoma and testicular tumors, urinary steroids in adrenal carcinoma and paraneoplastic Cushing's syndrome, 5-hydroxyindoleacetic acid in carcinoid syndrome, and prostatic acid phosphatase in prostatic carcinoma. Secreted tumor antigens such as alpha-fetoprotein can be found in hepatoma, in teratoembryonal carcinoma, and in occasional cases of gastric carcinoma and the carcinoembryonic antigen in carcinomas of the colon, lung, and breast. Techniques for measurement of these 2 fetal proteins are now generally available.

C. Organ Function: Normalization of function of organs that were previously impaired as a result of the presence of a tumor is a useful indicator of drug effectiveness. Examples of such improvement include the normalization of liver function (eg, increased serum albumin) in patients known to have liver metastases and improvement in neurologic findings in patients with cerebral metastases. Disappearance of the signs and symptoms of the paraneoplastic syndromes often falls in this general category and can be taken as an indication of tumor response.

D. General Well-Being and Performance Status: A valuable sign of clinical improvement is the general well-being of the patient. Although this finding is a combination of subjective and objective factors and may be subject to placebo effects, it nonetheless serves as an obvious and useful sign of clinical improvement and can be used in reassessment of some of the objective observations listed above. Factors included in the assessment of general well-being include improved appetite and weight gain and improved "performance status" (eg, ambulatory versus bedridden). Evaluation of factors such as activity status has the advantage of summarizing beneficial and toxic effects of chemotherapy and enables the physician to judge whether the net effect of chemotherapy is worthwhile palliation.

SECOND MALIGNANCIES & CANCER CHEMOTHERAPY

Second malignancy is a late complication of some types of cancer chemotherapy. The most frequent second malignancy is acute myelogenous leukemia (AML). Aside from AML, other second malignancies are sporadic. AML has been observed in up to 15% of patients with Hodgkin's disease who have received radiotherapy plus MOPP, or patients with multiple myeloma, ovarian, or breast carcinoma treated with melphalan. Several alkylating agents (as well as ionizing radiation) are considered to be leukemogenic. Additionally, procarbazine (a component of the MOPP combination) is known to be mutagenic to bacteria and carcinogenic in animals. The mechanisms of carcinogenesis with these other agents remain poorly understood. While the risk of AML is relatively small, the benefit of complete remission or cure of Hodgkin's disease or remission in other neoplasms is considerable. However, the benefit/risk ratio of adjuvant therapy of stage I breast cancer with melphalan could be relatively small if over 5% of women developed AML, because only 15–20% of women treated would be likely to have recurrent cancer. As further advances are made in chemical control and cure of cancer, the problem of the second malignant tumor assumes greater importance. There are already hints that certain alkylating agents (eg, cyclophosphamide) may be less carcinogenic than others. Systematic testing of carcinogenicity of anticancer drugs in several animal species allows selection of agents to be substituted for other more carcinogenic ones in chemotherapy regimens. In this fashion, the risk of second tumors should be reduced without sacrifice of therapeutic benefit.

• • •

References

General

Becker FF (editor): *Cancer: A Comprehensive Treatise*. Plenum Press, Vols 1, 2, 1975; Vols 3, 4, 5, 1976.

Capizzi RL (editor): The pharmacological basis of cancer chemotherapy. *Semin Oncol* 1977;**4:**131.

Chabner B et al: The clinical pharmacology of antineoplastic agents. (2 parts.) *N Engl J Med* 1975;**292:**1107, 1159.

Chen H-SG, Gross JF: Physiologically based pharmacokinetic models for anticancer drugs. *Cancer Chemother Pharmacol* 1979;**1:**85.

DeVita VT Jr: The evolution of therapeutic research in cancer. *N Engl J Med* 1978;**298:**907.

DeVita VT Jr, Hellman S, Rosenberg SA (editors): *Principles and Practice of Oncology*. Lippincott, 1982.

DeVita VT et al: The drug development and clinical trials program of the Division of Cancer Treatment, National Cancer Institute. *Cancer Clin Trials* 1979;**2:**195.

Dorr RT, Fritz WL: *Cancer Chemotherapy Handbook*. Elsevier/North Holland, 1980.

Goldie JH, Coldman AJ: A mathematical model for relating drug sensitivity of tumors to their spontaneous mutation rate. *Cancer Treat Rep* 1979;**63:**1727.

Haskell CM: *Cancer Treatment*. Saunders, 1980.

Kennedy KA et al: The hypoxic tumor cell: A target for selective cancer chemotherapy. *Biochem Pharmacol* 1980;**29:**1.

Pharmacological Basis of Cancer Chemotherapy: A Symposium. Williams & Wilkins, 1975.

Salmon SE (editor): *Cloning of Human Tumor Stem Cells*. A.R. Liss, 1980.

Salmon SE: Immunotherapy of cancer: Present status of trials in man. *Cancer Res* 1977;**37:**1245.

Salmon SE: Malignant disorders. Chap 32, pp 1013–1027, in: *Current Medical Diagnosis & Treatment 1982*. Krupp MA, Chatton MJ (editors). Lange, 1982.

Salmon SE et al: Quantitation of differential sensitivity of human-tumor stem cells to anticancer drugs. *N Engl J Med* 1978;**298:**1321.

Sartorelli AC, Johns DG (editors): *Antineoplastic and Immunosuppressive Agents*. 2 vols. Springer, 1975.

Sartorelli AC et al (editors): *Molecular Actions and Targets for Cancer Chemotherapeutic Agents*. Academic Press, 1981.

Skipper HE: Biochemical, biological, pharmacologic, toxicologic, kinetic and clinical relationships. *Cancer* 1968;**21:**600.

Skipper HE et al: Implications of biochemical, pharmacologic and toxicologic relationships in the design of optimal therapy. *Cancer Chemother Rep* 1970;**54:**431.

Von Hoff DD et al: Association between human tumor colony-forming assay results and response of an individual patient's tumor to chemotherapy. *Am J Med* 1981;**70:**1027.

Antimetabolites

Bloch A (editor): Chemistry, biology and clinical uses of nucleoside analogs. *Ann NY Acad Sci* 1975;**255:**1.

Erlichman et al: Phase I trial of n-(phosphonacetyl)-L-aspartate. *Cancer Res* 1979;**39:**3992.

Frei E et al: New approaches to cancer chemotherapy with methotrexate. *N Engl J Med* 1975;**292:**845.

Haghbin M: Antimetabolites in the prophylaxis and treatment of central nervous system leukemia. *Cancer Treat Rep* 1977;**61:**661.

Proceedings of the High-Dose Methotrexate Therapy Meeting. *Cancer Chemother Rep* 1975;**6(part 3):**1.

Stoller RG et al: Use of plasma pharmacokinetics to predict and prevent methotrexate toxicity. *N Engl J Med* 1977;**297:**630.

Alkylating Agents

Carter SK (editor): Proceedings of the 7th New Drug Seminar: Nitrosoureas. *Cancer Treat Rep* 1976;**60:**645.

Connors TA et al: Regression of human lung tumor xenografts induced by water-soluble analogs or hexamethylmelamine. *Cancer Treat Rep* 1977;**61:**927.

Cox PJ, Farmer PB, Jarman M (editors): Proceedings of the Symposium on the Metabolism and Mechanism of Action of Cyclophosphamide. *Cancer Treat Rep* 1976;**60:**299.

Hayes DM et al: High dose cis-platinum diammine dichloride: Amelioration of renal toxicity by mannitol diuresis. *Cancer* 1977;**39:**1372.

Rosenberg B: Possible mechanisms for antitumor activity of platinum coordination complexes. *Cancer Chemother Rep* 1975;**59:**589.

Van Duuren BL (editor): Biological effects of alkylating agents. *Ann NY Acad Sci* 1969;**163:**589.

Von Hoff DD et al: Estramustine phosphate: A specific chemotherapeutic agent? *J Urol* 1977;**117:**464.

Antibiotics & Other Natural Products

Alberts DS et al: Bleomycin pharmacokinetics in man: 2. Intracavitary administration. *Cancer Chemother Pharmacol* 1979;**2:**127.

Carter SK et al (editors): *Bleomycin: Current Status and New Developments*. Academic Press, 1978.

Creagan ET, Moertel CG, O'Fallon JR: Failure of high dose vitamin C to benefit patients with advanced cancer. *N Engl J Med* 1979;**301:**687.

Garnik MB, Ensminger WD, Israel M: A clinical-pharmacological evaluation of hepatic arterial infusion. *Cancer Res* 1979;**39:**4105.

Gralla RJ et al: Phase II evaluation of vindesine in patients with non-small cell carcinoma of the lung. *Cancer Treat Rep* 1979;**63:**1343.

Marmor JB, Kozak D, Hahn G: Effects of systemically administered bleomycin or adriamycin with local hyperthermia on primary tumor and lung metastases. *Cancer Treat Rep* 1979;**63:**1279.

Proceedings of 5th New Drug Seminar: Adriamycin. *Cancer Chemother Rep* 1975;**6(part 3):**83.

Radice PA, Bunn PA Jr, Idhe DC: Therapeutic trials with VP-16-213 and VM-26. *Cancer Treat Rep* 1979;**63:**1231.

Rozencweig M et al: VM26 and VP16-213: A comparative analysis. *Cancer* 1977;**40:**334.

Vindesine International Workshop (multiple authors). *Cancer Chemother and Pharmacol* 1979;**2:**229.

Young RC et al: The anthracycline antineoplastic drugs. *N Engl J Med* 1981;**305:**139.

Steroids & Steroid Antagonists

Allegra JC et al: Association between steroid hormone receptor status and disease-free interval in breast cancer. *Cancer Treat Rep* 1979;**63:**1271.

Eckman P et al: Steroid receptor content in human prostatic carcinoma and response to endocrine therapy. *Cancer* 1979;**44:**1173.

Jensen EV et al: The role of estrophilin in estrogen action. *Vitam Horm* 1974;**32:**89.

Kaiser N et al: Glucocorticoid receptors and the mechanisms of resistance in the cortisol-sensitive and resistant lines of lymphosarcoma. *Cancer Res* 1974;**34:**621.

Lippman M et al: In vitro models for the study of hormone-dependent human breast cancer. *N Engl J Med* 1977;**296:**154.

McGuire W, Carbone P, Vollmer E (editors): *Estrogen Receptors in Human Breast Cancer*. Raven, 1975.

Tamoxifen Workshop. *Cancer Treat Rep* 1976;**60:**1409.

Yamomoto K, Stampfer M, Tomkins GM: Receptors from glucocorticoid-sensitive lymphoma cells: Physical and DNA-binding properties. *Proc Natl Acad Sci USA* 1974;**71:**3901.

Clinical Oncology: Combined Modality or Drug Combinations

Alberts DS, Durie BGM, Salmon SE: Doxorubicin/BCNU chemotherapy for multiple myeloma in relapse. *Lancet* 1976;**1:**926.

Bagley CW et al: Advanced lymphosarcoma: Intensive cyclical combination chemotherapy with cyclophosphamide, vincristine, and prednisone. *Ann Intern Med* 1972;**76:**227.

Bonadonna G, Veronesi V (editors): Breast cancer. *Semin Oncol* 1978;**5:**341. [Entire issue.]

Bonadonna G, Mathé G, Salmon SE (editors): Adjuvant therapies and post surgical markers of minimal residual disease. In: *Recent Results in Cancer Research*. Vols 67 and 68. Springer-Verlag, 1979.

Bonadonna G et al: Combination chemotherapy as an adjuvant treatment in operable breast cancer. *N Engl J Med* 1976;**294:**405.

Bonadonna G et al: Combination chemotherapy (MOPP or ABVD)—radiotherapy approach in advanced Hodgkin's disease. *Cancer Treat Rep* 1977;**61:**7169.

Cortes EP et al: Amputation and adriamycin in primary osteosarcoma. *N Engl J Med* 1974;**291:**998.

De Vita VT Jr, Young RC, Canellos G: Combination versus single agent chemotherapy: A review of the basis for selection of drug treatment of cancer. *Cancer* 1975;**35:**98.

De Vita VT Jr et al: Combination chemotherapy in the treatment of advanced Hodgkin's disease. *Ann Intern Med* 1970;**73:**881.

Einhorn LH, Donohue J: Cis-diammine-dichloroplatinum, vinblastine and bleomycin combination chemotherapy in disseminated testicular cancer. *Ann Intern Med* 1977;**87:**293.

Einhorn LH, Williams SD: Current concepts in cancer: The

role of cisplatinum in solid tumor chemotherapy. *N Engl J Med* 1979;**300:**289.

Fisher B et al: L-Phenylalanine mustard (L-PAM) in the management of primary breast cancer: A report of early findings. *N Engl J Med* 1975;**292:**117.

Greenspan EM: Combination cytotoxic chemotherapy in advanced disseminated breast carcinoma. *J Mt Sinai Hosp* 1966;**33:**1.

Jaffe N: The potential of combined modalities approaches for the treatment of malignant bone tumors in children. *Cancer Treat Rev* (March) 1975;**2:**33.

Jones SE: Non-Hodgkin lymphomas. *JAMA* 1975;**234:**633.

Jones SE, Durie BGM, Salmon SE: Combination chemotherapy with adriamycin and cyclophosphamide for advanced breast cancer. *Cancer* 1975;**36:**90.

Kaplan HS: *Hodgkin's Disease*. Harvard Univ Press, 1972.

Kaplan HS: Hodgkin's disease: Multidisciplinary contributions to the conquest of a neoplasm. *Radiology* 1977;**123:**551.

Macdonald JS et al: 5-Fluorouracil, adriamycin, and mitomycin C (FAM) combination chemotherapy in the treatment of advanced gastric cancer. *Cancer* 1979;**44:**42.

Miller TP, Jones SE: Chemotherapy of localized histiocytic lymphoma. *Lancet* 1979;**1:**358.

Proceedings of the Conference on Breast Cancer. *Cancer* 1977;**39(Suppl):**2697.

Rainey JM, Jones SE, Salmon SE: Combination chemotherapy for advanced breast cancer utilizing vincristine, adriamycin and cyclophosphamide (VAC). *Cancer* 1979;**43:**66.

Rhomes JA et al: Central nervous system therapy and combination chemotherapy of childhood lymphocytic leukemia. *Blood* 1971;**37:**272.

Salmon SE, Jones SE (editors): *Adjuvant Therapy of Cancer III*. Grune & Stratton, 1981.

Santoro A et al: Alternating drug combinations in the treatment of advanced Hodgkin's disease. *N Engl J Med* 1982;**306:**770.

Young RC et al: Advanced ovarian carcinoma: A prospective clinical trial of melphalan (L-PAM) versus combination chemotherapy (Hexa-CAF). *N Engl J Med* 1978;**299:**1261.

Clinical Oncology: Miscellaneous

Alexanian R et al: Treatment of multiple myeloma: Combination chemotherapy with different melphalan dose regimens. *JAMA* 1969;**208:**1685.

Blum RH, Carter SK, Agre K: A clinical review of bleomycin: A new antineoplastic agent. *Cancer* 1973;**31:**903.

Bodey GP: Infections in cancer patients. *Cancer Treat Rev* (June) 1975;**2:**89.

Brennan M: Total parenteral nutrition in the cancer patient. *N Engl J Med* 1981;**305:**375.

Dean JC, Salmon SE, Griffith KS: Prevention of doxorubicin-induced alopecia with scalp hypothermia. *N Engl J Med* 1979;**301:**1427.

DeVita VT Jr: The consequences of the chemotherapy of Hodgkin's disease: The 10th David A. Karnofsky Lecture. *Cancer* 1981;**47:**1.

Durie BGM, Salmon SE: A clinical staging system for multiple myeloma. *Cancer* 1975;**36:**842.

Fisher B et al: Treatment of primary breast cancer with chemotherapy and tamoxifen. *N Engl J Med* 1981;**305:**1.

Gale RP: Advances in the treatment of acute myelogenous leukemia. *N Engl J Med* 1979;**300:**1189.

Glucksberg H et al: Combination chemotherapy (CMFVP) versus L-phenylalanine mustard (L-PAM) for operable breast cancer with positive axillary nodes. *Cancer* 1982;**50:**423.

Gottlieb JA, Hill CS Jr: Chemotherapy of thyroid cancer with adriamycin. *N Engl J Med* 1974;**290:**193.

Hamburger AW, Salmon SE: Primary bioassay of human tumor stem cells. *Science* 1977;**197:**461.

Hutter AM, Kayhoe DE: Adrenal cortical carcinoma: Results of treatment with o,p'DDD in 138 patients. *Am J Med* 1966;**41:**572.

Li MC, Hertz R, Spencer DB: Effect of methotrexate therapy upon choriocarcinoma. *Proc Soc Exp Biol Med* 1956;**93:**361.

Macdonald JS et al: 5-Fluorouracil, adriamycin, and mitomycin C (FAM) combination chemotherapy in the treatment of advanced gastric cancer. *Cancer* 1979;**44:**42.

McIntyre OR: Current concepts in cancer: Multiple myeloma. *N Engl J Med* 1979;**301:**193.

Merrigan TC, Sikora K, Breeder JH: Preliminary observations on the effects of human leukocyte interferon in non-Hodgkin's lymphoma. *N Engl J Med* 1979;**299:**149.

Miller RA, Levy R: Response of cutaneous T cell lymphoma to therapy with hybridoma monoclonal antibody. *Lancet* 1981;**2:**226.

Phillips TL et al: The hypoxic cell sensitizer programme in the United States. *Br J Cancer* 1978;**37(Suppl 3):**276.

Reifenstein E: Hydroxyprogesterone caproate therapy in advanced endometrial cancer. *Cancer* 1971;**27:**485.

Seyberth HS et al: Prostaglandins as mediators of hypercalcemia associated with cancer. *N Engl J Med* 1975;**293:**1283.

Storring RA et al: Oral non-absorbed antibiotics prevent infection in acute non-lymphoblastic leukaemia. *Lancet* 1977;**2:**837.

Veronesi U et al: Inefficacy of immediate node dissection in stage I melanoma of the limbs. *N Engl J Med* 1977;**297:**627.

Warren RD, Bender RA: Drug interactions with antineoplastic agents. *Cancer Treat Rep* 1977;**61:**1231.

Wilson CB: Current concepts in cancer: Brain tumors. *N Engl J Med* 1979;**300:**1469.

Ziegler JL, Magrath IT, Olweny CLM: Cure of Burkitt's lymphoma. *Lancet* 1979;**2:**936.

Drugs & the Immune System | 57

Sydney E. Salmon, MD

IMMUNOSUPPRESSIVE AGENTS

THE IMMUNE MECHANISM

With the increase in understanding of normal mechanisms of immunity and the role of immunologic abnormalities in the pathophysiology of certain disorders, agents that suppress the immune response now play an important role in tissue transplantation procedures and in certain diseases associated with disorders of immunity. Although some of the details of the overall immune mechanism are still uncertain, a general scheme of the steps involved in the genesis of specific immunity can be sketched (Figs 57–1 and 57–2) as a means of placing the effects and toxicities of immunosuppressive agents in perspective.

Specific immunity appears to result from the interaction of antigens (substances the host normally recognizes as foreign) with mononuclear cells that circulate in the blood and lymph. The nature of self-recognition, or "tolerance," is complex, but it appears to be defined in utero, during development of the lymphoid tissues. Mechanisms that have been impli-

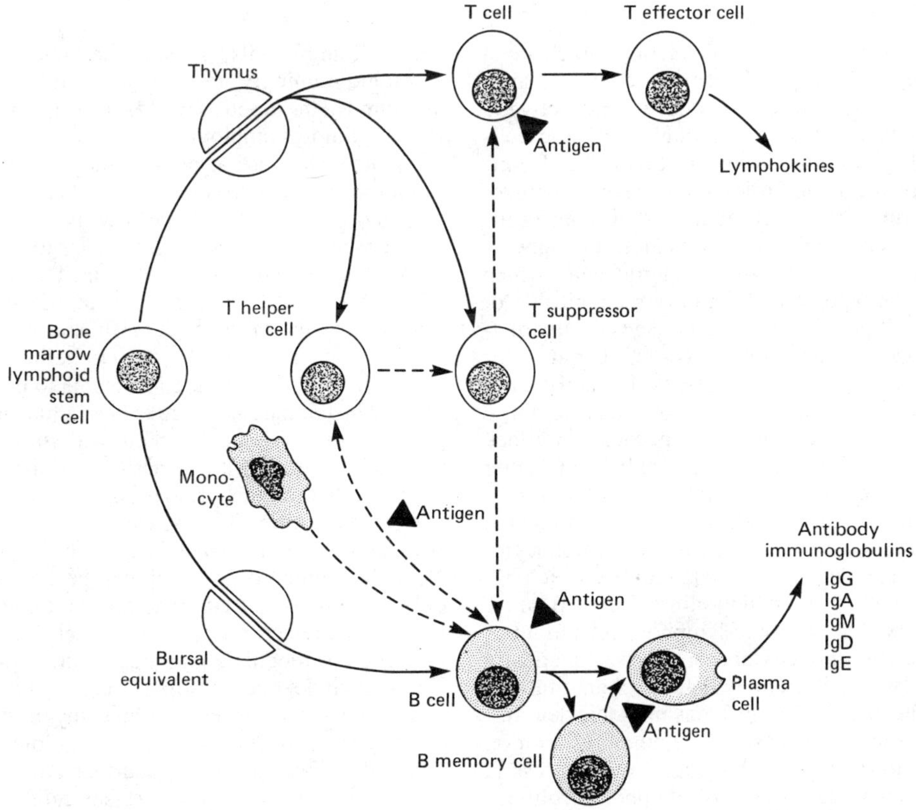

Figure 57–1. Genesis and interactions of the immune system. Solid arrows denote stimulation or development. Dashed arrows indicate inhibition.

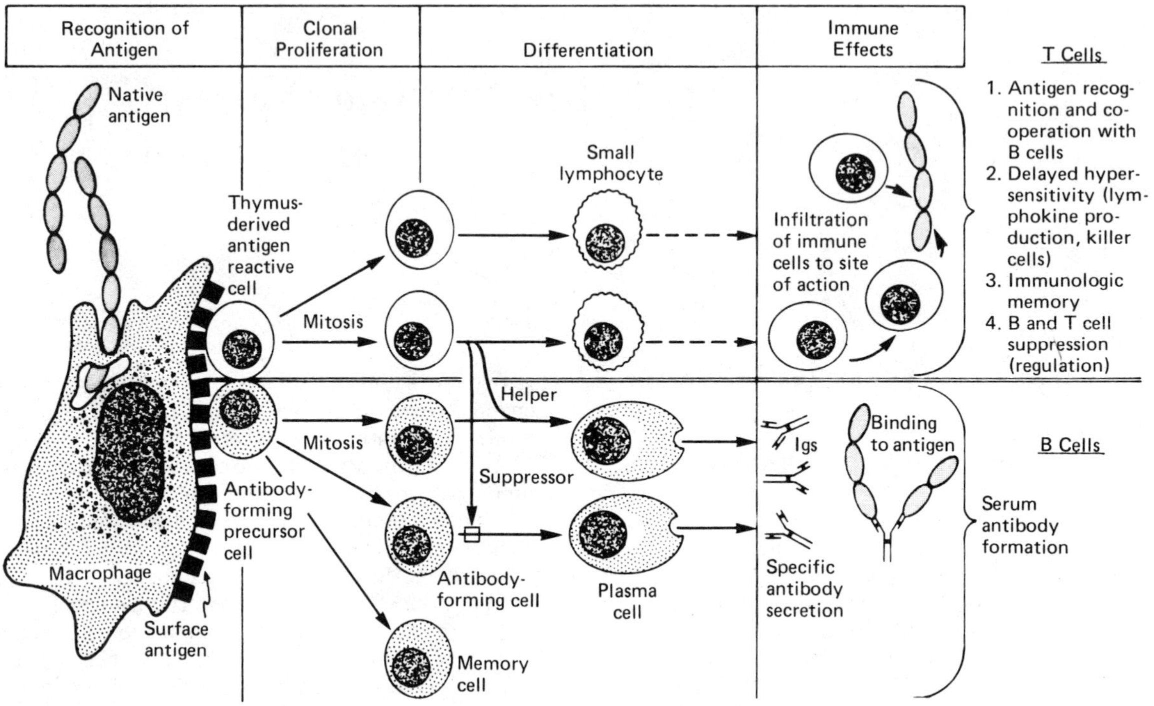

Figure 57–2. A theoretical scheme of cellular and humoral immunity.

cated in tolerance include clonal deletion, blockade of antigen receptor by antigen-antibody complex, antibody to cell surface immunoglobulin, and active T cell-mediated suppression. Although lymphoid cells derived embryologically from the thymus and bone marrow play the major role in the development of specific immunity, a critical initial "antigen-processing" step occurs in the mononuclear phagocyte (the blood monocyte or the tissue macrophage), which then makes the antigen more readily recognizable or available to lymphoid cells. Macrophages or supernatants from macrophage cultures also can stimulate or inhibit immunoproliferative reactions. Recently it has been established that macrophages secrete large amounts of thymidine, apparently because they lack thymidine kinase. It remains to be established whether local excess thymidine concentrations can block proliferative reactions in vivo, although this phenomenon has been observed in vitro. Additionally, monocytes and macrophages secrete prostaglandin E_2, which has been found to inhibit immunoproliferation of B and T cell precursors. The ability of lymphoid cells to interact with specific antigens appears to be genetically determined, with different lymphoid clones having individual specificities for different antigenic determinants. The genetic regulation of immunoproliferation also appears to reside in macrophages that express Ia antigens which signal or control lymphoid proliferation.

A basic dualism seems to govern the function of the lymphoid system. Two different types of lymphoid cells—T and B cells—mediate cellular immunity and serologic immunity, respectively. Both types of cells are found in the blood as well as in peripheral lymphoid tissues. Studies employing scanning electron microscopy have shown that both B and T cells may have numerous microvilli on their surfaces. Long-lived clones of small lymphoid cells derived from or influenced by the thymus (T cells) appear to recognize the antigen and presumably bind to it. The T cell specificity of this line of cells appears to arise from a bone marrow progenitor under the influence of thymic hormone, which is produced by the epithelioid component of the thymus. T cell function seems to be modulated also by histamine, and T cells bear a histamine type 2 receptor that can be blocked with burimamide or metiamide but not with "classic" antihistamines such as diphenhydramine. The proliferation of clones of antigen recognition T cells, which occurs after contact with antigen, is responsible for the development of "cellular immunity," which can be demonstrated in delayed hypersensitivity reactions and is important in tissue graft rejection. Specific subsets of T cells also influence or modulate antibody synthesis by B cells. These include both "helper" and "suppressor" T cells. The T cell subsets can be assayed functionally, but they are also identified with monoclonal antibodies directed against specific cell surface antigens that differ on the T helper and suppressor cells. T cells also have surface receptors that allow them to recognize a foreign antigen and react to it. T cells appear to exert their effects by direct cytotoxic interaction (eg, with

Table 57–1. The lymphokines produced by lymphocytes.

Substance	Effect
Transfer factor (TF)	Transfer of cutaneous hypersensitivity.
Migration inhibitory factor (MIF)	Inhibits macrophage migration.
Interleukin II	Stimulates growth of T lymphocytes.
Lymphotoxin (LT)	Cytotoxicity against target cells.
Chemotactic factor	Stimulates chemotactic migration of macrophages.
Interferon	Inhibits intracellular viral replication and immunoproliferation.
Immunoglobulin (Ig)	Specific antibody molecules.

tumor cells or transplants) and by release of various effector substances, or lymphokines (Table 57–1). In the case of most lymphokines (except immunoglobulins), it is not yet certain whether they are secreted by T cells, B cells, or both. The genesis of specific antibody immunoglobulins resides in the progeny of a second type of lymphoid cell, the antibody precursor cell (B cell), derived from the bone marrow. B cells can be identified by the presence of monoclonal immunoglobulins on their surfaces that are located in "spots" on the cell membrane and, through their antibody function, appear to serve as antigen receptors. B cells also have receptors for complement components and immune complexes as well as having cell surface "Ia-like" receptors that relate to the genetics of the immune response and are linked to the major histocompatibility complex. Prior to contact with antigen, lymphocyte surface immunoglobulin is predominantly of the IgD and IgM classes. By the time of birth, lymph node and splenic architecture includes parafollicular cuffs of thymus-derived lymphocytes and follicular nests of immunoglobulin-synthesizing cells that form germinal centers. Intimate cell-cell interaction between macrophages bearing the antigen in an immunogenic form on the cell surface and complementary clones of T cells and B cells are thought to be required before the clonal proliferation of T cells can develop cellular immunity and the B cells can form antibody-forming cells (Figs 57–1 and 57–2). The primary immunoproliferative response is augmented or inhibited by T cells with helper or suppressor function. A recently described natural killer (NK) cell may play an important role in tumor rejection. NK cells are surface immunoglobulin-negative, Fc receptor-positive lymphocytes with low affinity for sheep red blood cells. Studies with monoclonal antisera suggest that NK cells may be of T cell or monocytic origin, but they may represent an entirely separate lineage of lymphoid cells. NK cells have bred reactivity against tumor and normal cells and may play an important role in host defense. However, their in vivo relevance remains uncertain. Antibody-forming cells can increase their synthetic capacity by further differentiation into plasma cells, clones of which specifically secrete large amounts of antibody of one of the immunoglobulin classes—IgG, IgA, IgM, IgD, or IgE. During the course of this differentiation, individual clones may "switch" their immunoglobulin type from IgD to IgM to IgG or IgA, even though the active site of the secreted antibody retains the identical structure after this "switch." Finally, specific antibody binds to the foreign antigen, leading to its precipitation, inactivation (eg, virus), lysis (eg, red cells), or phagocytosis (eg, bacteria). In some of these circumstances, complement is bound to the antigen-antibody complex and facilitates the destruction or phagocytosis of the antigen. Once an antibody response is established, reexposure to antigen leads to an immediate chemical combination of antigen and antibody and also serves to provide a "booster" for a rapid secondary wave of cell proliferation and antibody synthesis. The dual nature of immunity is underscored by certain "experiments of nature," or genetic diseases. For example, DiGeorge's syndrome, resulting from absence of the third branchial cleft, is associated with absent thymic development and impaired delayed hypersensitivity but normal antibody formation, whereas delayed hypersensitivity is usually normal in X-linked congenital agammaglobulinemia, which presents as an antibody deficiency syndrome. Infants with DiGeorge's syndrome or those with severe combined immunodeficiency (missing both cellular and humoral immunity) lack circulating thymic hormone activity. Studies of circulating T and B cells in the blood have shown that patients with DiGeorge's syndrome lack T cells, whereas those with congenital agammaglobulinemia lack B cells. Patients with later onset of agammaglobulinemia may have circulating B cells that seem to be inhibited from undergoing terminal differentiation into plasma cells. This inhibition may be due to the action of suppressor T cells.

The complexity of the immune system appears to provide a sufficient number of control points to render the emergence of a "forbidden clone," which is reactive against the host's own constituents, a relatively rare event. Normally, most components of the lymphoid system remain in a highly "repressed" state until they are selectively activated for a specific immune response. The numerous steps of the process also imply that immunosuppressive agents can be directed at various steps along this pathway (Fig 57–3), including the induction of specific tolerance. Because the immune system provides a major barricade against invading microorganisms (including oncogenic viruses), toxins, and foreign cells, generalized immunosuppression can potentially be very dangerous to the host.

With only one notable exception—Rh_0 (D) immune globulin—the clinically useful immunosuppressive agents that are now available may have general immunosuppressive properties and must be used with caution. Generalized immunosuppression increases the risk of infection and may also increase the risk of development of lymphoreticular and other forms of cancer. In general, it is easier to block or attenuate a primary immune response with immunosuppressive drugs than to suppress an established immune response.

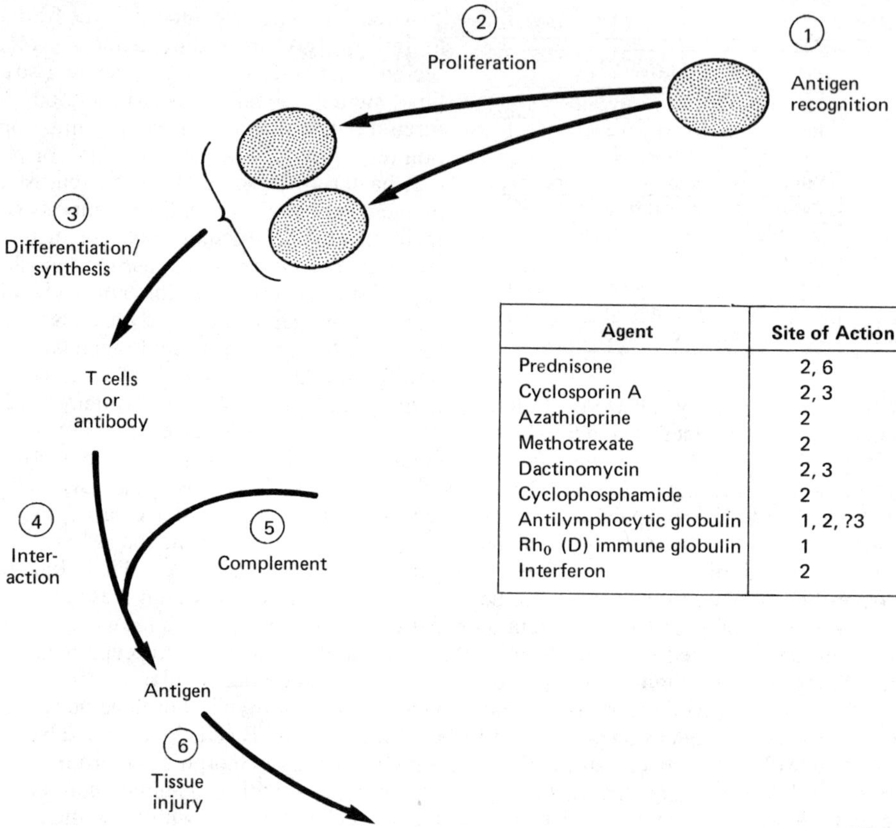

Agent	Site of Action
Prednisone	2, 6
Cyclosporin A	2, 3
Azathioprine	2
Methotrexate	2
Dactinomycin	2, 3
Cyclophosphamide	2
Antilymphocytic globulin	1, 2, ?3
Rh_0 (D) immune globulin	1
Interferon	2

Figure 57–3. The sites of action of immunosuppressive and immunomodulating agents on the immune response.

Even with these limitations and cautions, immunosuppression is of proved usefulness in a number of acquired immune disorders as well as in organ transplantation.

TESTS OF IMMUNOCOMPETENCE

A wide variety of techniques have been used to test immunologic competence and its drug-induced suppression. The simplest tests that can be used to detect the effects of immunosuppressive or immunostimulating agents include the following:

(1) Delayed hypersensitivity testing with skin test antigens to detect the ability to respond to mumps, streptokinase-streptodornase, *Candida albicans*, and other antigens to which most individuals have been exposed or to respond to sensitizing chemicals such as dinitrochlorobenzene.

(2) Measurement of serum immunoglobulins, serum complement, and specific antibodies to various natural and acquired antibodies.

(3) Serial measurements of antibody response after primary immunization or a secondary booster injection (Fig 57–4).

(4) Absolute circulating lymphocyte counts.

(5) Measurement of the percentages of B cells and T cells (''rosette testing'') and ''null cells'' that comprise the circulating blood lymphocyte count.

These relatively simple tests plus the evaluation of clinical responses in organ transplantation and autoimmune disorders have provided most of the current information on the in vivo effects of the immunosuppressive agents in humans. However, evidence of immunosuppression as measured by these tests of immune response does not always correlate well with the clinical response of the disease state being treated. The relevance to in vivo events of cell responses in various in vitro tests of lymphoid function, such as lymphocyte transformation testing, is less clear. Lymphocyte stimulation with phytohemagglutinin (PHA) measures the proliferative capacity of T cells; pokeweed mitogen measures the response of both B and T cells. Nonetheless, it is clear that once the in vitro tests are well standardized and made quantitative, they will take on an increasing importance and may supplant some of the in vivo studies.

RELATIONSHIP BETWEEN IMMUNOSUPPRESSIVE THERAPY & CANCER CHEMOTHERAPY

Although there is definite overlap between the drugs used for immunosuppression (Fig 57–3) and those used in cancer chemotherapy (see Chapter 56),

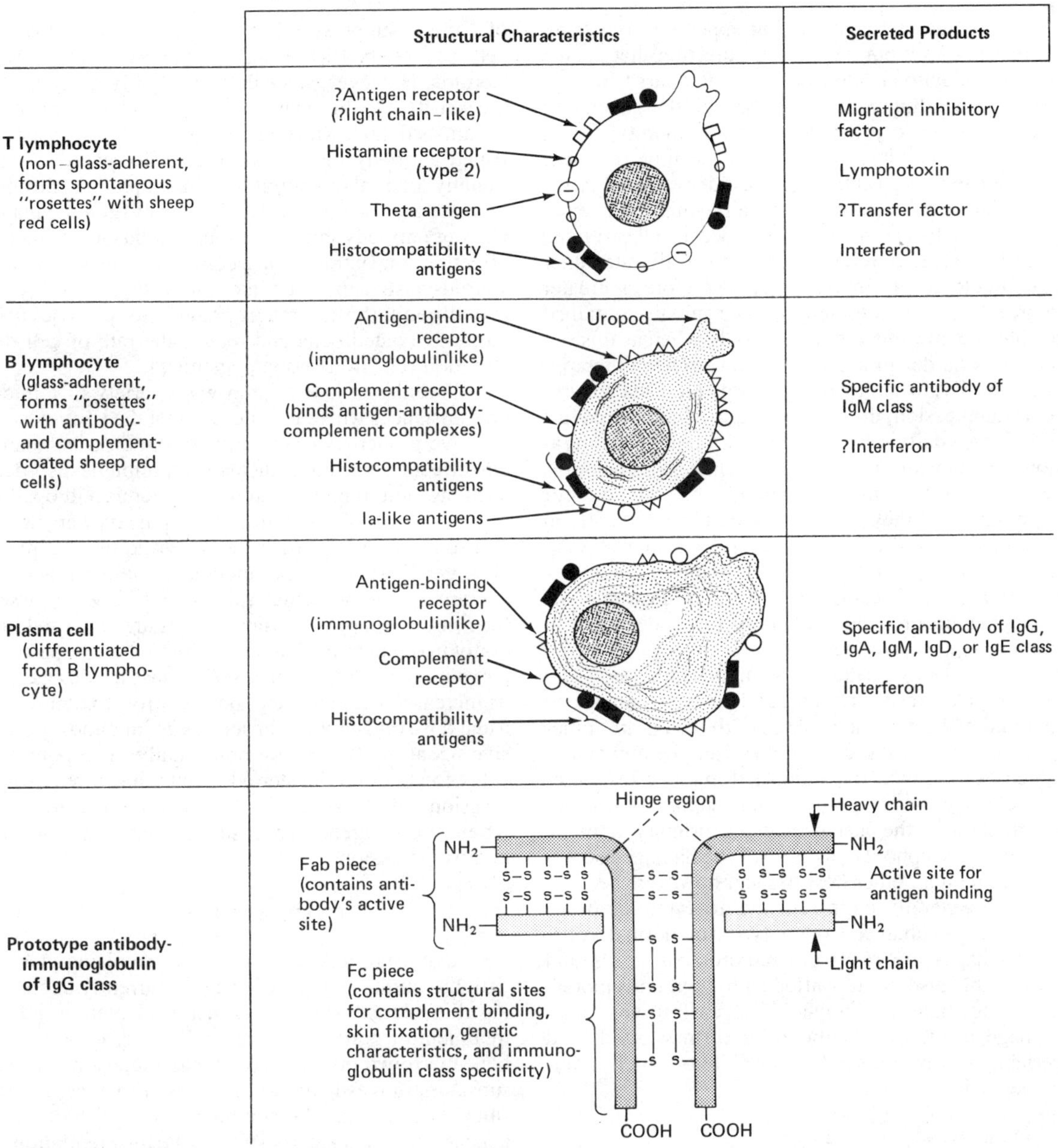

Figure 57–4. Effectors in the immune response. Specific cell types including T lymphocytes, B lymphocytes, and plasma cells—as well as secreted antibody-immunoglobulin—have binding sites for specific antigen as well as differential genetic and functional characteristics. Membrane features as well as secreted products can thus be seen to have important functions in the immune response.

different principles govern their use in these 2 disease categories. The general pharmacologic properties and toxicities of several of these agents (corticosteroids, alkylating agents, and certain structural analogs) were described in Chapter 56. The unique applications of these and other immunosuppressive drugs will be reviewed in this chapter in relationship to the action of these agents on the immune system and their effects in specific disease states. Since many cytotoxic drugs (eg, structural analogs) act primarily on proliferating cells, there is, in a sense, a similarity between their uses against proliferating cancer cells and against proliferating immune cells. However, the character and kinetics of cancer cell proliferation (see Chapter 56) are rather dissimilar to immune cell proliferation and allow different features to be exploited in immunosuppression. For example, whereas cancer cell proliferation appears to be "unstimulated," immune cell proliferation usually occurs in response to the presence of a specific antigen. While division of individual malignant cells within a large cancer cell population appears to occur randomly in an apparently unsynchronized way, immune cell proliferation appears to be "synchronized" in a burst of mitotic division that occurs after introduction of the antigen, with a large fraction of the responding cells going through the generation cycle in order to produce specific immunity. Thus, when cytotoxic drugs are used at the time of initial exposure to foreign antigen (eg, a kidney transplant), a very high percentage of an initially small number of precursor cells can be destroyed, because the antigen stimulates selected relevant clones to proliferate rather than all clones of immune cells. Therefore, a greater degree of selective toxicity can be initially obtained against the unwanted immune clone, whereas this objective is harder to achieve in cancer chemotherapy. Additionally, when cytotoxic drugs are used for immunosuppression, they are generally administered in a low-dosage daily schedule to block immunoproliferation continuously. In contrast, when these same drugs (eg, cyclophosphamide) are used for cancer chemotherapy, they are administered intermittently in high-dosage "pulse" courses every 3–6 weeks. Such "pulse" administration permits rapid immune rebound between treatments, which is desirable for augmentation of tumor immunity but undesirable in immunosuppressive therapy.

The selective nature of immunosuppression in a synchronized response can result in less damage to other normal cells, and dosages of the drugs are sometimes lower than those used in cancer chemotherapy. When dealing with an established immune response, the selective advantage in immunosuppression is not so great as in the instance of the primary immune response. Lymphoid cells can still be damaged somewhat more than other host tissues, however, because they are generally more sensitive to cytotoxic drugs and radiation than are other types of normal cells. Macrophages are relatively radioresistant cells and presumably also are less affected by immunosuppressive drugs than are lymphoid cells. However, macrophage function is inhibited by corticosteroids and perhaps also by prostaglandin inhibitors such as indomethacin.

CORTICOSTEROIDS

Corticosteroids were the first class of hormonal agents that were recognized to have lympholytic properties. Administration of a glucocorticoid (eg, prednisone, dexamethasone) reduces the size and lymphoid content of the lymph nodes and spleen, although it has essentially no toxic effect on proliferating myeloid or erythroid stem cells in the bone marrow. Glucocorticoids are thought to interfere with the cell cycle of activated lymphoid cells. The mechanism of their action is described in Chapter 56. Prednisone is quite cytotoxic to certain subsets of T cells but can suppress both cellular immunity and antibody as well as prostaglandin and leukotriene synthesis. Limited data currently available suggest that some of the diverse effects of prednisone may be attributable to lysis of either "suppressor" or "helper" T cells. Plasma cells seem to be less sensitive to the effects of corticosteroids. However, since the precursor lymphoid cells are sensitive to this agent, the primary response can be diminished, and, with continued use, previously established antibody responses are also decreased. Additionally, continuous administration of prednisone does increase the fractional catabolic rate of IgG, the major class of antibody immunoglobulins, thus lowering the effective concentration of specific antibodies. Corticosteroids also appear to interfere with the ability of reticuloendothelial macrophages to phagocytose antibody-coated cells and reduce the rate of cell destruction (eg, in hemolytic anemias).

Prednisone is used in a wide variety of clinical circumstances where it is thought that the immunosuppressive properties of the drug account for its beneficial effects. Indications include autoimmune disorders such as autoimmune hemolytic anemia, idiopathic thrombocytopenic purpura, and lupus erythematosus and some cases of Hashimoto's thyroiditis. Additionally, corticosteroids also modulate allergic reactions and are used in bronchial asthma, as will be discussed later in this chapter. Corticosteroids are also used liberally in organ transplant recipients and are of particular value during rejection crises because the dosage can be increased without fear of bone marrow toxicity. The usual dose range for prednisone as an immunosuppressive agent is 10–100 mg orally daily. The potential side-effects of corticosteroids, including adrenal suppression (see Chapters 37 and 56), are also relevant when these agents are used chronically for immunosuppression.

CYCLOSPORIN A

Cyclosporin A (Fig 57–5) is a promising investigational immunosuppressive agent currently undergoing clinical trial in human organ transplantation and for treatment of graft-versus-host (GVH) syndrome after bone marrow transplantation. It has already undergone substantial investigation in animals with excellent results. The drug is a fat-soluble peptide antibiotic that appears to act at an early stage in the differentiation of T cells and has been hypothesized to cause clonal deletion. Recent in vitro studies have indicated that cyclosporin A inhibits the *production* of factors that stimulate T lymphocyte growth, but it does not block the *effect* of such factors on primed T cells. However, its exact mechanism of action is unknown.

Cyclosporin A has been given orally on a daily basis at a dosage of 10–25 mg/kg. Toxicities have included nephrotoxicity (which may be preventable with mannitol diuresis), some increase in incidence of viral infections, and transient liver dysfunction. There is very little bone marrow toxicity. While an increased incidence of lymphoma has been seen in transplant recipients receiving cyclosporin A, there is also an increased incidence of lymphoma in other transplant recipients who have received other immunosuppressive agents.

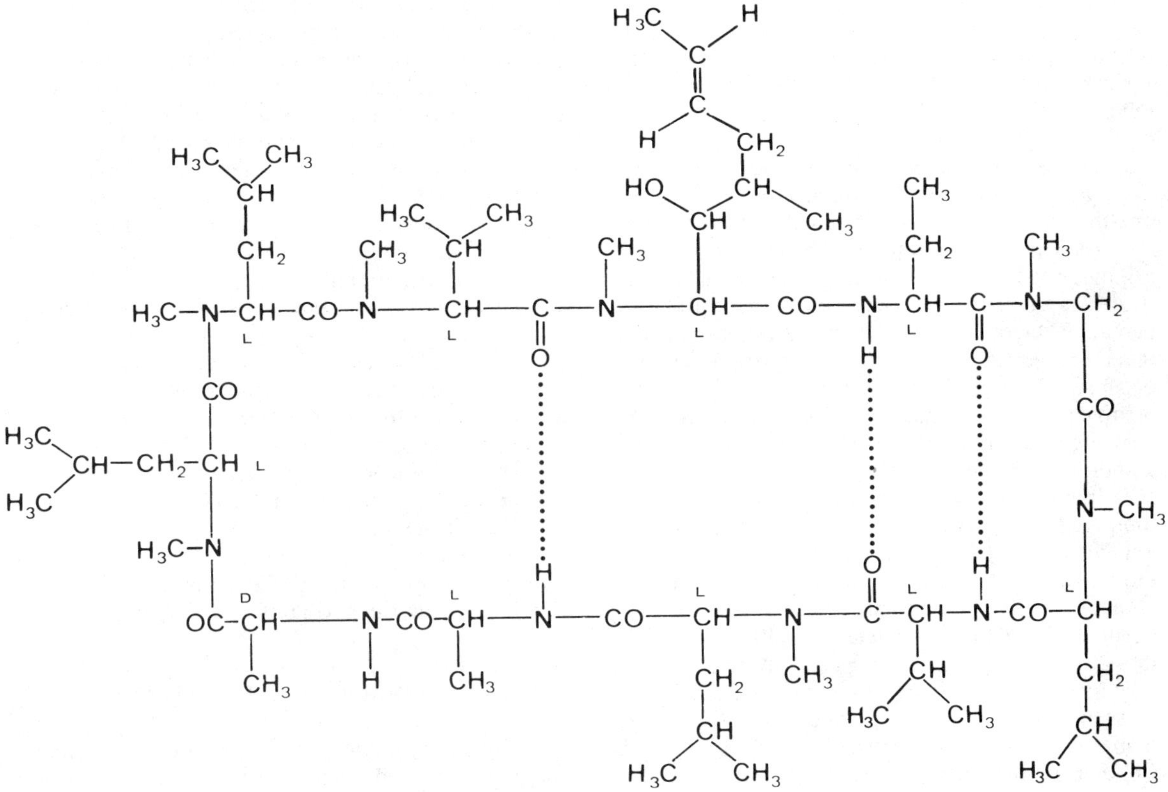

Figure 57–5. Cyclosporin A. "L" and "D" refer to levo- and dextrorotation forms of the indicated specific amino acids in the molecule.

Recent reports suggest that cyclosporin A may be of sufficient potency and efficacy to obviate the need for simultaneous use of corticosteroids, azathioprine, cyclophosphamide, or other immunosuppressive drugs. It has been used with apparent success as the sole immunosuppressant for cadaveric transplants of the kidney, pancreas, and liver.

Little is known about the pharmacokinetics of this agent at present. Cyclosporin A appears to be a step in the direction of a more specific and selective agent effective against a subpopulation of lymphocytes, but its side-effects are still considerable—although perhaps less than those of corticosteroids and other cytotoxic agents used for immunosuppression. Experimental studies suggest that the effects of cyclosporin A for suppression of GVH syndrome may be greater if the agent is begun prior to grafting.

CYTOTOXIC AGENTS

1. AZATHIOPRINE

Azathioprine is an imidazolyl derivative of mercaptopurine (6-mercaptopurine, 6-MP) and functions as a structural analog or "antimetabolite" (see Chapter 56). Although its action is presumably mediated by mercaptopurine as the active form, it has received more widespread use than mercaptopurine for immunosuppression in humans. These agents may represent prototypes of the structural analog or cytotoxic types of immunosuppressive drugs, and many other agents that kill proliferative cells seem to work at a similar level in the immune response.

Azathioprine is absorbed well from the gastrointestinal tract and is metabolized in vivo, primarily into mercaptopurine (portion below the dashed line in figure). Xanthine oxidase splits much of the active material to 6-thiouric acid prior to excretion in the urine.

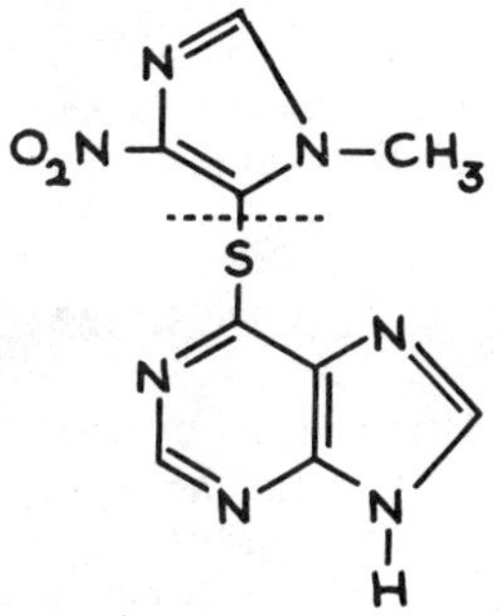

Azathioprine

After administration of azathioprine, small amounts of unchanged drug and mercaptopurine are also excreted by the kidney, and as much as a 2-fold increase in toxicity may occur in anephric or anuric patients. Since much of the drug's inactivation depends on xanthine oxidase, patients who are also receiving allopurinol (see Chapter 56) for control of hyperuricemia should have the dose of azathioprine reduced to one-fourth to one-third the usual dose to prevent excessive toxicity.

As with mercaptopurine, the chief toxicity of azathioprine is bone marrow depression, usually manifest as leukopenia, although anemia, thrombocytopenia, and bleeding may also occur. Skin rashes, drug fever, nausea and vomiting, and sometimes diarrhea occur, with the gastrointestinal symptoms seen mainly at higher dosages. Hepatic dysfunction, manifested by very high serum alkaline phosphatase levels and mild jaundice, occurs occasionally.

Immunosuppression with azathioprine or mercaptopurine therapy seems to result from interference with nucleic acid metabolism at steps that are required for the wave of cell proliferation that follows antigenic stimulation. The purine analogs are thus cytotoxic agents and destroy stimulated lymphoid cells. Although continued messenger RNA synthesis is necessary for sustained antibody synthesis by plasma cells, these analogs appear to have less effect on this process than on nucleic acid synthesis in proliferating cells. Cellular immunity as well as primary and secondary serum antibody responses can be blocked by these cytotoxic agents. Animal studies have shown that, if a course of mercaptopurine therapy is completed prior to exposure to a new antigen, the subsequent antibody response may actually be potentiated rather than suppressed. Although this latter phenomenon has yet to be substantiated clinically, such observations emphasize the need for precise timing of therapy relative to organ transplantation.

Azathioprine and mercaptopurine appear to be of definite benefit in maintaining renal homografts and may also be of value in transplantation of other tissues. These analogs have also been used with some success in the management of acute glomerulonephritis and in the renal component of systemic lupus erythematosus.

Although these agents are potentially toxic to bone marrow elements, including the megakaryocytes and red cell precursors, the favorable effects sometimes outweigh the toxic effects. The drugs have been of occasional use in prednisone-resistant antibody-mediated idiopathic thrombocytopenic purpura and autoimmune hemolytic anemias.

2. CYCLOPHOSPHAMIDE

The alkylating agent cyclophosphamide (Cytoxan) has recently been the focus of considerable interest as an immunosuppressive agent in animals and humans. It is perhaps the most potent immunosuppressive drug that has been synthesized. Cyclophosphamide destroys proliferating lymphoid cells but also appears to alkylate some resting cells. It has been observed that very large doses (eg, > 120 mg/kg intravenously over several days) may induce an apparent specific tolerance to a new antigen if the drug is administered simultaneously with—or shortly after—the antigen. In smaller doses, it has been very effective in autoimmune disorders (including systemic lupus erythematosus), in patients with acquired factor XIII antibodies and bleeding syndromes, in those with antibody-induced pure red cell aplasia, and in patients with Wegener's granulomatosis.

Although treatment with large doses of cyclophosphamide carries considerable risk of pancytopenia and hemorrhagic cystitis, the drug has aided in "takes" of bone marrow transplants and may have value in other types of organ transplantation also. Although cyclophosphamide appears to induce tolerance for marrow or immune cell grafting, its use does not prevent the subsequent GVH syndrome, which may be serious or lethal if the donor is a poor histocompatibility match. Highly specialized medical care and supportive facilities are mandatory for patient survival during the period of intensive therapy.

3. OTHER CYTOTOXIC AGENTS

Other cytotoxic agents, including vincristine, methotrexate, and cytarabine (see Chapter 56), also have immunosuppressive properties. Although these agents can be used for immunosuppression, they have not received as widespread use as the purine antagonists and their indications for immunosuppression are less certain. The use of methotrexate (which can be given orally) appears reasonable in patients with idiosyncratic reactions to purine antagonists. The antibiotic dactinomycin has also been used with some success at the time of impending renal transplant rejection. Vincristine appears to be quite useful in idiopathic thrombocytopenic purpura refractory to prednisone, but it is not yet certain whether this effect is immunologically mediated. The related vinca alkaloid vinblastine has been shown to prevent mast cell degranulation in vitro by binding to microtubule units within the cell and to prevent release of histamine and other vasoactive compounds.

ANTIBODIES AS IMMUNOSUPPRESSIVE AGENTS

Until recently, development of specific antibodies required immunization and collection of antisera with subsequent purification of the gamma globulin or IgG fraction. The recent development of "hybridoma" technology by Milstein and Köhler will revolutionize this field and radically increase the purity and specificity of antibodies used for immunosuppression and other applications. Hybridomas consist of antibody-forming cells fused to plasmacytoma cells. Hybrid cells that are stable and produce the required antibody can be cloned for mass culture for antibody production.

1. ANTILYMPHOCYTE GLOBULIN

Although antisera directed against lymphocytes have been prepared sporadically since Metchnikoff's first observations just before the turn of the century, detailed evaluation was not made of antilymphocytic serum until the 1960s. With the arrival of the era of human organ homotransplantation, heterologous antilymphocytic globulin (ALG) suddenly took on new importance. It has subsequently been the subject of many basic and clinical studies. ALG remains an investigational agent in the USA, but it is used in many medical centers that have organ transplantation programs.

The antiserum is usually obtained by immunization of large animals (eg, horses) with human lymphoid cells. Recently, extremely potent antisera have been obtained by immunization with human fetal thymus. The IgG fraction of the antiserum is prepared by cold alcohol precipitation or chromatographic fractionation. The potency of each batch of ALG is determined by lymphocyte agglutination and cytotoxicity testing in vitro. Cytotoxicity titers correspond somewhat to the clinical responses, but the activity of ALG has yet to be adequately standardized.

Antilymphocytic antibody acts primarily on the small, long-lived peripheral lymphocytes that circulate between the blood and lymph. With continued administration, the "thymus-dependent" lymphocytes from the cuffs of lymphoid follicles are also depleted, as they normally participate in the recirculating pool. Antilymphocytic antibody binds to the surface of these small "antigen recognition" T cells (Fig 57–2), with cytotoxic destruction of the cells mediated by serum complement. As a result of the destruction of the T cells, a rather specific impairment of delayed hypersensitivity and cellular immunity occurs while humoral antibody formation remains relatively intact. The pattern of immunosuppression obtained with ALG is similar to that which occurs when circulating small lymphocytes are depleted by prolonged thoracic duct drainage. The selectivity of ALG for the cellular immune system accounts for its usefulness in preventing rejection of transplanted organs. Although ALGs produced by immunization with fetal thymus are not yet widely available, they appear to be the most effective anti-T cell immunosuppressive agents. Application of the hybridoma technology to production of anti-T cell antibodies is now well under way, and various immunologic specificities have been identified. Murine hybridoma monoclonal antibodies directed against T cell antigens have just entered clinical trial for T cell leukemias and lymphomas. They will be tested also for immunosuppressive properties and for prevention of graft rejection.

Since heterologous ALG has still not been adequately standardized, only generalizations about dosage and treatment can be given. After transplantation of an organ such as the kidney, ALG is often administered (by intramuscular injection) first on a daily basis and subsequently cut back in frequency. Because ALG is usually administered along with azathioprine and prednisone, it has not been possible to assess the effects of ALG alone in human kidney transplants. Investigators who treat their renal transplant recipients with ALG believe that it reduces the dosage requirements for the other immunosuppressive drugs and improves survival in patients who receive kidneys from unrelated or cadaver donors. There has been some limited success in the use of ALG alone for recipient preparation for bone marrow transplantation. In this procedure the recipient is treated with ALG in large doses for 7–10 days, followed by transplantation of $1-3 \times 10^{10}$ bone marrow cells from the donor. Residual ALG appears to destroy the T cells in the donor marrow graft, and the severe GVH syndrome has not been observed. These limited data do indicate that ALG given alone is a potent immunosuppressive agent in humans.

The side-effects of ALG are mostly those of the injection of a foreign protein obtained from horse serum. Local pain and erythema often occur at the injection site. Since the humoral antibody mechanism remains active, skin-reactive and precipitating antibodies can be formed against the horse IgG. Similar reactions can be anticipated with monoclonal antibodies of murine origin. For this reason, development of human-human hybridomas is a major current research objective, as it should eliminate heterologous protein reactions.

Anaphylactic and serum sickness reactions have been observed and usually require cessation of ALG therapy. In addition, complexes of host antibodies with horse ALG may precipitate and localize in the glomerulus of the transplanted kidney. Even more disturbing has been the development of histocytic lymphoma in the buttock at the site of ALG injection. The incidence of lymphoma as well as other forms of cancer is increased in kidney transplant patients, and may be as high as 2% in long-term survivors. It appears likely that part of the increased risk of cancer is related to the suppression of a normally potent defense system against oncogenic viruses or transformed cells. Thus, it remains to be seen whether ALG is any more carcinogenic than the other immunosuppressive agents.

Antilymphocytic antibody has great potential as an immunosuppressive agent but presents significant problems in its present form. Standardization with antithymocyte globulin (ATG) of monoclonal origin would be an improvement, because some of these antisera are selective for T cell subsets and are potentially available in unlimited quantities with very well defined specificity. Some investigators now hope that a monoclonal antibody can be developed that would have activity against just those clones which respond to transplantation antigens rather than all antigen recognition cells.

2. Rh_0 (D) IMMUNE GLOBULIN

One of the major advances in medicine during the past decade has been the development of a technique for preventing Rh hemolytic disease of the newborn. The technique is based on the observation that a primary antibody response to a foreign antigen can be blocked if specific antibody is administered passively at the time of exposure to antigen.

Rh_0 (D) immune globulin (RhoGAM) is a concentrated (15%) solution of human IgG globulin containing a high titer of antibodies against the Rh_0 (D) antigen of the red cell. The IgG is prepared by cold alcohol fractionation of carefully selected plasma from Rh_0 (D)-negative, D^u-negative mothers sensitized by repeated Rh-incompatible pregnancies or from Rh-negative volunteers who have been deliberately immunized for plasma collection.

Sensitization of Rh-negative mothers to the D antigen occurs usually at the time of birth of an Rh_0 (D)-positive or D^u-positive infant, when fetal red cells may leak into the mother's bloodstream. Sensitization might also occur occasionally with miscarriages or ectopic pregnancies. With subsequent pregnancies, maternal antibody against Rh-positive cells is transferred to the fetus during the third trimester, leading to the development of erythroblastosis fetalis or hemolytic disease of the newborn.

If an injection of Rh_0 (D) antibody is administered to the mother within 72 hours after the birth of an Rh-negative baby, the mother's own antibody response to the foreign Rh_0 (D)-positive cells is suppressed. When the mother has been treated in this fashion, Rh hemolytic disease of the newborn has not been observed in the subsequent pregnancy. For this prophylactic treatment to be successful, the mother must be Rh_0 (D)-negative and D^u-negative and must not already be immunized to the Rh_0 (D) factor. Treatment is also often advised for Rh-negative mothers who have had miscarriages, ectopic pregnancies, or abortions in which the blood type of the fetus is unknown.

Note: Rh_0 (D) immune globulin is administered to the mother and must not be given to the infant.

The usual dose of RhoGAM is 2 mL intramuscularly. Adverse reactions are infrequent and consist of local discomfort at the injection site or, rarely, a slight temperature elevation.

The mechanism of suppression of the immune response by passive administration of specific antibody may consist of prompt elimination of the foreign antigen after combination with the antibody or may be a type of "feedback immunosuppression" in which a change in the antigen results from its combination with antibody, so that it is no longer recognized as foreign. If antibody produces "feedback" immunosuppression, it presumably acts on the macrophage, the T lymphocyte, or the B lymphocyte (Figs 57–1 to 57–3).

CLINICAL USES OF IMMUNOSUPPRESSIVE DRUGS

Immunosuppressive agents are currently used in 3 clinical circumstances: (1) organ transplantation, (2) autoimmune disorders, and (3) isoimmune disorders (Rh hemolytic disease of the newborn). The agents used differ somewhat for the specific disorders treated (see specific agents and Table 57–2), as do administration schedules also. Optimal treatment schedules have yet to be established in many clinical situations in which these drugs are used, and objective evaluations of their relative efficacy are uncertain in many instances, especially with agents such as ALG. Other considerations related to the conditions to be treated also affect the evaluation of effectiveness of the immunosuppressive agents.

Organ Transplantation

In organ transplantation, tissue typing, based on donor and recipient histocompatibility matching with the HLA haplotype system and in vitro mixed lymphocyte culture (MLC), is of definite value. Close histocompatibility matching reduces the likelihood of

Table 57–2. Clinical uses of immunosuppressive agents.

Disease	Immunosuppressive Agents Used	Response
Autoimmune		
Idiopathic thrombocytopenic purpura	Prednisone,* vincristine, occasionally mercaptopurine or azathioprine, high-dose gamma globulin	Usually good
Autoimmune hemolytic anemia	Prednisone,* cyclophosphamide, chlorambucil, mercaptopurine, azathioprine	Usually good
Acute glomerulonephritis	Prednisone,* mercaptopurine, cyclophosphamide	Usually good
Acquired factor XIII antibodies	Cyclophosphamide plus factor XIII	Usually good
Miscellaneous "autoreactive" disorders†	Prednisone, cyclophosphamide, azathioprine	Often good
Isoimmune		
Hemolytic anemia of the newborn	Rh_0 (D) immune globulin*	Excellent
Organ transplantation		
Renal	Azathioprine, prednisone, antilymphocytic globulin, dactinomycin, cyclophosphamide, cyclosporin A	Very good
Heart		Good
Liver	Cyclosporin A, prednisone	Fair
Bone marrow (HLA-matched)	Cyclophosphamide, prednisone, methotrexate, ALG, total body irradiation, cyclosporin A	Increasing success with well-matched donors

*Drug of choice.
†Systemic lupus erythematosus, rheumatoid arthritis, Wegener's granulomatosis, chronic active hepatitis, lipoid nephrosis, inflammatory bowel disease.

graft rejection and may also reduce the requirements for intensive immunosuppressive therapy. Response to transplantation and immunosuppressive drugs in renal disease may be dependent on the nature of the primary renal lesions in patients undergoing transplant.

Primary renal disease itself is frequently immunologic in nature. Two major types of glomerular injury are mediated by immune mechanisms. The first type results from the passive deposition of antigen-antibody complexes from the circulation as blood is filtered through the glomerulus. Deposition of antigen-antibody complexes, which may fix complement, in a "lumpy-bumpy" or discontinuous pattern, is associated with the renal disease of systemic lupus erythematosus and with most cases of acute glomerulonephritis. The second form of glomerulonephritis is associated with linear deposition of specific anti-basement membrane antibody in the glomerulus.

Although immunosuppressive therapy may be of benefit in both of these circumstances, the data are incomplete. Since patients with severe glomerulonephritis are often candidates for kidney transplantation, pathogenetic factors that might persist and also damage the transplanted kidney are of great importance. It has been observed that patients with anti-basement membrane antibody may experience an acute graft rejection when they receive a kidney transplant. Patients with anti-basement membrane antibodies are likely to need immunosuppressive therapy for 6–8 weeks after bilateral nephrectomy, being maintained on a dialysis program, before transplantation of a donor kidney can be considered. Similarly, patients with a disease such as systemic lupus erythematosus are poor candidates for renal transplant until the systemic cause of the renal injury is under control.

Even with all these considerations, the response to renal transplantation has become increasingly gratifying, including that with unmatched kidneys from cadaver donors. At present, over 80% of carefully selected but nonrelated recipients may survive beyond 2 years after the transplant, and 5-year survival is not an unrealistic hope.

Recently, increasing success has been achieved with bone marrow transplantation in patients with aplastic anemia, refractory acute leukemia, or severe combined immunodeficiency disease (congenital) who have an HLA- and MLC-matched donor. Patients with aplastic anemia or leukemia require intensive immunosuppression prior to transplantation. Monoclonal antibodies to leukemia-associated antigens in childhood acute lymphocytic leukemia have been used to "clean up" patients' bone marrow for autologous bone marrow storage and reinfusion after high-dose chemotherapy. Patients who do not receive autologous bone marrow or a graft from an identical twin require postengraftment immunosuppression to minimize the GVH syndrome attributable to donor immunocytes in the marrow graft. Recent investigations indicate that anti-T cell antiserum or cyclosporin A can modify or abrogate established GVH syndrome in a significant proportion of cases.

Transplantation of liver, heart, pancreas, and lungs (in order of decreasing success), has also been performed. In some cases, technical problems account for the poorer results. However, the results of cardiac transplantation are gradually improving.

Autoimmune Disorders

The effectiveness of immunosuppressive drugs in autoimmune disorders varies widely. Most of these disorders are of unknown cause and the rationale for immunosuppression is sometimes strained, although it is usually thought that faulty recognition mechanisms of antibody cross-reactivity account for the proliferation of unneeded lymphoid clones. Recent data obtained in studies of the NZB/NZW mouse strain suggest that there may be a deficiency in a soluble immune response suppressor substance (SIRS) in some autoimmune disorders. In the autoimmune diseases, unlike the situation in immunosuppression for transplantation, the unwanted immune response is already established when the disease is diagnosed, and a large proliferating mass of lymphoid cells must be dealt with. Nonetheless, with immunosuppressive therapy, remissions can be obtained in most instances of autoimmune hemolytic anemia, idiopathic thrombocytopenic purpura, Hashimoto's thyroiditis, and temporal arteritis. Apparent improvement is also often seen in patients with systemic lupus erythematosus, acute glomerulonephritis, acquired factor VIII inhibitors (antibodies), and certain other autoimmune states. Some cases of idiopathic aplastic anemia also appear to have an autoimmune etiologic basis. A recent series of aplastic anemia patients showed significant clinical improvement and prolonged survival with ALG alone. Some prior cases treated with bone marrow transplantation after conditioning with cyclophosphamide or ALG have also shown prolonged improvement in blood counts even though there was evidence of graft rejection and recovery of recipient marrow function, again supporting an autoimmune basis for some cases of aplastic anemia. Recently, the use of high doses of normal gamma globulin (administered intravenously) has been found useful in therapy of refractory idiopathic thrombocytopenic purpura. The presumed mechanism of action is through reticuloendothelial cell blockade, thus reducing the distribution of antibody-damaged platelets.

In most instances it is only assumed that it is the immunosuppressive properties of drugs such as prednisone, cyclophosphamide, mercaptopurine, or ALG that produce these improvements. Anti-inflammatory effects of some of these drugs may also contribute to their efficacy. Once the cause of these autoreactive states is defined, therapy may become more rational.

Hemolytic Disease of the Newborn

Prevention of Rh hemolytic disease of the newborn is a landmark in immunosuppressive therapy. It is hoped that this example of precise suppression without side-effects will also apply to other disease states once the offending antigens can be identified.

IMMUNOMODULATING AGENTS

A new frontier in pharmacology—still in the stage of exploration and debate—is the development of agents that modulate the immune response rather than suppress it. The rationale for the development of these agents is that they can be used to increase the immunoresponsiveness of patients who have either selective or generalized immunodeficiency. The major potential uses are in (1) immunodeficiency disorders, (2) chronic infectious disease, and (3) cancer. At present, all immunostimulating or immunomodulating agents are classed as investigational drugs.

Thymosin

This protein hormone, which is synthesized by the epithelioid component of the thymus, has recently been isolated and purified from bovine and human thymus glands. Thymosin, which has a molecular weight of approximately 10,000, appears to convey T cell specificity to uncommitted lymphoid stem cells. Lower molecular weight fractions may also have thymic hormone-like activity. Thymosin levels are high through normal childhood and early adulthood, begin to fall in the third to fourth decades, and are low in elderly people. Serum levels are also low in DiGeorge's syndrome of T cell deficiency. In vitro treatment of lymphocytes with thymosin increases the number of cells that manifest T cell surface markers and function. Mechanistically, thymosin is considered to induce the maturation of pre-T cells. The effects of fetal thymus transplantation in DiGeorge's syndrome are probably attributable to the action of thymosin. The purified hormone therefore has potential therapeutic applications in DiGeorge's syndrome and other T cell deficiency states. Over 60 children with various immunodeficiencies have been treated with thymosin, and favorable responses are reported in over half of cases.

Interferons & Interferon Inducers*

Interferons were first described as antiviral proteins produced by host cells. Subsequently, the interferons were found to have antiproliferative activity and to modulate the function of other immune cells (eg, macrophages and natural killer [NK] cells). Significant amounts of interferon have been extracted from leukocytes harvested at the time of routine blood donation using a process developed in Finland by Cantrell. This material has a purity of 0.1%. Interferon might be useful in the treatment of certain infections (eg, hepatitis; see p 527) as well as certain forms of cancer, particularly myelomas and lymphomas arising from B cells (see Chapter 56). At present, 3 types of interferon are being produced (see p 527). Several pharmaceutical firms are currently producing standardized natural interferon in adequate quantities for clinical trial. What is more, recombinant DNA cloning technology has been successfully applied to several subtypes of leukocyte interferon, yielding products at least 95% pure. The cloned interferons have also just been introduced into clinical trials.

*Interferons and interferon inducers are discussed also in Chapter 48 as antiviral agents.

Transfer Factor (TF)

This agent is a small RNA molecule or peptide (MW about 5000) derived from normal human lymphoid cells. Transfer factors are apparently immunologically specific for given antigens, although they may serve as adjuvants or "superantigens." Transfer factors also appear to be species-specific. Cell-mediated immunity to the specific antigen required should be present in the potential transfer factor donor. TF often converts negative delayed hypersensitivity skin tests to positive. The effect of a TF dose lasts for up to 6 months. The effects of transfer factor therapy may be dramatic in some cases of chronic mucocutaneous candidiasis. Claims also have been made for the possible usefulness of transfer factor in the treatment of leprosy, Wiskott-Aldrich syndrome, and osteogenic sarcoma. These latter reports are all preliminary and will require detailed confirmation before a clear role for transfer factor therapy can be established for any of these disease states. Transfer factor dosage is based on the number of lymphocytes from which the TF has been prepared. Therapeutic doses require that at least 10^9 lymphocytes be used for TF preparation, although the TF from as many as 40×10^9 lymphocytes has been administered as a single dose without incident. The TF is not immunogenic, and only very rare reactions have occurred on repeated injection.

Levamisole

This chemical agent was first synthesized for the treatment of parasitic infections. Recent studies suggest that it increases the magnitude of delayed hypersensitivity or T cell-mediated immunity in humans. In immunodeficiency associated with Hodgkin's disease, levamisole has been noted to increase the number of E rosette-forming lymphoid cells (T cells) in vitro and to enhance skin test reactivity in vivo. Levamisole has also been widely tested in rheumatoid arthritis and found to have some efficacy but not without toxicity (see Chapter 33). Its mechanism of action is unknown, and its significance as an immunostimulant is still quite controversial.

BCG & Other Adjuvants

BCG is a viable strain of *Mycobacterium bovis* that has been used for immunization against tuberculosis. Recently, it has been employed as a nonspecific adjuvant or immunostimulant in cancer therapy. BCG appears to act—at least in part—via activation of macrophages to make them more "effective" killer cells in concert with lymphoid cells in the efferent limb of the immune response. Macrophage activation with BCG also appears to increase the rate of clearance of immune complexes (eg, antibody-soluble tumor antigen) from the blood, and thereby may overcome "tolerance" to the tumor. Immune T cells are also necessary for BCG's anticancer action, since, in animals pretreated with anti-T cell sera, the immunotherapeutic effect of BCG is blocked. It is being tried in studies of melanomas, lung and ovarian cancer, and other neoplasms. Some beneficial "local" immunotherapy effects appear likely. Systemic effects are unproved. Lipid extracts of BCG (eg, methanol-extractable residue) as well as nonviable preparations of *Corynebacterium parvum* may also have similar nonspecific immunostimulant properties.

IMMUNOLOGIC REACTIONS TO DRUGS & DRUG ALLERGY

The basic immune mechanism and the ways in which it can be suppressed or stimulated by drugs are discussed in the foregoing sections of this chapter. Drugs often serve also to *activate* the immune system in undesirable ways that appear as adverse drug reactions. These reactions are generally lumped in a broad classification as "drug allergy." Indeed, many drug reactions such as those to penicillin, iodides, phenytoin, and sulfonamides are allergic in nature. These drug reactions are manifested as skin eruptions, edema, anaphylactoid reactions, fever, and eosinophilia. The underlying mechanism of the allergic sensitization to drugs was clarified by the discovery of the IgE class of immunoglobulins by the Ishizakas and by a better understanding of the process of sensitization and activation of blood basophils and tissue mast cells.

Other drug reactions mediated by immune mechanisms may have different mechanisms. Thus, any one of the 4 major types of hypersensitivity can be associated with an allergic drug reaction:

Type I: Allergic reactions to drugs, including anaphylaxis, urticaria, and angioedema (IgE-mediated).

Type II: Allergic reactions are complement-dependent and therefore involve IgG or IgM antibodies in which the antibody is fixed to a circulating blood cell subject to complement-dependent lysis.

Type III: Drug reactions are exemplified by serum sickness, which involves IgG and is a multisystem complement-dependent vasculitis.

Type IV: Cell-mediated allergy is the mechanism involved in allergic contact dermatitis from topically applied drugs.

Some adverse reactions to drugs may be mistakenly classified as allergic or immune when they are in reality genetic deficiency states or are idiosyncratic and not mediated by immune mechanisms (eg, hemolysis due to primaquine in glucose-6-phosphate dehydrogenase deficiency, or aplastic anemia due to chloramphenicol).

MECHANISMS OF IMMEDIATE (TYPE I) DRUG ALLERGY

The mechanisms of immune activation that are operative in drug allergy are similar to the normal humoral antibody responses to foreign macromolecules. These mechanisms can now be placed in a theoretical construct that includes an afferent limb of the immune response (Fig 57–6) as well as an efferent limb that includes the pharmacologic mediators of allergy (Fig 57–7). Landsteiner and his associates first demonstrated that animals could be sensitized to simple chemicals such as picric acid (a hapten) if the chemical was linked to a carrier protein. This linkage can occur in the body with a normal tissue or serum protein serving as the carrier. The subsequent immune response will be specific for the hapten even though linkage to a carrier is necessary for immune recognition. Surprisingly, carrier recognition is genetically determined even though the host does not produce antibodies against the carrier protein. When drugs serve as haptens, the antibody-forming precursor cells.

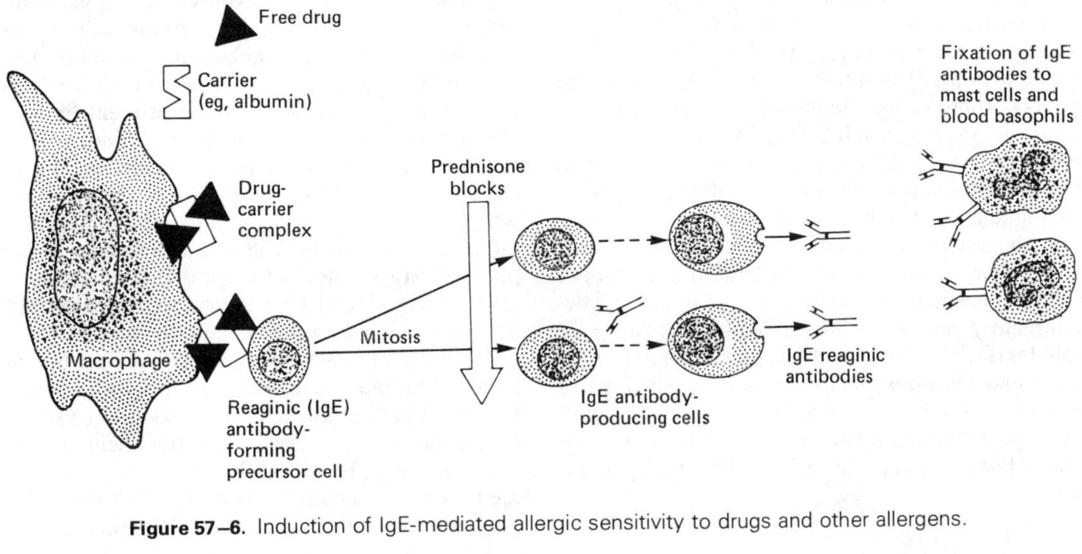

Figure 57–6. Induction of IgE-mediated allergic sensitivity to drugs and other allergens.

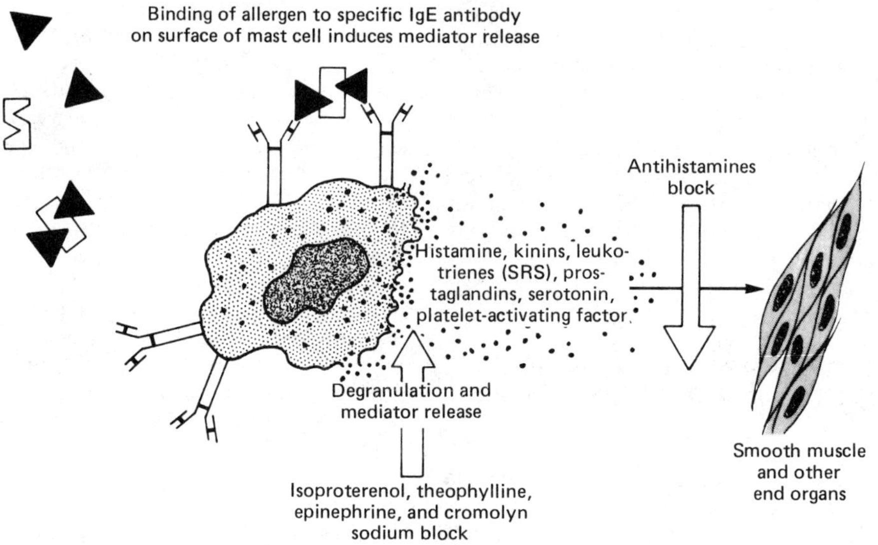

Figure 57–7. Response of IgE-sensitized cells to subsequent exposure to allergens.

that respond are often the precursors of cells which produce antibodies of the IgE class. IgE class-specific antibody responses are very dependent on helper T cell effects. Suppressor T cells may also function in modulating or inhibiting the IgE response. In nonallergic individuals, IgE globulin levels are the lowest of any immunoglobulin (< 1 μg/mL), whereas in allergy they may be increased 10-fold or more. IgE antibodies have the interesting property of fixing to blood basophils and tissue mast cells and are described as skin-sensitizing or reaginic antibodies.

The fixation of the IgE antibody to blood basophils or their tissue equivalent (mast cells) sets the stage for an acute allergic reaction. When the offending drug is reintroduced into the body, IgE antibody molecules on the surface of sensitized basophilic leukocytes bind to the antigenic form of the drug (Fig 57–7). Sensitized tissue mast cells or blood basophils are stimulated to release mediators (eg, histamine, leukotrienes) from granules. Mediator release is associated with a fall in intracellular cAMP within the mast cell. Many of the drugs that block mediator release appear to act through the cAMP mechanism (eg, catecholamines, corticosteroids, theophylline), with different loci of action in the pathway of cAMP synthesis or degradation. Other vasoactive substances such as kinins may also be generated during histamine release. These mediators initiate immediate skin and smooth muscle responses and thus initiate tissue injury and the inflammatory response. Slow-reacting substance of anaphylaxis (SRS) has recently been shown to consist of the leukocyte lipoxygenase products designated as leukotrienes. Mediator-induced reactions can be devastating or lethal to the patient, especially when they produce laryngospasm, bronchospasm, or hypotension.

DRUG TREATMENT OF IMMEDIATE ALLERGY

One can test an individual for possible sensitivity to a drug by a simple scratch test, ie, by applying an extremely dilute solution of the drug to the skin. If allergy is present, an immediate wheal and flare will often occur. However, in many instances the skin test may be negative in spite of marked hypersensitivity to a hapten or to a metabolic product of the drug, or at times when the antibody may be of a class other than IgE. Skin reactivity to a specific drug can also be transferred from an allergic individual to a normal recipient (human or primate) with serum that contains the reaginic IgE antibodies (the Prausnitz-Küstner reaction).

Drugs that modify allergic responses act at several links in this chain of events. Prednisone, which is often used in severe allergic reactions, is immunosuppressive and probably blocks proliferation of the IgE-producing clones and could inhibit function of helper T cells in the IgE response. In the efferent limb of the allergic response, isoproterenol, epinephrine, and theophylline block the release of mediators from mast cells and basophils and produce bronchodilation, whereas antihistamines competitively inhibit histamine, which would otherwise produce increased permeability in the end organ. Corticosteroids may also act to reduce tissue injury and edema in the inflamed tissue, as well as "unblocking" β-blocked cells, thereby facilitating the actions of catecholamines in cells that may have become refractory to epinephrine or isoproterenol. Cromolyn sodium (Aarane, Intal), a drug that is useful for treatment of allergic asthma, appears to inhibit the liberation of the mediators of anaphylaxis that are released after antibody-antigen interaction (see Chapter 17).

DESENSITIZATION TO DRUGS

When reasonable alternatives are not available, certain drugs (eg, penicillin) must be used for life-threatening illnesses even in the presence of known allergic sensitivity. In such cases, desensitization can sometimes be accomplished by starting with minute dosages of the drug and gradually increasing the dose over a period of hours or days to the full therapeutic range. This practice is hazardous, and one must always be ready to treat the patient for an episode of acute anaphylactic shock before desensitization has been achieved. This form of desensitization differs from immunosuppression in that the immune mechanism often appears to be stimulated and reactivity is only predictably diminished while the treatment is continued.

The exact mechanism of desensitization to drugs is complex and incompletely understood. It may be due to controlled anaphylaxis (with gradual depletion of mast cells and basophils) while symptoms are suppressed or to antigen excess, which can under certain circumstances block mediator release. In some instances, allergic desensitization appears to be accomplished by the stimulation of competing clones of cells that produce "blocking" antibodies, often of the IgG or IgA immunoglobulin class. Additionally, desensitization with antigen could induce the generation of specific suppressor T cells.

AUTOIMMUNE (TYPE II) REACTIONS TO DRUGS

Certain autoimmune syndromes can be induced by drugs. Examples of this phenomenon include systemic lupus erythematosus following hydralazine or procainamide therapy, "lupoid hepatitis" due to cathartic sensitivity; autoimmune hemolytic anemia resulting from methyldopa administration, thrombocytopenic purpura due to quinidine, and agranulocytosis due to a variety of drugs. In these drug-induced autoimmune states, antibodies to tissue constituents or to the drug can be demonstrated. Immune mechanisms also appear to be involved in many additional cases of so-called idiopathic thrombocytopenic purpura, but it is more difficult to demonstrate the specific antibodies. The blood platelet or granulocyte is sometimes an innocent bystander to an immunologic reaction to a drug but manages to be damaged or activated by antigen-antibody complexes or destroyed by the reticuloendothelial system, leading to the development of "idiopathic" thrombocytopenic purpura or agranulocytosis.

Fortunately, autoimmune reactions to drugs usually subside within several months after the offending drug is withdrawn. Immunosuppressive therapy is warranted only when the autoimmune response is unusually severe.

SERUM SICKNESS & VASCULITIC (TYPE III) REACTIONS

Serum sickness reactions to drugs are more common than immediate anaphylactic responses. The clinical features of serum sickness include urticarial skin eruptions, arthralgia or arthritis, lymphadenopathy, and fever. The reactions generally last 6–12 days and usually subside once the offending drug is eliminated. Although IgE antibodies may play some role, complement-fixing antibodies of the IgM or IgG class are usually involved. Corticosteroids are useful in attenuating severe serum sickness reactions to drugs.

Immune vasculitis can also be induced by drugs. The sulfonamides, penicillin, thiouracil, anticonvulsants, and iodides have all been implicated in the initiation of hypersensitivity angiitis. Erythema multiforme is a relatively mild vasculitic skin disorder that may be secondary to drug hypersensitivity. Stevens-Johnson syndrome is probably a more severe form of this hypersensitivity reaction and includes erythema multiforme, arthritis, nephritis, central nervous system abnormalities, and myocarditis. It has frequently been associated with sulfonamide therapy.

CLINICAL IDENTIFICATION OF IMMUNOLOGIC REACTIONS TO DRUGS

In view of the multiplicity of drugs that hospitalized patients frequently receive, it is not always easy to determine which drug has initiated an allergic or immune syndrome of drug sensitivity. Careful questioning about the history of prior drug sensitivities is an important part of every patient's medical record, and errors of omission can be dangerous. In almost all instances, once an offending drug is identified, its use is discontinued. If an alternative drug is to be used (eg, an antibiotic), it is important to select one from a different class of agents to avoid cross-sensitivity reactions. Since certain commonly used drugs such as the penicillins are frequent offenders, direct questions about penicillin sensitivity should always be included in the patient's history. Skin testing may be very useful in confirming drug allergy when the history is equivocal and the proper antigens are available. Skin testing is considerably less hazardous than a therapeutic trial and is usually indicated where there is an equivocal allergic history and a strong clinical indication for treatment with the drug. An alternative to skin testing that is sometimes available is the radioallergosorbent test (RAST), a form of radioimmunoassay procedure. In selected rare instances, use of a drug may be needed for lifesaving purposes despite well-documented allergy to the agent.

Warnings of known sensitivities should be prominently displayed in the patient's record or hospital chart. When drug intolerance is suspected, an assessment of the patient's anaphylactic potential should be made, since delayed rashes carry a different prognosis than urticaria and angioedema. Once a drug allergy is defined, this information should always be conveyed to the patient in clear language to prevent repeated challenges with the same agent in the future, when the reaction may be much more severe. In the case of known severe sensitivity to common drugs, the patient should be advised to carry a clearly written notice of the sensitivity to lessen the chance of being given the agent during incapacitation, as after an accident.

• • •

References

Current Concepts in Immunology

Bockman RS, Rothschild M: Prostaglandin E inhibition of T-lymphocyte colony formation. *J Clin Invest* 1979;**64:**812.

Hymes JL et al: Macrophages synthesize and release prostaglandins in response to inflammatory stimuli. *Nature* 1977;**269:**149.

Kiesling R, Haller O: Natural killer cells in the mouse: An alternative immune surveillance mechanism. *Contemp Top Immunobiol* 1978;**8:**171.

Köhler O, Milstein C: Continuous cultures of fused cells secreting antibody of defined specificity. *Nature* 1975;**55:**495.

Ledbetter J et al: Evolutionary conservation of surface molecules that distinguish T lymphocyte helper/inducer and cytotoxic/suppressor subpopulation in mouse and man. *J Exp Med* 1981;**153:**310.

Marchalonis JJ: Lymphocyte surface immunoglobulins. *Science* 1975;**190:**20.

Melchers F, Potter M, Warner NL (editors): *Lymphocyte Hybridomas*. Springer, 1978.

Origins of Lymphocyte Diversity. (2 parts.) *Cold Spring Harbor Symp Quant Biol* 1977;**41:1, 417.**

Ortaldo JR et al: Determination of surface antigens on highly purified human NK cells by flow cytometry with monoclonal antibodies. *J Immunol* 1981;**127:**2401.

Stites DP et al (editors): *Basic & Clinical Immunology,* 4th ed. Lange, 1982.

Unanue ER: The regulation of lymphocyte function by the macrophage. *Immunol Rev* 1978;**40:**227.

Vietta ES, Uhr JW: Immunoglobulin receptors revisited. *Science* 1975;**189:**964.

Waldmann TA, Broder S: Suppressor cells in the regulation of the immune response. Pages 155–199 in: *Progress in Clinical Immunology*. Schwartz RS (editor). Grune & Stratton, 1977.

Immunosuppressive Agents

Calne RY et al: Cyclosporin A initially as the only immunosuppressant in 34 recipients of cadaveric organs: 32 kidneys, 2 pancreases, and 2 livers. *Lancet* 1979;**2:**1033.

Fehr J, Hofmann V, Kappeler CM: Transient reversal of thrombocytopenia in idiopathic thrombocytopenia purpura by high-dose intravenous gamma globulin. *N Engl J Med* 1982;**306:**1254.

Freda VJ et al: Prevention of Rh hemolytic disease: Ten years' experience with Rh immune globulin. *N Engl J Med* 1975;**292:**1014.

Goodwin JS, Messner RP: Sensitivity of lymphocytes to prostaglandin E_2 increases over the age of 70. *J Clin Invest* 1979;**64:**434.

Gordon MY, Singer JW: Selective effects of cyclosporin-A on colony-forming lymphoid and myeloid cells in man. *Nature* 1979;**279:**433.

Hess AD, Tutschka PJ, Santos GW: Effect of cyclosporin A on human lymphocytes in vitro. *J Immunol* 1982;**128:**355.

Kaplan SR, Calabresi P: Drug therapy: Immunosuppressive agents. *N Engl J Med* 1973;**289:**952.

Marwick JR et al: Timing of cyclosporin-A therapy for abrogation of HGV and GVH responses in rats. *Lancet* 1979;**2:**1037.

Nossal GJV, Abbott A, Mitchell J: Antigens in immunity. 14. Electron microscopic radioautographic studies of antigen capture in the lymph node medulla. *J Exp Med* 1968;**127:**263.

Powles RL et al: Cyclosporin-A in patients receiving renal allografts from cadaver donors. *Lancet* 1978;**2:**1327.

Ramsay NK et al: A randomized study of the prevention of graft-versus-host disease. *N Engl J Med* 1982;**306:**392.

Salmon SE, Krakauer RS, Whitmore WF: Lymphocyte stimulation: Selective destruction of cells undergoing the blastogenic response to transplantation antigens. *Science* 1971;**172:**490.

Speck B et al: Treatment of aplastic anemia by antilymphocytic globulin with and without allogeneic bone marrow infusions. *Lancet* 1977;**2:**1145.

Stadecker MJ et al: Synthesis and release of thymidine by macrophages. *J Immunol* 1977;**119:**1738.

Starzl TE et al: Liver transplantation with the use of cyclosporin A and prednisone. *N Engl J Med* 1981;**305:**266.

Thomas ED et al: Bone marrow transplantation. *N Engl J Med* 1975;**292:**895.

Uhr JW, Moller G: Regulatory effects of antibody on antibody formation. *Adv Immunol* 1968;**8:**81.

Winkelstein A: Effects of immunosuppressive drugs on T and B lymphocytes in guinea pigs. *Blood* 1977;**50:**81.

Immunostimulating Agents

Baron S, Diazani F (editors): The interferon system: A current review to 1978. *Texas Rep Biol Med* 1977;**35.**

Goldstein G: Isolation of bovine thymin: A polypeptide hormone of the thymus. *Nature* 1974;**247:**11.

Kirkpatrick CH et al: Treatment of chronic mucocutaneous candidiasis by immunologic reconstitution. *Clin Exp Immunol* 1971;**9:**733.

Lawrence HS: Transfer factor in cellular immunity. *Harvey Lect* 1974;**8:**239.

Lewis V: Circulating thymic-hormone activity in congenital immunodeficiency. *Lancet* 1977;**2:**471.

Vilcek J, Gresser I, Merrigan TC (editors): Regulatory functions of interferons. *Ann NY Acad Sci* 1980;**350:**1. [Entire issue.]

White A, Goldstein AL: Thymosin. Page 465 in: *Control Processes in Multicellular Organisms*. Vol 1. Ciba Foundation Symposium. Litwak G (editor). Academic Press, 1970.

Immunologic Reactions to Drugs & Allergy

Blumenstein GI: Drug treatment of allergies. 1. The pathophysiologic basis of allergy. *Semin Drug Treat* 1973; **2:**353.

Ishizaka T et al: Release of histamine and slow reacting substance of anaphylaxis by E system from sensitized monkey lung. *J Allergy* 1969;**43:**168.

Lichtenstein LM, Norman PS: Human allergic reactions. *Am J Med* 1969;**46:**163.

Parker CW: Drug allergy. *N Engl J Med* 1975;**292:**732.

Patterson R: *Allergic Diseases: Diagnosis and Management.* Lippincott, 1972.

Plaut M, Lichtenstein LM, Henney C: Properties of a subpopulation of T cells bearing histamine receptors. *J Clin Invest* 1975;**55:**856.

Russell AS, Lessoff MH: Hypersensitivity to drugs. *Clin Allergy* 1971;**1:**179.

Spiegelberg HL et al: Lymphocytes with immunoglobulin E FC receptors in patients with atopic disorders. *J Clin Invest* 1979;**64:**714.

Tjio AH, Hull WM, Gleich JG: Production of human immunoglobulin E in vitro. *J Immunol* 1979;**122:**2131.

58 | Management of the Poisoned Patient

Charles E. Becker, MD, & Kent R. Olson, MD

Acute poisoning is rarely fatal if good supportive care is given, but diagnosis and treatment must be based on sound pharmacologic principles. Common poisons include chemicals of industrial, medicinal, or natural (including biologic) origin that are encountered in the environment. Many therapeutic agents in excess dosage cause cellular injury or death, and the variable that distinguishes therapy from poisoning is the size of the dose. Poisoning may be acute, subacute, or chronic depending on the dose and the time course of the injury to tissues. Rational management of poisoning thus requires knowledge of the dose and time of administration of the toxin. Unfortunately, this information is often not available.

This chapter reviews some of the basic principles of poisoning as well as methods of diagnosis, routine and specialized laboratory procedures, and methods of enhancing elimination of toxins. Mention will be made also of common errors in management of poisoning.

Toxicologic problems are best viewed in a classic pharmacologic model. This model is based on the pharmacologic properties of physical and chemical agents and the effects of "normal" doses on "normal" people. Toxicology extends this information base to excessive doses. The history, physical examination, routine and specialized laboratory procedures, and responses to treatment are compared with the expected outcome from a given dose as estimated by clinical and laboratory criteria. It is essential in such a model to appreciate differences in neonates, infants, children, adults, and the elderly. Assessment of organs essential for detoxification must also be carried out. Especially important in toxicology are the theoretic and practical methods of removing or binding toxins before they are absorbed into or otherwise injure the body. This process is called decontamination.

In the common toxicologic problems such as sedative-hypnotic drug overdose, the physician's clinical experience is useful in management. However, in estimating subtle long-term effects following acute or subacute poisoning, care must be exercised in reviewing the toxicology literature because it often lacks information about specific dose-response criteria or the appropriate means of laboratory confirmation of a specific toxin.

TOXICOKINETICS & TOXICODYNAMICS

The term "toxicokinetics" has been coined to denote the absorption, distribution, excretion, and metabolism of toxins, toxic doses of therapeutic agents, and their metabolites. "Toxicodynamics" can be used to denote the injurious effects of these substances on vital function. Although there are many similarities between the pharmacokinetics and toxicokinetics of most substances, there are also important differences. The same caution applies to pharmacodynamics and toxicodynamics.

SPECIAL ASPECTS OF TOXICOKINETICS

Volume of Distribution

If a potential toxin, eg, digoxin, is sequestered outside the blood and bound avidly to tissue, its volume of distribution will be very great (see Chapter 3, Part I). A large volume of distribution requires unique strategies for management—eg, dialysis will be of little value, but specific binding antibodies will be of considerable value.

Clearance

Knowledge about total body clearance and half-life of a toxin makes it possible to evaluate strategies variously directed at combating immediate toxicity (which may be sufficient for toxins that are rapidly cleared) or enhancing clearance (which may be essential for toxins that would otherwise have very long half-lives).

Organ clearance is another important toxicokinetic variable. For example, a toxin may be 90% metabolized by the liver and 10% excreted in the urine. In such a case, it is possible to have a dramatic increase in urinary excretion and yet have relatively little effect on total body clearance if liver metabolism is the primary method of detoxification.

In cases of large oral overdose, dissolution of tablets or gastric emptying time may be altered so that the peak effects of the toxin are delayed. Toxins may also injure the gastrointestinal tract and thereby alter absorption. If the liver's finite capacity to metabolize a toxin is exceeded, a dose-dependent increase in the delivery of the agent to the systemic circulation may occur. Normally, the rate at which toxins are distributed to tissues depends on the rate of administration. Toxins enter the blood after absorption, bind to proteins, and then partition to tissues. With a dramatic increase in the concentration of a toxin in the blood, protein-binding capacity may be exceeded (eg, in aspirin overdose), so that the fraction of free toxin dramatically increases and thus confuses clearance calculations. Changes of half-life in toxic situations can thus reflect changes in volume of distribution owing to changes in protein binding or to alteration of the toxin-metabolizing systems themselves. Most toxins are eliminated at a rate that is directly proportionate to the plasma concentration (first-order elimination); however, if large quantities of a toxin are ingested, elimination capacity may be exceeded, thereby enhancing toxicity. Oral forms of some toxins can decrease gastrointestinal motility, leading to slowed transit through the gut. Under these circumstances, toxin may remain and absorption continue over a prolonged period. In such circumstances, induction of emesis, lavage, and administration of charcoal (a binding agent) or a cathartic are important factors in reducing the amount of toxin that is absorbed.

SPECIAL ASPECTS OF TOXICODYNAMICS

Knowledge of basic pharmacology may also help the physician anticipate important toxicodynamic problems in the diagnosis and management of the intoxicated patient. The general dose-response principles described in Chapter 2 are of crucial importance in determining the severity of the intoxication. When considering **quantal dose-response** data, both the therapeutic index and the overlap of therapeutic and toxic response curves must be considered. The standardized safety margin, if known, takes the latter factor into account. For instance, as shown in Fig 58–1, drugs A and B have the same therapeutic index. However, drug B is much more liable to cause inadvertent intoxication, because its toxic response curve overlaps the therapeutic dose range much more than in the case of drug A. For some drugs, eg, sedative-hypnotics, the major toxic effect is a direct extension of the therapeutic action, as shown by their **graded dose-response curves** (Fig 58–2). In the case of a drug with a flat dose-response curve (drug 1), lethal effects may require 100 times the normal therapeutic dose. In contrast, a drug with a steeper curve (drug 2) may be lethal at 10 times the normal dose.

For many drugs, at least part of the toxicity may be distinct from the therapeutic action yet interact with it. For example, intoxication with drugs that have atropinelike effects (eg, tricyclic antidepressants) will block sweating, making it more difficult to dissipate heat. In tricyclic antidepressant intoxication, there may also be increased muscular activity or seizures; the body's production of heat is thus enhanced, and lethal hyperpyrexia may result. Overdoses of drugs that depress the cardiovascular system, eg, beta-adrenergic blocking agents or barbiturates, can profoundly alter not only target organ function but all functions that are dependent on blood flow. These include renal and hepatic elimination of the toxin and any other drugs that may be given.

Conversely, lack of tissue perfusion with falling blood pressure may lead to a transient decrease in target organ drug levels. When the blood pressure is restored, enhanced delivery of the toxin can lead to an increase in the degree of intoxication. The result is a confusing waxing and waning of the signs and symptoms. Thus, an appreciation of the toxicodynamics of an agent will allow for better understanding of changes in the clinical course of intoxicated patients.

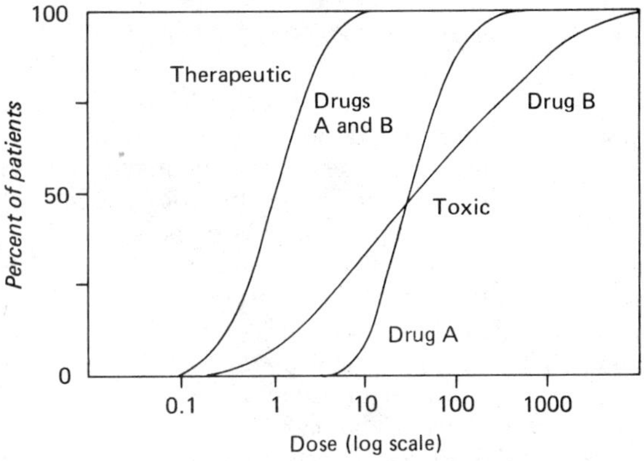

Figure 58–1. Quantal dose-response comparison of 2 drugs with differing safety margins. Both drugs have the same therapeutic index (TD50/ED50). However, at the dose required for therapeutic effects in 90% of patients, less than 1% of patients receiving drug A have toxicity, but 20% of those taking drug B are toxic.

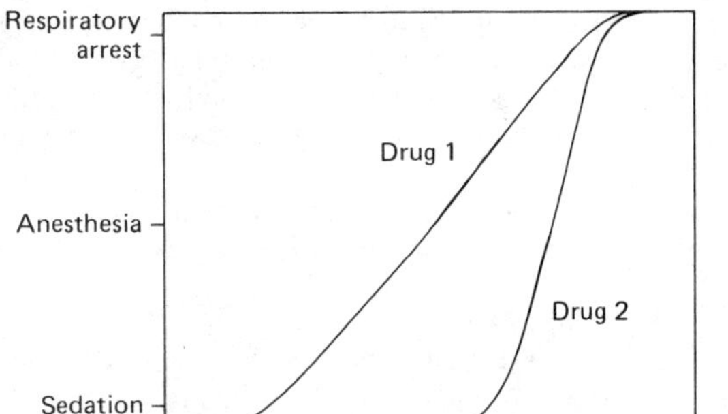

Figure 58–2. Graded dose-response comparison of 2 sedative-hypnotic drugs. A much larger multiple of the normal prescription dose of drug 1 is required to cause respiratory arrest, ie, it is safer than drug 2.

APPROACH TO THE POISONED PATIENT

History & Physical Examination

A. History: Oral statements about the amount and even the type of drug ingested in toxic emergencies are often unreliable. Family members, police, and fire department or paramedical personnel should nonetheless be asked to describe the environment in which the toxic emergency occurred and should bring to the emergency room all syringes, empty bottles, household products, or over-the-counter medications in the immediate vicinity of the possibly poisoned patient.

B. Initial Physical Examination: A brief but thorough physical examination should be performed with special emphasis on vital signs, eyes, skin, breath, mouth, and abdomen. The initial approach to the toxic emergency is to seek answers to 4 questions: (1) Based on the preliminary physical examination, can one arrive at a tentative diagnosis of the toxin ingested? (2) Will any routine or specialized laboratory procedures define the toxic emergency? (3) Will unique treatment have diagnostic importance (eg, naloxone treatment of narcotic overdose)? (4) Based on knowledge of toxicology, how severe (dose) is the overdose?

The answers to these questions provide a rational basis for initial decontamination, supportive care, and use of antidotes. However, one must always treat the patient and not the poison; eg, with a history of a large ingestion but no physical or laboratory evidence of toxicity, one must be cautious about giving potentially dangerous antidotes.

C. Assessment of Vital Signs: Careful observation of vital signs (respiration, pulse, blood pressure, and temperature) is essential in all toxic emergencies and should be done before decontamination procedures are initiated.

1. Respirations should be carefully counted to detect evidence of respiratory insufficiency induced by a toxin.

2. Pulse and blood pressure–Alteration of blood pressure and the pulse should be assessed in all toxic emergencies. Amphetamines and hallucinogenic drugs frequently raise the blood pressure, whereas sedative-hypnotic drugs usually lower it. Discrepancies between blood pressure and pulse (eg, both reduced) point to toxins that block autonomic reflexes.

3. Temperature–

a. Hyperthermia–Sympathomimetics (amphetamines), atropinelike medications (tricyclic antidepressants), and uncouplers of oxidative phosphorylation (aspirin) may cause hyperthermia.

b. Hypothermia–Sedative-hypnotic drugs, hypothyroidism, and hypoglycemia may cause hypothermia. In sedative-hypnotic drug overdose, vasodilatation may occur and lead to lowering of the core temperature, especially when there is exposure to low environmental temperatures. Hypothermia itself may mimic severe cardiovascular complications such as bradyarrhythmias.

D. Eye Examination: Among the most important physical findings in toxic emergencies are those associated with the eyes.

1. Constriction of pupils–Many toxins, especially central nervous system depressants, cause pupillary constriction; opiates, organophosphates, phenothiazines, pilocarpine, and clonidine are specific examples. Heat stroke and structural neurologic lesions, especially infarction of the pontine angle, also cause the pupils to constrict.

2. Dilatation of pupils–The pupils may be large when drugs releasing catecholamines, such as cocaine or amphetamine, are ingested. Drugs with atropinelike effects such as the tricyclic antidepressants also dilate the pupil. With brain death, pupils are fixed and dilated.

3. Nystagmus may be present with phencyclidine poisoning and in various states of barbiturate intoxication. Overdosage with phenytoin also causes nystagmus.

4. Ophthalmoplegia occurs with botulism, Wernicke's syndrome, and carbamazepine overdose.

5. Optic neuritis may be observed by ophthalmoscopic examination in many but not all patients with methanol poisoning.

6. Retinal hemorrhages may be present in cases of carbon monoxide poisoning and hypertensive emergencies.

E. Central Nervous System and Mental Status Examination: Careful recording of the mental status of the patient in toxic emergencies is essential. Specific description of the level of coma or agitation is most important. Blood behind the tympanic membranes or other evidence of head trauma must also be sought, since head trauma may be present in any toxic emergency. Focal neurologic findings are uncommon in toxic-metabolic emergencies. Muscular hyperactivity, rigidity, posturing, and tremor are common findings with many overdoses.

F. Examination of the Skin: Flushing may occur with atropine poisoning, apparent cyanosis with methemoglobinemia, icterus with acetaminophen poisoning, desquamation of the palms and soles with arsenic ingestion, bullae with sedative-hypnotic or carbon monoxide poisoning, sweating with catecholamine poisoning, and dry skin with poisoning due to atropinelike drugs. Needlemarks indicate parenteral injection.

G. Mouth Examination:

1. Ulceration of mucous membranes may occur with corrosive or acid injury.

2. Odors–Identifying odors may be detected on the breath, eg, alcohol, ammonia, tobacco, disinfectants, camphor, glue, paraldehyde, acetone, and hydrogen sulfide. Organophosphate pesticides and arsenic may yield a garlic breath odor, cyanide a bitter almond or silver polish odor, methyl salicylate a wintergreen odor, and chloral hydrate a pearlike odor.

Table 58–1. Drug-induced anion gap acidosis.

The normal anion gap calculated from ($Na^+ + K^+$) − ($HCO_3^- + Cl^-$) is 12–16 mEq/L; calculated from (Na^+) − ($HCO_3^- + Cl^-$), it is 8–12 mEq/L.

Type of Elevation of the Anion Gap	Agents
Metabolic acidosis	Methanol, ethylene glycol, salicylates, paraldehyde.
Lactic acidosis	Any drug-induced seizures, iron, phenformin, hypoxia.
Ketoacidosis	Ethanol, diabetes mellitus.

Laboratory & X-Ray Procedures

Once a tentative clinical diagnosis has been arrived at, based on the history and physical examination, laboratory procedures can be used to achieve greater diagnostic specificity and precision.

A. Blood Gases: Arterial blood gases should be measured to evaluate respiratory function and determine appropriate tissue perfusion. Often it is difficult to count respirations accurately; respiratory failure is quantitated by noting alterations in arterial P_{CO_2}.

B. Blood Chemistry: Serum sodium, potassium, chloride, and bicarbonate should be measured to estimate anion gap abnormalities. Table 58–1 lists some drugs that may induce anion gap metabolic acidosis. Diabetic ketoacidosis can be excluded by appropriate testing for blood sugar and ketone bodies. With kidney function abnormalities (see below) and diabetes mellitus excluded, other common causes of anion gap metabolic acidosis include aspirin, methanol, ethylene glycol, isoniazid, and ethanol overdose. Factitious elevated serum chloride levels may be reported in bromide poisoning.

C. Renal Function Tests: Kidney function measurement should include, in addition to urinalysis, blood urea nitrogen, and serum creatinine, a test for myoglobin in urine if there is potential for muscle destruction. Oxalate crystals may be present in the urine in cases of ethylene poisoning. Red blood cells in the urine and proteinuria suggest nephrotoxins.

D. Blood Osmolality: Calculated and observed osmolalities of serum will provide valuable clues to some life-threatening toxins. Calculated osmolality is dependent mainly on sodium, glucose, and blood urea nitrogen levels.

The calculated serum osmolality from

$$2 \times Na^+ \text{ (mEq/L)} + \text{Blood sugar (mg/dL)} \div 18 + \text{BUN (mg/dL)} \div 2.8$$

is 285 ± 4 mosm/L. The difference between the directly measured osmolality and that calculated from the above expression is normally zero. Since low-molecular-weight substances can significantly increase the directly measured value but are not included in the calculation, patients with high levels of alcohol, ethylene glycol, etc, will manifest an osmolar gap, corresponding to the concentration of the toxin:

$$\text{mg/dL Serum concentration} \simeq \text{Osmolar gap} \times \text{MW} \div 10$$

These abnormalities will be detected only when freezing point methods are used for determining osmolality. Table 58–2 lists the molecular weight, lethal dose, and expected contribution to total osmolality in lethal ethanol, methanol, ethylene glycol, and isopropanol poisonings.

E. Electrocardiogram: A widened QRS complex is a useful predictor of the severity of tricyclic antidepressant poisoning. Q–T interval may be prolonged in phenothiazine and tricyclic poisonings. The ECG may show evidence of hypothermia or altered electrolyte balance, especially hypokalemia. With chemical asphyxiants, acute elevations of the ST segment may be present in all leads of the ECG.

F. X-Ray Findings: A plain film of the abdomen to detect radiopaque toxins and capsules is most useful when obtained soon after ingestion. If hydrocarbon ingestion is suspected or if there is evidence of respiratory abnormalities, chest x-ray is required. If there is evidence of head trauma, blood behind the tympanic membrane, or cerebrospinal fluid rhinorrhea, skull x-rays should be obtained.

Screening Tests

Toxicologic screening techniques and assays for specific toxins in gastric juice, blood, or urine should not be relied on for major therapeutic decisions until they are verified by other more specific toxicologic laboratory tests.

A. Methemoglobinemia: The blood on filter paper test determines methemoglobin content. Blood that is chocolate-brown indicates at least 15% methemoglobin.

B. Aspirin Poisoning: Ferric chloride tests of urine and blood may detect aspirin qualitatively if the patient is excreting significant amounts of salicylate. It should be noted that unless the patient has an alkaline urine pH, he may not excrete detectable amounts of

Table 58–2. Substances that cause osmolar gap.

	Molecular Weight (mg/mol)	Lethal Level (mg/dL)	Corresponding Osm (mosm/L)
Ethanol	46	350	75
Methanol	32	80	25
Ethylene glycol	62	200	35
Isopropanol	60	350	60

Example: For ethanol (the commonest cause of osmolar gap), a gap of 30 mosm/L would indicate an ethanol level of 30 × 46 ÷ 10 = 138 mg/dL. See text for the basis of this calculation.

Note: Most laboratories use the freezing point method of determining osmolality. If the vaporization point method is used, the alcohols will be driven off and their contribution to osmolality will be lost.

salicylate, even with very high serum levels. This test may also suggest the presence of phenothiazines and isoniazid in the urine.

Other Examinations

If it is likely that the toxin was taken orally, a gastric aspirate should be sent to the toxicology laboratory. Empty bottles, syringes, or needles from the scene may also be helpful in diagnosis. The physician must know the specificity and sensitivity of the tests used. It is sometimes important to know whether or not the laboratory methods used distinguish the parent toxin from metabolites.

Time of Ingestion of Poison

To estimate the severity of poisoning, it is important to estimate the time since ingestion and compare it with the plasma level. The importance of time in evaluating plasma levels has been particularly well demonstrated for aspirin poisoning. An aspirin concentration of 50 mg/dL 4–6 hours after ingestion is associated with only mild intoxication; the same level obtained 36 hours after ingestion is associated with very severe poisoning. The basis for this relationship lies in the fact that the clinical manifestation of toxic effects in some target organs such as the brain may lag significantly behind the peak levels in the blood.

Blood Levels of Toxins

Note: Treatment should not be delayed while waiting for laboratory reports.

There are 5 acute toxic emergencies in which measurement of blood levels is necessary to monitor treatment: acetaminophen, aspirin, lithium, carbon monoxide, and theophylline poisoning. Poisoning with ethanol, methanol, ethylene glycol, and digoxin can usually be diagnosed on clinical grounds but must be confirmed by the toxicology laboratory. Quantitative analysis of blood and urine for sedative-hypnotic drugs is important when simple supportive procedures do not appear adequate and especially when dialysis is being considered, eg, in phenobarbital poisoning. Table 58–3 lists common sedative-hypnotic drugs, their kinetic parameters, and treatment methods.

A special role of the toxicology laboratory involves forensic toxicology and confirmation of brain death. Some toxic emergencies can mimic brain death. Therefore, decisions about depth and length of supportive care must be reviewed in light of thorough toxicology laboratory assessments.

Decontamination

Decontamination procedures should be undertaken after initial diagnostic assessment and laboratory evaluation. Decontamination involves removing toxins from the skin or gastrointestinal tract.

A. Skin: Contaminated clothing should be completely removed and saved for analysis. Percutaneous penetration of toxins has been poorly studied but should be anticipated. Vigorous washing with copious amounts of water and soap should be carried out.

B. Gastrointestinal Tract: ***Caution:*** It is essential to protect the airway. All necessary emergency equipment such as suction must be readily available. Seizures, absence of the gag reflex, and ulcerated oral mucous membranes are contraindications to emesis. Gastric lavage is contraindicated if the airway is at risk (eg, unconscious patient with no gag reflex). Acid and alkaline corrosives should be diluted but not neutralized.

Table 58–3. Toxicologic features of sedative-hypnotic overdose.

Drug	V_d (L/kg)	$t_{1/2}$ (Hours) Normal Doses	$t_{1/2}$ (Hours) Overdoses	Maximum Therapeutic Level (μg/mL)	Treatment	Comments
Phenobarbital	0.75	60–100	70–120	20	Supportive; hemoperfusion. Repeat administrations of charcoal by nasogastric tube are useful.	Avoid fluid overload.
Pentobarbital	1–2	20–30	50	50	Supportive.	Short-acting.
Chloral hydrate	0.6	4–8	10–20	15	Supportive.	Gastritis, arrhythmias. Radiopaque pills.
Glutethimide (Doriden)	20–25	8–12	24–40	0.5	Supportive.	Cyclic variation in coma; mydriasis.
Ethchlorvynol (Placidyl)	3–4	10–20	20–100	100	Supportive; hemoperfusion(?).	Pink or green gastric aspirate with pungent odor. Prolonged coma with overdose.
Methaqualone (Quaalude)	1–2	10–40	?	20	Supportive.	With severe overdose, muscular rigidity and myoclonus may occur.
Diazepam (Valium)	1–2	30–70	50–140	5	Supportive.	Severe overdose uncommon unless combined with other drugs.

Decontamination procedures have important clinical consequences. "Universal antidote" is not an antidote and certainly not a universal one. Therapists should not put their fingers in the patient's throat and should not use salt water or mustard as emetic agents.

1. Emesis–If the airway is protected by a gag reflex, there is no ulceration of mucous membranes, and the patient is not having seizures, induce emesis by oral administration of **ipecac syrup,** 30 mL for adults or 10–15 mL (in fruit juice) for children, repeated once after 15 minutes if necessary. (Ipecac fluid extract should be avoided because of its cardiac toxicity.) Home use of ipecac, an emetinelike alkaloid, has been documented to be safe and effective and should be part of the home treatment of children in poisoning emergencies. Ipecac is effective even when antiemetic medications have been taken in overdose. Apomorphine is much more toxic than ipecac, especially in children, because of its persistent emetic effects and the central nervous system depression it causes.

2. Gastric lavage–In adults, if the airway is protected by an endotracheal tube, gastric lavage may be performed. Gastric lavage is usually not successful in children, because of the necessity of using small-bore tubes; as large a tube as possible should be used in adults. Lavage solutions (usually 0.9% saline) should be at body temperature to prevent hypothermia.

3. Catharsis–Administration of a cathartic agent should hasten removal of toxins from the gastrointestinal tract and reduce absorption, though no controlled studies have been done. Pediatricians have reported finding whole tablets—especially enteric-coated ones—in stools after administration of cathartic agents. If charcoal is also administered, this procedure marks the stool with charcoal, so that total gastrointestinal transit time can be estimated. **Sodium sulfate** is the preferred cathartic agent if heart failure is not present. **Magnesium sulfate** may be used if renal function is unimpaired. Cathartic agents with an oil base are of no value and are potentially harmful. Table 58–4 lists some common cathartics.

Table 58–4. Usual doses of cathartics in decontamination.*

Magnesium citrate (10%) (magnesium = 1.6 mEq/mL)	Adult: 150–250 mL Child: 1–2 mL/kg
Magnesium sulfate (10%) (magnesium = 0.8 mEq/mL)	Adult: 150–250 mL Child: 1–2 mL/kg
Milk of magnesia	Adult: 15–60 mL Child: 0.1–0.2 mL/kg
Sodium sulfate (10%) (sodium = 1.4 mEq/mL)	Adult: 150–250 mL Child: 1–2 mL/kg
Sorbitol (70%)	Adult: 100–150 mL Child: 1–2 mL/kg

*Modified and reproduced, with permission, from Riegel JM, Becker CE: Use of cathartics in toxic ingestions. *Ann Emerg Med* 1981;**10**:254.

Note:

1. Avoid magnesium cathartics in renal disease and cases of nephrotoxin ingestion.
2. Avoid sodium cathartics in congestive heart failure and hypertension.
3. *Never* use oil-based cathartics.

4. Activated charcoal–Administration of activated charcoal is a valuable decontamination procedure if given in sufficient quantity because it binds many toxins. It is best to give it in a ratio of at least 10:1 of charcoal to estimated dose of toxin. It is believed that charcoal does not bind cyanide, iron, or alcohols. Generally, charcoal is underutilized and given in insufficient doses. Charcoal should not be administered simultaneously with ipecac, because it binds ipecac. In most studies in humans, charcoal was administered after normal therapeutic doses of drug; controlled studies of the use of charcoal after overdose are few. Recent studies suggest that serial administration of charcoal every 4 hours may be of value in shortening coma in sedative-hypnotic poisoning, especially in cases of phenobarbital overdose.

Specific Antidotes

There is a popular misconception that there is an antidote for every poison. The opposite is true—relatively selective antidotes are available for only 8 classes of toxins. The major antidotes and their characteristics are listed in Table 58–5. These drugs are supplemented by the immunologic agents such as snake antivenin (see below) and digoxin antibodies.

Methods of Enhancing Elimination of Toxins

After appropriate diagnostic and decontamination procedures and administration of antidotes, it is important to consider measures for enhancing elimination, such as forced diuresis, dialysis, or exchange procedures. If a patient is able to eliminate a toxin rapidly, the period of coma will be shortened, metabolites removed, and organ damage reduced. It is thus important to have knowledge of the toxicokinetics of the poison.

In cases of massive overdose, elimination pathways often involve enzyme and carrier systems with limited capacities. Elimination of even normal doses of ethanol, salicylate, and phenytoin is limited by saturation of the elimination mechanism. Drugs that have been demonstrated to exhibit concentration-dependent toxicokinetics in the overdose setting are chloral hydrate, ethchlorvynol, some barbiturates, theophylline, and acetaminophen. In cases of toxic ingestion of these drugs, methods of enhancing elimination that contribute to total body clearance can significantly improve the clinical outcome.

A. Techniques Available:

1. Dialysis procedures, including peritoneal dialysis, hemodialysis, and hemoperfusion, are theoretically appealing as a means of removing toxins that are eliminated through metabolic mechanisms that cannot be enhanced.

2. Renal elimination of a few toxins is enhanced by forced diuresis or alteration of urinary pH. Forced alkaline diuresis is useful in cases of salicylate or phenobarbital overdose. Forced acid diuresis has been

Table 58–5. Specific antidotes.

Antidote	Poison(s)	Comments
Naloxone (Narcan)	Narcotic drugs, propoxyphene, pentazocine, diphenoxylate.	A specific antagonist of narcotics. 0.4 mg (1 mL) may be given by IV, IM, or subcutaneous injection and repeated every 2–3 minutes for 2 or 3 doses. Larger doses may be needed to reverse the effects of overdose with propoxyphene.
Atropine	Anticholinesterases, organophosphates, physostigmine.	A test dose of 2 mg (for children, 0.05 mg/kg) is given IV until symptoms of atropinism appear (dilated pupils, ileus, tachycardia). Dose may be repeated every 10–15 minutes, with decrease of secretions as therapeutic end point.
Pralidoxime (2-PAM)	Anticholinesterases, organophosphates.	Adult dose is 1 g IV, which may be repeated every 8–12 hours as needed. Pediatric dose is approximately 250 mg. Benefit in carbamate poisoning is controversial.
Physostigmine salicylate	"Suggested" for antimuscarinic anticholinergic agents.	Adult dose is 1 mg IV slowly (usually 0.5 mg first) and wait for changes in diarrhea, urination, miosis, increased bronchial secretions, bradycardia, fasciculations, lacrimation, or salivation. Maximum initial doses: 4 mg for adults and 2 mg for children. The effects are transient (30–60 minutes), and the lowest effective dose may be repeated when symptoms return. Have atropine ready to reverse excess effects. Nonspecific central nervous system stimulation may occur.
Ethanol	Methanol, ethylene glycol.	Ethanol therapy is begun before laboratory diagnosis is confirmed. A loading dose is calculated so as to give a blood level of at least 100 mg/dL (42 g/70 kg in adults).
Sodium nitrite, sodium thiosulfate, amyl nitrite	Cyanide, hydrogen sulfide.	Nitrites cause production of methemoglobin, which has a greater affinity for cyanide than oxyhemoglobin. Sodium nitrite 3% (10 mL) is given IV over 5 minutes. Sodium thiosulfate 25% (50 mL) is given IV over 10 minutes. Reduce doses for children. Amyl nitrite is inhaled.
Deferoxamine (Desferal)	Iron salts. (Toxic dose, 60–70 mg/kg; lethal dose, 60–180 mg/kg.) Judge severity by white blood count, elevated blood sugar, severe vomiting and diarrhea, central nervous system depression, and plain film of abdomen.	If poisoning is severe, give 15 mg/kg hour IV *after* blood has been drawn for serum iron and iron-binding capacity determination. Maximum dose: 80 mg/kg/d. Urine will become wine-red. 100 mg of deferoxamine binds 8.5 mg of iron.
Metal chelators		
Dimercaprol (BAL)	Arsenic, gold, mercury.	Give 3–5 mg/kg every 4 hours IM for 2 days, then 2.5–3 mg/kg every 6 hours for 7 days. When urine arsenic falls below 50 μg/24 hours, antidote may be stopped. After 5 days off all chelation, repeat urine arsenic determination. Not effective for arsine gas. Side-effects: increased blood pressure, burning lips. Try to keep urine pH alkaline.
Calcium disodium ethylenediamine-tetraacetate (CaEDTA)	Lead.	Give 50–75 mg/kg/d IM or IV in 3–6 divided doses for up to 5 days in cases of lead encephalopathy. Modify dose in renal failure. Toxicity: zinc depletion and vitamin B_6 deficiency. Avoid oral therapy.
Penicillamine	Copper, lead, gold.	Give 1 g orally daily in 4 divided doses before meals.
N-Acetyl-D,L-penicillamine	Mercury.	Excreted rapidly by kidney. Side-effects: loss of taste, nephrotic syndrome, trace metal deficiencies.
Acetylcysteine (Mucomyst)	Acetaminophen.	Acetylcysteine binds to charcoal but may diffuse into blood. Best results if given within 12 hours of overdose. Follow liver function tests and acetaminophen blood levels. Little recognized toxicity. Dose: 140 mg/kg orally as loading dose, then 70 mg/kg orally every 4 hours for 17 doses in severe cases.

demonstrated to be useful in strychnine and amphetamine intoxication. (Acid diuresis has been proposed to be of value also in cases of phencyclidine [PCP] poisoning, but this requires further study.) Increasing renal elimination of most sedative-hypnotic drugs may increase the urinary concentration of the drug but contributes little to total body clearance. Such forced diuresis also enhances the risk of fluid and electrolyte imbalance and of worsening pulmonary function.

B. Dialyses:

1. Peritoneal dialysis–This is a relatively simple and available technique but is inefficient in removing most drugs.

2. Hemodialysis–Hemodialysis is more efficient than peritoneal dialysis and has been well studied. It assists in correction of fluid and electrolyte imbalance and may also enhance removal of toxic metabolites, eg, formate in cases of methanol poisoning. The efficiency of both peritoneal dialysis and hemodialysis is a function of the molecular weight, water solubility, protein binding, endogenous clearance, and distribution in the body of the specific toxin. Removal of drug with these procedures can be enhanced by increasing the time on dialysis or by altering the dialysis medium to bind the toxin. However, the complications of these procedures also increase with the length of time of dialysis. Hemodialysis is especially useful in overdose cases in which fluid and electrolyte imbalances are present or when toxic byproducts are removable.

a. Salicylate, methanol, and ethylene glycol are 3 toxins in which hemodialysis is the preferred method of treatment.

b. Because lithium overdose is extremely dangerous when sufficient to cause seizures and prolonged coma, prolonged hemodialysis is probably valuable but has not been adequately studied.

C. Hemoperfusion: Hemoperfusion for treatment of drug intoxication has been used increasingly in the past 5 years. Blood is pumped from the patient via a venous catheter through a column of adsorbent material and then recirculated to the patient. Systemic anticoagulation with heparin is required to prevent the blood from clotting in the cartridge. Hemoperfusion does not alter fluid and electrolyte balance and does not remove all toxic products. However, it does remove many high-molecular-weight toxins that have poor water solubility, because the perfusion cartridge has a large surface area for adsorption that is directly perfused with the blood and is not impeded by a membrane. The rate-limiting factors in removal of toxins by hemoperfusion are the affinity of the adsorbent resin for the drug, the rate of blood flow through the cartridge, and the rate of equilibration of the drug from the peripheral tissues to the blood. Many different hemoperfusion cartridges are now being studied for use in various toxic circumstances.

Although relatively few toxins have been studied, there is evidence that hemoperfusion may enhance whole body clearance of salicylate, phenytoin, ethchlorvynol, phenobarbital, and, in the early stages, theophylline and paraquat. Complications such as embolization of adsorbed particles, depletion of blood cells, and removal of proteins, solutes, and steroids have been minimized with increasing clinical experience.

D. Selection of Technique to Be Used: Drugs or toxins with extremely large volumes of distribution such as tricyclic antidepressants and digoxin are poorly removed by hemodialysis or resin hemoperfusion. Toxins with large volumes of distribution and intense protein binding would also be expected to be poorly removed by these methods. Therefore, critical review of kinetic parameters and dialysis capability is required before undertaking dialysis procedures. Table 58–6 lists intoxications requiring immediate dialysis, those used only if supportive measures fail, and those for which dialysis is not indicated. The toxicology laboratory should monitor methanol, ethylene glycol, salicylate, theophylline, phenobarbital, paraquat, and lithium blood levels during dialysis.

Table 58–6. Indications for hemodialysis (HD) and hemoperfusion (HP).

	Toxin	Procedure
Indicated immediately if significant intoxication	Ethylene glycol	HD
	Lithium	HD
	Methanol	HD
	Salicylate	HD
	Theophylline	HP
	Paraquat	HP
Indicated if supportive measures fail or if prolonged coma is expected	Digitoxin	HP
	Ethchlorvynol	HP
	Phenobarbital	HP, then HD if HP unsuccessful
	Tricyclic antidepressants	HP
Not indicated	Amphetamines, PCP, cocaine	
	Benzodiazepines (chlordiazepoxide, diazepam)	
	Chlorpromazine, haloperidol, other antipsychotics	
	Digoxin	
	Glutethimide	
	Narcotics	
	Quinidine, procainamide	
	Short-acting barbiturates	

The problems of enhancing elimination are well illustrated in PCP intoxication. Studies in laboratory animals suggest that there is limited renal clearance and little effect of blood pH changes on the distribution of the drug. However, urinary acidification has been demonstrated to increase the renal clearance of phencyclidine. Gastric acidification and gastric suction increase the diffusion of phencyclidine into gastric contents. Based on these preliminary data, large numbers of patients have been treated by acidification of the urine and gastric suction but with little documentation of the effectiveness of these techniques. Because intoxication with PCP has a waxing and waning clinical response, it has been difficult to evaluate improvement in the clinical status. Because phencyclidine poisoning is associated with muscle destruction and excretion of myoglobin in the urine, inappropriate acidification of the urine may increase the likelihood of precipitation of myoglobin, thereby increasing the likelihood of renal failure.

"Toxidromes"

Based on preliminary physical examination, routine and specialized laboratory tests, and response to antidotes, it is usually possible to estimate the dose and severity in the overdose setting. Table 58–7 is a

Table 58–7. "Toxidromes."

Acetaminophen
Mild anorexia, nausea, vomiting, delayed jaundice, renal failure.

Alcohol
Depressed sensorium, odor on breath, metabolic acidosis, osmolar and anion gap.

Amphetamines
Toxic psychosis, hyperthermia, flushing, increased blood pressure, dilated pupils, hallucinations, seizures, tachycardia, rhabdomyolysis.

Antifreeze (ethylene glycol)
Renal failure, crystals in urine, anion and osmolar gap, initial central nervous system excitation, normal eye examination.

Arsenic
Garlic on breath, vomiting, profuse bloody diarrhea, delayed hair loss, lines on nails, delayed neuropathy, increased skin pigmentation (arsine gas: hemolysis), burning tears.

Barbiturates
Bullae on skin, nystagmus, fluid accumulation in the lung. Prognosis depends on systolic blood pressure on admission and blood pH.

Botulism
Mimicking poisoning syndrome: vertigo, normal to dilated pupils, ptosis, ophthalmoplegia, muscle weakness. Incubation period 12–36 hours.

Bromide
Increased pigmentation, acne, dementia, psychosis, hyperchloremia.

Cadmium
Metallic taste, delayed pulmonary edema; late, kidney and lung disease.

Carbon monoxide
Bullae on skin, metabolic acidosis, normal P_{aO_2}, retinal hemorrhages.

Chloral hydrate
Pearlike odor, cardiac arrhythmias, abnormal plain film of abdomen.

Clonidine
Miosis, decreased blood pressure, decreased pulse, no response to naloxone.

Cocaine
Perforated nasal septum, dilated pupils, psychosis, tachycardia, scarred veins (cocaine burns).

Cyanide
Bitter almond odor, convulsions, coma, abnormal ECG.

Digitalis
Visual disturbances, delirium, abnormal ECG, nausea, increased serum potassium levels, normal kidney function.

Ethchlorvynol (Placidyl)
Deep coma, pungent aromatic odor, slow pulse, decreased blood pressure, pink gastric aspirate.

Gasoline
Distinctive odor, choking, pulmonary infiltrates.

Glutethimide (Doriden)
Dilated pupils, coma, prolonged respiratory depression, laryngeal spasms.

Heroin
Coma, decreased blood pressure, bradycardia, hypoventilation, miosis, needle marks, rapid response to narcotic antagonist.

Hydrocarbons
Pulmonary edema, lipid pneumonia, tinnitus, convulsions, ventricular fibrillation, unique odor.

Hydrogen sulfide
Rotten egg smell, sudden collapse, olfactory fatigue, conjunctivitis.

Iron
Bloody diarrhea, coma, radiopaque material on x-ray film, hypotension, pallor out of proportion to gastrointestinal bleeding, high leukocyte count, high blood glucose level.

Isoniazid
Coma, seizures, severe acidosis.

Isopropyl alcohol
Gastritis, acetonemia with normoglycemia, osmolar gap.

Lead
Abdominal pain, increased blood pressure, milky vomitus, convulsions, muscle weakness, metallic taste, anorexia, encephalopathy, delayed motor neuropathy, subtle changes in renal and reproductive function.

Lithium
Tremor, seizures, polyuria, delayed central nervous system and renal toxicity, prolonged coma.

LSD
Hallucinations, dilated pupils, hypertension.

Manganese
Patient is a steel or glass worker with parkinsonism.

Mercury
Acute renal failure, tremor, salivation, gingivitis, colitis, erethism (fits of crying, irrational behavior), nephrotic syndrome.

Methadone
Miosis, coma, slow pulse, decreased blood pressure and respiration, transient response to narcotic antagonist.

Methaqualone (Quaalude)
Increased reflexes, tonic-clonic spasms.

Table 58–7 (cont'd). "Toxidromes."

Methyl alcohol (methanol)
History of alcoholism; hyperventilation, visual symptoms, osmolar gap.

Methylene chloride
History of paint stripping exposure; confusion, increased carbon monoxide level, sudden death.

Methylphenidate (Ritalin)
Eosinophilia, wheezing, scarred veins, abscesses.

Mushrooms
Severe nausea and vomiting 8 hours after ingestion; delayed hepatic and renal failure with *Amanita phalloides.*

Nitrites (Rush)
Postural hypotension, flushing, anemia, methemoglobinemia.

Nitrogen and its oxides
History of silo or cave exposure; sudden collapse, no response to cardiopulmonary resuscitation, delayed pulmonary edema.

Organophosphates or carbamate
Miotic pupils, abdominal cramps, salivation, lacrimation, urination, defecation, increased bronchial secretions, muscle fasciculations, bradycardia.

Paraquat
Oropharyngeal burning, headache, vomiting, delayed pulmonary edema.

Phencyclidine (PCP)
Coma with eyes open, hyperacusis, myoclonic jerks, vertical nystagmus, analgesia, violent behavior.

Phenothiazines
Postural hypotension, hypothermia, miosis, tremor, radiopaque material on abdominal film, increased Q–T interval.

Phosgene
History of exposure to burning plastics; pulmonary edema.

Phosphorus, yellow
Garlic odor, necrosis of jaw ("phossy-jaw").

Plants, poisonous

Dieffenbachia and philodendron
Burning and swelling of mouth and tongue.

Nightshade family, Jimson weed
Hallucinations, dilated pupils, seizures (contain atropine-like alkaloids).

Oleander and foxglove
Digitalislike poisoning.

Predatory bean (rosary pea)
Delayed severe gastrointestinal distress, seizures, hemolytic anemia, death.

Propoxyphene (Darvon)
Pink gastric aspirate, seizures, miosis, limited response to naloxone.

Salicylates
Hyperventilation, vomiting, fever, bleeding, acidosis, tinnitus.

Scopolamine
Tachycardia, decreased secretions, urinary retention, dilated pupils, hallucination, confusion, dry skin, fever.

Strychnine
Stiff neck, status epilepticus, hyperacusis.

Thallium
Alopecia, gastrointestinal distress, rat poison, normal heme system, motor and sensory neuropathy.

Theophylline
Gastrointestinal distress, seizures, asthma patient.

Tricyclic antidepressants
Coma, convulsions, conduction disturbances, prolonged QRS.

Vacor (rat poison)
Sudden ketoacidosis, postural hypotension.

Vanadium
Green tongue, severe pulmonary irritation.

list of common poisons and the syndromes or "toxidromes" that result.

Supportive Care

Management of poisoning requires thorough knowledge of how to treat hypoventilation, coma, shock, seizures, and psychosis. Sophisticated toxicokinetic considerations are of little value if vital functions are not maintained. Hypoventilation and coma require particular attention to airway management. Arterial blood gases must be checked frequently, and aspiration of gastric contents must be prevented.

Fluid and electrolyte management may be complex. Monitoring body weight, central venous pressure, pulmonary capillary wedge pressure, and arterial blood gases is necessary to ensure adequate but not excessive administration of fluid.

Control of seizures may require lowering of body temperature or medications such as diazepam or phenytoin.

With appropriate support for coma, shock, seizures, and agitation, additional areas of supportive care may be checked. If bowel sounds are decreased or if excessive quantities of toxin are noted on the plain abdominal film, serial administration of activated charcoal may be required. Monitoring of renal and hepatic function is essential. Muscle destruction (rhabdomyolysis) may result in acute renal failure. Inadvertent acidification of the urine may increase the likelihood of renal insufficiency resulting from myoglobin destruction and excretion. Catheters in veins and arteries or in the bladder may become sources of infection. Large amounts of fluid at room temperature or dialysis procedures may lower body temperature and worsen cardiovascular function. Apparent worsening of the patient's status may follow administration of an antidote with a short half-life such as physostigmine or naloxone. Appropriate supportive treatment may on occasion result in physiologic survival of a neurologically impaired patient, so that lumbar puncture, CT scans, and electroencephalograms may be required to confirm brain death. One must be extremely cautious in diagnosing brain death, however, especially in cases of sedative-hypnotic drug overdose.

Treatment of Snake, Spider, & Scorpion Envenomation

The venoms of several snakes and scorpions and (in very small children) that of black widow spiders are important toxicologic emergencies. In the USA, rattlesnake bite is by far the most important, because of the amount of venom that may be injected, its intrinsic toxicity, and the fact that victims may be far from medical help when the bite occurs.

Evidence of envenomation includes local bleeding, severe pain, superficial edema of rapid onset, hemorrhagic bleb formation, lymphadenitis, and obvious fang marks. Many studies have shown that emergency field remedies such as incision and suction, tourniquets, and ice packs are far more damaging than useful. Avoidance of unnecessary motion, on the other hand, does help to limit the spread of the venom. Definitive therapy relies on antivenins and should be started as soon as possible.

Three antivenins are available in the USA: (1) mixed crotalid snake antivenin, (2) coral snake antivenin (used rarely), and (3) black widow spider antivenin (of little therapeutic value).

Blood should be typed and cross-matched before antivenin is administered. Clotting and bleeding times should be monitored. Dose of the antivenin should be adjusted according to the presence or absence of signs of systemic intoxication, including nausea, vomiting, paresthesias, bleeding disorder, shock, arrhythmias, renal failure, and pulmonary edema. For rattlesnake bite, at least 5 vials of mixed crotalid antivenin should be administered; if envenomation is severe, 10–20 vials may be required. Skin testing is important because the antivenins are made in horses; signs of serum sickness usually develop 10–12 days after treatment. It is important to avoid ice packs, incisions, tourniquets, fasciotomies, and steroids in snakebite management. Steroids are useful only for severe serum sickness.

Common Errors in Management of Poisoning

"Universal antidote" (burnt toast, magnesium oxide, tannic acid) is of no value and may be harmful. If ipecac syrup is to be used, it should be given at once and not postponed until arrival at the hospital or during the evaluation procedure in the emergency room. Clinical experience, especially in pediatrics, suggests that ipecac can be administered as instructed by the physician over the telephone.

In the past, ingested acid and alkaline substances were neutralized; this liberates heat and increases tissue destruction. Dilution of caustics or acid substances is preferred. Inducing emesis by placing a finger in the throat or with copper salts or hypertonic salt solution is hazardous to the mouth and esophagus. Use of oil-based cathartic agents may cause lipid pneumonia. Lavage fluids containing large quantities of sodium and phosphate may cause severe adverse reactions. Excessive hydration may worsen pulmonary function. Large amounts of glucose may lower phosphate and potassium. Respiratory stimulants and analeptic agents are of no value and are harmful in toxic emergencies.

• • •

References

Basic Texts

Arena JM (editor): *Poisoning: Toxicology, Symptoms and Treatment,* 3rd ed. Thomas, 1974.

Casarett LJ, Doull J (editors): *Toxicology: The Basic Science of Poisons.* Macmillan, 1980.

Gosselin RE et al: *Clinical Toxicology of Commercial Products,* 4th ed. Williams & Wilkins, 1976.

Proctor NH, Hughes JP: *Chemical Hazards of the Workplace.* Lippincott, 1978.

Other Sources

Berg GL (editor): *Farm Chemicals Handbook 1982.* Meister, 1982.

Rumack BH (editor): *Poisindex.* Micromedex, Inc., 1982.

Winchester JF et al: Dialysis and hemoperfusion of poisons and drugs: Update. *Trans Am Soc Artif Intern Organs* 1977;**23:**762.

Handbooks of Poisoning

Dreisbach RH: *Handbook of Poisoning: Prevention, Diagnosis, & Treatment.* Lange, 1980.

Hanenson IB (editor): *Quick Reference to Clinical Toxicology.* Lippincott, 1980.

Matthew H, Lawson AAH: *Treatment of Common Acute Poisonings,* 4th ed. Churchill Livingstone, 1979.

Useful Phone Numbers

Poison Control Centers:

San Francisco: (415) 666–2845

Denver: (303) 629–1123

Boston: (617) 232–2120

Teratogen Registry (California): (714) 294–3584

Chelators & Heavy Metal Intoxication | 59

Charles E. Becker, MD, & Maria Almira Correia, PhD

Heavy metals in the environment have posed a hazard to biologic organisms since life began. Some of the oldest diseases of humans can be traced to heavy metal poisoning associated with the development of metal mining, refining, and use. Even with the present recognition of the hazards of heavy metals, the incidence of intoxication remains significant and the need for effective therapy remains high.

I. PHARMACOLOGY OF CHELATORS

Chelating agents are the most versatile and effective antidotes for metal intoxication. These compounds are usually flexible molecules with 2 or more electronegative groups that form stable coordinate-covalent bonds with the cationic metal atom. The complexes thus formed are then excreted by the body. The action of these drugs provides an excellent application of the principle of chemical antagonism.

The efficiency of the chelator is partly determined by the number of ligands available for metal binding. Edetate (ethylenediamine-tetraacetate, Fig 59–1) is an important example. The greater the number of these ligands, the more stable the metal-chelator complex. Depending on the number of metal-ligand bonds, the complex may be referred to as mono-, bi-, or polydentate. The chelating ligands include functional groups such as –OH, –SH, and –NH, which can donate electrons for coordination with the metal. Such bonding effectively prevents interaction of the metal with similar functional groups of enzymes, coenzymes, cellular nucleophiles, and membranes. Unfortunately, chelators are often nonspecific and may chelate essential metals such as Ca^{2+} and Zn^{2+}, which are vital for body function. Such interactions are determined by the relative affinities of the toxic metal and the essential metal for the chelator. Thus, the toxicity associated with administration of some chelators may be associated with chelation of essential metals. This problem may be circumvented by judicious administration of the essential metal along with the chelating agent.

The relative efficacy of various chelators in facilitating excretion of metals from the body is also determined in part by the pharmacokinetics of the

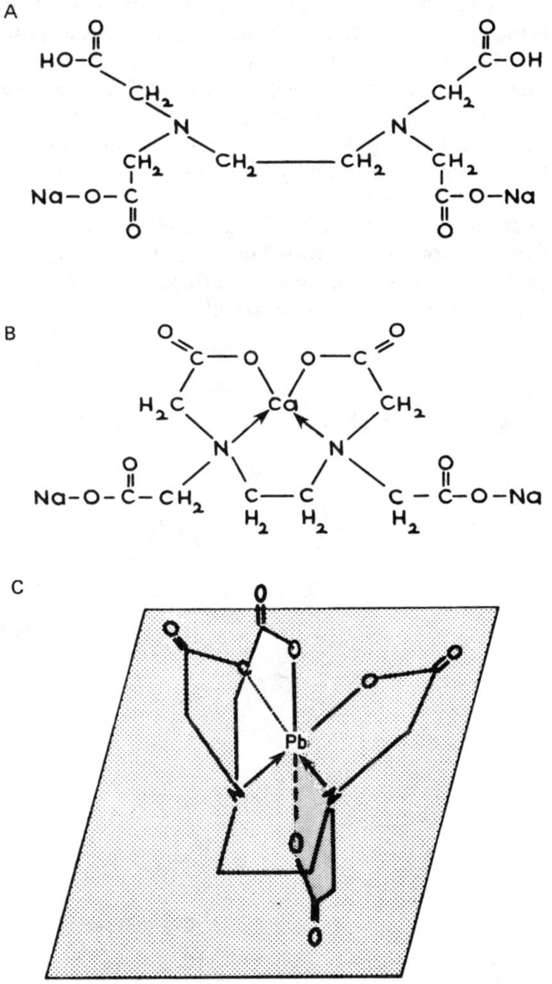

Figure 59–1. Salt and chelate formation with ethylene-diamine-tetraacetate (EDTA). *A:* In a solution of the disodium salt of EDTA, the sodium and hydrogen ions are chemically and biologically available. *B:* In solutions of calcium disodium edetate, calcium is bound by coordinate-covalent bonds with nitrogen as well as by the usual ionic bonds. Calcium ions are effectively removed from solution. *C:* In the lead-edetate chelate, lead is incorporated into 5 heterocyclic rings. (Modified and reproduced, with permission, from Meyers FH, Jawetz E, Goldfien A: *Review of Medical Pharmacology,* 7th ed. Lange, 1980.)

chelator in vivo. For any significant metal sequestration to occur, the affinity of the metal for the chelator must be greater than its affinity for endogenous ligands, and the relative rate of exchange of the metal between the endogenous ligands and the chelator must be faster than the rate of elimination of the chelator. If a chelator is eliminated more rapidly than the dissociation of the metal-endogenous ligand complex, it may not be present in sufficient concentrations for effective competition with the endogenous binding sites. This would be particularly critical if sequestration occurred via a ternary complex (endogenous ligand-metal-exogenous chelator). The above considerations also dictate that efficient mobilization can be accomplished only when the physiologic distribution of the chelator is the body compartment containing the metal. Following absorption, the tissue distribution profile of the metal may change markedly with time. For example, lead is first distributed to soft tissue such as bone marrow, liver, kidneys, and testes. Distribution to bone occurs subsequently. Therefore, the choice of chelator may also be determined on the basis of its distribution to primary and secondary tissue sites. Combination therapy with 2 or more chelating agents, each capable of permeating different target tissue compartments, may prove useful.

SPECIFIC AGENTS

Bidentate

DIMERCAPROL (BAL; 2,3-Dimercaptopropanol)

Dimercaprol (Fig 59–2) is a colorless oily liquid with an offensive odor of rotten eggs. It is soluble in water, but aqueous solutions are unstable and oxidize readily. Dimercaprol is therefore dispensed in 10% solution in peanut oil and must be administered intramuscularly. It interacts directly with metals in blood and tissue fluids and reactivates cellular sulfhydryl-containing enzymes. However, it is most efficient if administered immediately following exposure to the metals. This indicates that its salutary effects may be due primarily to *prevention* of metal binding to cellular constituents rather than *removal* of metal already bound.

Indications & Toxicity

Dimercaprol is a useful antidote in arsenic, mercury, lead, and cadmium poisoning. Given intramuscularly, it is readily absorbed, metabolized, and excreted within 4 hours. It produces a variety of side-

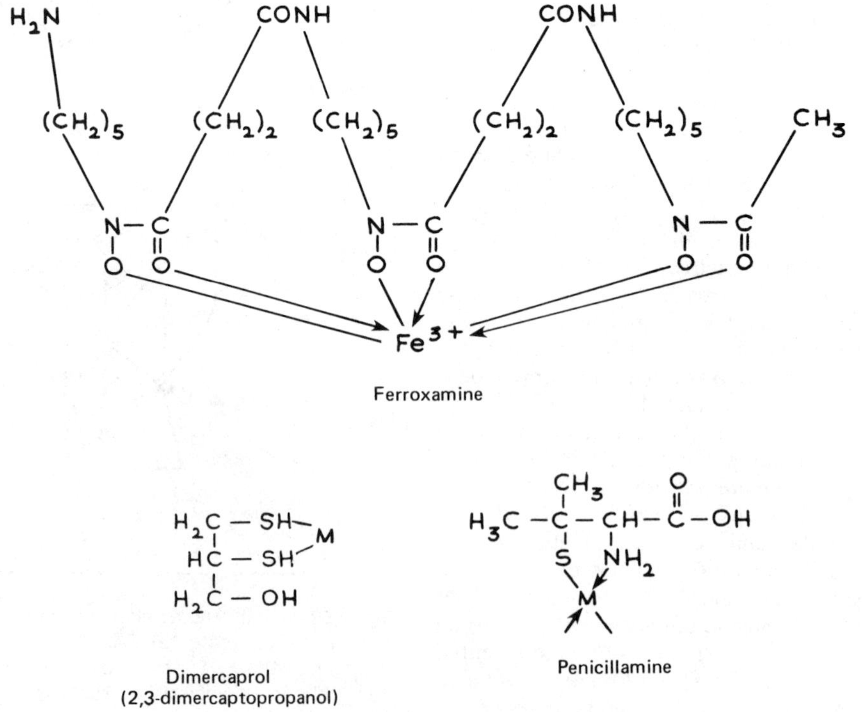

Figure 59–2. Chemical structures of several metal chelates. Ferroxamine without the chelated iron is deferoxamine. It is represented here to show the functional groups; the iron is actually held in a caged system. Dimercaprol incorporates the metal into a stable heterocyclic ring by covalent bonding. A single molecule of copper or other metal may be held by 2 molecules of penicillamine. M = metal molecules. (Modified and reproduced, with permission, from Meyers FH, Jawetz E, Goldfien A: *Review of Medical Pharmacology,* 7th ed. Lange, 1980.)

effects of which the cardiovascular are most significant. It also causes headache, nausea, vomiting, lacrimation, salivation, paresthesias, and pain. Because of the high incidence of these untoward side-effects, several congeners are currently being investigated. One of them is the 2,3-dimercaptopropane-1-sulfonate, which, owing to its relatively greater polarity, may remain confined to the extracellular space to a greater extent and thus reduce cellular toxicity. However, for the same reason, its relative efficacy as compared to BAL may also prove to be inferior. A second analog is 2,3-dimercaptosuccinic acid, which has been found to be relatively less toxic than BAL and effective by the oral route.

PENICILLAMINE (D-β,β-Dimethylcysteine)

Penicillamine (Cuprimine) (Fig 59–2) is a white crystalline, water-soluble product of degradation of penicillin. The D isomer is relatively nontoxic compared to the L form and consequently is the preferred form of the antidote. Penicillamine is readily absorbed from the gut and is resistant to metabolic degradation. Greater resistance to metabolic degradation has also been achieved by N-acetylation, as in N-acetylpenicillamine.

Indications & Toxicity

Penicillamine is used chiefly for poisoning with copper or to prevent copper accumulation, as in Wilson's disease. It is also used as adjunctive therapy in the treatment of lead and arsenic poisoning.

Pyridoxine deficiency is a frequent toxic effect of other forms of the drug but is rarely seen with the D form. Acute allergic reactions may, however, preclude the continued use of the drug. Nephrotoxicity with proteinuria has also been reported and with protracted use of the drug may result in renal insufficiency. Bone marrow toxicity resulting in aplastic anemia has been associated with prolonged drug intake. Autoimmune diseases, including lupus erythematosus and hemolytic anemia have been reported also.

Polydentate

EDETATE CALCIUM DISODIUM

Ethylenediamine-tetraacetic acid (EDTA, Versenate) (Fig 59–1) is an efficient chelator of many divalent and trivalent metals in vitro. However, chelation of essential calcium in vivo—due to this very property—limits its clinical use. This limitation has been partially circumvented by administration of its calcium disodium salt.

EDTA penetrates cell membranes relatively poorly, thus serving primarily as an extracellular rather than an intracellular chelator.

The highly polar ionic character of EDTA precludes significant oral absorption, and consequently the chelator (calcium disodium salt) is administered either by slow intravenous infusion or intramuscularly. It is excreted by glomerular filtration in the urine almost completely unchanged over 24 hours.

Indications & Toxicity

Metals such as lead and a few other heavy metals capable of binding EDTA and displacing Ca^{2+} are effectively chelated. EDTA-induced mobilization of mercury, in contrast to that of lead, is unsuccessful, perhaps owing to the relatively poor distribution of the chelator into tissue compartments where mercury is found as well as to the less successful competition of mercury with the chelated calcium.

EDTA is toxic to the kidney, and the renal tubules appear relatively sensitive to its toxic effects, which include hydropic degeneration of the proximal tubules, progressing into total destruction. These effects disappear with cessation of therapy. Other toxic effects have been observed also, including chills, fever, nausea, vomiting, myalgia, allergic reactions, and glycosuria.

DEFEROXAMINE

Deferoxamine mesylate (Desferal) is isolated from *Streptomyces pilosus*. It binds iron avidly but essential trace metals poorly. Furthermore, while competing for loosely bound iron in iron-carrying proteins (hemosiderin and ferritin), it fails to compete with biologically chelated iron, as in microsomal and mitochondrial cytochromes and hemoproteins. Consequently, it is the chelator of choice for iron poisoning.

Deferoxamine is poorly absorbed when administered orally. To be effective, it must be administered intramuscularly or intravenously. It is believed to be metabolized, but the pathways are unknown. The products are excreted almost completely in the urine. Intravenous administration may result in hypotensive shock due to histamine release.

Use of deferoxamine in iron poisoning is described in Chapter 30.

II. TOXICOLOGY OF HEAVY METALS

LEAD

The toxic effects of lead probably constitute the oldest occupational disease in the world. Lead is now widely distributed in air, food, and water, so that a completely lead-free environment would be difficult or impossible to achieve. With a greater understanding of the kinetics and toxicology of lead, acute lead poisoning is fortunately much less frequent than in the past. Hazardous working conditions have been improved, exposure of children to flaking lead-base paints has been reduced, and adult exposure to illicit whiskey and battery casings is less frequent. However, important public health questions remain concerning environmental pollution and the hazard to reproductive, hematopoietic, and neurologic function imposed by chronic lead exposure.

Pharmacokinetics

Metallic lead is slowly but consistently absorbed by all routes except through the skin. Absorption of lead dust via the respiratory tract is the most common cause of industrial poisoning. The intestinal tract is the primary route of entry in nonindustrial exposure (Table 59–1). Absorption via the gastrointestinal tract varies with the nature of the lead compound, but in general, about 10% of ingested inorganic lead is absorbed. Dietary calcium, iron, and phosphorus may alter gastrointestinal lead absorption. Studies in laboratory animals demonstrate that a diet low in calcium increases lead retention and that there are associated biochemical and morphologic manifestations of enhanced lead toxicity.

Once absorbed from the respiratory or gastrointestinal tract, lead is bound to erythrocytes and widely distributed initially to soft tissues such as bone marrow, liver, kidney, and testes. Its half-life in these tissues is about 30 days. Lead also crosses the placenta and poses a potential hazard to the fetus. Most lead entering the body is eventually bound in the skeleton; the half-life of elimination from bone is in excess of 20 years. Lead is also bound in hair and nails, which could theoretically be a useful method of estimating the body burden. However, external contamination creates special problems in interpreting these levels. Ingested lead is excreted in the stool (over 90%) and urine. Most of the absorbed lead is excreted via renal elimination. Lead is also eliminated through sweat and in mother's milk.

Pharmacodynamics

Lead is capable of forming complex ligands with many compounds. It interferes with the activity of enzymes and affects a variety of organ systems.

A. Blood: The organ system most sensitive to lead is the hematopoietic system. Hypochromic microcytic anemia is common, but not all patients with

Table 59–1. Toxicology of lead, mercury, and arsenic.

	Form Entering Body	Route of Absorption	Distribution	Target Organs for Toxicity	Metabolism	Elimination
Lead	Inorganic lead oxides and salts.	Gastrointestinal, respiratory, skin (minor).	Bone (90%), teeth, hair, blood (erythrocytes), liver, kidney.	Hematopoietic tissues and liver, CNS, kidney, neuromuscular junction.	Dissociation and binding of lead to critical tissue sulfhydryl groups.	Urine and feces (major); sweat (minor).
	Organic (tetraethyl lead).	Skin (major), gastrointestinal.	Liver.	CNS.	Hepatic dealkylation (fast) → trialkylmetabolites (slow) → dissociation to lead.	Same as above.
Mercury	Elemental mercury.	Respiratory tract.	CNS (where it is trapped as Hg^{2+}), kidney (following conversion of elemental Hg to Hg^{2+}).	CNS (neuropsychiatric due to elemental Hg and its Hg^{2+} metabolite), kidney (substantial due to conversion of elemental Hg to Hg^{2+}).	Elemental Hg converted to Hg^{2+}.	Urine (major); feces (minor).
	Inorganic: Hg^{+} (less toxic); Hg^{2+} (more toxic).	Gastrointestinal, skin (minor).	Kidney (predominant), blood, brain (minor).	Kidney, GI.	Hg^{2+} plus R–SH converted to Hg^{+}–S–R, $Hg(S{-}R)_2$.	Urine.
	Organic: alkyl, aryl, alkoxy-alkyl.	Gastrointestinal, skin (substantial).	Kidney, brain, blood.	CNS.	R–Hg^{+} converted to Hg^{2+} plus R (slow).	Urine.
Arsenic	Inorganic arsenic salts.	Gastrointestinal, skin, respiratory (all mucous surfaces).	Red cells (95–99% bound to globin) 24 hours, then to liver, lung, kidney, wall of gastrointestinal tract, spleen, muscle, nerve tissue (2 weeks), then to skin, hair, and bone (years).	Increased vascular permeability leading to vasodilatation and vascular collapse. Uncoupling of oxidative phosphorylation resulting in impaired cellular metabolism.	Binds avidly to cellular sulfhydryl groups of various critical enzymes to form stable cyclic thioarsenicals. Substitutes for inorganic phosphorus in synthesis of high-energy phosphates.	Principally renal. Sweat and feces minor.

lead poisoning are anemic. Lead induces critical derangements in heme biosynthesis, leading to excretion of porphyrins and their precursors in urine. The enzymes most sensitive to lead inhibition are delta-aminolevulinic acid dehydratase and ferrochelatase. Inhibition of the first enzyme blocks conversion of delta-aminolevulinic acid to porphobilinogen. Delta-aminolevulinic acid is excreted in the urine, and the urine concentration can be used as a diagnostic test. Inhibition of ferrochelatase results in decreased production of heme and accumulation of its precursor, protoporphyrin IX. In addition, the shortened life span of erythrocytes contributes to lead-induced anemia.

B. Nervous System: Lead also affects the peripheral and central nervous systems. The lowest concentration of lead associated with neurologic damage is still uncertain. Even at very high blood levels and marked alterations of hematopoietic function, some individuals may have no neurologic manifestations. The most common sign of peripheral neuropathy is painless weakness of the extensor muscles of the hand (wristdrop). The lower limb is less often involved. Sensory function is usually not affected. Lead-induced neuropathy usually develops after months of chronic exposure but may occur subacutely in 2–3 weeks.

Lead encephalopathy is an important acute disorder usually seen in children who have eaten lead-base paints. It is rare in adults. Encephalopathy most often begins with convulsions and is associated with increased intracranial pressure and brain edema. The mortality rate is high, and urgent chelation therapy is required.

C. Kidneys: Lead may cause kidney damage. Acutely, lead may affect uric acid metabolism and cause both acute gout and gouty nephropathy. Lead nephropathy itself develops only after years of prolonged lead exposure.

D. Reproductive Organs: Lead also affects reproductive function. It has long been known that lead poisoning is associated with decreased fertility in women and an increased incidence of stillbirths. Little is known about the effects of lead on male reproductive function, though sterility and testicular atrophy have been noted in severe cases, and asymptomatic lead exposure has been associated with dose-related alteration of sperm.

E. Gastrointestinal Tract: Lead poisoning causes loss of appetite, epigastric distress, abdominal colicky pains, and constipation. The mechanism of lead colic is unclear but involves contraction of smooth muscles of the intestinal wall. The gastrointestinal symptoms are reversible with chelation therapy.

Major Forms of Lead Intoxication

A. Inorganic Lead Poisoning:

1. Acute–Acute inorganic lead poisoning is very uncommon. It usually results from industrial inhalation of large quantities of lead oxide or, in small children, from ingestion of a large oral dose of lead in lead-based paints. Acute intoxication is associated with severe gastrointestinal distress that progresses to marked central nervous system abnormalities and anemia. If absorption of lead is slower, abdominal colic and encephalopathy may develop over days. The diagnosis of acute inorganic lead poisoning may be difficult. Disorders that simulate lead poisoning include appendicitis, peptic ulcer, and pancreatitis.

2. Chronic–The most common manifestations of chronic inorganic lead poisoning are weakness, anorexia, nervousness, tremor, weight loss, headache, and gastrointestinal symptoms. The association of recurrent abdominal pain and extensor muscle weakness without sensory disturbances suggests the possibility of lead poisoning. The most characteristic neurologic finding in chronic lead poisoning is wristdrop.

The diagnosis is confirmed by measuring lead in the blood and identifying abnormalities of porphyrin metabolism. The zinc erythrocyte protoporphyrin test is especially valuable if iron deficiency anemia can be ruled out. Peripheral blood smears may show basophilic stippling. Lead deposits in long bones are uncommon, as are lead lines on the gums.

Treatment is discussed below.

B. Organic Lead Poisoning: Organic lead poisoning is usually caused by tetraethyl or tetramethyl lead, which is used as an "antiknock" agent in gasoline. Organic lead is highly volatile and lipid-soluble. Thus, it can be readily absorbed through the skin and respiratory tract. Acute central nervous system disorders result. These can progress rapidly, causing hallucinations, insomnia, headache, and irritability (similar to severe alcohol withdrawal). Organic lead causes relatively few hematologic abnormalities. Tetraethyl and tetramethyl lead are metabolized by the liver to trialkyl lead and inorganic lead. Trialkyl lead is thought to be responsible for the acute poisoning syndrome. Chronic poisoning with organic lead is fortunately uncommon. Most organic lead exposures occur in the course of cleaning gasoline storage tanks. With massive organic lead exposure, seizures may terminate in coma and death. Blood and urine lead levels are relatively unreliable in organic lead poisoning but may be elevated.

Treatment is discussed below.

Treatment

A. Inorganic Lead Poisoning: Treatment of inorganic lead poisoning involves immediate termination of exposure and use of chelation therapy. The more severe the symptoms, the more urgent the need for chelation therapy. For severe intoxication, use an intravenous infusion of calcium disodium EDTA in a dose of approximately 8 mg/kg; dimercaprol, 2.5 mg/kg/dose intramuscularly, may also be given. Blood and urine levels of lead should be monitored as a guide to therapy. For less severe acute intoxication, chronic therapy with penicillamine (Cuprimine), 1 g over 24 hours orally in divided doses, may be repeated until blood and urine lead levels are reduced. Treating asymptomatic patients with chelating agents is not recommended. Prophylactic use of chelating agents in workers exposed to lead is contraindicated. After discontinuing chelation therapy, blood lead and porphyrin function should be assessed by serial analysis in order to identify a rebound increase in lead as lead is mobilized from bone.

B. Organic Lead Poisoning: Initial treatment consists of decontaminating the skin and preventing further exposure. Treatment of seizures requires judicious use of anticonvulsants.

ARSENIC

Elemental arsenic and arsenic compounds are widely distributed in nature. Arsenic is a common contaminant of coal and of many metal ores, especially copper, lead, and zinc. The 2 largest sources of industrial arsenic are coal-burning power plants and smelters. Approximately 1.5 million employees in the USA are potentially exposed to arsenic compounds.

The chemical forms of arsenic of toxicologic importance are elemental arsenic, inorganic arsenic, organic arsenicals, and arsine gas (AsH_3).

Arsenic was used as both a therapeutic agent and poison in ancient Greek and Roman times. More recently (until the advent of penicillin), arsenic was used in the treatment of syphilis and as a tonic in Fowler's solution. Its only therapeutic use today is in the treatment of trypanosomiasis involving the central nervous system. The most common nonmedical uses of arsenic compounds are as insecticides, herbicides, fungicides, algicides, and wood preservatives. Arsenic is also used for doping semiconductors, alloying, and in glassmaking.

Pharmacokinetics

Environmental and dietary exposure to arsenic and its compounds is possible, since arsenic is present in ocean water, especially near the mouths of estuaries draining industrial areas. Alcoholic beverages when improperly prepared occasionally contain large amounts of arsenic. Many types of seafood contain high levels of pentavalent arsenic. These environmental contaminants may account for elevated urinary arsenic levels. The average daily intake of arsenic from environmental sources is less than 1 mg. The total body burden of arsenic in adults is about 20 mg, mostly in bone and to a lesser extent in hair and skin. Inorganic arsenic can be absorbed from the lungs, the gut, and occasionally through intact skin (Table 59–1).

Gastrointestinal absorption of arsenic compounds is a function of their water solubility. Trivalent arsenites are poorly soluble and pentavalent arsenates more soluble. Organic arsenicals are usually poorly absorbed from the gastrointestinal tract. Arsenic can cross the placenta and may cause fetal damage. The trivalent form of arsenic is excreted slowly, chiefly by the fecal route, whereas the pentavalent form is more rapidly excreted in urine in a methylated form. Absorption of arsenic through the skin is a function of lipid solubility, with the trivalent form being more lipid-soluble than the pentavalent form. Trivalent inorganic arsenicals are partially oxidized in the body to the pentavalent form, and some is methylated.

Pharmacodynamics

All of the major toxicologic effects of inorganic arsenical compounds are attributable to the trivalent form of arsenic. Trivalent arsenic inhibits sulfhydryl enzymes and is corrosive to epithelium lining the respiratory and gastrointestinal tracts, to skin, and to other tissues. The primary target organs for trivalent arsenic are the nervous system, bone marrow, liver, skin, and respiratory tract.

Major Forms of Arsenic Intoxication

A. Acute and Subacute Inorganic Arsenic Poisoning: Acute and subacute forms of inorganic arsenic poisoning may produce acute violent nausea, vomiting, abdominal pain, skin irritation, laryngitis, and bronchitis. The gastroenteritis may be so severe as to be hemorrhagic. A sweet metallic garlicky odor is imparted to breath and feces. Vomiting may be severe, and diarrhea may be characterized as "rice water stool." The trivalent form of arsenic also damages capillaries, causing increased permeability, dehydration, shock, and death. If patients survive the acute episodes, bone marrow depression, encephalopathy, and a crippling sensory neuropathy may follow.

Treatment of acute arsenic poisoning includes induction of emesis or gastric lavage, correction of dehydration and electrolyte imbalance, and supportive care for liver and other tissue injury. In severe cases, give also immediate chelation therapy with dimercaprol, 3–5 mg/kg intramuscularly every 4 hours for 48 hours. Dimercaprol is continued every 12 hours for 10 days while monitoring urinary excretion of arsenic. Occasionally, oral penicillamine therapy may be used as an adjunctive measure if dimercaprol injections cause intolerable pain.

B. Chronic Inorganic Arsenic Poisoning: Chronic inorganic arsenic poisoning may present as perforation of the nasal septum, irritation of the skin, sensory neuropathy, hair loss, bone marrow depression, fatty infiltration of the liver, or renal damage. The skin manifestations include cutaneous vasodilatation and pallor (from anemia), resulting in a characteristic "milk and roses" complexion. Prolonged arsenic exposure may lead to hyperkeratosis of the palms and soles, increased skin pigmentation, hair loss, and white lines over the nails. Patients may become cachectic owing to chronic nausea and gastrointestinal complaints. Conjunctivitis and irritation of the mucous membranes, larynx, and respiratory passages are common.

Laboratory diagnosis of inorganic arsenic poisoning may be difficult. Urinary arsenic measurements and hair and nail analysis are indications of exposure but not intoxication. Urinary arsenic levels are influenced by intake of seafood. Most unexposed persons taking an average amount of seafood in the diet will excrete less than 100 μg of arsenic per 24 hours in the urine. Laboratory evidence of bone marrow suppression, abnormal liver function tests, proteinuria, and hematuria may also be diagnostically useful.

C. Organic Arsenic Poisoning: Organic arsenical poisoning is rare. Organic arsenicals are absorbed to a varying extent depending on their valences and are usually rapidly excreted. Benzene arsenicals are not converted to inorganic arsenic compounds under most circumstances. The mechanism of organic arsenical toxicity involves inhibition of sulfhydryl enzymes, especially in the central nervous system. Cerebral lesions are occasionally observed in both gray and white matter. Symptoms of encephalopathy, headache, convulsions, and coma may occur with organic arsenical poisoning.

D. Arsine Gas Poisoning: Arsine gas (AsH_3) is one of the most powerful hemolytic agents known. It is absorbed primarily through inhalation. Arsine combines with hemoglobin and is oxidized to a hemolytic compound. Dramatic destruction of red blood cells leads to hemoglobinuria, causing acute renal failure. Extensive renal tubular damage occurs, along with thickening of glomerular basement membranes. Initial symptoms are dark urine, jaundice, and severe abdominal pain. Severe arsine exposure will lead to high arsenic levels in the urine. Laboratory findings consist of hemolysis and severe anemia. Chelation therapy is generally not useful to prevent red cell destruction. Supportive care, including exchange transfusion and hemodialysis for renal failure, determines the outcome with acute arsine poisoning.

E. Other Manifestations of Arsenic Poisoning: Increased incidence of skin cancer is recognized in patients undergoing prolonged treatment for psoriasis and other skin disease with inorganic arsenicals, especially Fowler's solution. A study of smelter workers in the USA suggests an increased risk of respiratory system cancer that is probably dose-related. Since smelter workers have multiple exposures and confounding variables for enhanced risk of respiratory cancer, further studies are required to define the risk. Attempts to demonstrate the carcinogenic potential of arsenic compounds in animals have generally been unrewarding. Mutagenic testing, especially with the Ames test, has failed to show any mutagenic effects of arsenic compounds.

MERCURY

Metallic mercury as "quicksilver"—the only metal that is liquid under ordinary conditions—has attracted scholarly and scientific interest from earliest times. It was quickly recognized that the mining of mercury was hazardous to health. As industrial uses of mercury became common during the past 200 years, new forms of toxicity were recognized that were found to be associated with inorganic compounds of the element or of the metal itself. In 1953, a mysterious epidemic occurred in the Japanese fishing village of Minamata. The village is located near the effluent of a large factory in which vinyl plastic is manufactured. The epidemic of poisoning was traced to the consumption of fish contaminated by the effluent discharged by the factory. The causative agent was methyl mercury, formed in ocean water by bacterial action on inorganic mercury from the effluent.

The main sources of inorganic mercury as a toxic hazard include materials used in dental laboratories, wood preservatives, herbicides, insecticides, spermicidal jellies, fireworks, batteries, thermometers, barometers, gauges, and preparations of chlorine and sodium hydroxide. Organic mercury compounds are used as seed dressings, as fungicides, and in preventing mold.

Pharmacokinetics

The absorption of mercury varies considerably depending on the chemical form of the metal. Elemental mercury is poorly absorbed from the gastrointestinal tract but is quite volatile and can be absorbed from the lungs (Table 59–1). Inhaled mercury is the primary source of occupational exposure. Organic short-chain alkyl mercury compounds are volatile and potentially harmful by the same route. After absorption, mercury is distributed to the tissues in a few hours, with the highest concentration occurring in the proximal renal tubules. Mercury is readily bound to sulfhydryl groups. Excretion of mercury is primarily through the urine, although some is removed through the gastrointestinal tract and the sweat glands. Most inorganic mercury gaining entrance into the body is excreted over a 1-week period, but the kidney and the brain retain mercury for longer periods.

The acute and chronic poisoning syndromes with mercury depend on the form of the metal. Oral metallic mercury has little effect. Oral mercurous chloride has relatively low toxicity. Mercuric chloride is very toxic and causes acute kidney damage. Organic mercurials, especially methyl mercury, are more completely absorbed from the gastrointestinal tract. The short-chain organic mercury compounds are usually distributed to the central nervous system and are devoid of renal toxicity.

Major Forms of Mercury Intoxication

A. Acute: Acute mercury poisoning most frequently occurs from inhalation of high concentrations of mercury vapor. Symptoms include chest pain and shortness of breath, metallic taste, and nausea and vomiting. Acute damage to the kidney occurs next. If the patient survives, severe gingivitis and gastroenteritis occur on the third to fourth days. In the most severe cases, severe muscle tremor and psychopathology develop.

B. Chronic: Chronic mercury poisoning may be difficult to diagnose. Complaints of mouth and gastrointestinal disorders may be reported, and signs of renal insufficiency may be present. Gingivitis, discolored gums, and loosening of the teeth are common. The salivary glands may be enlarged. Tremor involving the fingers, arms, and legs is often present. Chronic mercury poisoning may also simulate drug intoxication, cerebellar dysfunction, or Wilson's disease. An alteration of handwriting is frequently observed. Ocular changes, including deposition of mercury in the lens, are reported. Personality changes with unusual fearfulness, inability to concentrate, and irritability have been described. This psychologic disorder is known as erethism.

Diagnosis of chronic mercury poisoning depends primarily on a history of exposure. Assays of mercury in the body vary widely, apparently due to pharmacokinetic factors.

Treatment

A. Acute: Treatment of acute mercury poisoning consists of removal from exposure and chelation treatment with dimercaprol, usually in a dosage of 3–5 mg/kg intramuscularly every 4 hours for 48 hours and then every 12 hours for 10 days. If renal damage occurs, hemodialysis will be required. Oral charcoal therapy is probably not useful in binding mercury in the gastrointestinal tract.

B. Chronic: With chronic mercury poisoning, oral penicillamine or N-acetylpenicillamine (250–500 mg orally 4 times a day for 10 days) is usually required. Urinary mercury levels should be monitored to observe enhanced removal. Treatment of organic mercury poisoning has been poorly studied. Administration of chelating agents requires further study.

• • •

References

Chelating Agents

Catsch A, Hartmuth-Hoehne AE: Pharmacology and therapeutic applications of agents used in heavy metal poisoning. *Pharmacol Ther* [*A*] 1976;**1:**1.

Gordon MH: Penicillamine for treatment of rheumatoid arthritis. *JAMA* 1974;**229:**1342.

Penicillamine: More lessons from experience. *Br Med J* 1975; **3:**120.

Lead

Brangstrup-Hanse JP: Chelatable lead burden by calcium disodium EDTA and blood lead concentration in man. *J Occup Med* 1981;**93:**39.

Hernberg SL: Lead in occupational medicine. Chap 30, pp 715–769, in: *Principles and Practical Approach of Occupational Medicine*. Zenz C (editor). Year Book, 1975.

Oheme FW: Mechanism of heavy metal toxicity. *J Clin Toxicol* 1972;**5:**151.

Settle DM: Lead in albacore: Guide to lead pollution in America. *Science* 1980;**207:**1167.

Arsenic

Martin DW Jr, Woeber KA: Arsenic poisoning. *Calif Med* (March) 1973;**118:**13.

National Institute of Safety and Health: *Occupational Exposure to Inorganic Arsenic, New Criteria*. US Department of Health, Education, and Welfare Publication No. 75–140, 1975.

Peterson RG, Rumack BH: D-Penicillamine therapy of acute arsenic poisoning. *J Pediatr* 1977;**91:**661.

Mercury

Done AK: The toxic emergency: The many faces of mercurialism. *Emerg Med* (Jan) 1980;**12:**137.

Jung RC, Aaronson J: Death following inhalation of mercury vapor at home. *West J Med* 1980;**132:**539.

Kahn A, Denis R, Blum D: Accidental ingestion of mercuric sulphate in a 4-year-old child. *Clin Pediatr* 1977;**16:**956.

Krohn IT et al: Subcutaneous injection of metallic mercury. *JAMA* 1980;**243:**548.

Snodgrass W et al: Mercury poisoning from home gold ore processing. *JAMA* 1981;**246:**1929.

Special Aspects of Perinatal & Pediatric Pharmacology | 60

Martin S. Cohen, MD

The effects of drugs in the fetus and newborn infant are based on the general principles set forth in Chapters 1–3 of this book. However, the contexts in which these pharmacologic laws operate are different in pregnant women and in rapidly maturing infants. At present, the special pharmacokinetic factors are beginning to be understood, whereas information regarding pharmacodynamic differences (eg, receptor affinities and number) is still quite fragmentary.

This chapter presents the basic principles of pharmacology in the special context of perinatal and pediatric therapeutics.

DRUG THERAPY IN PREGNANCY

Many drugs taken by pregnant women can cross the placenta and expose the developing embryo and fetus to their pharmacologic and teratogenic effects. Critical factors affecting placental drug transfer and drug effects on the fetus include the following: (1) The physicochemical properties of the drug. (2) The rate at which the drug crosses the placenta and the amount of drug reaching the fetus. (3) The duration of exposure to the drug. (4) How the drug is distributed in different fetal tissues. (5) The stage of placental and fetal development at the time of exposure to the drug. (6) The effects of drugs used in combination.

As is true also of other biologic membranes, drug passage across the placenta is dependent on the lipid solubility and degree of drug ionization. Lipophilic drugs tend to diffuse readily across the placenta and enter the fetal circulation. For example, thiopental, a drug commonly used for cesarean sections, crosses the placenta almost immediately and can produce sedation or apnea in the newborn infant. Highly ionized drugs such as succinylcholine and d-tubocurarine, also used for cesarean sections, cross the placenta slowly and achieve very low concentrations in the fetus.

Impermeability of the placenta to polar compounds is relative rather than absolute. If high enough maternal-fetal concentration gradients are achieved, polar compounds can cross the placenta. Salicylate, which is almost completely ionized at physiologic pH, crosses the placenta rapidly. This occurs because the small amount of salicylate that is not ionized is highly lipid-soluble.

The molecular weight of the drug also influences the rate and amount of drug transferred across the placenta. Drugs with molecular weights of 250–500 can cross the placenta easily, depending upon their lipid solubility and degree of ionization; those with molecular weights of 500–1000 cross the placenta with more difficulty; and those with molecular weights greater than 1000 cross very poorly. The apparent exceptions of maternal antibody globulins and certain polypeptides cross the placenta by some selective mechanism as yet unknown.

The degree to which a drug is bound to plasma proteins (particularly albumin) also affects the rate and amount transferred. If a compound is very lipid-soluble (eg, anesthetic gases), it is not affected to any great extent by protein binding. Transfer of these drugs and their overall rates of equilibration are more dependent on (and proportionate to) placental blood flow. This is because very lipid-soluble drugs diffuse across placental membranes so rapidly that their overall rates of equilibration do not depend on the free drug concentrations becoming equal on both sides.

If a drug is poorly lipid-soluble and is ionized, its transfer is slow and will probably be impeded by its binding to maternal plasma proteins. Protein binding is also important, since some drugs exhibit greater protein binding in maternal plasma than in fetal plasma because of a lowered binding affinity of fetal proteins: This has been shown for sulfonamides, barbiturates, phenytoin, and local anesthetic agents.

Two mechanisms help to protect the fetus from drugs in the maternal circulation: (1) The placenta itself plays a role both as a semipermeable barrier and as a site of metabolism of some drugs passing through it. Several different types of aromatic oxidation reactions (eg, hydroxylation, N-dealkylation, demethylation) have been shown to occur in placental tissue. Ethanol and pentobarbital are oxidized in this way. (2) Drugs that have crossed the placenta enter the fetal circulation via the umbilical vein. About 40–60% of umbilical venous blood flow enters the fetal liver; the remainder bypasses the liver and enters the general fetal circulation. A drug that enters the liver may be metabolized there before it enters the fetal circulation. In addition, a large proportion of drug present in the umbilical artery (returning to the placenta) may be shunted through the placenta back to the umbilical vein and into the liver again. It should be noted that metabolites of some drugs may be more active than the parent compound and may affect the fetus adversely.

A single intrauterine exposure to a drug can affect structures undergoing rapid development at the time of exposure. Thalidomide is an example of a drug that profoundly affects the development of the limbs after only brief exposure. This exposure, however, must be at a critical time in the development of the limbs. Continued exposure may produce cumulative effects or may affect several organs going through varying stages of development.

Chronic consumption of ethanol during pregnancy, particularly during the first and second trimesters, results in the fetal alcohol syndrome (Chapter 20). In this syndrome, the central nervous system, growth, and facial development are all affected. Another example of the effects of continued exposure is chronic use of opiate narcotics by the mother, which produces narcotic dependence in the fetus. This dependence is manifested after delivery as narcotic withdrawal syndrome.

Some drugs with known adverse effects in pregnancy are listed in Table 60–1.

Fetal therapeutics is an emerging area in perinatal pharmacology. This involves drug administration to the pregnant woman with the fetus as the target of the drug. At present, corticosteroids are used to stimulate fetal lung maturation when premature birth is expected. Phenobarbital, when given to pregnant women near term, can induce fetal hepatic enzymes responsible for the glucuronidation of bilirubin, and the incidence of jaundice is lower in newborns whose mothers are given phenobarbital than when phenobarbital is not used. Drugs have also been given to mothers for treatment of fetal cardiac arrhythmias.

Table 60–1. Drugs with significant adverse effects on the fetus.

Drug	Trimester	Effect
Aminopterin	First	Multiple gross anomalies.
Barbiturates	All	Chronic use leads to neonatal dependence.
Chloramphenicol	Third	Increased risk of gray baby syndrome.
Chlorpropamide	All	Prolonged symptomatic neonatal hypoglycemia.
Cortisone	First	Increased risk of cleft palate.
Diazepam	All	Chronic use leads to neonatal dependence.
Diethylstilbestrol	All	Vaginal adenosis, clear cell vaginal adenocarcinoma.
Ethanol	All	High risk of fetal alcohol syndrome.
Heroin	All	Chronic use leads to neonatal dependence.
Iodide	All	Congenital goiter, hypothyroidism.
Methadone	All	Chronic use leads to neonatal dependence.
Methyltestosterone	Second and third	Masculinization of female fetus.
Methylthiouracil	All	Hypothyroidism.
Norethindrone	All	Masculinization of female fetus.
Phenytoin	All	Cleft lip and palate.
Propylthiouracil	All	Congenital goiter.
Tetracycline	All	Discoloration of teeth.
Thalidomide	First	Phocomelia.
Trimethadione	All	Multiple congenital anomalies.
Warfarin	First	Hypoplastic nasal bridge, chondrodysplasia.
	Third	Risk of bleeding. Discontinue use 1 month before delivery.

DRUG DISPOSITION IN INFANTS & CHILDREN

Drug Absorption

Drug absorption in infants and children follows the same general principles as in adults. Unique factors that influence drug absorption include blood flow at the site of administration as determined by the physiologic status of the infant or child; and (for orally administered drugs) gastrointestinal function, which changes rapidly during the first few days after birth. The effects of age after birth on gastrointestinal function also influence the regulation of drug absorption.

A. Blood Flow At the Site of Administration: Absorption after intramuscular or subcutaneous injection depends mainly, in neonates as in adults, on the rate of blood flow to the muscle or subcutaneous area injected. Physiologic conditions that might reduce blood flow to these areas are cardiovascular shock, vasoconstriction due to sympathomimetic agents, and heart failure. However, many sick premature infants require intramuscular injections yet have very little muscle mass. This is further complicated by diminished peripheral perfusion to these areas. In this case, absorption becomes irregular and difficult to predict, because the drug may remain in the muscle and be absorbed more slowly than expected. In this way, it acts like a reservoir. However, if perfusion suddenly improves, there can be a sudden and unpredictable increase in the amount of drug entering the circulation, resulting in high and often toxic concentrations of drug. Examples of drugs especially hazardous in this situation are cardiac glycosides, aminoglycoside antibiotics, and anticonvulsants.

B. Gastrointestinal Function: Significant biochemical and physiologic changes occur in the neonatal gastrointestinal tract shortly after birth. Within the first 24 hours of life, there is a marked increase in gastric acidity. Therefore, drugs that are partially or totally inactivated by the low pH of gastric contents should not be administered orally.

Gastric emptying time is prolonged in the neonate (up to 6 or 8 hours). Therefore, drugs that are absorbed primarily in the stomach may be absorbed more completely than anticipated. However, in the case of drugs absorbed in the small intestine, absorption—and therefore therapeutic effect—is delayed. Peristalsis in the neonate is irregular and may be slow. The amount

Table 60–2. Oral drug absorption (bioavailability) of various drugs in the neonate compared with older children and adults.

Drug	Oral Absorption
Acetaminophen	Decreased
Ampicillin	Increased
Diazepam	Normal
Digoxin	Normal
Gentamicin	Decreased
Nafcillin	Increased
Penicillin G	Increased
Phenobarbital	Decreased
Phenytoin	Decreased
Sulfonamides	Normal

of drug absorbed in the small intestine is therefore unpredictable in neonates; eg, more than the usual amount of drug may be absorbed if peristalsis is slowed, and this could result in toxicity from an otherwise normal dose. Table 60–2 lists the absorption of various drugs in the neonate as compared with older children and adults.

An increase in peristalsis, as in diarrheal conditions, tends to decrease overall absorption, since contact time with the large absorptive surface of the intestine is decreased.

Drug Distribution

As body composition changes with development, the relative volume into which a drug is distributed also changes. The neonate has a higher percentage (70–75%) of its body weight in the form of water than does the adult (50–60%). Differences can also be observed between the full-term neonate (70% of body weight as water) and the small premature neonate (85% of body weight as water). In addition, extracellular water is 40% of body weight in the neonate, compared with 20% in the adult. Since most drugs become distributed throughout the extracellular water space in order to reach their receptors, the size (volume) of the extracellular water compartment is important in determining the concentration of drug at the receptor sites.

Premature infants have much less fat than full-term infants. Total body fat in premature infants is about 1% of total body weight, compared with 15% in full-term neonates. Therefore, organs that generally accumulate high concentrations of lipid-soluble drugs in adults and older children may accumulate smaller amounts of these drugs in more immature infants.

Another major factor determining drug distribution is drug binding to plasma proteins. Albumin is the plasma protein with the greatest binding capacity. In general, protein binding of drugs is reduced in the neonate. This has been seen with local anesthetic drugs, phenytoin, ampicillin, and phenobarbital. Therefore, the concentration of free (unbound) drug in plasma is increased. This can result in a greater drug effect or toxicity despite a normal or even low plasma concentration of total drug (bound plus unbound.).

As a practical example, consider 100 mg of drug X given to a patient. The concentration of total drug in the plasma is 100 μg/mL. If the drug is 50% protein-bound in an older child or adult, then 50 μg/mL is the concentration of free drug. Assume that this concentration of free drug produces the desired effect in the patient without producing toxicity. However, if this drug is given to a premature infant in a dosage adjusted for body weight and it produces a total drug concentration of 100 μg/mL, the concentration of free drug could be as high as 75 μg/mL because of reduced plasma protein binding. This concentration might be toxic.

Some drugs compete with serum bilirubin for binding to albumin. Drugs given to a neonate with jaundice can displace bilirubin from albumin. Because of the greater permeability of the premature blood-brain barrier, significant amounts of bilirubin may enter the brain and cause kernicterus. This was in fact observed when sulfonamide antibiotics were given to premature neonates as prophylaxis against sepsis. Conversely, as the serum bilirubin rises for physiologic reasons or because of a blood group incompatibility, bilirubin can displace a drug from albumin and significantly raise the free drug concentration. This would occur without altering the total drug concentration and would result in greater drug effects or toxicity at normal drug concentrations.

Drug Metabolism

The metabolism of most drugs occurs in the liver (Chapter 3). The drug-metabolizing activities of the cytochrome P-450-dependent, mixed-function oxidases and the conjugating enzymes are substantially lower in early neonatal life than later. The point in development at which enzymatic activity is maximal depends upon the specific enzyme system in question. Because of the neonate's decreased ability to metabolize drugs, many drugs have slow clearances and prolonged half-lives in the body. If drug doses and dosing schedules are not altered accordingly, this immaturity predisposes the neonate toward adverse drug responses from drugs that are metabolized by the liver.

The data in Table 60–3 demonstrate how neonatal

Table 60–3. Approximate half-lives of various drugs in neonates and adults.

Drug	Neonatal Age	$t_{1/2}$ (Neonates) (hours)	$t_{1/2}$ (Adults) (hours)
Acetaminophen		2.2–5	1.9–2.2
Diazepam		25–100	15–25
Digoxin		60–107	30–60
Phenobarbital	0–5 days	200	64–140
	5–15 days	100	
	1–30 months	50	
Phenytoin	0–2 days	80	12–18
	3–14 days	18	
	14–50 days	6	
Salicylate		4.5–11	2–4
Theophylline	Neonate	13–26	5–10
	Child	3–4	

and adult drug half-lives can differ and how the half-lives of phenobarbital and phenytoin decrease as the neonate gets older. The process of maturation must be considered when administering drugs to this age group, especially if the drug or drugs are administered over long periods.

Another consideration for the neonate is whether or not the mother was receiving a drug such as phenobarbital, which can induce early maturation of fetal hepatic enzyme. In this case, the ability of the neonate to metabolize certain drugs will be greater than expected, and one may see less therapeutic effect and lower plasma drug concentrations when the normal neonatal dose is given.

Drug Excretion

The glomerular filtration rate is much lower in newborns than in older infants, children, or adults, and this limitation persists during the first few days of life. Calculated on the basis of 1.73 m^2 of surface area, glomerular filtration in the neonate is only 30–40% and tubular secretion 20–30% of adult values. Function improves substantially during the first week of life. At that time, the glomerular filtration rate and renal plasma flow have increased 50% from the first day. By the end of the third week, glomerular filtration is 50–60% of the adult value; by 6–12 months, it reaches adult values. Therefore, drugs that depend on renal function for elimination are cleared from the body very slowly in the first weeks of life.

Penicillins, for example, are cleared from premature infants at 17% of the adult rate based on comparable surface area and 34% of the adult rate when adjusted for body weight. A decreased rate of renal elimination in the neonate has also been observed with aminoglycoside antibiotics (kanamycin, gentamicin, neomycin, streptomycin). Total body clearance of digoxin is directly dependent upon adequate renal function, and accumulation of digoxin can occur when glomerular filtration is decreased.

Since renal function in a sick infant may not improve at the predicted rate during the first weeks and months of life, appropriate adjustments in dose and dosing schedules may be very difficult. In this situation, adjustments are best made on the basis of plasma drug concentrations, determined at intervals throughout the course of therapy.

In summary, physiologic processes in the infant change significantly in the first year of life and particularly in the first few weeks. These changes must be considered when any drug is administered in the neonatal period.

PEDIATRIC DOSAGE FORMS & COMPLIANCE

The form in which a drug is manufactured and the way in which the parent dispenses the drug to the child determine the actual dose administered. Many drugs prepared for children are in the form of elixirs or suspensions. Elixirs are usually alcoholic solutions in which the drug molecules are evenly distributed. No shaking is required, and the first dose from the bottle and the last dose should contain equivalent amounts of drug.

Suspensions contain undissolved particles of drug that must be distributed throughout the vehicle by shaking. If shaking is not thorough each time a dose is given, the first doses from the bottle will contain far less drug than the last doses, with the result that less than the expected plasma concentration or effect of drug may be achieved early in the course of therapy. Conversely, toxicity may occur late in the course of therapy when not expected. It is thus essential that the prescriber know the form in which the drug will be dispensed.

Compliance may be more difficult to achieve in pediatric practice than otherwise, since it involves not only the parent's conscientious effort to follow directions but such practical matters as measuring errors, spilling, and spitting out. (The measured volume of "teaspoons" ranges from 2.5 to 7.8 mL.) When evaluating compliance, it is often helpful to ask if an attempt has been made to give a further dose after the child has spilled half of what was offered. The parents may not always be able to say with confidence how much of a dose the child actually received. The parents must be told whether or not to wake the baby for its every-6-hour dose day or night. In the first 3 days of antibiotic therapy for otitis media, it may be important to maintain a relatively constant concentration of antibiotic in the blood and middle ear. If that is the goal, it is important that the parent give the medication on schedule no matter who is sleeping at the time. During the second week of treatment, since a constant concentration of antibiotic is then less important, a strict 6-hour schedule is not obligatory. These matters should be discussed with the parents and made clear to them, and no assumptions should be made about what the parents may or may not do. Noncompliance frequently occurs when antibiotics are prescribed to treat otitis media or urinary tract infections and the child feels well after 4 or 5 days of therapy. The parents may not feel there is any reason to continue giving the medicine even though it was prescribed for 10 or 14 days. This common situation should be anticipated so the parents can be told why it is important to continue the medicine for the prescribed period even if the child seems to be "cured."

Practical and convenient dosage forms and dosing schedules should be chosen to the extent possible. The easier it is to administer and take the medicine and the easier the dosing schedule is to follow, the more likely it is that compliance will be achieved.

Consistent with their ability to comprehend and cooperate, children should also be given some responsibility for their own health care and for taking medications. This should be discussed in appropriate terms both with the child and the parents. Possible side-effects and drug interactions with over-the-counter medicines or foods should also be discussed.

DRUG USE DURING LACTATION (Table 60–4.)

Drugs should be used conservatively during lactation, and the physician must know which drugs enter breast milk and are potentially dangerous to nursing infants (Table 60–4). Most drugs administered to lactating women are detectable in breast milk. Fortunately, the concentration of drug achieved in breast milk is usually low. Therefore, the total amount the infant would receive in a day is likely to be less than what would be considered a "therapeutic dose." If the nursing mother must take medication and the drug is a relatively safe one, she should take it 30–60 minutes after nursing and 3–4 hours before the next feeding. This allows time for many drugs to be cleared from the mother's blood, and the concentrations in breast milk will be relatively low. Drugs for which there are no data on safety during lactation should be avoided or breast feeding discontinued while they are given.

Most antibiotics taken by nursing mothers can be detected in breast milk. Sulfonamides should not be taken in the early neonatal period, because they compete with bilirubin for binding to plasma albumin and increase the risk of kernicterus. Tetracycline concentrations in breast milk are approximately 70% of maternal serum concentrations and present a risk of permanent tooth staining in the infant. Chloramphenicol concentrations in breast milk are not sufficient to cause gray baby syndrome, but there is a remote possibility of causing bone marrow suppression, and chloramphenicol should be avoided during lactation. Isoniazid

Table 60–4. Commonly used drugs and their excretion into breast milk.

Drug	Effect on Infant	Comments
Ampicillin	Minimal	No significant side-effects; possible occurrence of diarrhea or allergic sensitization.
Aspirin	Minimal	Occasional doses probably safe; high doses may produce significant concentration in breast milk.
Caffeine	Minimal	Caffeine intake in moderation is safe; concentration in breast milk is about 1% of total dose taken by mother.
Chloral hydrate	Significant	May cause drowsiness if fed at peak concentration in milk.
Chloramphenicol	Significant	Concentrations too low to cause gray baby syndrome; possibility of bone marrow suppression does exist; recommend not taking chloramphenicol while breast feeding.
Chlorothiazide	Minimal	No side-effects reported.
Chlorpromazine	Minimal	Appears insignificant.
Codeine	Minimal	No side-effects reported.
Diazepam	Significant	Will cause sedation in breast-fed infants; accumulation can occur in newborns.
Dicumarol	Minimal	No adverse side-effects reported; may wish to follow infant's prothrombin time.
Digoxin	Minimal	Insignificant quantities enter breast milk.
Ethanol	Moderate	Moderate ingestion by mother unlikely to produce effects in infant; large amounts consumed by mother can produce alcohol effects in infant.
Heroin	Significant	Enters breast milk and can prolong neonatal narcotic dependence.
Iodine (radioactive)	Significant	Enters milk in quantities sufficient to cause thyroid suppression in infant.
Isoniazid (INH)	Minimal	Milk concentrations equal maternal plasma concentrations. Possibility of pyridoxine deficiency developing in the infant.
Kanamycin	Minimal	No adverse effects reported.
Lithium	Significant	Avoid breast feeding.
Methadone	Significant	(See heroin.) Under close physician supervision, breast feeding can be continued. Signs of opiate withdrawal in the infant may occur if mother stops taking methadone or stops breast feeding abruptly.
Oral contraceptives	Minimal	Will suppress lactation in high doses.
Penicillin	Minimal	Very low concentrations in breast milk.
Phenobarbital	Moderate	Hypnotic doses can cause sedation in the infant.
Phenytoin	Moderate	Amounts entering breast milk may be sufficient to cause side-effects in infant.
Prednisone	Moderate	Low maternal doses probably safe. Doses 2 or more times physiologic amounts should probably be avoided.
Propranolol	Minimal	Very small amounts enter breast milk.
Propylthiouracil, thiouracil	Significant	Can suppress thyroid function in infant.
Spironolactone	Minimal	Very small amounts enter breast milk.
Tetracycline	Moderate	Possibility of permanent staining of developing teeth in the infant. Should be avoided during lactation.
Theophylline	Moderate	Can enter breast milk in moderate quantities but not likely to produce significant effects.
Thyroxine	Minimal	No adverse effects in therapeutic doses.
Tolbutamide	Minimal	Low concentrations in breast milk.
Warfarin	Minimal	Very small quantities found in breast milk.

reaches a rapid equilibrium between breast milk and maternal blood. The concentrations achieved in breast milk are high enough so that pyridoxine deficiency may occur in the infant if the mother is not given pyridoxine supplements.

Most sedatives and hypnotics achieve concentrations in breast milk sufficient to produce a pharmacologic effect in the infant. Barbiturates taken in hypnotic doses by the mother can produce lethargy, sedation, and poor suck reflexes in the infant. Chloral hydrate can produce sedation if the infant is fed at peak milk concentrations. Diazepam can have a sedative effect on the nursing infant, but most importantly, its long half-life can result in significant drug accumulation.

Narcotics such as heroin, methadone, and morphine enter breast milk in quantities sufficient to prolong neonatal narcotic dependence if the drug was taken chronically during pregnancy. If conditions are well controlled and there is a good relationship between the mother and the physician, an infant could breast-feed while the mother is taking methadone. She should not, however, stop taking the drug abruptly; the infant will be tapered off the methadone as the mother's dose is tapered. The infant should be watched for signs of narcotic withdrawal.

Moderate use of alcohol by the mother should not be harmful to a nursing infant. Large amounts, however, can produce alcohol effects in the infant. Nicotine concentrations in the breast milk of smoking mothers are low and do not produce effects in the infant. Very small amounts of caffeine are excreted in the breast milk of coffee-drinking mothers.

Lithium enters breast milk in concentrations equal to those in maternal serum. Clearance of this drug is almost completely dependent upon renal elimination, and women who are receiving lithium should not breast-feed.

Drugs that can alter endocrine function such as thiouracil and tolbutamide enter breast milk in quantities sufficient to affect endocrine function in the infant. They should be avoided if possible or breast feeding discontinued.

Radioactive substances such as iodinated I 125 albumin and radioiodine can cause thyroid suppression in infants and may increase the risk of subsequent thyroid cancer as much as 10-fold. Breast feeding is contraindicated after large doses and should be withheld for days to weeks after small doses.

In general, drug use by nursing mothers should be avoided if possible, and they should be cautioned against excessive use of over-the-counter medications, since the effects on nursing infants have not been studied extensively.

PEDIATRIC DRUG DOSAGE

Because of differences in pharmacokinetics in infants and children, simple linear reduction in the adult dose is rarely adequate in achieving a safe and effective pediatric dose. If specific pediatric dosage information is not available in the package insert for a given product, an approximation can be made by any of several methods based on age, weight, or surface area.

Age

Young's rule:

$$\text{Dose} = \text{Adult dose} \times \frac{\text{Age (years)}}{\text{Age} + 12}$$

Weight

Somewhat more precise is Clark's rule:

$$\text{Dose} = \text{Adult dose} \times \frac{\text{Weight (kg)}}{70}$$

or

$$\text{Adult dose} \times \frac{\text{Weight (lb)}}{150}$$

Surface Area

Both of the above rules are conservative and tend to underestimate the required dose. Doses based on surface area are more likely to be adequate (Table 60–5).

Table 60–5. Determination of drug dosage from surface area.*†

Weight		Approximate Age	Surface Area (m^2)	Percent of Adult Dose
kg	lb			
3	6.6	Newborn	0.2	12
6	13.2	3 months	0.3	18
10	22	1 year	0.45	28
20	44	5.5 years	0.8	48
30	66	9 years	1	60
40	88	12 years	1.3	78
50	110	14 years	1.5	90
65	143	Adult	1.7	102
70	154	Adult	1.76	103

*Reproduced, with permission, from Silver HK, Kempe CH, Bruyn HB: *Handbook of Pediatrics,* 13th ed. Lange, 1980.

†If adult dose is 1 mg/kg, dose for 3-month-old infant would be 2 mg/kg.

• • •

References

Hansten PD: *Drug Interactions,* 4th ed. Lea & Febiger, 1979.

McCracken HH, Nelson JD: *Antimicrobial Therapy for Newborns*. Grune & Stratton, 1977.

Mirkin BL (editor): *Clinical Pharmacology and Therapeutics: A Pediatric Perspective*. Year Book, 1978.

Mirkin BL (editor): *Perinatal Pharmacology and Therapeutics*. Academic Press, 1976.

Pagliaro LA, Levin RH (editors): *Problems in Pediatric Drug Therapy*. Drug Intelligence, 1979.

Rementeria JL (editor): *Drug Abuse in Pregnancy and Neonatal Effects*. Mosby, 1977.

Shirkey HC: *Pediatric Drug Handbook*. Saunders, 1977.

Yaffe SJ (editor): *Pediatric Pharmacology: Therapeutic Principles in Practice*. Grune & Stratton, 1980.

61 | Dermatologic Pharmacology

Dirk B. Robertson, MD, & Howard I. Maibach, MD

The skin offers a number of special problems and opportunities to the therapist. Because of its location, topical therapy is especially appropriate for diseases of the skin, although some dermatologic diseases respond as well or better to drugs administered systemically.

The general pharmacokinetic principles governing the use of drugs applied to the skin are the same as those involved in other routes of drug administration (Chapters 1 and 3). However, human skin, though often depicted as a simple 3-layered structure, is a complex series of diffusion barriers. Quantitation of the flux of drugs and drug vehicles through these barriers is the basis of pharmacokinetic analysis of dermatologic therapy; techniques for making such measurements are rapidly increasing in number and sensitivity.

Major variables that determine pharmacologic response to drugs applied to the skin include the following:

(1) Regional variation in drug penetration: For example, the scrotum, face, axilla, and scalp are far more permeable than the forearm and may require less drug for equivalent effect.

(2) Concentration gradient: Increasing the concentration gradient increases the mass of drug transferred per unit time, just as in the case of diffusion across other barriers (Chapter 1). Thus, resistance to topical corticosteroids can sometimes be overcome by use of higher concentrations of drug.

(3) Dosing schedule: Because of its physical properties, the skin acts as a reservoir for many drugs. As a result, the "local half-life" may be long enough to permit once-daily application of drugs with short systemic half-lives. For example, once-daily application of corticosteroids appears to be just as effective as multiple applications.

(4) Vehicles and occlusion: An appropriate vehicle maximizes the ability of the drug to penetrate the outer layers of the skin. In addition, through its physical properties (moistening or drying effects), vehicles may themselves have important therapeutic effects.

Occlusion (application of a plastic wrap to hold the drug and its vehicle in close contact with the skin) is extremely effective in maximizing absorption of many drugs.

DERMATOLOGIC VEHICLES

Topical medications usually consist of active ingredients incorporated in a vehicle that facilitates cutaneous application. Important considerations in selection of a vehicle include the solubility of the active agent in the vehicle; the rate of release of the agent from the vehicle; the ability of the vehicle to hydrate the stratum corneum, thus enhancing penetration; the stability of the therapeutic agent in the vehicle; and interactions, chemical and physical, of the vehicle, stratum corneum, and active agent. Vehicles have traditionally been considered pharmacologically inert; however, owing to their unique physical properties, many are therapeutically beneficial themselves.

Depending upon the vehicle, dermatologic formulations may be classified as tinctures, wet dressings, lotions, gels, aerosols, powders, pastes, creams, and ointments. The ability of the vehicle to retard evaporation from the surface of the skin increases in this series, being least in tinctures and wet dressings and greatest in ointments. In general, acute inflammation with oozing, vesiculation, and crusting is best treated with drying preparations such as tinctures, wet dressings, and lotions, while chronic inflammation with xerosis, scaling, and lichenification is best treated with more lubricating preparations such as creams and ointments. Tinctures, lotions, gels, and aerosols are convenient for application to the scalp and hairy areas. Emulsified vanishing type creams may be used in intertriginous areas without causing maceration.

Emulsifying agents are used to provide homogeneous, stable preparations when mixtures of immiscible liquids such as oil-in-water creams are compounded. Examples include alkyl sulfates (sodium lauryl sulfate), glyceryl monostearate, polyoxyethylene sorbitan monostearate and monooleate (Polysorbate 80), and polyethylene glycols (Carbowax). These emulsifying agents are commonly found in lotions, creams, and ointments containing oily constituents and water. Some patients develop irritation from these agents. Substituting a preparation that does not contain them or using one containing a lower concentration may resolve the problem. Other additives widely used in dermatologic preparations include cetyl palmitate and related esters, which improve the consistency and appearance of creams; stearic acid and stearyl alcohol, which act as lubricants, emollients, and antifoaming agents; and methylcellulose and gum tragacanth, which are inert compounds used as suspending agents in pastes and ointments. The methyl and propyl esters of *p*-aminobenzoic acid (methylparaben and propylparaben) frequently are added as preservatives.

ANTIBACTERIAL AGENTS

Topical Antibacterial Preparations

Topical antibacterial agents may be useful in preventing infections in clean wounds, in the early treatment of infected dermatoses and wounds, in reducing colonization of the nares by staphylococci, in axillary deodorization, and in the management of acne vulgaris. The efficacy of antibiotics in these topical applications is not uniform. The general pharmacology of the antimicrobial drugs is discussed in Chapters 41–53.

Numerous topical anti-infectives contain corticosteroids in addition to antibiotics. There is no convincing evidence that topical corticosteroids inhibit the antibacterial effect of antibiotics when the 2 are incorporated in the same preparation. In the treatment of secondarily infected dermatoses, which are usually colonized with streptococci, staphylococci, or both, combination therapy may prove superior to corticosteroid therapy alone. Antibiotic-corticosteroid combinations may be useful in treating diaper dermatitis, otitis externa, and impetiginized eczema.

The selection of a particular antibiotic depends of course upon the diagnosis and, whenever possible, in vitro culture and sensitivity studies of clinical samples. The pathogens isolated from most infected dermatoses are group A beta-hemolytic streptococci, *Staphylococcus aureus,* or both. The pathogens present in surgical wounds will be those resident in the environment. Information about regional epidemiologic data and the prevailing patterns of drug resistance is therefore important in selecting a therapeutic agent. Prepackaged topical antibacterial preparations that contain multiple antibiotics are available in fixed dosages well above the therapeutic threshold. These formulations offer the advantages of efficacy in mixed infections, broader coverage for infections due to undetermined pathogens, and delayed microbial resistance to any single-component antibiotic.

BACITRACIN & GRAMICIDIN

Bacitracin and gramicidin are polypeptide antibiotics, active against gram-positive organisms such as streptococci, pneumococci, and staphylococci. In addition, most anaerobic cocci, neisseriae, tetanus bacilli, and diphtheria bacilli are sensitive. Bacitracin is compounded in an ointment base alone or in combination with neomycin, polymyxin B, or both. The use of bacitracin in the anterior nares temporarily decreases colonization by pathogenic staphylococci. Microbial resistance may develop following prolonged use. Bacitracin-induced contact urticaria syndrome occurs rarely. Allergic contact dermatitis occurs more frequently. Bacitracin is poorly absorbed through the skin, so systemic toxicity is rare.

Gramicidin is available only for topical use, in combination with other antibiotics such as neomycin, polymyxin, bacitracin, and nystatin. Systemic toxicity limits this drug to topical use. The incidence of sensitization following topical application is exceedingly low in therapeutic concentrations.

POLYMYXIN B SULFATE

Polymyxin B is a polypeptide antibiotic effective against gram-negative organisms, including *Pseudomonas aeruginosa, Escherichia coli, Enterobacter,* and *Klebsiella*. Most strains of *Proteus* and *Serratia* are resistant, as are all gram-positive organisms. Topical preparations may be compounded in either a solution or ointment base. Numerous prepackaged antibiotic combinations containing polymyxin B are available. Detectable serum concentrations are difficult to achieve from topical application, but the total daily dose applied to denuded skin or open wounds should not exceed 200 mg in order to reduce the likelihood of neurotoxicity and nephrotoxicity. Hypersensitivity to topically applied polymyxin B sulfate is uncommon.

NEOMYCIN & GENTAMICIN

Neomycin and gentamicin are aminoglycoside antibiotics active against gram-negative organisms, including *E coli, Proteus, Klebsiella,* and *Enterobacter*. Gentamicin generally shows greater activity against *P aeruginosa* than neomycin. Gentamicin is also more active against staphylococci and group A beta-hemolytic streptococci. Widespread topical use of gentamicin, especially in a hospital environment, should be avoided to slow the appearance of gentamicin-resistant organisms.

Neomycin is available in numerous topical formulations, both alone and in combination with polymyxin, bacitracin, and other antibiotics. It is also available as a sterile powder for topical use. Gentamicin is available as an ointment or cream.

Topical application of neomycin rarely results in detectable serum concentrations. However, in the case of gentamicin, serum concentrations of 1–18 μg/mL are possible if the drug is applied in a water-miscible preparation to large areas of denuded skin, as in burned patients. Both drugs are water-soluble and are excreted primarily in the urine. Renal failure may permit the accumulation of these antibiotics, with possible nephrotoxicity, neurotoxicity, and ototoxicity.

Neomycin frequently causes sensitization, particularly if applied to eczematous dermatoses or if compounded in an ointment vehicle. When sensitization occurs, cross-sensitivity to streptomycin, kanamycin, paromomycin, and gentamicin is possible.

TOPICAL ANTIBIOTICS IN ACNE

Several parenteral antibiotics that have traditionally been used in the treatment of acne vulgaris have been shown to be effective when applied topically. Currently, 3 antibiotics are so utilized: clindamycin phosphate, erythromycin base, and tetracycline hydrochloride. The effectiveness of topical therapy is less than that achieved by systemic administration of the same antibiotic. Therefore, topical therapy is generally effective only in mild to moderate cases of inflammatory acne.

Clindamycin

Clindamycin has in vitro activity against *Propionibacterium (Corynebacterium) acnes;* this has been postulated as the mechanism of its beneficial effect in acne therapy. Approximately 10% of an applied dose is absorbed, and rare cases of bloody diarrhea and pseudomembranous colitis have been reported following topical application. The hydroalcoholic vehicle may cause drying and irritation of the skin, with complaints of burning and stinging. Allergic contact dermatitis is uncommon.

Erythromycin

In topical preparations, the base of erythromycin rather than a salt is used to facilitate penetration. Although the mechanism of action of topical erythromycin in inflammatory acne vulgaris is unknown, it is presumed to be due to its inhibitory effects on *P acnes*. One of the possible complications of topical therapy is the development of antibiotic-resistant strains of organisms, including staphylococci. If this occurs in association with a clinical infection, topical erythromycin should be discontinued and appropriate systemic antibiotic therapy started. Adverse local reactions may include a burning sensation at the time of application and drying and irritation of the skin. Allergic hypersensitivity appears to be uncommon.

Tetracycline

Two topical tetracycline antibiotics are currently available for topical treatment of acne vulgaris: (1) tetracycline hydrochloride in a hydroalcoholic base containing *n*-decyl methyl sulfoxide and (2) meclocycline sulfosalicylate in a cream base. The pharmacology of the tetracycline antibiotics is presented in Chapter 43. Serum levels of tetracycline obtained from continued twice-daily topical use of hydroalcoholic preparations are 0.1 μg/mL or less, and no demonstrable absorption has been reported following extensive twice-daily topical application of the meclocycline sulfosalicylate preparation over 4 weeks.

The beneficial effect of these preparations on acne vulgaris has been attributed to their inhibitory action on *P acnes*. Their use is associated with temporary yellow staining of the skin, which is most noticeable in fair-skinned individuals. Although photosensitivity has not been a problem, this hazard should be considered when using these potentially phototoxic antibiotics. As with all tetracycline derivatives, these agents should not be used in patients who are pregnant or have a history of significant renal or hepatic dysfunction.

ANTIFUNGAL AGENTS

Topical Antifungal Preparations

The treatment of superficial fungal infections caused by dermatophytic fungi may be accomplished (1) with topical antifungal agents, eg, clotrimazole, miconazole, tolnaftate, and haloprogin; or (2) with orally administered agents, eg, griseofulvin and ketoconazole. Superficial infections caused by *Candida* sp may be treated with topical applications of clotrimazole, miconazole, nystatin, or amphotericin B. Chronic generalized mucocutaneous candidiasis is responsive to long-term therapy with oral ketoconazole.

CLOTRIMAZOLE & MICONAZOLE

Clotrimazole and miconazole have a wide range of activity against dermatophytes *(Epidermophyton, Microsporum,* and *Trichophyton)* and yeasts, including *Candida albicans* and *Pityrosporon orbiculare,* the cause of tinea versicolor (see Chapter 47).

Miconazole (Micatin) is available for topical application and in an injectable form for intravenous administration in the treatment of potentially fatal systemic fungal infections. Clotrimazole (Lotrimin, Mycelex) is available for topical application to the skin and as vaginal cream and tablets for use in vulvovaginal candidiasis.

Twice-daily application to the affected area will generally result in clearing of superficial dermatophyte infections in 2–3 weeks, although the medication should be continued until eradication of the organism is confirmed. Paronychial and intertriginous candidiasis can be treated with either agent applied 3–4 times daily.

Adverse local reactions to clotrimazole and miconazole may include stinging, pruritus, erythema, and local irritation. Allergic contact dermatitis appears to be uncommon.

TOLNAFTATE

Tolnaftate is a synthetic antifungal compound that is effective topically against dermatophyte infections caused by *Epidermophyton, Microsporum,* and *Trichophyton*. It is also active against *P orbiculare* but not against *Candida*.

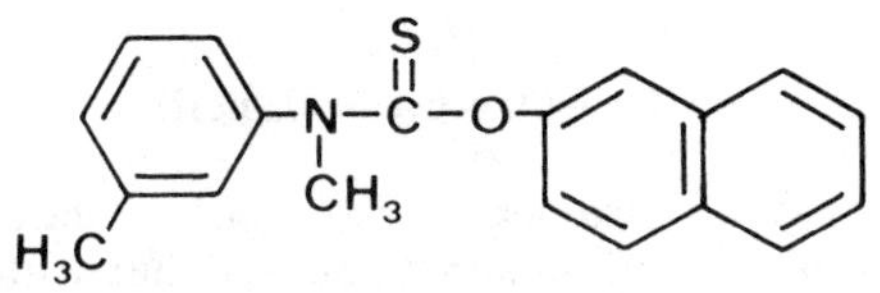

Tolnaftate

Tolnaftate (Aftate, Tinactin) is available as a cream, solution, powder, or powder aerosol for application twice daily to infected areas. Recurrences following cessation of therapy are common, and infections of the palms, soles, and nails are usually unresponsive to tolnaftate alone. The powder or powder aerosol may be used chronically following initial treatment in patients susceptible to tinea infections. Tolnaftate is generally well tolerated and rarely causes irritation or allergic contact sensitization.

HALOPROGIN

Haloprogin is a synthetic halogenated phenolic ether, active against *Epidermophyton, Microsporum,* and *Trichophyton* as well as *P orbiculare*. Although this compound does exhibit in vitro activity against *Candida,* its use is generally restricted to the treatment of dermatophyte infections and tinea versicolor.

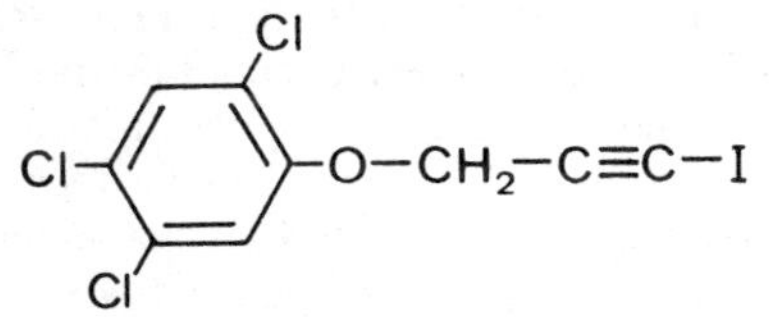

Haloprogin

Haloprogin (Halotex) is available as cream or solution. There is only slight penetration through intact skin, and systemic toxicity following topical application has not been observed. The small amounts of drug that are absorbed are converted to trichlorophenol, which is excreted predominantly in the urine. Twice-daily application to the affected area usually results in clearing in 2–3 weeks. Infections of the palms, soles, and nails are generally resistant to topical therapy. Adverse reactions include local irritation, burning sensations, vesiculation, increased maceration, and exacerbation of the preexisting lesion. Contact with the eyes must be avoided. Allergic contact hypersensitivity is uncommon.

NYSTATIN & AMPHOTERICIN B

Nystatin and amphotericin B are useful in the topical therapy of *C albicans* infections but ineffective against dermatophytes. Nystatin is limited to topical treatment of cutaneous and mucosal *Candida* infections because of its narrow spectrum and negligible absorption from the gastrointestinal tract following oral administration. Amphotericin B has a broader antifungal spectrum and is used intravenously in the treatment of many systemic mycoses and to a lesser extent in the treatment of cutaneous *Candida* infections.

The recommended dosage for topical preparations of nystatin in treating paronychial and intertriginous candidiasis is application 2 or 3 times a day. Oral candidiasis (thrush) is treated by holding 5 mL (infants, 2 mL) of nystatin oral suspension in the mouth for several minutes 4 times daily before swallowing. An alternative therapy for thrush is to retain a vaginal tablet in the mouth until dissolved 4 times daily. Recurrent or recalcitrant perianal, vaginal, vulvar, and diaper area candidiasis may respond to oral nystatin, 0.5–1 million units in adults (100,000 units in children) 4 times daily in addition to local therapy. Vulvovaginal candidiasis may be treated by insertion of 1 vaginal tablet twice daily for 14 days, then nightly for an additional 14–21 days.

Amphotericin B (Fungizone) is available for topical use in cream, ointment, and lotion form. The recommended dosage in the treatment of paronychial and intertriginous candidiasis is application 2–4 times daily to the affected area.

Adverse side-effects associated with oral administration of nystatin include mild nausea, diarrhea, and occasional vomiting. Topical application is nonirritating, and allergic contact hypersensitivity is exceedingly uncommon. Topical amphotericin B is well tolerated and only occasionally locally irritating. Hypersensitivity is exceedingly rare. The drug may cause a temporary yellow staining of the skin, especially when the cream vehicle is used.

Oral Antifungal Agents

GRISEOFULVIN

Griseofulvin is effective orally against dermatophyte infections caused by *Epidermophyton, Microsporum,* and *Trichophyton* (Chapter 47). It is ineffective against *Candida* and *P orbiculare*.

Griseofulvin's antifungal activity has been attributed to inhibition of hyphal cell wall synthesis, effects on nucleic acid synthesis, and inhibition of mitosis. Griseofulvin interferes with microtubules of the mitotic spindle and with cytoplasmic microtubules. The destruction of cytoplasmic microtubules may result in impaired processing of newly synthesized cell wall constituents at the growing tips of hyphae. Griseofulvin is active only against growing cells.

Following the oral administration of 1 g of griseofulvin, peak serum levels of 1.5–2 μg/mL are obtained in 4–8 hours. The drug can be detected in the stratum corneum 4–8 hours following oral administration, with the highest concentration in the outermost layers and the lowest in the base. Topical application has not been found to be efficacious.

The usual adult dose of the micronized (''microsize'') form of the drug is 500 mg daily in single or divided doses with meals; occasionally, 1 g/d is indicated in the treatment of recalcitrant infections. The pediatric dose is 10 mg/kg of body weight daily in single or divided doses with meals. An oral suspension is available for use in children.

Griseofulvin is most effective in treating tinea infections of the scalp and glabrous (nonhairy) skin. In general, infections of the scalp respond to treatment in 4–6 weeks, and infections of glabrous skin will respond to 3–4 weeks. Dermatophyte infections of the nails respond only to prolonged administration of griseofulvin. Fingernails may respond to 6 months of therapy, whereas toenails are quite recalcitrant to treatment and may require 8–18 months of therapy; relapse almost invariably occurs.

Adverse side-effects seen with griseofulvin therapy include headaches, nausea, vomiting, diarrhea, photosensitivity, peripheral neuritis, and occasionally mental confusion. Griseofulvin is derived from a *Penicillium* mold, and cross-sensitivity with penicillin may occur. It is contraindicated in patients with porphyria or hepatic failure or those who have had hypersensitivity reactions to it in the past. Its safety in pregnant patients has not been established. Leukopenia and proteinuria have occasionally been reported, and in patients undergoing prolonged therapy, routine evaluation of hepatic, renal, and hematopoietic systems may be desirable. Coumarin anticoagulant activity may be altered by griseofulvin, and anticoagulant dosage may require adjustment.

KETOCONAZOLE

Ketoconazole is a water-soluble synthetic antifungal imidazole derivative active against many fungi and yeasts, including dermatophytes, *Candida, P orbiculare,* and numerous dimorphic fungi responsible for systemic mycoses.

As explained in Chapter 47, imidazole derivatives, including ketoconazole, act by affecting the permeability of the cell membrane of sensitive cells through alterations of the biosynthesis of lipids, especially sterols, in the fungal cell.

Ketoconazole (Nizoral) is the first imidazole derivative available for oral treatment of systemic mycoses. In the USA, its use in dermatology is restricted to chronic mucocutaneous candidiasis and chromomycosis. Patients with chronic mucocutaneous candidiasis respond well to a once-daily dose of 200 mg of ketoconazole, with a median clearing time of 16 weeks. Most patients require long-term maintenance therapy. Variable results have been reported in treatment of chromomycosis. Preliminary reports suggest that ketoconazole will be effective against dermatophytosis and tinea versicolor.

ECTOPARASITICIDES

LINDANE (Hexachlorocyclohexane)

The gamma isomer of hexachlorocyclohexane is commonly called gamma benzene hexachloride (GBHC), which is a misnomer, since no benzene ring is present in this compound. Lindane is an effective pediculicide and scabicide.

Percutaneous absorption studies using a solution of lindane in acetone have shown that almost 10% of a dose applied to the forearm is absorbed, to be subsequently excreted in the urine over a 5-day period. Serum levels following the application of a commercial lindane lotion reach maximum at 6 hours and decline thereafter with a half-life of 24 hours. After absorption, lindane is concentrated in fatty tissues, including the brain.

Lindane is available as a shampoo, lotion, or cream. For pediculosis capitis or pubis, 30 mL of shampoo is worked into a lather and left on the scalp or genital area for 5 minutes and then rinsed off. If living lice are present 1 week after treatment, reapplication may be required. Recent concerns about the toxicity of lindane have altered treatment guidelines for its use in scabies; the current recommendation calls for a single application to the entire body from the neck down, left on for 8–12 hours, and then washed off. Patients should be re-treated only if active mites can be demonstrated, and never within 1 week of initial treatment.

Much controversy exists about the possible systemic toxicities of topically applied lindane used for medical purposes. Concerns about neurotoxicity, hematotoxicity, and mutagenicity have resulted in warnings that lindane should be used with caution in infants, children, and pregnant women. The current USA package insert recommends that it not be used as an antiscabetic in children under age 10 years, during pregnancy, or during lactation. The risk of adverse systemic reactions to lindane appears to be minimal when it is used properly and according to directions in adult patients. However, local irritation may occur, and contact with the eyes and mucous membranes should be avoided.

CROTAMITON

Crotamiton, N-ethyl-*o*-crotonotoluidide, is a scabicide with some antipruritic properties. Its mechanism of action is not known, and studies on percutaneous absorption have not been performed.

Crotamiton (Eurax) is available as cream or lotion. Suggested guidelines for scabies treatment call for 2 applications to the entire body from the chin down at 24-hour intervals, with a cleansing bath 48 hours after the last application. Crotamiton is an effective agent that can be used as an alternative to lindane. Allergic contact hypersensitivity and primary irritation may occur, necessitating discontinuation of therapy. Application to acutely inflamed skin or to the eyes or mucous membranes should be avoided.

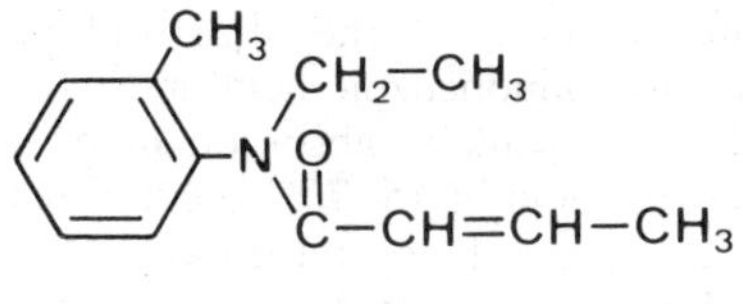

Crotamiton

BENZYL BENZOATE

Benzyl benzoate is effective as a pediculicide and scabicide. It has generally been supplanted by lindane. The mechanism of action of benzyl benzoate is unknown. Although it appears to be relatively nontoxic after topical application, there are no studies of its toxic potential in the treatment of scabies.

SULFUR

Sulfur has a long history of use as a scabicide. Although it is nonirritating, it has an unpleasant odor, is staining, and is disagreeable to use. It has been replaced by more aesthetic and effective scabicides in recent years, but it remains a possible alternative drug for use in infants and pregnant women. The usual formulation is 5% precipitated sulfur in petrolatum.

AGENTS AFFECTING PIGMENTATION

HYDROQUINONE & MONOBENZONE

Hydroquinone and monobenzone, the monobenzyl ether of hydroquinone, are used to *reduce hyperpigmentation* of the skin. Topical hydroquinone usually results in temporary lightening, whereas monobenzone causes irreversible depigmentation.

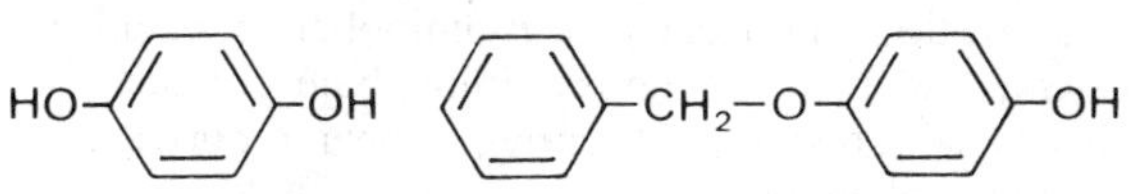

Hydroquinone Monobenzone

The mechanism of action of these compounds appears to involve inhibition of the enzyme tyrosinase, thus interfering with the biosynthesis of melanin. In addition, monobenzone may be toxic to melanocytes, resulting in permanent depigmentation. Some percutaneous absorption of these compounds takes place, because monobenzone may cause hypopigmentation at sites distant from the area of application.

Hydroquinone may be useful in treating melasma, lentigines, and ephelides but is of minimal benefit in treating postinflammatory hyperpigmentation, particularly when the melanin is no longer confined to the epidermis but has dropped down into the dermis. Most lesions treated with hydroquinone will respond with only a temporary lightening; when the medication is discontinued, the lesions return to their original color. Patients should be encouraged to use an opaque sunscreen to block the melanogenic long wavelengths of ultraviolet light. Hydroquinone is usually applied twice daily to the area to be lightened.

Monobenzone is used only when permanent irreversible depigmentation is desired, ie, in patients with disseminated vitiligo who have a few remaining areas of normal pigmentation. It is applied to the area to be depigmented twice daily until all pigmentation has resolved. As noted above, monobenzone has been reported to cause depigmentation at sites distant from the treatment area, and this should be explained to any patient in whom only local depigmentation is desired.

Both hydroquinone and monobenzone may cause local irritation. Allergic sensitization to these compounds does occur, and it is advisable to do a patch test on a small area of the body prior to use on the face. Contact of the drug with the eyes must be avoided. An unusual ochronosislike syndrome of hyperpigmentation has been reported in black South African patients who were using 6–8% hydroquinone creams in areas of intense sunlight exposure.

TRIOXSALEN & METHOXSALEN

Trioxsalen and methoxsalen are members of the naturally occurring tricyclic furocoumarins used for centuries in India for the *repigmentation* of depig-

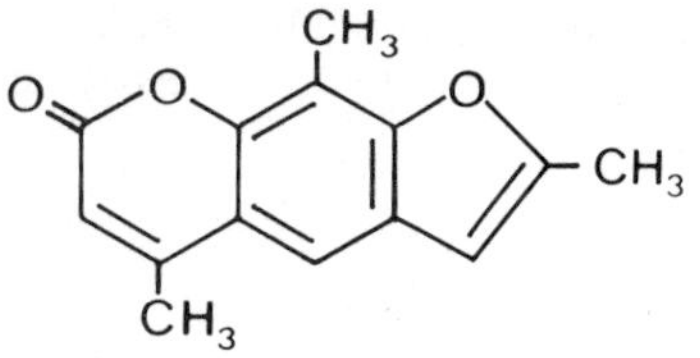

Trioxsalen

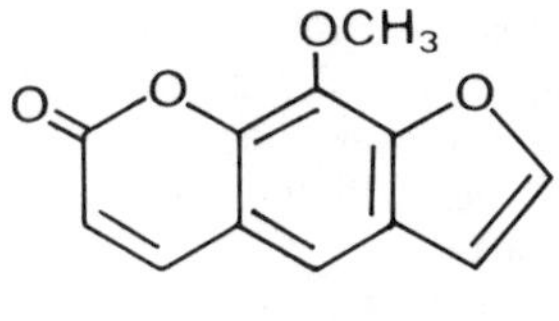

Methoxsalen

mented macules of vitiligo. With the recent development of high-intensity long-wave ultraviolet fluorescent lamps, photochemotherapy with oral methoxsalen for psoriasis and with oral trioxsalen for vitiligo has been under intensive investigation. The drugs are not yet available for general use.

Psoralens must be photoactivated by long-wavelength ultraviolet light in the range of 320–400 nm (UVA) to produce a beneficial effect. Psoralens intercalate with DNA and, with subsequent UVA irradiation, cyclobutane adducts are formed with pyrimidine bases. Both monofunctional and bifunctional adducts may be formed, the latter causing interstrand cross-links. These DNA photoproducts may inhibit DNA synthesis.

In the treatment of vitiligo, 10 mg of trioxsalen (Trisoralen) is given orally 2 hours prior to measured periods of ultraviolet exposure, either from sunlight or an artificial light source. Methoxsalen (Oxsoralen) may be used in the treatment of vitiligo in a dosage of 20 mg orally 2 hours prior to light exposure. Topical methoxsalen may be used to treat small vitiliginous lesions, but extreme caution is necessary to prevent severe erythema and blistering. Dilution of the 1% lotion to a concentration of 1:1000 or 1:10,000 is helpful to avoid excessive reactions. The use of oral and topical methoxsalen in the treatment of psoriasis is still investigational. Any UVA light source used for photochemotherapy should be calibrated regularly to prevent excessive exposure.

The major long-term risks of psoralen photochemotherapy are cataracts and skin cancer. Therefore, when oral psoralens are given, patients should wear UVA-opaque sunglasses and avoid exposure to sunlight from the time of ingestion, during their light treatment, and through the remaining hours of daylight on treatment days. The psoralens are contraindicated in persons under 12 years of age and in those who have received ionizing radiation or have porphyria, discoid or systemic lupus erythematosus, or xeroderma pigmentosum. Acute side-effects include erythema, pruritus, severe burns from excessive exposure, and nausea from orally administered psoralens. In view of the delayed erythema caused by psoralens and UVA, treatments should never be given less than 48 hours apart.

SUNSCREENS

Topical medications useful in protecting against sunlight contain either chemical compounds that absorb ultraviolet light, called *sunscreens;* or opaque materials such as titanium dioxide that reflect light, called *sunshades*. The 2 classes of chemical compounds most commonly used in sunscreens are *p*-aminobenzoic acid (PABA) and its derivatives and the benzophenones.

Most sunscreen preparations are designed to absorb ultraviolet light in the "B" ultraviolet wavelength range from 280 to 320 nm, which is the range respon-

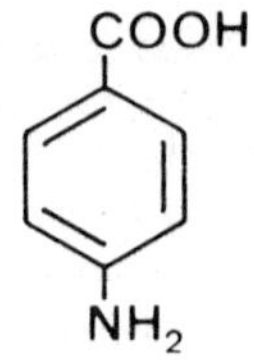

p-Aminobenzoic acid

sible for most of the erythema and tanning associated with sun exposure. Chronic exposure to light in this range induces aging of the skin and photocarcinogenesis. *p*-Aminobenzoic acid and its esters are the most effective available absorbers in the B region. *p*-Aminobenzoic acid in 55–70% alcohol is the most efficient agent, while padimate A (pentyl *p*-dimethylaminobenzoate), padimate O (2-ethylhexyl-dimethyl-*p*-aminobenzoate), and glyceryl *p*-aminobenzoate are somewhat less efficient but often utilized for their other qualities. *p*-Aminobenzoic acid may photo-oxidize to produce a yellow stain on light-colored fabrics, while the *p*-aminobenzoic acid esters do not stain as easily.

The benzophenones include oxybenzone, dioxybenzone, and sulisobenzone. These compounds provide a broader spectrum of absorption from 250 to 360 nm, but their effectiveness in the UVB erythema range is less than that of *p*-aminobenzoic acid. Several of the newer ultraprotective suncreens contain a combination of *p*-aminobenzoic acid, its esters, and a benzophenone.

The protection factor (PF) of a given sunscreen is a measure of its effectiveness in absorbing erythrogenic ultraviolet light. It is determined by measuring the minimal erythema dose (MED) with and without the sunscreen in a group of normal people. The ratio of the minimal erythema dose with sunscreen to the minimal erythema dose without sunscreen is the protection factor. If the protection factor value is determined in field tests using sunlight rather than an artificial light source, it may be called the sun protection factor (SPF). Fair-skinned individuals who sunburn easily are advised to use a product with a high protection factor of 10–15; those with darker skins may use a sunscreen with a lower protection factor of 6–8.

Sunscreens should be applied 1 hour before sun exposure, and reapplication is advised after swimming or profuse sweating. Some recently introduced products have greater resistance to removal, thereby reducing the need for reapplication. Tingling and stinging sometimes occur with application of *p*-aminobenzoic acid preparations. Allergic contact and photocontact sensitization can occur with *p*-aminobenzoic acid, its esters, and benzophenones. Immediate contact sensitivity with resulting urticaria has been reported with the benzophenones.

ACNE PREPARATIONS

RETINOIC ACID

Retinoic acid, also known as tretinoin or *trans*-retinoic acid, is the acid form of vitamin A. It is an effective topical treatment for acne vulgaris. Several analogs of vitamin A, eg, 13-*cis*-retinoic acid (isotretinoin), have recently been shown to be effective in various dermatologic diseases when given *orally*. Vitamin A alcohol is the physiologic form of vitamin A. The topical therapeutic agent, retinoic acid, is formed by the oxidation of the alcohol group, with all 4 double bonds in the side chain in the *trans* configuration as shown.

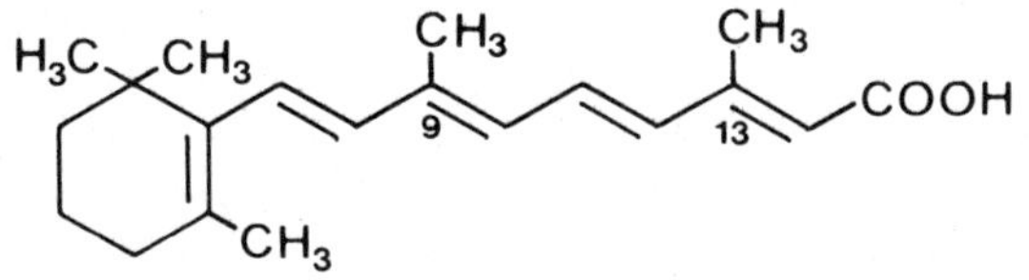

Retinoic acid

Retinoic acid is insoluble in water but soluble in many organic solvents. It is susceptible to oxidation and ester formation, particularly when exposed to light. Topically applied retinoic acid remains chiefly in the epidermis, with less than 10% absorption into the circulation. The small quantities of retinoic acid absorbed following topical application are metabolized by the liver and excreted in bile and urine.

Retinoic acid has several effects on epithelial tissues. It stabilizes lysosomes, increases ribonucleic acid polymerase activity, increases prostaglandin E_2, cAMP, and cGMP levels, and increases the incorporation of thymidine into DNA. Its action in acne has been attributed to decreased cohesion between epidermal cells and increased epidermal cell turnover. This is thought to result in the expulsion of open comedones and the transformation of closed comedones into open ones.

Topical retinoic acid (Retin-A) is applied initially in a concentration sufficient to induce slight erythema with mild peeling. The concentration or frequency of application may be decreased if too much irritation is produced. Topical retinoic acid should be applied to dry skin only, and care should be taken to avoid contact with the corners of the nose, eyes, mouth, and mucous membranes. During the first 4–6 weeks of therapy, comedones not previously evident may appear and give the impression that the acne has been aggravated by the retinoic acid. However, with continued therapy, the lesions will clear, and in 8–12 weeks optimal clinical improvement should occur.

The most common adverse side-effects of topical retinoic acid are the erythema and dryness that occur in the first few weeks of use, but these can be expected to resolve with continued therapy. Patients using retinoic acid are at increased risk for sunburn, and they should be advised to limit their sun exposure and use a protective sunscreen. Allergic contact dermatitis to topical retinoic acid is rare.

ISOTRETINOIN

Isotretinoin (Accutane) is given orally at a dosage of 1–2 mg/kg/d for 4–5 months. The drug is well absorbed, extensively bound to plasma albumin, and has a half-life of 10–20 hours. It is effective in severe acne, and remissions may persist for years after 1–2 courses of treatment. Common adverse effects resemble hypervitaminosis A and include dryness and itching of the skin and mucous membranes. Less common side-effects are headache, anorexia, alopecia, and muscle and joint pains. These effects are all reversible on discontinuation of therapy. Lipid abnormalities (triglycerides, HDL) are frequent; their clinical relevance is unknown at present.

BENZOYL PEROXIDE

Benzoyl peroxide is an effective topical agent in the treatment of acne vulgaris. It penetrates unchanged through the stratum corneum or follicular openings and is converted metabolically to benzoic acid within the epidermis and dermis. Less than 5% of an applied dose is absorbed from the skin in an 8-hour period.

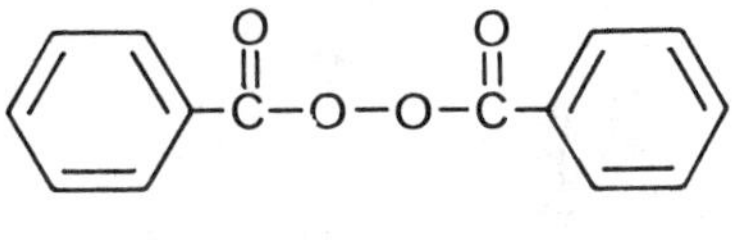

Benzoyl peroxide

It has been postulated that the mechanism of action of benzoyl peroxide in acne is related to its antimicrobial activity against *P acnes* and to its peeling and comedolytic effects.

To decrease the possibility of irritation, application should be limited to a low concentration (2.5%) once daily for the first week of therapy and increased in frequency and strength if the preparation is well tolerated.

Benzoyl peroxide is a potent contact sensitizer in experimental studies, and this adverse effect may occur in up to 1% of acne patients. Care should be taken to avoid contact with the eyes and mucous membranes. Benzoyl peroxide is an oxidant and may rarely cause bleaching of the hair or colored fabrics.

ANTI-INFLAMMATORY AGENTS

TOPICAL CORTICOSTEROIDS

The remarkable efficacy of topical corticosteroids in the treatment of inflammatory dermatoses was noted soon after the introduction of hydrocortisone in 1952. Subsequently, numerous analogs have been developed that offer extensive choices of potencies, concentrations, and vehicles. The therapeutic effectiveness of topical corticosteroids is based primarily on their anti-inflammatory activity. Definitive explanations of the effects of corticosteroids on endogenous mediators of inflammation such as histamine, kinins, lysosomal enzymes, and prostaglandins await further experimental clarification. The antimitotic effects of corticosteroids on human epidermis may account for an additional mechanism of action in psoriasis and other dermatologic diseases associated with increased cell turnover. The general pharmacology of these endocrine agents is discussed in Chapter 37.

The original topical glucocorticosteroid was hydrocortisone, the natural glucocorticosteroid of the adrenal cortex (Fig 61–1). Prednisolone and methylprednisolone are active to the same extent as hydrocortisone. The 9α-fluoro derivatives of hydrocortisone were active topically, but their salt-retaining properties made them undesirable even for topical use. The 9α-fluorinated steroids dexamethasone and betamethasone subsequently developed did not have any advantage over hydrocortisone. However, triamcinolone and fluocinolone, the acetonide derivatives of the fluorinated steroids, had a distinct advantage in topical therapy. Similarly, betamethasone is not very active topically, but attaching a 5-carbon valerate chain to the 17-hydroxyl position results in a compound over 300 times as active as hydrocortisone for topical use. Fluocinonide is the 21-acetate deriva-

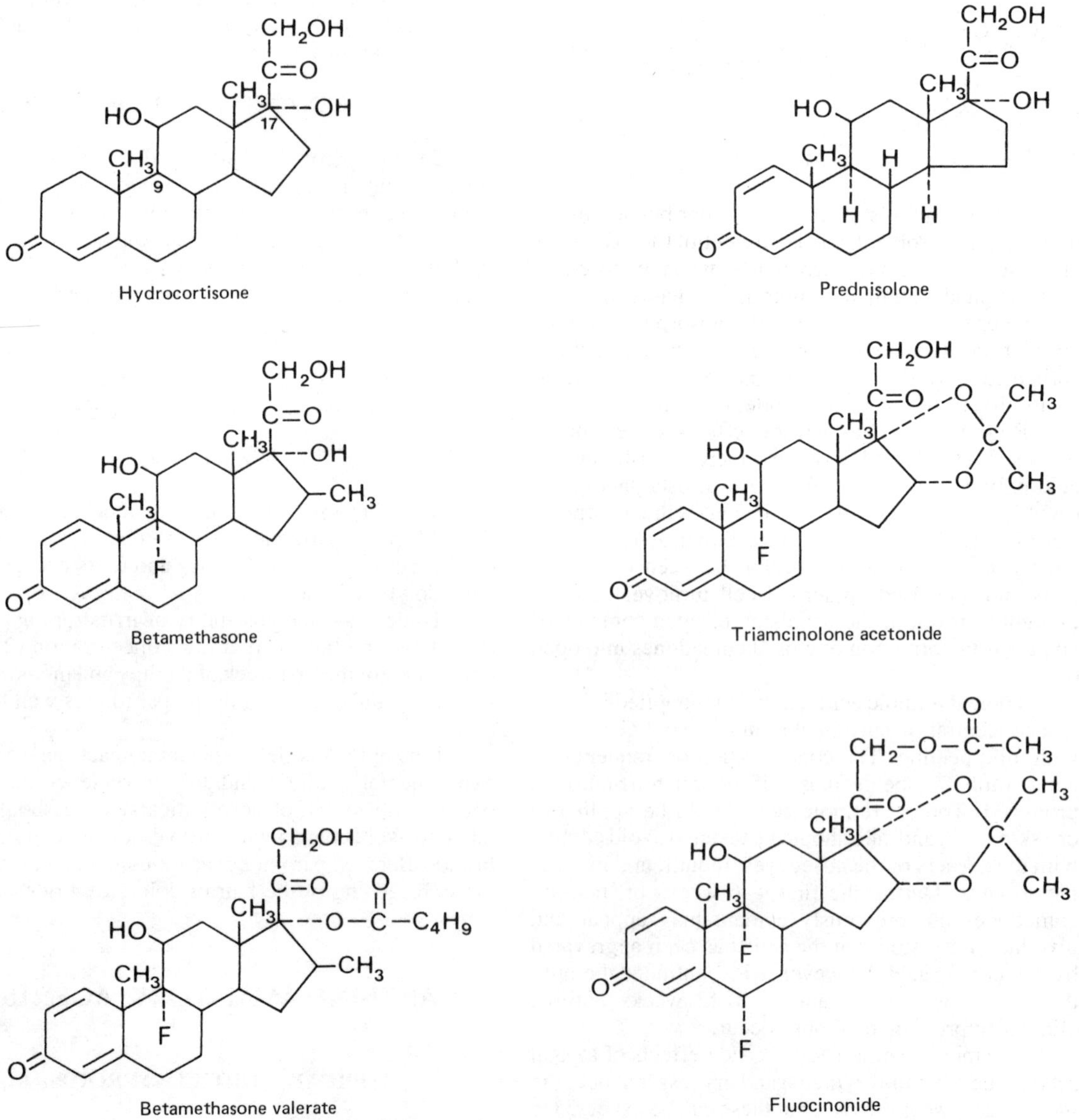

Figure 61–1. Chemical structures of several glucocorticoids.

Table 61–1. Relative efficacy of topical corticosteroids in various formulations.

Lowest efficacy	
0.25–2.5%	Hydrocortisone
0.25%	Methylprednisolone acetate (Medrol)
0.04%	Dexamethasone* (Hexadrol)
0.1%	Dexamethasone* (Decaderm)
1.0%	Methylprednisolone acetate (Medrol)
0.5%	Prednisolone (Meti-Derm)
0.2%	Betamethasone* (Celestone)
Low efficacy	
0.01%	Fluocinolone acetonide* (Fluonid, Synalar)
0.01%	Betamethasone valerate* (Valisone)
0.025%	Fluorometholone* (Oxylone)
0.025%	Triamcinolone acetonide* (Aristocort, Kenalog, Triacet)
0.1%	Clocortolone pivalate* (Cloderm)
0.03%	Flumethasone pivalate* (Locorten)
Intermediate efficacy	
0.2%	Hydrocortisone valerate (Westcort)
0.025%	Betamethasone benzoate* (Benisone, Flurobate, Uticort)
0.025%	Flurandrenolide* (Cordran)
0.1%	Betamethasone valerate* (Valisone)
0.05%	Desonide (Tridesilon)
0.025%	Halcinonide* (Halog)
0.05%	Desoximetasone* (Topicort L.P.)
0.05%	Flurandrenolide* (Cordran)
0.1%	Triamcinolone acetonide*
0.025%	Fluocinolone acetonide*
High efficacy	
0.05%	Betamethasone dipropionate* (Diprosone)
0.1%	Amcinonide* (Cyclocort)
0.25%	Desoximetasone* (Topicort)
0.5%	Triamcinolone acetonide*
0.2%	Fluocinolone acetonide* (Synalar-HP)
0.05%	Diflorasone diacetate* (Florone)
0.1%	Halcinonide* (Halog)
0.05%	Fluocinonide* (Lidex, Topsyn)

*Fluorinated steroids.

tive of fluocinolone acetonide; the addition of the 21-acetate enhances the topical activity about 5-fold. Fluorination of the steroid is not required for high potency; hydrocortisone valerate and butyrate have activity similar to that of triamcinolone acetonide.

Corticosteroids are only minimally absorbed following application to normal skin, eg, approximately 1% of a dose of hyrocortisone solution applied to the ventral forearm is absorbed. The newer analogs may not owe their increased efficacy to enhanced penetration. Those corticosteroids for which published data exist are absorbed to no greater—and perhaps to a lesser—degree than hydrocortisone. However, occlusion with an impermeable film, such as plastic wrap, is an effective method of enhancing penetration, yielding a 10-fold increase in absorption for all these agents. There is a marked regional anatomic variation in corticosteroid penetration. Compared to the absorption from the forearm, hydrocortisone is absorbed 0.14 times as well through the plantar foot arch, 0.83 times as well through the palm, 3.5 times as well through the scalp, 6 times as well through the forehead, 9 times as well through vulvar skin, and 42 times as well through scrotal skin. Penetration is increased severalfold in the inflamed skin of atopic dermatitis; and in severe exfoliative diseases, such as erythrodermic psoriasis, there appears to be little barrier to penetration.

Experimental studies on the percutaneous absorption of hydrocortisone fail to reveal a significant increase in absorption when applied on a repetitive basis compared to a single dose, and a single daily application may be effective in most conditions. Ointment bases tend to give better activity to the corticosteroid than do cream or lotion vehicles. Novel vehicles, including gels, may not retain their optimal drug delivery qualities if they are diluted, even with the same base. Increasing the concentration of a corticosteroid increases the penetration but not to the same degree. For example, approximately 1% of a 0.25% hydrocortisone solution is absorbed from the forearm. A 10-fold increase in concentration causes a 4-fold increase in absorption.

Table 61–1 groups topical corticosteroid formulations according to approximate relative efficacy. Table 61–2 lists major dermatologic diseases in order of their responsiveness to these drugs. In the first group, low- to medium-efficacy corticosteroid preparations often produce clinical remission. In the second group, it is often necessary to use high-efficacy preparations, occlusion therapy, or both. Once a remission

Table 61–2. Dermatologic disorders responsive to topical corticosteroids ranked in order of sensitivity.

Very responsive
Atopic dermatitis
Seborrheic dermatitis
Lichen simplex chronicus
Pruritus ani
Later phase of allergic contact dermatitis
Later phase of irritant dermatitis
Nummular eczematous dermatitis
Stasis dermatitis
Psoriasis, especially of genitalia and face
Less responsive
Discoid lupus erythematosus
Psoriasis of palms and soles
Necrobiosis lipoidica diabeticorum
Sarcoidosis
Lichen striatus
Pemphigus
Familial benign pemphigus
Vitiligo
Granuloma annulare
Least responsive: intralesional injection required
Keloids
Hypertrophic scars
Hypertrophic lichen planus
Alopecia areata
Acne cysts
Prurigo nodularis
Chondrodermatitis nodularis helicus

has been achieved, every effort should be made to maintain the patient with a low-efficacy corticosteroid.

The limited penetration of topical corticosteroids can be overcome in certain clinical circumstances by the intralesional injection of relatively insoluble corticosteroids, eg, triamcinolone acetonide, triamcinolone diacetate, triamcinolone hexacetonide, and betamethasone acetate-phosphate. When these agents are injected into the lesion, measurable amounts remain in place and are gradually released for 3–4 weeks. This form of therapy is often effective for the lesions listed in Table 61–2 that are generally unresponsive to topical corticosteroids. The dosage of the triamcinolone salts should be limited to 1 mg per treatment site, ie, 0.1 mL of 10 mg/mL suspension, to decrease the incidence of local atrophy (see below).

Adverse Effects

All absorbable topical corticosteroids possess the potential to suppress the pituitary-adrenal axis (Chapter 37). Although most patients with pituitary-adrenal axis suppression demonstrate only a laboratory test abnormality, cases of severely impaired stress response can occur. Iatrogenic Cushing's syndrome may occur as a result of protracted use of topical corticosteroids in large quantities. Applying potent corticosteroids to extensive areas of the body for prolonged periods, with or without occlusion, increases the likelihood of systemic side-effects. Fewer of these factors are required to produce adverse systemic effects in children, and growth retardation is of particular concern in the pediatric age group.

Adverse local effects of topical corticosteroids include the following: atrophy, which may present as depressed, shiny, often wrinkled "cigarette paper"-appearing skin with prominent telangiectases and a tendency to develop purpura and ecchymosis; steroid rosacea, with persistent erythema, telangiectatic vessels, pustules, and papules in central facial distribution; perioral dermatitis, steroid acne, alterations of cutaneous infections, hypopigmentation, hypertrichosis, and increased intraocular pressure; and allergic contact dermatitis, which may be confirmed by patch testing with high concentrations of corticosteroids, ie, 1% in petrolatum, because topical corticosteroids are not irritating. Topical corticosteroids are contraindicated in individuals who demonstrate hypersensitivity to them.

TAR COMPOUNDS

Coal tar preparations have been used in dermatologic practice since the late 19th century, chiefly in the treatment of psoriasis. Coal tar is the principal byproduct of the destructive distillation of bituminous coal and an exceedingly complex mixture, containing about 10,000 compounds. These include naphthalene, phenanthrene, fluoranthrene, benzene, xylene, toluene, phenol, cresols, other aromatic compounds, pyridine bases, ammonia, and peroxides. Chiefly because of the complexity of coal tar and the difficulties of isolating topically active fractions, analyses of the rates of absorption, blood levels, and excretion of specific compounds have been inadequate. Dermatologically useful tar compounds are also derived from the destructive distillation of shale rock, yielding ichthammol, and the heartwood of *Juniperus oxycedrus,* yielding juniper tar. Coal tar is available in many over-the-counter preparations in the form of bath additives, shampoos, and hydroalcoholic base gels. Coal tar may also be compounded in accordance with *United States Pharmacopeia, National Formulary,* or other formulations in concentrations ranging from 2 to 10%.

Liquor carbonis detergens (LCD) is a coal tar solution prepared by extracting coal tar with alcohol and an emulsifying agent, such as polysorbate 80. This solution contains 20 g of coal tar per 100 mL and may be compounded in concentrations of 2–10% in creams, ointments, or shampoos.

Tar preparations are used mainly in the treatment of psoriasis, dermatitis, and lichen simplex chronicus. The phenolic constituents endow these compounds with antipruritic properties, making them particularly valuable in the treatment of chronic lichenified dermatitis. Acute dermatitis with vesiculation and oozing may be irritated by even weak tar preparations, which should be avoided. However, in the subacute and chronic stages of dermatitis and psoriasis, these preparations are quite useful and offer an alternative to the use of topical corticosteroids.

The most common adverse reaction to coal tar compounds is an irritant folliculitis, necessitating discontinuation of therapy to the affected areas for a period of 3–5 days. Phototoxicity and allergic contact dermatitis may also occur. Tar preparations should be avoided in patients who have previously exhibited sensitivity to them. Care should be exercised when using tar compounds in patients with erythrodermal or generalized pustular psoriasis, because of the risk of total body exfoliation.

KERATOLYTIC & DESTRUCTIVE AGENTS

SALICYLIC ACID

Salicylic acid was chemically synthesized in 1860 and has been extensively used in dermatologic therapy as a keratolytic agent. It is a white powder quite soluble in alcohol but only slightly soluble in water.

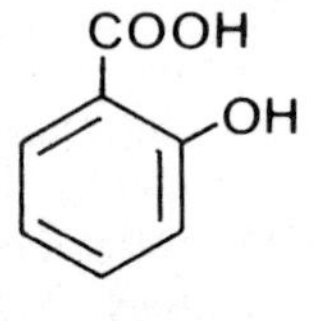

Salicylic acid

Salicylic acid is absorbed percutaneously and distributed in the extracellular space, with maximum plasma levels occurring 6–12 hours after application. Since 50–80% of salicylate is bound to albumin, transiently increased serum levels of free salicylates are found in patients with hypoalbuminemia. The urinary metabolites of topically applied salicylic acid include salicyluric acid and acyl and phenolic glucuronides of salicylic acid; only 6% of the total recovered is unchanged salicylic acid. About 95% of a single dose of salicylate is excreted in the urine within 24 hours after its absorption.

The mechanism by which salicylic acid produces its keratolytic and other therapeutic effects is poorly understood. The drug may solubilize cell surface proteins that keep the stratum corneum intact, thereby resulting in desquamation of keratotic debris. Salicyic acid is keratolytic in concentrations of 3–6%. In concentrations greater than 6%, it can be destructive to tissues.

Salicylism and death have occurred following topical application. In an adult, 1 g of a topically applied 6% salicylic acid preparation will raise the serum salicylate level not more than 0.5 mg/dL of plasma; the threshold for toxicity is 30–50 mg/dL. Higher serum levels are possible in children, who are therefore at a greater risk to develop salicylism. It is advisable to limit both the total amount of salicylic acid applied and the frequency of application. Urticarial, anaphylactic, and erythema multiforme reactions may occur in patients allergic to salicylates. Topical use may be associated with local irritation, acute inflammation, and even ulceration with the use of high concentrations of salicylic acid. Particular care must be exercised when using the drug on the extremities of diabetics or patients with peripheral vascular disease.

PROPYLENE GLYCOL

Propylene glycol is extensively used in topical preparations because it is an excellent vehicle for organic compounds. Propylene glycol has recently been used alone as a keratolytic agent in 40–70% concentrations, with plastic occlusion, or in gel with 6% salicylic acid.

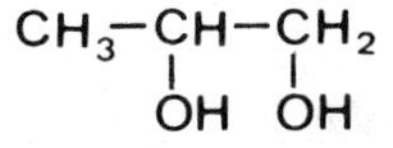

Propylene glycol

Only minimal amounts of a topically applied dose are absorbed through normal stratum corneum. Percutaneously absorbed propylene glycol is oxidized by the liver to lactic acid and pyruvic acid, with subsequent utilization in general body metabolism. Approximately 12–45% of the absorbed agent is excreted unchanged in the urine. Propylene glycol is an effective keratolytic agent for the removal of hyperkeratotic debris. This keratolytic effect is attributed to reversible and irreversible changes in epidermal structural proteins. Propylene glycol increases the solubility of proteins in water and also denatures proteins, with the maximum effect seen in a concentration range of 61–77%. The addition of salicylic acid to propylene glycol may augment the keratolytic effect of propylene glycol by lowering the pH of the preparation, thus enhancing subsequent protein denaturation.

Propylene glycol is also an effective humectant and increases the water content of the stratum corneum. The hygroscopic characteristics of the agent may help it to develop an osmotic gradient through the stratum corneum, thereby increasing hydration of the outermost layers by drawing water out from the inner layers of the skin.

Propylene glycol is used under polyethylene occlusion or with 6% salicylic acid for the treatment of ichthyosis, palmar and plantar keratodermas, psoriasis, pityriasis rubra pilaris, keratosis pilaris, and hypertrophic lichen planus.

In concentrations greater than 10%, propylene glycol may act as an irritant in some patients; those with eczematous dermatitis may be more sensitive. Allergic contact dermatitis occurs with propylene glycol, and at present a 4% aqueous propylene glycol solution is recommended for the purpose of patch testing.

UREA

Urea in a compatible cream vehicle or ointment base has a softening and moisturizing effect on the stratum corneum. It has the ability to make creams and lotions feel less greasy, and this has been utilized in dermatologic preparations to decrease the oily feel of a preparation that otherwise might feel unpleasant. It is a white crystalline powder with a slight ammonia odor when moist.

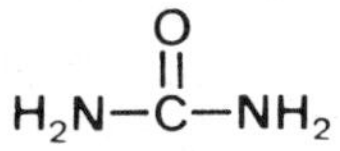

Urea

Urea is absorbed percutaneously, although the precise amount absorbed is not well documented. It is predominantly distributed in the extracellular space and excreted in urine. Urea is a natural product of metabolism, and systemic toxicities with topical application do not occur.

Urea allegedly increases the water content of the stratum corneum, presumably as a result of the hygroscopic characteristics of this naturally occurring molecule. Urea is also keratolytic. The mechanism of action appears to involve alterations in prekeratin and keratin, leading to increased solubilization. In addition, urea may break hydrogen bonds that keep the stratum corneum intact.

As a humectant, urea is used in concentrations of 2–20% in creams and lotions. As a keratolytic agent, it is used in 20% concentration in diseases such as ichthyosis vulgaris, hyperkeratosis of palms and soles, xerosis, and keratosis pilaris. Concentrations of 30–50% in ointment base applied to the nail plate under occlusion have been useful in softening the nail prior to avulsion. Concentrations of 10–20% applied to the diaper area, groin, or areas of eczematous dermatitis may be associated with an unpleasant stinging sensation that may necessitate discontinuation of the preparation.

PODOPHYLLUM RESIN

Podophyllum resin, an alcoholic extract of *Podophyllum peltatum,* commonly known as mandrake root or May apple, is used in the treatment of condyloma acuminatum and other verrucae. It is a mixture of podophyllotoxin, alpha and beta peltatin, desoxypodophyllotoxin, dehydropodophyllotoxin, and other compounds. It is soluble in alcohol, ether, chloroform, and compound tincture of benzoin.

Percutaneous absorption of podophyllum resin occurs, particularly in intertriginous areas and from applications to large moist condylomas. It is soluble in lipids and therefore is distributed widely throughout the body, including the central nervous system.

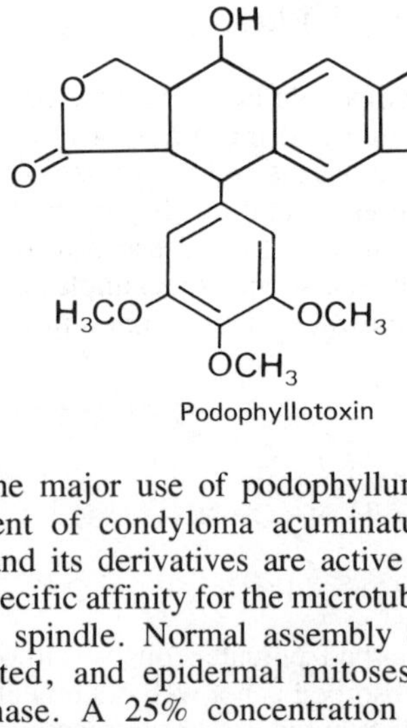

Podophyllotoxin

The major use of podophyllum resin is in the treatment of condyloma acuminatum. Podophyllotoxin and its derivatives are active cytotoxic agents with specific affinity for the microtubule protein of the mitotic spindle. Normal assembly of the spindle is prevented, and epidermal mitoses are arrested in metaphase. A 25% concentration of podophyllum resin in compound tincture of benzoin is recommended for the treatment of condyloma acuminatum. Application should be restricted to wart tissue only, to limit the total amount of medication used and to prevent severe erosive changes in adjacent tissue. In treating cases of large extensive condylomas, it is advisable to limit application to sections of the affected area to minimize systemic absorption. The patient is instructed to wash off the preparation 2–3 hours after the initial application, since the irritant reaction is variable. Depending on the individual patient's reaction, this period can be extended to 6–8 hours on subsequent applications. If 3–5 applications have not resulted in significant resolution, other methods of treatment should be considered.

Toxic symptoms associated with excessively large applications include nausea, vomiting, alterations in sensorium, muscle weakness, neuropathy with diminished tendon reflexes, coma, and even death. Local irritation is common, and inadvertent contact with the eye may cause severe conjunctivitis. Use during pregnancy is contraindicated in view of possible cytotoxic effects on the fetus.

CANTHARIDIN

Cantharidin is the active irritant isolated from cantharides, or dried blister beetles—*Lytta (Cantharis) vesicatoria,* also known as Russian fly or Spanish fly. The ability of insects of the *Cantharis* type to produce vesicles and bullae on human skin led to the investigation of possible therapeutic uses of the vesicant cantharidin in dermatology. The major clinical use is in the treatment of molluscum contagiosum and verruca vulgaris, particularly periungual warts.

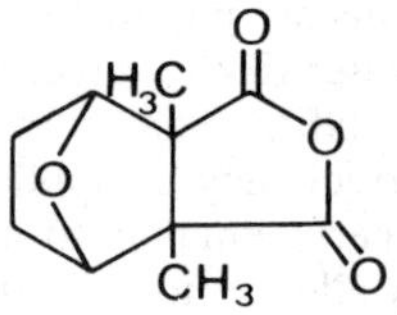

Cantharidin

The amount of cantharidin absorbed following cutaneous application is unknown. It is excreted by the kidney, and in cases of oral ingestion of significant amounts, marked irritation of the entire urinary tract has resulted, with pain, urinary urgency, and priapism.

Cantharidin acts on mitochondrial oxidative enzymes, resulting in decreased ATP levels. This leads to changes in the epidermal cell membranes, acantholysis, and blister formation. This effect is entirely intraepidermal, and no scarring ensues.

The main use of cantharidin is in the treatment of verruca vulgaris. Periungual warts are treated by applying this mixture to the wart surface, allowing it to dry, and occluding it with a nonporous plastic tape. A blister will form that will resolve in 7–14 days, at which time the area is debrided and any remaining wart is re-treated. Several applications may be required to effect a cure. Plantar warts are treated by paring and then applying several layers of cantharidin. An occlusive plastic tape is then applied. The resulting blister is removed in 10–14 days, and any residual wart is re-treated. Molluscum contagiosum will often respond to a single application without occlusion. Painless application and lack of residual scarring make cantharidin ideally suited for treatment of children.

A ring of warts may develop at the periphery of a cantharidin-treated wart as a result of intraepidermal inoculation. These may be re-treated with cantharidin or by an alternative method. Systemic toxic effects have not been observed with topical therapy, although ingestion of as little as 10 mg has resulted in abdominal pain, nausea, vomiting, and shock.

FLUOROURACIL

Fluorouracil is a fluorinated pyrimidine antimetabolite that resembles uracil, with a fluorine atom substituted for the 5-methyl group. Its systemic pharmacology is described in Chapter 56. Fluorouracil is used topically for the treatment of multiple actinic keratoses and intralesionally for keratoacanthomas.

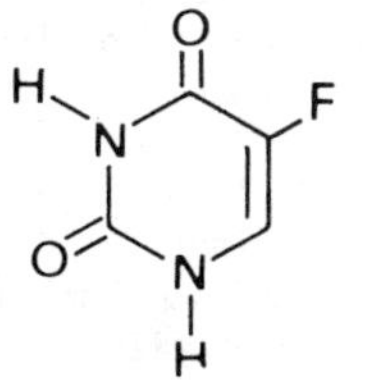

Fluorouracil

The pharmacokinetics of intralesional therapy have not been determined. Approximately 6% of a topically applied dose is absorbed—an amount insufficient to produce adverse systemic effects. Most of the absorbed drug is metabolized and excreted as carbon dioxide, urea, and α-fluoro-β-alanine. A small percentage is eliminated unchanged in the urine. Fluorouracil inhibits thymidylate synthetase activity, interfering with the synthesis of deoxyribonucleic acid and to a lesser extent ribonucleic acid. These effects are most marked in atypical, rapidly proliferating cells.

The response to treatment begins with erythema and progresses through vesiculation, erosion, superficial ulceration, necrosis, and finally reepithelialization. Fluorouracil should be continued until the inflammatory reaction reaches the ulceration and necrosis stage, usually in 2–4 weeks, at which time treatment should be terminated. The healing process may continue for 1–2 months after therapy is discontinued. Local adverse reactions may include pain, pruritus, a burning sensation, tenderness, and residual postinflammatory hyperpigmentation. Excessive exposure to sunlight during treatment may increase the intensity of the reaction and should be avoided. Allergic contact dermatitis to fluorouracil has been reported, and its use is contraindicated in patients with known hypersensitivity. Intralesional injections of keratoacanthomas with a 5% aqueous solution of fluorouracil has recently been advocated. Weekly injections of 25–50 mg are given until a 70–80% involution of the lesion is noted. If the lesion does not involute after 5 injections, excisional surgery is performed. Local reactions include erythema, inflammation, and subsequent necrosis of the tumor. Systemic adverse effects have not been observed and are not anticipated in view of the comparatively small amounts of fluorouracil administered on a weekly basis.

• • •

References

General

Wester R, Maibach H: Ten steps in percutaneous penetration. *Drug Metab Rev* (Feb) 1983. [In press.]

Anti-Bacterial Drugs

Eady EA, Holland KT, Cunliffe WJ: Topical antibiotics in acne therapy. *J Am Acad Dermatol* 1981;**5**:455.

Leyden JJ et al: Topical antibiotics and topical antimicrobial agents in acne therapy. *Acta Derm Venereol* [Suppl] (Stockh) 1980;**89**:75.

Meleney FL, Johnson BA: Bacitracin. *Am J Med* 1949;**7**:794.

Milstone EM, McDonald AJ, Scholhamer CF: Pseudomembranous colitis after topical application of clindamycin. *Arch Dermatol* 1981;**117**:154.

Newton BA: The properties and mode of action of the polymyxins. *Bacteriol Rev* 1956;**20**:14.

Rasmussen JE: Topical antibiotics. *J Dermatol Surg* 1976;**2**:69.

Wachs GN, Maibach HI: Cooperative double blind trial of an antibiotic corticoid combination in impetiginized atopic dermatitis. *Br J Dermatol* 1976;**95**:323.

Antifungal Drugs

Borgers M: Mechanism of action of antifungal drugs, with special reference to the imidazole derivatives. *Rev Infect Dis* 1980;**2**:520.

Codish SD, Tobias JS, Monaco AP: Systemic mycotic infections–Part 1. *Hosp Med* (June) 1978;**14**:6.

Graybill JR et al: Ketoconazole treatment of chronic mucocutaneous candidiasis. *Arch Dermatol* 1980;**116**: 1137.

Hermann HW: Clinical efficacy studies of haloprogin, a new topical antimicrobial agent. *Arch Dermatol* 1972;**106**:839.

Jones HE, Simpson JG, Artis WW: Oral ketoconazole: An effective and safe treatment for dermatophytosis. *Arch Dermatol* 1981;**117**:129.

Katz R, Cahn B: Haloprogin therapy for dermatophyte infections. *Arch Dermatol* 1972;**106**:837.

Knight AG: The activity of various griseofulvin preparations and the appearance of oral griseofulvin in the stratum corneum. *Br J Dermatol* 1974;**91**:49.

Robinson HM Jr, Raskin J: Tolnaftate, a potent topical antifungal agent. *Arch Dermatol* 1965;**94**:372.

Sawyer PR et al: Miconazole: A review of its antifungal activity and therapeutic efficacy. *Drugs* 1975;**9:**406.

Shah VP, Epstein WL, Riegelman S: Role of sweat in accumulation of orally administered griseofulvin in skin. *J Clin Invest* 1974;**53:**1673.

Stritzler C: Cutaneous candidiasis treated with topical amphotericin B. *Arch Dermatol* 1966;**93:**101.

Weber K, Wehland J, Herzog W: Griseofulvin interacts with microtubules both in vivo and in vitro. *J Mol Biol* 1976;**102:**817.

Weinstein MJ, Oden EM, Moxx E: Antifungal properties of tolnaftate in vitro and in vivo. *Antimicrob Agents Chemother* 1964;**1964;**595.

Zalias N, Battistini F: Superficial mycoses: Treatment with a new broad spectrum antifungal agent: 1% Clotrimazole solution. *Arch Dermatol* 1977;**113:**307.

Ectoparasiticides

Cubela V, Yawalkar SJ: Clinical experience with crotamiton cream and lotion in the treatment of infants with scabies. *Br J Clin Pract* 1978;**32:**229.

Konstantinou D, Stanoeva L, Yawalkar SJ: Crotamiton cream and lotion in the treatment of infants and young children with scabies. *J Int Med Res* 1979;**7:**443.

Orkin M, Epstein E Jr, Maibach HI: Treatment of today's scabies and pediculosis. *JAMA* 1976;**236:**1136.

Orkin M et al (editors): *Scabies and Pediculosis.* Lippincott, 1977.

Rasmussen JE: The problem of lindane. *J Am Acad Dermatol* 1981;**5:**507.

Schacter B: Treatment of scabies and pediculosis with lindane preparation: An evaluation. *J Am Acad Dermatol* 1981;**5:**517.

Agents Affecting Pigmentation

Engasser PG, Maibach HI: Cosmetics and dermatology: Bleaching creams. *J Am Acad Dermatol* 1981;**5:**143.

Kaidbey KH, Kligman AM: An appraisal of the efficacy and substantivity of the new high-potency sunscreens. *J Am Acad Dermatol* 1981;**4:**566.

Mosher DB, Parrish JA, Fitzpatrick TB: Monobenzylether of hydroquinone: A retrospective study of treatment of 18 vitiligo patients and a review of the literature. *Br J Dermatol* 1977;**97:**669.

Pathak MA, Kramer DM, Fitzpatrick TB: Photobiology and photochemistry of furocoumarins (psoralens). In: *Sunlight and Man: Normal and Abnormal Photobiologic Responses.* Tokyo University Press, 1974.

Sayre RM et al: Performance of six sunscreen formulations on human skin. *Arch Dermatol* 1979;**115:**46.

Acne Preparations

Heel RC et al: Vitamin A acid: A review of its pharmacological properties and therapeutic use in the topical treatment of acne vulgaris. *Drugs* 1977;**14:**401.

Isotretinoin. *Med Lett Drugs Ther* (Sept 3) 1982;**24:**79.

Nacht S et al: Benzoyl peroxide: Percutaneous penetration and metabolic disposition. *J Am Acad Dermatol* 1981;**4:**31.

Plewig G, Kligman AM: *Acne Morphogenesis and Treatment.* Springer-Verlag, 1975.

Thomas JR, Doyle MB: The therapeutic uses of topical vitamin A acid. *J Am Acad Dermatol* 1981;**4:**505.

Anti-inflammatory Agents

Grupper C: The chemistry, pharmacology and use of tar in the treatment of psoriasis. In: *Psoriasis: Proceedings of the International Symposium, Stanford University.* Farber E, Cox AJ (editors). Stanford University Press, 1971.

Maibach HI, Stoughton RB: Topical corticosteroids. Chap 13, p 174, in: *Steroid Therapy.* Arzanoff DL (editor). Saunders, 1975.

Miller JA, Munro DD: Topical corticosteroids: Clinical pharmacology and therapeutic use. *Drugs* 1980;**19:**119.

Robertson DB, Maibach HI: Topical corticosteroids: A review. *Int J Dermatol* 1982;**21:**59.

Keratolytic & Destructive Agents

Ashton H, Frenk E, Stevenson CJ: Urea as a topical agent. *Br J Dermatol* 1971;**84:**194.

Chamberlain MJ, Reynolds AL, Yeoman WB: Toxic effects of podophyllum applications in pregnancy. *Br Med J* 1972;**3:**391.

Epstein WL, Kligman AM: Treatment of warts with cantharidin. *Arch Dermatol* 1958;**77:**508.

Fine JD, Arndt KA: *Propylene glycol: A Review.* Excerpta Medica, 1980.

Geotte DK: Topical chemotherapy with 5-fluorouracil. *J Am Acad Dermatol* 1981;**4:**633.

Geotte DK, Odom RB: Successful treatment of keratoacanthoma with intralesional fluorouracil. *J Am Acad Dermatol* 1980;**2:**212.

Goldsmith LA, Baden HP: Propylene glycol with occlusion for treatment of ichthyosis. *JAMA* 1972;**220:**579.

Taylor JR, Halprin KM: Percutaneous absorption of salicylic acid. *Arch Dermatol* 1975;**111:**740.

Ward J et al: Fatal systemic poisoning following podophyllin treatment of condyloma acuminata. *South Med J* 1954;**47:**1204.

Dermatotoxicology

Maibach H (editor): *Dermatotoxicology,* 2nd ed. Hemisphere Press, 1982.

Drugs Used in Gastrointestinal Diseases | 62

David F. Altman, MD

Many drugs discussed elsewhere in this book have applications in the treatment of gastrointestinal diseases. Anticholinergic drugs inhibit the food-stimulated secretion of gastric acid and also affect intestinal smooth muscle; these drugs are useful in some forms of functional bowel disease. Cholinergic agonists stimulate smooth muscle and are used to promote gastrointestinal motility. Some phenothiazines have excellent antiemetic properties, and narcotic analgesics and some of their derivatives are useful antidiarrheal medications by virtue of their ability to inhibit intestinal motility.

Several other groups of medications are used almost exclusively in gastrointestinal disease; these are grouped and discussed according to their therapeutic uses below.

DRUGS USED IN PEPTIC ULCER DISEASE

The pathogenesis of peptic ulcer disease is not completely understood. It is clear that gastric acid and pepsin secretion are necessary for the development of a peptic ulcer. However, factors relating to mucosal resistance to acid and pepsin are also important, particularly in gastric ulcer disease. Currently, drugs are available that have some effect on each of these factors.

ANTACIDS

Gastric antacids are weak bases that react with gastric hydrochloric acid to form a salt and water. Their usefulness in peptic ulcer disease thus lies in their ability to reduce gastric acidity and, since pepsin is inactive in solutions above pH 4, to reduce peptic activity.

Most antacids in current use are combinations of aluminum, magnesium, and calcium salts (Table 62–1). The differences among antacids relate to the rapidity of their reaction with gastric acid, their neutralizing capacity, their gastrointestinal side-effects, and their systemic complications. Price to the consumer varies widely.

Sodium bicarbonate, the active ingredient in baking soda, is highly soluble and reacts almost instantaneously with hydrochloric acid:

$$NaHCO_3 + HCl \rightarrow NaCl + H_2O + CO_2$$

Table 62–1. Representative liquid antacids.

Proprietary Preparation	Ingredients	Acid-Neutralizing Capacity (mEq/mL)	Volume Containing 140 mEq (mL)	Sodium Content (mg/5 mL)	Cost of High-Dose Regimen*
Maalox T.C.	Aluminum hydroxide, magnesium hydroxide	4.2	33	1.2	$ 46.58
Titralac	Calcium carbonate	4.2	33	11.0	40.99
Delcid	Aluminum hydroxide, magnesium hydroxide	4.1	34	1.5	45.72
Mylanta-II	Aluminum hydroxide, magnesium hydroxide, simethicone	3.6	39	1.1	58.39
Gelusil-II	Aluminum hydroxide, magnesium hydroxide, simethicone	3.0	47	1.3	60.52
Riopan	Magaldrate	2.7	50	0.7	60.93
Maalox Plus	Aluminum hydroxide, magnesium hydroxide, simethicone	2.3	61	2.5	71.28
ALternaGEL	Aluminum hydroxide	2.4	60	2.0	89.44
Amphojel	Aluminum hydroxide	1.4	100	7.0	168.53

*Cost to the pharmacist of 1 month's treatment with high-dose regimen (see text) based on manufacturers' listings in *Drug Topics Red Book 1982.*

However, this compound is highly soluble and is absorbed rapidly from the gut. Thus, it may promote systemic alkalosis and fluid retention and is not recommended for long-term use.

Calcium carbonate reacts more slowly than sodium bicarbonate but is very effective in neutralizing gastric acid:

$$CaCO_3 + 2HCl \rightarrow CaCl_2 + H_2O + CO_2$$

However, approximately 10% of the calcium chloride produced is absorbed, with the potential side-effects of hypercalcemia, milk-alkali syndrome, and acid rebound. This antacid is therefore not recommended for long-term use.

Aluminum hydroxide reacts with hydrochloric acid in similar fashion:

$$Al(OH)_3 + 3HCl \rightarrow AlCl_3 + 3H_2O$$

However, there is wide variability in the solubility of various aluminum hydroxide preparations and therefore wide variations in the rate of acid neutralization. The aluminum chloride formed is generally insoluble and often causes constipation. It also binds certain drugs (eg, tetracycline) and phosphate, preventing their absorption. This effect on phosphate absorption is used to therapeutic advantage in patients with chronic renal failure and bone diseases.

Magnesium hydroxide (milk of magnesia) reacts with acid almost as promptly as does sodium hydroxide:

$$Mg(OH)_2 + 2HCl \rightarrow MgCl_2 + 2H_2O$$

Unlike sodium hydroxide, however, the relative insolubility of magnesium hydroxide slows its emptying from the stomach, thus prolonging its neutralizing effect. Magnesium salts produced are poorly absorbed and are responsible for the well-known cathartic effect of this compound. A small amount of magnesium is absorbed, but this is of clinical significance only when renal insufficiency impairs its urinary excretion.

After a meal, gastric acid is produced at a rate of about 45 mEq/h. A single dose of 156 mEq of antacid given 1 hour after a meal effectively neutralizes gastric acid for 2 hours. A second dose given 3 hours after eating maintains the effect for over 4 hours after the meal. The dose-response relationship of antacids is variable, depending on the gastric secretory capacity (some individuals are "hypersecretors," some "hyposecretors") and the rate at which the antacid is emptied from the stomach.

In addition, as implied by the discussion of the individual antacid compounds, antacids vary widely in their potency. The relative amounts of the various compounds and their reactivity will not be clear on the product label. However, commercially available antacids vary as much as 7-fold in acid-neutralizing capacity.

Antacids can be effective in promoting healing of duodenal ulcers. Their benefit in gastric ulcers is less clear. In the best controlled trial of duodenal ulcer therapy, 140 mEq of antacid given 1 and 3 hours after each meal and at bedtime accelerated the healing of duodenal ulcers, although pain relief was not much better than that seen with placebo. Different doses of antacid are required to achieve this degree of neutralizing capacity, depending on the commercial product used (Table 62–1). Tablet antacids are generally weak in their neutralizing capacity, and a large number of tablets would be required for this high-dose regimen. They are not recommended for the treatment of active peptic ulcer.

Thus, an appropriate antacid regimen for peptic ulcer disease—one that would maximally neutralize gastric acid throughout a 24-hour period—would use 140 mEq of a liquid antacid given 1 and 3 hours after meals and at bedtime. The actual volume of antacid given should be adjusted to provide 140 mEq of acid-neutralizing effect. A final important factor in such a regimen is palatability. Patients will often state a preference for one antacid over another.

Adverse reactions to antacids often include a change in bowel habits. As has been mentioned, magnesium salts have a cathartic effect, and aluminum hydroxide may be constipating. These problems can be managed by either combining or alternating compounds with these effects. Other potential problems with antacids relate to cation absorption (sodium, magnesium, aluminum, calcium) and systemic alkalosis. Fortunately, these become clinical problems only in patients with renal impairment. In large doses, the sodium content of some antacids may become an important factor in patients with congestive heart failure.

Antacids have been used for pain relief from esophagitis, gastric ulcer, and duodenal ulcer. However, placebo-controlled trials have shown no effect of a single "effective" antacid dose for pain relief in any of these conditions.

H_2 RECEPTOR ANTAGONISTS

Since their introduction in the mid 1970s, these compounds have gained wide acceptance. The 2 major drugs in use are **cimetidine** and **ranitidine** (Chapter 14). These agents are capable of over 90% reduction in basal, food-stimulated, and nocturnal secretion of gastric acid after a single dose. Many trials have demonstrated their effectiveness in promoting the healing of duodenal ulcers and preventing their recurrence. The efficacy of these drugs in gastric ulcer has been less impressive. However, they are important in the medical management of Zollinger-Ellison syndrome and gastric hypersecretory states seen in systemic mastocytosis.

The usual adult dose of cimetidine is 300 mg 4 times daily with meals and at bedtime. The drug can be given intravenously at the same dose. Occasionally, larger doses are necessary—up to 2400 mg per 24 hours—particularly in patients with Zollinger-Ellison syndrome. The dose should be reduced in patients with renal insufficiency, in whom the drug's half-life is prolonged.

Although the H_2 receptor antagonists have been generally well tolerated, with few side-effects reported, several adverse reactions have occurred with cimetidine, for which there has been longer experience. Confusional states have been seen particularly in older patients. Antiandrogenic properties have been blamed for the occasional gynecomastia and male sexual dysfunction seen. Rare cases of leukopenia are reported. Cimetidine also delays hepatic microsomal metabolism of some drugs, such as warfarin, theophylline, diazepam, and phenytoin.

The dosage and toxicity of ranitidine, which is still investigational, have not yet been established.

ANTICHOLINERGICS

Anticholinergic drugs are discussed in more detail in Chapter 6. They are able to reduce gastric acid secretion in the basal state by up to 50% and in the postprandial period by up to 30%. However, their use is limited by side-effects such as dry mouth and sedation. They cannot be used in patients with gastric retention, partial gastric outlet obstruction, prostatism, or glaucoma. They probably should not be used in patients with gastroesophageal reflux disease. However, anticholinergic drugs may potentiate the suppression of acid secretion obtained with H_2 receptor antagonists, and they may have a role as adjunctive therapy in peptic ulcer disease.

MUCOSAL PROTECTIVE AGENTS

Sucralfate

Sucralfate (Carafate), or aluminum sucrose sulfate, is a sulfated disaccharide recently developed for use in peptic ulcer disease.

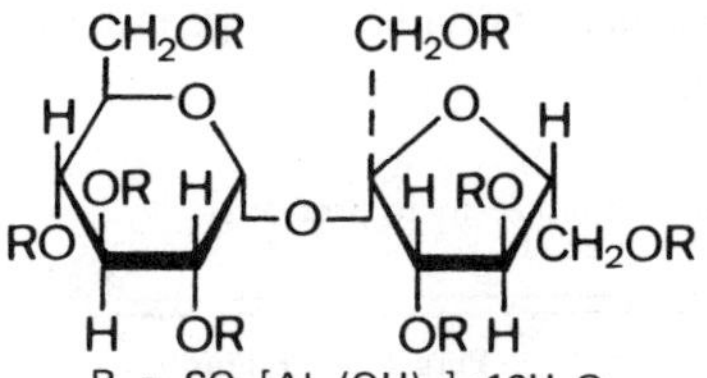

$R = SO_3[Al_2(OH)_5] \cdot 16H_2O$

Sucralfate

Its mechanism of action is thought to involve selective binding to necrotic ulcer tissue, where it may act as a barrier to acid, pepsin, and bile. In addition, sucralfate may directly adsorb bile salts. The drug has been shown to be effective in the healing of duodenal ulcers. It is not absorbed systemically, and few side-effects have been reported. The dosage is 1 g 4 times daily on an empty stomach (at least 1 hour before meals). It also requires an acid pH to be activated and so should not be administered simultaneously with antacids or an H_2 receptor antagonist.

Colloidal Bismuth Compounds

These compounds also appear to work by selective binding to an ulcer and by coating it to protect the ulcer from acid and pepsin. **Tripotassium dicitrato bismuthate (De-Nol)** has been extensively tested in Europe and shown to be superior to placebo in the healing of both duodenal and gastric ulcers. Side-effects have been minimal, and the encephalopathy reported with long-term use of other bismuth compounds has not been noted.

Carbenoxolone

This derivative of glycyrrhizic acid (an agent extracted from licorice) has been shown to be effective in healing both gastric and duodenal ulcers. The mechanism of action of carbenoxolone is not clear but is thought to involve an increase in the production, secretion, and viscosity of intestinal mucus. Although its ulcer-healing properties are evident, the drug has a major aldosteronelike side-effect, so that hypertension, fluid retention, and hypokalemia have limited its clinical usefulness. The concurrent administration of spironolactone controls the fluid retention but also abolishes the ulcer-healing effect; thiazides prevent sodium retention without abolishing the beneficial effect in peptic disease.

Carbenoxolone, although widely used in Europe, is investigational in the USA.

Prostaglandins

These derivatives of arachidonic acid are discussed in detail in Chapter 16. Certain prostaglandins, especially prostaglandin E_2, are produced by the gastric mucosa and are thought to have a major role in gastric cytoprotection. When administered orally, methyl analogs of prostaglandin E_2 have been shown to be effective in healing not only peptic ulcers but also gastric lesions produced in experimental animals by the administration of aspirin and indomethacin. The mechanism of cytoprotection by prostaglandin E_2 is not known but may be related to stimulation of gastric mucus secretion. The clinical usefulness of prostaglandins is limited by the diarrhea they induce. Newer prostaglandin derivatives without this effect are being developed; none of those presently available are approved for use in peptic disease.

DRUGS PROMOTING GASTROINTESTINAL MOTILITY

Cholinergic mechanisms are responsible for modulating motor phenomena in the gut; thus it is not surprising that cholinergic agents such as **bethanechol** are effective in promoting gastrointestinal motility.

Metoclopramide (Reglan), recently promoted as a gut stimulant, also has cholinergic properties, apparently sensitizing intestinal smooth muscle to the action of acetylcholine rather than acting directly on cholinergic receptors. In addition, the drug is a potent dopamine antagonist, particularly at central dopamine receptors.

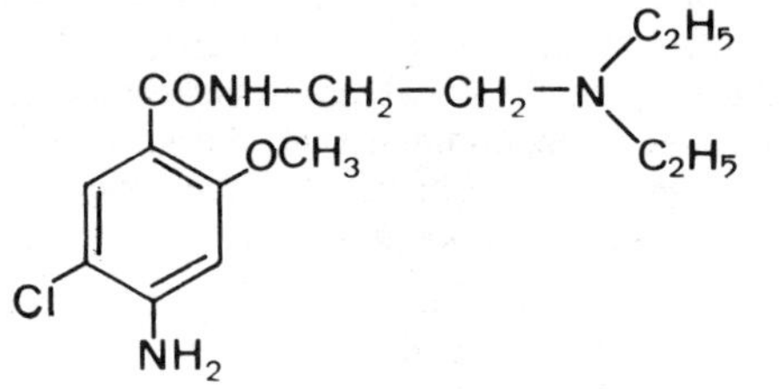

Metoclopramide
(methoxychloroprocainamide)

These properties contribute to the stimulant effects of metoclopramide in the gastrointestinal tract. The drug acts to hasten esophageal clearance, raise lower esophageal sphincter pressure, accelerate gastric emptying, and shorten small bowel transit time. The central dopamine antagonist effect is principally responsible for its antiemetic properties.

Clinical applications follow these effects. Metoclopramide is useful for facilitating small bowel intubation. In addition, in patients with gastric motor failure—particularly diabetic gastroparesis but possibly also after vagotomy and in other disorders of gastric emptying—metoclopramide can produce significant symptomatic relief. In patients with chronic gastroesophageal reflux disease, metoclopramide has been effective in decreasing the incidence of heartburn, although long-term effects are uncertain. Finally, the drug is an effective antiemetic, particularly useful in association with cancer chemotherapy and in emergency surgery or labor and delivery to prevent aspiration of gastric contents.

Metoclopramide is rapidly absorbed, with peak concentrations after a single oral dose seen in 40–120 minutes. Its plasma half-life is about 4 hours, and the drug is excreted mainly by the kidneys. The usual dose is 10 mg 4 times daily with meals and at bedtime. Larger doses, up to 1–2 mg/kg, have been used in conjunction with cancer chemotherapy. A dose of 20 mg given by slow intravenous infusion is used for small bowel intubation.

The most common side-effects of metoclopramide are somnolence, nervousness, and dystonic reactions. Parkinsonism and tardive dyskinesia have also been reported. The drug also causes increased pituitary prolactin release, and galactorrhea and menstrual disorders have been reported.

PANCREATIC ENZYME REPLACEMENT PRODUCTS

Steatorrhea occurs in pancreatic insufficiency when lipase output is reduced below 10% of normal. It is estimated that in the postprandial period, approximately 100,000 units of lipase are delivered to the intestinal lumen per hour. Thus, the goal of pancreatic enzyme replacement should be to deliver at least 10,000 units per hour. However, because of inactivation of the enzyme below pH 4, only about 8% of the ingested lipase activity reaches the distal duodenum.

Different pancreatic enzyme preparations vary markedly in enzyme activity. Manufacturers' listings of enzyme content may not always match a well-standardized in vitro laboratory assay. Two major types of preparation in use are pancreatin, an alcoholic extract of hog pancreas, and pancrelipase, a lipase-enriched hog pancreas preparation. The enzyme content of several pancreatic enzyme preparations as measured by in vitro assay is given in Table 62–2. As indicated in the table,variation in enzyme content can be partly compensated for by increases in dosage; the in vivo response—measured as reduction in stool fat and nitrogen—can be appreciable.

Various dosage schedules have been recommended for pancreatic enzyme replacement, but there appears to be little difference between giving the medication with meals and giving it every 2 hours through the day. Because individual dosage requirements vary,

Table 62–2. Enzyme activities in some pancreatic enzyme replacement products. (nd = data not available.)

Proprietary Preparation	Amount (Units per Tablet or Capsule)			Number of Tablets or Capsules per Meal	Percentage Reduction in Fecal	
	Lipase	Trypsin	Amylase		Fat	Nitrogen
Ilozyme*	3600	3444	329,600	3	48	nd
Cotazyme*	2014	2797	499,200	5	nd	35
Pancrease*	2005	nd	nd	3	73	40
Viokase†	1636	1828	277,333	6	49	40
Phazyme	210	620	15,800	nd	nd	nd

*Generic pancrelipase.
†Generic pancreatin.

it is essential that the result of therapy—the daily stool fat excretion—be monitored and the number of capsules or tablets increased until a therapeutic effect is seen. Supplementing the regimen with cimetidine enhances the effectiveness of the enzymes, presumably by decreasing the destruction of enzyme activity by gastric acid.

Because the enzyme preparations have a high purine content, uric acid renal stones have been seen as a side-effect. Also, the lactose in the pills may be sufficient to cause symptoms in lactose-intolerant patients. Finally, pancreatic enzyme replacement is expensive, costing up to $1500 per year for adequate therapy.

LAXATIVES

Laxatives of various types are widely prescribed and more widely purchased without prescription, indicating a cultural preoccupation with "regularity." Laxatives are best classified by their mechanism of action as irritants or stimulants, bulking agents, and stool softeners.

IRRITANT OR STIMULANT LAXATIVES

Castor oil is hydrolyzed in the upper small intestine to ricinoleic acid, a local irritant that increases intestinal motility. The onset of action is prompt and continues until the compound is excreted via the colon.

Cascara, senna, and **aloes** contain emodin alkaloids that are liberated after absorption from the intestine and are excreted into the colon, where peristalsis is stimulated. Thus, their onset of activity is delayed for 6–8 hours. Chronic stimulation of the colon is thought to lead to chronic colonic distention and perpetuation of the perceived need for laxatives.

Phenolphthalein and **bisacodyl,** which are chemically similar, are also potent colonic stimulants. Their action may be prolonged by an enterohepatic circulation.

BULK LAXATIVES

Hydrophilic colloids, prepared from the indigestible parts of fruits, vegetables, and seeds, form gels within the large intestine, distending the intestine and thereby stimulating its peristaltic activity. Agar, psyllium seed, and methylcellulose all act in this manner as well. Bran and other forms of vegetable fiber have the same effect.

Saline cathartics such as magnesium citrate and magnesium hydroxide also distend the bowel and stimulate its contractions. These nonabsorbable salts hold water in the intestine by osmotic force and cause distention.

STOOL SOFTENERS

Agents that become emulsified with stool serve to soften it and make passage easier. Examples are **mineral oil, glycerin suppositories,** and detergents such as **dioctyl sodium sulfosuccinate (docusate).**

ANTIDIARRHEAL DRUGS

The 2 most widely used prescription drugs for diarrhea—**diphenoxylate** and **loperamide**—are weak analogs of meperidine, and their mechanism of action is similar to that of other opiates (Chapter 28). Loperamide (Imodium) may not cross the blood-brain barrier and thus may cause less sedation than diphenoxylate.

Adsorbents such as **kaolin** and **pectin** are also widely used. Their action is through their ability to adsorb compounds from solution, presumably binding potential intestinal toxins.

DRUGS USED FOR THE DISSOLUTION OF GALLSTONES

Cholesterol is solubilized in aqueous bile by the combined effect of bile acids and lecithin, which, together with cholesterol, form the mixed micelle. When cholesterol is secreted in bile in relative excess to lecithin and bile acids, cholesterol crystals precipitate and may coalesce into cholesterol gallstones. Patients with cholesterol gallstones have a diminished total body bile acid pool, and consequently their bile is saturated with cholesterol. Subsequently, it has been found that oral administration of the investigational drug **chenodeoxycholic acid** (chenodiol), a primary bile acid, can reduce the concentration of cholesterol in bile; the mechanism is inhibition of hepatic cholesterol synthesis. Chronic therapy with chenodiol is capable of causing gallstone dissolution in some patients.

The usefulness of chenodiol in the medical treatment of gallstones was elucidated by the National Cooperative Gallstone Study, the results of which were published in 1981. In this study, patients were assigned to either a "high-dose" (750 mg/d), "low-dose" (350 mg/d) or placebo group. Over a 2-year period of high-dose therapy, 13.5% of patients had complete dissolution of stones and 41% had partial dissolution. Dissolution was more successful in women and thin people. Diarrhea occurred in 41% of patients receiving the high dose of chenodiol. It was pointed out later that few of the patients in the high-dose group received the recommended dose of 15 mg/kg, but such a dose would presumably cause even more severe diarrhea.

Ursodeoxycholic acid, the 7β epimer of

chenodiol, may be a more potent desaturating agent for cholesterol in bile. It has also been reported to cause fewer side-effects. It is investigational.

The role of medical therapy in the treatment of gallstones remains to be defined. Gallstone dissolution by the oral administration of bile acids is only useful for cholesterol gallstones. Radiopaque stones are rarely if ever cholesterol stones; however, fewer than 75% of radiolucent stones are cholesterol stones. In addition, this therapy is successful only in patients with functioning gallbladders. Several studies have shown a high recurrence rate for stones after treatment was stopped, presumably committing patients to lifelong therapy. These factors, together with the relatively low incidence of complete dissolution and the potentially high incidence of side-effects, suggest that surgery will remain the favored therapeutic approach except in highly selected patients.

DRUGS USED IN THE TREATMENT OF CHRONIC INFLAMMATORY BOWEL DISEASE

The principal drugs used in the treatment of chronic inflammatory bowel disease (ulcerative colitis, Crohn's disease) are corticosteroids and other immunosuppressive agents, which are discussed elsewhere, and **sulfasalazine.** Sulfasalazine was introduced in the 1940s for the treatment of rheumatoid arthritis. It has subsequently been shown to be effective in ulcerative colitis, Crohn's colitis, and less so in Crohn's disease of the small intestine. In ulcerative colitis, it is more effective in maintaining than in obtaining clinical remission.

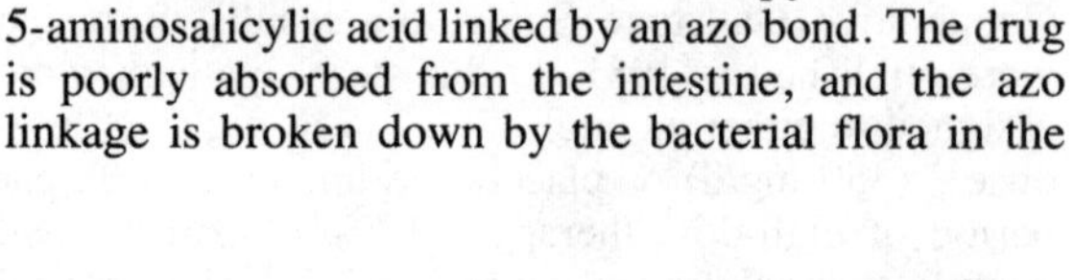

Sulfasalazine

Sulfasalazine combines sulfapyridine with 5-aminosalicylic acid linked by an azo bond. The drug is poorly absorbed from the intestine, and the azo linkage is broken down by the bacterial flora in the colon. Most evidence suggests that the nonabsorbed salicylate moiety is the most active part of the drug. The mechanism of action of sulfasalazine is unknown. Recent studies have suggested either a cytoprotective role, perhaps by inhibition of breakdown of prostaglandin $F_{2\alpha}$, or a suppressant effect on immune function.

The usual therapeutic dose of sulfasalazine is 3–4 g daily in divided doses. Smaller doses, usually 2 g/d, are needed to maintain remission in ulcerative colitis. Dose-related side-effects such as malaise, nausea, abdominal discomfort, or headache occur in up to 20% of patients given 4 g/d. Some of these effects may be avoided by beginning at a lower dose and slowly increasing to the desired dosage level or by using enteric-coated or liquid suspension preparations. The inhibition of folic acid absorption by sulfasalazine has been reported, so that supplemental folate should be administered. Finally, as with other sulfonamides, serum sickness-like reactions and severe bone marrow suppression have occasionally been seen.

DRUGS IN THERAPY OF PORTAL-SYSTEMIC ENCEPHALOPATHY

The broad-spectrum, nonabsorbable antibiotic neomycin (Chapter 44) has been combined with dietary restriction of protein for the treatment of portal-systemic encephalopathy. **Lactulose (Cephulac),** a synthetic disaccharide (galactose-fructose) that is not absorbed, is also effective in this condition.

The mechanism of action of lactulose is unclear. It is apparently degraded by intestinal bacteria to lactic acid, acetic acid, and other organic acids. It is thought that this may facilitate the "trapping" of ammonium ion or other putative central nervous system toxins in the intestinal tract. Modification of the normal intestinal flora by lactulose has been suggested as another mechanism of action, but this has not been demonstrated with certainty.

Lactulose is available as a syrup and is given in doses of 15–30 mL 4 times daily or until the patient has 4 or 5 soft bowel movements daily. The drug is well tolerated and may be given in combination with neomycin, although this combination has no clear advantage over lactulose alone. Lactulose may also be administered as an enema.

• • •

References

Peptic Ulcer Disease

Drake D, Hollander D: Neutralizing capacity and cost effectiveness of antacids. *Ann Intern Med* 1981;**94:**215.

Grossman MI et al: Peptic ulcer: New therapies, new diseases. *Ann Intern Med* 1981;**95:**609.

Peterson WL et al: Healing of duodenal ulcer with an antacid regimen. *N Engl J Med* 1977;**297:**341.

Gastrointestinal Motility

Schulze-Delrieu K: Drug therapy: Metoclopramide. *N Engl J Med* 1981;**305:**28.

Pancreatic Insufficiency

DiMagno EP et al: Fate of orally ingested enzymes in pancreatic insufficiency: Comparison of two dosage schedules. *N Engl J Med* 1977;**296:**1318.

Graham DY: Enzyme replacement therapy of exocrine pancreatic insufficiency in man: Relation between in vitro enzyme activities and in vivo potency in commercial pancreatic extracts. *N Engl J Med* 1977;**296:**1314.

Laxatives

Binder HJ, Donowitz M: A new look at laxative action. *Gastroenterology* 1975;**69:**1001.

Gallstone Therapy

Danziger RG et al: Dissolution of cholesterol gallstones by chenodeoxycholic acid. *N Engl J Med* 1972;**286:**1.

Schoenfield LJ et al: Chenodiol (chenodeoxycholic acid) for dissolution of gallstones: The National Cooperative Gallstone Study. *Ann Intern Med* 1981;**95:**257.

Thistle JL, Hofmann AF: Efficacy and specificity of chenodeoxycholic acid therapy for dissolving gallstones. *N Engl J Med* 1973;**289:**655.

Inflammatory Bowel Disease

Goldman P, Peppercorn MA: Sulfasalazine. *N Engl J Med* 1975;**293:**20.

Klotz U et al: Therapeutic efficacy of sulfasalazine and its metabolites in patients with ulcerative colitis and Crohn's disease. *N Engl J Med* 1980;**303:**1499.

Portal-Systemic Encephalopathy

Conn HO, Lieberthal MM: *The Hepatic Coma Syndromes and Lactulose*. Williams & Wilkins, 1978.

63 | Clinical Interpretation of Drug Concentrations

Nicholas H.G. Holford, MSc, MRCP (UK)

Improvements in drug analysis methods during the past 15 years have greatly increased the number of drugs that can be measured in body fluids, and the development of pharmacokinetics has defined the use of such measurements in therapeutics. The rationale for making such measurements lies in the fact that for many therapeutic situations, drug concentration *in the blood* determines the clinical response; variations in clinical response, eg, treatment failure, often result from variations in drug concentration that are predictable from pharmacokinetic considerations.

Pharmacokinetic & Pharmacodynamic Correlations

The basic principles outlined in Chapters 1–3 can be applied to the interpretation of clinical drug concentration measurements on the basis of 3 major pharmacokinetic variables—absorption, clearance, and volume of distribution—and 2 pharmacodynamic variables of maximum effect attainable in the target tissue and the sensitivity of the tissue to the drug.

Pharmacokinetic Variables

A. Absorption: The amount of drug that enters the body depends on the patient's compliance with the prescribed regimen and on the rate and extent of transfer from the site of administration to the blood.

B. Clearance: The ability of the body to eliminate drug is a function of total body clearance, the sum of all elimination pathways (renal excretion, liver metabolism, etc). The exact mechanism of elimination may not be known in all cases. Clearance is conveniently expressed in liters per hour (L/h), ie, the volume of plasma the body can completely clear of drug per hour.

C. Volume of Distribution: The apparent volume of distribution depends on the extent of drug penetration and binding to tissues. The smallest possible value for a drug injected into the blood is the plasma volume. Very large volumes may result if there is extensive tissue binding; eg, digoxin has an apparent volume of distribution of over 640 L per 70 kg.

Table 3–1 gives typical values of drug absorption, clearance, and volume of distribution in healthy adults.

Pharmacodynamic Concepts

A. Maximum Effect: All pharmacologic responses must have a maximum effect (E_{max}). No matter how high the drug concentration goes, a point will be reached beyond which no further increment in response is achieved.

B. Sensitivity: The sensitivity of the target organ to drug concentration is reflected by the concentration required to produce 50% of maximum effect. This concentration, known as the EC50, can be used to define the potency of one drug with respect to another.

The Target Concentration Strategy

Recognition of the essential role of concentration in linking pharmacokinetics and pharmacodynamics has led to the target concentration strategy. Pharmacodynamic principles can be used to predict the concentration required to achieve a particular degree of therapeutic effect. This "target concentration" can then be achieved by using pharmacokinetic principles to arrive at a suitable dosing regimen.

INDICATIONS FOR DRUG CONCENTRATION MEASUREMENT

Drug concentration measurements are required in clinical practice for estimating individual pharmacokinetic parameters and for determining the target concentration in order to prescribe appropriate doses.

Pharmacokinetic Indications

A. Absorption: Overdosage and underdosage—both aspects of failure of compliance—can frequently be detected by concentration measurements when gross deviations from expected values are obtained. If compliance is found to be adequate, malabsorption abnormalities in the small bowel may be the cause of abnormally low concentrations. Variations in the extent of bioavailability are rarely caused by irregularities in the manufacture of the particular drug formulation. More commonly, variations in bioavailability are seen with drugs such as propranolol that undergo extensive metabolism during absorption.

B. Clearance: Abnormal clearance may be anticipated when there is major impairment of the function of the heart, kidney, or liver. The extent of the abnormality will depend upon the predominant route of elimination as well as the extent of functional loss. Creatinine clearance is a useful quantitative indicator of renal function. Drug clearance may be a useful indicator of the functional consequences of heart or liver failure, with greater precision than clinical findings or other laboratory tests. For example, when renal function is changing rapidly, estimation of the clearance of aminoglycoside antibiotics may be a more accurate indicator of glomerular filtration than serum creatinine.

C. Volume of Distribution: The volume of distribution may be overestimated in obese patients if based on total body weight and the drug does not enter fatty tissues well, as is the case with digoxin. In contrast, abnormal accumulation of fluid—edema, ascites, pleural effusion—can markedly increase the volume of distribution of drugs such as tobramycin that are hydrophilic and have small volumes of distribution (10–20 L/70 kg).

Pharmacodynamic Indications

A. Maximum Effect: If increasing the dose does not lead to a further clinical response, it is possible that the maximum effect has been reached. This can be verified by demonstrating that an increase in dose results in increased drug concentration without further drug effect. Recognition of maximum effect is helpful in avoiding ineffectual increases of dose with the attendant risk of toxicity.

B. Sensitivity: Failure of response that is due to diminished sensitivity to the drug can be detected by measuring drug concentrations that are usually associated with therapeutic response in a patient who is not getting better. This may be a result of abnormal physiology—eg, hyperkalemia diminishes responsiveness to digoxin; or drug antagonism—eg, propranolol impairs the response to theophylline. Increased sensitivity to the drug is usually signaled by exaggerated responses to small or moderate doses. The pharmacodynamic nature of this sensitivity can be confirmed by drug concentrations that are low in relation to the observed effect.

THE SPECTRUM OF DRUG ELIMINATION

Most drug elimination pathways will become saturated if the dose is high enough. The relation between dose rate and average steady-state concentration (C_{ss}) is shown in Fig 63–1 and is expressed mathematically in equation (1):

$$\text{Dose rate} = \frac{EC \times C_{ss}}{K_m + C_{ss}} \quad \ldots(1)$$

This equation is similar to the Michaelis-Menten statement of enzyme kinetics. The maximum elimination capacity (EC) corresponds to V_{max} of the

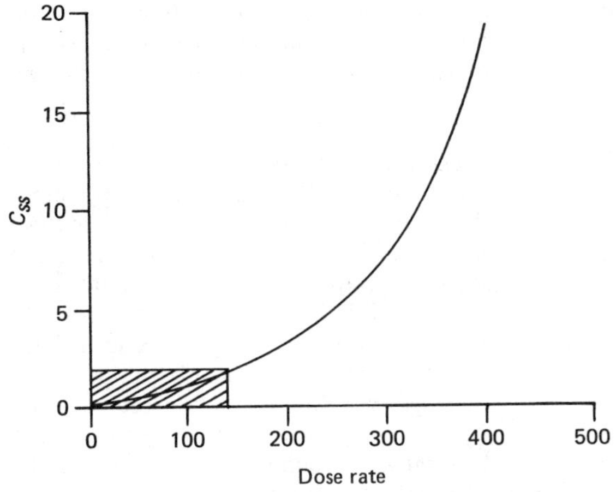

Figure 63–1. The relationship between dose rate and steady-state concentration (C_{ss}). Drugs with linear elimination occupy the shaded area. Drugs with nonlinear elimination encompass the whole curve. The units of dose rate and C_{ss} are arbitrary but are typical of phenytoin (EC = 500 mg/d, K_m = 5 mg/L).

Michaelis-Menten equation, and K_m is the concentration at which the rate of elimination is 50% of EC. It is important to note that in the nonlinear region (the right-hand side of Fig 63–1), the increase in steady-state concentration is much faster than the increase in dose rate. If dose rate exceeds elimination capacity, steady state cannot be achieved: the concentration will keep on rising as long as dosing continues. This kind of capacity-limited elimination becomes important when steady-state concentration is greater than K_m. It is an example of nonlinear pharmacokinetics caused by concentration-dependent clearance. This pattern of drug elimination is important for 3 drugs in common clinical use: propranolol, phenytoin, and aspirin.

Fortunately, the target concentration for most drugs used in clinical practice is usually less than their K_m, and steady-state concentration is always proportionate to the dose rate (shaded area in Fig 63–1). This is the region of linear pharmacokinetics. One major pathway of elimination, glomerular filtration, is never capacity-limited, and drugs excreted only by this route will have linear pharmacokinetics. Equation (1) reduces to a simpler form when steady-state concentration is much less than K_m:

$$\text{Dose rate} = \text{Clearance} \times C_{ss} \quad \ldots(2)$$

This equation is often used to estimate total body clearance.

Clearance & Blood Flow

Drug elimination from liver and kidney may be dependent upon blood flow if blood clearance is similar to organ blood flow—about 90 L/h for the liver and 70 L/h for the kidneys (Table 1–3). Clearance of drugs such as lidocaine and propranolol approaches hepatic blood flow, and they are said to have a high extraction ratio. Excretion of drugs with high extraction ratios is largely dependent upon blood flow to the eliminating organ.

Clearance & Protein Binding

Many drugs are avidly bound by plasma proteins. This is not detected in clinical drug concentration determinations, because bound and unbound drug are measured together by most routine analytical methods. Clearance of drugs with high extraction ratios is unaffected by changes in protein binding, because these drugs are stripped completely from plasma proteins. Clearance of drugs with low extraction ratios, however, will appear to be inversely proportionate to the degree of drug-protein binding. This is because the elimination mechanism (filtration, secretion, or metabolism) is available only to unbound drug. Clearance of unbound drug is unaffected by protein binding changes, but total drug concentration will vary with the extent of binding. Clearance estimated from total drug concentration will therefore appear to vary with changes in protein binding. (See Chapter 3, Part I for more detailed discussion.)

Factors Affecting Protein Binding

A. Albumin Concentration: Drugs such as phenytoin, salicylates, and disopyramide are extensively bound to plasma albumin. Albumin levels are low in many disease states, resulting in lower total drug concentrations.

B. Orosomucoid Concentration: Orosomucoid (α_1-acid glycoprotein) is an important protein-binding site for drugs such as quinidine, lidocaine, and propranolol. It is increased in acute inflammatory disorders and causes major changes in total plasma concentration of these drugs even though drug elimination is unchanged.

C. Drug Concentration: The binding of drugs to plasma proteins is capacity-limited. Therapeutic concentrations of salicylates, disopyramide, and prednisolone show concentration-dependent protein binding. Because unbound drug concentration is determined by clearance—which is not altered, in the case of these low-extraction-ratio drugs, by protein binding—increases in dose will cause proportionate changes in the pharmacodynamically important unbound concentration, but total drug concentration will increase less rapidly because protein binding approaches saturation at higher concentrations.

THE VALUE OF DRUG CONCENTRATION MEASUREMENTS

A single drug concentration measurement typically costs about 20 times as much as a common laboratory test such as serum sodium or blood glucose. This is because the procedures are technically demanding and are performed in relatively small numbers. However, the information generated by a drug concentration measurement is potentially of more value than that provided by a serum sodium or blood glucose determination, because the amount of drug intake is often known more precisely than sodium or glucose intake, and drug distribution and elimination mechanisms are often simple and well understood. A single drug concentration measurement may often be relied upon to predict the consequences of dosing changes for days or even weeks.

Assessment of dosing regimen compliance and drug identification in suspected poisoning or overdose are sometimes possible only by measuring drug concentrations in the blood. Estimation of clearance and volume of distribution, prediction of future drug concentrations, rational design of dosing regimens, and assessment of functional impairment due to disease are also greatly facilitated by appropriate drug concentration measurements.

INTERPRETATION OF DRUG CONCENTRATION REPORTS

Dosing History

An accurate dosing history is essential to obtain maximum value from a drug concentration measurement. In fact, if the dosing history is unknown or incomplete, a drug concentration measurement loses all predictive value.

Timing

Quantitative interpretation of drug concentrations relies upon appropriately timed blood samples and accurate recording of time of collection. Blood samples should be drawn at a time (specified below) that provides maximum pharmacokinetic information about the patient.

Expected Concentration

The information to be gained from a drug concentration measurement must be interpreted in light of its expected value. The expected value is calculated from the dosing history, the condition of the patient, and the timing of the blood samples. Comparison of the expected value with the drug concentration measurement permits rational adjustment of future dosing.

TIMING OF DRUG CONCENTRATION MEASUREMENTS

Absorption

Information about the rate and extent of drug absorption in a particular patient is rarely of great clinical importance. Absorption usually occurs during the first 2 hours after a drug dose but varies according to food intake, posture, and activity. Therefore, it is important to avoid drawing blood until absorption is complete (about 2 hours after an oral dose). Attempts to measure peak concentrations early after oral dosing are usually unsuccessful and compromise the validity of the measurement, because one cannot be certain whether absorption is complete.

Clearance

The commonest pharmacokinetic indication for concentration measurements is to estimate clearance. Individual variations in clearance are much greater than variations in absorption or volume of distribution and are the single most important factor in successful pursuit of the target concentration strategy. Because the average steady-state concentration is most commonly used to predict drug effect (Table 3–1), the required dosing rate can be easily calculated from equation (2) above if clearance is known.

Conversely, clearance is readily estimated from the dosing rate and steady-state concentration. Blood samples should be appropriately timed to estimate steady-state concentration. Provided steady state has been reached (at least 3 half-lives of constant dosing), a sample obtained near the midpoint of the dosing interval will usually be close to steady-state concentration.

Volume of Distribution

Estimation of volume of distribution is sometimes feasible, especially if more than one measurement is available or if the drug is given intravenously. However, it is seldom important in individual cases to revise the expected value for volume of distribution. Plasma concentrations can be used to estimate volume of distribution when measured at the start of dosing, before extensive elimination has occurred (equation [1], Chapter 3, Part I), or—in combination with predosing (trough) concentration—immediately after a dose when input is complete (equations [9] and [10], Chapter 3, Part I).

THE INFLUENCE OF DOSING INTERVAL & HALF-LIFE ON OPTIMAL SAMPLING TIMES

Dosing Interval Much Longer Than Half-Life

Drugs given at intervals that are much longer than one half-life (eg, tobramycin, penicillin, prednisolone) are almost completely eliminated by the time the next dose is given (Fig 63–2). The timing of the blood sample is crucial to its interpretation. For example, tobramycin concentrations measured soon after the dose has been given reflect the volume of distribution and are little affected by clearance. Just before the next dose, however, the concentration is affected by both volume and clearance. Small errors in knowledge of the sample time can produce large errors in revising volume or clearance estimates. It is usually advisable to draw 2 samples, one just before the dose and another after the dose has been given, so that both volume and clearance can be accurately determined.

Dosing Interval About Equal to Half-Life

The great majority of drugs are given about once every half-life (Fig 63–3). This is because many have half-lives between 4 and 8 hours and traditionally are given 3 or 4 times a day. The typical peak-to-trough drug concentration ratio is 2:1 when the dosing interval equals the half-life. A sample drawn in the middle of the dosing interval will be a good estimate of steady-state concentration if more than 3 half-lives have elapsed since starting regular dosing.

Dosing Interval Much Less Than Half-Life

Some drugs with small clearances (eg, phenobarbital) or large volumes of distribution (eg, digoxin) have half-lives longer than a day. To encourage patient

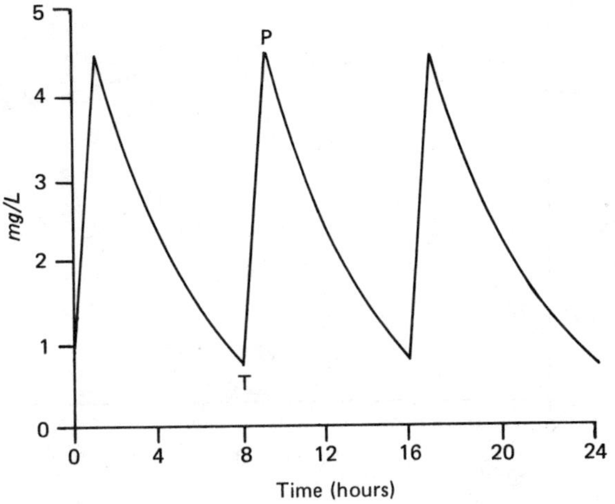

Figure 63–2. Time course of drug concentration in plasma for a drug when dosing interval is greater than half-life. A typical plasma concentration time curve is shown for tobramycin (half-life 2.2 hours) given every 8 hours by infusion over 1 hour. Ideal sampling times are just before the next dose (T, trough) and at the end of the infusion (P, peak).

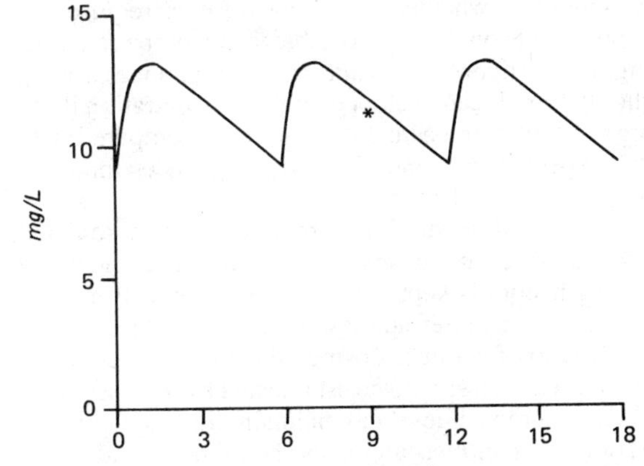

Figure 63–3. Dosing interval about equal to half-life. Typical plasma concentration time curve for theophylline (half-life 9 hours) given every 6 hours by mouth. Ideal sampling time is at the midpoint of the dosing interval (*).

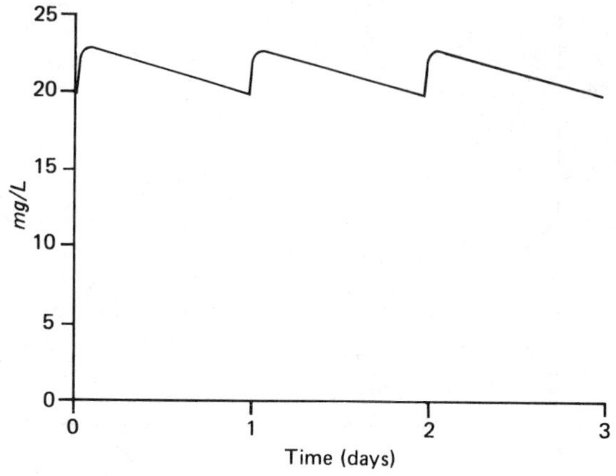

Figure 63–4. Dosing interval much less than half-life. A typical plasma concentration time curve is shown for phenobarbital (half-life 110 hours) given every 24 hours by mouth. Ideal sampling time is anywhere in the dosing interval.

compliance, they are usually given once a day; the peak-to-trough variation is therefore usually quite small (Fig 63–4). For example, phenobarbital has a half-life of 5 days, and trough concentrations at steady state are only 10% lower than the peak. Blood samples drawn within a few hours after the first dose will accurately reflect the volume of distribution, and at steady state a sample drawn at any time will closely estimate steady-state concentration and allow clearance to be calculated.

FREQUENCY OF DRUG CONCENTRATION MEASUREMENTS

It is often valuable to obtain a drug concentration measurement on admission to hospital. This has 2 purposes: First, if the measurement is made rapidly, it can indicate whether a loading dose is required to supplement concentrations achieved by outpatient dosing or, conversely, whether maintenance dosing should be reduced or stopped if the concentration is too high. Second, the actual measurement compared with the expected concentration provides an estimate of outpatient compliance.

Hospital admissions are frequently associated with rapid, erratic dosing adjustments. If an accurate dosing history is kept, a second measurement made 2 or 3 half-lives after admission may provide essential information for future dosing adjustment. A constant dosing regimen should be established as soon as possible in order to achieve and maintain the target concentration. Further measurements should be considered if the clinical state of the patient, especially clearance, is changing, eg, in heart failure. Measurements taken at intervals less than one half-life apart are of little value. At least 3 half-lives should be allowed to elapse after establishing a constant dosing regimen to obtain the most information about clearance.

OTHER BIOLOGIC FLUIDS

Therapeutic drug concentrations are most commonly measured in serum, plasma, or blood. The choice among these 3 is usually dictated by analytical requirements, and there is no pharmacokinetic or pharmacodynamic reason to prefer one over the other.

Saliva has been used instead of blood in order to avoid venipuncture. Unfortunately, salivary concentrations are influenced by factors such as saliva flow rate and pH that are not readily controlled and that result in an unacceptable variability in the ratio of concentration in saliva to concentration in blood. Reliable salivary concentrations usually impose more inconvenience on the patient than blood sampling and have found little favor except in pediatric practice.

Cerebrospinal fluid drug concentration measurements are sometimes useful for monitoring penetration of antibiotics into this compartment during treatment of intrathecal infections. However, their use for this purpose is semiquantitative and can give only rough guidance for future dosing. Concentrations of methotrexate in cerebrospinal fluid have been related to central nervous system toxicity and may be used in predicting when the target concentration for stopping leucovorin rescue therapy will be reached.

THE IMPORTANCE OF KNOWING THE EXPECTED VALUE

Interpretation of drug concentrations and their application to therapeutics hinges on knowing the expected values for the pharmacokinetic parameters of absorption, volume, and clearance and the pharmacodynamic parameters of maximum effect and sensitivity.

Pharmacokinetic parameters can be used to predict the drug concentration in a blood sample. Comparison of the measured concentration with the predicted one can then be used to decide if compliance was good, if the sample was drawn at the indicated time, if an error was made by the laboratory in measuring or reporting the result, or if revision of the expected pharmacokinetic parameters is required.

If pharmacokinetic revision is performed, deviations from the expected values for volume or clearance should be critically examined for reasonableness in direction and magnitude. For example, if tobramycin is administered to an emaciated patient, the expected tobramycin clearance using a prediction of creatinine production rate based on body weight (see equation [3], below) is likely to be too high because the actual creatinine production rate (per unit of body weight) will be lower as a result of muscle wasting.

Pharmacodynamic parameters can be used to predict whether a symptom or sign is drug-related. For example, a patient taking phenytoin who has a posterior fossa tumor may have nystagmus because of the drug or because of the tumor. Phenytoin-induced nystagmus usually does not appear until blood concentrations exceed 15 mg/L; a low phenytoin level may be used to identify the tumor as the more likely cause. However, withdrawal of phenytoin altogether may be required to resolve the issue, because the patient may have an unusually high sensitivity to this effect.

If a patient continues to have seizures and if repeated measurements after increasing doses have confirmed that concentrations are increasing and higher than those usually required, it should be assumed that the maximum effect has been achieved and another agent should be added or substituted.

Caution should be exercised in using drug concentrations in diagnosis. The inherent individual variability in pharmacodynamics should be recognized and weighed with other clinical features before a decision is made.

PREDICTION OF PHARMACOKINETIC PARAMETERS

The commonsense approach to the interpretation of drug concentrations uses predictions of pharmacokinetic parameters and expected concentrations. For example, if a patient is taking 0.25 mg of digoxin a day, a physician may expect (from application of equation [2]) the digoxin concentration to be about 1 ng/mL. This is based on the assumptions of typical bioavailability of 65% and total clearance of about 7 L/h. If the patient has heart failure, the concentration is expected to be about 1.5 ng/mL (expected clearance of 4.5 L/h). Suppose that the concentration actually measured is 2 ng/mL. Common sense would suggest halving the daily dose to achieve a target concentration of 1 ng/mL. This approach has used a revised clearance of 3.5 L/h (using equation [2], p 731).

This technique will often be misleading if steady state has not been reached. For example, if a loading dose of 1 mg of digoxin is given intravenously and the concentration is measured before a second dose hours later, it may be 1 ng/mL. However, this measurement says little about clearance and should not be used to determine the required maintenance dose. At least a week must elapse before the implicit method will be reliable. Failure to compare the expected concentration with the measured value in patients taking digoxin and quinidine explains why the major pharmacokinetic interaction between these 2 drugs went unnoticed for over 10 years, yet the doubling of steady-state concentrations by the action of quinidine on digoxin clearance can be detected in almost every patient taking this drug combination.

Typical values for absorption, clearance, and volume of distribution for many drugs measured by clinical laboratories are presented in Table 3–1. However, these values must sometimes be adjusted to reflect the clinical status of the patient.

Absorption

Quantitative adjustment of absorption parameters is rarely required. Patients with small bowel malabsorption can be expected to have reduced absorption. Digoxin bioavailability may be impaired in some patients by bacterial metabolism in the gut; this is difficult to identify in advance but may account for a marked increase in bioavailability that sometimes occurs when antibiotics are given.

Clearance

Drugs cleared by the renal route often require adjustment of clearance in proportion to renal function. This can be conveniently estimated from the creatinine clearance, determined from a single blood sample. It is done using the patient's weight, age, and sex to calculate the creatinine production rate:

$$\text{Creatinine production rate} = \frac{140 - \text{Age (years)} \times \text{Weight (kg)}}{72} \quad (\times\ 0.85 \text{ if female}) \qquad \ldots(3)$$

It is then easy to find the creatinine clearance (in milliliters per minute) by dividing the creatinine production rate by the serum creatinine (in milligrams per deciliter). Because of the difficulty of obtaining complete urine collections, creatinine clearance calculated in this way is at least as reliable as estimates of production rate based on urine collection. Ideal body weight should be used for obese patients, and correction should be made for muscle wasting in severely ill patients.

The clearance of drugs excreted only by glomerular filtration is expected to be the same as the estimated creatinine clearance. If tubular secretion or reabsorption is important, renal clearance of the drug can often be estimated from creatinine clearance, eg, renal clearance of procainamide is about 3 times that of creatinine clearance. Congestive heart failure impairs the functional ability of the liver to metabolize drugs. Both theophylline total clearance and digoxin nonrenal clearance are reduced nearly 60% by severe heart failure, and this effect is not due to a change in liver blood flow, since both drugs have low extraction ratios. Drugs such as lidocaine with high extraction ratios have their clearance reduced in proportion to the reduction in liver blood flow.

Liver failure will impair drug clearance, but there are few reliable estimates of the quantitative effect. The presence of liver disease (eg, acute viral hepatitis, alcoholic cirrhosis) does not usually change drug elimination until liver dysfunction is severe enough to produce signs of neurologic impairment.

Volume of Distribution

Volume of distribution is commonly calculated from total body weight. If a patient is obese, drugs that do not readily penetrate fat (eg, tobramycin and digoxin) should have their volumes calculated from ideal body weight as shown below:

$$\text{Ideal body weight (kg)} = 43 + 2.3 \times (\text{Height in inches} - 60) \quad (+\ 7 \text{ kg if male}) \qquad \ldots(4)$$

Patients with edema, ascites, or pleural effusions offer a larger volume of distribution to the aminoglycoside antibiotics (eg, tobramycin) than is predicted by total body weight. In such patients, the total weight should be corrected as follows: Subtract an estimate of the weight of the excess fluid accumulation. Use the resultant "normal" body weight to calculate the normal volume of distribution. Finally, this normal volume should be increased by 1 L for each estimated kilogram of excess fluid. This correction is important because of the relatively small volumes of distribution of these water-soluble drugs.

Half-Life

Once the volume of distribution and clearance are known, the expected half-life can be calculated as follows:

$$\text{Half-life} = \frac{0.7 \times \text{Volume}}{\text{Clearance}} \qquad \ldots(5)$$

It is important to understand that volume of distribution and clearance are quite independent. A change in volume will not influence clearance, nor will a change in clearance alter volume. The half-life of a drug is determined by these 2 independent factors: volume of distribution, reflecting body size and composition; and clearance, reflecting organ size and function (mainly liver and kidney).

Time to Steady State

A practical guide to the time it will take for drug concentrations to reach steady state can be obtained by multiplying the half-life by 4. This is very close to the time it will take to reach 90% of the steady-state value.

Elimination Capacity

Drugs with capacity-limited elimination are difficult to study in patients with disease. As a consequence, little quantitative information is available to guide adjustment of elimination capacity estimates in a particular individual. Enzyme induction, eg, by anticonvulsants, may raise the elimination capacity substantially in some patients.

Percent Unbound in Plasma

Changes in protein binding may be caused by alterations in plasma protein concentration (albumin, orosomucoid), affinity to plasma proteins (phenytoin affinity is decreased in renal failure), or drug displacement interactions (valproic acid increases unbound phenytoin by half, from 10% to 15%).

Bioavailability & Drug Formulation

The bioavailability of intravenous doses, by definition, is always 100%. Care must be taken to adjust doses for the actual amount of active drug when the dose is given as a complex or salt. For example, theophylline is always given intravenously as aminophylline, a complex containing 85% theophylline.

REVISING PHARMACOKINETIC PARAMETER ESTIMATES

The first thing to be done with a measured drug concentration is to compare it with the expected value. Gross deviations recognized at this point raise the possibility of errors in sample collection, concentration measurement, or reporting of the result. The most common explanation, however, is an error in calculation of the expected value—either in computation of the pharmacokinetic parameters, eg, a smoking history was neglected in predicting theophylline clearance; or in the equations used to describe each dose, eg, the bioavailability of oral digoxin (65%) was neglected.

After it is clear that the discrepancy between observed and expected concentrations is probably due to the pharmacokinetics of the particular patient, the observed concentration should be used to revise one or more pharmacokinetic parameters from their initial expected values. In general, if only one reliable measured concentration is available, only one parameter can be adjusted. Depending on the timing of the sample, as discussed above, the concentration will reflect either volume or clearance. If 2 concentrations have been obtained, separated by at least one half-life (or before and after a dose at steady state with a dosing interval of at least one half-life), it is possible to revise both volume and clearance and obtain values that will exactly predict measured concentrations.

Procedures for revising pharmacokinetic parameters that can be performed with a simple hand calculator must assume that there is no error in the timing or measurement of samples. Occasionally, quite unrealistic revised values for volume or clearance are obtained. This is particularly likely if the timing of doses or samples is uncertain or if the interval between samples is too short. Interpretation of measured concentrations should realistically take into account expected errors in timing and measurement. Furthermore, expected variability in volume or clearance must be considered in order to exclude unlikely values. Individual variability in volume of distribution is usually smaller than variability in clearance. This is to be expected when one considers the generally similar structure (which determines volume of distribution) of one person to another compared with the variations in organ function (which determines clearance) both among and within individuals. For example, the coefficient of variation of theophylline volume of distribution is about 25%, compared with 50% coefficient of variation of clearance in the same hospitalized patient.

The technique of revising parameter estimates in the light of their typical values in the population and their relative variability is known as Bayesian feedback. Computer programs are available to perform this analysis either over a time-sharing network or with a microcomputer. Use of a computer reduces the risk of computational errors in the process of drug concentration interpretation and allows several measured concentrations to be incorporated in the analysis, including allowance for timing and measurement errors.

• • •

References

Azarnoff DL: Use of pharmacokinetic principles in therapy. (Editorial.) *N Engl J Med* 1973;**289:**635.

Benet LZ: Effect of route of administration and distribution on drug action. *J Pharmacokinet Biopharm* 1978;**6:**559.

Holford NHG, Sheiner LB: The digoxin concentration: Before and after the fact. *Am Heart J* 1977;**94:**529.

Holford NHG, Sheiner LB: Understanding the dose-effect relationship. *Clin Pharmacokin* 1981;**6:**429.

Peck CC et al: A micro-computer drug (theophylline) dosing program which assists and teaches physicians. Proceedings of the Fourth Annual Conference. *Comput Appl Med Care* 1980;**2:**988.

Sokolow M, Edgar AL: Blood quinidine concentrations as a guide to the treatment of cardiac arrhythmias. *Circulation* 1950; **1:**576.

Winter ME: *Basic Clinical Pharmacokinetics*. Applied Therapeutics, 1980.

Zito RA, Reid PR: Lidocaine kinetics predicted by indocyanine green clearance. *N Engl J Med* 1978;**298:**1160.

64 | Therapeutic & Toxic Potential of Over-the-Counter Agents

Mary Anne Koda-Kimble, PharmD

In the United States, drugs are divided by law into 2 classes: those restricted to sale by prescription only and those for which directions for safe use by the public can be written. The latter category constitutes the nonprescription or over-the-counter (OTC) drugs. The American public spends approximately $5 billion annually on an estimated 300,000 OTC products to medicate themselves for self-diagnosed ailments ranging from warts to psoriasis. These 300,000 products represent about 500 active ingredients in various forms and combinations. It is thus apparent that many are no more than ''me too'' products advertised to the public in ways that suggest that there are significant differences between them. For example, the current (sixth) edition of *Handbook of Nonprescription Drugs* lists 82 different internal analgesic products almost all of which contain aspirin, acetaminophen, phenacetin, or a combination of these agents as their primary ingredients. They are made different from one another by the addition of questionable ingredients such as caffeine or antihistamines; by brand names chosen to suggest a specific use (''feminine pain,'' ''night-time pain,'' ''arthritis''); or by their special dosage form (enteric-coated tablets, liquids, sustained-release products, powders, seltzers). There is a price attached to all of these gimmicks, and in most cases a less expensive generic product can be equally effective. It is probably safe to assume that the public is generally overwhelmed and confused by the wide array of products presented and will probably use those that are most heavily advertised.

There are 3 reasons why it is critical for the clinician to be familiar with this class of products. First, many of the ingredients contained in these products are effective in treating common ailments, and it is important to be able to help the patient select a safe, effective product. (See Table 64–1.) Second, many of the active ingredients contained in OTC drugs may worsen existing medical conditions or interact with prescription medications. (See Appendix I, Drug Interactions.) Finally, the misuse or abuse of OTC products may actually produce significant medical complications. A general awareness of these products and their formulation will enable clinicians to more fully appreciate the potential for OTC drug-related problems in their patients.

Table 64–1 lists examples of OTC products that may be used effectively to treat medical problems commonly encountered in ambulatory patients. The selection of one ingredient over another may be important in patients with certain medical problems or in patients taking certain prescription medications. These are discussed in detail in other chapters. The recommendations listed in Table 64–1 are based upon the efficacy of the ingredients and on the principles set forth in the following paragraphs:

(1) Select the product that is simplest in formulation with regard to ingredients and dosage form. In general, single-ingredient products are preferred. Although some combination products contain effective doses of all ingredients, others contain therapeutic doses of some ingredients and subtherapeutic doses of others. Furthermore, there may be differing durations of action among the ingredients, and there is always a possibility that the clinician or patient will be unaware of the presence of certain active ingredients in the product. Aspirin, for example, is present in many cough and cold preparations; a patient unaware of this may take separate doses of analgesic in addition to that contained in the cold preparation.

(2) Select a product that contains a therapeutically effective dose.

(3) Select a product that lists its ingredients and their amounts. The label of a product should always be read carefully, since ingredients may be changed without public notification or change in brand name.

(4) Recommend a generic product if one is available.

(5) Be wary of ''gimmicks'' or advertising claims that claim specific superiority over similar products.

(6) For children, the dose, dosage form, and palatability of the product will be prime considerations.

Certain ingredients in OTC products should be avoided or used with caution in selected patients because they may exacerbate existing medical problems or interact with prescription medications the patient is taking. Many of the more potent OTC ingredients are ''hidden'' in products where their presence would not ordinarily be expected (Table 64–2). This lack of awareness of the ingredients present in OTC products and the belief by many physicians that OTC products are ''ineffective and harmless'' may cause diagnostic confusion and perhaps interfere with therapy.

Table 64–1. Ingredients of choice for selected over-the-counter (OTC) classes.

OTC Category	Ingredient and Dosage	Product Examples	Comments
Analgesics and antipyretics	Aspirin 300–600 mg every 4–6 hours.	Generic, Bayer Aspirin (325 mg/tablet).	There are numerous product modifications, including the addition of antacid, caffeine, and methapyriline; enteric-coated tablets and seltzers; long-acting or extra-strength formulations; and various mixtures of analgesics. None have any substantial advantage over a single-ingredient product. Acetaminophen lacks anti-inflammatory activity. Aspirin should be used cautiously in certain individuals (see text). Avoid products that contain phenacetin, eg, A.S.A. Compound, Bromo-Seltzer, A.P.C. Capsules. Extra-strength formulations contain 400–600 mg of active ingredient.
	Acetaminophen 300–600 mg every 4–6 hours.	Generic, Datril, Nebs, Tylenol (325 mg/tablet—various strengths available).	
Allergy preparations	Chlorpheniramine 4 mg every 4–6 hours.	Chlor-Trimeton (4 mg/tablet or 10 mL syrup).	Antihistamines alone relieve most symptoms associated with allergic rhinitis or hay fever. Chlorpheniramine and brompheniramine cause less drowsiness than methapyriline, pyrilamine, doxylamine, and phentoloxamine. Occasionally, symptoms unrelieved by the antihistamine respond to the addition of a sympathomimetic.
	Brompheniramine 4 mg every 4–6 hours.	Symptom 3 (4 mg/10 mL).	
	Chlorpheniramine (4 mg) with pseudoephedrine (60 mg).	Chlor-Trimeton Decongestant (per tablet), Novafed A Syrup (per 10 mL).	
	Chlorpheniramine (4 mg) with phenylpropanolamine (37.5 mg).	Novahistine, elixir and tablets (per 10 mL or 2 tablets); Triaminicin Allergy (per tablet).	
Antitussives	Codeine 10–20 mg every 4–6 hours (with guaifenesin).	Cheracol, Robitussin A-C (both contain 2 mg/mL).	In doses required for cough suppression, the addictive liability associated with codeine is low. Codeine is a Schedule V narcotic, and its OTC sale is restricted in some states. The efficacy of expectorants, which are included in almost all antitussives, is questionable. Guaifenesin has the least potential for toxicity. Watch for hidden ingredients in these products.
	Dextromethorphan 10–20 mg every 4 hours (with guaifenesin).	Cheracol D (2 mg/mL), 2/G-DM (3 mg/mL), Pertussin 8-Hour Cough Formula (1.5 mg/mL), Robitussin-DM (3 mg/mL).	
Decongestants	Topical Oxymetazoline.	Afrin.	Topical sympathomimetics are effective in the acute management of rhinorrhea associated with common colds and allergies. Long-acting agents (oxymetazoline and xylometazoline) are generally preferred, although phenylephrine is equally effective. Oral decongestants have a prolonged duration of action but may cause more systemic effects. Pseudoephedrine has the least CNS stimulatory effect. Phenylpropanolamine is also effective. Phenylephrine is unpredictably absorbed.
	Xylometazoline.	Dristan Long Lasting Nasal Mist, Sinex-L.A., Sinutab Nasal Spray, Neo-Synephrine II.	
	Phenylephrine.	Allerest, Contac Nasal Mist, Coricidin Nasal Spray, Neo-Synephrine, NTZ.	
	Oral Pseudoephedrine 60 mg every 4 hours.	Sudafed (30 mg/tablet or 5 mL), Novafed (30 mg/5 mL), Symptom 2 (30 mg/5 mL).	
	Phenylpropanolamine 25 mg every 4 hours.	No single-ingredient product available.	
Laxatives	Bulk-formers.	Metamucil, Serutan.	The safest laxatives for chronic use include the bulk-formers and stool softeners. Saline laxatives and stimulants may be used acutely but not chronically (see text).
	Stool softeners—docusate sodium.	Generic, Colace, Coloctyl, Doxinate.	
	Saline laxatives.	Phillips' Milk of Magnesia.	
Antacids	Magnesium hydroxide and aluminum hydroxide combinations.	Gelusil, Gelusil II, Maalox No. 1, Maalox No. 2, Mylanta, Mylanta-II, Wingel.	Combinations of magnesium and aluminum hydroxide are less likely to cause constipation or diarrhea and offer high neutralizing capacity. The "II" formulations are approximately twice as potent on a mL/mL basis. The products listed are liquid products with a low sodium content.

Table 64–2. Hidden ingredients in over-the-counter (OTC) products.

Hidden Drug or Drug Class	OTC Class Containing Drug	Product Examples
Alcohol	Cough syrups/cold preparations.	Breacol (10%), Broncho-Tussin (40%), Cotussis (20%), Formula 44-D (10%), Halls (22%), Novahistine DMX (10%), Pertussin 8-Hour Cough Formula (9.5%), Quiet Nite (25%), Romilar III (20%), Trind (15%), NyQuil (25%).
Anticholinergic agents	Antidiarrheals.	Donnagel, Donnagel-PG.
	Cold/allergy preparations.	Contac Timed Cold Capsules.
	Sleep aids.	Nite Rest Capsules, Seedate Capsules, Sominex Tablets and Capsules.
Antihistamines	Analgesics.	Excedrin PM, Cope, Percogesic.
	Cold/allergy products.	Many. Alka-Seltzer Plus, Allerest, Chlor-Trimeton, Contac, Coricidin, Co-Tylenol, Dristan, Novahistine, NyQuil, Sinarest, Sine-Off, Sinutab, Super Anahist, Triaminic, Triaminicin, 4-Way Cold Tablets.
	Sleep aids.	Compoz Tablets, Nervine, Nytol, Sleep-Eze, Sominex.
	Motion sickness products, antiemetics.	Bonine, Dramamine, Marezine.
	Asthma products.	Bronitin, Primatene M.
	Menstrual products.	Cardui, Pamprin, Sunril.
	Topical decongestants.	Contac Nasal Mist, Dristan, Sinex, 4-Way.
	Dermatologic preparations.	Pyribenzamine Cream or Ointment.
Aspirin and other salicylates	Cold/allergy preparations.	Alka-Seltzer Plus, Bayer Decongestant, Congespirin, Coricidin, Dristan Tablets, Sine-Off, Super Anahist, Triaminicin, 4-Way Cold Tablets.
	Analgesics.	Many. Alka-Seltzer, Anacin, Aspergum, Cope, Ecotrin, Excedrin, Fizrin Powder, Measurin, Persistin, Stanback Tablets and Powder, Vanquish.
	Antidiarrheals.	Pepto-Bismol (bismuth subsalicylate).
	Menstrual products.	Midol.
	Sleep aids.	Quiet World Tablets, Tranquil Capsules (sodium salicylate).
Caffeine	Systemic analgesics.	Anacin, Bromo-Seltzer, Cope, Excedrin, Stanback Tablets and Powder, Vanquish.
	Cold/allergy products.	Coryban D, Dristan, Super Anahist, Triaminicin.
	Weight control products.	Anorexin Capsules, Appedrine Tablets, Dexatrim Capsules, Prolamine Capsules, Spantrol Capsules.
	Menstrual/diuretic products.	Aqua-Ban, Midol, Pre-Mens Forte, Tri-Aqua.
Local anesthetics (usually benzocaine)	Antitussives.	Formula 44 Cough Disc, Silexin Cough Syrup and Tablets, Sucrets Cough Control Formula, Vicks Cough Silencer Tablets.
	Lozenges.	Cepacol Troches, Hold, Listerine Cough Control, Spec-T Sore Throat Products, Trokettes.
	Weight loss products.	Diet Trim Tablets, Slim Line Candy and Gum, Spantrol.
	Toothache, cold sore, and teething products.	Baby OraJel, Benzodent, Numzident, Orabase with Benzocaine, OraJel teething lotion, toothache drops.
	Dermatologic preparations.	Americaine First Aid Spray or Ointment, Dermoplast, Nupercainal Cream or Ointment, Medi-Quick, Solarcaine, Unguentine Spray, Unguentine Plus First Aid and Burn Cream.
Sodium (mg/tablet or mg/5 mL)	Antacids.	Alka-Seltzer Effervescent Antacid (276), Amphogel Liquid (7), A.M.T. (7), BisoDol (157), Phosphajel (12.5), Rolaids (53), Soda Mint (89), Trisogel (16).
	Analgesics.	Alka-Seltzer Effervescent Pain Reliever and Antacid (521), Bromo-Seltzer (717), Fizrin Powder (673), sodium salicylate (50 mg/300 mg).
	Laxatives.	Instant Mix Metamucil (250 mg/packet), Fleets Enema (5000 mg, of which 250–300 mg is absorbed), Phospho-Soda (55), Sal Hepatica (1000).
	Cough syrups.	Coryban D (31), Cerose (38), Dristan (59), Pertussin 8-Hour Cough Formula (24), Formula 44 (68), Vicks Cough Syrup (54).
Sympathomimetics	Asthma products.	Bronkaid, Bronkotabs, Primatene, Tedral.
	Cold/allergy preparations.	Many. Alka-Seltzer Plus, Allerest, Bayer Decongestant, Chlor-Trimeton Decongestant, Contac, Co-Tylenol, Novafed, Novahistine Sinus Tablets, Nyquil, Sinarest, Sine-Aid, Sine-Off, Sinutab, Sudafed, Super Anahist, Triaminicin, 4-Way Cold Tablets.
	Cough syrups.	Cerose, Cerose DM, Formula 44-D, Robitussin-CF, Robitussin-PE, Triaminic Expectorant, Triaminicol.
	Lozenges.	Spec-T Sore Throat/Decongestant.
	Menstrual products.	Femcaps, Fluidex-Plus with Diadax.
	Topical decongestants.	Many. Afrin, Benzedrex, Neo-Synephrine Hydrochloride, NTZ, Privine Sinex, Vicks Inhaler.
	Weight control products.	Appedrine Tablets, Dexatrim Capsules, Prolamine Capsules.

For example, innumerable OTC products, including cough and cold preparations, decongestants, and appetite control products, contain sympathomimetics. These agents should be avoided or used cautiously in insulin-dependent diabetics and patients with hypertension, angina, or hyperthyroidism. Aspirin should be avoided by individuals with active peptic ulcer disease, certain platelet disorders, or patients taking oral anticoagulants.

Finally, overuse or misuse of OTC products may induce significant medical problems. A prime example is rebound congestion from the regular use of nasal sprays for more than 3–4 days. The improper and chronic use of some antacids (eg, aluminum hydroxide) may cause constipation and even impaction in elderly people as well as hypophosphatemia. Laxative abuse (chiefly by older people) can result in abdominal cramping and fluid and electrolyte disturbances. Insomnia, nervousness, and restlessness can result from the use of sympathomimetics or caffeine hidden in many OTC products (Table 64–2). The chronic systemic use of some analgesics containing large amounts of caffeine may produce rebound headaches, and long-term use of analgesics, especially those containing phenacetin, has been associated with interstitial nephritis. Acute ingestion of large amounts of aspirin or acetaminophen by adults or children causes serious toxicity. Antihistamines may cause sedation or drowsiness, especially when taken concurrently with sedative-hypnotics, tranquilizers, alcohol, or other central nervous system depressants. Finally, antihistamines, local anesthetics, antibiotics, antibacterial agents, counterirritants, *p*-aminobenzoic acid (PABA), preservatives, and deodorants contained in a myriad of OTC topical and vaginal products may induce allergic reactions.

There are 3 major drug information sources for OTC products. *Handbook of Nonprescription Drugs* is the most comprehensive resource for OTC medications; it evaluates ingredients contained in major OTC drug classes and lists the ingredients included in many OTC products. *Physicians' Desk Reference for Nonprescription Drugs,* a compendium of manufacturers' information regarding OTC products, is somewhat incomplete with regard to the number of products included and the consistency of information provided. *The Medicine Show,* a consumer guide to the use of OTC products, critically evaluates these products and discusses their rational use. It is well written and factually correct. Any clinician who seeks more specific information regarding OTC products should find these references useful.

• • •

References

The Medicine Show, 5th ed. Editors of Consumer Reports Books, 1980.

Penna RP et al (editors): *Handbook of Nonprescription Drugs,* 6th ed. American Pharmaceutical Association, 1979.

Physicians' Desk Reference For Nonprescription Drugs, 2nd ed. Medical Economics, 1981.

Widger HN: *Widger's Guide to Over-the-Counter Products.* JP Tarcher, 1979.

65 | Drug Discovery & Evaluation

Barry A. Berkowitz, PhD

One hundred years ago, the useful life of a drug in medical practice could be measured in decades or even centuries. In the last 50 years, new drugs have proliferated so rapidly that the useful life of drugs now on the most-prescribed list can be stated in years or at most decades (Table 65–1).

One result of this rapid turnover is that most drugs are now discovered and characterized by the pharmaceutical industry rather than in academic laboratories. Over 80% of new drugs originate in the industrial environment—a marked change from 30 years ago, when industry played a lesser role. One reason for this trend is that contemporary drug discovery research often requires a greater commitment of multidisciplinary resources in biology, chemistry, pharmacology, toxicology, and clinical trials than any single academic laboratory or department could reasonably contemplate. The costs and potential financial gain involved have further contributed to the visibility of the industrial laboratory in the search for new drugs. Clinical trials of new drugs are still carried out chiefly in academic centers.

This chapter reviews the process whereby drugs are discovered, evaluated, and introduced as new therapeutic agents. The 4 primary scientific components of this process can be sketched as follows: (1) Drug discovery, either by synthesis or by extraction from natural sources. A function of medicinal chemists. (2) Definition of the drug's pharmacologic profile in animals. (Does it work? What does it do?) A function of preclinical pharmacologists. (3) Toxicologic testing in animals. (Is it safe?) A function of toxicologists, pharmacologists, and pathologists. (4) Evaluation in humans, ie, clinical testing. A process carried out in the USA in 4 phases by clinical pharmacologists and clinical practitioners.

Table 65–1. A century of drug discovery: Most frequently employed drugs.*

1885[1]	1980[2]
1. Iron (for anemia)	1. Diazepam
2. Quinine (for malaria)	2. Triamterene with hydrochlorothiazide
3. Ether	3. Furosemide
4. Opium	4. Acetaminophen
5. Sodium bicarbonate	5. Digoxin
6. Alcohol	6. Methyldopa
7. Bromide	7. Propoxyphene napsylate with acetaminophen
8. Mercury and iodides (for syphilis)	8. Cimetidine
9. Calomel (as laxative)	9. Flurazepam
10. Paregoric (for diarrhea)	10. Propranolol

*Based on extent of use or number of prescriptions.
[1] See Smith and Knapp reference on p 747.
[2] *Scrip World Pharm News* (Sept 10) 1980;**No. 522**:1.

DRUG DISCOVERY; DOES THE COMPOUND WORK?

Whether a drug will be useful in the diagnosis or treatment of a human disease can only be established in humans by carefully controlled clinical trials. Elements of the pathway a drug must take before this question can be answered are shown in Fig 65–1.

Seldom does the first agent synthesized by the medicinal chemist or tested by the pharmacologist meet the criteria of efficacy and safety necessary for further development. Modifications of the chemical structure are usually necessary to obtain a compound with a promising balance of efficacy in animal studies over apparent toxicity. These modifications are guided by structure-activity studies, using measures of both therapeutic and toxic activity, which are utilized to improve the therapeutic index of the group of compounds under study. Here the interplay and communication between medicinal chemist, biologist, and pharmacologist are essential elements in identifying a candidate drug and obtaining useful biologic quantitation of its action.

It has been estimated that for every 10,000 molecules tested, only 10 reach the stage where investigational new drug (IND) notification is filed with the Food and Drug Administration (FDA) and studies in humans are initiated to evaluate their safety and usefulness (Fig 65–2). Of these 10, it is likely that only one will ever become a new prescription drug.

Once a lead compound is identified as a potential drug with one or more clinical applications, a patent application is made. If the compound is found not

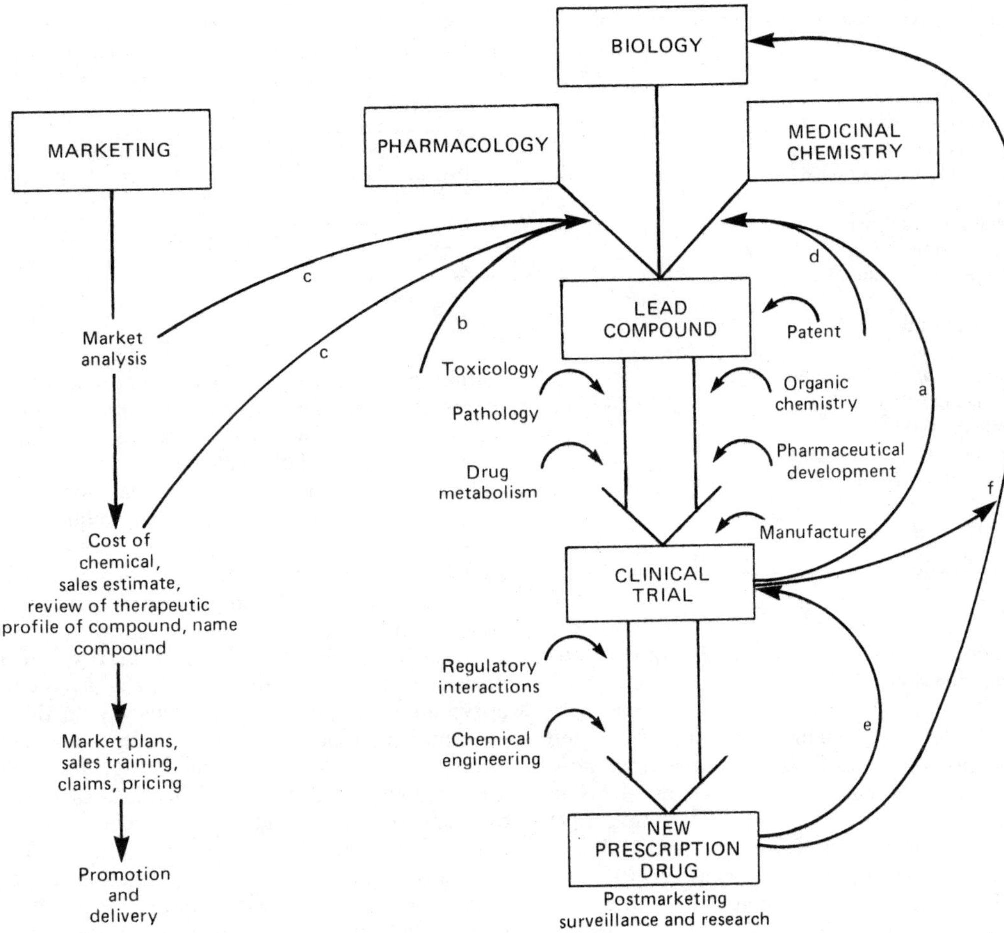

Figure 65–1. Pathway for a new prescription drug. Problems that may result in retrograde movement along this path are as follows: *a:* Clinical trials may reveal unacceptable side-effects, toxicity, or lack of efficacy in humans. *b:* Animal toxicologic studies or pathologic examination may reveal undesirable effects near therapeutic doses or unacceptable effects. *c:* Marketing review may indicate lack of need or unacceptable expense. *d:* The lead compound (ie, the most promising member of the chemical family under study) may be held not patentable. *e:* A new clinical indication may require additional studies. Some new drugs also return to the basic laboratory *(f)* if the agent is found to be useful as a tool in exploration of fundamental biologic processes, eg, cimetidine as a probe for H_2 histamine receptors.

patentable as a new chemical entity or new medical use, the commercial potential of the molecule is usually destroyed unless there are strong overriding forces such as unusual medical need.

The drug's **pharmacologic profile,** which is a composite of a wide range of screening studies followed by more intensive and narrower ones (Table 65–2), constitutes the major evidence upon which the decision is made to invest additional resources in a new agent. Such decisions are based on analysis of the effects of a drug on physiologic or biochemical responses believed to be predictive of clinical efficacy or on the observed effects of a drug on an animal with experimentally induced disease. As we better understand disease processes, better preclinical models can be devised. The availability of a good in vitro or animal model greatly facilitates development of new drugs for a disease.

While the scientific team is determining the pharmacologic properties of a new chemical, the corporate marketing group is investigating its economic potential: Is the drug needed, and how large is the market?

IS IT SAFE?

The greater the interest in the pharmacologic profile of a compound, the more rapid becomes the pace of safety evaluation. The goal of **preclinical toxicity testing** (Table 65–3) is the discovery and characterization of any significant harmful consequences following single or repeated dosing. It is hoped that the results will be predictive of events likely to occur in

Table 65–2. Typical tests involved in drug evaluation.

Pharmacology
- Cardiovascular hemodynamics
- Electrocardiography
- Respiratory function
- Gastrointestinal function
- Renal function
- Central nervous system action
- Drug interaction
- Endocrine gland function

Drug metabolism
- Pharmacokinetics
- Tissue distribution
- Metabolite identification and profile
- Enzyme induction
- Protein binding
- Placental transfer

Mechanism of action
- Molecular action
- Receptor interaction
- Action in relevant animal models of clinical disease

humans. The crucial features include both the results obtained and the dosage level at which they occurred.

The difference or spread between the toxic dose and the effective dose can be expressed by the therapeutic index (LD50/ED50). The lower this ratio, the greater the expectation of potential problems in other species. Major areas of toxicity testing are (1) effects of single doses, (2) effects of repeated doses, (3) effects on reproductive performance, (4) carcinogenicity, and (5) mutagenicity. Examples are summarized in Table 65–3.

EVALUATION IN HUMANS

Federal law in the USA requires that the study of new drugs in humans be conducted in accordance with certain stringent requirements. Scientifically meaningful results are not guaranteed simply by conforming to government regulations, however, and the design and execution of a good clinical trial require the efforts of a clinician-scientist or clinical pharmacologist, a statistician, a doctor of pharmacy, and frequently other personnel as well. The need for this research team is based upon 3 major factors inherent in the study of any therapeutic measure—pharmacologic or nonpharmacologic—in humans:

Table 65–4. Typical cross-over design for comparing a mythical new analgesic, "Novent," with placebo and a known active drug, aspirin, in the management of chronic pain. Each therapeutic period lasts 7 days.

	Medication Given		
Patient Group	**Week 1**	**Week 2**	**Week 3**
I	Aspirin	Placebo	"Novent"
II	Placebo	"Novent"	Aspirin
III	"Novent"	Aspirin	Placebo

(1) The variable natural history of most diseases: Most diseases tend to wax and wane in severity; some disappear spontaneously with time; and even malignant neoplasms may undergo spontaneous remissions. A good experimental design must take into account the natural history of the disease under study by evaluating a large enough population of subjects over a sufficiently long period of time. Additional protection against errors of interpretation induced by fluctuations in severity of the manifestations of disease is provided by utilizing a **cross-over design,** which consists of alternating periods of administration of test drug, placebo preparation, and standard drug control, if any, in each subject. These sequences are systematically varied so that different subsets of patients receive each of the possible sequences of treatment. An example of such a design is shown in Table 65–4.

(2) The presence of other diseases and risk factors: Known or unknown diseases and risk factors (including life-styles of subjects) may influence the

Table 65–3. Safety tests.

	Approach	Comment
Acute toxicity	Acute dose required to kill 50% of population of animals (LD50; mg/kg). Usually 2 species, 2 routes, single dose.	Calculate therapeutic index (LD50/ED50).
Subacute toxicity	Three doses, 2 species. Up to 6 months may be necessary prior to clinical trial. The longer the duration of expected clinical use, the longer the subacute test.	Clinical chemistry, symptoms and signs, autopsy studies, hematology, histology, electron microscopy.
Chronic toxicity	One to 2 years. Required when drug is intended to be used in humans for prolonged periods. Usually run concurrently with clinical trial.	Goals of subacute and chronic tests are to show which organs are susceptible to drug toxicity. Tests as noted above for subacute.
Effect on reproductive performance	Effects on animal mating behavior, reproduction, parturition, progeny, birth defects.	Examines fertility, teratology, perinatal and postnatal effects, lactation.
Carcinogenic potential	Two years, 2 species. Required when drug is intended to be used in humans for prolonged periods.	Hematology, histology, autopsy studies.
Mutagenic potential	Determine effects of drug on genetic structure of bacteria or mammalian cells in culture.	Increasing interest in this problem.

results of a clinical study. For example, some diseases alter the pharmacokinetics of drugs (Chapters 2 and 3). Levels of a blood component being monitored as a measure of the effect of the new agent may be influenced by other diseases or other drugs. Attempts to avoid this hazard usually involve the cross-over technique (when feasible) and proper selection of patients and assignment to each of the study groups. This requires that careful medical and pharmacologic histories (including use of recreational drugs) be obtained and that statistically valid methods of randomization be used in assigning subjects to particular study groups.

(3) Subject and observer bias: Most patients tend to perceive any therapeutic intervention by interested, caring, and enthusiastic personnel as a positive measure. The manifestation of this phenomenon in the subject is the **placebo response** (Latin "I shall please") and may involve objective physiologic and biochemical changes as well as changes in subjective complaints associated with the disease. It is usually quantitated by administration of an inert material, manufactured to give it (the placebo or "dummy" medication) exactly the same physical appearance and properties as the active dosage form. The magnitude of the response varies considerably with the condition being treated. However, the incidence of the placebo response is fairly constant, being observed in 20–40% of patients in almost all studies. Placebo "toxicity" also occurs but usually involves only subjective effects: stomach upset, insomnia, sedation, etc.

Observer bias includes the unconscious as well as any conscious tendency of the personnel evaluating the response of subjects to find an expected result.

Subject bias effects can be quantitated—and deducted from the response measured during active therapy—by the **single-blind** technique. This involves use of a placebo or dummy medication, as described above, which is administered to the same subjects in a cross-over design, if possible, or to a separate control group of subjects. Observer bias can be taken into account by disguising the identity of the medication being used—placebo or active form—from both the subjects and the personnel evaluating the subjects' responses (**double-blind** design). In this design, a third party holds the code identifying each medication packet, and the code is not broken until all of the clinical data have been collected.

The Food & Drug Administration

The Food and Drug Administration (FDA) is the administrative body that oversees the drug evaluation process in the United States and grants approval to market new drug products. The authority of the FDA to regulate drug marketing derives from several pieces of legislation (Table 65–5). If a drug has not been shown through adequately controlled testing to be safe and effective for a specified use, it cannot be marketed in interstate commerce for this use.

Of course it would be impossible except in very rare cases to prove that a drug is absolutely safe, ie, free of all risk. It is possible, however, to identify hazards associated with use of the drug and to place some statistical limits on the maximum frequency of occurrence of such hazards in the population under study. However, an operational and pragmatic definition of "safety" can usually be reached, based upon the nature and incidence of drug-associated hazards as compared to the hazard of nontherapy of the target disease.

Table 65–5. Major legislation pertaining to drugs in the USA.

Law	Purpose and Effect
Pure Food & Drug Act of 1906	Prohibited mislabeling and adulteration of drugs.
Opium Exclusion Act of 1909	Prohibited importation of opium.
Amendment (1912) to the Pure Food & Drug Act	Prohibited advertising claims if they were both false and fraudulent (which had the effect of legalizing false claims, since intent to defraud had to be proved).
Harrison Narcotics Act of 1914	Established regulations for the use of opium, opiates, and cocaine (marihuana added in 1937).
Food, Drug, & Cosmetic Act of 1938	Required that new drugs be **safe** as well as pure (but did not require proof of efficacy).
Durham-Humphrey Act of 1952	Vested in the FDA the power to determine which products could be sold without prescription.
Kefauver-Harris Amendment (1962) to the Food, Drug, & Cosmetic Act	Required proof of **efficacy** as well as safety for new drugs and for drugs released since 1938; established guidelines for reporting of information about adverse reactions, clinical testing, and advertising of new drugs.

THE IND & NDA

Once a drug is judged ready to be studied in humans, a Notice of Claimed Investigational Exemption for a New Drug (IND) is filed with the FDA. The IND includes (1) information on composition and source of the drug, (2) manufacturing information, (3) all data from animal studies, (4) clinical plans and protocols, and (5) names and credentials of physicians who will conduct the trials.

Clinical testing often requires 4–6 years to accumulate all required data and to fulfill regulatory requirements (Fig 65–2). In all phases of clinical trials, volunteers or patients are informed of the investigational status of the drug as well as possible risks and must consent to participate and receive the drug.

In phase 1, the effect of the drug as a function of dosage is established in a small number of healthy volunteers. Phase 1 trials are carried out to determine whether animals and humans show significantly different responses to the drug and to establish the probable limits of the clinical dosage range. These trials are

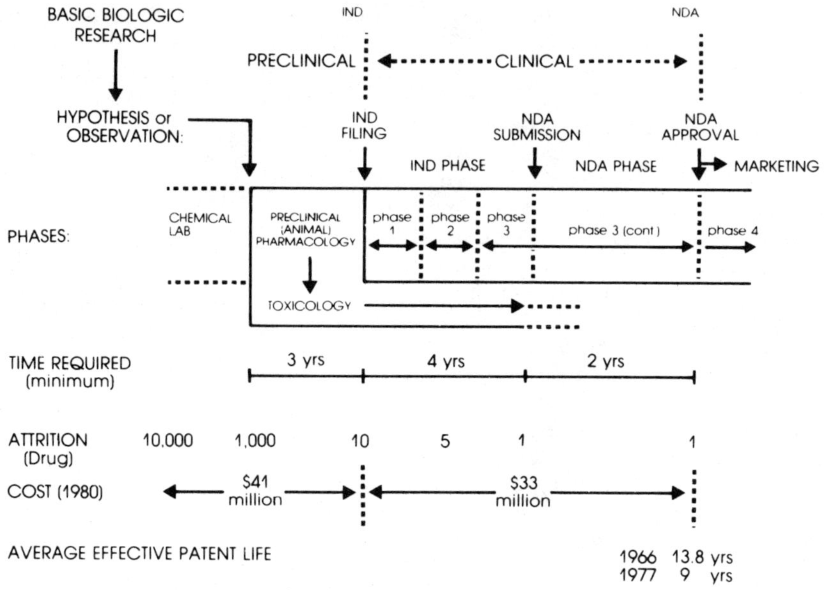

Figure 65–2. Drug development in the USA showing interrelationships of phases of drug development, time required, attrition rate of compounds evaluated, cost estimates, and average patent life. (Modified and reproduced, with permission, from Wardell W in: *Drug Assessment Criteria and Methods.* Bowers JZ, Velo GP [editors]. Elsevier/North Holland, 1979.)

nonblind, ie, both the investigators and the subjects know what is being given. Pharmacokinetic measurements of absorption, half-life, and metabolism are often done in phase 1. Such studies are usually performed in clinical research centers by specially trained clinical pharmacologists.

In phase 2, the drug is studied for the first time in patients with the target disease to determine safety and efficacy. A small number of patients (10–150) are studied in great detail. A single-blind design is often used, with an inert placebo medication and an older active drug (positive control) in addition to the investigational agent. Phase 2 trials also are usually done in special clinical centers.

In phase 3, the drug is evaluated in much larger numbers of patients, sometimes thousands. Using information gathered in phases 1 and 2, trials are designed (optimally) to minimize errors caused by placebo effects, variable course of the disease, etc. Therefore, double-blind and cross-over techniques (Table 65–4) are frequently employed. Phase 3 trials are usually carried out in clinical settings similar to those anticipated for the ultimate use of the drug. Phase 3 studies are difficult to design and execute and are usually very expensive, because of the large numbers of patients involved and the masses of data that must be collected and analyzed. The investigators are usually specialists in the disease being treated.

If phase 3 results are positive, application will be made for permission to market the new agent. The process of applying for marketing approval requires submission of a New Drug Application (NDA) to the FDA. The application contains, usually in hundreds of volumes, full reports of all preclinical and clinical data pertaining to the drug under review. A decision on approval by the FDA may take 1.5–3 years or longer. In areas of extreme need, eg, cancer chemotherapy, the process of preclinical and clinical testing may be considerably abbreviated.

Once approval to market a drug has been obtained, phase 4 begins. This constitutes an attempt to monitor the safety of the new drug under ordinary conditions of use in much larger numbers of patients. The importance of careful and complete reporting of toxicity after marketing approval by the FDA can be appreciated by noting that many important drug-induced effects have an incidence of 1:10,000 or less. Such low-incidence drug-effect associations will not generally be detected in phase 1–3 studies, no matter how carefully executed. Phase 4 has no fixed duration.

• • •

References

Beyer KH: *Discovery, Development and Delivery of New Drugs*. Spectrum, 1978.

Bowers JZ, Velo GP (editors): *Drug Assessment Criteria and Methods*. Elsevier/North Holland, 1979.

Hayes AH: Advances in cardiovascular pharmacology. *JAMA* 1982;**248:**537.

Kennedy D: Creative tension: FDA and medicine. *N Engl J Med* 1978;**298:**846.

Schwartzman D: *Innovation in the Pharmaceutical Industry*. Johns Hopkins Univ Press, 1976.

Smith M, Knapp D: *Pharmacy, Drugs, and Medical Care,* 2nd ed. Williams & Wilkins, 1976.

66 | Prescription Writing

Paul W. Lofholm, PharmD

A prescription is a physician's order to prepare or dispense a specific treatment—usually medication—for an individual patient. The physician's decision to prescribe a drug assumes that the patient has been evaluated and a diagnosis arrived at and that it is rational to prescribe drugs. Much of this book is devoted to discussions of the pharmacologic principles of drug action used to select the drug of choice. This chapter deals with the techniques of prescription writing once the therapeutic agent is selected and the legal, economic, and social factors involved in that process.

LEGAL FACTORS (USA)

The United States government recognizes 2 classes of drugs: (1) over-the-counter (OTC) drugs and (2) those that require a prescription from a licensed prescriber. OTC drugs are those that can be safely self-administered by the layman, that are for self-limiting conditions, and for which there can be appropriate labels written for use. Half of all drug doses consumed by the American public are OTC drugs.

Prescription drugs are controlled by the US Food and Drug Administration. They are identified by the federal legend statement: "Caution: Federal law prohibits dispensing without a prescription." This statement, as well as the package insert, is part of the packaging requirements for all prescription drugs. The package insert is the official brochure setting forth the indications, contraindications, warnings, and dosing for the drug.

The prescriber controls who may obtain prescription drugs by writing and signing a prescription order. The pharmacist may purchase these drugs, but they may only be dispensed on the order of a legally qualified prescriber. The patient may only legally possess these drugs when the drug vial or container has the pharmacist's label properly affixed to it. Thus, a "prescription" is actually 3 things: the physician's order, the written order to which the pharmacist refers when dispensing, and the patient's medication vial with a label affixed.

While the federal government controls the drugs and their labeling and distribution, the individual states control who may prescribe drugs through their licensing boards, ie, the Board of Medical Examiners. Physicians, dentists, veterinarians, and podiatrists acting within the scope of their practice are licensed to prescribe drugs. These prescribers must pass examinations, pay fees, and—in the case of some states and some professions—meet other requirements for relicensure such as continuing education. If these requirements are met, the prescriber is licensed to order dispensing of drugs.

The federal government and the states further impose special restrictions on drugs with a potential for abuse. Drugs with abuse potential include opiates, hallucinogens, stimulants, and depressants (Chapter 29). Special requirements must be met when these drugs are to be prescribed. The Controlled Drug Act requires prescribers and dispensers to register with the Drug Enforcement Agency (DEA), pay a fee, receive a personal registration number, and keep records of all controlled drugs prescribed or dispensed. The registration period is for 1 year. Every time a controlled drug is prescribed, a valid DEA number must appear on the prescription blank. Controlled drugs are classified according to their potential for abuse as shown in Table 66–1.

Prescriptions for substances with a high potential for abuse (class II) cannot be refilled. Prescriptions for class III, IV, and V drugs can be refilled, but there is a

Table 66–1. Classification of controlled substances. (See inside front cover for examples.)

	Potential For Abuse	Other
Class I	High	No accepted medical use; lack of accepted safety as drug.
Class II	High	Current accepted medical use. Abuse may lead to severe psychologic or physical dependence.
Class III	Less than I or II	Current accepted medical use. Moderate or low potential for physical dependence and high potential for psychologic dependence.
Class IV	Less than III	Current accepted medical use. Limited potential for dependence.
Class V	Less than IV	Current accepted medical use. Limited dependence possible.

5-refill maximum, and in no case may the prescription be refilled after 6 months from the date of writing. Class II drug prescriptions may not be transmitted over the telephone, and some states require a special state-issued prescription blank. These restrictive prescribing laws are intended to limit the amount of drugs of abuse that are made available to the public.

THE PRESCRIPTION

While a prescription can be written on any piece of paper (as long as all of the legal elements are present), it usually takes a particular form. A typical printed prescription form for outpatients is shown in Fig 66–1.

In the hospital setting, drugs are prescribed on a particular page of the patient's hospital chart called the physician's order sheet. Such a prescription order is known as a **chart order,** and the contents of that prescription are specified by the medical staff rules. The patient's name is typed or written on the form; therefore, the orders consist of the name and strength of the medication, the dose, the route and frequency of administration, other pertinent information, and the signature of the prescriber. Often the duration of therapy or the number of doses is not specified; therefore, medications are continued until the prescriber discontinues the order or until it is terminated as a matter of policy routine.

A typical chart order might be as follows:

6/14/82 (1) Ampicillin 500 mg IV q6h × 5 days
(2) ASA 0.6 g per rectum q4h prn temp over 101.

(Signed) John B. Doe, M.D.

Thus, the elements of the hospital chart order are equivalent to the central elements (8–11) of the outpatient prescription.

Whether in the hospital or in an office practice setting, the implications of each element of the prescription should be understood.

Elements of the Prescription

The first 4 elements of the outpatient prescription establish the identity of the prescriber: name, license classification (ie, professional degree), address, and office telephone number. Before dispensing a prescription, the pharmacist must establish the prescriber's bona fides and should be able to contact the prescriber by telephone should any question arise. Element 5 is the date the prescription was written. It should be near the top of the prescription form or at the beginning (left margin) of the order. Since the order has legal significance and usually has some temporal relationship to the date of the patient-physician interview, a pharmacist should refuse to fill a prescription without verification by telephone if too much time has elapsed since its writing.

Elements ⑥ and ⑦ identify the patient by name and address. The patient's name and full address should be clearly spelled out.

The body of the prescription contains the elements ⑧ to ⑪ that specify the medication, the quantity to be dispensed, the dose, and complete directions for use. When writing the drug name (element ⑧), either the brand name (proprietary name) or generic name (nonproprietary name) may be used. Reasons for using one or the other are discussed below. The strength of the medication (element ⑨) should be written in metric units. However, the prescriber should be familiar with both systems now in use: apothecary and metric. For practical purposes, the following approximate conversions are useful:

1 grain (gr) = 0.065 grams (g), or about 60 milligrams (mg)
15 gr = 1 g
1 ounce (oz) = 30 milliliters (mL)
1 teaspoonful (tsp) = 5 mL
1 tablespoonful (tbsp) = 15 mL
1 quart (qt) = 1000 mL
20 drops (gtt) = 1 mL
2.2 pounds (lb) = 1 kilogram (kg)
1 minim = 1 drop

The strength of a solution is usually expressed as the quantity of solute in sufficient solvent to make 100 mL; for instance, 20% potassium chloride solution is 20 grams per deciliter (g/dL).

The quantity of medication prescribed should reflect the anticipated length of therapy, the cost, the need for continued contact with the clinic or physician, the potential for abuse, and the potential for toxicity or overdose. Consideration should be given also to the standard sizes in which the product is available and whether this is the initial prescription of the drug or a repeat prescription or refill. If 10 days of therapy are required to effectively cure a streptococcal infection, an appropriate quantity for the full course should be prescribed. Birth control pills are often prescribed for 1 year or until the next examination is due; however, some patients may not be able to afford a year's supply at one time; therefore, a 3-month supply might be ordered, with refill instructions to renew 3 times or for 1 year (element ⑫). Finally, when first prescribing medications that are to be used for the treatment of a chronic disease, the initial quantity should be small, with refills for larger quantities. The purpose of beginning treatment with a small quantity of drug is to reduce the cost if the patient cannot tolerate the drug. Once it is determined that tolerance is not a problem, a larger quantity purchased less frequently is usually less expensive.

The directions for use (element ⑪) must be drug-specific and patient-specific. The simpler the directions, the better; and the fewer the number of doses (and drugs) per day, the better. Patient noncompliance (failure to adhere to the drug regimen) is a major cause of treatment failure. To help patients remember to take

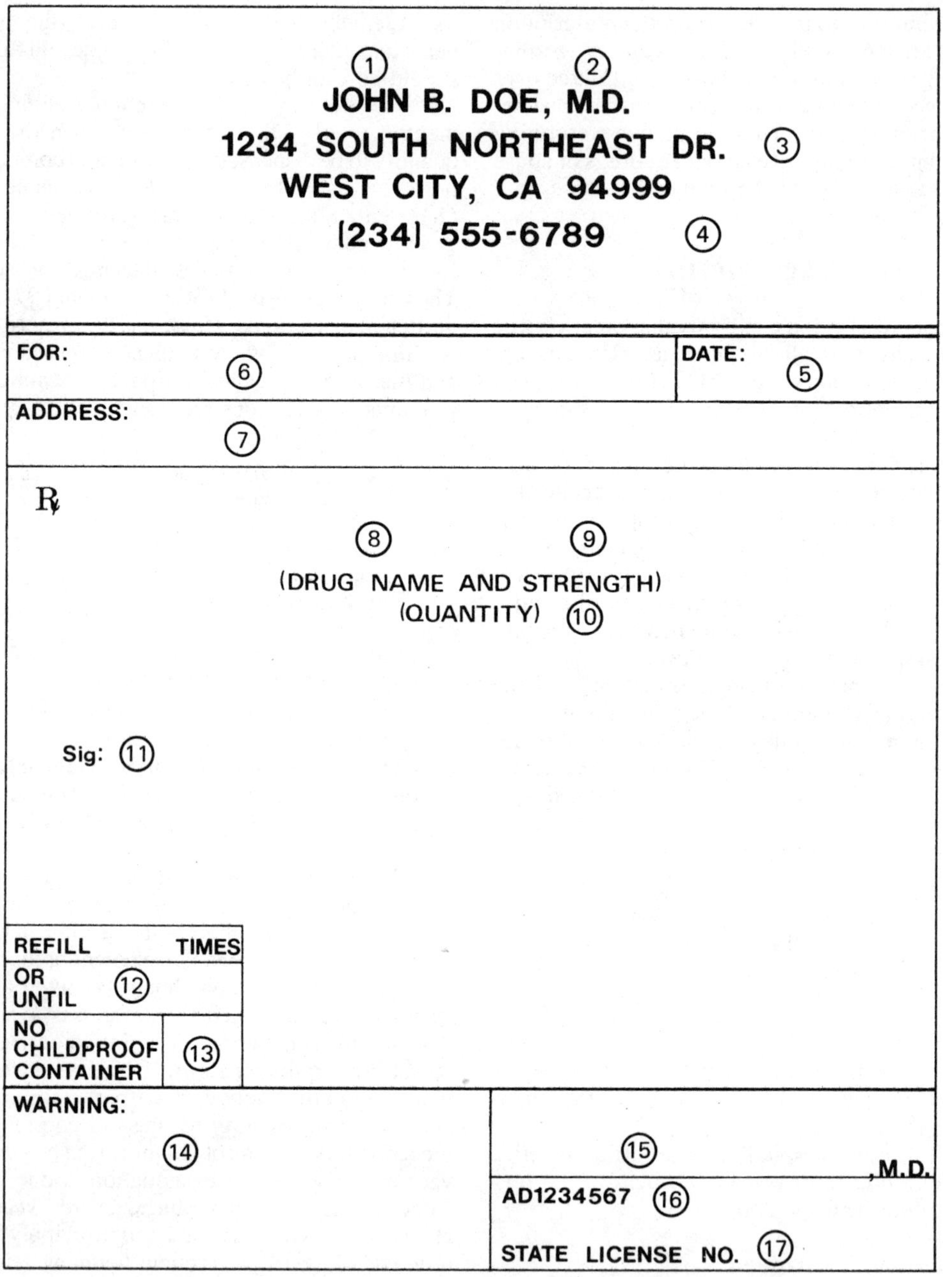

Figure 66–1. Common form of outpatient prescription. Circled numbers are explained in the text.

their medications, prescribers often give an instruction that medications be taken at or around mealtimes and at bedtime. However, it is important to inquire about the patient's eating habits and other life-style patterns, since many patients do not eat 3 regularly spaced meals a day, especially if they are sick or dieting.

The instructions on how and when to take medications, the duration of therapy, and the purpose of the medication must be explained to each patient by the physician and by the pharmacist. Furthermore, the drug name, the purpose for which it is given, and the duration of therapy should be written on each label so that the drug may be identified easily in case of overdose. An instruction to "take as directed" may save the time it takes to write the orders out but often leads to noncompliance, patient confusion, and medication error. The directions for use must be clear and concise to avoid toxicity and to obtain the greatest benefits from therapy.

Patient education has been of concern to the FDA and professional groups and has resulted in several experimental programs. The United States Pharmacopeial Convention (USP) annually publishes a 2-volume work entitled *USP-DI* [“dispensing information”]. The first volume contains information for the professional (prescriber) and the second consists of short informational notes prepared for patients' use in understanding the drugs they are given. About 300 medications are covered in the current (1983) edition. Information about *USP-DI* may be obtained from the USP Drug Information Division, 12601 Twinbrook Parkway, Rockville, MD 20852.

A new program sponsored by the American Medical Association has the potential for similar usefulness to patients. Patient medication instruction (PMI) sheets are being prepared that provide patient information about individual drugs or classes of drugs. The content of the PMI sheet is very similar to that of the *USP-DI* note for the same drug. It is hoped that PMI sheets for about 80 medications will be made available during the next 2 years. The PMI sheets will be distributed by prescribers at their discretion directly to patients.

Although directions for use are no longer written in Latin, many Latin apothecary abbreviations (and some others included below) are still in use. Knowledge of these abbreviations is essential for the dispensing pharmacist and often useful for the prescriber. Abbreviations still commonly used are listed below.

Dose
- **dr,** teaspoonful
- **g** or **gm,** gram
- **gr,** grain
- **gtt,** drops
- **mcg, μg,** microgram
- **mg,** milligram

Route
- **ad,** right ear
- **as,** left ear
- **au,** each ear
- **od,** right eye
- **os,** left eye
- **ou,** each eye
- **po,** by mouth
- **supp,** suppository
- **vag,** vaginally

Frequency
- **ac,** before meals
- **ad lib,** freely at pleasure
- **bid,** twice a day
- **h,** hour
- **hs,** at bedtime
- **pc,** after meals
- **prn,** as needed
- **q,** every
- **qd,** every day
- **qid,** four times daily
- **qod,** every other day
- **stat,** at once, immediately
- **tid,** three times daily
- **ut dict,** as directed

Miscellaneous
- **$\bar{a}\bar{a}$,** of each
- **cap,** capsule
- **$\bar{c}$,** with
- **n.r.,** no refill
- **qs ad,** add a sufficient amount to make
- **rep,** repeat, refill
- **$\bar{s}$,** without
- **$\overline{ss}$,** one-half
- **sig,** directions for use
- **tab,** tablet

Elements ⑫ to ⑭ of the prescription include refill information, waiver of the requirement for childproof containers, and additional labeling instructions (eg, name of drug on label, “may cause drowsiness,” “do not drink alcohol”). Most pharmacists now put the name of the medication on the label unless directed otherwise by the prescriber (some medications have the name of the drug stamped or imprinted on the tablet or capsule). Pharmacists should place the expiratory date for the drug on the label. If the patient or prescriber does not request waiver of childproof containers, the pharmacist or dispenser must place the medication in such a container. Pharmacists may not refill a prescription medication without authorization from the prescriber. Prescribers may grant authorization to renew prescriptions at the time of writing the prescription or over the telephone. Finally, the prescriber may request that special warning notices be placed on the label by the pharmacist.

Elements ⑮ to ⑰ are the prescriber's signature and other identification data.

SOCIOECONOMIC FACTORS

Generic Prescribing

Prescribing by generic name offers the pharmacist flexibility in selecting the particular drug product to fill the order and the patient a potential savings if there is price competition. The brand name of a popular diuretic is, eg, Esidrix by Ciba. The generic (public, nonproprietary) name of the same chemical substance adopted by United States Adopted Names (USAN) and approved by the Food and Drug Administration (FDA) is hydrochlorothiazide. All hydrochlorothiazide drug products in the USA meet the pharmaceutical standards expressed in *United States Pharmacopeia* (USP). However, there are many manufacturers, and prices vary as much as 2-fold. For other drugs, the difference in cost between the brand name product and generic products varies from less than 2-fold to more than 10-fold.

In some states and in many hospitals, pharmacists have the option of supplying a generically equivalent drug product even if a proprietary name has been specified in the order. In office practice, drug product selection laws enable the pharmacist to make that selection, and in many hospitals the pharmacy and therapeutics committee through its drug formulary policies establish the dispensing practices of the pharmacist. If the physician wants a particular brand of drug product dispensed, handwritten instruction to “dispense as written” or words of similar meaning are required. Some government-subsidized health care programs require that pharmacists dispense the cheapest generically equivalent product in the inventory. However, the principles of drug product selection by pharmacists do not permit substituting one therapeutic agent for another; ie, dispensing trichlormethiazide for hydrochlorothiazide would not be permitted without the prescriber's permission even though the 2 drugs may be considered pharmacodynamically equivalent.

It should not be assumed that all generic drug products are as satisfactory as brand-named products. Bioavailability—the effective absorption of the drug product—varies between manufacturers and sometimes between different lots of a drug produced by the same manufacturer. In the case of drugs with a low therapeutic index, poor solubility, or a high ratio of inert ingredients to active drug content, a specific manufacturer's product might well give superior results. In the case of life-threatening diseases, the advantages of generic substitution are probably outweighed by the clinical urgency so that the prescription should be filled as written.

Other Cost Factors

The private pharmacist bases his or her charges on the cost of the drug plus a fee for providing a professional service. Each time a prescription is dispensed, there is a fee. The prescriber controls the frequency of filling prescriptions by authorizing refills and specifying the quantity to be dispensed. Thus, the prescriber can save the patient money by prescribing standard sizes (so that drugs do not have to be repackaged) and, when chronic treatment is involved, by ordering the largest quantity consistent with safety and expense. Thus, optimal prescribing often involves consultation between the prescriber and the pharmacist.

• • •

References

Business and Professions Code, Chap 9, Div 2, Pharmacy Law. Department of Consumer Affairs, Sacramento, Calif, 1979.

Final Report: Task Force on Prescription Drugs. Department of Health, Education, and Welfare, 1969.

Hoover JE: *Dispensing of Medication*, 8th ed. Mack Publishing Co., 1976.

Hoover JE: *Remington's Pharmaceutical Sciences*, 16th ed. Mack Publishing Co., 1980.

Jerome JB, Sagan P: The USAN nomenclature system. *JAMA* 1975;**232:**294.

Kickoff for AMA's new PMI program. (Medical News.) *JAMA* 1982;**248:**1031.

United States Pharmacopeial Convention: *1983 USP-DI*. Vol 1: *Advice for the Health Care Provider;* Vol 2: *Advice for the Patient*. United States Pharmacopeial Convention, Inc., 1982.

Appendix I: Important Drug Interactions

Philip D. Hansten, PharmD

MECHANISMS OF DRUG INTERACTIONS

One of the factors that can alter the response to drugs is the concurrent administration of other drugs. There are several mechanisms by which drugs may interact, but most can be categorized as pharmacokinetic (absorption, distribution, metabolism, excretion), pharmadocynamic, or combined toxicity.

Pharmacokinetic Mechanisms

The gastrointestinal **absorption** of drugs may be affected by concurrent use of other agents that (1) have a large surface area upon which the drug can be adsorbed, (2) bind or chelate, or (3) alter gastrointestinal motility. One must distinguish between effects on absorption *rate* and effects on *extent* of absorption. A reduction in only the absorption rate of a drug is seldom clinically important, whereas a reduction in the extent of absorption may be clinically important if it is of sufficient magnitude to result in subtherapeutic serum levels of the drug.

The mechanisms by which drug interactions alter drug **distribution** include (1) competition for plasma protein binding and (2) displacement from tissue binding sites. Although competition for plasma protein binding can increase the free concentration (and thus the effect) of the displaced drug in plasma, the increase tends to be temporary owing to a compensatory increase in drug disposition. The importance of protein binding displacement has probably been overemphasized; only a few drugs are known to manifest clinically important interactions by this mechanism (eg, oral anticoagulants, sulfonylureas, hypoglycemics). Displacement from tissue binding sites would tend to increase the blood concentration of the displaced drug. Such a mechanism is partially responsible for the elevation of serum digoxin concentration by concurrent quinidine therapy.

The **metabolism** of drugs can be stimulated or inhibited by concurrent therapy. Induction (stimulation) of hepatic microsomal drug-metabolizing enzymes can be produced by drugs such as barbiturates, carbamazepine, phenytoin, primidone, and rifampin. Enzyme induction does not take place quickly; maximal effects usually occur after 7–10 days and require an equal or longer time to dissipate after the enzyme inducer is stopped. Drugs that may inhibit hepatic microsomal metabolism of other drugs include cimetidine, disulfiram, metronidazole, phenylbutazone, and sulfonamides. Inhibition of metabolism generally takes place more quickly than enzyme induction and may begin as soon as sufficient hepatic concentration of the inhibitor is achieved. However, if the half-life of the affected drug is long, it may take a week or more to reach a new steady-state serum level.

The renal **excretion** of active drug can also be affected by concurrent drug therapy. The renal excretion of certain drugs that are weak acids or weak bases may be influenced by other drugs that affect urinary pH. This is due to changes in ionization of the drug, thus altering its lipid solubility and therefore its ability to be reabsorbed back into the blood from the kidney tubule. For some drugs, active secretion into the renal tubules is an important elimination pathway. This process may be affected by concurrent drug therapy, thus altering serum drug levels and pharmacologic response.

Pharmacodynamic Mechanisms

When drugs with similar pharmacologic effects are administered concurrently, an additive or synergistic response is usually seen. The 2 drugs may or may not act on the same receptor to produce such effects. Conversely, drugs with opposing pharmacologic effects may reduce the response to one or both drugs. Pharmacodynamic drug interactions are relatively common in clinical practice, but adverse effects can be minimized if the interactions are anticipated and appropriate countermeasures taken.

Combined Toxicity

The combined use of 2 or more drugs, each of which has toxic effects on a given organ, can greatly increase the likelihood of organ damage. For example, concurrent administration of 2 nephrotoxic drugs can produce kidney damage even though the dose of either drug alone may have been insufficient to produce toxicity. Furthermore, some drugs can enhance the organ toxicity of another drug even though the enhancing drug has no intrinsic toxic effect on that organ.

PREDICTABILITY OF DRUG INTERACTIONS

The designations listed below will be used here to *estimate* the predictability of the drug interactions. These estimates are intended to indicate simply whether or not the interaction will occur and do not always mean that the interaction is likely to produce an adverse effect. Whether the interaction produces an adverse effect or not depends upon (1) the presence or absence of factors that predispose to the adverse effects of the drug interaction (diseases, organ function, dose of drugs, etc) and (2) *awareness* on the part of the prescriber, so that appropriate monitoring can be ordered or preventive measures taken.

HP	Highly predictable. Interaction occurs in almost all patients receiving the combination of 2 or more drugs.
P	Predictable. Interaction occurs in most patients receiving the combination.
NP	Not predictable. Interaction occurs only in some patients receiving the combination.
NE	Not established. Insufficient data available on which to base estimate of predictability.

ALCOHOL

Properties Promoting Interaction

(1) Chronic alcoholism results in enzyme induction.

(2) Acute alcohol intoxication tends to inhibit drug metabolism (whether person is alcoholic or not).

(3) Severe alcohol-induced hepatic dysfunction may inhibit ability to metabolize drugs.

(4) Alcohol may induce a disulfiramlike reaction in the presence of certain drugs.

(5) Additive central nervous system depression with other central nervous system depressants.

Clinically Documented Interactions

Acetaminophen: [NE] Increased formation of hepatotoxic metabolites.

Central nervous system depressants: [HP] Additive or synergistic central nervous system depression.

Insulin: [NE] Acute alcohol intake may increase hypoglycemic effect (especially in fasting patients).

Drugs that may produce a disulfiramlike reaction:

- Chloral hydrate: [NP] Mechanism not established.
- Disulfiram: [HP] Inhibits aldehyde dehydrogenase.
- Metronidazole: [NP] Mechanism not established.
- Sulfonylureas: [NE] Chlorpropamide is most likely to produce a disulfiramlike reaction; acute alcohol intake may increase hypoglycemic effect (especially in fasting patients).

ANTACIDS

Properties Promoting Interaction

(1) Antacids may adsorb drugs in gastrointestinal tract, thus reducing absorption.

(2) Antacids tend to speed gastric emptying, thus delivering drugs to absorbing sites in the intestine more quickly.

(3) Some antacids (eg, magnesium hydroxide + aluminum hydroxide) alkalinize the urine somewhat, thus altering excretion of drugs sensitive to urinary pH.

Clinically Documented Interactions

Digoxin: [NP] Reduced gastrointestinal absorption of digoxin.

Sodium polystyrene sulfonate: [NE] Binds antacid cation in gut, resulting in metabolic alkalosis.

Tetracyclines: [HP] Reduced gastrointestinal absorption of tetracyclines.

ANTICHOLINERGICS

Properties Promoting Drug Interaction

(1) Decreased gastrointestinal motility. This may increase bioavailability of poorly soluble drugs and reduce bioavailability of drugs degraded in gut.

(2) Combined use of more than one anticholinergic increases likelihood of anticholinergic adverse effects.

Clinically Documented Interactions

Levodopa: [P] Increased degradation of levodopa in gut; serum levodopa levels lowered.

Combined anticholinergics: [P] Anticholinergic adverse effects (eg, paralytic ileus, urinary retention, blurred vision).

ANTICOAGULANTS, ORAL

Properties Promoting Drug Interaction

(1) Susceptible to enzyme induction.

(2) Susceptible to inhibition of metabolism.

(3) Highly bound to plasma proteins.

(4) Anticoagulant response altered by drugs that affect clotting factor synthesis or catabolism.

Clinically Documented Interactions

Drugs that may increase anticoagulant effect:

- Allopurinol: [P] Inhibits anticoagulant metabolism.
- Anabolic steroids: [P] Alter clotting factor disposition?
- Chloramphenicol: [NE] Inhibits dicumarol metabolism (possibly also warfarin).
- Cimetidine: [HP] Inhibits anticoagulant metabolism.
- Clofibrate: [P] Mechanism not established.
- Dextrothyroxine: [P] Enhances clotting factor catabolism?

Disulfiram: [P] Inhibits anticoagulant metabolism.
Metronidazole: [P] Inhibits anticoagulant metabolism.
Oxyphenbutazone: [HP] Inhibits anticoagulant metabolism.
Phenylbutazone: [HP] Inhibits anticoagulant metabolism.
Quinidine: [NP] Additive hypoprothrombinemia.
Salicylates: [HP] Platelet inhibition; [P] Large doses have hypoprothrombinemic effect.
Sulfinpyrazone: [NE] Mechanism not established.
Sulindac: [NP] Mechanism not established.
Sulfonamides: [NE] Inhibit anticoagulant metabolism; displace protein binding.
Thyroid hormones: [P] Enhance clotting factor catabolism.

Drugs that may decrease anticoagulant effect:
Barbiturates: [P] Enzyme induction.
Carbamazepine: [P] Enzyme induction.
Cholestyramine: [P] Reduces absorption of anticoagulant.
Glutethimide: [P] Enzyme induction.
Primidone: [P] Enzyme induction.
Rifampin: [P] Enzyme induction.

Effects of anticoagulants on other drugs:
Hypoglycemics, oral: [P] Dicumarol inhibits hepatic metabolism of tolbutamide and chlorpropamide.
Phenytoin: [P] Dicumarol inhibits metabolism of phenytoin.

BARBITURATES

Properties Promoting Interaction

(1) Induction of hepatic microsomal drug-metabolizing enzymes.

(2) Additive central nervous system depression with other central nervous system depressants.

Clinically Documented Interactions

Antidepressants, tricyclic: [P] Increased antidepressant metabolism.
Beta-adrenergic blockers: [P] Increased beta-blocker metabolism.
Central nervous system depressants: [HP] Additive central nervous system depression.
Corticosteroids: [P] Increased corticosteroid metabolism.
Doxycycline: [P] Increased doxycycline metabolism.
Estrogens: [P] Increased estrogen metabolism.
Phenothiazines: [P] Increased phenothiazine metabolism.
Quinidine: [P] Increased quinidine metabolism.
Valproic acid: [P] Decreased phenobarbital metabolism.
See also Anticoagulants, Oral.

BETA-ADRENERGIC BLOCKERS

Properties Promoting Drug Interaction

(1) Beta blockade (especially with nonspecific agents such as propranolol) alters response to sympathomimetics with beta-agonist activity (eg, epinephrine).

(2) Beta-blockers that undergo extensive first-pass metabolism may be affected by drugs capable of altering this process.

(3) Beta-blockers may reduce hepatic blood flow.

Clinically Documented Interactions

Drugs that may increase beta-blocker effect:
Chlorpromazine: [P] Reduces metabolism of propranolol.
Cimetidine: [P] Reduces metabolism of propranolol; additive bradycardia.
Furosemide: [P] Reduces metabolism of propranolol.
Hydralazine: [P] Reduces metabolism of propranolol.

Drugs that may decrease beta-blocker effect:
Enzyme inducers: [P] Barbiturates and phenytoin may enhance beta-blocker metabolism; other enzyme inducers may produce similar effects.
Indomethacin: [P] Reduces antihypertensive response; other prostaglandin inhibitors might also interact.

Effects of beta-blockers on other drugs:
Clonidine: [NE] Hypertensive reaction if clonidine is withdrawn while patient is taking propranolol.
Lidocaine: [NE] Reduced plasma clearance of intravenous lidocaine; increased plasma lidocaine levels.
Sympathomimetics: [P] Enhanced pressor response to epinephrine (and possibly other sympathomimetics); this is more likely to occur with nonspecific beta-blockers.

BILE ACID–BINDING RESINS
(Cholestyramine, Colestipol)

Properties Promoting Interaction

(1) Resins may bind with orally administered drugs in gastrointestinal tract.

(2) Resins may bind in gastrointestinal tract with drugs that undergo enterohepatic circulation, even if the latter are given parenterally.

Clinically Documented Interactions

Digitalis glycosides: [NE] Reduced gastrointestinal absorption of digitoxin (possibly also digoxin).
Thiazide diuretics: [P] Reduced gastrointestinal absorption of thiazides.
Thyroid hormones: [P] Reduced thyroid absorption.
See also Anticoagulants, Oral.

CARBAMAZEPINE

Properties Promoting Interaction

(1) Induces hepatic microsomal drug-metabolizing enzymes.

(2) Susceptible to inhibition of metabolism.

Clinically Documented Interactions

Doxycycline: [P] Increased doxycycline metabolism.
Estrogens: [P] Increased estrogen metabolism.
Propoxyphene: [HP] Decreased carbamazepine metabolism.
Troleandomycin: [P] Decreased carbamazepine metabolism.
See also Anticoagulants, Oral.

CHLORAMPHENICOL

Properties Promoting Interaction

Inhibits hepatic drug-metabolizing enzymes.

Clinically Documented Interactions

Sulfonylurea hypoglycemics: [P] Inhibited sulfonylurea metabolism.
Phenytoin: [P] Inhibited phenytoin metabolism.
See also Anticoagulants, Oral.

CIMETIDINE

Properties Promoting Drug Interaction

(1) Inhibits hepatic microsomal drug-metabolizing enzymes.

(2) May reduce hepatic blood flow, thus reducing first-pass metabolism of highly extracted drugs.

(3) May increase bone marrow suppression caused by other drugs.

Clinically Documented Interactions

Benzodiazepines: [P] Inhibit metabolism of chlordiazepoxide, diazepam, prazepam, and clorazepate but not oxazepam or lorazepam.
Lidocaine: [P] Inhibits metabolism of lidocaine; increased serum lidocaine.
Phenytoin: [NE] Inhibits phenytoin metabolism; increased serum phenytoin.
Theophylline: [P] Inhibits theophylline metabolism; increased plasma theophylline.

DIGITALIS GLYCOSIDES

Properties Promoting Drug Interaction

(1) Digoxin susceptible to inhibition of gastrointestinal absorption.

(2) Digitalis toxicity may be increased by drug-induced electrolyte imbalance (eg, hypokalemia).

(3) Digitoxin susceptible to enzyme induction.

(4) Renal excretion of digoxin susceptible to inhibition.

Clinically Documented Interactions

Drugs that may increase digitalis effect:
Nifedipine: [P] Increased serum digoxin levels.
Potassium depleting drugs: [P] Increased likelihood of digitalis toxicity.
Quinidine: [HP] Reduced renal digoxin excretion; displacement of digoxin from tissue binding sites; digitoxin may also be affected.
Verapamil: [P] Increased serum digoxin levels.

Drugs that may decrease digitalis effect:
Antacids: [NP] Reduced gastrointestinal digoxin absorption.
Kaolin-pectin: [P] Reduced gastrointestinal digoxin absorption.
Penicillamine: [NE] Decreased serum digoxin.
Sulfasalazine: [NE] Reduced gastrointestinal digoxin absorption.
See also Bile Acid-Binding Resins.

DISULFIRAM

Properties Promoting Interaction

(1) Inhibits hepatic microsomal drug-metabolizing enzymes.

(2) Inhibits aldehyde dehydrogenase.

Clinically Documented Interactions

Benzodiazepines: [P] Inhibits metabolism of chlordiazepoxide and diazepam but not lorazepam and oxazepam.
Phenytoin: [P] Inhibits phenytoin metabolism.
See also Alcohol; Anticoagulants, Oral.

ESTROGENS

Properties Promoting Interaction

(1) Susceptible to enzyme induction.

(2) Enterohepatic circulation of estrogen may be interrupted by alteration in bowel flora (eg, due to antibiotics).

Clinically Documented Interactions

Ampicillin: [NP] Interruption of enterohepatic circulation of estrogen; possible reduction in oral contraceptive efficacy.
Phenytoin: [NP] Increased estrogen metabolism; possible reduction in oral contraceptive efficacy.
Rifampin: [NP] Increased estrogen metabolism; possible reduction in oral contraceptive efficacy.
See also Barbiturates, Carbamazepine.

LEVODOPA

Properties Promoting Interaction

(1) Levodopa degraded in gut prior to reaching sites of absorption. Agents that alter gastrointestinal motility may alter degree of intraluminal degradation.

(2) Antiparkinsonism effect of levodopa susceptible to inhibition by other drugs.

Clinically Documented Interactions

Clonidine: [NE] Inhibits antiparkinsonism effect.
Monoamine oxidase inhibitors: [P] Hypertensive reaction (carbidopa prevents the interaction).
Papaverine: [NE] Inhibits antiparkinsonism effect.
Phenothiazines: [P] Inhibits antiparkinsonism effect.
Phenytoin: [NE] Inhibits antiparkinsonism effect.
Pyridoxine: [P] Inhibits antiparkinsonism effect (carbidopa prevents the interaction).
See also Anticholinergics.

LITHIUM

Properties Promoting Interaction

(1) Renal lithium excretion sensitive to changes in sodium balance. (Sodium depletion tends to cause lithium retention.)

(2) Susceptible to drugs enhancing central nervous system lithium toxicity.

Clinically Documented Interactions

Diuretics (sodium-depleting): [P] Reduced renal excretion of lithium; furosemide may be less likely to produce this effect than thiazide diuretics.
Haloperidol: [NP] Occasional cases of neurotoxicity in manic patients, especially with large doses of one or both drugs.
Methyldopa: [NE] Increased likelihood of central nervous system lithium toxicity.
Nonsteroidal anti-inflammatory drugs (NSAIDs): [NE] Indomethacin reduces renal lithium excretion; possibly other NSAID do the same.

MONOAMINE OXIDASE INHIBITORS (MAOI)

Properties Promoting Interaction

(1) Increase norepinephrine stored in adrenergic neuron. Displacement of these stores by other drugs may produce acute hypertensive response.

(2) MAOI have intrinsic hypoglycemic activity.

Clinically Documented Interactions

Antidiabetic agents: [P] Additive hypoglycemic effect.
Guanethidine: [P] Reversal of the hypotensive action of guanethidine.
Narcotic analgesics: [NP] Some patients develop hypertension, rigidity, excitation; Meperidine may be more likely to interact than morphine.
Phenylephrine: [P] Hypertensive episode, since phenylephrine is metabolized by monoamine oxidase.
Sympathomimetics (Indirect Acting): [HP] Hypertensive episode due to release of stored norepinephrine.
See also Levodopa.

NONSTEROIDAL ANTI-INFLAMMATORY DRUGS (NSAIDs)

Properties Promoting Interaction

(1) Prostaglandin inhibition may result in reduced renal sodium excretion, impaired resistance to hypertensive stimuli, and reduced renal lithium excretion.

(2) Most NSAIDs inhibit platelet function; may increase likelihood of bleeding due to other drugs that impair hemostasis.

(3) Most NSAIDs are highly bound to plasma proteins.

(4) Phenylbutazone may inhibit hepatic microsomal drug metabolism (also seems to act as enzyme inducer in some cases).

(5) Phenylbutazone may alter renal excretion of some drugs.

Clinically Documented Interactions

Furosemide: [P] Reduced diuretic, natriuretic, and antihypertensive response to furosemide with indomethacin (possibly also other NSAIDs).
Lithium: [P] Reduced renal lithium excretion with indomethacin (possibly also other NSAIDs).
Phenytoin: [P] Reduced hepatic phenytoin metabolism.
Thiazides: [P] Reduced antihypertensive response to thiazides.
Triamterene: [NE] Reduced renal function noted with triamterene plus indomethacin; effect was reversible.
See also Anticoatulants, Oral; Beta-Adrenergic Blockers.

PHENYTOIN

Properties Promoting Interaction

(1) Induces hepatic microsomal drug metabolism.

(2) Susceptible to inhibition of metabolism.

Clinically Documented Interactions

Drugs whose metabolism is stimulated by phenytoin:
- Corticosteroids: [P] Reduced serum corticosteroid levels.
- Doxycycline: [P] Reduced serum doxycycline levels.
- Methadone: [P] Reduced serum methadone levels; withdrawal symptoms.
- Quinidine: [P] Reduced serum quinidine levels.

See also Estrogens.

Drugs that inhibit phenytoin metabolism:
- Chloramphenicol: [P] Increased serum phenytoin.
- Isoniazid: [NP] Increased serum phenytoin; problem primarily with slow acetylators of isoniazid.
- *See also* Disulfiram; Phenylbutazone.

PROBENECID

Properties Promoting Interaction

(1) Interference with renal excretion of drugs that undergo active tubular secretion, especially weak acids.

(2) Inhibition of glucuronide conjugation of other drugs.

Clinically Documented Interactions
- Clofibrate: [P] Reduced glucuronide conjugation of clofibric acid.
- Methotrexate: [P] Reduced renal methotrexate excretion.
- Penicillin: [P] Reduced renal penicillin excretion.
- Salicylates: [P] Reduced uricosuric effect of probenecid (interaction unlikely with less than 1.5 g of salicylate daily).

QUINIDINE

Properties Promoting Interaction

(1) Susceptible to enzyme induction.

(2) Renal excretion susceptible to changes in urine pH.

Clinically Documented Interactions
- Acetazolamide: [P] Reduced renal quinidine excretion due to increased urinary pH; elevated serum quinidine.
- Rifampin: [P] Enhanced hepatic quinidine metabolism.
- *See also* Anticoagulants, Oral; Barbiturates; Digitalis Glycosides; Phenytoin.

THEOPHYLLINE

Properties Promoting Interaction

(1) Susceptible to inhibition of hepatic metabolism.

(2) Susceptible to enhanced hepatic metabolism.

Clinically Documented Interactions
- Erythromycin: [P] Inhibition of hepatic theophylline metabolism.
- Smoking: [HP] Enhanced hepatic theophylline metabolism.
- Troleandomycin: [P] Inhibition of hepatic theophylline metabolism.
- *See also* Cimetidine.

• • •

References

Cluff LE, Petrie JC: *Clinical Effects of Interaction Between Drugs*. Excerpta Medica, 1974.

Cohen SN, Armstrong MF: *Drug Interactions: A Handbook for Clinical Use*. Williams & Wilkins, 1974.

Hansten PD: *Drug Interactions*. Lea & Febiger, 1979.

Smith NT, Miller RD, Cobascio AN: *Drug Interactions in Anesthesia*. Lea & Febiger, 1981.

Appendix II: Drug Effects on Laboratory Tests

Philip D. Hansten, PharmD, & Lisa A. Lybecker, RPh

THE EFFECTS OF DRUGS ON COMMON CLINICAL LABORATORY PROCEDURES (Table 1)

With the increasing number of available drugs and the increasing number and complexity of tests performed by the clinical laboratory, drug-induced interference with test results is occurring with greater frequency. Table 1 has been prepared to assist clinicians and laboratory personnel in identifying such drug effects. In an effort to keep the information clinically relevant, no information from in vitro or animal studies has been included.

Although an effort has been made to cover each area thoroughly, it is inevitable that a listing of this type will be incomplete. The reader may wish to add to the chart on the basis of personal reading and experience.

Types of Drug Interference

Alterations in clinical laboratory results caused by drugs may be grouped into 2 general categories:

A. Effects Due to Pharmacologic or Toxic Properties of Drugs: Here, a true change is produced in the level of the parameter being measured. In Table 1, changes of this nature are designated as increase (+) or decrease (−). The magnitude of the change depends upon a variety of factors such as dosage of drug, duration of administration, condition of patient, etc.

B. Effects Due to Interference With the Testing Procedure: In this case, the drug or its metabolite becomes a contaminant that may alter the value obtained or interfere with the measurement. This type of interference is indicated in Table 1 as increase (●) or decrease (○). It should be noted that drugs may affect one method of performing a given laboratory procedure and have no effect on another. For this reason, the specific testing method affected has been specified whenever possible.

Arrangement of Table 1

Table 1 lists the drugs that may affect the results of the laboratory tests indicated at the top. Tests less commonly influenced by drug administration are included in the column headed Other Tests.

All drugs are listed alphabetically by generic name, with common trade names and other names in parentheses. Some general drug classifications have been used. If a drug falls into one of the categories listed below, it should be sought under that general classification.

- Aluminum antacids
- Aminoglycosides
- Anabolic steroids
- Barbiturates
- Calcium antacids
- Cephalosporins
- Contrast media, iodine-containing
- Corticosteroids
- Digitalis glycosides
- Estrogens
- Gold salts
- Inorganic iodides
- Iron, oral
- Mercurial diuretics
- Monoamine oxidase inhibitors
- Oral contraceptives
- Phenothiazines
- Progestogens
- Salicylates
- Sulfonamides
- Tetracyclines
- Thiazide diuretics
- Tricyclic antidepressants

Table 1. Effects of drugs on common laboratory tests.

+ = Increase (pharmacologic or toxic effect)
– = Decrease (pharmacologic or toxic effect)
N = See notes (below)
● = Increase (test interference)
○ = Decrease (test interference)
★ = Present or positive

	BLOOD, SERUM, OR PLASMA													URINE										OTHER TESTS
	Amylase	Bilirubin	Cholesterol	Coombs (Direct)	CPK	Glucose	Thyroxine	Phosphatase, Alk.	Potassium	Prothrombin Time	SGOT and SGPT	Urea Nitrogen	Uric Acid	Color	Catecholamines	Glucose (Benedict)	5-HIAA	Ketones	Porphyrins	Protein	Steroids	Urobilinogen	VMA	
Acetaminophen		N		★		N					+						N							
Acetazolamide (Diamox)									–				+							●		+		Blood ammonia +
Acetohexamide (Dymelor)		+				–		+			+		–											
Alcohol, ethyl	+	–			N	–				N	N		+	N	+		–		N					Serum aldolase (N); plasma cortisol +; serum lactate +
Allopurinol (Zyloprim)		+						+		N	+	+	–											
Aluminum antacids																								Serum phosphate –
Aminocaproic acid (Amicar)					+				+															
Aminoglycosides			N									+								★		N		Blood ammonia (N); serum magnesium (N); urine estriol (N)
Aminosalicylic acid (PAS)	N		–				–		–	+	+			N		●			N					
Amphotericin B (Fungizone)		+			+				–			+								★				
Ampicillin				★	N						+													Urine estriol –
Anabolic steroids		+				N	–			N	N										N			
Ascorbic acid													N			N					N			
Asparaginase (Elspar)	+	+	–			+	–	+		+	+													Blood ammonia +; serum albumin –
Azathioprine (Imuran)	N	+						+			+		N											
Barbiturates	N	–						N		N									N					Metyrapone response –
Bromsulphalein (BSP)								N										N				●		
Caffeine						+							N		+								●	
Calcium antacids																								Serum calcium (N)
Captopril (Capoten)			+	★					+											★				Serum albumin –
Carbamazepine (Tegretol)		N						+		N	+										N			Serum sodium –

Acetaminophen:

Overdose may produce liver damage with hyperbilirubinemia.

Hypoglycemia has been reported with large doses, but false decreases have also been reported (glucose oxidase-peroxidase method).

May cause false increases in urinary 5-HIAA (screening methods using nitrosonaphthol reagent).

Alcohol, ethyl:

Acute intoxication may produce myopathy, with elevation of serum aldolase, CPK, and SGOT.

Acute intoxication may enhance hypoprothrombinemic effect of oral anticoagulants.

The diuresis produced results in a lighter urine.

Attacks of acute intermittent porphyria may be precipitated by ethanol.

Allopurinol:

May enhance hypoprothrombinemic effect of oral anticoagulants.

Aminoglycosides:

Oral aminoglycosides may decrease serum cholesterol.

Oral aminoglycosides may reduce urinary urobilinogen.

Oral aminoglycosides may decrease blood ammonia in patients with hepatic disease.

Gentamicin has been associated with decreased serum magnesium.

Oral aminoglycosides may decrease urinary estrogen excretion.

Aminosalicylic acid:

Reportedly may produce acute pancreatitis with elevated serum amylase.

May cause reddening of the urine if toilet bowl recently cleaned with hypochlorite bleach.

Will produce yellow color with Ehrlich's reagent test for porphobilinogen or urobilinogen.

Ampicillin:

Intramuscular ampicillin may result in increased serum CPK levels.

Anabolic steroids:

May decrease blood glucose in diabetic patients.

May enhance hypoprothrombinemic effect of oral anticoagulants.

Norethandrolone (Nilevar) may elevate SGOT.

Testosterone treatment increases urinary excretion of 17-ketosteroids, whereas methyltestosterone does not appear in the urine.

Ascorbic acid:

May produce false elevations in uric acid determinations (except enzymatic methods).

Large doses may produce false-positives by copper reduction methods (eg, Clinitest), and false negatives by glucose oxidase methods (eg, Clinistix, Tes-Tape).

May interfere with the determination of urinary 17-hydroxycorticosteroids by a modification of the Reddy, Jenkins, Thorn procedure (*Metabolism* 1952; **1**:511 and 1954;**3**:489).

Azathioprine:

Pancreatitis has been reported following azathioprine administration.

May decrease serum uric acid in patients with gout.

Barbiturates:

Serum amylase may be decreased in barbiturate poisoning.

Prolonged use of barbiturates as anticonvulsants has resulted in osteomalacia with elevated serum alkaline phosphatase.

May inhibit hypoprothrombinemic effect of oral anticoagulants.

Attacks of acute intermittent porphyria may be precipitated by barbiturates.

Bromsulphalein (BSP):

May interfere with alkaline phosphatase determinations.

May produce false-positive tests for acetone by reacting with sodium nitroprusside (as found in some reagent strips).

Caffeine:

Coffee reportedly may result in spurious elevations in serum uric acid as done by an adaptation of the method of Bittner (*Am J Clin Pathol* 1963;**40**:423).

Calcium antacids:

Large doses of calcium carbonate may produce hypercalcemia.

Carbamazepine:

Jaundice has occurred; incidence must await further trials.

May inhibit hypoprothrombinemic effect of oral anticoagulants.

May produce false-positive Zimmermann reaction for 17-ketosteroids and 17-hydroxycorticosteroids.

Table 1 (cont'd). Effects of drugs on common laboratory tests.

+ = Increase (pharmacologic or toxic effect)
– = Decrease (pharmacologic or toxic effect)
N = See notes (below)
● = Increase (test interference)
○ = Decrease (test interference)
★ = Present or positive

	BLOOD, SERUM, OR PLASMA													URINE										OTHER TESTS
	Amylase	Bilirubin	Cholesterol	Coombs (Direct)	CPK	Glucose	Thyroxine	Phosphatase, Alk.	Potassium	Prothrombin Time	SGOT and SGPT	Urea Nitrogen	Uric Acid	Color	Catecholamines	Glucose (Benedict)	5-HIAA	Ketones	Porphyrins	Protein	Steroids	Urobilinogen	VMA	
Carbenicillin (Geopen, Pyopen)					N				–															Bleeding time +
Cephalosporins				★				+			+	N				N				★	N			
Chloral hydrate (Noctec)										N		N			N	●			N		N			
Chloramphenicol (Chloromycetin)																●						–		
Chlordiazepoxide (Librium)		+									+													
Chloroquine (Aralen)														N					N					
Chlorpropamide (Diabinese)		+	–	★		–	–	+			+								N					
Chlorthalidone (Hygroton)	N				N	+			–				+											Serum calcium +; blood ammonia +
Chlorzoxazone (Paraflex)		+												N										
Cholestyramine (Cuemid)			–				N			+														Serum chloride (N)
Cimetidine (Tagamet)										N				N										Serum creatinine +; serum prolactin +
Cisplatin (Platinol)									–			+	+											Serum magnesium –; serum calcium –
Clindamycin (Cleocin)					N																			
Clofibrate (Atromid-S)			–		+	N		–		N	+		–											Serum aldolase +
Clonidine (Catapres)															N								–	Plasma growth hormone +
Cloxacillin (Tegopen)											+													
Codeine	N										N													
Colchicine			–				N																	
Colistin (Coly-Mycin)												+								★				
Contrast media, iodine-containing	N	N											–		N	N				N	N			
Corticosteroids	N		+			+	–		–	N			N			+					N			Urine estriol –
Cyclophosphamide (Cytoxan)									N															Serum cholinesterase –

Carbenicillin:
Intramuscular administration may result in increased serum CPK levels.

Cephalosporins:
Larger doses may adversely affect renal function, with elevation of the BUN.
Cephalothin may form an interfering dark color in Benedict's test for urinary glucose.
Large doses of cephalothin may produce false increases in urinary 17-ketosteroids (Zimmermann reaction).

Chloral hydrate:
May transiently increase the hypoprothrombinemic response to oral anticoagulants.
Large doses reportedly may cause false elevation of BUN (nesslerization technique), but more study is needed.
Attacks of acute intermittent porphyria may be precipitated.
May interfere with fluorimetric test for urine catecholamines.
May interfere with the determination of urinary 17-hydroxycorticosteroids by a modification of the Reddy, Jenkins, Thorn procedure (*Metabolism* 1952;**1**:511 and 1954;**3**:489).

Chloroquine:
May color urine rusty yellow or brown.
May be a precipitating factor in porphyria.

Chlorpropamide:
May be a precipitating factor in porphyria.

Chlorthalidone:
Has produced pancreatitis, with resultant increase in serum amylase.
Excessive use has produced hypokalemic myopathy with elevated CPK.

Chlorzoxazone:
May color urine orange or purplish-red.

Cholestyramine:
Has produced hyperchloremic acidosis in children.
Absorption of orally administered thyroid hormones is decreased if cholestyramine is given within several hours.

Cimetidine:
May enhance hypoprothrombinemic effect of oral anticoagulants.
Phenol in intravenous cimetidine may turn urine green.

Clindamycin:
Intramuscular administration of clindamycin appears to increase serum CPK levels in a majority of patients.

Clofibrate:
Glucose tolerance tends to improve in diabetics receiving clofibrate.
May enhance the hypoprothrombinemic effect of oral anticoagulants.

Clonidine:
Chronic therapy reduces urine catecholamines, but abrupt withdrawal may increase them.

Codeine:
May elevate serum amylase, but less potent than other opiates (eg, morphine) in this regard.
May produce elevated transaminase levels in certain patients.

Colchicine:
Reported to have an unpredictable antithyroid effect.

Contrast media, iodine-containing:
Cholangiography may result in transient elevations of serum amylase.
Cholecystographic media can result in increased serum bilirubin.
May see false decreases in urinary metanephrines (Crout modification of Pisano method).
Sodium diatrizoate (Hypaque) may form a black color in Benedict's tests for glucose.
Iodoalphionic acid (Priodax), iopanoic acid (Telepaque), and sodium diatrizoate (Hypaque) may give false-positives with sulfosalicylic acid and nitric acid, but not with heat and acetic acid.
May decrease values for 17-ketogenic steroids (Rutherford-Nelson method).

Corticosteroids:
Have produced pancreatitis, with resultant increase in serum amylase.
May increase the requirement for coumarin anticoagulants.
Corticosteroids are weak uricosurics but may produce severe hyperuricemia in patients with acute leukemia.
Potent corticosteroids decrease urinary 17-ketosteroid and 17-hydroxycorticosteroid excretion.

Cyclophosphamide:
Rapid lysis of tumor cells in patients with lymphomas or leukemias may result in hyperkalemia.

Table 1 (cont'd). Effects of drugs on common laboratory tests.

\+ = Increase (pharmacologic or toxic effect)
— = Decrease (pharmacologic or toxic effect)
N = See notes (below)
● = Increase (test interference)
○ = Decrease (test interference)
★ = Present or positive

	BLOOD, SERUM, OR PLASMA													URINE										OTHER TESTS
	Amylase	Bilirubin	Cholesterol	Coombs (Direct)	CPK	Glucose	Thyroxine	Phosphatase, Alk.	Potassium	Prothrombin Time	SGOT and SGPT	Urea Nitrogen	Uric Acid	Color	Catecholamines	Glucose (Benedict)	5-HIAA	Ketones	Porphyrins	Protein	Steroids	Urobilinogen	VMA	
Cyproheptadine (Periactin)	+					N																		
Dapsone (Avlosulfon)		N						N			N													Serum albumin (N)
Dextrothyroxine (Choloxin)			—			+	+			N						+								
Diazoxide (Hyperstat)						+							+			+								
Digitalis glycosides					N																			Serum estrogen +
Disopyramide (Norpace)		N				N		N			N													
Disulfiram (Antabuse)		+	N					+		N	+				—								—	
Epinephrine						+							+		N								N	
Erythromycin		N						+			N				N									
Estrogens	N	+	N			+	+	+								+					N			Serum ceruloplasmin +; serum iron +; plasma cortisol +
Ethacrynic acid (Edecrin)	N					N			—				N								N			
Ethambutol (Myambutol)													+											
Ethchlorvynol (Placidyl)										N														
Ethinamate (Valmid)																					N			
Ethionamide (Trecator)		+					—	+			+													
Ethoxazene (Serenium)														N					N					Urine bilirubin (N)
Furazolidone (Furoxone)														N										
Furosemide (Lasix)	N					+		+	—			+	+											Blood ammonia +
Glucagon						+				N														Serum calcium —
Glucose infusions						+			—				—			N								Blood ammonia (N)
Glutethimide (Doriden)								N		N														
Glyceryl guaiacolate (Robitussin)													—				●						N	

Cyproheptadine:
Although depression of fasting blood glucose has been reported, subsequent studies have not confirmed this.

Dapsone:
Occasional hepatotoxicity with elevated bilirubin, alkaline phosphatase, and transaminases.
Occasional reports of hypoalbuminemia.

Dextrothyroxine:
Enhances hypoprothrombinemic effect of oral anticoagulants.

Digitalis glycosides:
Intramuscular digoxin may increase serum CPK.

Disopyramide:
Occasional hepatotoxicity with elevated serum bilirubin, alkaline phosphatase, and transaminases.
Fasting hypoglycemia may occur, especially in elderly.

Disulfiram:
Inhibits decrease in serum cholesterol that normally occurs when alcoholics abstain.
Enhances hypoprothrombinemic effect of oral anticoagulants.

Epinephrine:
Epinephrine and related agents used in asthma by inhalation may increase urinary catecholamines and urinary VMA.

Erythromycin:
The estolate salt may produce cholestatic hepatitis with elevated bilirubin levels.
May cause false increase of transaminases done by colorimetric methods. The estolate salt may produce true increases in transaminase owing to hepatic toxicity.
May produce false elevation in fluorimetric determinations for urinary catecholamines.

Estrogens:
Oral contraceptives have been associated with pancreatitis and elevated serum amylase.
Cholesterol usually unchanged or decreased in postmenopausal women. Massive elevation of cholesterol and triglyceride occasionally reported.
May increase cortisol-binding proteins, resulting in moderate decrease in urinary 17-ketosteroids and 17-hydroxycorticosteroids.

Ethacrynic acid:
Has been implicated in the production of pancreatitis, with resultant increase in serum amylase.
Both hypoglycemia (in uremic patients) and hyperglycemia (in diabetics) have been reported.
May cause uricosuria if given intravenously and urate retention if given orally.
May slightly decrease urinary cortisol excretion.

Ethchlorvynol:
May depress the anticoagulant activity of the coumarin anticoagulants.

Ethinamate:
May markedly increase the absorption in 17-ketosteroid determinations (modified Zimmermann reaction).

Ethoxazene:
May color urine orange to orange-red.
May produce falsely high readings in the assay of porphyrins by spectrophotofluorimetry.
May produce interfering color for urine bilirubin by Bili-Labstix or Ictotest.

Furazolidone:
May color urine brown.

Furosemide:
Has precipitated pancreatitis, with resultant increase in serum amylase. (Also, small increases in serum amylase occur regularly.)

Glucagon:
May enhance response to oral anticoagulants.

Glucose:
Intravenous glucose may produce glycosuria in some patients.
Some studies have shown that a large glucose load may increase blood ammonia in patients with cirrhosis and portasystemic shunts; however, further studies have indicated that this effect is small.

Glutethimide:
Long-term use occasionally results in osteomalacia with elevated alkaline phosphatase.
May enhance metabolism of coumarin anticoagulants.

Glyceryl guaiacolate:
May cause a color change during screening methods for VMA, but final measurement apparently is not affected.

Table 1 (cont'd). Effects of drugs on common laboratory tests.

+ = Increase (pharmacologic or toxic effect)
– = Decrease (pharmacologic or toxic effect)
N = See notes (below)
● = Increase (test interference)
○ = Decrease (test interference)
★ = Present or positive

	BLOOD, SERUM, OR PLASMA													URINE										OTHER TESTS
	Amylase	Bilirubin	Cholesterol	Coombs (Direct)	CPK	Glucose	Thyroxine	Phosphatase, Alk.	Potassium	Prothrombin Time	SGOT and SGPT	Urea Nitrogen	Uric Acid	Color	Catecholamines	Glucose (Benedict)	5-HIAA	Ketones	Porphyrins	Protein	Steroids	Urobilinogen	VMA	
Gold salts		+						+												★				Serum proteins (N)
Griseofulvin (Fulvicin, Grifulvin)										N									N	★				
Guanethidine (Ismelin)						N						+			–								–	
Heparin			–	N		N			N	+							N							
Hydralazine (Apresoline)		N		★				N			N													
Hydroxyzine (Atarax, Vistaril)																					N			
Imipramine (Tofranil)		+						+									–						–	
Indomethacin (Indocin)	N			★				+	N		+	+												
Insulin						–			–						N									Serum calcium –
Iodides, inorganic							N														N			
Iron, oral																								Stool blood (N)
Isoniazid (INH)				★		+					+					N	–	N						Blood ammonia (N); blood lactate (N)
Levodopa (L-dopa)				★									N	N		N	–	N					N	
Levothyroxine (Synthroid)							N			N														
Lidocaine					N																			
Lithium carbonate						+	–									+				★			N	
Mefenamic acid (Ponstel)				N						N										★				Urine bilirubin ●
Meperidine (Demerol)	+	+									N													
Mephenesin (Sinan, Tolserol)																	●						N	
Meprobamate (Equanil, Miltown)																					N			Metyrapone response –

Gold:
Gold-induced nephrotic syndrome of colitis may lower serum albumin, globulins, or both.

Griseofulvin:
May depress anticoagulant activity of coumarin anticoagulants.
May precipitate acute attack in patients with porphyria.

Guanethidine:
Has antidiabetic activity and may decrease insulin requirements.

Heparin:
In acquired hemolytic anemia, heparin may cause the direct Coombs test to become negative.
Reportedly may increase blood glucose; confirmation is needed.
Hyperkalemia in predisposed patients, due to heparin-induced decrease in aldosterone synthesis.
May decrease urinary 5-HIAA excretion in patients with carcinoid syndrome.

Hydralazine:
Occasional hepatotoxicity with elevated bilirubin, alkaline phosphatase, and transaminase.

Hydroxyzine:
May falsely increase the reading for 17-hydroxycorticosteroids (modified Glenn-Nelson technique).

Indomethacin:
Has produced pancreatitis, with resultant increase in serum amylase.
Hyperkalemia has occurred in some patients, and in others the hypokalemia of Bartter's syndrome has improved.

Inorganic iodides:
Occasionally produce thyrotoxicosis with elevated serum thyroxine.
May interfere with the determination of urinary 17-hydroxycorticosteroids by a modification of the Reddy, Jenkins, Thorn procedure (*Metabolism* 1952;**1**:511 and 1954;**3**:489).

Insulin:
Insulin-induced hypoglycemia results in release of epinephrine, thus increasing urinary excretion.

Iron, oral:
Administration of ferrous sulfate and ferrous fumarate has resulted in false-positive benzidine tests for occult blood in the stools.

Isoniazid:
Both true glycosuria and false-positive Benedict's tests have been reported.
Acetonuria may occur with isoniazid intoxication.
Although isoniazid is reported to increase blood ammonia, some studies have failed to confirm this.
Isoniazid intoxication may increase serum lactate.

Levodopa:
May produce false increases for serum uric acid by colorimetric methods but not when uricase is used. True increases also reported.
Urine may darken on standing.
Both false-positive Clinitest and false-negative glucose oxidase reactions may occur, especially with large doses.
May interfere with ferric chloride tests for urine ketones, Ketostix, and possibly Acetest.
Small increase in urinary VMA excretion, but VMA measured by Pisano method may be falsely decreased.

Levothyroxine:
Serum thyroxine levels increased to normal or above normal in adequately treated patients.
Increasing thyroid hormone activity enhances anticoagulant effect of coumarins.

Lidocaine:
Intramuscular lidocaine may increase serum CPK.

Lithium carbonate:
Preliminary studies indicate that urinary VMA excretion may be somewhat increased.

Mefenamic acid:
Autoimmune hemolytic anemia may occur after prolonged therapy.
May increase response to oral anticoagulants.

Meperidine:
May elevate transaminase levels in certain patients.

Mephenesin:
May cause color changes during screening methods for VMA, but final measurement apparently is not affected.

Meprobamate:
May increase the absorbance in measurements for 17-ketosteroids (Zimmermann reaction).

Table 1 (cont'd). Effects of drugs on common laboratory tests.

+ = Increase (pharmacologic or toxic effect)
– = Decrease (pharmacologic or toxic effect)
N = See notes (below)
● = Increase (test interference)
○ = Decrease (test interference)
★ = Present or positive

	BLOOD, SERUM, OR PLASMA													URINE										OTHER TESTS
	Amylase	Bilirubin	Cholesterol	Coombs (Direct)	CPK	Glucose	Thyroxine	Phosphatase, Alk.	Potassium	Prothrombin Time	SGOT and SGPT	Urea Nitrogen	Uric Acid	Color	Catecholamines	Glucose (Benedict)	5-HIAA	Ketones	Porphyrins	Protein	Steroids	Urobilinogen	VMA	
Mercurial diuretics													+			N								
Metaxalone (Skelaxin)																●				N				
Methenamine (Mandelamine, Uritone)															●		○				N	N		Urine estriol ○
Methicillin (Dimocillin, Staphcillin)												+								★				
Methocarbamol (Robaxin)												N		N			●						N	
Methotrexate		+						+			+	N	N											
Methyldopa (Aldomet)	N	+		★				+			+	+		N	●		–						N	
Methylene blue														N										
Metronidazole (Flagyl)										N				N										
Miconazole (Monistat i.v.)			+							N														Serum triglycerides +
Monoamine oxidase inhibitors (MAOI)		+				–											–						–	Blood ammonia (N); metyrapone response (N); serum cholinesterase (N)
Morphine	+	+									N					●			N					
Nafcillin (Unipen)											+									N				
Nalidixic acid (NegGram)						N					+	+				●					N			Serum lactate +
Nicotinic acid (large doses)		+	–			+		+			+	+	+		●	N								
Nitrofurantoin (Furadantin)		N						+			+			N										
Nitroglycerin															+								+	
Novobiocin (Albamycin)		N																						
Oral contraceptives	N	+	N			+	+	+		N	+								N		N			Metyrapone response –
Oxacillin (Prostaphlin)								+			+	N								N				
Pargyline (Eutonyl)						–											–						–	
Penicillamine (Cuprimine)																				★				
Penicillin G				★					N							●				N	N			
Pentamidine	N					N					+	+												

Mercurial diuretics:

Meralluride (Mercuhydrin) may produce false-negatives for urinary glucose as measured by glucose oxidase methods (eg, Clinistix, Tes-Tape).

Metaxalone:

Implicated in the production of proteinuria.

Methenamine:

Produces false elevation in urinary 17-hydroxycorticosteroids by method of Reddy (*Metabolism* 1954;**3**:489).

May interfere with tests for urinary urobilinogen.

Methocarbamol:

Parenteral preparations may contain polyethylene glycol, which may increase urea retention in patients with renal impairment.

Urine may darken on standing.

May produce false increases in urinary VMA by screening method of Gitlow but not in quantitative procedure of Sunderman.

Methotrexate:

Nephropathy with elevated urea nitrogen has been reported.

Hyperuricemia may occur due to rapid lysis of tumor cells.

Methyldopa:

May produce sialadenitis with increased amylase.

Urine may darken on standing.

Does not appreciably affect VMA determinations.

Methylene blue:

Colors the urine blue.

Metronidazole:

Enhances hypoprothrombinemic effect of oral anticoagulants.

May cause darkening of urine.

Miconazole:

May enhance hypoprothrombinemic effect of oral anticoagulants.

Monoamine oxidase inhibitors:

Although MAO inhibitors have been reported to reduce blood ammonia, some of these agents have produced hepatotoxicity and thus could be dangerous in patients with impaired liver function.

Nialamide may decrease the response to metyrapone.

Phenelzine (Nardil) may decrease serum cholinesterase levels.

Morphine:

May elevate transaminase levels in certain patients.

Attacks of acute intermittent porphyria may be precipitated.

Nafcillin:

Large doses may produce false-positives for urine protein (sulfosalicylic acid method) and interfere with the interpretation of the trichloroacetic acid method.

Nalidixic acid:

Large doses or overdoses may produce false elevations in blood glucose (Somogyi-Nelson procedure).

May cause false elevation of urinary 17-ketosteroids (Zimmermann reaction).

Nicotinic acid:

May impair glucose tolerance, resulting in glycosuria.

Nitrofurantoin:

Cholestatic jaundice occasionally occurs following nitrofurantoin.

May tint urine brown.

Novobiocin:

May produce jaundice with an increase in unconjugated but not conjugated bilirubin in plasma; also, a yellow pigment may occur in the plasma that interferes with icterus index and bilirubin determinations.

Oral contraceptives:

Hyperlipidemic patients have developed pancreatitis following initiation of oral contraceptive use.

Oral contraceptives have been reported to elevate serum cholesterol.

A decrease in the hypoprothrombinemic effect of bishydroxycoumarin may occur.

May affect the handling of porphyrins by the liver; urinary coproporphyrin excretion may be increased.

The estrogenic component may increase cortisol-binding proteins, resulting in a moderate decrease in urinary 17-ketosteroids and 17-hydroxycorticosteroids.

Oxacillin:

High doses in infants may cause azotemia and proteinuria.

Penicillin G:

Massive intravenous doses of penicillin G sodium may produce hypokalemia. Penicillin G potassium can produce hyperkalemia.

Massive doses may yield false-positive results for proteinuria when turbidity measures are used (eg, heat and acetic acid, sulfosalicylic acid).

Intravenous doses may produce false elevations of 17-ketogenic steroids (Norymberski method) and a less marked increase in 17-ketosteroid determinations (Zimmermann reaction).

Pentamidine:

Isolated reports of acute pancreatitis with elevated serum amylase.

Tends to produce hypoglycemia but rarely may produce hyperglycemia.

Table 1 (cont'd). Effects of drugs on common laboratory tests.

+ = Increase (pharmacologic or toxic effect)
– = Decrease (pharmacologic or toxic effect)
N = See notes (below)
● = Increase (test interference)
○ = Decrease (test interference)
★ = Present or positive

	BLOOD, SERUM, OR PLASMA													URINE										OTHER TESTS
	Amylase	Bilirubin	Cholesterol	Coombs (Direct)	CPK	Glucose	Thyroxine	Phosphatase, Alk.	Potassium	Prothrombin Time	SGOT and SGPT	Urea Nitrogen	Uric Acid	Color	Catecholamines	Glucose (Benedict)	5-HIAA	Ketones	Porphyrins	Protein	Steroids	Urobilinogen	VMA	
Pentazocine (Talwin)	N																							
Phenazopyridine (Pyridium)														N				N	N	N		N		Urine bilirubin ●
Phenolphthalein														N										
Phenothiazines		+	+		N	+		+	–		+		N	N	N		○	N			N	●	N	Metyrapone response –; serum albumin –
Phensuximide (Milontin)														N										
Phenylbutazone (Butazolidin)	N	N						+		N	+		N											
Phenytoin (Dilantin)		N				+	–	+			+			N							N			Metyrapone response –; serum calcium –
Polymyxin B (Aerosporin)												+								★				
Primaquine														N										
Probenecid (Benemid)													–			●					N			
Procainamide (Pronestyl)		+						+			+													
Procaine																			N			N		
Progestogens								+																
Propoxyphene (Darvon)		+				N		+			+										N			
Propranolol (Inderal)		N				–					+	+			N									
Propylthiouracil		+					–			+	+													
Pyrazinamide (PZA)		+								N	+		+								N			
Quinacrine (Atabrine)														N										
Quinethazone (Hydromox)													+											
Quinidine		+		★				+		+	+				●						N			
Reserpine															N		N				N		N	
Riboflavin														N	●									
Rifampin (Rifadin, Rimactane)	+	+		★				+		N	+	N		N										

Pentazocine:
Causes sphincter of Oddi spasm, indicating that elevations of serum amylase may occur.

Phenazopyridine:
May color urine orange to orange-red.
May produce interfering colors for urine ketones by Ketostix or Gerhardt ferric chloride method.
May produce falsely high readings in the assay of porphyrins by spectrophotofluorimetry.
May interfere with Ames reagent strips for urine protein as well as the nitric acid ring test.
May yield a pink to red color in Ehrlich's test for urobilinogen.

Phenolphthalein:
May impart a red to purple color to an alkaline urine.

Phenothiazines:
Intramuscular chlorpromazine may result in increased CPK levels.
Chlorprothixene may result in significant uricosuria.
May color urine pink to red or red-brown.
Chlorpromazine may result in high apparent values for urine metanephrines (Pisano method).
May interfere with diacetic acid determinations.
May cause false increases in 17-ketosteroids (Zimmermann reaction).
Chlorpromazine may produce moderate decreases in urinary VMA excretion.

Phensuximide:
May color urine pink to red or red-brown.

Phenylbutazone:
May occasionally produce hepatitis with hyperbilirubinemia.
Parotitis, with resultant elevation of serum amylase, is a rare complication of phenylbutazone therapy.
Markedly enhances hypoprothrombinemic effect of oral anticoagulants.
Phenylbutazone is a weak uricosuric.

Phenytoin:
Serum bilirubin tends to be low (due to phenytoin-induced enzyme induction), but hepatotoxicity with jaundice occasionally occurs.
May color urine pink or red to red-brown.
Slightly decreases excretion of 17-ketosteroids and 17-hydroxycorticosteroids.

Probenecid:
May decrease urinary 17-ketosteroid excretion.

Procaine:
May react with Ehrlich's reagent in test for porphyrins or urobilinogen.

Propoxyphene:
Has produced hypoglycemia in a patient with impaired renal function.
Preliminary evidence indicates that propoxyphene may cause false decreases in urinary 17-hydroxycorticosteroids (Porter-Silber) and 17-ketosteroids (Zimmermann reaction).

Propranolol:
False increases in serum bilirubin (by SMA 12/60) in uremic patients taking propranolol.
False decrease in urine metanephrines (Pisano method).

Pyrazinamide:
May decrease plasma prothrombin levels owing to its hepatotoxicity.
Urinary 17-ketosteroids may be decreased, followed by a return to normal.

Quinacrine:
May color the urine yellow.

Quinidine:
May interfere with the determination of urinary 17-hydroxycorticosteroids by a modification of the Reddy, Jenkins, Thorn procedure.

Reserpine:
May cause slight initial increase in excretion of 5-HIAA.
May cause slight increase in absorbance in 17-hydroxycorticosteroid measurements (modified Glenn-Nelson technique).
Chronic administration decreases urinary catecholamine and VMA excretion; however, increases in both may be seen during the first day or 2 of therapy.

Riboflavin:
Large doses may produce yellow discoloration in urine.

Rifampin:
Inhibits hypoprothrombinemic effect of oral anticoagulants.
May produce acute renal failure with elevated urea nitrogen.
May produce red-orange color in urine.

Table 1 (cont'd). Effects of drugs on common laboratory tests.

+ = Increase (pharmacologic or toxic effect)
– = Decrease (pharmacologic or toxic effect)
N = See notes (below)
● = Increase (test interference)
○ = Decrease (test interference)
★ = Present or positive

	BLOOD, SERUM, OR PLASMA													URINE										OTHER TESTS
	Amylase	Bilirubin	Cholesterol	Coombs (Direct)	CPK	Glucose	Thyroxine	Phosphatase, Alk.	Potassium	Prothrombin Time	SGOT and SGPT	Urea Nitrogen	Uric Acid	Color	Catecholamines	Glucose (Benedict)	5-HIAA	Ketones	Porphyrins	Protein	Steroids	Urobilinogen	VMA	
Salicylates	N	+	N		N	N	–	+	–	+	+		N		–	●	N	N		★			N	Urine estriol –
Spironolactone (Aldactone)									+			+												Plasma cortisol ●
Succinylcholine (Anectine)									+															
Sulfinpyrazone (Anturane)													–											
Sulfonamides	N	N						+		N	+			N		●			N	N		N		
Sulindac (Clinoril)	N							N			N									N				
Tetracyclines	N		N			N				N	+	+			●	N						–		
Thiabendazole (Mintezol)						N					+													
Thiazide diuretics	+		+			+			–			+	+			N					N			Blood ammonia +; serum calcium +
Thyroglobulin (Proloid)			–				N			N														
Thyroid, desiccated			–				N			N														
Tolazamide (Tolinase)						–		+			+													
Tolbutamide (Orinase)						–	–													N				
Triamterene (Dyrenium)						+			+			+	+	N	N									
Tricyclic antidepressants		+						+			+						–						–	
Triiodothyronine (Cytomel)			–				–			N														
Trimethadione (Tridione)																				★				
Troleandomycin (TAO)		+									+										N			
Valproic acid (Depakene)	N																							Blood ammonia +
Verapamil						N																		Serum prolactin +
Viomycin (Vanactane, Viocin)									–											★				Serum calcium –
Vitamin A		N						N			N													Serum calcium (N)

Salicylates:

Salicylism has resulted in pancreatitis, with resultant increase in serum amylase.

Large doses may decrease serum cholesterol.

Salicylate overdose may increase serum CPK.

The salicylates have variable effects on blood glucose; a hypoglycemic action may be seen (especially in diabetics), and both hyperglycemia and hypoglycemia have occurred from salicylate intoxication.

Large doses (eg, 3–5 g/d) can cause uricosuria; smaller doses result in urate retention.

Aspirin may interfere with fluorescence methods for urinary 5-HIAA.

May produce an interfering color in ferric chloride test for acetoacetic acid.

False increases with various methods for urinary VMA, but false *decreases* may occur with Pisano method.

Sulfonamides:

Reports have appeared describing pancreatitis with elevated serum amylase following sulfasalazine and sulfamethizole.

Jaundice has been produced, owing to both acute hemolytic anemia and hepatotoxicity.

Some sulfonamides enhance the hypoprothrombinemic effect of oral anticoagulants.

May color urine rusty yellow or brownish.

May react with Ehrlich's reagent in test for porphyrins or urobilinogen. May also precipitate an attack of acute intermittent porphyria.

Sulfisoxazole may lead to false-positive results for proteinuria by turbidity and by heat and acid methods; also, many sulfonamides may result in crystalluria with true proteinuria.

Sulindac:

Isolated cases of pancreatitis with elevated serum amylase.

Isolated cases of liver function abnormalities (eg, increased alkaline phosphatase, transaminases).

Isolated cases of proteinuria have occurred.

Tetracyclines:

Prolonged high doses have resulted in pancreatitis in certain patients.

Oral chlortetracycline may reduce serum cholesterol.

Oxytetracycline has produced hypoglycemic effects in diabetics but apparently not in normal subjects.

Intravenous tetracycline may decrease plasma prothrombin activity; also, tetracyclines may reduce the vitamin K–producing bacteria in the gut.

Parenteral forms containing ascorbic acid may cause false-negatives in urinary glucose by glucose oxidase methods (eg, Clinistix, Tes-Tape).

Thiabendazole:

Hyperglycemia may occur (incidence is low).

Thiazide diuretics:

May cause hyperglycemia and glycosuria in patients predisposed to diabetes.

May cause slight decrease in urinary cortisol excretion.

Thyroglobulin; desiccated thyroid:

Effects on serum thyroxine should be consistent with metabolic effects.

Increasing thyroid hormone activity increases anticoagulant effect of coumarins.

Tolbutamide:

A metabolite may cause false-positive tests for proteinuria when turbidity procedures are used (eg, heat and acetic acid, sulfosalicylic acid).

Triamterene:

May produce a pale blue fluorescence in the urine.

False increases in urinary metanephrines (Sandhu and Freed method).

Triiodothyronine:

Increasing thyroid hormone activity increases hypoprothrombinemic effect of coumarins.

Troleandomycin (triacetyloleandomycin):

May cause false elevations of 17-ketosteroids (Drekter) and 17-hydroxycorticosteroids (Porter-Silber).

Valproic acid:

Isolated cases of pancreatitis with increased serum amylase.

Verapamil:

May improve glucose tolerance in patients with non–insulin-dependent diabetes.

Vitamin A:

Intoxication may produce hepatotoxicity with increased bilirubin, alkaline phosphatase, and transaminase.

Intoxication may produce hypercalcemia.

CONVERSION TABLES

Fahrenheit/Celsius Temperature Conversion

(°F = 9/5 °C + 32; °C = 5/9 [°F − 32])

°F	°C	°F	°C
90	= 32.2	100	= 37.8
91	= 32.8	101	= 38.3
92	= 33.3	102	= 38.9
93	= 33.9	103	= 39.4
94	= 34.4	104	= 40.0
95	= 35.0	105	= 40.6
96	= 35.6	106	= 41.1
97	= 36.1	107	= 41.7
98	= 36.7	108	= 42.2
99	= 37.2	109	= 42.8

Milliequivalent Conversion Factors

mEq/L of:	Divide mg/dL or vol% by:
Calcium	2.0
Chloride (from Cl)	3.5
(from NaCl)	5.85
CO_2 combining power	2.222
Magnesium	1.2
Phosphorus	3.1 (mmol)
Potassium	3.9
Sodium	2.3

Metric System Prefixes (Small Measurement)

In accordance with the decision of several scientific societies to employ a universal system of metric nomenclature, the following prefixes have become standard in many medical texts and journals.

k	kilo-	10^3
c	centi-	10^{-2}
m	milli-	10^{-3}
μ	micro-	10^{-6}
n	nano- (formerly millimicro, mμ)	10^{-9}
p	pico- (formerly micromicro, $\mu\mu$)	10^{-12}
f	femto-	10^{-15}
a	atto-	10^{-18}

Household Equivalents (Approximate)

1 tsp = 6 mL
1 tbsp = 15 mL
1 oz (eg, medicine glass) = 30 mL
1 cup = 8 fluid oz = 240 mL
1 quart = 946 mL

Apothecary Equivalents

Metric	Approximate Apothecary Equivalents	Metric	Approximate Apothecary Equivalents
30 g	... 1 oz	20 mg	... 1/3 gr
6 g	... 90 gr	15 mg	... 1/4 gr
5 g	... 75 gr	12 mg	... 1/5 gr
4 g	... 60 gr	10 mg	... 1/6 gr
3 g	... 45 gr	8 mg	... 1/8 gr
2 g	... 30 gr	6 mg	... 1/10 gr
1.5 g	... 22 gr	5 mg	... 1/12 gr
1 g	... 15 gr	4 mg	... 1/15 gr
0.75 g	... 12 gr	3 mg	... 1/20 gr
0.6 g	... 10 gr	2 mg	... 1/30 gr
0.5 g	... 7½ gr	1.5 mg	... 1/40 gr
0.4 g	... 6 gr	1.2 mg	... 1/50 gr
0.3 g	... 5 gr	1 mg	... 1/60 gr
0.25 g	... 4 gr	0.8 mg	... 1/80 gr
0.2 g	... 3 gr	0.6 mg	... 1/100 gr
0.15 g	... 2½ gr	0.5 mg	... 1/120 gr
0.12 g	... 2 gr	0.4 mg	... 1/150 gr
0.1 g	... 1½ gr	0.3 mg	... 1/200 gr
75 mg	... 1¼ gr	0.25 mg	... 1/250 gr
60 mg	... 1 gr	0.2 mg	... 1/300 gr
50 mg	... 3/4 gr	0.15 mg	... 1/400 gr
40 mg	... 2/3 gr	0.12 mg	... 1/500 gr
30 mg	... 1/2 gr	0.1 mg	... 1/600 gr
25 mg	... 3/8 gr		

Pounds to Kilograms
(1 kg = 2.2 lb; 1 lb = 0.45 kg)

lb	kg	lb	kg	lb	kg	lb	kg	lb	kg
5	2.3	50	22.7	95	43.1	140	63.5	185	83.9
10	4.5	55	25.0	100	45.4	145	65.8	190	86.2
15	6.8	60	27.2	105	47.6	150	68.0	195	88.5
20	9.1	65	29.5	110	49.9	155	70.3	200	90.7
25	11.3	70	31.7	115	52.2	160	72.6	205	93.0
30	13.6	75	34.0	120	54.4	165	74.8	210	95.3
35	15.9	80	36.3	125	56.7	170	77.1	215	97.5
40	18.1	85	38.6	130	58.9	175	79.4	220	99.8
45	20.4	90	40.8	135	61.2	180	81.6		

Feet and Inches to Centimeters
(1 cm = 0.39 in; 1 in = 2.54 cm)

ft	in	cm	ft	in	cm	ft	in	cm	ft	in	cm	ft	in	cm
0	6	15.2	2	4	71.1	3	4	101.6	4	4	132.0	5	4	162.6
1	0	30.5	2	5	73.6	3	5	104.1	4	5	134.6	5	5	165.1
1	6	45.7	2	6	76.1	3	6	106.6	4	6	137.1	5	6	167.6
1	7	48.3	2	7	78.7	3	7	109.2	4	7	139.6	5	7	170.2
1	8	50.8	2	8	81.2	3	8	111.7	4	8	142.2	5	8	172.7
1	9	53.3	2	9	83.8	3	9	114.2	4	9	144.7	5	9	175.3
1	10	55.9	2	10	86.3	3	10	116.8	4	10	147.3	5	10	177.8
1	11	58.4	2	11	88.8	3	11	119.3	4	11	149.8	5	11	180.3
2	0	61.0	3	0	91.4	4	0	121.9	5	0	152.4	6	0	182.9
2	1	63.5	3	1	93.9	4	1	124.4	5	1	154.9	6	1	185.4
2	2	66.0	3	2	96.4	4	2	127.0	5	2	157.5	6	2	188.0
2	3	68.6	3	3	99.0	4	3	129.5	5	3	160.0	6	3	190.5

Desirable Weights (Pounds)

Men (Age 25 and Over)					Women (Age 25 and Over)*				
Height* Feet	Inches	Small Frame	Medium Frame	Large Frame	Height† Feet	Inches	Small Frame	Medium Frame	Large Frame
5	2	112–120	118–129	126–141	4	10	92– 98	96–107	104–119
5	3	115–123	121–133	129–144	4	11	94–101	98–110	106–122
5	4	118–126	124–136	132–148	5	0	96–104	101–113	109–125
5	5	121–129	127–139	135–152	5	1	99–107	104–116	112–128
5	6	124–133	130–143	138–156	5	2	102–110	107–119	115–131
5	7	128–137	134–147	142–161	5	3	105–113	110–122	118–134
5	8	132–141	138–152	147–166	5	4	108–116	113–126	121–138
5	9	136–145	142–156	151–170	5	5	111–119	116–130	125–142
5	10	140–150	146–160	155–174	5	6	114–123	120–135	129–146
5	11	144–154	150–165	159–179	5	7	118–127	124–139	133–150
6	0	148–158	154–170	164–184	5	8	121–131	128–143	137–154
6	1	152–162	158–175	168–189	5	9	126–135	132–147	141–158
6	2	156–167	162–180	173–194	5	10	130–140	136–151	145–163
6	3	160–171	167–185	178–199	5	11	134–144	140–155	149–168
6	4	164–175	172–190	182–204	6	0	138–148	144–159	153–173

*With shoes with 1-inch heels.

*For women between 18 and 25, subtract 1 lb for each year under 25.
†With shoes with 2-inch heels.

This table was derived primarily from data on the Build and Blood Pressure Study, 1959, Society of Actuaries. A useful discussion is presented in Seltzer CC, Mayer J: How representative are the weights of insured men and women? *JAMA* 1967;201:221.

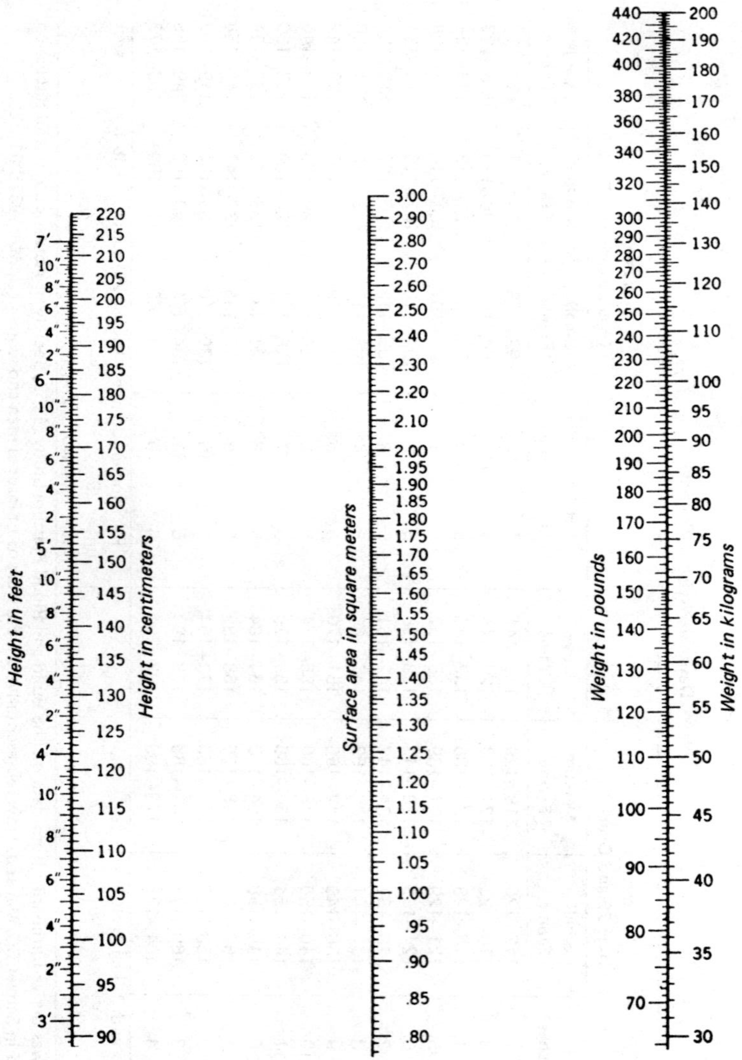

Nomogram for the determination of body surface area of children and adults. (Reproduced, with permission, from Boothby & Sandiford: *Boston MSJ* 1921;**185**:337.) [Revised 1979.]

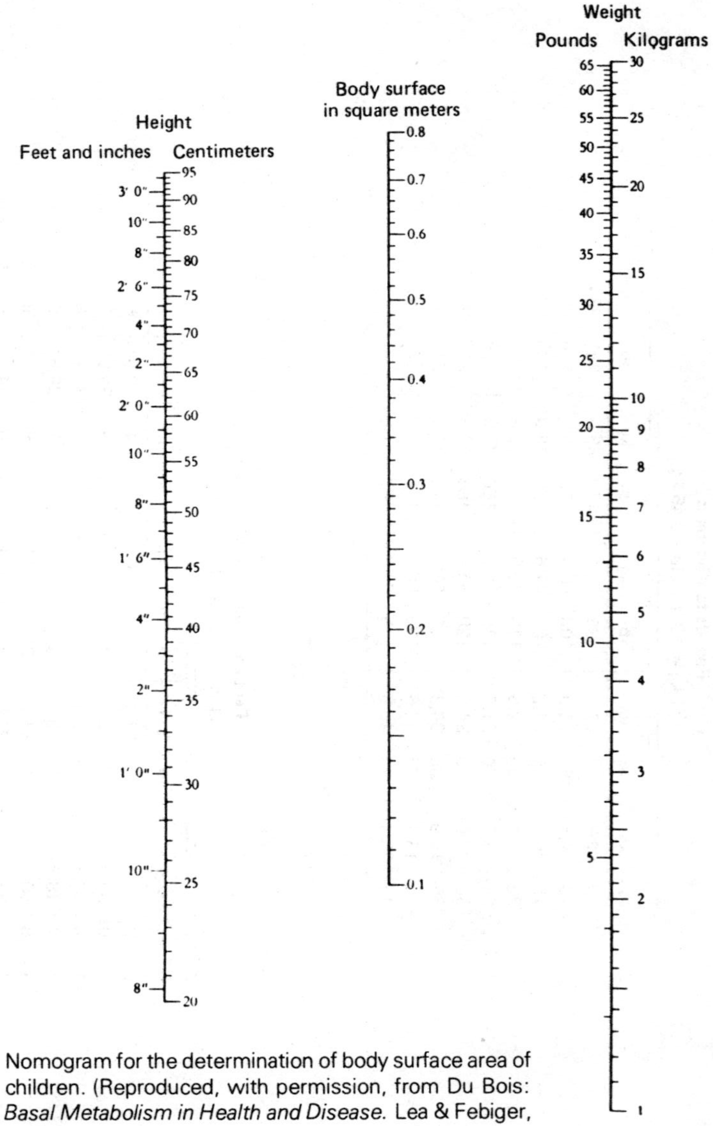

Nomogram for the determination of body surface area of children. (Reproduced, with permission, from Du Bois: *Basal Metabolism in Health and Disease.* Lea & Febiger, 1936.)

Index

The indexers have tried to emphasize major discussions of drugs and drug groups, so that drugs mentioned in passing or in minor applications may not be listed. Disease names are indexed also, however, so that it should be possible to locate every mention of a drug the reader is interested in. Trade names are indexed with the generic name in parentheses, and in most cases the listing under the generic name will be more complete. Trade names of combination remedies are indexed without generic components in most cases, but the components are listed on the page cited. British readers should note that only American generic and trade names are indexed, but the indexers feel that the differences are either trivial (phenobarbit*al*, -barbit*one*) or both rare and well known (meperidine, pethidine).